PSYCHIATRIE DER GEGENWART

FORSCHUNG UND PRAXIS

HERAUSGEGEBEN VON

H. W. GRUHLE† · BONN · R. JUNG · FREIBURG / BR.
W. MAYER-GROSS† · BIRMINGHAM · M. MÜLLER · BERN

BAND I/1B

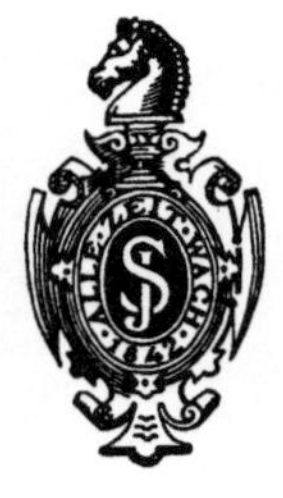

SPRINGER-VERLAG

BERLIN · GÖTTINGEN · HEIDELBERG

1964

GRUNDLAGENFORSCHUNG ZUR PSYCHIATRIE

TEIL B

BEARBEITET VON

M. BLEULER · W. A. GILJAROWSKY† · G. HUBER
D. PLOOG · C. RIEBELING† · H. WAELSCH
H. WEIL-MALHERBE

MIT 85 ABBILDUNGEN

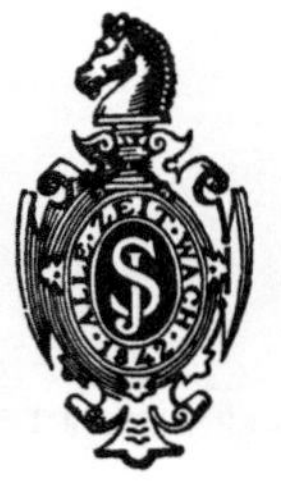

SPRINGER-VERLAG

BERLIN · GÖTTINGEN · HEIDELBERG

1964

ISBN-13: 978-3-642-94903-6   e-ISBN-13: 978-3-642-94902-9
DOI: 10.1007/978-3-642-94902-9

Titel Nr. 6596

Inhaltsverzeichnis

GRUNDLAGENFORSCHUNG
ZUR PSYCHIATRIE
TEIL B

Neurochemistry and Psychiatry[1]

By

HEINRICH WAELSCH, New York (USA), and

HANS WEIL-MALHERBE, Washington (USA)

Table of contents

---

[1] In the original manuscript the literature was covered up to and including 1959. Because of the delay in publication some of the aspects of the review have been revised and brought up to date.

A. Introduction
I. General remarks

The inclusion of a chapter on neurochemistry in a handbook of psychiatry attests to the ever-increasing appreciation of the need for understanding biochemical mechanisms in order to interpret disease processes of the nervous system. The interest in neurochemistry, fostered in some isolated centers of psychiatric research for many years, has become more general during the last decade.

To make the position of neurochemistry clear in its relation to neurophysiology and clinical problems, it may be useful to consider briefly the background of this aspect of biochemistry. Dynamic neurochemistry came into its own only after the main outlines of intermediary metabolism had been established by the work on a variety of organs such as muscle, liver, kidney, and brain. This work proved that the intermediary metabolism of nerve tissue differs from that of other organs only in detail. Its enzymatic and metabolic potentialities are essentially the same as those of other organs, some specialized enzymatic processes occurring preferentially in the nervous tissue. What, therefore, makes a brain a brain? It is obvious, and perhaps unnecessary to point out, that it is the structure which provides the tridimensional framework for the processes of intermediary metabolism which, as in other tissues, gives the nerve tissue its unique aspects.

The fact that expression of cerebral function is not biochemical in nature has influenced not only the approach of biochemists to the problem of brain metabolism but has for many years impeded the appreciation and acceptance of an "organic basis" of mental disease. The major obstacle was the emergence of psychoanalysis as a self-contained intellectual system instead of as a companion of the "organic approach". Once the basic ideas had been accepted, psychoanalysis appeared to offer the psychiatrist and medical scientist an integrated interpretation of normal and abnormal functioning of the brain. It should be mentioned that the "organic approach" does not hold out hope for an early understanding of organically anchored psychodynamics.

Neurochemistry, in relation to function, will become increasingly productive after the functional correlatives of cerebral metabolism have been found in behavioral phenomena. This study is in its infancy and the underlying ideas are at present no more than working hypotheses, but they represent a new approach to problems of the function of the central nervous system in health and disease.

During the last few years support for this approach has gained ground. Before that, the probable hereditary basis of schizophrenia appeared to many psychiatrists as the only indication of an organic basis of mental disease, although it did not seriously shake their belief in the environmental origin of the major psychoses.

While genetic investigation has shown that certain types of mental disease have a hereditary background, this finding has not resolved the question as to the type and extent of environmental influence necessary to bring about a mental disease of a particular phenotype. Biochemical and genetic studies of so-called inborn errors of metabolism have given the neurochemist confidence that the search for metabolic abnormalities may be rewarding also in the major psychoses.

II. Scope of review

For the present discussion, those aspects of brain metabolism have been selected which appear most promising for our understanding of, and for the therapeutic approach to, the problems of mental disease. This choice is biased by the authors' acquaintance with and interest in these particular aspects.

Cerebral energy metabolism will be discussed, since, in conjunction with the metabolism of glucose, it has attracted and will continue to attract many investigators. Quite often it has been assumed that disturbances in cerebral energy metabolism may be the essential biochemical feature of mental disease.

Other sections will be devoted to the blood-brain barrier, lipid metabolism, inborn errors of metabolism, and the biochemistry of the developing brain. The metabolism of amino acids, and especially of glutamic acid and of the metabolic derivatives of amino acids — the biogenetic amines and proteins —, will also be considered.

III. Structure and neurochemistry

It is necessary before discussing the biochemical aspects of cerebral metabolism to recall some of the structural features of the nervous system in order to understand the magnitude of the problem that the biochemist must face. In the central nervous system, the study of metabolism without consideration of structure is meaningless, particularly if one intends to interpret cerebral metabolism in functional terms.

The mammalian central nervous system is composed of about 45% white and 55% grey matter. The white matter, containing the tracts, is characterized by its high lipid content, which on a dry weight basis amounts to 50% or more, the remainder being proteins, salts, etc.

The specific cell population of grey matter, and particularly of the cerebral cortex, consists of a variety of neuronal cell bodies, their dendrites, parts of the axons, and the glial cells. Recent estimates show that the cell bodies of the neurons comprise only 5% of the volume of the cortex, the remaining volume being taken up by dendrites, axons, glia, and the elusive extracellular space (POPE, 1955). If the number of cells is based on counts of nuclei, a ratio which can only be approximate, one gram of human cerebral cortex contains about $1.6 \cdot 10^7$ neuronal nuclei and $7.7 \cdot 10^7$ glial nuclei (rat: $1.4 \cdot 10^7$ and $8.4 \cdot 10^7$ respectively), whereas the white matter, such as the corpus callosum, contains about $8 \cdot 10^7$ glial and endothelial nuclei (NURNBERGER and GORDON, 1957). These figures are considered approximate and are quoted mainly to show the complexity of the composition of the central nervous system. We have been accustomed to assume that cerebral functional activity is carried on by the neurons. For biochemical investigations on the other hand, the whole brain, perfused brain, tissue slices, or homogenates are taken. Even in experiments with isolated tissue preparations, such as cortex or any functionaly or anatomically well-defined area, the metabolism of the neurons including dendrites and parts of the axons can only be a varying function of the total sample.

The recent visualization of subcellular structures has had a powerful impact on the direction and formulations of problems of general biochemistry, but in particular of neurochemistry. Classical neurohistology, owing to the low resolution of the light microscope and to the vagaries of the staining techniques, could only in rare cases penetrate to the degree where biochemical and/or functional processes could be assigned to specific subcellular structures. To the advantage of an integrated picture of biochemical structure, the establishment of the basic framework of intermediary metabolism coincided with the development of the techniques of X-ray diffraction, ultraviolet microscopy, and electron microscopy.

Electron microscopy particularly is exerting, and will exert increasingly, a powerful influence on neurochemical concepts, and it is on this level of subcellular organization that an integration of metabolism and function is being attempted.

While electron microscopy has not solved all of its technical problems and preparative artifacts cannot always be distinguished from in vivo situations, results obtained by this technique, supplemented by observations with other optical methods, have already produced many significant points of interest to the neurochemist. Since some of these observations will form the basis of later discussions, they will be briefly summarized.

Electron microscopy appears to indicate that in the central nervous system there is no significant extracellular fluid space as found in muscle or liver. Although the extracellular fluid phase may have shrunk as a consequence of the preparation of the tissue, it is now thought probable that ground substance, (myelin, glia, etc.), or the content of the endoplasmic reticulum, may represent the chloride space (cf. section on blood-brain barrier).

The endoplasmic reticulum of the neurons has been demonstrated as being arranged to a large extent in an orderly fashion of superimposed cisterns or sacs. The reticulum may be divided into two types, one having the basophilic granules of nucleoproteins attached, and the other being free of these granules (agranular reticulum). The endoplasmic reticulum containing attached nucleoprotein granules represents the Nissl bodies (see PALAY und PALADE, 1955), while the agranular reticulum is assumed to correspond to the Golgi apparatus. As will be discussed later, the nucleoprotein-containing reticulum, or Nissl granules of the neurons, corresponds to the microsomal preparations of other cells and is involved in processes of protein synthesis. Therefore, the behavior of Nissl granules under physiological and pathological conditions is of particular interest to the neurochemist.

It may be speculated by analogy with findings in other cell types that the channels and sacs of the endoplasmic reticulum may supply routes of transportation, in addition to playing a possible role in the separation of intracellular components such as potassium and sodium.

Mitochondria are found, not only in the cell body and dendrites, but also in the axoplasm and are particularly numerous in the synaptic knobs. Since mitochondria are the carriers of the enzymatic systems of oxidative phosphorylation, they provide, in the form of adenosine triphosphate, the major portion of energy for biosynthetic processes of functional and structural significance. Their occurrence in the cytoplasm, axoplasm, and synaptic knobs points to the likelihood of autonomous biosynthetic processes occurring in the various structures of the neuron.

Electron microscopy has been particularly illuminating in the study of the synapse, whether we are dealing with the neuromuscular junction or the axo- or somato-dendritic synapses. The cytoplasm of the synaptic buds is filled with small vesicles of a diameter of 150 to 500 Ångstrom. These synaptic vesicles are supposed to contain transmitter substances such as acetylcholine. It is assumed that they attach themselves to the pre-synaptic membranes and on stimulation release the transmitter substances in "quantal" amounts. The synaptic vesicles are not only found in the synaptic buds, but, according to recent pictures, their presence extends also throughout the axoplasm of the nerve fiber. It has already been noted that there is a considerable accumulation of mitochondria in the pre-synaptic as opposed to the post-synaptic region. Great effort has been directed towards the localization of enzymes, in particular cholinesterase, in pre- or post-synaptic structures with the aid of cytochemical methods.

Considerably less information is available at present as to the morphological fine-structure of the glial elements of the nervous system. The interest of the neurochemist in these cells arises from their participation in the formation of myelin, as suggested sites of the blood-brain barrier, as well as their possible symbiotic relationship to the neurons.

As is apparent from the preceding discussion, our knowledge of the subcellular organization of the nervous system has advanced rapidly during recent years. We are now able to assign basic metabolic processes to different structures of the cell. This approach is of course only in its preliminary stage.

Simultaneously with the optical methods, micromethods have been developed for the determination of cell constituents and enzymatic activities on the cellular and subcellular level. The neurochemist is increasingly interested in the analysis of smaller and smaller morphological units; whereas the isolation and characterization of compounds from the brain serves, today, more the purpose of clarifying their chemical constitution and less that of supplying data for the interpretation of functional states.

The application of quantitative histochemistry and microanalysis — admirable from the technical point of view — has given us new and essential insight into the chemoarchitectonics of the nervous system and promises to attract increasing attention among neurochemists.

In these investigations either thin sections or single neurons or glia cells are analyzed. Many of the methods applied are based on the pioneering work of LINDERSTRØM-LANG and his laboratory.

The analysis of six layers of the rabbit Ammon's horn (LOWRY et al., 1954) and eight layers of the monkey retina (LOWRY et al., 1956b) demonstrated the constancy of the constituents, such as lipids or proteins, as well as of the enzyme activities, which vary within a relatively small range and are characteristic of the layer analyzed, be it cell bodies, dendrites, myelinated fibers, or other structures.

The in vitro measurement of the activities of a number of enzymes of cerebral glucose metabolism shows that these are greatly in excess (sometimes more than 50 times) over the activities needed for the metabolism of glucose in vivo (McILWAIN, 1953; LOWRY, 1955). The sensitivity of the method has been extended to the point where it is possible to measure a number of enzymes in some dorsal root ganglion cells and their capsules and in other structures of similar size (0.005 to 0.03 μg dry weight), as shown in Table 1 (LOWRY et al., 1956a; LOWRY, 1957).

In one series of studies the distribution pattern of certain enzymes determined quantitatively within the cortical cytoarchitectonic layers and sublayers was correlated with the anatomical fine structure (POPE, 1955). Studies of this type on the somatosensory isocortex of the rat indicated that intracellular oxidation is localized principally in the neuronal cell bodies and dendrites (POPE et al., 1956). Acetylcholinesterase and Ca^{++}-activated adenosine triphosphatase were primarily associated with layers rich in dendrites and in plexus of axons (POPE, 1955).

Measurements of cytochrome oxidase in human frontal isocortex show a parallelism between enzyme activity and density of cell bodies and dendrites (POPE et al., 1956) in conformity with the localization of respiratory enzymes in structures of the Ammon's horn (LOWRY et al., 1954). On the other hand the distribution of cell dipeptidase suggests its relation to cell density irrespective of whether the cells are neurons or glia, since the enzymatic activity is similar in cortical grey and in subcortical white (POPE et al., 1957).

In gliomas, particularly astrocytomas, cytochrome oxidase activity is low, while tumors with an admixture of oligodendrocytes show a higher enzyme content, a finding in accord with the relatively high oxygen uptake of oligodendrogliomas (HELLER and ELLIOTT, 1955).

Table 1. *Methods available for single cell analysis* (LOWRY, 1957)

Component	Dry brain mμg	Component	Dry brain mμg
Malic dehydrogenase	1 (0.002)	P-fructokinase	5
Lactic dehydrogenase	1 (0.01)	DPNase	1
Glutamic dehydrogenase	5 (0.2)	Nu. phosphorylase	20
		Alkaline phosphatase	20
Transaminase	1 (0.02)	DPN	10
Hexose isomerase	10	Total lipid	5
Aldolase	20	Dry weight	2
Fumarase	5		
Hexokinase	20		

Weight of dry brain required in millimicrograms (10^{-9} g.). Figures in parenthesis: amounts of brain needed if present methods were used at the limits of their sensitivity. One anterior horn cell body has a dry weight of 5 to 30 mμg.

In continuation of studies of protein and nucleic acid metabolism in nerve cells during rest and activity, with the aid of the ultraviolet microscope and specific staining techniques (HYDEN, 1943), X-ray microphotometry has been utilized for the analysis of nerve cell sections and quantitative determination of the intracellular mass, lipids and proteins in amounts of 10^{-12} g (HYDEN, 1955). By refinement of analytical methods it became possible to analyze the ribose nucleic acid content and the component mononucleotides of single nerve cells (EDSTRÖM and HYDEN, 1954). X-ray microphotometry as well as a variety of micromethods has led to a determination of the composition of neurons and glia of spinal ganglia and DEITER's nucleus, and the activity of certain enzymes. These studies suggest a high metabolic activity of oligodendrocytes (HYDEN, 1959).

The outstanding importance of all these quantitative histochemical studies lies in the fact that they narrow the conceptual gap between morphology and biochemistry. They pave the way toward a definition of the dynamics of intermediary metabolism in terms of metabolic pools or compartments. These are the only terms which include morphological and biochemical data on all levels of cellular organization and make structure and metabolism inseparable. Only by a development in this direction can neurochemistry become a link between neuroanatomy and neurophysiology and hope to approach the problem of function of the nervous system in health and disease (WAELSCH, 1960; WAELSCH and LAJTHA, 1961). A beginning has been made recently by investigations in vivo of the cerebral compartments of glutamic acid metabolism (BERL et al., 1961a, 1962; WAELSCH, 1961). In order to demonstrate the potentialities of this approach, it may be mentioned that of the high concentration of cerebral glutamic acid (150 to 180 mg/ 100 gm tissue) only a small fraction, less than 20 per cent, is present in a compartment with a half-life time of less than 60 minutes while the bulk of this amino acid is distributed over compartments with half-life times in excess of 6 hours. It is apparent that the glutamic acid in the various compartments will have a different metabolic and functional significance. Similar conclusions have been drawn as to the metabolic compartments of cerebral γ-aminobutyric acid (BERL et al., 1961b).

B. The brain barrier systems

The central nervous system obtains its nutrients from and releases metabolites into the circulating blood and the cerebrospinal fluid. Without knowledge of the mechanism which governs the entrance of substances into and their release from the central nervous system, a definitive understanding of cerebral metabolism in vivo is not possible.

Since the original observation of EHRLICH (1885) establishing the presence of a permeability barrier in the central nervous system more pronounced than in any other organ, systematic investigations of the blood-brain barrier, as well as of the blood-cerebrospinal fluid barrier, have been few, although incidental observations have brought their importance to the attention of the investigator whenever he was dealing with the uptake and metabolism of cerebral constituents. The anatomical and biochemical concepts of the location and dynamics of the permeability barriers have at the present time not reached a stage of development where a rational correlation between structure and transport mechanism is possible.

The basic phenomenon of the blood-brain barrier was originally established when it was shown that acidic dyes did not penetrate into the nervous system of the living animal. Since then it has been demonstrated that the rate of entrance from the circulating blood into the brain, of cations as well as anions, organic or inorganic, is slowed down sometimes to such a degree that a net uptake of the substance cannot be demonstrated (BAKAY, 1957; DAVSON, 1955; cf. sections C, D IV, and G. No permeability barrier appears to exist for lipid-soluble substances and gases. Although with some substances no net uptake by the brain can be shown, there may be a rapid exchange of such substances between blood and the brain (cf. section on amino acids). Whether a net uptake is blocked by the barrier acting as a protective mechanism only when "unphysiological" situations are created by an increase of the respective metabolites in the blood, or whether the same holds true in cases where the concentration of the metabolites in the brain is depleted, as for example, in an amino deficiency, ist not known. For normal metabolites, the systems of permeability barriers may represent a homeostatic mechanism for maintenance of a relatively constant metabolic environment for the functional units of the central nervous system.

The significance of the blood-brain barrier is apparent from the fact that it permits only glucose on substrate levels to enter the central nervous system, and thereby makes this carbohydrate the main fuel of the brain.

There are certain areas in the central nervous system, such as the choroid plexus, the posterior pituitary, the pineal gland, and the area postrema etc., which show a less effective blood-brain barrier (WISLOCKI and LEDUC, 1952). Indication of a lowered blood-brain barrier has also been obtained for the hypothalamic area (WEIL-MALHERBE et al., 1959). It seems as if certain parts of the brain, some exerting an endocrine function, have a lowered blood-brain barrier. Such endocrine function may require rapid exchange of and reaction to metabolites supplied by the circulating blood.

In the immature brain the blood-brain barrier is apparently not fully effective and a rapid uptake of substances from the blood by the brain can be demonstrated (cf. section on development, amino acids, lipid metabolism; WAELSCH, 1955).

The location of the blood-brain barrier has been discussed for many years. Recently it has been assumed to be located in the feet of the astrocytes enveloping the capillaries. A consequence of the last interpretation is that the enzymatic make-up of the astrocytes would be a factor in determining the rate at which a substance might penetrate into the brain (for a discussion and literature of the location of the barrier, see BRIERLEY, 1957).

The question of the occurrence and extent of the extracellular space has played an increasing role in the interpretation of the brain barrier systems. Since electron microscopic evidence points to a very close packing of the elements of the central nervous system (in contrast to liver and muscle), the absence of a significant extracellular space is proposed. In this concept the chloride space has been assigned to the glial elements. As a consequence of a virtual absence of extracellular space, it has been argued that the blood-brain barrier represents nothing more than an expression of the rate of entrance of substances into the cells from the circulating blood, while in liver and muscle the extracellular space is the first recipient of any substance leaving the blood (cf. EDSTRÖM, 1958).

It does not seem justified to draw conclusions as to the presence or absence of extracellular space in the brain solely on the result of electron microscopic evidence since the technical problems of shrinkage, etc. are not resolved definitely. There is sufficient reason to assume on physiological grounds that there will be an extracellular space also in the central nervous system although the determination of its exact size probably requires a new methodological approach.

Whatever the location of the blood-brain barrier turns out to be, it appears that we are not dealing with a barrier but with a transport mechanism dependent on the metabolic events in a hitherto undetermined location of the central nervous system. It is of major interest to ascertain whether or not there exist gradations in the blood-brain barrier in different functional areas of the brain because such variations may make different areas dependent, in various degrees, upon the metabolic and hormonal influences of the body.

While we know little about the blood-brain barrier in the direction of blood to brain, we know still less about the reverse direction from brain to blood. There are various indications that substances administered intracerebrally appear at different rates in the blood, suggesting that the blood-brain barrier acts in both directions.

An injury to the brain results in a localized decreased efficiency of the blood-brain barrier as indicated by the staining of the damaged areas after systemic administration of dye, the uptake of labeled substances (BAKAY, 1956; QUADBECK and HELMCHEN, 1955), and the effect of otherwise non-penetrating drugs on the electroencephalogram of frozen areas of the brain (e. g., γ-aminobutyric acid, BERL et al., 1961b). After infarction of the brain, some enzymes appear in the cerebrospinal fluid but not in the blood, a fact which suggests that the spinal fluid-blood barrier is not penetrable by these enzyme proteins (WAKIM and FLEISHER, 1956; GREEN, 1958).

Although the interstitial fluid of the brain and the cerebrospinal fluid are in rapid equilibrium, the production of the cerebrospinal fluid is apparently not restricted to the choroid plexus alone and its final composition is the result of diffusion and active transport mechanism dependent on the metabolism of the linings of the respective cavities of the central nervous system (SWEET et al., 1954; SWEET and LOCKSLEY, 1953).

C. Energy metabolism

I. Oxygen consumption of the brain in vivo

The brain has an oxygen consumption which is one of the highest among the tissues of the body, and it is the first organ to succumb to oxygen deprivation. The energy requirements of the nervous cell, therefore, are high even in a state of apparent mental rest. The metabolic function in which most of the energy is presumably consumed is the maintenance of selective distributions of sodium and potassium ions. The highly unstable state of disequilibrium thus established is responsible for the creation of the membrane potentials essential for nervous excitability.

It is possible to measure the oxygen consumption of the brain in vivo (or for that matter, the consumption or production of any other substance) if two factors are known, the blood flow (ml blood/100 g brain/min) and the arteriovenous difference (e.g., ml O_2/ml blood). According to the Fick formula their product equals uptake (or output) in the tissue:

$$\text{Substrate consumption} = \text{blood flow} \cdot A-V \text{ difference}$$
$$\text{Substrate output} \qquad = \text{blood flow} \cdot V-A \text{ difference.}$$

In primates, including man, almost pure cerebral blood with only slight admixture of cranial or facial venous blood may be obtained from the superior bulb of the internal jugular vein. The A−V difference can thus be determined by direct analysis of arterial and cerebral venous blood. The determination of cerebral blood flow is again based on Fick's formula, in the form:

$$\text{Blood flow} = \frac{\text{Substrate taken up}}{\text{Arteriovenous difference of substrate}}$$

The "substrate" in this case is an indifferent gas, such as nitrous oxide (KETY, 1948) or radioactive krypton (LASSEN and MUNCK, 1955), which, when inhaled, diffuses into the brain until its tension is the same in arterial and cerebral venous blood (KETY and SCHMIDT, 1948). This equilibrium is reached within 10 minutes in the nitrous oxide method where a gas mixture consisting of 15% N_2O, 20% O_2 and 65% N_2 is administered. In the case of ^{85}Kr equilibration is more rapid and blood analysis is simpler and more accurate.

Cerebral blood flow has been shown to be very variable. It is in fact an essential factor in the homoeostatic control of oxygen consumption. Before methods for the determination of cerebral blood flow were available numerous data on arteriovenous differences were collected. Although these studies were very valuable in allowing comparisons of the utilization or production of different metabolites relative to each other, they can not legitimately be used for the estimation of metabolic rates.

In spite of great variability of cerebral blood flow, the oxygen consumption of the adult human brain has been found to be remarkably constant, with an average value of 3.5 ± 0.6 ml/100 g/min or 49 ml/min for a brain of 1400 g. The rate is unaffected by changes of activity within the physiological range. Thus, neither the increase of mental activity elicited by solving arithmetical problems nor the decrease of mental activity during natural sleep produces any noticeable change of cerebral oxygen consumption. It should be realized however that with the methods available at present only global values appertaining to the brain as a whole may be obtained and changes in circumscribed locations might go unnoticed.

Under experimental or pathological conditions, however, changes may be observed which indicate a reduced oxygen consumption in states of impaired consciousness and a rise of oxygen consumption during convulsive activity (Table 2). Moderate depression of consciousness, such as might be observed in confusional states or in superficial anaesthesia, has been found to be associated with a moderate depression of oxygen consumption, while in deep anaesthesia or in comatose states of varying origin oxygen consumption may fall by 40—50%. An increase of cerebral oxygen consumption by about 100% has been observed in monkeys during convulsions. In the postconvulsive state oxygen consumption is depressed.

Pathological processes leading to a loss of neurons often cause a decrease in cerebral oxygen consumption, e.g. arteriosclerosis, brain tumor, cerebral atrophy, neurosyphilis. Occurrences of low oxygen consumption in cases of congenital mental deficiency are probably also attributable to anatomical lesions.

Rates of oxygen consumption are normal in epilepsy (during interictal period) and in pyrexia. No changes were found in LSD-intoxication. The question as to whether there is a depression of oxygen consumption in schizophrenia is still controversial. According to KETY et al. (1948) cerebral oxygen consumption in schizophrenia, including the advanced stages is, on the average, normal, while GORDAN et al. (1955) report that there are two groups of schizophrenics, one with normal and one with lowered oxygen consumption. The latter consisted of patients with a history of more than 4 years.

Other factors

1. *Age:* Cerebral oxygen consumption is probably constant throughout adult life, even at extreme old age, unless vascular, degenerative or other pathological changes intervene, but it is considerably higher in infants and children up to the age of puberty (KENNEDY, 1956). In adults, the cerebral oxygen consumption accounts for 20—25% of that of the body as a whole; in children this figure is 50%. But as the weight of the brain is 2—3% of the body weight in the adult and 7—8% in a 7 year old child, the relative oxygen consumption of the brain compared with the rest of the body is higher in the adult than in the child. The changeover to the adult pattern occurs just prior to puberty, presumably brought on by gonadal hormones. In eunuchoidism and related hypogonadal dysfunctions where there is no puberty a high cerebral oxygen consumption may persist into adult life. On the other hand, castration after puberty in the male does not cause the rate of cerebral oxygen consumption to revert to the prepubertal pattern. Once established, the change appears to be irreversible (GORDAN, 1956).

2. *Other hormones:* Thyroid hormone, even though it accelerates the metabolism of the body as a whole, does not affect the rate of cerebral metabolism.

Table 2. *Cerebral blood flow and oxygen consumption in man [mean values $\pm$ standard errors: standard deviations are followed by (σ)]*

	No. of observation	Cerebral blood flow (ml/100 g/min)	Cerebral respiratory rate (ml O$_2$/100 g/min)	Ref.
Normal adults	14	54 $\pm$ 12 (σ)	3.3 $\pm$ 0.4 (σ)	[1]
Normal adults	20	65 $\pm$ 2.14	3.8 $\pm$ 0.09	[2]
Normal adults	20	52 $\pm$ 1.9	3.4 $\pm$ 0.13	[3]
Schizophrenics	30	54. $\pm$ 7.6 (σ)	3.3 $\pm$ 0.43 (σ)	[4]
Epileptics	12	55	3.5	[5]
Essential hypertension	13	54	3.4	[6]
Children below age 10	6	104.3 $\pm$ 4.0	5.1 $\pm$ 0.32	[7]
Old age (mean age 71)	"large group"		3.4	[8]
{ Sleep	6	65.0 $\pm$ 5.3	3.4 $\pm$ 0.39	
{ controls	6	59.2 $\pm$ 4.9	3.5 $\pm$ 0.020	
{ Mental arithmetic	12	66.8 $\pm$ 3.6	4.0 $\pm$ 0.07	[9]
{ controls	12	69.2 $\pm$ 4.0	3.9 $\pm$ 0.12	
{ Epinephrine infusion	7	60.7 $\pm$ 5.2	4.16 $\pm$ 0.34	
{ controls	7	50.1 $\pm$ 3.0	3.4 $\pm$ 0.14	
Cerebrovascular disease, acute .	22	40	2.7	[10]
chronic	17	35	2.1	
Organic dementia	10		2.2	[11]
Brain tumor	12	44	2.9	[12]
Pentothal anaesthesia	10	61	2.1	[13]
Myxoedema	8	40 $\pm$ 3.7	2.8 $\pm$ 0.2	[14]
Coma of various origin			1.6 — 2.5	[15]

References to Table 2.

[1] KETY, S. S., and C. F. SCHMIDT: J. clin. Invest. **27**, 476 (1948).

[2] SCHEINBERG, P., and E. A. STEAD: J. clin. Invest. **28**, 1163 (1949).

[3] LASSEN, N. A., and O. MUNCK: Acta physiol. scand. **33**, 30 (1955).

[4] KETY, S. S., R. B. WOODFORD, M. H. HARMEL, F. A. FREYHAN, K. E. APPEL and C. F. SCHMIDT: Amer. J. Psychiat. **104**, 765 (1948).

[5] SCHMIDT, C. F.: Pflügers Arch. ges. Physiol. **251**, 571 (1949).

[6] KETY, S. S., J. H. HAFKENSCHIEL, W. A. JEFFERS, I. H. LEOPOLD and H. A. SHENKIN: J. clin. Invest. **27**, 511 (1948).

[7] KENNEDY, C.: Neurochemistry. p. 230. (Ed. S. R. KOREY and J. I. NURNBERGER) London: Cassell and Co. Ltd. 1956.

[8] SOKOLOFF, L., D. K. DASTUR, M. H. LANE and S. S. KETY: Unpublished data quoted by N. A. LASSEN. Physiol. Rev. **39**, 183 (1959).

[9] SOKOLOFF, L.: Neurochemistry. p. 216. (Ed. S. R. KOREY, and J. I. NURNBERGER). London: Cassell and Co. Ltd. 1956.

[10] HEYMAN, A., J. L. PATTERSON, T. W. DUKE and L. L. BATTEY: New Engl. J. Med. **249**, 223 (1953).

[11] LASSEN, N. A., O. MUNCK and E. R. TOTTEY: Arch. Neurol. Psychiat. **77**, 126 (1957).

[12] KETY, S. S., H. A. SHENKIN and C. F. SCHMIDT: J. clin. Invest. **27**, 493 (1948).

[13] WECHSLER, R. L., R. D. DRIPPS, and S. S. KETY: Anaesthesiology **12**, 308 (1951).

[14] SCHEINBERG, P., E. A. STEAD, E. S. BRANNON, and J. V. WARREN: J. clin. Invest. **29**, 1139 (1950).

[15] LASSEN, N. A.: Physiol. Rev. **39**, 183 (1959).

This is probably due to the restraining effect of the blood-brain barrier since an effect of thyroid hormones on cerebral oxygen consumption is observed in newborn rats where the blood-brain barrier is not yet fully effective (REISS, REISS, and WYATT, 1956). ACTH, cortisone and deoxycorticosterone have no significant effects on cerebral oxygen consumption. Adrenaline if infused in relatively high dosage may cause a rise in cerebral oxygen consumption and it is possible that a discharge of endogenous adrenaline, such as might occur in severe anxiety, would have a similar effect (SOKOLOFF, 1956).

3. *Hypoxia:* When the oxygen tension of air is reduced by 50% (corresponding to an altitude of 18,000 feet) cerebral oxygen consumption remains unimpaired, although mental changes are usually pronounced. The subjects complain of lassitude, headache and inability to concentrate; failure of memory, loss of visual acuity and changes in the EEG can be recorded objectively. Presumably this lack of correlation between oxygen consumption and mental changes is again due to localized effects.

4. *Hypoglycaemia:* In the normal human being cerebral oxygen consumption essentially depends on 3 factors: a normal supply of oxygen, a normal circulation and a normal supply of the principal substrate, glucose. Cerebral oxygen consumption is therefore decreased in hypoglycaemia. The effects of hypoglycaemia will be further discussed in a subsequent section.

II. Carbon dioxide fixation in nervous tissue

Contrary to various experimentally unfounded statements, the mammalian central nervous system shows a significant fixation of carbon dioxide as demonstrated by the appearance of labeled carbon in glutamic acid, glutamine and aspartic acid after the intracarotid infusion of ^{14}C bicarbonate to cats (BERL et al., 1961, 1962). This finding is in agreement with the demonstration of the occurrence of the respective enzymes in brain tissue. Carbon dioxide fixation is not a metabolic characteristic of the mammalian brain only, but seems to be a property of nervous tissue as such, since it has also been demonstrated in preparations such as lobster nerve (CHENG and WAELSCH, 1962). The finding of a significant CO_2 fixation in nervous tissue raises the interesting question whether or not some effects of CO_2 ascribed to its influences on the physico-chemical environment may not be due to its direct participation in metabolism via the citric acid cycle mediated by carbon dioxide fixation.

III. Regional differences in cerebral respiration

Macroscopically and microscopically the brain is an organ comprising a number of disparate structures and elements. The in vivo measurement of the metabolism of circumscribed cerebral areas would be of great importance, but the methods at present available are of only limited usefulness. Local changes in blood flow have been recorded by a thermoelectric method; although the results were only comparative, an increase of blood flow could be demonstrated when specific regions were stimulated, for instance in the visual cortex of cat brain after illuminating the eye (SCHMIDT and HENDRIX, 1938). LANDAU et al. (1955) have developed a method for the quantitative evaluation of regional blood flow in absolute terms; the method is based on the degree of radioactivity attained in frozen brain slices after the intravenous injection of a radioactive gas. Valuable as these methods are they do not give information on oxygen consumption, except by inference. DAVIES and REMOND (1947) measured the oxygen tension at the surface of cat cerebral cortex by inserting an oxygen cathode. They were able to demonstrate a decrease of oxygen tension during convulsive activity, but their results are not of a quantitative nature.

Our present knowledge regarding the respiration of different brain areas is largely derived from in vitro measurements on surviving tissue preparations. The respiration of grey matter is about 5 times as high as that of white matter; since human brain contains about 50% grey matter the oxygen consumption of grey matter in vivo is calculated as 6.0 ml/100 g/min, that of white matter as 1.2 ml/100 g/min. Differences are also found when the respiration of different areas of grey matter is compared, but they are not large (Table 3).

The greater part of white matter respiration is presumably attributable to interspersed glia cells. The respiratory enzymes are located in the mitochondria; these are present in high concentration in the cytoplasm surrounding the nucleus and also in the terminals of the synaptic junction, but they are relatively sparse in axoplasm. In the case of the giant axon of the squid it has been possible to show that the metabolism of extruded axoplasm is very low, while the slit sheath with its associated Schwann cells respires at a rate very similar to that of the intact fibre (SCHMITT, 1957).

Cellular density is however not solely responsible for the respiratory rate of nervous tissue. Great differences were found when respiration was related to the number of nuclei (HELLER and ELLIOTT, 1955), due not only to differences between neuronal and glial cells but also to those between different kinds of neurons. On the basis of cellular density, respiration in vitro is highest in cerebral cortex, followed by corpus callosum and cerebellar cortex in that order (Table 4 — ELLIOTT and HELLER, 1957). Thus, although corpus callosum contains only glial cells, these have higher respiration than the cells of cerebellar cortex the majority of which are presumably neurons.

If it is assumed that the glia cells in the cerebral cortex respire at the same rate as the glia cells in the corpus callosum, and if it is further assumed that the respiration of the axonal elements of the corpus callosum is negligible, it is possible to calculate the relative contribution of neuronal and glial elements to the observed respiration of

Table 3. *Rates of respiration of slices from various areas of the central nervous system. Incubation at 37° in glucose-containing medium and in atmosphere of oxygen*

Species	Area	Medium[1]	$-QO_2$ (μl O_2/mg dry weight/hour)	Ref.
Rabbit	Cerebral cortex	P	8.8	1
	White matter	P	3.7	
Cat	Cerebral cortex	P	10.5	2
	Medulla oblongata	P	3.5	
	Spinal cord	P	1.3	
	Cerebral cortex	B	8.8	3
		P	12.4	
	Cerebellar cortex	P	10.6	
	Corpus callosum	B	2.2	
		P	2.5	
	Cerebral cortex	P	6.6	4
	Cerebellar cortex	P	7.1	
	Caudate nucleus	P	8.6	
	Thalamus	P	5.4	
	Hypothalamus	P	5.0	
	Ammon's horn	P	5.2	
	Septal area	P	6.6	
Dog	Cerebral cortex	B	8.5	3
		P	13.1	
	Cerebellar cortex	P	10.8	
	Corpus callosum	P	2.2	
Ox	Cerebral cortex	P	8.5	5
	Cerebellar cortex	P	12.7	
	Corpus striatum	P	9.7	
	Thalamus	P	5.8	
	Ammon's horn	P	6.3	
	Globus pallidus	P	1.8	
Man	Cerebral cortex	B	6.7	3
		P	10.6	
	White matter	P	1.2—2.7	

[1] B: Ringer solution buffered with bicarbonate
P: Ringer solution buffered with phosphate

References to Table 3.

[1] KREBS, H. A., and H. ROSENHAGEN: Z. ges. Neurol. **134**, 643 (1931).
[2] CRAIG, F. N., and H. K. BEECHER: J. Neurophysiol. **6**, 135 (1943).
[3] HELLER, I. H., and K. A. C. ELLIOTT: Canad. J. Biochem. **33**, 395 (1955).
[4] WEIL-MALHERBE, H.: Unpublished data.
[5] DIXON, T. F., and A. MEYER: Biochem. J. **30**, 1577 (1936).

cerebral cortex, since it is known that the proportion of neurons in human cortex is about 23% of the total number of cells (NURNBERGER and GORDON, 1957). A method has recently been described for the preparation of a highly purified fraction of glia cells and a second fraction of myelinated axon fragments, poor in cells (KOREY and ORCHEN, 1959). The study of the respiration of these fractions in a medium fortified with essential co-factors revealed that the respiration of the axonal fraction was by no means negligible, but accounted for about a third of the respiration of white matter. On this basis it was calculated that the respiration of cerebral cortex is 76% neuronal, 22% non-neuronal (glial) and 2% "axoplasmic". If the whole brain is considered the figures are 55%, 34% and 11%, or 27, 16.5 and 5.5 ml O_2/min, respectively.

Table 4. *Comparison of respiratory rate per unit of weight and per cellular nucleus in the brain (from ELLIOTT and HELLER,1957)*

Species	Area	Oxygen uptake (μl/hr.)	
		per mg dry wt.	per 10^6 nuclei
Cat	Cerebral cortex	12.4	19.0
	Cerebellar cortex	10.6	2.6
	Corpus callosum	2.5	5.7
Dog	Cerebral cortex	13.1	14.5
	Cerebellar cortex	10.8	3.0
	Corpus callosum	2.2	4.8

HYDEN (1958) studied the activities of cytochrome oxidase and succinoxidase in oligodendrocytes isolated from those neuroglia cells intimately surrounding the ganglion cells. The concentration of these respiratory enzymes was 2—7 times higher in the glia cells than in the nerve cells, presumably indicating a higher respiratory rate in the former. The discrepancy between these results and those based on measurements of tissue respiration may be due to differences in the respiratory activity of different types of glia cells or to differences in sample preparation.

The study of human glial tumors has given valuable clues to the relative rates of respiration of different glia cell species. Oligodendroglioma was shown to respire more actively than astrocytoma. The rate per nucleus of even the actively respiring oligodendroglioma was only about the same as for human white matter (HELLER and ELLIOTT, 1955).

IV. The utilization of substrates by the brain in vivo

It is generally agreed that under normal conditions glucose is utilized as the principal source of energy by nervous tissue. What is still under discussion is the question of whether other substrates are utilized when sufficient glucose is not available or when energy demands are abnormal.

The evidence for a predominant utilization of glucose by the brain is based on the following facts:

1. The respiratory quotient of the brain in vivo is close to unity (GIBBS, LENNOX and GIBBS, 1945). This is also true for brain slices in vitro, whether respiring in glucose-saline or in a substrate-free medium (DICKENS, 1936). With brain suspensions lower values have been reported, especially in the absence of glucose; these may be partly due to a non-enzymatic autoxidation of unsaturated lipids.

2. The only substrate for which a consistently significant cerebral arteriovenous difference can be demonstrated is glucose. The average uptake of glucose, on its passage through the brain, is 5.5 mg/100 g/min (77 mg/min for the whole brain). Not all of it is completely oxidized to CO_2 and water; about 15% leaves the brain in the form of lactic and pyruvic acids, the end products of glycolysis. Out of 5.5 mg of glucose taken up, 4.7 mg or 26.1 μmoles are therefore oxidized, requiring

$26.1 \cdot 6 = 156$ μmoles of oxygen. Now 156 μmoles $= 3.5$ ml of oxygen, which is the amount normally consumed; in other words, the utilization of oxygen in cerebral metabolism is, within the experimental error, quantitatively accounted for by the utilization of glucose (HIMWICH and HIMWICH, 1946).

Efforts to demonstrate the utilization of α-ketoacids or of total ketones by the normal human brain or by the brain of subjects in ketosis were unsuccessful (KETY, 1957). ADAMS and coworkers (1955) claimed a significant cerebral uptake of glutamic acid in 16 out of 19 normal subjects, at the rate of 0.4 mg/100 g/min. Glutamic acid was apparently utilized for a quantitative conversion into glutamine which was released at the rate of 0.6 mg/100 g/min. No such amidation was found in 14 out of 16 patients with multiple sclerosis. The amidation of glutamic acid will be discussed in a subsequent section. In any case, the utilization of glutamic acid, observed by ADAMS et al., does not appear to be for the supply of energy.

SACKS (1956, 1957) showed the formation of $^{14}CO_2$ by the human brain after an injection of ^{14}C-labelled fumaric or butyric acid. The utilization of these acids, however, may have resulted from an exchange mechanism rather than from a net uptake, a probability which must be considered especially in view of the work of LAJTHA, BERL and WAELSCH (1959) with labelled amino acids.

RODNIGHT, MCILWAIN, and TRESIZE (1959) have examined cerebral arterio-venous differences for a number of substances in the rabbit. They found a small release of lactic acid but no change in ketoacids, twenty amino acids, nucleotides, creatine, ascorbic acid or glutathione.

3. *If the brain is deprived of its normal supply of glucose both its metabolism and its function are gravely impaired.* When hypoglycaemia reaches a certain degree of severity (about 20 mg glucose/100 ml), cerebral oxygen consumption begins to fall and continues to fall as hypoglycaemia progresses. In hypoglycaemia the glucose oxidized by the brain is not only removed from blood but also from "extracellular" fluid and from the glycogen stores of the brain. The arteriovenous difference is therefore no longer a reliable indicator of glucose utilisation, which may continue at a much reduced level even when the arteriovenous difference has reached zero; nor is there a strict correlation between the reduction of oxygen consumption and the degree of hypoglycaemia, but the fact that, during hypoglycaemic coma, the respiratory quotient remains at unity for some time shows that the brain continues to metabolize carbohydrate. KETY (1953) has estimated that the carbohydrate reserves of the brain are sufficient to last for about 60—90 minutes after the blood sugar has disappeared, taking into account the reduced rate of cerebral oxygen consumption in hypoglycaemia coma[1]. This period coincides with the length of time through which it is usually safe to keep the patient in deep insulin coma.

HIMWICH (1951) distinguishes five phases of hypoglycaemia, corresponding to a progressive failure of cerebral centres from superficial, phylogenetically new layers, which are most sensitive, to deeper, phylogenetically older layers which are more resistant to hypoglycaemia. Death ensues when respiratory and other essen-

---

[1] If the carbohydrate reserves (glycogen, glucose, lactic acid) of a human brain of 1400 g + 120 ml of cerebrospinal fluid are calculated from figures given in the literature (see MCILWAIN, 1955) the result is 2.8—2.9 g. At the reduced rate of consumption of 3 mg/100 g/min this amount would be utilized in about 70 min. The glucose concentration used for this computation is that found in cat brain (76 mg/100 g). However, there are great species differences: thus, in rabbit brain a glucose concentration of 37 mg/100 g (KERR and GHANTUS, 1936) and in rat brain one of 20 mg/100 g have been found by reduction methods. THORN et al. (1959) found 90 mg/100 g in the brain of anesthetized rabbits by a specific enzymatic procedure. Of the reducing substances in rat brain only 40%, or 8 mg/100 g tissue, was actually glucose (GEY, 1956). If we substitute this figure in our calculation the carbohydrate reserves of human brain would be exhausted in about 45 min.

tial autonomic centres become impaired. In support of his hypothesis Himwich found that glycogen disappeared from the brain of hypoglycaemic dogs in a sequence progressing from the cortex to the deeper centres. Death coincided with the disappearance of glycogen from the medulla oblongata, while glycogen in the spinal cord remained largely intact.

Many substances have been studied with regard to their ability to relieve symptoms of hypoglycaemia in animals and man, but only mannose and maltose were found to be effective substitutes for glucose. The substances tested and found inactive included sugars, viz. fructose, galactose, hexosediphosphate, lactose, and inulin, and metabolites of glucose, such as lactate, pyruvate, ethanol, glycerol, succinate, fumarate, acetate, and glutamate (Mann and Magath, 1922; Maddock, Hawkins and Holmes, 1939; Goldfarb and Wortis, 1941; Wortis et al., 1941). Some of these, particularly fructose, lactate, pyruvate, glutamate and succinate, are able to sustain the respiration of brain slices in the absence of glucose; the discrepancy is accounted for by the intervention of the blood-brain barrier (Klein, Hurwitz and Olsen, 1946; Klein and Olsen, 1947; Schwerin, Bessman and Waelsch, 1950).

It has been shown by Mayer-Gross and Walker (1949) that hypoglycaemic coma is terminated, in a proportion of patients, by an intravenous injection of L-glutamate. The arousal is however only temporary and the patients soon slip back into coma unless given glucose. The effect of glutamate could be duplicated by injection of arginine or p-aminobenzoate, and, in a somewhat smaller proportion of cases, by that of glycine or succinate; injection of adrenaline was at least as effective as that of glutamate. The transient nature of the effect, the variety of effective agents and the impermeability of the blood-brain barrier to glutamate suggest that the effect of glutamate is not that of an energy-producing substrate but mediated by an adrenergic mechanism (Weil-Malherbe, 1949, 1952).

Although fructose was previously found to be ineffective in the relief of hypoglycaemic symptoms in hepatectomized animals, Tagnon and Corvilain (1959) have reported that it may alleviate symptoms of hypoglycaemia, such as sweating, malaise, confusion, eosinopenia and electroencephalographic changes, in the human; a total of 90 g of fructose in 10% solution was given by intravenous infusion for 1 hour. It is claimed that the level of blood glucose remained unaffected. However, Seltzer, Eisenberg and Sensenbach (1957) who also found an alleviation of hypoglycaemic symptoms after the infusion of fructose consider that fructose is converted to glucose in the liver at a rate sufficient to satisfy the needs of the brain.

V. The utilization of substrates by perfused nervous tissue

The metabolism of the perfused cat brain has been studied particularly by Geiger and his colleagues (1947, 1952). When cat brain was perfused with a "simplified blood" containing 36—38% of washed bovine erythrocytes, 7% serum albumin and 0.1% glucose in bicarbonate Krebs-Ringer solution the glucose content of the brain fell to very low levels and its lactate content rose. It was assumed that the transfer of glucose from blood to brain and that of lactate from brain to blood had ceased. The galactoside and phospholipid content of the brain decreased and the perfused brain gradually lost its electrical activity and its response to chemical, electrical or afferent stimulation. These changes could be avoided by inserting the isolated liver into the perfusion circuit or by adding fresh liver extract to the perfusion fluid (Geiger, Magnes, Taylor and Veralli, 1954). Later it was found that liver extract could be replaced by cytidine and uridine (Geiger and Yamasaki, 1956); the addition of a few mg of these substances to perfusion blood maintained the function of perfused cat brain for over 4 hours. Uridine which is part of a co-enzyme involved in galactose metabolism restored the normal cerebroside content; cytidine which is a component of a co-factor for phospholipid synthesis restored the normal phospholipid content.

ALLWEIS and MAGNES (1958), using an improved perfusion technique and radioactive glucose, were able to show that the perfused cat brain, in spite of its low glucose content and in the absence of the liver or liver extract, continues to utilize glucose at a rapid rate. However, only about one-quarter of the glucose taken up was oxidized to CO_2, the remainder being converted to lactic acid. The oxidation of glucose accounted for only about one-fifth of the respiratory CO_2, while the remainder presumably originated from non-carbohydrates. The respiratory quotient, accordingly, was well below unity. Fructose was not significantly utilized. The addition of uridine and cytidine did not improve the oxidation of glucose.

The fate of radioactive glucose in the perfused cat brain has also been studied by GEIGER (1958). As in the experiments of ALLWEIS and MAGNES, only a third of the glucose taken up by the brain "at rest" was oxidized, and less when the brain was stimulated. Since the oxygen consumption agreed with that expected from the complete oxidation of the glucose taken up, GEIGER assumed that the oxygen not accounted for by glucose actually oxidized to CO_2 was used up in the oxidation of non-carbohydrate material which was subsequently resynthesized from glucose. This assumption is based on a "steady state" having been reached; the results could however also have been due to an incomplete equilibration between the labelled glucose and its metabolites on the one hand and pre-formed carbohydrates and carbohydrate metabolites on the other.

There was considerable labelling in the soluble and insoluble fractions of brain tissue in which amino acids, lipids and proteins were taking part. Labelling was increased in the post-convulsive period, indicating an increased rate of resynthesis of lipids and proteins from glucose.

It thus appears that in the perfused cat brain non-carbohydrates are metabolized to a large extent. It is not surprising, therefore, that this preparation can survive and continues to show certain aspects of function for up to an hour in the complete absence of glucose, provided the rate of blood flow is increased two- to threefold. Oxygen consumption is maintained at about the same rate as in the presence of glucose. The respiratory quotient, which is 1.0 initially, decreases gradually to values as low as 0.5 (GEIGER, MAGNES and GEIGER, 1952). During this time there is a loss of up to 60% of phospholipids and 50% of nitrogen from the microsomal and supernatant fractions of brain cortex, while amino acids and nucleotides appear in the perfusion fluid in increased amounts (ABOOD and GEIGER, 1955).

In a preliminary note which was never followed up by a more detailed publication, TSCHIRGI et al. (1949) reported that reflex responses of the perfused spinal cord of the rat disappeared after withholding glucose for 2—4 minutes and returned after renewal of the glucose supply. Glucose could be replaced by pyruvate, isocitrate, α-ketoglutarate, glutamate and glutamine and, partly, by oxaloacetate, while acetate, lactate, succinate, fumarate, malate, β-hydroxybutyrate and several amino acids were ineffective.

It is difficult to reconcile these results with the conclusion, arrived at on the basis of in vivo observations, that glucose is irreplaceable for the maintenance of normal brain functions. It should be pointed out, however, that although certain elementary functions continue during the glucose-free perfusion of cat brain, the possibility of irreversible damage cannot be excluded in this type of experiment.

VI. The utilization of substrates by preparations of isolated nervous tissue in vitro

Preparations of isolated nervous tissue whose metabolism may be studied in vitro range from the intact superior cervical ganglion of the rat to solutions of purified enzymes. Brain slices, brain homogenates, suspensions of mitochondria or other intracellular fractions occupy intermediate positions on the scale of disintegration. Experiments with these preparations have the advantage that the blood-brain barrier and, according to the degree of disintegration, other membrane barriers have been eliminated. On the other hand, quite apart from the structural damage which is inevitably inflicted even upon such well-integrated preparations as brain slices, the very absence of the circulation imposes certain limitations and "unphysiological" conditions, since the supply of oxygen and nutrients and the removal of waste products is by diffusion only. Experiments with brain slices are usually carried out in an atmosphere of 96—100% oxygen so as to increase the oxygen tension in the tissue. This in itself is not entirely harmless, particularly for brain tissue. Oxygen at several atmospheres pressure may lead to "oxygen poisoning", in vivo and in vitro; prolonged exposure to an atmosphere of pure oxygen may cause damage even at normal pressure, probably due to the oxidation of sulphydryl groups and a resulting inhibition of enzymatic functions.

The destruction of membrane barriers attendant upon the slicing or mincing of the tissue facilitates not only the access of substrates but also the loss of essential metabolites, coenzymes and minerals and of soluble enzymes which may escape into the suspension medium. Moreover, coenzymes become exposed to the action of catabolizing enzymes, normally restrained by the intact cellular structure. This difficulty can be overcome in part by suitably supplementing or "fortifying" the suspension medium with cofactors, substrates and inhibitors of autolytic enzymes. It is not clear at present to what degree metabolic compartmentation — responsible to a large extent for the control of metabolism — has broken down in tissue slices (see Waelsch, 1960).

The in vitro experiments which have perhaps come closest to in vivo conditions are those of Larrabee (1958) who studied the metabolism and the activity of superior cervical ganglia excised from young rats. In resting ganglia the consumption of glucose was completely accounted for by the formation of lactate and the consumption of oxygen. When glucose was withdrawn oxygen uptake fell by 15—20% within 90 minutes. Impulse conduction and synaptic transmission failed progressively during the following 60 minutes in spite of an oxygen uptake which increased. In ganglia adequately supplied with glucose, activity was induced by preganglionic nerve stimulation; this caused increased consumption of both glucose and oxygen. However, the increased consumption of glucose was completely accounted for by conversion to lactic acid. The extra oxygen uptake must therefore have been due to the metabolism of endogenous substrate. This, at any rate, was the situation when the experiments were carried out at a temperature of 37° and a pH of 7.4. When temperature was lowered to 23° and the pH to 7.0, activity still caused an increase of both glucose and oxygen consumption, but there was less formation of lactic acid, with the result that under these conditions the increment in oxygen uptake could be accounted for by glucose oxidation. It was considered likely that the results obtained at 37° were caused by the existence of an anoxic zone in the centre of the ganglion (Dolivo and Larrabee, 1958).

The respiration of brain slices is maintained not only by glucose but also by fructose, glutamate and some metabolites of glucose, notably lactate, pyruvate, oxaloacetate and α-ketoglutarate. Others, such as the phosphorylated intermediates and some di- and tricarboxylic acids, are only oxidized if the cell structure is broken down further.

Of particular interest is the fact that brain contains enzymes for the synthesis or oxidation of fatty acids, albeit in lower concentration than in several other tissues tested (LYNEN, 1957). Accordingly, the ability of rat brain slices (GEYER, MATTHEWS and STARE, 1949; VOLK, MILLINGTON and WEINHOUSE, 1952) and of rat brain mitochondria (VIGNAIS, GALLAGHER and ZABIN, 1958) to form radioactive CO_2 from carboxyl-labelled long-chain fatty acids has been demonstrated; the activity is low compared with that of liver.

In vitro studies therefore lead to the conclusion that the potential of nervous tissue for metabolizing substrates is more diversified than one might have expected from the results of the in vivo experiments. It appears that the enzymatic equipment is available but that the access of foodstuffs is limited by the blood-brain barrier and by cellular membranes. The presence of enzymes metabolizing substrates which arise in the intermediary metabolism of glucose is of course not in disagreement with the thesis that glucose is the principal source of energy in nervous tissues. Those reacting with nitrogenous and lipid material presumably have functions which are not primarily aimed at the supply of energy.

There has been much speculation on the reasons for the exclusive reliance of the brain on glucose as energy source. Is it to be regarded as a kind of metabolic streamlining permitting the development of specialized functions at the expense of the greater latitude in the choice of oxidizable substrates enjoyed by less highly differentiated cells ? Is its purpose an easier control of the metabolic rate ? Or does it facilitate the maintenance of a favourable internal and external environment ?

VII. Mechanisms and pathways

During the past 30 years the principal pathways of intermediary metabolism have been fairly well elucidated. The fundamental pattern varies little from tissue to tissue or even from organism to organism. The reaction sequences of glycolysis and the citric acid cycle, the mechanisms of electron transport and oxidative phosphorylation are the same in nervous as in other tissues and apparent discrepancies have, in most cases, found a satisfactory explanation. For information on these topics, therefore, a textbook of general biochemistry may be consulted.

Where the metabolic pathways in the brain differ from those in other tissues, the differences are either of a quantitative nature or they concern subsidiary pathways or specialized mechanisms. Brain contains the enzymes required for the oxidation of glucose through the so-called pentose shunt, but, like the enzymes involved in fatty acid metabolism, they are present in low concentration. Comparison of the formation of $^{14}CO_2$ from glucose-1-^{14}C and from glucose-6-^{14}C (cf. Fig. 1) has given no indication of a significant role of this pathway in the glucose metabolism of brain (BLOOM, 1955; DIPIETRO and WEINHOUSE, 1959; TOWER, 1958). It has been reported (HOSKIN, 1960) that the oxidation of glucose via the pentose shunt by guinea pig brain slices is greatly stimulated by the addition of 10^{-5}—10^{-3} M synkavite (vitamin K_3 diphosphate) to the medium. Some enzymes occur mainly in nervous tissue, such as choline acetylase, glutamic decarboxylase and glutamine synthetase. They are presumably closely related to nervous function. Others are widespread in other tissues but are not found in brain. One of these is fructose-1-phosphokinase which forms fructose-1-phosphate from fructose and adenosine triphosphate (ATP) in liver and muscle. In brain, fructose is converted into fructose-6-phosphate by the enzyme hexokinase which is relatively unspecific. MEYERHOF (1947) has shown that, at low concentrations of ATP, glucose is phosphorylated at a much faster rate than fructose. This observation explained a heretofore puzzling inconsistency: while glucose and fructose are both capable of maintaining the respiration of brain slices, only glucose, but not fructose, is broken down to lactic acid anaerobically. This has led to the assump-

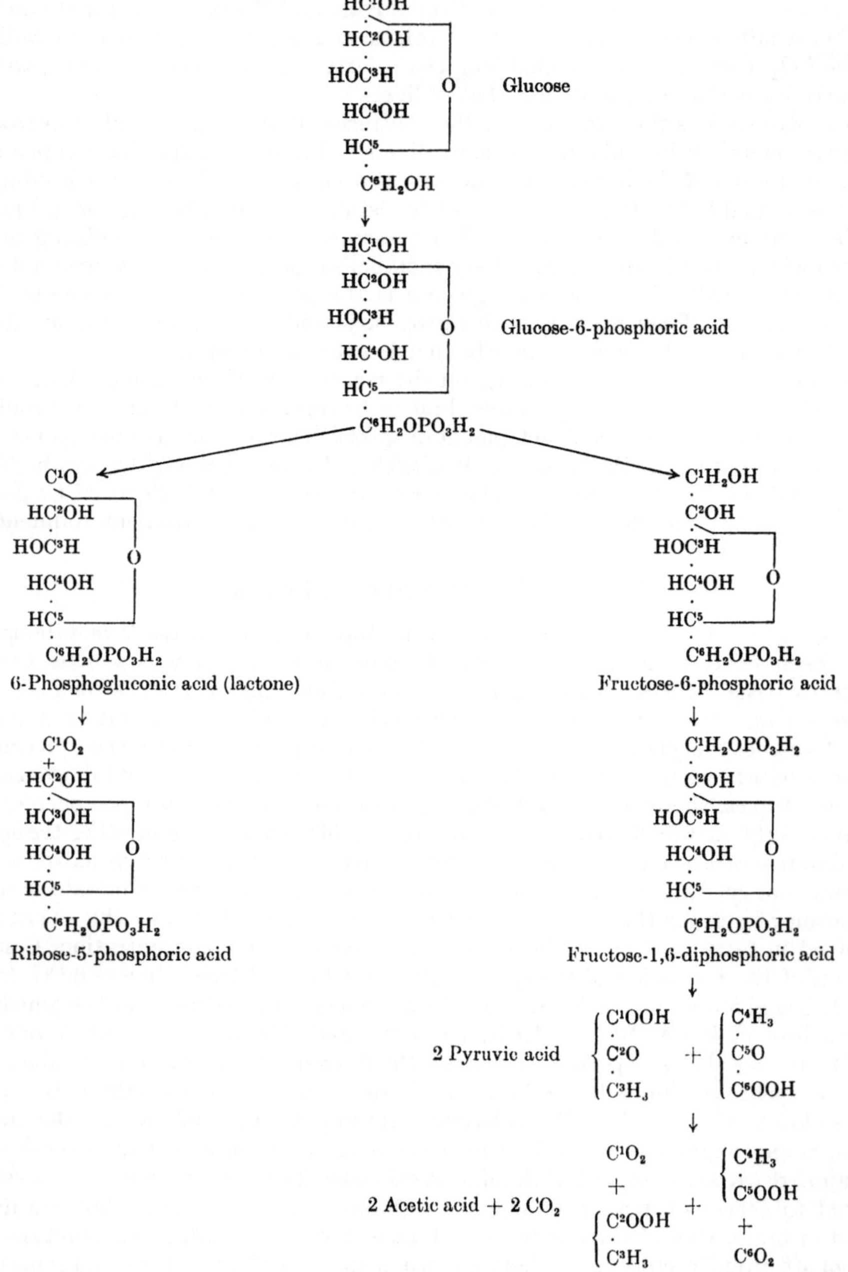

Fig 1. Breakdown of glucose (simplified) by the pentose shunt (left) and by the "glycolytic" pathway (right) In the latter equal amounts of CO_2 are derived from C^1 and C^6 of glucose while in the former CO_2 is primarily derived from C^1 of glucose

tion that the oxidative metabolism of fructose does not follow the glycolytic pathway in its initial stages. However, since the concentration of ATP in brain slices is higher aerobically than anaerobically it is probable that aerobically the ATP-level is adequate for the phosphorylation of both glucose and fructose while anaerobically it is only adequate for the phosphorylation of glucose. In fact, in a brain extract or homogenate suitably fortified with ATP, fructose forms lactic acid anaerobically at a rate equal to glucose (MEYERHOF, 1947). Even in brain slices an active anaerobic "fructolysis" can be demonstrated if the slices are suspended in a hypertonic sucrose medium containing ATP (SPIRTES and BRUNNER, 1959). Apparently the penetrability of ATP is increased in hypertonic sucrose medium.

It has recently been shown that cell nuclei isolated from brain tissue contain glycolytic enzymes and several dehydrogenases in concentrations similar to those in unfractionated brain (SIEBERT, BAESSLER, HANNOVER, ADLOFF and BEYER, 1961). Apart from the nuclear fraction, and with the exception of hexokinase of which about 70% is bound to mitochondria, the glycolytic enzymes of the brain, as in other tissues, are located in the cytoplasm (JOHNSON, 1960). Contrary observations (HESSELBACH and DU BUY, 1953; GALLAGHER, JUDAH and REES, 1956; ABOOD, BRUNNGRABER and TAYLOR, 1959) were due to insufficient disintegration of cellular fragments, particularly of axonal elements. Magnesium ions, are retained more tenaciously in the mitochondria of brain than in those of liver (KUNZ, 1958) and more chlorpromazine is absorbed by the former than by the latter (BERGER, 1957). It thus seems that the mitochondrial membrane in brain is different from that in liver. This is further borne out by the observation that the swelling of brain mitochondria is prevented by calcium ions, but not by ATP while exactly the opposite is found in liver mitochondria (GAYET, 1958).

VIII. Metabolism during activity

Large and rapid fluctuations in states of activity is a characteristic feature of all excitable tissues. To cope with the commensurate fluctuations of energy requirements special mechanisms have been evolved. A state of increased nervous activity is accompanied by an acceleration of metabolism, as manifested in an increased consumption of oxygen and glucose, an increased output of lactic acid and ammonia and an increased hydrolysis of the so-called "high-energy phosphate bonds".

Of these changes the increase in lactic acid formation, due to an increased glycolytic breakdown of glucose, is perhaps the most dramatic. While the consumption of oxygen can rise at the most to twice its normal level, the formation of lactic acid has been found to increase from a resting value of about 30 μmoles/g/hr to rates of 600 μmoles/g/hr in vivo (THORN, 1951; THORN and RASZKOWSKI, 1952) and about 400 μmoles/g/hr in vitro (MACFARLANE and WEIL-MALHERBE, 1941; MCILWAIN and TRESIZE, 1956), especially under anoxic conditions. These rates are, however, only of short duration, lasting for periods of 0.5—1 minute; they are then replaced by a lower but steady rate of glycolysis, at least in vitro, at a level of 5—10 times normal.

Glycolysis is a wasteful process since it delivers only $^1/_{12}$ of the free energy and only $^1/_{16}$—$^1/_{18}$ of the number of high-energy phosphate bonds obtainable from the complete oxidation of glucose. On the other hand it is less complicated than oxidation and is independent of the diffusion of oxygen, which, on a neurophysiological time scale, may be a slow process. Its retention by the nervous cell as a special activity mechanism suggests that glycolysis offers particular advantages although they are not fully understood at present.

Hand in hand with bursts of glycolysis goes the breakdown of phosphocreatine and adenosine triphosphate; reactions which also proceed with extraordinary speed. Thus the breakdown of phosphocreatine has been measured to reach a rate of 1,500 μmoles/g/hr during a period of 3 seconds while inorganic phosphate increased at a rate of 800 μmoles/g/hr (HEALD, 1954). These rates may be compared with the normal rate of oxygen uptake for the whole brain which is 100 μmoles/g/hr, equivalent to a maximum synthesis of 600 μmoles of high-energy phosphate bonds per gram per hour.

It is now generally assumed that the energy for all the manifestations of cellular activity is ultimately derived from the breakdown of adenosine triphosphate (ATP), resulting eventually, probably over several intermediate steps, in the appearance of adenosine diphosphate (ADP) and inorganic phosphate (P_i):

$$ATP \to ADP + P_i \, . \tag{1}$$

In the respiring cell ATP is resynthesized at the expense of chemical energy derived from the oxidation of a substrate (X). The ratio of phosphate esterified to atoms of oxygen reduced varies according to the substrate; from thermodynamic considerations a value of 3 may be assumed for most substrates. The net result of this "oxidative phosphorylation" may be represented by the equation:

$$3\,ADP + 3\,P_i + XH_2 + {}^1\!/_2 O_2 \to 3\,ATP + X + H_2O \, . \tag{2}$$

If the rate of breakdown of ATP exceeds the rate of resynthesis by oxidative phosphorylation, be it owing to excessive energy requirements or to impaired respiration, a second mechanism of resynthesis takes over, in which phosphocreatine (P−Cr) reacts with ADP to form ATP and creatine (Cr):

$$P-Cr + ADP \to ATP + Cr \, . \tag{3}$$

The net result of reaction (1) minus (3) is:

$$P-Cr \to Cr + P_i \, . \tag{4}$$

Phosphocreatine therefore disappears before ATP. The concentration of the latter begins to decrease when the reservoir of phosphocreatine has been emptied.

In a state of increased activity we may assume that not only reactions 1 and 3 are accelerated but also reaction 2. If the cell contains radioactive phosphorus its incorporation into ATP, its subsequent transfer to other acceptors, its eventual hydrolysis and reincorporation into ATP, in other words its "turnover", will be accelerated. This has been verified in vivo (VLADIMIROV and RUBEL, 1957) and in vitro (HEALD, 1956).

If the hydrolysis of ATP were to proceed as formulated in equation (1), the energy liberated would be degraded in the form of heat. Conversion of the free energy of hydrolysis into a form utilizable by the cell must involve intermediate steps in which energy is transferred to suitable acceptors. It has in fact been shown, in vivo (LISOVSKAYA, 1954; STREICHER, 1954) as well as in vitro (HEALD, 1957), that the incorporation of ^{32}P into the phosphoprotein fraction of the brain is greatly increased during activity. The incorporation of phosphate into phosphoprotein may be the end result of an energy-consuming process which may be connected with excitation. Phosphoproteins contain phosphate in ester linkage and not in the form of high-energy phosphate. One might postulate a primary formation of high-energy bonds subsequently transformed into ester bonds with liberation of energy.

If the rate of reaction (2) is inadequate to counterbalance the rate of ATP breakdown, a state of exhaustion will eventually be reached in which the "energy-rich" phosphate bonds have been depleted, the inorganic phosphate has correspondingly increased and as a result of increased glycolysis large amounts of lactic acid have accumulated. This state is of course reached not only as a result of excessive activities but also as a result of anoxia, ischaemia or intoxication by inhibitors of respiratory enzymes.

Changes in the opposite direction, viz. a decreased oxygen consumption, a decreased formation of lactic acid, decreased levels of inorganic phosphate and ammonia and an enrichment in ATP and phosphocreatine, are observed during anaesthesia (cf. RICHTER, 1952). This is of importance in connection with the mechanism of action of narcotics. There has been a great deal of discussion as to whether the impairment of nervous function is the result of respiratory inhibition or whether, conversely, the diminished oxygen consumption is the consequence of reduced energy requirements. The evidence at present favours the second alternative, since a pattern of exhaustion might have been expected to follow a primary inhibition of respiration, rather than an enrichment of the stores of energy-rich compounds.

1. In vivo investigations

The results outlined above were obtained by studies on the living organism as well as by experiments with excised nervous tissue. For the in vivo studies two methods have been used: one of them is based on the analysis of venous cerebral blood and several of the results have already been discussed in preceding sections. These investigations demonstrated changes in oxygen and glucose consumption and of lactic acid formation: decreases in anaesthesia and increases during convulsive activity (for summary and references see KETY, 1957). A rise in the hydrogen ion concentration of cerebral tissue, due to the formation of lactic acid, has also been recorded in the living rabbit during ischaemia (OPITZ, 1952) and in cats during convulsive cortical activity (JASPER and ERICKSON, 1941; WANG and SONNENSCHEIN, 1955), with the aid of electrodes inserted into the cerebral cortex.

Results concerning the concentration of phosphate esters and of inorganic phosphate were obtained in animal experiments by the analysis of cerebral tissue itself. In view of the great speed of the reactions affecting these substances, methods were required for rapid fixation of cerebral tissue in situ. For this purpose freezing in liquid air has been widely employed.

It should be realized that in most experiments extreme conditions were chosen; thus, anaesthesia was used to achieve a decrease of nervous activity and generalized convulsions were produced to study increased nervous activity. No changes in oxygen consumption of the human brain could be demonstrated within a more physiological range of activity, i.e., sleep on the one hand and mental arithmetic on the other. But, as pointed out before, changes in circumscribed areas of the brain may well have escaped detection. RICHTER and DAWSON (1948), however, were able to demonstrate, in rats, a decrease of the lactic acid concentration of brain in sleep and an increase during excitement. More extensive literature references are to be found in review articles of RICHTER (1952), WEIL-MALHERBE (1952) and McILWAIN (1956).

2. Experiments in vitro

McILWAIN has developed a method for exposing slices of cerebral cortex to electrical pulses at an optimal frequency of 100 per second in the Warburg respirometer. Application of electrical impulses elicited a series of metabolic responses: oxygen uptake was doubled and glucose utilization increased threefold. Lactic acid formation rose by a factor of 5—6, even more when the rate occurring during the first few seconds of stimulation was measured. At the same time phosphocreatine was broken down to inorganic phosphate. All the changes were reversible on cessation of the stimulus. In fact, the capacity of brain slices to replenish their stores of potassium and energy-rich phosphates (KREBS, EGGLESTON and TERNER, 1951; ÁCS, BALÁZS and STRAUB, 1953; McILWAIN, BUCHEL and CHESHIRE, 1951), after an initial loss, proved to be the prerequisite for their response to electrical impulses.

Doubts have been expressed as to the validity of comparing the electrical stimulation of brain slices in vitro with nervous activity in vivo. Certainly the two phenomena are not identical, but the following facts suggest that they may well be analogous in many respects (McILWAIN, 1956): 1. Response to electrical stimulation in vitro is restricted to excitable tissues, i.e. brain and muscle. It is absent in slices of liver and kidney, in cerebral tumors and in areas of gliosis. 2. The development of the respiratory response of brain slices to applied pulses in the young rat and guinea pig coincides with the appearance of spontaneous electrical activity and other signs of cerebral function. 3. The metabolic responses of brain slices depend on the presence of glucose. Glucose may be replaced by pyruvate and by high concentrations of lactate or fructose, but other substrates yield little or no response. The ability of a substrate to support response is correlated with its ability to restore and maintain the high-energy phosphates of the tissue. 4. Response depends on the integrity of cellular structure. Reports to the contrary (ABOOD, GERARD and OCHS, 1952) appear to be attributable to artefacts (NARAYANASWAMI and McILWAIN, 1954; McILWAIN, 1956). 5. The metabolic increments evoked by electrical pulses are much more sensitive to the action of certain drugs than the metabolism of unstimulated brain slices, effects being caused at concentrations comparable to those effective in vivo. Thus barbiturates and other depressants which inhibit the respiration of unstimulated brain slices only at relatively high concentrations were found to increase the threshold to electrical stimulation in concentrations which reproduce those reached in anaesthesia. They prevented not only the increase in respiration and glycolysis but also the energy-consuming processes leading to the breakdown of high-energy phosphate esters (McILWAIN, 1953). Similarly, anticonvulsants, including trimethadione and diphenylhydantoin, inhibited responses to electrical stimuli, but only those produced by alternating current at 500 or 2,000 cycles/sec. This parallels the absence of their effects on a normal EEG and their effectiveness in repressing the high-frequency, high-voltage bursts of the epileptic EEG (GREENGARD and McILWAIN, 1955). Finally, mescaline, dibenamine and ergot alkaloids, including lysergic acid diethylamide, were shown to inhibit metabolic responses at concentrations about 30 times lower than those which affected metabolism in the absence of pulses (LEWIS and McILWAIN, 1954).

The electrical excitability of brain slices is lost when they have been stored for some time at 0°. It has been shown that this is due to the fact that basic histones diffusing out of the cellular nucleus combine with acidic components in the membranes of the endoplasmic reticulum (McILWAIN, 1961). It may be mentioned in this connection that phosphatidic acids in the membranes of microsomes apparently play a part in sodium transport (HOKIN and HOKIN, 1959a and b).

Metabolic changes, similar in many respects to those produced by electric pulses, may be induced in brain slices, though not in other tissues, by an increase in the potassium concentration of the suspension medium to about 40 mM: respiration and glycolysis increase (ASHFORD and DIXON, 1935), phosphocreatine disappears and inorganic phosphate rises (GORE and McILWAIN, 1952); the incorporation of ^{32}P into phospholipids and nucleic acids is inhibited (FINDLAY, MAGEE and ROSSITER, 1954), that into phosphoproteins is accelerated (TSUKADA, TAKA-GAKI and HIRANO, 1958). It may be assumed that a high extracellular potassium concentration imposes an extra burden on the activities of the cell, thus increasing its energy expenditure. Of special interest is the fact that the metabolic response to extracellular potassium is much more sensitive to the action of inhibitors, such as narcotics (GHOSH and QUASTEL, 1954), azide and malonate (KIMURA and ITO, 1954; KIMURA and NIWA, 1953), than the metabolism of brain slices in the usual media.

It is a well-known fact that the electrical activity of cerebral tissue is arrested when its axonal connections are severed. Similarly, isolated brain slices, deprived of afferent impulses, may be at a lower level of activity than that prevailing in vivo. It is probable that the activity induced by electrical impulses or by high extracellular potassium concentrations more closely approaches the conditions in the living brain.

Negative membrane potentials have been observed in vitro in slices of tissues, including cerebral cortex; they were shown to depend on metabolic energy since they were reversibly diminished by anoxia, glucose lack or increased extracellular potassium concentration (LI and McILWAIN, 1957).

3. The Pasteur effect and the regulation of metabolic rates

The adaptation of metabolic rates to the varying energy demands is controlled by special mechanisms. It is true that an accelerated heart rate, a dilatation of blood vessels, an opening-up of capillaries may improve the supply of oxygen and nutrients to a tissue, but these mechanisms are second-line defences; the problem is not so much how the metabolic rate of the cell is accelerated as why the metabolism is restrained in spite of an abundant supply of oxygen and glucose.

An example of a regulatory mechanism is the phenomenon known as the Pasteur effect consisting of the suppression of fermentation or glycolysis by respiration. A higher rate of glucose utilization partly compensates for the smaller energy yield of the glycolytic as compared with the respiratory process. Replacement of glycolysis by respiration therefore results in a decreased utilization of glucose. While brain tissue has a high capacity for glycolysis it also has a strong Pasteur effect; thus in well-oxygenated brain slices in a glucose medium, lactic acid formation is slight.

In the older theories of the Pasteur effect oxygen itself was thought to intervene in some way, either by inactivating an enzyme or coenzyme, by decreasing the permeability of the cell, or by forming an inhibitory combination. Newer concepts have developed, however, with the growth of our knowledge of oxidative phosphorylation and with the realization that, in the intact cell as well as in suspensions of isolated mitochondria, phosphorylation and oxidation are "tightly coupled". This means not only that phosphorylation depends on oxidation but also that oxidation cannot proceed without phosphorylation. From the equation for oxidative phosphorylation (reaction 2, page 22) it is apparent that the reaction depends on the presence of inorganic phosphate and adenosine diphosphate (ADP). Their concentrations in the intact cell are relatively low; if the level of either or both of them falls, the rate of phosphorylation, and with it that of oxidation (respiration), is decelerated. The end product of oxidative phosphorylation is adenosine triphosphate (ATP). ATP is at the same time a source of energy and a source of inorganic phosphate and ADP, and again these two reactions are "tightly coupled", i.e. in the intact cell ATP is mainly hydrolysed in reactions releasing utilizable energy. The rate of ATP-breakdown therefore depends on the energy requirements of the cell and in the course of its breakdown ATP sets free the two components, ADP and inorganic phosphate, needed to speed up respiration: a perfect example of a biochemical feedback mechanism. To obtain maximum rates of respiration in vitro it is necessary to increase the energy requirements, e.g. by exposing brain slices to electrical pulses or to high potassium concentration; or, if working with suspended mitochondria, one can increase the rate of ATP-breakdown by adding adenosine triphosphatase or hexokinase.

Maximum rates of respiration are also observed in the presence of so-called "uncoupling" agents, i.e. drugs which break the tight coupling between respiration and phosphorylation and thus enable respiration to proceed without phosphorylation. The classical example is 2:4-dinitrophenol, but many other substances with similar action have been found. In fact, the coupling between respiration and phosphorylation seems to be one of the most sensitive vital activities. Uncoupling properties have been described, for instance, for barbiturates (BRODY and BAIN, 1954) and chlorpromazine, though the latter substance inhibited oxidative phosphorylation in the mitochondria of liver but not in those of brain (BERGER, 1957). It is doubtful, whether this effect has any bearing on the pharmacological action of these drugs: the gaseous anaesthetics have been shown to have no uncoupling activity (LEVY and FEATHERSTONE, 1954). Moreover, neither the accumulation of high-energy phosphate esters during the action of anaesthetics (see above) or chlorpromazine (GRENELL, MENDELSON and McELROY, 1955) nor the increased incorporation of ^{32}P into phospholipids by brain slices in the presence of chlorpromazine (MAGEE, BERRY and ROSSITER, 1956) conforms with an uncoupling mechanism.

When energy requirements of nervous cells are greatly increased, in vitro by electrical pulses or by a high extracellular potassium concentration, or in vivo during convulsive activity, there is an increase of glycolysis together with an increase of respiration, even though there is no lack of oxygen. These procedures, therefore, eliminate the Pasteur effect. The decisive factor is a disproportion of energy requirements and energy supply, resulting in an accelerated consumption of ATP. Anoxia is only a special case leading to a disproportion between supply and demand of energy: the restriction of oxygen supply reduces oxidative phosphorylation which is replaced by glycolytic phosphorylation. But this is a less efficient mechanism, and the deficiency can only be partly compensated by a greatly increased consumption of glucose.

This interpretation of the Pasteur effect is supported by experiments with cell-free preparations. A well-preserved Pasteur effect is observed in brain homogenates prepared in isotonic salt solutions (ELLIOTT and HENDERSON, 1948). Such preparations contain intact mitochondria capable of oxidative phosphorylation. If however brain homogenates are prepared in distilled water the mitochondria lose their capacity for oxidative phosphorylation; these preparations if suitably fortified with cofactors have a high rate of glycolysis which is the same in the presence and absence of oxygen (REINER, 1947). A Pasteur effect has also been demonstrated in a reconstructed system consisting of a particle-free brain extract and liver mitochrondria and shown to be due to competition of the two systems for ADP and inorganic phosphate (GATT and RACKER, 1959; see also TERNER, 1956).

Competition for ADP and inorganic phosphate is not the only mechanism regulating metabolic rates, though probably the most important one. There may also be competition for other cofactors which take part in more than one reaction, e.g. di- and triphosphopyridine nucleotides (DPN and TPN) and their reduced forms. It is inherent in the coupling mechanism that the oxidation of the reduced coenzymes cannot proceed without phosphorylation; therefore if the ratio of ATP:ADP is high, that of DPN^+:DPNH is low and vice versa. A high ratio of oxidized:reduced coenzymes favours oxidative reactions while a low ratio favours synthetic processes.

Another regulatory mechanism to which RAAFLAUB (1956) has drawn attention is based on the fact that the metal-complexing, or chelating, capacity of ATP is greater than that of ADP. The metals which, in physiological media, are mainly affected by this change are calcium and magnesium: the concentrations of their ionized forms increase when ATP is transformed to ADP, and the action of some enzymes, particularly kinases and phosphatases, will thereby be accelerated.

Although the synthesis and utilization of high-energy phosphate bonds is the basic mechanism for the regulation of metabolic rates, other regulatory and feedback mechanisms operate at every level of metabolism. The rate and direction of reversible reactions is controlled by the concentration of the reaction partners. Irreversible reactions, on the other hand, are practically independent of the concentration of the reaction product. A significant exception is the hexokinase reaction which, in animal tissues, is subject to non-competitive inhibition by the reaction product, glucose-6-phosphate (WEIL-MALHERBE and BONE, 1951). In view of the strategic position of hexokinase in glucose metabolism this inhibition may have an important regulatory function.

IX. Energy metabolism and mental disease

States of hypoxia, whether caused by a decrease of oxygen tension, by ischaemia, anaemia or respiratory poisons, are accompanied by mental symptoms similar in many ways to those observed in mental disease. The same is true of some vitamin deficiencies which, as we now know, affect the functioning of enzyme systems connected, directly or indirectly, with electron transport or dehydrogenation. Deficiencies of thiamin, riboflavin, pantothenic acid or niacin may result in neurological or psychotic disorders (SEBRELL, 1943; SPILLANE, 1947; SEBRELL and SCHWARZ, 1953). It is hardly surprising, therefore, that theories were put forward, particularly with regard to schizophrenia, postulating an aetiology based on a lesion of oxygen transport or utilization; anoxia, it was claimed, "is a necessary as well as a sufficient condition for the development of mental disorder" (DANZIGER, 1945). Abnormalities of peripheral circulation in schizophrenic patients, as manifested by cyanosis of the extremities (SHATTOCK, 1950), structure of cutaneous capillaries (OLKON, 1939) and a decreased oxygen saturation of capillary blood (LOVETT DOUST, 1952), seemed to lend support to such a mechanism. However, with the advent of a method for the estimation of cerebral oxygen consumption, normal values were found in schizophrenic patients by most observers (KETY et al., 1948; WILSON et al., 1952; SOKOLOFF et al., 1957); lower values found by one group (GORDAN et al., 1955) in cases of long-standing disease were presumably the result of secondary changes.

In view of its predominance in the energy supply of brain, the carbohydrate metabolism in mental disease has attracted the attention of many observers. Among much conflicting evidence a reduction of the rate of glucose utilization or "glucose tolerance" in cases of severe depression stands out as perhaps the most significant and constant finding (McFARLAND and GOLDSTEIN, 1939; HOLMGREN and WOHLFAHRT, 1944). Although glucose tolerance is influenced by extraneous factors of which the rate of intestinal absorption and the presence of malnutrition are the most important, significant deviations from the norm remain even after these two factors have been eliminated (PRYCE, 1958). A low glucose tolerance is presumed to be indicative of a preponderance of plasma hormones of pituitary and adrenocortical origin, a state characteristic of the stress syndrome.

In schizophrenia a decrease of glucose tolerance has been described by some (e.g. Freeman and Zaborenke, 1949) and an increase, as indicated by a low fasting blood sugar and a flat blood sugar curve after a glucose test dose, by others (e.g. Shattock, 1950). Such variations may be interpreted as representing different phases of the general adaptation syndrome to stress (Selye, 1950).

Plasma from depressive patients with lowered glucose tolerance was found to cause inhibition of the hexokinase reaction in rat brain extracts; frequently the peak of the blood sugar curve coincided with the maximum of inhibition. A similar factor was present in some specimens of diabetic plasma (Weil-Malherbe and Bone, 1951). Haavaldsen, Lingjaerde and Walaas (1958) found a globulin fraction in the serum of some female schizophrenics which inhibited the glucose uptake of the isolated rat diaphragm. These results are compatible with the assumption that hormones which inhibit glucose utilization are circulating in some cases of mental disease in increased amounts.

A similar explanation may also apply to the increased insulin tolerance frequently found in schizophrenics (Freeman et al., 1943; Braceland et al., 1945; Nadeau and Rouleau, 1953). The phenomenon has been studied particularly by Meduna (1950) who concluded that it occurred in a special type of schizophrenia ("oneirophrenia") characterized by a clouding of the sensorium ranging from mild disorders of perception and orientation to confusional states and florid hallucinosis. Meduna, Gerty and Urse (1942) demonstrated an anti-insulin factor in the blood of schizophrenics; such blood, when injected into rabbits, reduced their response to insulin. Later, a factor was found in the urine of schizophrenics (Meduna and Vaichulis, 1948) which caused a rise of blood sugar after its injection into test animals. This hyperglycaemic factor was further concentrated and purified and shown to consist largely of protein (Morgan and Pilgrim, 1952). The excretion of a urinary hyperglycaemic factor is, however, not confined to schizophrenics, or even psychotics (Mayer-Gross, 1952). Moya et al. (1956; see also Löhr and Schümann, 1953) isolated a hyperglycaemic factor from normal urine. In their opinion the factor is identical with kallikrein and the hyperglycaemia is due to adrenaline discharge secondary to the hypotensive effect of kallikrein. The hyperglycaemic response to schizophrenic urine is much stronger than that to normal urine and the time-response curves are also different. In addition, extracts of schizophrenic urines were toxic to rabbits while those of normal urines were well tolerated (Moya et al., 1958).

According to Lingjaerde (1953, 1956) the abnormal tolerance responses of schizophrenics to glucose as well as to insulin disappear after prolonged administration of a high-carbohydrate diet, which is more drastic than that required to repair the disorders caused by acute carbohydrate deficiency in normal subjects.

The overall glucose utilization of the whole brain was found to be normal in schizophrenics (Sokoloff et al., 1957). On the other hand, a difference in the carbohydrate metabolism of frontal lobe cortex between schizophrenics and non-schizophrenics has been claimed by Utena and Ezoe (1951). These workers studied tissue samples removed during lobotomy operations by in vitro techniques; while oxygen uptake and carbon dioxide output were the same in the two groups, glucose consumption and lactic acid production were significantly lower in the samples from the schizophrenic patients than in those from psychopaths, manic-depressives and compulsive neurotics, pointing to a depression of aerobic glycolysis in schizophrenics. The same abnormality was found in two chronic methamphet-amine addicts with paranoid hallucinatory symptoms closely resembling schizophrenia. Later experiments showed that chronic administration of methamphet-amine to guinea pigs produced a similar depression of the glycolytic activity of brain tissue (UTENA, EZOE and KATO, 1955).

Little is known concerning a possible abnormality of intermediate carbohydrate metabolism in mental disease. HENNEMAN, ALTSCHULE and GONCZ (1954) studied the plasma levels of various glucose metabolites after a glucose test meal and claimed significant differences between psychotic patients and normal controls. Most of their patients showed a decrease of glucose tolerance and it is possible that the other changes were related to this fact.

DAWSON et al. (1954, 1956) observed fluctuations in the blood levels of acetoin and its reduction product, 2,3-butylene glycol. Acetoin arises in a side reaction of the metabolism of pyruvic acid. The concentration of acetoin in plasma was found to be raised in depressed patients and reduced below normal in manic patients; the decrease sometimes preceded the manic phase or was associated with its early stages. Since the blood levels of acetoin are raised in diabetics and in fasting subjects, it seems reasonable to assume an inverse correlation with the level of glucose tolerance. Increased physical activity was without effect on the blood levels of acetoin and butylene glycol.

Several authors have studied the metabolism of blood cells. According to BOSZORMENYI-NAGY and GERTY (1955) differences are apparent in haemolysates prepared from normal and schizophrenic blood pre-incubated with insulin in vitro. Addition of hexosediphosphate and pyruvate to the haemolysate induces the for-mation of acid-labile phosphate. In blood from normal controls pre-incubation with insulin reduces, in blood from schizophrenics it increases the formation of acid-labile phosphate. The same authors (BOSZORMENYI-NAGY, GERTY and KUEBER, 1956) studied the incorporation of ^{32}P into ATP and ADP in blood samples incubated with pyruvate and citrate. The further addition of methylene blue to the incubation mixture led to an increase of relative specific activity in the ADP-fraction which was significantly greater in blood from schizophrenics than in normal blood.

GOTTLIEB et al. (1959) also studied the incorporation of ^{32}P into ATP of red blood cells in vitro. They compared the rate of reaction in blood samples collected before and after an injection of insulin. Insulin caused a large increase of specific activity in controls and in remissions from schizophrenia of recent onset, a smaller rise in acute cases and a fall in chronic cases. More recent developments from the same group indicate the presence of a factor in the serum of schizophrenics which affects the metabolism of glucose in human as well as in chicken erythrocytes in such a way that it depresses the formation of pyruvate and raises the ratio of lactate/pyruvate. Another criterion claimed to differentiate schizophrenic from normal plasma is based on the fact that the formation of $^{14}CO_2$ from glucose-6-^{14}C is increased and the ratio, CO_2 from C^1 to CO_2 from C^6, is decreased in normal blood after insulin stress while it remains unchanged in schizophrenic blood (FROHMAN, LATHAM, BECKETT and GOTTLIEB, 1960; FROHMAN, CZAJKOWSKI, LUBY, GOTTLIEB and SENF, 1960; FROHMAN, TOURNEY, BECKETT, LEES, LATHAM and GOTTLIEB, 1961; FROHMAN, LUBY, TOURNEY, BECKETT and GOTTLIEB, 1960).

When ^{32}P was injected intravenously the specific activity of ATP in the blood of controls was six times as high as in the blood of chronic schizophrenics. Schizo-phrenic blood contained two radioactive components of which one was identified as metaphosphate (ORSTROM and SKAUG, 1950).

Although the concentrations of inorganic phosphate, lipid phosphate and total phosphate were the same in schizophrenic and control plasmas, injection of ^{32}P produced an increase of the specific activity of the lipid phosphate fraction in schizophrenics over that in normals (PERUTZ, 1951).

These observations are at present difficult to evaluate. They do not fall into an easily recognizable pattern and are, in some respects, contradictory, some indicating a decrease, others an increase of phosphate turnover in schizophrenia. Caution in accepting these claims seems advisable until they have been confirmed.

D. Metabolism of nitrogenous compounds

The metabolism of nitrogenous compounds has moved into the center of attention during recent years. The nitrogenous compounds of interest comprise amino acids, amines, and proteins.

I. The pool of free amino acids (cf. WAELSCH 1957)

The pool of free amino acids of the brain is the source from which both amines and proteins are derived and to which amino acids liberated in the breakdown of proteins are returned. Its composition is unique for the central nervous system. In Table 5 the composition of the free amino acid pool of cat and rat brain is reported on the basis of the analyses by TALLAN et al. (1954), SCHURR et al. (1950), ANSELL and RICHTER (1954) and BERL and WAELSCH (1958).

The pool is characterized in all mammals by a concentration of glutamic acid higher than in any other organ (0.01 molar), and by a high concentration of glu-

Table 5. *Concentrations of free amino acids in the brain of cat and rat*

Amino acid	Rat				Cat			
	μmoles/g	% IC	F_L	F_P	μmoles/g	% IC	F_L	F_P
Leucine	0.2	150	3.0	1.0	0.14	100	2.0	1.5
Phenylalanine	0.06	110	5.0	1.0	0.07	90	1.5	0.7
Tryptophan	0.03		3.0					
Valine	0.1	200	5.0	2.0	0.18	80	2.0	0.7
Histidine	0.08	220	4.0	0.5	0.06	160	10.0	1 5
Lysine	0.02	105	2.5	1.3	0.14	140	1.8	1.5
Isoleucine					0.09	110	1.5	0.7
Tyrosine	0.1	90	3.0	0.8	0.06	70	2.0	0.7
Methionine	0.08	80	3.0	1.3	0.1			0.3
Threonine	1.0	90	1.3	0.3	0.22		1.2	0.5
Arginine	0.2	80	0.3	1.0	0.08	110	0.14	1.0
Aspartic acid					2.2	400	0.3	0.003
Asparagine					0.1		2.0	0.7
Acetyl aspartic acid	5.0				6.0		0.03	
Glutamic acid	10.0		0.4		8.7	150	0.5	0.014
Glutamine	4.0		1.0		3.4		1.0	0.1
Glycine	1.3				1.3	250	1.0	0.2
Alanine	0.6				1.0	100	2.0	0.8
γ-Aminobutyric acid	2.0				2.3	100	0.04	0.001
Proline					0.14		1.6	1.5
Cystine					0.04			0.5
Serine	1.1				0.72		0.5	0.3
Glutathione	1.0				0.9		4.5	
Cystathionine					2.5[1]			

[1] human brain.

% IC: increase after hydrolysis, amino acid before hydrolysis = 100

F_L and F_P: factors by which concentration in brain has to be multiplied to arrive at concentrations in liver (L) or blood plasma (P).

tamine (0.004 molar). In addition, brain has a high concentration of γ-aminobutyric acid (0.002 molar), of acetyl aspartic acid (0.006 molar), and, in man, of cystathionine (up to 0.0025 molar, TALLAN et al. 1958), the condensation product of serine and homocysteine. The three last mentioned compounds do not occur in any significant concentration in other tissues of the mammalian body. In addition to the role of amino acids as mother substances of amines and proteins, the dicarboxylic amino acids in particular have the function of compensating partially for the anionic deficit in tissues. In the invertebrate nerve, this is accomplished by a large concentration of aspartic acid (133 μmoles/g in lobster nerve, SILBER 1941). or of the hydroxyl analogue of taurine, isethionic acid (220 μmoles/g in axon of giant squid, KOECHLIN 1955).

II. Peptides

Since the amounts of amino acids other than those derived from glutathione and acetyl aspartic acid liberated upon hydrolysis of protein-free filtrates of brain tissue of the cat are small (Table 5), it is unlikely that peptides of unknown composition occur in brain tissue in high concentration. The possibility of the presence of low concentrations of peptides as yet not identified is suggested by the occurrence of homocarnosine and possibly of carnosine in cattle brain (PISANO et al., 1961). Whereas the presence of peptide bound amino acids could not be shown in the hypothalamus, the occurrence of considerable amounts of peptides beyond those accounted for by oxytocin, vasopressin or intermedin was demonstrated in the tissue of the posterior pituitary (WINNICK et al., 1955). This observation is of some interest since it has been suggested that neurohormones of peptide nature are synthesized in the hypothalamus and are stored in the posterior pituitary (BARGMANN and SCHARRER, 1951). Recent experiments on the in vivo synthesis of vasopressin appear to be inconsistent with such a simple two-compartment relationship (SACHS, 1959).

III. Origin of the amino acids (Fig. 2)

The carbon skeleton of the non-essential amino acids is derived, as in other organs, through the citric acid cycle and ultimately from glucose. There are powerful transaminases present in the brain which reversibly aminate and deaminate essential as well as non-essential amino acids (AWAPARA and SEALE, 1952).

$$R.CO.COO^- + \text{glutamate} \longleftrightarrow \text{Amino acids} + \text{Ketoglutarate}$$

The keto acid-catalyzed deamidation of glutamine by liver and kidney extracts has been shown to be due to the participation of the amide in transamination reactions (MEISTER and TICE, 1950). Recent experiments suggest a similar participation of glutamine in transamination reactions in cerebral tissue (GUHA and GHOSH, 1959).

IV. Uptake of amino acids by the brain from the blood

In animal experiments where the concentration of various amino acids in the blood was raised, the analysis of brain at different time intervals showed that after glutamine administration there was an increase in the glutamine content of the brain (SCHWERIN et al., 1950, KAMIN and HANDLER, 1951) but no comparable net uptake of glutamic acid from the circulating blood could be demonstrated. Also in the case of lysine (LAJTHA, 1958), leucine (LAJTHA, 1959) and proline (DINGMAN and SPORN, 1959), a net uptake of the amino acids by the brain is found only when the blood concentration is increased significantly and the experiments extended for a considerable period of time. It seems, therefore, that any net uptake of the amino acids tested (glutamic acid, leucine and lysine) is too small to be measured by the available micromethods. Apparently

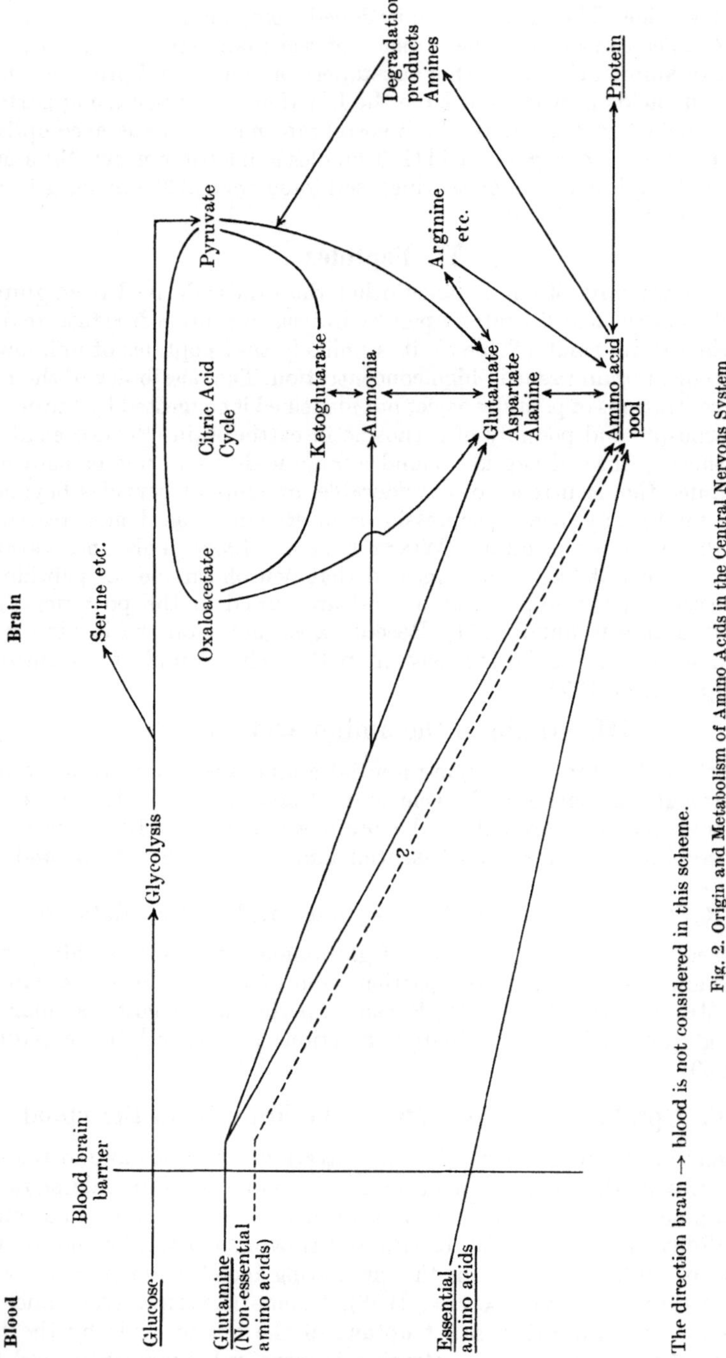

Fig. 2. Origin and Metabolism of Amino Acids in the Central Nervous System

The direction brain → blood is not considered in this scheme.

only the fully developed blood-brain barrier of the mature brain is able to protect the brain from increased concentration of blood amino acids since net uptake of

amino acids by the immature brain can be demonstrated (LAJTHA, 1958; HIM-
WICH and HIMWICH, 1955). On the other hand, the exchange of the amino acids
between blood and brain may be quite rapid even if the blood-brain barrier
slows down the net uptake of amino acids to a non-measurable rate. It can be
shown with the aid of isotopically labeled amino acids that half of the free lysine
of the brain is replaced by blood lysine within one hour (LAJTHA et al., 1957).
Similar findings were made with leucine (LAJTHA, 1958) and glutamic acid (LAJTHA
et al., 1959). It has also been shown for other cells that exchange of amino acids
may be considerably more rapid than one-directional active transport (HEINZ,
1957; HEINZ and WALSH, 1958). These findings do not exclude the possibility that
slow changes of the pool of free amino acids can be effected despite the restraining
action of the blood-brain barrier, otherwise the replenishment of the essential
amino acids of the pool would be impossible. Since it is difficult to ascertain
what fraction of amino acids liberated from protein breakdown is re-used for protein
synthesis and other purposes, the extent of this net uptake has not been estimated.
The finding of a rapid exchange of amino acids between blood plasma and brain
despite a barrier to net uptake (WAELSCH, 1958; WAELSCH and LAJTHA, 1961)
indicates that diffusion cannot be the controlling mechanism. Evidence is accumulating which would suggest that an active metabolic process underlies the transfer of some amino acids into and out of the brain. This evidence includes transport
against a diffusion gradient (LAJTHA and TOTH, 1961) and metabolic specificity,
different carriers probably transporting different substrates (CHIRIGOS et al.,
1960; LAJTHA and MELA, 1961).

These findings demonstrate the homeostatic mechanism which protects the
brain from sudden changes of its metabolic environment. The question arises
whether the amino acids or any other metabolites are in a homogeneous pool
throughout the brain, or whether their concentrations vary in the different
anatomical and functional areas, or differ in different cells or parts of them.
There is good evidence for considerable heterogeneity of the amino acid pools
(LAJTHA et al., 1959).

V. Glutamic acid and its metabolic derivatives (Fig. 2)

It has been mentioned previously that glutamic acid occurs in the brain in
concentrations exceeding those found in other organs. Together with the
glutamic acid occurring in glutamine and glutathione, the amino acid accounts
for close to 50 per cent of the α-amino nitrogen of the protein-free filtrates of
brain tissue (WAELSCH, 1951). Aside from this fact, many other observations
point to the important role of this dicarboxylic amino acid and its metabolic
derivatives — glutamine and γ-aminobutyric acid — in the metabolism of nervous
tissue in relation to function in health and disease.

The carbon skeleton of glutamic acid — in the form of ketoglutaric acid — is
derived from glucose through the citric acid cycle; the keto acid is aminated to
the amino acid either by transamination with other amino acids or by free ammonia
in a reductive amination catalyzed by glutamic dehydrogenase. Both transaminases and glutamic dehydrogenase are very active in brain tissue. The latter
enzyme is responsible for one of the two principal mechanisms for the removal
of ammonia in the central nervous system.

$$\text{Ketoglutarate} + \text{Ammonia} \xleftarrow{\quad} \frac{\text{Dehydrogenase}}{\text{DPN (TPN)}} \xrightarrow{\quad} \text{Glutamic acid}$$

The origin of the carbon skeleton (ketoglutaric acid) of a major portion of
cerebral glutamic acid from glucose through the citric acid cycle is supported by

the results of in vitro and in vivo experiments in which the incorporation of the carbon atoms of C^{14}-labeled glucose or pyruvic acid was studied. The glutamic acid content of cortex slices exhausted by prior incubation in glucose-free medium is increased upon incubation with added glucose (Waelsch, 1949).

Brain slices, supplied with ^{14}C-glucose, incorporate 10—20% of ^{14}C into non-carbohydrates, principally amino acids. Of the incorporated ^{14}C about 75% is found in glutamic acid and its associated derivatives, glutamine and γ-aminobutyric acid, with aspartic acid and alanine accounting for the rest (Beloff-Chain et al., 1955).

After 20 minutes of incubation with pyruvate-2-^{14}C as substrate, 42% of the metabolized pyruvate was recovered in glutamic acid in in vitro studies with rat cerebral cortex and 53% in vivo 3 minutes after the intravenous administration of pyruvic acid (Busch, 1955; Busch et al., 1956; Tower, 1959). If the citric acid cycle is interrupted and the flow of ammonia acceptors stopped, an increase of the ammonia level in the brain results (Benitez et al., 1954).

Although there is evidence, as mentioned above, that at least in animal experiments glutamic acid cannot penetrate the blood-brain barrier, it has been claimed that arterio-venous differences are observed in man, a fact which may suggest glutamic acid uptake by the human brain (Adams et al., 1955).

VI. Glutamic acid as a substrate in nervous tissue

Early experiments with brain cortex slices suggested a unique position for glutamic acid in cerebral metabolism since it was the only amino acid oxidized of thirteen tested (Weil-Malherbe, 1936). In the intact animal rapid metabolism of other amino acids (proline, alanine, aspartic acid, arginine) can be demonstrated (Sporn et al., 1959).

Whereas the presence of active transaminases implies that the carbon skeleton of other amino acids would be made available for oxidation by brain tissue, up to the present time no clear picture has emerged as to the oxidation by slices fortified by various essential cofactors of amino acids other than glutamic acid. The oxidation of glutamic acid by brain cortex slices from guinea pig does not support the regeneration of creatine phosphate (and therefore these do not respond to electrical stimulation in the presence of glutamic acid), while under the same experimental conditions slices from human cortex are able to do so (McIlwain, 1951; McIlwain et al., 1952; McIlwain, 1953). One might speculate on whether this finding points to a special role of glutamic acid in the metabolism of the human brain and suggests the possibility that, from the evolutionary point of view, the efficacy of glutamic acid utilization may be a parameter of the functional refinement of the central nervous system. This possibility is of more than passing interest in view of the claim quoted above of the ability of the human brain to take up glutamic acid and of the still controversial effects of glutamic acid administration to man.

When glutamic acid is incubated with brain slices it is oxidized without the appearance of free ammonia; instead the concentration of amide-N increases (Weil-Malherbe, 1936). The underlying reaction may be formulated thus:

$$2 \text{ Glutamic acids} + \tfrac{1}{2} O_2 \rightarrow \text{Glutamine} + \alpha\text{-Ketoglutaric acid} + H_2O$$

indicating that the rate of deamination is limited by the rate of glutamine synthesis under these experimental conditions. This limitation is explained by the fact that the equilibrium of the glutamic dehydrogenase system is strongly in favor of the reductive amination of ketoglutarate (Strecker, 1953). Other mechanisms for the metabolism of glutamic acid involve transamination reactions directly or after decarboxylation to γ-aminobutyric acid and are not accompanied by the appearance of ammonia.

Since glutamic acid can serve as substrate of respiration for brain cortex slices, the question arises as to whether it may have a similar function in vivo. Decreases of glutamic acid concentration have been reported in the rat brain after strychnine convulsions (HABER and SAIDEL, 1948), in hypoglycaemic coma, in thiopenthal anaesthesia with a slight increase in glutamine (DAWSON, 1950, 1951) and in epileptogenic foci in cat cortex produced by freezing (BERL et al., 1959).

Slices of cerebral cortex of aminals after induced epileptogenic seizures and of human epileptogenic cerebral cortex show upon incubation a decrease in glutamic acid levels in contrast to control slices where a significant increase is observed under the same conditions (TOWER, 1955, 1959).

While in hypoglycemia the decrease of glutamic acid may be suggestive of its function as respiratory substrate, the decrease was only relatively minor and less than in situations where no deprivation of glucose could be assumed such as anaesthesia or experimentally-induced epilepsy. In order to act as a substrate of respiration, ketoglutaric acid originating from glutamic acid would have to be channeled through the citric acid cycle; there are no indications that, even at levels of increased activity, glucose metabolized by the same pathway is unable to furnish all the energy required.

VII. Glutamine metabolism

$$\text{Glutamic Acid} + \text{Ammonia} \xrightarrow[\text{ATP, Mg.}]{\text{Synthetase}} \text{Glutamine}$$

The second major and biologically more important mechanism (DU RUISSEAU et al., 1957; TAKAGAKI et al., 1961; WAELSCH, 1961; BERL et al., 1962). for the fixation of free ammonia in the central nervous system is the formation of glutamine from glutamic acid and ammonia, an adenosine triphosphate-requiring reaction catalyzed by glutamine synthetase (KREBS, 1935; SPECK, 1949; ELLIOTT, 1951). This enzyme is highly active in the brain and appears to be concentrated in the microsomal and mitochondrial fraction, as identified by fractional centrifugation (WAELSCH, 1959). Glutamine synthetase from brain tissue cannot be separated from glutamotransferase which catalyzes the replacement of the amide group by hydroxylamine or hydrazine (LAJTHA et al., 1953). A possible function of the transferase system in peptide synthesis has been considered (WAELSCH, 1957). There is evidence that glutamine synthesis from administered glutamic acid occurs either in the surface of the cells or within the endoplasmic reticulum (LAJTHA et al., 1959, 1960). Glutamine penetrates the blood-brain barrier of adult animals with greater ease than glutamic acid (SCHWERIN et al., 1950) and may therefore serve as a supply of ammonia and glutamic acid in the central nervous system.

The concentration of amide nitrogen in brain slices remains steady in the absence of glucose but rises in its presence (WEIL-MALHERBE and GREEN, 1955a). The effect is even more pronounced if the medium contains, in addition to glucose, ammonium ions and either ketoglutarate or pyruvate (WEIL-MALHERBE, 1936). An increase of the level of cerebral glutamine in vivo with or without a corresponding decrease of that of glutamic acid has been observed in rats after physical exercise (VRBA, 1955), after tumbling in a revolving drum (GRAY et al., 1956) and after electrical stimulation of the extremities (TSUKADA et al., 1958). These conditions are likely to lead to increased ammonia production in the brain. A significant increase of glutamine concentration was found in rat and dog brain after an infusion of ammonium salts (DU RUISSEAU et al., 1957; CLARK and EISEMAN, 1958; TAKAGAKI et al., 1960). In epileptogenic foci produced in the cortex of cats, a comparable decrease of glutamic acid as well as of glutamine was found (BERL et al., 1959).

VIII. Glutamic acid uptake by tissue slices

A considerable leakage of potassium ions from brain slices occurs during their preparation, especially if the slices are stored at temperatures below 37°. This process is stopped and to some extent reversed on subsequent incubation of the slices in a glucose-bicarbonate medium under aerobic conditions. The uptake of potassium is accelerated if the medium contains, in addition, glutamic acid (TERNER et al., 1950). This effect of glutamic acid is dependent on the buffers used and has been related to an increase of the intracellular space (ELLIOTT, 1955).

Brain slices respiring in a medium containing glucose and glutamic acid are capable of accumulating glutamic acid against the concentration gradient (STERN et al., 1949). The accumulation of L-glutamic acid in cortex slices is accompanied by an approximately equivalent migration of potassium (TERNER et al., 1950). No equivalence between the uptake of D-glutamic acid and potassium is found (TAKAGAKI et al., 1959). These observations cannot be transposed to in vivo conditions in which the bloodbrain barrier regulates potassium migration between blood and brain, since the half-life time of brain potassium has been estimated as approximately 24 hours (KATZMAN and LEIDERMAN, 1953), a figure indicating a rate of migration considerably lower than that obtained with tissue slices. On the other hand, these observations suggest a possible role of the dicarboxylic acid in the maintenance of the intracellular ionic milieu.

IX. Ammonia

It has been pointed out above that glutamic acid metabolism provides two effective mechanisms for the removal of ammonia. Upon infusion the base has shown to be a powerful irritant with strychnine-like action on cord and medulla, followed by convulsions. Electroencephalographic records after ammonia infusion suggested a spinal rather than a cortical origin of the convulsions (AJMONE-MARSAN et al., 1949). In rats convulsions occur at a concentration of 9 mg/g of brain tissue while the normal concentration, depending on the speed of freezing of the brain, varies from 0.28 to 1 mg/100 g (RICHTER and DAWSON, 1948).

It is now well established that nervous activity is accompanied by a liberation of ammonia. Since the original observations of TASHIRO (1922) and WINTERSTEIN (1925), made on nerve tissue of frog and rabbit, several authors using the technique of rapid freezing found that a convulsive stimulus caused the concentration of ammonia to rise by about 50 per cent in rat brain (RICHTER and DAWSON, 1948; TORDA 1953; TSUKADA and TAKAGAKI, 1954) and by about 400 per cent in cerebral cortex of dogs (BENITEZ et al., 1954). During ischaemia the ammonia concentration in rabbit cerebral cortex increased linearly by 0.0337 μmol/g/min up to 15 minutes (THORN and HEIMANN, 1958). Among the various convulsive agents methyl-fluoroacetate was especially effective, raising the ammonia concentration seven-fold (BENITEZ et al., 1954). This is probably due to a specific effect of this drug on the utilization of ammonia.

Changes in the opposite direction are produced by anaesthesia and sleep. RICHTER and DAWSON (1948) found a progressive drop and finally a practically complete disappearance of ammonia in the brain of rats under nembutal anaesthesia for periods of up to 90 minutes. According to VLADIMIROVA (1954, 1957) the ammonia concentration of rat brain decreases by about 50 per cent during normal sleep. Although it would be intriguing to consider ammonia one of the functionally active components of the nervous tissue, particularly in view of the action of its organic derivatives — the quaternary ammonium bases —, present evidence does not give definite indication of such a function.

In hepatic coma, the symptoms have been claimed to be closely related to the high level of ammonia and its toxicity, although it should be noted that the severity of symptoms does not always parallel the ammonia concentration in blood (EISEMAN et al., 1956; BESSMAN and BESSMAN, 1955). In cases where the ammonia level in plasma is raised, significant amounts of ammonia are taken up by the brain (BESSMAN and BESSMAN, 1955; WEBSTER and GABUZDA, 1958). It is of interest that in hepatectomized dogs a considerable increase of glutamine is found in the brain, attesting to the function of the glutamic acid-glutamine system as an ammonia removal mechanism (FLOCK et al., 1953).

X. Ammonia formation by brain tissue in vitro

Rapid fixation of the brain is essential to avoid any post mortem formation of ammonia. If the freezing of the severed heads is delayed, the concentration of ammonia rises from about 20 to 50 μmoles/100 g within a few seconds. But this initial burst is followed by a further output of ammonia. Three minutes after death a value of 200 μmoles/100 g has been found in cat brain (KREBS et al., 1949). In slices of rat brain cortex fixed about 20 minutes after death it is usual to find about 500 μmoles/100 g (WEIL-MALHERBE and GREEN, 1955).

The origin of ammonia formed in cortex slices has not been clarified. Neither the deamination of nucleosides and nucleotides (WEIL-MALHERBE and GREEN, 1955b; DAWSON and PETERS, 1955; KORANSKY, 1956) which is responsible for the formation of free ammonia in muscle, nor the deamination of glutamine, glutamic acid or hexosamine, nor the deamidation of the amide can account quantitatively for the ammonia liberated (WEIL-MALHERBE and GREEN, 1955b, WEIL-MALHERBE and DRYSDALE, 1957).

While it had been claimed that physical exhaustion lowers the level of protein-bound amide in brain (VRBA, 1955) and although a Ca^{++} dependent enzymatically catalyzed deamidation of protein-bound glutamine has been reported recently (CLARKE et al., 1957), there is at present no clear-cut evidence that the cleavage of protein amide groups may account for all the ammonia liberated in tissue slices (WEIL-MALHERBE and DRYSDALE, 1957).

The changes in cytoplasmic lipids, proteins and nucleoproteins associated with nervous activity are considered elsewhere in this chapter. It is shown there that these constituents are no longer to be regarded as mere structural units, but that they have a rapid turnover and actively participate in the various functional activities of the cell. GEIGER, MAGNES and DOBKIN (1954) and GEIGER (1959) found that increased activity of cat brain cortex increased the non-protein nitrogen (NPN) in the active area. An increase of NPN was also found in incubated brain slices. Like ammonia formation, it was inhibited by anoxia and abolished by destruction of cellular structure (WEIL-MALHERBE and GREEN, 1955a).

In summary it may be said that there are indications that the formation of ammonia by nervous tissue in vivo and in vitro is due to reactions involving proteins and nucleoproteins but that detailed information about the nature of the precursors and the mechanism of its liberation is lacking.

XI. Some consequences of the ammonia-binding mechanism

The synthesis of glutamine depends on a supply of energy in the form of ATP (ELLIOTT, 1951). Its consumption and the disturbance of the ATP:ADP ratio in this reaction is probably the explanation for some effects observed when brain slices are incubated in media containing either ammonium ions or glutamate. Synthetic and other reactions depending on ATP, such as anaerobic glycolysis, incorporation of labeled phosphate into various phosphate esters, fixation of CO_2 and responses to electrical pulses, are inhibited (WEIL-MALHERBE, 1938; FINDLAY et al., 1954; CRANE and BALL, 1951; GORE and McILWAIN, 1952; McILWAIN, 1951). The synthesis of acetylcholine is inhibited by ammonia but not by glutamic acid (BRAGANCA et al., 1953), and possibly formation of glutamylcholine may occur (KOREY et al., 1951) which was analyzed as acetylcholine. As might be expected, the concentration of high-energy phosphates is depressed by ammonium ions as well as by glutamate (McILWAIN 1952; Acs et al., 1953), resulting in an ATP:ADP ratio favorable to an increased rate of respiration and glycolysis (WEIL-MALHERBE, 1936, 1938).

A further consequence of the ammonia-binding mechanism may be the withdrawal of ketoglutarate from the citric acid cycle (BESSMAN, 1956). Since it was postulated that brain tissue is unable to fix carbon dioxide and thereby to replenish the intermediates of the citric acid cycle, the toxicity of ammonia, particularly in hepatic coma, was assumed to be based on a depletion of these intermediates leading to a slowing down of glucose oxidation and a decrease in the generation of energy rich phosphate bonds (BESSMAN, 1961). The demonstration of a significant CO_2 fixation in nervous tissue (cf. C. II.) throws considerable doubt on the validity of the above hypothesis although it is too early to state whether or not the rate of CO_2 fixation would be sufficient to compensate for the ketoglutarate removed from the cycle by the increased glutamine formation.

XII. γ-Aminobutyric acid (Fig. 3)

Discovered ten years ago in the brain (ROBERTS and FRANKEL, 1950; AWAPARA et al., 1950), γ-aminobutyric acid moved into the center of interest when it was found to be a component of Factor I, a fraction isolated from mammalian brain and inhibitory for the stretch receptor reflex in the crayfish (FLOREY, 1953; BAZEMORE et al., 1957). Upon application to the mammalian cortex, its action suggests an inhibition of the excitatory synapses (PURPURA et al., 1957, 1958).

γ-Aminobutyric acid is formed from glutamic acid by the action of a decarboxylase dependent on pyridoxal phosphate. It is further metabolized by transamination with ketoglutaric acid catalyzed by a pyridoxal phosphate dependent transaminase (BESSMAN et al., 1953; ROBERTS et al., 1953). The succinic semialdehyde formed is oxidized to succinic acid (ALBERS and SALVADOR, 1958) which enters the citric acid cycle.

The sequence of glutamic acid, γ-aminobutyric acid, succinic acid, represents a metabolic bypass of the direct metabolism of ketoglutaric acid to succinic acid. The enzymes for γ-aminobutyric acid formation and metabolism are restricted to the grey matter, and the presence of alternate pathways for ketoglutaric acid is of particular interest in an organ, whose function expresses itself in an interplay of excitation and inhibition. γ-Aminobutyric acid can serve as acceptor of the amidine group from arginine with the formation of γ-guanidinobutyric acid (PISANO et al., 1957), the presence of which has been demonstrated in cerebral tissue (IRREVERRE and EVANS, 1959). It acts as excitatory agent in the cerebral

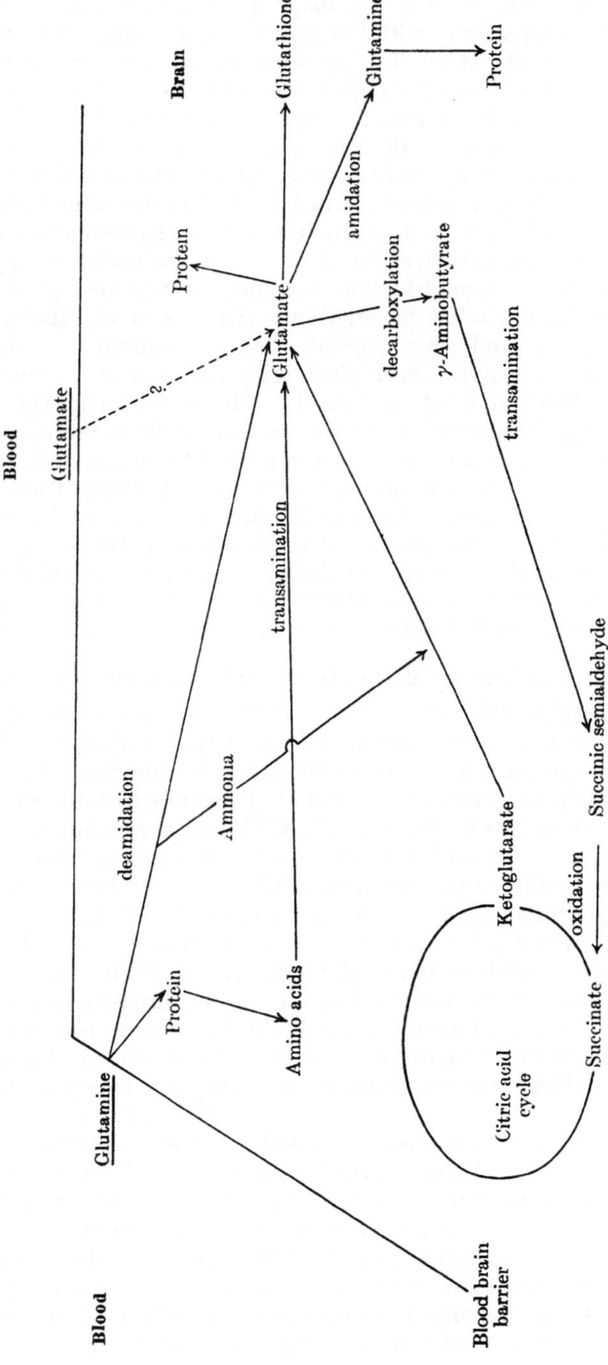

The direction brain → blood is not considered in this scheme.

Fig. 3. Glutamic Acid Metabolism in the Brain

cortex (Purpura et al., 1959). In contrast to acetylcholine, catecholamines and serotonin, γ-aminobutyric acid occurs in high concentration in the nervous system, and it has been suggested that a major portion of ketoglutaric acid is metabolized through this pathway with the production of energy-rich phosphate bonds (cf. McKhann, et al., 1959). The question arises, therefore, whether γ-aminobutyric acid has a direct action on the synaptic receptor sites or is a precursor of a neurohormone, or sets the metabolic stage for the action of neurohormones.

The involvement of γ-aminobutyric acid in nervous excitation and inhibition is suggested by the action of hydrazides which precipitate convulsions with a concomitant decrease of the γ-aminobutyric acid content of the brain (Killam and Bain, 1957). The action of the convulsant hydrazide is interpreted as arising from inhibition of glutamic decarboxylase by blocking of its coenzyme pyridoxal phosphate. Intraventricular administration of γ-aminobutyric acid or of vitamin B_6 prevented the hydrazine-induced convulsions (Killam et al., 1960). On the other hand biochemical and physiological changes induced by convulsant pyridoxine analogues are not reversed after administration of γ-aminobutyric acid (Purpura et al., 1960). It should be noted that the concentrations of γ-aminobutyric acid inhibiting the excitatory synapse as well as those normalizing paroxysmal electric activity in epileptogenic foci in the cat brain are far below those actually occurring in the central nervous system (Berl et al., 1960). These findings add to the observations suggesting that γ-aminobutyric acid as well as glutamic acid, glutamine and other metabolites occur in tissues in specific pools and that the concentration measured by analysis of the whole organ or part of it does not give an estimate of the concentration at the site of action. Without such knowledge interpretation of the action of metabolites and drugs is obviously very difficult.

XIII. Glutamic acid and its derivatives and the convulsive states

The apparent participation of γ-aminobutyric acid in the mechanism of suppression of seizures is the most recent indication that glutamic acid and its metabolic derivatives play a role in the metabolic mechanism related to the convulsive state. More than 15 years ago an effect of glutamic acid administration on petit mal attacks was reported (Price et al., 1943). As a consequence of these observations, the action of glutamic acid in mental defectives was tested (Albert et al., 1951). This was followed by attempts to influence epileptic seizures by the administration of glutamine and asparagine (Tower, 1955), and a trial with γ-aminobutyric acid in epileptics has been reported recently (Tower, 1960). The clinical efficacy of the administration of glutamic acid, which has been extended to other diseases of the nervous system, has been under discussion since its first clinical trials (Waelsch, 1951; Klingmüller, 1955). The results are contradictory, and at present it appears that, despite the large amount of biochemical and physiological work stimulated by these observations, the therapeutic effects are mainly of theoretical interest.

Animal experimentation also has suggested a close connection between glutamic acid metabolism and the convulsive state. After the discovery of the effect of glutamic acid on petit mal epilepsy, attempts were made to design antimetabolites blocking the metabolism of glutamic acid. The methionine sulfoxide developed for this purpose (Waelsch et al., 1946) was superseded when it was found that methionine sulfoximine was the agent in bleached flour which produced running fits in dogs. The sulfoximine has since become a useful tool for the production of convulsions in animals (Misani and Reiner, 1950; Peters and Tower, 1959). Its action, as that of methionine sulfoxide, is overcome by glutamine as well as by methionine.

The question arises whether the effects of glutamic acid, glutamine etc. may all be explained by the final conversion to γ-aminobutyric acid which is the real anticonvulsive agent. While this question cannot be answered at present, it may be noted that both glutamic acid and γ-aminobutyric acid are kept out of the brain by the blood-brain barrier, and it might be speculated that glutamic acid was effective only in such cases where a lesion with lowered barrier permitted the entrance of dicarboxylic acid. Similarly in mental defectives, those with secondary deficiency seemed to be more susceptible to its action (ALBERT et al., 1951).

XIV. Protein metabolism (cf. WAELSCH and LAJTHA 1961)

1. The turnover of brain proteins

The solution of the problem of the rate of replacement or turnover of proteins in the central nervous system has been hampered by the lack of methodological approach — a fact which has led to the denial of the dynamic state of brain proteins. This notion was made unlikely by the indirect observations of HYDEN (1943) which, on the basis of absorption measurements and staining with acidophilic dyes, suggested a rapid protein metabolism in the anterior horn cells of the guinea pig after exhausting exercise and in spinal ganglion cells after electric stimulation. An active turnover of brain proteins was definitely established by the results of studies carried out in various laboratories during recent years (PALLADIN and VERTAIMER, 1955; GAITONDE and RICHTER, 1955; WAELSCH, 1958; LAJTHA et al. and FURST et al. 1957—1959). These findings may be summarized by the statement that the proteins of the central nervous system have a rapid turnover which is not much below that of the liver proteins. On the basis of evidence obtained by radio autography it has been suggested that ganglion cells may have a protein turnover surpassing that of liver cells (MAURER, 1957). Proteolipids on the other hand have a turnover 10 to 40 times slower than the average turnover of brain proteins. Their half-life times varies between 90 and 600 days and may even be longer if calculated from experiments of longer duration. This finding suggests that some brain proteins may not be replaced during the life time of the animal (FURST et al., 1958; DAVISON, 1961; GAITONDE, 1961). In the experiments carried out with the aid of isotopic lysine (LAJTHA, FURST, WAELSCH loc. cit.), it was found that by varying the time period between intravenous administration of the amino acid and sacrifice of the animals, it was possible to measure the differing turnover rates of the different protein fractions. Thus a whole spectrum of turnover rates could be observed in brain as well as in liver (Table 6). The fastest protein fraction of total mouse brain has a turnover corresponding to a half-life time of three days while, in the same experiment, the fastest protein fraction of liver has a half-life time of one day. These results underscore the fact that the proteins of the brain, as of any other organ, are heterogeneous in their turnover rates. The question now arises as to whether or not the different functional areas of the brain contain proteins with different turnover rates. In the experiments with monkey brain, it was surprising to find that the corpus callosum and its radiation contained the proteins with the highest rate of turnover (for a discussion of this observation, see WAELSCH, 1958, WAELSCH and LAJTHA, 1961). followed by the proteins of the cortex and cerebellum, thalamus, hypothalamus, pons and finally of the cord. When the cells of the cortex of the monkey brain were fractioned into nuclei, mitochondria, microsomes and soluble proteins, the microsomal fraction showed by far the highest rate of turnover of isotopic lysine (Table 7). The rate of incorporation into microsomal fractions was three to five times the average value for the total cortex proteins (FURST et al., 1958; CLOUET and RICHTER, 1959). One may therefore suspect that some of the brain cortex proteins, e.g. those of the microsomal fraction, turn over with a half-life time of 15 hours or considerably less since these fractions are in themselves not homogeneous but mixtures of fast and slowly metabolizing proteins. Microsomal preparations from brain tissue incubated with labeled amino acids under appropriate conditions also show a higher rate of incorporation of amino acids than any other fraction of the cell (LAJTHA, 1960). Brain ribosomes exhibit a rate of incorporation of amino acids equal to, if not surpassing, that of liver ribosomes (ACS et al., 1961). It is, of course, of interest that the microsomal

Table 6. (WAELSCH 1958) *Half-life time (days) of proteins of mouse organs*

Time, after injection of ^{14}C-lysine minutes	Brain	Liver	Muscle
2	2.8	0.9	3.5
5	3.5	1.3	7.6
10	5.5	2.6	7.6
30	6.9		13.2
60	15.2		23.6

Table 7. (WAELSCH 1958). *Incorporation of ^{14}C-lysine into the proteins of different cell fractions of brain cortex (Macacus irus)* (30 min after injection)

Composition of fraction	Counts/mg protein-lysine/min
Cell debris, whole cells, nuclei, large mito-chondria	500
Mitochondria . . .	400
Microsomes	800—1400
Supernatant fluid .	600

proteins of the brain show such a rapid turnover since modern electron microscopy has equated the microsomes of the cortex with Nissl granules (PALAY and PALADE, 1955). These findings are in keeping with the observations of rapid changes in the appearance of Nissl granules in situations of stress.

The overall picture of the metabolism of the proteins of brain suggests that their rapid metabolism may contribute to some of the functional properties of this organ beyond their importance as structural components.

2. The origin of the proteins of the axoplasm

The synthesis of the proteins of the axoplasm may either occur locally or in the corresponding cell body from which the protein would then move out into the axonal sheath. WEISS and HISCOE (1948), SAMUELS et al. (1951) and OCHS and BURGER (1958) have accumulated circumstantial evidence for axonal flow. With the aid of isotopic lysine, a proximal-distal gradient in time of radioactivity of the protein of the sciatic plexus and sciatic nerve of the frog could be established (Table 8) (WAELSCH, 1958; LAJTHA, 1960). On the other hand, acetylcholinesterase, irreversibly inhibited, recovers in a distal-proximal direction in the sciatic nerve of the frog (CLOUET and WAELSCH, 1961) and evenly in various cat nerves (KOENIG and KOELLE, 1961). At present it cannot be decided whether the protein already synthesized or a component of the protein synthesizing system moves from the cell body through the axon. The latter possibility would also satisfy the experimental results obtained so far. It is furthermore difficult to decide on the basis of our present knowledge as to the contribution made by the Schwann or glia cells to the biosynthetic processes within the axon, just as

Table 8. (WAELSCH 1958). *Lysine ^{14}C incorporation into sciatic nerve proteins*
(Rana p.)
Cts/min/100 γ protein-lysine; upper portion plexus = 100

Days	Liver	Cord	Sciatic plexus		Sciatic nerve	
			upper	lower	upper	lower
8	220		100	51	28	25
17	150		100	73	29	35
28	260	130	100	83	63	63
38	300	170	100	100	100	116

there is no clear evidence whether the axon contains the machinery for protein synthesis or that mitochondria take part in it. It is undoubtedly attractive to speculate that the endoplasmic reticulum of the cell body might be continuously extended into the axon and that therefore axonal flow would be microsomal protein synthesis channeled into the extensions of the perikaryon. The determination of the origin of nerve axoplasm protein is of major significance not only as a possible clue to the origin of neurohormones of peptide nature, but also because it has important bearings on the problem of pharmacological effects on the nerve through influence on local protein synthesis or flow of axoplasm.

3. General significance of protein metabolism

Our interest in protein metabolism of the central nervous system is manifold. If we assume that the functional activity of an organ is carried by its enzymatic activity, there is no necessity to assume a turnover of proteins since the enzyme proteins may be permanently deposited. On the other hand, if the dynamic state of body constituents is a general biological law, we may expect all proteins to turn over, some at a very slow rate.

In brain macromolecules such as proteins or ribose nucleic acids may be considered as the organic basis of stored information. Such a possibility has been discussed (HYDEN, 1959; DINGMAN and SPORN, 1961) but it seems likely that if these macromolecules are involved in such processes, memory would probably express itself less in their varying composition than in changes of their orientation or type of folding in relation to each other.

The changes of composition or of amino acid sequence, or of the presence or absence of enzymatic activity, probably belong to the realm of gene-determined hereditary changes in the protein makeup of the cell.

XV. The amine incorporating system

The recent discovery (SARKAR et al., 1957; CLARKE et al., 1957) of an enzyme system present in mammalian organs, which catalyzes in vitro the fixation to proteins of a variety of primary amines, raises the possibility of the occurrence of tissue proteins modified by stably bound amines. According to present data, the enzyme catalyzes the exchange of the amide groups of protein-bound glutamine by a primary amine and has, therefore, been named "transglutaminase" (MYCEK et al., 1959). The enzyme action is Ca^{+r} dependent. The acceptor proteins which fix the amines occur in all organs in various amounts and the brain is among the organs with a high concentration of such proteins. Other purified proteins such as casein, lactoglobulin or insulin may also serve as acceptor proteins. Aliphatic primary mono- and diamines, such as putrescine, cadaverine, and spermine, are incorporated as well as histamine, serotonin, noradrenaline or mescaline etc. (CLARKE et al., 1959).

It appears possible that transglutaminase is responsible for the reported incorporation of mescaline into the liver proteins of mice in vivo (BLOCK et al., 1952; BLOCK, 1954). In this case oxidation of the administered amine and formation of melanin-like products may have simulated at least in part an incorporation of mescaline into proteins (CLOUET, 1958).

Since transglutaminase catalyzes the exchange of the amine with the amide group of protein-bound glutamine, ammonia is evolved in this reaction usually in excess of the amine incorporated. Also, in the absence of added amine, transglutaminase catalyzes a Ca^{++} dependent liberation of ammonia from the acceptor proteins (MYCEK and WAELSCH, 1960). This ammonia liberation is in part due to a hydrolysis of the amide groups and in part to a replacement of the amide group of protein-bound glutamine by free protein amino groups such as the ε-amino group of protein-bound lysine. Protein amide groups have, therefore, to be counted among the possible sources of tissue ammonia (see section D, X). A reversible de- and reamidation of proteins may establish a metabolic cycle of significance for a functional role of ammonia in the nervous system. The importance of proteins modified by incorporated amines cannot be assessed today but the possibility of such proteins acting as antigens in autoimmunization reactions has to be kept in mind. Autoimmunization has been considered as a possible etiological factor in psychoses as well as in neurological diseases such as multiple sclerosis.

XVI. Protein metabolism in various experimental and pathological conditions

Since the first observation by HYDEN on the changes of nucleic acid and protein content of neurones upon stimulation, a considerable number of studies have been concerned with the rate of protein metabolism in the nervous system under various conditons of stress. In HYDEN's experiments intense acoustic stimulation decreased the neuronal proteins, a decrease lasting for several weeks (CASPERSSON, 1947; HAMBERGER and HYDEN, 1945; HYDEN, 1947, 1959) while moderate stimulation led to an increase of nucleoproteins (HAMBERGER and HYDEN, 1949a, 1949b). Apparently the synthetic and degradative processes, balancing each other under resting conditions, do not do so under stimulation.With moderate stimulation the rate of synthesis is greater than that of degradation of protein while, at strong stimulation, degradation exceeds synthesis. It is of interest to note that in moderate stimulation increased protein synthesis expresses itself also in an increased concentration of enzymes related to energy metabolism [cytochrome and succinic oxidase (HYDEN, 1959; HYDEN et al., 1958; BRATTGARD, 1952)]. It is of considerable interest that the oligodendroglia showed the reverse changes, a fact which suggested to the authors that nerve cells and surrounding glia cells represent a metabolic unit (HYDEN and PIGON, 1960).

With the aid of histochemical techniques, changes in the concentration of nucleoproteins and lipoproteins in nervous tissue were found in exhaustion, after administration of various drugs, in vitamin E deficiency, hypoxia, insulin and metrazol shock, and as the result of disease processes (EINARSON, 1954, 1957).

In a considerable number of recent investigations the rate of the incorporation of labeled amino acids into brain protein as measured by radioautography has been taken as a measure of the rate of protein metabolism in various conditions of stress. It should be noted that in these studies the precursor-product relationship, i.e. the specific activity of the labeled amino acid, was not established. Therefore it cannot be decided whether any change in rate of protein metabolism observed is not secondary to changes in the concentration of the precursor amino acid due to changes in the properties of the permeability barriers or of the rate of metabolism of the free amino acid itself under the particular conditions. No change (DINGMAN et al., 1959) as well as an increase (PALLADIN et al., 1955) and a decrease (GAITONDE and RICHTER, 1956) of the rate of incorporation of labeled amino acid into brain proteins was found upon electrical stimulation. The data on amino acid incorporation into proteins in narcosis are similarly equivocal (GAITONDE and RICHTER, 1956; PALLADIN, 1957). Upon exhaustion the rate of incorporation of methionine dropped to one third and increased twofold in subsequent sleep (SHAPOT, 1957).

The phosphate moiety of phosphoprotein shows high metabolic activity, but the turnover of this group probably does not reflect the rate of turnover of the protein portion but rather the amount of energy available for phosphorylation (MAGEE and ROSSITER, 1954). In convulsions there is an increased uptake of P^{32} phosphate into brain phosphoprotein while in combined anesthesia and hypothermia a decrease of the rate of incorporation, not only of phosphate but also of labeled amino acids, was found (VLADIMIROV, 1953; VLADIMIROV and URINSON, 1957; NECHAEVA et al., 1957).

It has been claimed that the ratio of brain protein amide groups to total protein nitrogen decreases during excitation and strenuous physical exercise (VRBA, 1955; VRBA and FOLBERGROVA, 1959). Since these experiments have been carried out on non-fractionated protein mixtures the small changes observed may be due to a depletion of a particular protein species. During stimulation an increase of protein SH has been found, and changes of protein configuration have been suggested under such conditions (UNGAR et al., 1957; UNGAR and ROMANO, 1958).

In line with HYDEN's observation, strong stimulation leads to a decrease in the protein, lipid and nucleic acid content in the brain of the intact animal. The same results were obtained in cat brain perfused with glucose-free fluid (ABOOD et al., 1955; GEIGER, 1959). Despite many equivocal observations the findings in cerebral protein metabolism under conditions of stimulation, metabolic depression and various stresses suggest that the proteins of the brain participate actively and rapidly in the over-all metabolism of the organ under normal and abnormal conditions.

XVII. Proteins and mental disease

In the field of mental disease, aspects of abnormal protein metabolism have attracted the attention of several laboratories. About 35 years ago GJESSING (1938, 1939) started the study of nitrogen retention and excretion in periodic catatonics. The etiological basis of this disease was considered to be the retention of toxic products of protein metabolism, a variant of the old so-called "toxic amine hypothesis". GJESSING studied his patients only after the establishment of nitrogen balance. In the first group of patients he found a retention of about 15—25 g of nitrogen during the quiet period. When this level was reached, they started to excrete more nitrogen than they absorbed and went into the catatonic phase. These results seemed to indicate a rhythm of mental and metabolic symptoms. In a later group of patients the rhythm was reversed, nitrogen retention being accompanied by the catatonic phase and a negative nitrogen balance by the quiet one. In still another group the mental and metabolic rhythms did not coincide. One may conclude that in this work the mental changes were removed from nitrogen metabolism by a considerable chain of metabolic events; unfortunately as yet the intervening links are unknown. This work represents an example of critical investigative work in psychiatry of the highest order.

During the last few years, the search has been revived for an abnormal protein or enzyme in schizophrenics (for review of previous work see KEUP, 1954). It was speculated that the genetic background modified the enzymatic pattern in this disease which shows a high concordance in monozygotic twins. First, it was claimed that the quantity of ceruloplasmin, the copper-containing protein which catalyzes the oxidation of N,N-dimethyl-p-phenylene diamine, was increased in the blood of schizophrenic patients (AKERFELDT, 1957; ABOOD et al., 1957; LEACH et al., 1956) and that the rate of adrenaline oxidation in the blood of schizophrenics was increased. These observations proved to be unspecific and probably related to dietary influences which would lower the ascorbic acid content of the blood (Scheinberg et al., 1957). In the course of similar investigations a protein fraction (taraxein) was isolated from blood of schizophrenics, the administration of which is supposed to elicit schizophrenia episodes of short duration (Heath et al., 1957, 1958). Up to the present this claim could not be confirmed in other laboratories (Robins et al., 1957), and the whole problem is unresolved. (For a detailed discussion and review of the data see Kety, 1959).

E. Lipids

In contrast to the biochemistry of carbohydrates and nitrogenous compounds, that of the lipids of the nervous system has not found direct consideration in the etiology of mental disease. The biochemistry of lipids, however, has played an important role in our understanding of some inborn errors of metabolism, i. e. hereditary abnormalities of metabolism accompanied by abnormal mentation, in particular mental deficiency. Myelination, characterized by the deposition of large amounts of lipids during maturation of the nervous system, attracted the attention of neurochemist and pathologist very early, and it is conceivable that minor aberrations of this process may have considerable significance in the function of the mature brain. Attempts were made early to correlate the degree of myelination with the functional development of the brain (Watson, 1903). Therefore, a short review of the basic aspects of lipid metabolism appears appropriate.

Conventionally, the lipid components of the nervous system are divided into phosphatides, glycosphingosides, mucolipids, and steroids.

I. Phosphatides

According to the alcohol moiety present the phosphatides are classified as phosphoglycerides, phosphoinositides and phosphosphingosides.

The two main representatives of phosphoglycerides were assumed to be lecithin (phosphatidyl choline) and kephalin (phosphatidyl ethanolamine) until a study of the kephalin fraction led to the isolation of phosphatidyl serine (Folch, 1942, 1948). Plasmalogen, an additional member of the class of phosphoglycerides was considered an acetal phosphatide containing a fatty acid moiety and one aldehyde moiety bound in acetal linkage to glycerol. It has now been shown to contain an ether of an α-β unsaturated alcohol probably produced by rearrangement of the corresponding aldehyde (Rapport and Franzl, 1957).

The phosphoinositides from brain tissue contain, in addition to fatty acids and glycerol, inositol and phosphate in molar ratios of 1:3, mixtures of mono- and diphosphates are being formed during alkaline hydrolysis. The inositides in the original brain lipid are probably mainly present as the triphosphates (Dittmer and Dawson, 1961; Tomlinson and Ballou, 1961).

The phosphosphingosides (sphingomyelin) contain, in addition to sphingosine, phosphocholine and fatty acids (Carter and Greenwood, 1952; Chibnall et al., 1936).

II. Glycosphingosides and mucolipids

The galactosphingosides (cerebrosides) contain galactose and fatty acids (Klenk, 1927; Klenk and Faillard, 1953).

Although cerebrosides containing glucose have been isolated from other sources, only galactocerebrosides have been found in brain tissue. In the white matter, a cerebroside has been found in which the primary hydroxyl of the galactose moiety is esterified with sulfate. This sulfur-containing cerebroside has been given the name sulfatide (Blix, 1933; Lees et al., 1959).

Much effort has been concentrated during recent years on sphingosine-containing lipids which comprise a group of complex high polymer substances all characterized by a high content of sialic acid (ROSENBERG et al.; 1956; BLIX, 1936, 1938; BLIX et al., 1952; KLENK, 1941), the substituted form of neuraminic acid (GOTTSCHALK, 1956). This acid constitutes 21% of a crystalline lipid. The name gangliosides had been proposed for these lipids (KLENK, 1941). A substance containing up to 30% sialic acid was isolated as a high-molecular water-soluble complex obtained in long birefringent strands (strandin) (FOLCH et al., 1951). In addition to sialic acid, the gangliosides contain sphingosine, fatty acids, galactose, glucose, and galactosamine (BRANTE, 1948).

III. Cholesterol

Cholesterol occurs in the non-saponifiable fraction of brain lipids as the free sterol. In this respect, the brain differs from other organs which contain cholesterol esters in addition. There are derivatives and isomers of cholesterol present in the unsaponifiable fraction of brain but no definite conclusion as to the native occurrence of these compounds can be drawn at present.

IV. Synthesis and degradation of fatty acids

By sheer bulk, fatty acids make up the largest portion of the lipid components of the nervous system. In a 30 day old rat brain the fatty acids compose 19% of the dry weight corresponding to about 40% of the total lipid content (WAELSCH et al., 1941). The fatty acids of the brain are not only those characteristic of depot fat such as palmitic, stearic, and oleic acids, but there are present saturated, unsaturated, and hydroxylated fatty acids containing 20—26 carbon atoms. The degradation of fatty acids has been elucidated (LYNEN and OCHOA, 1953; LYNEN, 1957) by the discovery of acetyl coenzyme A as the reactive derivative of acetic acid participating in fatty acid metabolism as well as in the citric acid cycle. The synthetic pathway proceeding by condensation of acyl CoA and malonyl CoA (GIBSON et al., 1958) also accounts for the synthesis of unsaturated fatty acids which comprise up to 30% of the total fatty acids of the lipids of the nervous system.

The close relationship between the citric acid and the fatty acid cycles becomes apparent since, depending on available enzyme activities, substrate, and coenzyme concentration, acetyl CoA will either condense with oxaloacetic acid to citric acid, the acetyl moiety thereby being oxidized to CO_2 and water, or will condense with another malonyl CoA derivative to form the building stones for fatty acid synthesis. Enzymes catalyzing various steps of the fatty acid cycle have been found in the human brain, a fact which indicates that the central nervous tissue has the enzymatic equipment for the metabolism of its fatty acids (LYNEN, 1957). The enzymes of fatty acid metabolism are located within the mitochondria (SCHNEIDER, 1959) and their close proximity to the enzymes of the citric acid cycle is noteworthy.

The mechanism of synthesis of phosphatides has been established in part by experiments on tissue other than brain and has been shown to occur through phosphatidic acids (KORNBERG and PRICER, 1953a and b). The phosphate group is split off by a phosphatase and the diacyl glycerol may add another acyl moiety from acyl CoA, phosphoryl choline or phosphoryl ethanolamine, whereby neutral fat (KENNEDY and WEISS, 1956a), lecithin (WEISS and KENNEDY, 1956), and kephalin (KENNEDY and WEISS, 1956b) respectively are formed. In the transfer of phosphoryl choline and ethanolamine, cytidine coenzymes act as carriers

(Kennedy and Weiss, 1956). Phosphorylcholine and phosphorylethanolamine are synthesized by an adenosine triphosphate-dependent reaction (Wittenberg and Kornberg, 1953), and these compounds occurring in the brain and other organs are now assumed to arise by synthetic pathways rather than by degradation of phosphatides (Dawson, 1956; Ansell and Dawson, 1951). Our knowledge of the metabolism of sphingolipids has not progressed as far as that of the phosphatides. It has been proposed that sphingosine is synthesized from serine and from palmityl CoA by an enzyme system from brain (Brady and Koval, 1958).

V. Cerebral fatty acid metabolism in vivo

In earlier attempts to study the turnover of fatty acids in the central nervous system with fatty acids such as elaidic acid used as markers, it could not be decided whether such fatty acids were not incorporated into the brain lipids because of the inability of this substance to penetrate the blood-brain barrier or because of the lack of turnover of the brain lipids (McConnell and Sinclair, 1937). The same argument holds true for the lack of incorporation of deuterium-labeled fatty acid into brain lipids of adult animals (Sperry et al., 1940). When, on the other hand, the turnover of fatty acids is estimated in animals the body water of which was enriched with deuterium oxide, the incorporation of deuterium may be taken as a measure of the amount of hydrogen derived from body water, and of the extent of replacement of fatty acids by newly synthesized fatty acids (Waelsch et al., 1940). Such experiments indicated that about 20% of the fatty acids of the adult rat brain was replaced within one week. Since these analyses were carried out on the whole brain without differentiation between grey and white matter, it appears possible that most of the fatty acid metabolism found would occur in the former, with hardly any fatty acid turnover in the latter. The fatty acid metabolism of the central nervous system appears not to be a very active process when compared whith that of the liver. It is also possible that the turnover observed refers to fatty acid metabolism of glial elements in both grey and white matter. The indicated lack of turnover of the fatty acids in the myelin of the central nervous system would support the supposition that this structure once formed is separated from the enzymes responsible for its biosynthesis, a fact of considerable significance for the mechanism of demyelination under pathological conditions (cf. R. Adams, 1960).

The presence of higher fatty aldehydes in the lipids of the nervous tissue raises the question as to their position in fatty acid metabolism. Earlier experiments with animals, whose body water was enriched with deuterium oxide or to which labeled fatty acids were administered, suggested that the fatty aldehydes were derived from the corresponding acids and not *vice versa* (Ehrlich and Waelsch, 1946). These findings are supported by more recent experiments in which the incorporation of ^{14}C labeled acetate into the fatty acids and aldehydes of brain or liver of adult rats or into the corresponding compounds of slices from the same organs was studied. Hardly any incorporation of ^{14}C acetate into the aldehydes of the brain tissue slices was found although isotope was incorporated into the fatty acid fractions (Klenk, 1957; Korey and Orchen, 1959).

VI. Cerebral cholesterol synthesis and metabolism

In the adult brain the rate of turnover of cholesterol is so low as to suggest that this steroid is metabolically inert once deposited during growth and myelination of the nervous system (Sperry et al., 1940). Recent experiments which seem to show that brain cholesterol incorporates labeled precursors but that once labeled the steroid does not disappear (McMILLAN et al., 1957) may be an indication of the fact that the brain of the rat — the outstanding laboratory animal used in these studies — grows for a considerable period of postnatal life (DONALDSON, 1924).

VII. Cerebral metabolism of phosphatides (cf. ROSSITER, 1957)

In vivo (FRIES et al., 1940) as well as in vitro (TAUROG et al., 1942) ^{32}P phosphate is incorporated into the phosphatides of brain and nerve. In vivo, after systemic administration of the phosphate, the incorporation of ^{32}P phosphate is considerably lower into phosphatides of the brain than into those of other organs, while in vitro (STRICKLAND, 1954; McMURRAY et al., 1957) or after intracerebral administration (DAWSON, 1954; LINDBERG and ERNSTER, 1950), rapid labeling of the brain phosphatides takes place. These findings emphasize again the significance of the blood-brain barrier for the uptake by the brain of substances from the circulating blood. Also choline and serine, appropriately labeled with ^{14}C, entered the phosphatide fraction when incubated with brain slices and were found in the corresponding non-fatty acid fraction of the phosphatides (PRITCHARD, 1956). In the intact animal, brain takes up much less choline or ethanolamine than other organs (STETTEN, 1941).

Qualitative results similar to those found for the incorporation of precursors into the brain lipids were demonstrated with lipids of peripheral nerve (BODIAN and DZIEWIATKOWSKI, 1950; FRIES et al., 1942; MAGEE and ROSSITER, 1954; MAJNO and KARNOVSKY, 1958). The incorporation of glucose or galactose into cerebrosides has been studied in young and adult animals in vivo and in vitro (BURTON et al., 1958; MOSER and KARNOVSKY, 1958).

At one step or another in lipid synthesis, the synthetic pathways depend on the participation of adenosine triphosphate which has, therefore, to be generated at a sufficient rate (STRICKLAND, 1954). It is thus not surprising that agents affecting the main ATP generating process — oxidative phosphorylation — influence the incorporation of phosphate or the rate of other biosynthetic processes leading to synthesis of lipids.

Therefore glutamic acid, high potassium concentrations, electric stimulation or dinitrophenol, which deplete the energy-rich phosphate stores or uncouple oxidative phosphorylation, decrease the incorporation of ^{32}P phosphate into phosphatides in vitro (STRICKLAND, 1954; FINDLAY et al., 1954; DAWSON and RICHTER, 1950).

On the other hand, chlorpromazine, which in relatively high concentrations (10^{-3} moles) has the same effect, stimulates at lower concentrations (10^{-4} moles) (MAGEE et al., 1956) the incorporation of ^{32}P phosphate into lipids.

An interesting but also hitherto unexplained observation is the finding that the addition of carbamyl choline or acetylcholine (+ eserine) increased the labeling of brain lipids when brain slices were incubated with ^{32}P phosphate (HOKIN and HOKIN, 1955, 1953).

VIII. The turnover of lipids in the brain

Since the brain lipids are divided between those occurring in grey and white matter, different metabolic rates may be shown by the same compound according to its location. While in the immature brain rapid incorporation of lipid constituents and a fast synthesis of cholesterol can be demonstrated, some of these reactions slow down to a rate variously considered negligible or significant according to the method used (WAELSCH, 1959).

It has been suggested that the decrease of lipid nitrogen found in brain cortex of the anaesthetized cat after stimulation of the brachial plexus (GEIGER et al., 1956) or the loss of lipid phosphorus from isolated cat brain perfused with glucose-free fluid (ABOOD and GEIGER, 1955) is an indication of a metabolic utilization of lipids.

The lipid constituents of myelin may show only incorporation in the immature brain, the label persisting during life (DAVISON et al., 1960). If the brain grows slowly also during young adulthood as suggested, an incorporation of labeled lipid constituent has to be expected without subsequent disappearance of the label (see discussion of Cholesterol Metabolism). It is of major significance to ascertain whether or not the lipids of the myelin sheath are metabolically inert or are rejuvenated in vivo once deposited. In vitro experiments showing incorporation of labeled lipid components into lipid of peripheral nerve have not up to now been able to differentiate as to whether we are dealing with the metabolic activity of Schwann cells or with deposited myelin.

F. Neurohumors

In the preceding sections the metabolism of carbohydrates, proteins and lipids in the central nervous system has been surveyed. The picture that emerged showed that the fundamental economy of the nerve cell does not greatly differ from that of other living cells. It must be admitted, however, that our present biochemical knowledge is still removed by many steps from an understanding of the chemical correlates of such phenomena as sensory perception, motor impulses or memory engrams, let alone speech or abstract thought.

The area where biochemistry has so far made its deepest penetration into the realm of neurophysiology is that dealing with chemical transmission of nerve impulses. The protagonists in this story are certain organic bases, notably acetyl-choline, catechol amines and serotonin.

The intervention of chemical mediators in the transmission of nervous impulses had been postulated even before the discontinuous structure of interneuronal and neuromuscular junctions was recognized. The similarity of effects of sympathetic nerve impulses with those of adrenaline was pointed out by T. R. ELLIOTT (1905) who first suggested that adrenaline might act as a chemical transmitter at sympathetic nerve endings. DALE (1914) noted the remarkable fidelity with which acetylcholine mimicked the effects of parasympathetic stimulation and the transient nature of the action of acetylcholine. He proposed that an esterase in the tissues rapidly splits acetylcholine. However, it was through the famous experiments of OTTO LOEWI (1921, 1922, 1924) that the theory of chemical transmission was put on a secure foundation. LOEWI's "Vagus-stoff" was soon identified with acetylcholine. LOEWI also showed that adrenaline, or an adrenaline-like substance, was released on stimulation of cardiac sympathetic nerves.

I. Acetylcholine
1. The function of acetylcholine

The pharmacological activity of the autonomic transmitter agents greatly facilitated the acceptance of the concept of chemical transmission of impulses from postganglionic autonomic nerve endings to the effector organs. Its extension to synaptic transmission (KIBJAKOW, 1933; FELDBERG and GADDUM, 1934) and to the transmission of impulses from somatic motor nerves to striated muscle (DALE et al.,

1936; BROWN et al., 1936) was a natural development. Evidence for these functions of acetylcholine was provided by the following observations among others: 1. liberation of acetylcholine after stimulation of preganglionic or motor nerve fibres, 2. response of ganglion cells or striated muscle to acetylcholine, and 3. potentiation by eserine and other anticholinesterases of response to stimulation, whether produced electrically or by application of acetylcholine.

A similar function of acetylcholine in at least some of the synapses of the central nervous system is an attractive hypothesis, though much less amenable to experimental verification. However, the available evidence is in support of such a mechanism. 1. Acetylcholine has been detected in the venous blood leaving the brain (CHANG et al., 1937; CHUTE et al., 1940) or the spinal cord (BÜLBRING and BURN, 1941); it also appears in cerebrospinal fluid (FELDBERG and SCHRIEVER, 1936; CHANG et al., 1938; ADAM et al., 1938) and in saline pools placed next to the exposed cerebral cortex (MACINTOSH and OBORIN, 1953). 2. Topical application of acetylcholine seems to have a direct excitatory action on neurons. Other central actions of acetylcholine and of anticholinesterases have been described (cf. the reviews of BURGEN and MACINTOSH, 1955; and of FELDBERG, 1957). 3. The functional activity of the brain is related to changes in the concentration of acetylcholine. Anaesthesia produces a pronounced increase (RICHTER and CROSSLAND, 1949; MCLENNAN and ELLIOTT, 1951; CROSSLAND and MERRICK, 1954; HERKEN and NEUBERT, 1953). According to several authors (RICHTER and CROSSLAND, 1949; MCLENNAN and ELLIOTT, 1951) convulsions have the opposite effect, though this has been denied by HERKEN and NEUBERT (1953). A decrease in the acetylcholine content of rat brain was also found as a result of insulin hypoglycaemia (CROSSLAND et al., 1955).

Marked differences in the distribution of acetylcholine and the synthesizing enzyme, choline acetylase, throughout the central nervous system, have led to the conclusion that not all central neurons are cholinergic. FELDBERG and VOGT (1948) have pointed out that in the optic pathway, leading from the retina to the visual areas of the occipital cortex, neurons with high concentrations of acetylcholine and choline acetylase alternate with others where these concentrations are low, and they suggested that a similar pattern may exist elsewhere in the central nervous system. KOELLE (1957) showed histologically that in the optic nerve a small number of fibres containing cholinesterase exist among a majority of fibres containing little or none.

It is generally accepted that impulses are propagated along the axon by electrical currents. The currents are generated by movements of sodium and potassium ions across the conducting membrane. In the unexcited state the membrane is the seat of an electric potential which is maintained by the unequal distribution of ions, particularly potassium ions, in the intracellular and extracellular fluids. An active, energy-consuming metabolic process assures a continuous removal of sodium ions which have diffused through the membrane into the intracellular fluid; the high intracellular concentration of potassium ions is simply the electrostatic consequence of this process, which has been called the sodium pump. In a state of excitation the polarization of the membrane is reversed due to a rapid and transient increase of the membrane permeability for sodium, resulting in an inward flow of sodium, and a slower and delayed increase of the membrane permeability for potassium, resulting in an outward flow of potassium. The inflow of sodium corresponds by and large to the rising phase of the action potential, the outflow of potassium to the falling phase (HODGKIN, 1951; KEYNES, 1957). According to the prevailing theory the permeability change in the axonal membrane is produced by the depolarization spreading ahead of the active region.

4*

A contrary view has been proposed by Nachmansohn (1947, 1955); he believes that the depolarization is secondary to the change in permeability and that the latter is dependent on the release of bound acetylcholine. Axonal conduction, synaptic and motor endplate transmissions are supposed to be essentially identical phenomena initiated by the reaction of acetylcholine with specific receptors and rapidly terminated by the action of acetylcholinesterase. These processes are entirely intracellular; leakage of acetylcholine into extracellular fluids is held to be the result of experimental artefacts. The actual transmitting agent is the flow of current, not only on the axonal surface but also across the synaptic gap, aided by the greater surface at the end-arborization and the resulting decrease of resistance. The hypothesis has the attraction of being unitary and it explains some facts for which a satisfactory explanation is otherwise lacking, for instance the presence of cholinesterase in the nerve fibre. Nachmansohn has adduced other circumstantial evidence which he has presented in several reviews (1947, 1948, 1955, 1959).

Numerous objections have been raised against Nachmansohn's hypothesis, among which the following may be mentioned: 1. On the basis of the theory it is to be expected that a conduction block induced by anticholinesterases would be associated with a long-lasting depolarization of the axonal membrane. This could not be verified (Toman et al., 1947). 2. There is evidence that the postsynaptic membrane is not excitable electrically (Grundfest, 1957). 3. Cholinesterase may be inhibited completely in brain slices (Strickland and Thompson, 1955) and almost completely in red blood cells (Taylor et al., 1952; Goodman et al., 1955) without an increase of potassium leakage. 4. Acetylcholine and choline acetylase are present in non-cholinergic nerve fibres only in traces or not at all and, although cholinesterase is found in non-cholinergic as well as in cholinergic nerves, it is not equally distributed among the fibres. These differences would be difficult to explain if the acetylcholine system were uniformly involved in axonal conduction. Moreover, there would be no justification to distinguish between cholinergic and adrenergic nerves.

With reference to the last point, Cohen (1956) working in Nachmansohn's laboratory pointed out that although sensory fibres, such as dorsal roots or optic nerve, contain much smaller concentrations of choline acetylase than, for instance, ventral roots, they nevertheless contain the enzyme in sufficient quantity to restore the acetylcholine content in the space of a minute. Cohen assumes that the amount of acetylcholine released per impulse is exceedingly small, so that there is no need for a particularly active rate of synthesis.

2. Synthesis of acetylcholine

In vitro synthesis of acetylcholine by brain slices was first demonstrated by Quastel, Tennenbaum and Wheatley (1936); the synthesis depended on the presence of eserine to prevent enzymatic hydrolysis and of an oxidizable substrate, such as glucose, lactate or pyruvate. Mann, Tennenbaum and Quastel (1938. 1939) showed the existence of acetylcholine in two forms: a free, active, soluble form and an inactive, insoluble or bound form. The inactive form could be converted to the free form by the action of acids or organic solvents. It is now known that this can also be done by mechanical grinding, by freezing and thawing or by treatment with distilled water (Stone, 1955). Potassium, calcium (in low concentration) and bicarbonate ions stimulate acetylcholine synthesis by brain slices (Mann et al., 1939; McLennan and Elliott, 1950).

Subsequent work (Nachmansohn and Machado, 1943; Feldberg and Mann. 1946; Lipmann and Kaplan, 1946; Nachmansohn and Berman, 1946) has established the existence of an enzyme, choline acetylase, which could be extracted and to some extent purified. It catalyses the following reaction:

$$\text{Choline} + \text{acetyl-coenzyme A} \rightarrow \text{acetylcholine} + \text{coenzyme A (Co A)}.$$

Acetyl-coenzyme A arises in the course of the oxidation of pyruvic acid and of long-chain fatty acids (cf. NOVELLI, 1953; GREEN, 1954). It can also be formed from acetic acid and adenosine triphosphate by the enzyme acetic thiokinase in the following reaction:

$$\text{ATP} + \text{acetate} + \text{CoA} \rightleftarrows \text{AMP} + \text{Pyrophosphate} + \text{acetyl CoA}$$

or from citric acid by "condensing enzyme" according to the equation:

$$\text{Citrate} + \text{CoA} \rightleftarrows \text{Acetyl CoA} + \text{oxaloacetate}.$$

Choline, in free form, is available in blood plasma and in brain tissue in sufficient quantity. However, being a quaternary ammonium base, it is unable to diffuse through the cellular membranes. There is now evidence that choline is rapidly transported into ganglion cells by a specific carrier mechanism (MACINTOSH, BIRKS and SASTRY, 1956). The question arises whether choline transport is related to the effect described by HOKIN and HOKIN (1958, 1959). These workers found that acetylcholine stimulates the incorporation of phosphate into phospholipids, particularly into phosphatidic acid. Such an effect might conceivably regulate the availability of a carrier for choline.

Choline acetylase is contained in particles which can be separated from the mitochondria by centrifugation in a density gradient and seem to be identical with the vesicles containing acetylcholine (WHITTAKER, 1959). There is some evidence for choline acetylase being synthesized in the ganglion cell and migrating along the axon towards the nerve endings (BERRY and ROSSITER, 1958).

3. Cholinesterases

Acetylcholine is hydrolyzed by two types of cholinesterases, both powerful and widespread enzymes. "Specific" or acetylcholinesterase occurs throughout the nervous system. Its concentration is greater in grey than in white matter; it is particularly high in the caudate nucleus (BURGEN and CHIPMAN, 1951). Histochemically the enzyme has been found to be localized principally in zones rich in end arborizations (POPE et al., 1952). It has been claimed that in the giant axon of the squid the enzyme is present in the membrane but not in the extruded axoplasm.

Outside of the nervous system, acetylcholinesterase occurs in red blood cells, placenta, muscle and other tissues. In muscle the enzyme is probably localized mainly in the motor endplate.

Unspecific or pseudo-cholinesterase occurs mainly in liver, pancreas and serum. It is also present in brain where it is localized mainly in the glial elements.

The two enzymes may be differentiated by their different specificities. The most useful substrates are acetyl-β-methylcholine, cleaved by acetylcholinesterase but not by pseudo-cholinesterase, and benzoylcholine, split by pseudo-cholinesterase but not by acetylcholinesterase. The two enzymes also differ in their susceptibility to inhibitors (HAWKINS and MENDEL, 1946, 1947, 1949).

While it is agreed that the physiological function of acetylcholinesterase is the hydrolysis of acetylcholine, it is usually assumed that that of pseudocholinesterase is directed towards other, at present unknown, substrates.

Rapid destruction of acetylcholine is essential in order to re-establish the resting potential of the excitable membranes. The high activity of the enzyme and its great concentration at the synapses and neuromuscular junctions assure the necessary speed. Interference with the activity of acetylcholinesterase profoundly affects both the central and peripheral nervous system.

The concept of competitive enzyme inhibition is applicable to most inhibitors of acetylcholinesterase, such as eserine and prostigmine. Other inhibitors, such as alkyl phosphates, inhibit cholinesterases (and also proteinases and peptidases) irreversibly, presumably by phosphorylation of protein-bound serine. Phosphorylated acetylcholinesterase can be reactivated by substituted oximes (WILSON, 1954, 1958).

Acetylcholinesterase is enriched in and synthesized by microsomal fractions of the neuron (endoplasmic reticulum) (FUKUDA and KOELLE, 1959; TOSCHI, 1959). It has been suggested that the enzyme located along the nerve fiber is synthesized in the cell body and travels to the synapse (DALE, 1955; LEWIS and HUGHES, 1957) where its function is seen as the destruction of the acetylcholine continuously liberated during the resting stage (KOELLE and KOELLE, 1959). In recent studies the cholinesterase concentration in rat brain was correlated to age, genetic strain and adaptive behavior (BENNETT et al., 1958a, 1958b; ROSENZWEIG et al., 1958.

4. Storage and release of acetylcholine

The electron microscope has revealed the existence of characteristic vesicular particles in efferent nerve endings and particularly in the immediate neighbourhood of the presynaptic membrane. It is now generally assumed that these synaptic vesicles act as storage depots of acetylcholine and that the acetylcholine thus sequestered constitutes the "bound" fraction of acetylcholine. With the arrival of an impulse a large number of these vesicles discharge their contents. It has been calculated (MACINTOSH, 1959) that each vesicle contains about 400 molecules of acetylcholine and that the concentration of acetylcholine in the vesicular fluid is 0.11 M, i. e. approaching isotonicity. Acetylcholine therefore must be the most abundant cation in that fluid.

Under certain conditions the acetylcholine concentration of nervous tissues can be elevated much above its usual level, viz. when brain slices are incubated in an eserinized medium containing 27 mM potassium (MANN et al., 1939) or when ganglia are perfused with eserinized plasma (MACINTOSH, 1959). It is noteworthy that the "surplus" acetylcholine is present entirely in the "free" form, presumably in the cytoplasm or axoplasm.

II. Catecholamines

1. Distribution and localisation

Just as acetylcholine is released upon stimulation of cholinergic nerve fibres, an adrenaline-like substance is released from adrenergic fibres and presumably mediates the stimulation of the effector organ. The specific neurohormone of adrenergic nerves has been identified as noradrenaline by EULER (1946, 1948).

Postsynaptic sympathetic fibres are rich in noradrenaline. Most organs contain noradrenaline in relation to the density of adrenergic fibres present therein. If the sympathetic nerve supply to an organ is severed noradrenaline disappears. Regeneration of the adrenergic nerves is followed by a reappearance of noradrenaline (EULER, 1956).

In addition to noradrenaline many tissues other than the adrenal medulla contain adrenaline though in smaller amounts than noradrenaline. Adrenaline is assumed to be localized in chromaffine cells which are widely scattered in many organs.

$$HO{-}\hspace{-2pt}\bigcirc\hspace{-2pt}{-}CHOH{-}CH_2NH \cdot CH_3 \qquad HO{-}\hspace{-2pt}\bigcirc\hspace{-2pt}{-}CHOH{-}CH_2NH_2$$

Adrenaline   Noradrenaline

$$HO{-}\hspace{-2pt}\bigcirc\hspace{-2pt}{-}CH_2{-}CH_2NH_2$$

Dopamine

In the adrenal medulla adrenaline and noradrenaline are produced by two different types of cells (HILLARP and HÖKFELT, 1953, 1954, 1955). Since the secretion of the adrenal medulla contains various proportions of noradrenaline, depending on the specific stimulus applied, it may be assumed that discharge from the two types of cells is controlled by separate centres. The proportion of noradrenaline in the adrenal medulla varies greatly from one species to another. It also varies with age; the adrenal medulla of newborn animals and of human embryos contains predominantly noradrenaline (EULER, 1956).

In the brain noradrenaline, with an admixture of about 5% of adrenaline, occurs in characteristic distribution (VOGT, 1954; SANO et al., 1959). The highest concentration was found in the hypothalamus and in the area postrema (about 1 μg/g in the dog.) Other parts of the diencephalon, mesencephalon and medulla oblongata also contained high concentrations, especially those bordering on the ventricles and aqueduct and those containing the reticular formation. Although noradrenaline was found in all parts of the brain examined, concentrations were low (0.01—0.2 μg/g) in the grey matter of cerebral and cerebellar cortex, in some basal nuclei and in white matter.

A third catecholamine, dopamine, has recently been found in several tissues (MONTAGU, 1957; EULER and LISHAJKO, 1957). In the brain its concentration is of the same order as that of noradrenaline (WEIL-MALHERBE and BONE, 1957; CARLSSON et al., 1958) but its distribution seems to be different since the highest concentration is found in the putamen and caudate nucleus (BERTLER and ROSEN-GREN, 1959; SANO et al., 1959).

Like acetylcholine, a large proportion of tissue catecholamines is associated with particulate cell constituents. In the adrenal medulla the catecholamines are contained in spherical granules, smaller but denser than the mitochondria (BLASCH-KO, HAGEN and HAGEN, 1957). It is possible to separate two types of granules by centrifugation through a concentration gradient, one which contains noradrenaline and settles in the bottom layer, and another fraction above the bottom layer which contains mainly adrenaline (SCHÜMANN, 1957). These granules are probably more closely related to the microsomes, since they contain a microsomal enzyme, cyto-chrome-m (SPIRO and BALL, 1958). They also contain a high concentration of ATP (FALCK et al., 1956). Since the molar ratio of ATP to amines has an approximately constant value of 1:4, it is assumed that the two compounds form a salt-like combination. The granules are stable in neutral isotonic salt solution, but they release their content of amines and ATP if subjected to treatments capable of disrupting their membranes, such as acid, heat, hypotonic solutions, surface-active agents, freezing and thawing.

EULER and HILLARP (1956) showed that noradrenaline in splenic nerve is partly associated with particles, usually accounting for 20—30% of the total amount. According to SCHÜMANN (1958) the particles contain no dopamine, all of which was found in the soluble fraction. On the other hand, all three catecholamines occurring in brain are distributed about evenly between a particulate and a soluble fraction (WEIL-MALHERBE and BONE, 1957).

2. Synthesis of catecholamines

The pathway of catecholamine synthesis has been well established and consists of a number of distinct steps. The parent substance is the amino acid tyrosine from which 3 : 4-dihydroxyphenylalanine (dopa) is formed by oxidation. Dopa is converted to dopamine by the enzyme dopa-decarboxylase, with pyridoxal phosphate acting as co-enzyme. The enzyme occurs in sympathetic ganglia and nerves and also in the grey matter of the central nervous system (HOLTZ and WESTERMANN, 1956).

The next step is the oxidation of dopamine to noradrenaline which has been demonstrated with the aid of isotopically labelled precursors, in vivo (UDENFRIEND and WYNGAARDEN, 1956), in perfusion experiments (ROSENFELD et al., 1957) and in vitro (NERI et al., 1956; HAGEN, 1956; GOODALL and KIRSHNER 1957; PELLERIN and D'IORIO, 1957). The enzyme, dopamine β-oxidase, has been extracted from bovine adrenal medulla and purified. It requires ascorbic acid as cofactor; its activity is enhanced by fumarate and inhibited by 10^{-2} M imipramine (LEVIN, LEVENBERG and KAUFMAN, 1960; GOLDSTEIN and CONTRERA, 1961). Finally, noradrenaline is N-methylated to adrenaline. Adenosylmethionine acts as methyl donor in the reaction (KIRSHNER and GOODALL, 1957).

It has been shown that tritium-labelled adrenaline does not readily cross the blood-brain barrier (WEIL-MALHERBE et al., 1959). On the other hand, dopa seems to be able to penetrate into the central nervous system, since it has marked central effects (HOLTZ et al., 1957; CARLSSON et al., 1957). In rabbits pretreated with pheniprazine, an inhibitor of monoamine oxidase, the intravenous injection of dopa led to an increase of the noradrenaline and particularly of the dopamine concentration in both the cytoplasmic and granular fractions of brain tissue. After pretreatment with pyrogallol, an inhibitor of catechol-O-methyl transferase dopa injection increased the concentration of dopamine only (WEIL-MALHERBE, POSNER and BOWLES, 1961).

3. Inactivation and breakdown of catecholamines

It is inherent in the concept of chemical transmission of impulses that there must be a mechanism by which the action of the transmitter is rapidly terminated. Such a mechanism is essential if the receptor cell is to regain its excitability. In the acetylcholine system this is assured by the extremely rapid action of acetylcholinesterase, as a result of which the life time of free acetylcholine is of the order of microseconds.

A similar mechanism has been postulated for the adrenergic system and it has been suggested that the enzyme monoamine oxidase fulfills the function performed by acetylcholinesterase in the cholinergic system. Monoamine oxidase acts according to the following general equation:

$$R' \cdot CH_2 \cdot NH.R'' + {}^1/_2 O_2 \rightarrow R'.CHO + NH_2.R''$$

Ammonia is formed from primary amines, such as dopamine and noradrenaline; adrenaline gives rise to methylamine. The aldehyde formed in the primary reaction is usually further oxidized to the corresponding carboxylic acid; the latter, in the case of noradrenaline and adrenaline, is 3 : 4-dihydroxymandelic acid (doma) while dopamine is converted into 3 : 4-dihydroxyphenylacetic acid (dopac).

If the main function of amine oxidase were the termination of the activity of adrenaline and noradrenaline one would expect its reaction with these amines to be more rapid than, or at least as rapid as, its reactions with other substrates. This is however not so. Adrenaline and noradrenaline are both oxidized by amine oxidase at a comparatively sluggish rate, whereas the reaction with dopamine is quite brisk.

Moreover, inhibition of amine oxidase by iproniazid failed to potentiate the effects of administered adrenaline or noradrenaline in several instances (CORNE and GRAHAM, 1957; SCHMITT and GONNARD, 1955; KAMIJO, KOELLE and WAGNER, 1956). These observations raised some doubt as to the physiological significance of the oxidation of adrenaline and noradrenaline by monoamine oxidase.

Mainly through the brilliant work of J. AXELROD it has now become clear that the principal reaction leading to the inactivation of adrenaline and noradrenaline is O-methylation at position 3 of the benzene ring. The enzyme, catechol-O-methyl transferase, catalyses the transfer of a methyl group from the methyl donor, S-adenosylmethionine, to the catechol according to the equation:

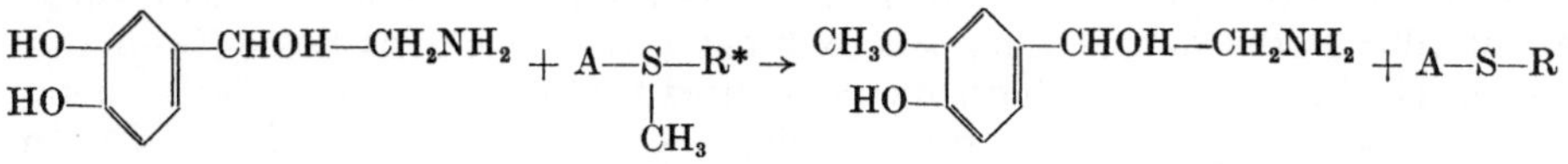

$$\text{HO-}\bigcirc\text{-CHOH-CH}_2\text{NH}_2 + \text{A-S-R*} \rightarrow \text{CH}_3\text{O-}\bigcirc\text{-CHOH-CH}_2\text{NH}_2 + \text{A-S-R}$$

| Noradrenaline | Adenosylmethionine | 3-O-methylnoradrenaline (normetanephrine) | Adenosylhomocysteine |

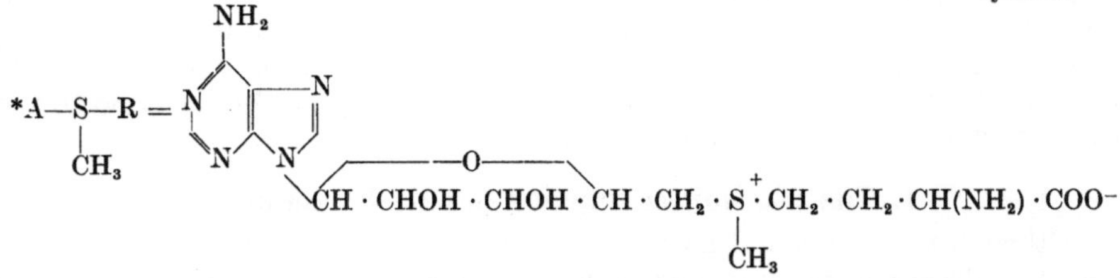

$$\text{*A-S-R} = \text{(adenine)} \cdots \text{CH} \cdot \text{CHOH} \cdot \text{CHOH} \cdot \text{CH} \cdot \text{CH}_2 \cdot \overset{+}{\text{S}} \cdot \text{CH}_2 \cdot \text{CH}_2 \cdot \text{CH(NH}_2) \cdot \text{COO}^-$$

Catechol-O-methyl transferase was found to occur in the soluble fraction of many tissues, including the brain (AXELROD and TOMCHICK, 1958). The great speed with which this reaction occurs was demonstrated in experiments in which ^{3}H-adrenaline was infused or injected (AXELROD, WEIL-MALHERBE and TOMCHICK, 1960). A high concentration of ^{3}H-3-O-methyladrenaline (^{3}H-metanephrine) was reached in many tissues and in plasma in a very short time. It was estimated that more than half of the injected adrenaline was O-methylated within two minutes, during which period its physiological effects had subsided. When ^{3}H-adrenaline was injected intravenously into mice almost all of the adrenaline which had disappeared after 10 minutes could be accounted for as metanephrine. The disappearance of adrenaline from the whole animal showed a rapid initial phase followed by a more gradual decline. This suggests that inactivation of the hormone is due to two different processes: (1) enzymatic inactivation, presumably mainly by O-methylation and (2) binding to receptor sites in many tissues from which unchanged adrenaline is slowly released.

The "binding" mechanism is as yet obscure; sequestration by membrane barriers or formation of electrovalent or covalent bonds with receptor molecules must be considered. In this connection the enzyme transglutaminase, mentioned in a preceding section (p. 43) may well have an important function by linking biologically active amines to proteins.

The methylated metabolites, metanephrine and normetanephrine, are oxidized by monoamine oxidase (AXELROD, 1959; AXELROD et al., 1958); in fact, they are better substrates than adrenaline and noradrenaline. The acid formed from both methylated metabolites on oxidation is 3-methoxy-4-hydroxymandelic acid (vanillyl mandelic acid, VMA, Armstrong et al., 1957).

It is probable that catecholamines are, for the greater part, O-methylated before they are oxidized, but there is no reason to assume that the reverse process is impossible. There are indeed various observations which are difficult to explain except on the assumption that amine oxidase has some part to play in the control of sympathetic activity. Thus, Biel et al. (1958) found that, after treating rabbits with iproniazid or with another powerful inhibitor of amine oxidase, 1-phenyl-2-isopropylhydrazine (JB 516), for five days, the level of noradrenaline in the brain was more than doubled. It has further been shown that an injection of iproniazid in rabbits will prevent the breakdown of catecholamines when the brain is homogenized (Weil-Malherbe and Bone, 1959). Zile and Lardy (1959) studied the effects of hyperthyroidism in rats and found an association of low monoamine oxidase activity with high levels of circulating noradrenaline.

After an infusion of ^{14}C-d,l-adrenaline or ^{14}C-d,l-noradrenaline in human beings about 70% of the radioactivity was excreted in the urine in 24 hours (Goodall, 1959). The bulk of the products was accounted for by two compounds: 1. metanephrine or normetanephrine, respectively, in conjugated form and 2. VMA. In addition, unchanged catecholamine, free O-methylated amine, dihydroxymandelic acid and several unidentified compounds were detected.

Rats injected with dopamine excreted a small amount of 3-methoxytyramine in free and conjugated form and considerable quantities of its deaminated product, homovanillic acid (Axelrod et al., 1958). Goldstein et al. (1959) found that 6.4% were excreted as unchanged dopamine, 2—3% as 3-methoxytyramine, 6.25% as dopac and 60% as homovanillic acid.

4. The transmitter function of catecholamines

Although the function of noradrenaline as the transmitter released from postsynaptic adrenergic nerve endings is well-established, there is so far no definite evidence for a transmitter function of catecholamines elsewhere in the nervous system. The fact that noradrenaline is concentrated at the cerebral autonomic centres and along the reticular formation suggests that it is implicated in the activity of these structures, but exactly in which way is not known. Various drugs were found to deplete the noradrenaline level in the hypothalamus, but their pharmacological effects were very different, some causing convulsions and others anaesthesia or tranquillization. They all had, however, a similar depleting effect on the catecholamine content of adrenal medulla (Vogt, 1957). Reserpine which had previously been shown to cause depletion of brain serotonin (Brodie et al., 1955) also has a strong depleting action on brain catecholamines (Holzbauer and Vogt, 1956). Muscholl and Vogt (1958) have shown that peripheral organs with adrenergic innervation no longer respond to electrical stimulation of pre- or postganglionic fibres, when the loss of noradrenaline is severe and has persisted for several hours. This is in accordance with a transmitter function of noradrenaline. On the other hand, after depletion of cerebral noradrenaline the brain was still found to be discharging normally into the preganglionic fibres of the cervical sympathetic nerve (Iggo and Vogt, 1959). It must be concluded, therefore, either that noradrenaline is not essential for the firing of sympathetic centres in the brain or is only required in minute amounts. As to the possible correlation of the central effects of reserpine with the lowering of the noradrenaline concentration in the brain one can only speculate; present knowledge does not yet permit any detailed interpretation.

III. Serotonin

The name serotonin was originally applied to a vasoconstrictor substance occurring in serum. It was obtained in crystalline form by RAPPORT, GREEN and PAGE (1948) who showed that it was a complex consisting of creatinine, sulphuric acid and 5-hydroxytryptamine. Serotonin turned out to be identical with enteramine, a substance previously isolated from intestinal mucous membrane by ERSPAMER (1940, 1952). The term serotonin is now generally employed as a synonym of 5-hydroxytryptamine.

The candidacy of serotonin (5-hydroxytryptamine) as a neurohumor rests on three sets of observations: 1. serotonin occurs in the brain in a specific pattern of localisation; 2. serotonin has central effects and 3. links have been found between serotonin and the action of drugs with potent effects on the nervous system, notably reserpine and lysergic acid diethylamide (LSD).

1. Serotonin in the central nervous system

The occurrence of serotonin in brain was first shown by TWAROG and PAGE (1953). Its distribution has been studied by AMIN et al. (1954), BOGDANSKI and UDENFRIEND (1956), BOGDANSKI et al. (1957) and PAASONEN et al. (1957). Serotonin was found to be distributed similarly to noradrenaline, with highest concentrations in the hypothalamus, area postrema and central grey substance. High values were also found in the midbrain, amygdala and thalamus. PAASONEN et al. (1957) stress the association of serotonin with the limbic system: in contrast to its low concentration in other cortical areas, high values of serotonin were found in those belonging to the limbic system, i. e. the hippocampal gyrus, orbital gyrus, cingulate and retrosplenial cortex. All limbic nuclei, such as amygdala, septal nuclei, hypothalamus, thalamus and habenula, contained high concentrations of serotonin. In order of magnitude the concentrations of serotonin are similar to those of noradrenaline, both reaching values of $1-1.5\ \mu g/g$ in the areas of greatest concentration.

Studies of the intracellular distribution of serotonin in whole rat brain have given the following result: 22% in the low-speed sediment (containing coarse debris and nuclei), 63% in the mitochondrial fraction and 12% in the supernatant fraction (WALASZEK and ABOOD, 1959; GIARMAN and SCHANBERG, 1959; WHITTAKER, 1959). A large proportion of serotonin, as of other neurohumors, is therefore associated with particles.

2. Synthesis of serotonin

The parent substance of serotonin is the amino acid tryptophan from which the immediate precursor, 5-hydroxytryptophan, is formed by oxidation. Tryptophan-5-hydroxylase activity has been demonstrated in extracts of rat intestinal mucosa (COOPER and MELCER, 1961) and rat liver (FREEDLAND et al., 1961a). The tryptophan hydroxylating system of rat liver is identical with L-phenylalanine hydroxylase (RENSON et al., 1961) and is inhibited competitively by L-phenylalanine (FREEDLAND et al., 1961). The conversion of 5-hydroxytryptophan to serotonin is brought about by the enzyme 5-hydroxytryptophan decarboxylase. In properties, distribution, requirement for pyridoxal phosphate as coenzyme and occurrence in the cytoplasmic fraction of brain homogenates this enzyme closely resembles dopa-decarboxylase. The two enzymes are now thought to be identical (ROSENGREN, 1960).

Injection or infusion of animals with serotonin does not produce any increase of its concentration in the brain, indicating that it does not penetrate across the blood-brain barrier to a significant extent. Likewise, no central symptoms are usually seen in cases of carcinoid tumours, in spite of greatly increased levels of serotonin in the blood. On the other hand, the blood-brain barrier seems to be freely permeable to 5-hydroxytryptophan, since brain serotonin levels were significantly increased when the precursor was administered intravenously to animals.

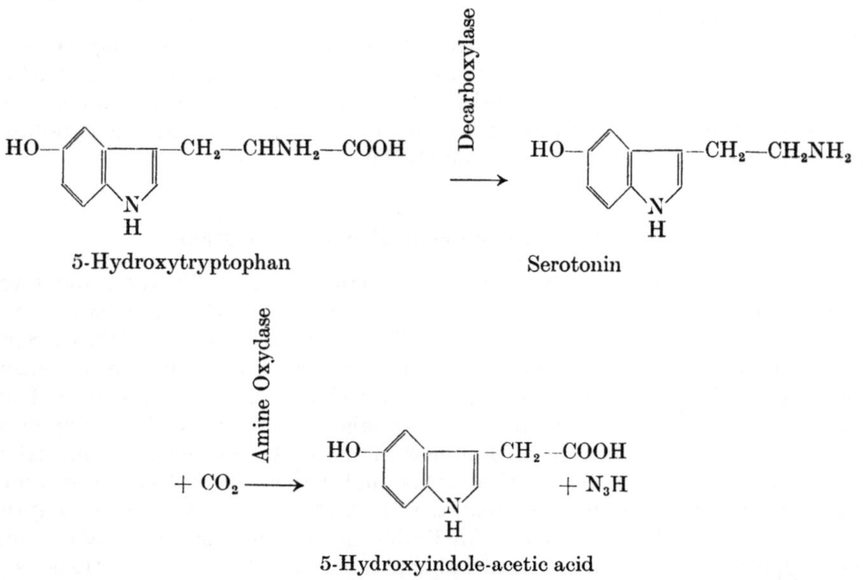

Formation and Metabolism of Serotonin

The areas of the brain showing the largest increase of serotonin were those rich in the decarboxylase and where serotonin is normally found in high concentration. The injection of 5-hydroxytryptophan induced dramatic effects pointing to excitation of autonomic centres: the animals showed generalized muscular tremor, ataxia and incoordination of movements, lacrimation, salivation, piloerection, hyperpnoea, tachycardia, pupillary dilatation, loss of light reflexes and loss of response to visual stimuli suggesting a temporary state of blindness (UDENFRIEND, WEISSBACH and BOGDANSKI, 1957). These effects are reminiscent of those produced in monkeys by high doses of bufotenine (a serotonin derivative with a dimethylamino group) or LSD (EVARTS, 1956). It was found, moreover, that 5-hydroxytryptophan had a hyperpyretic effect like LSD in rabbits. Both effects were attenuated by the LSD-analog, bromo-lysergic acid diethylamine (BOL). and by the development of tolerance to LSD (HORITA and GOGERTY, 1958).

3. Metabolism of serotonin

Unlike adrenaline and noradrenaline, serotonin is oxidized rapidly by monoamine oxidase. The reaction is probably the principal route of serotonin metabolism, since 1. inhibition of amine oxidase by iproniazid and other agents produces an increase in brain serotonin levels (UDENFRIEND et al., 1957; SHORE et al., 1957; BIEL et al., 1958) and 2. the product of deamination, 5-hydroxyindoleacetic acid, is the main urinary metabolite of serotonin; after intravenous infusion of serotonin

30—60% are excreted in the form of the acid within 4 hours (ERSPAMER, 1954). The concentration of 5-hydroxyindoleacetic acid in urine is greatly increased in cases of carcinoid.

After inhibition of amine oxidase by iproniazid in cats the proportion of infused serotonin accounted for by urinary 5-hydroxyindoleacetic acid fell from 52 to 18% (CORNE and GRAHAM, 1957). The drop in excretion of 5-hydroxyindoleacetic acid after a test dose of serotonin has been used as a method of evaluating the efficiency of amine oxidase inhibitors in man (SJOERDSMA et al., 1958).

The increase of serotonin concentration in the brain produced by inhibitors of amine oxidase has central effects similar to those observed after 5-hydroxy-tryptophan injection. Combining both procedures produces the largest increase in brain serotonin and the strongest central effects (UDENFRIEND, WEISSBACH and BOGDANSKI, 1957). The hyperpyretic effect of 5-hydroxytryptophan in rabbits is greatly enhanced by the amine oxidase inhibitor phenylisopropylhydrazine (JB-516) and may be lethal (HORITA, 1958).

Experiments with amine oxidase inhibitors revealed an unsuspectedly rapid rate of increase in brain serotonin levels: these were doubled within a few minutes, suggesting a very rapid turnover of brain serotonin (UDENFRIEND and WEISS-BACH, 1958). In rabbits injected with JB-516 the serotonin level in the brain stem rose from 0.65 to 1.02 μg/g in 20 min., indicating a half-life time of brain serotonin of 10—15 min. (BRODIE et al., 1958).

4. Serotonin, reserpine and LSD

Reserpine potentiates the hypnotic effects of hexobarbital and ethanol in mice and, in this respect, resembles the effect of serotonin in large doses (BRODIE et al., 1955). Both actions are antagonized by LSD (SHORE, SILVER and BRODIE, 1955). When this observation was followed up, it was found that reserpine induced the release of large amounts of serotonin from body depots, such as brain or small intestine. The sedative effects persisted after reserpine had disappeared from brain and correlated much better with the changes in serotonin concentration than with the presence of reserpine (BRODIE, PLETSCHER and SHORE, 1955).

During the period of low cerebral levels of serotonin the excretion of 5-hydroxy-indoleacetic acid was increased. It was suggested that in the reserpinized animal serotonin continues to be formed at the normal rate, but that the tissues are unable to retain it in bound form. After its release from its bound form serotonin is presum-ably open to rapid oxidation by amine oxidase. If this reaction is inhibited by iproniazid the serotonin concentration in the brain remains unchanged after reserpine administration. In that case reserpine, far from acting as a tranquillizer, actually leads to enhanced excitement, the animals showing motor unrest, dilated pupils, rapid breathing, etc. (BRODIE, PLETSCHER and SHORE, 1956; PLETSCHER, SHORE and BRODIE, 1956).

The effect of reserpine is specific. It is only obtained by those other Rauwolfia alkaloids and reserpine congeners which show tranquillizing effects. Tranquillizers which are chemically unrelated to reserpine, such as chlorpromazine, do not affect the serotonin concentration of the brain (PLETSCHER et al., 1956; PAASONEN and GIARMAN, 1958).

Iproniazid not only blocks the tranquillizing effect of reserpine but also its potentiating effect on barbiturate narcosis. The hypothesis has been put forward that serotonin itself acts as a stimulant, whereas the aldehyde formed from it by the action of amine oxidase acts as a depressant; reserpine iproniazid would increase the level of free serotonin, whereas reserpine alone would cause increased formation of the aldehyde (Holtz et al., 1957). A similar theory had been proposed many years ago by Mann and Quastel (1940) who found that the oxidation of amines to aldehydes had a depressant action on the metabolism of brain slices and suggested that the analeptic effects of amphetamine were due to its action as an inhibitor of amine oxidase.

The situation has become even more complicated when it was found that reserpine causes depletion not only of serotonin but also of catecholamines (Holz-bauer and Vogt, 1956). The time curve of noradrenaline disappearance and re-appearance in brain tissue is practically identical with that relating to serotonin (Brodie et al., 1957). The pharmacological effects of reserpine may thus be due, wholly or partly, to serotonin, catecholamines or any of their metabolites. Recent observations suggest that the sedative effects of reserpine are associated with the depletion of brain serotonin rather than of brain noradrenaline. Reserpine when administered to cold-stressed rats did not induce sedation or appreciably lower the brain serotonin level, but its effect in depressing the level of brain nor-adrenaline was not diminished. When the animals were brought into a warm room, the levels of brain serotonin declined slowly; sedation appeared when the serotonin level had declined by about 50% (Orlans et al., 1960). A selective depletion of brain noradrenaline is also attained by the drugs α-methyldopa and α-methyl-metatyrosine; they produce a rapid and transient fall of brain serotonin and brain dopamine and a prolonged depression of brain noradrenaline (Porter et al., 1961; Hess et al., 1961).

After the administration of reserpine to rats serotonin disappears more rapidly from the particulate than the soluble fraction of the brain, in accordance with the postulated releasing action of the drug (Giarman and Schanberg, 1959). The catecholamines, on the other hand, were found to disappear from the soluble fraction at a faster rate than from the particulate fraction (Weil-Malherbe and Bone, 1959). Whether this indicates a difference in the mechanism of action of reserpine or is due to the fact that different enzymes are involved in the metabolism of serotonin and catecholamines, is not clear at present.

A relationship between the function of serotonin and the action of LSD was suggested by the discovery that the action of serotonin on the rat's uterus and other tissues was specifically inhibited by LSD (Gaddum and Hameed, 1954). A certain resemblance in the chemical structures of serotonin and LSD lent support to the view that LSD was acting as an antimetabolite of serotonin. It was further supported when it was found that LSD inhibited the potentiating effect of reserpine and serotonin on hexobarbital hypnosis (*vide supra*).

Gradually, however, the view is gaining ground that the psychological effects of LSD, at any rate in small doses, are due, not to antagonism, but to synergism with serotonin. The facts on which this view is based are as follows:

1. Small doses of LSD, similar to those producing hallucinations in man, enhanced, rather than blocked the potentiation of hexobarbital hypnosis by serotonin, while the potentiation produced by reserpine was blocked by both small and large doses of LSD. Other hallucinogens (bufotenine, mescaline and ibogaine) acted like LSD (Salmoiraghi and Page, 1957).

2. While doses of LSD of 1 μg/l inhibited the action of serotonin on the isolated rat uterus, still lower doses, 0.05—0.2 μg/l, potentiated it. Mescaline had the same effect, while tranquillizers (reserpine, chlorpromazine and azacyclonol) inhibited the serotonin effect (Costa, 1956).

3. LSD has a serotonin-like effect on the isolated heart of the clam, *Venus Mercenaria* (Shaw and Woolley, 1956).

4. Injection of LSD in high doses (1 mg/kg) produces symptoms in animals similar to those produced by the administration of 5-hydroxytryptophan or iproniazid which is known to elevate the brain serotonin level (EVARTS, 1956). Moreover, both 5-hydroxytryptophan and LSD have a similar hyperpyretic effect (HORITA and GOGERTY, 1958).

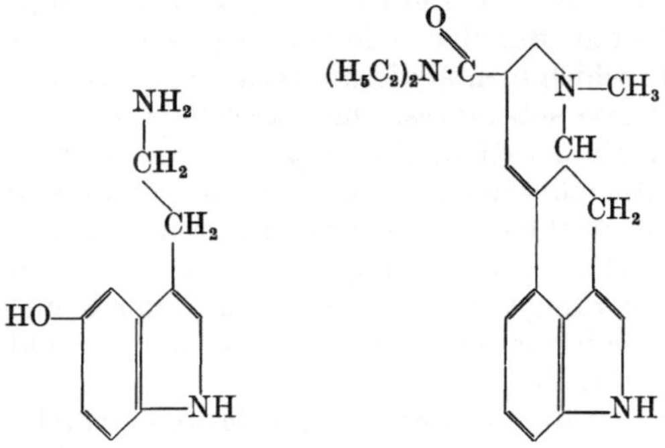

Serotonin   LSD

5. MARRAZZI and HART (1955) studied the potentials produced in one optic cortex of the cat by stimulation of the contralateral optic cortex and found that both LSD and serotonin inhibited transcallosal synaptic transmission in similar fashion when injected into the carotid at the side of the transmitted potential. However, in view of the inability of serotonin to cross the blood-brain barrier, the possibility must be considered that the effects were elicited by reflexes from vasomotor or other peripheral receptors. In any case the specificity of the observed inhibitions does not appear to be very high. BULLE and KONCHEGUL (1957) have also reported that the intracarotid injection of serotonin and LSD produces similar effects in dogs.

To add to the confusion it has been found that the LSD-analog, 2-brom-d-lysergic acid diethylamide (BOL 148), resembles LSD in acting as a serotonin antagonist in the rat's uterus test (CERLETTI and ROTHLIN, 1955) and in potentiating the sedative effect of serotonin, while blocking that of reserpine in mice treated with hexobarbital (SALMOIRAGHI and PAGE, 1957). Yet, unlike LSD, BOL has no psychological effects in man, except in very high doses (SCHNECKLOTH et al., 1957). This observation is a serious obstacle to the acceptance of the theory that the psychological effects of LSD are connected with the function of serotonin unless it can be shown that BOL does not have the same access to the sites of serotonin action as LSD. CERLETTI and ROTHLIN have shown that BOL does penetrate into mouse brain; whether the same holds good for human brain, and if so, whether access to the active receptors is the same for LSD and BOL, once they have passed the blood-brain barrier, is not known at present.

IV. Other possible neurohumors

The evidence for acetylcholine, catecholamines and serotonin acting as neurohumors in the central nervous system is, at present, tentative and circumstantial. This is even more so in the case of some other substances occurring in the brain and possessing pharmacological activities. One of these, γ-aminobutyric acid, has already been briefly discussed in a preceding chapter. Two other substances, histamine and substance P, are frequently mentioned in this context. However, the paucity of our present knowledge regarding their connection with nervous function is such that any discussion would be largely conjectural and might profitably be deferred.

V. Neurohumors and mental disease

Since the neurohumors constitute an actual or presumptive link between body chemistry and brain function it is not surprising that theories have been proposed according to which mental disease is caused by an abnormal metabolism or a dysfunction of these substances. The catecholamines and serotonin, particularly, have been incriminated in this way; in spite of the central effects of atropine and some anticholinesterases the possibility of a disturbed acetylcholine metabolism as an etiological factor in mental disease has so far received less attention. Acetylcholine has, however, been implicated in convulsive disorders, although earlier observations according to which focal epileptogenic tissue in human cerebral cortex is deficient in the formation of bound acetylcholine could not be confirmed (Pappius and Elliott, 1958).

In view of the fact that the theories and speculations revolving around serotonin and adrenaline are presently the focal points of a great deal of interest and of much active research, they will be briefly presented, although in this rapidly changing field the views of the day are bound to be short-lived.

1. The adrenaline hypothesis of schizophrenia

This hypothesis which has attracted a great deal of attention suggests that schizophrenia, or on entity among the group of schizophrenic diseases, is caused by an aberrant type of adrenaline metabolism leading to the production of an abnormal metabolite with hallucinogenic properties. In their first publication Osmond and Smythies (1952) discussed the similarity in structure between adrenaline and the hallucinogenic drug, mescaline.

$HO-C_6H_3-CHOH-CH_2-NHCH_3$ (with two HO groups)

Adrenaline

$H_3CO-C_6H_2(OCH_3)-CH_2-CH_2-NH_2$ (with two H_3CO groups and OCH_3)

Mescaline

Methylation of phenolic hydroxyl groups was held to be a reaction of which the animal organism was incapable. We now know that it does occur and that, in fact, O-methylation of catecholamines represents the major route of metabolism. The methylated derivative of dopamine which has been found in urine and in brain (Axelrod et al., 1958; Goldstein et al., 1959) differs from mescaline only by the absence of a methyl group in position 4 and a methoxy group in position 5.

$H_3CO-C_6H_3(HO)-CH_2-CH_2NH_2$

3-Methyldopamine

Although the gap between mescaline and endogenous metabolites has narrowed it is still a considerable one and it is useful to bear in mind that none of the physiological methoxy-compounds has yet been shown to have pharmacological activities similar to mescaline.

Perhaps because O-methylation of catecholamines seemed improbable OSMOND and SMYTHIES who meanwhile had joined forces with HOFFER shifted their emphasis on to another derivative of adrenaline, adrenochrome. Adrenochrome is formed from adrenaline by autoxidation in vitro, catalysed by heavy metals or by heavy metal enzymes, such as coeruloplasmin or cytochrome oxidase.

$$HO-C_6H_3(OH)-CHOH-CH_2-NH-CH_3 \longrightarrow O=C_6H_3=O-CHOH-CH_2-N(CH_3) \longrightarrow HO-C_6H_2(OH)-OH-N-CH_3$$

Adrenaline   Adrenochrome   Adrenolutine

An analogue of adrenochrome, "dopachrome", is formed in vivo as an intermediary in the formation of melanin from dopa (RAPER, 1927). Although adrenaline can be converted to a melanin-like product in vitro, presumably via adrenochrome, evidence for the occurrence of such a reaction in vivo is lacking. Adrenochrome has a ring configuration with an indole skeleton; it is easily converted to adrenolutine (N-methyl-3:5:6-trihydroxyindole) which has a fully aromatic indole ring. The fact that many hallucinogens, such as harmine, ibogaine, bufotenine, dimethyl- and diethyltryptamine and, last but not least, LSD are indole derivatives suggested to HOFFER, OSMOND and SMYTHIES (1954) that adrenochrome, too, might be hallucinogenic and might, in fact, be the hypothetical substance arising in schizophrenics. They were encouraged by reports of hallucinatory experiences and other mental phenomena among patients treated with adrenaline for asthmatic or allergic disorders, especially when the adrenaline solutions had deteriorated and assumed a pink tint. Subsequent trials with adrenochrome administered intravenously showed psychological effects similar to those of mescaline or LSD. It has further been claimed that adrenolutine produces the same changes as adrenochrome (HOFFER, 1957). These changes are summarized by HOFFER and OSMOND (1959) as follows: 1. changes in thought similar to those seen in schizophrenia; i.e. blocking, referential thinking, delusions, slowing of thought, lack of insight, decrease in level of abstraction, 2. depression, often long sustained, often with a paranoid tinge, 3. changes in personality from pleasant mild mannered individuals to hostile difficult states, 4. changes in visual perception and, rarely, hallucinations, 5. decreases in anxiety and 6. marked increases in fatigue and irritability.

Adrenochrome semicarbazone, which, unlike adrenochrome, is a stable substance, has no hallucinogenic effects (RINKEL, HYDE and SOLOMON, 1955). TAUBMANN and JANTZ (1957) are of the opinion that the psychological effects are due neither to adrenochrome nor to adrenolutine but to small amounts of an unknown oxidation product of adrenaline.

The greatest obstacle to the acceptance of the adrenochrome hypothesis is the fact that there is no evidence for adrenochrome being a metabolite of adrenaline in vivo. SCHAYER and SMILEY (1953) compared the metabolism of radioactive adrenaline and adrenochrome respectively; the excretion patterns were found to be quite different. More recent work by AXELROD, GOODALL and their colleagues which was reviewed in a preceding section (p. 56—58) has shown that 70—90% of infused radioactive adrenaline or noradrenaline can be accounted for in the urine in the form of free or conjugated metabolites produced by the action of the enzymes catechol-O-methyl transferase and/or amine oxidase. These results conclusively exclude the possibility that adrenochrome is a major metabolite of adrenaline; they do not exclude the possibility that it is formed in trace amounts or under pathological conditions. However, RESNICK and ELMADJIAN (1956) found no difference in the pattern of adrenaline metabolites in the urine from schizophrenic patients as compared with normal controls. If we concede the possibility that trace amounts of adrenochrome may be formed from adrenaline in vivo these could hardly account for more than 10% of the total metabolites of adrenaline. The daily production of adrenaline in man under normal conditions may be estimated to be of the order of 0.5—1 mg. Under conditions of stress the secretion of adrenaline may increase 100—200 fold, but the periods of increased discharge are usually brief. In the light of these considerations the concentrations of adrenochrome required to produce psychological effects, viz. 10 mg given by rapid intravenous injection, are larger than those that could be expected to arise in vivo. The assumption that adrenochrome is only produced in circumscribed regions of the brain has little intrinsic probability and would be difficult to prove or disprove at present.

HOFFER (1958) claimed to have shown the presence of adrenochrome in the plasma of normal subjects and an increase in its level following the administration of LSD. Schizophrenics were reported to have normal amounts of adrenochrome in blood plasma, but increased amounts in cerebrospinal fluid; in addition, after the injection of adrenochrome the substance was found to persist longer in the plasma of schizophrenics and of normals treated with LSD than in the plasma of untreated controls (HOFFER and OSMOND, 1959).

HOFFER found about 50 μg of adrenochrome per litre of plasma. Even if it were assumed that adrenochrome is the principal metabolite of adrenaline, a concentration as high as this could hardly be expected. After an injection of radioactive adrenaline the concentration in plasma of metanephrine, which actually is the principal metabolite of adrenaline, was found to be about the same as that of adrenaline within 2 minutes and to decrease at a similar rate thereafter (AXELROD et al., 1960). SZARA et al. (1958), using a different method of assay, failed to confirm the occurrence of adrenochrome in the plasma of normal or schizophrenic subjects.

The in vitro oxidation of adrenaline to adrenochrome by the plasma protein, coeruloplasmin, has sometimes been cited as evidence in favour of the formation of adrenochrome in vivo. However, in the experiments of LEACH and HEATH (1956) the concentration of adrenaline was about 10^6 times the physiological concentration of adrenaline in plasma. When adrenaline is used in concentrations as high as this it is probable that normal protective mechanisms are swamped. Catecholamines present in plasma or added in small, physiological quantities were found to be stable in plasma from both normal and schizophrenic subjects (WEIL-MALHERBE and BONE, 1958; COHEN, HOLLAND and GOLDENBERG, 1958).

2. Other aspects of catecholamine metabolism in mental disease

Whatever the final verdict on the theory of HOFFER and colleagues will be, there is no doubt that problems connected with the formation, release and metabolism of the catecholamines will command the attention of the clinically oriented neurochemist in increasing measure. Although it is now well recognized that adrenaline is one of the most important links in the psychosomatic relationship and its association with tension and anxiety has become proverbial, the actual evidence, in terms of discharge rates or blood levels of adrenaline, is surprisingly slight. The short life time of circulating adrenaline, the difficulties of producing true emotions in an experimental setting and the limited suitability of animals for the study of emotional reactions, let alone the technical difficulties of estimation, have been serious obstacles to progress, especially with regard to the estimation of adrenaline in blood. Urinary excretion rates to some extent reflect the rates of discharge; on the other hand, the proportions of catecholamines which are excreted unchanged are variable and small, accounting for only 1—5% of the amounts secreted. To obtain a more quantitative picture of the rate of catecholamine release it would be necessary to estimate a number of metabolites; methods suitable for reliable routine use are now becoming available.

On the whole the results, as far as they go, are in accordance with expectations. EULER and LUNDBERG (1954), in a study on air force personnel, showed that flying, whether in the capacity of passenger or pilot, induced a marked increase of adrenaline excretion, while noradrenaline excretion was only increased in pilots doing advanced flying. GODDARD (1958) found an increased excretion of noradrenaline though not of adrenaline in glider pilot apprentices. ELMADJIAN, HOPE and LAMSON (1957, 1958) found a rise in the excretion of adrenaline and noradrenaline in hockey players after a game; boxers had an elevated adrenaline excretion before and after the match while the noradrenaline excretion varied. Physical exercise without emotional involvement led to only moderate increases in the rate of catecholamine excretion. Administration of LSD had no mental effects in chronic schizophrenics and did not change their catecholamine output, but it caused an increase in the excretion of adrenaline, and sometimes also of noradrenaline, in depressed patients. Urinary adrenaline was found to be elevated in psychiatric patients after they had attended a staff conference. During psychotherapeutic interviews a rise of adrenaline excretion or noradrenaline excretion or both was sometimes observed, in the therapist as well as in the patient.

High rates of catecholamine excretion probably unrelated to motor unrest were observed in cases of mania by STRÖM-OLSEN and WEIL-MALHERBE (1958) and BERGSMAN (1959). An increased output of adrenaline was found in cases of acute schizophrenia (BERGSMAN, 1959).

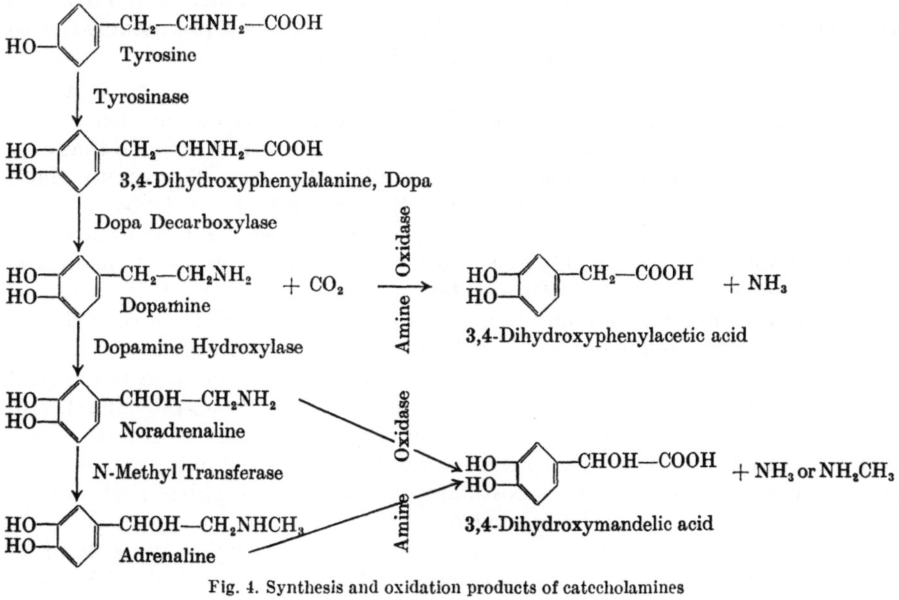

Fig. 4. Synthesis and oxidation products of catecholamines

In depression the rate of excretion of both adrenaline and noradrenaline is normal or below normal (Ström-Olsen and Weil-Malherbe, 1958; Bergsman, 1959). Cases of senile dementia have a low rate of adrenaline excretion. Increases of adrenaline output in response to a test dose of insulin were below normal in cases of depression and senile dementia, while schizophrenics, on the average, reacted normally. In chronic schizophrenics the excretion rates of adrenaline and noradrenaline were normal (Bergsman, 1959).

Convulsive treatment whether by electroshock or by the injection of convulsant drugs causes a strong but transient increase of the adrenaline and noradrenaline levels in plasma. If the treatment is modified by premedication with a barbiturate and/or a paralysant, the rise of the noradrenaline concentration, but not that of the adrenaline concentration, is suppressed (Weil-Malherbe, 1955).

3. The serotonin hypothesis of schizophrenia

As reviewed above (p. 61—63), two drugs with pronounced psychological effects, reserpine and LSD, were recently shown to be functionally related to serotonin. These discoveries greatly stimulated speculations on a possible role of serotonin in the genesis of psychosis, more particularly of schizophrenia. Other observations pointed in the same direction: serotonin shares the indole ring configuration with many hallucinogenic drugs; bufotenin and dimethyltryptamine, especially, have a close chemical similarity with serotonin. The action of these drugs might therefore be due to their competition with serotonin in the manner of antimetabolites; alternatively, they might act as spurious substrates capable of stimulating serotonin receptors.

Furthermore, it has been reported that iproniazid treatment provoked psychotic or near-psychotic reactions in some cases (Pleasure, 1954; Crane, 1956). Since iproniazid is an inhibitor of amine oxidase and causes a rise of the serotonin concentration in brain it seemed plausible to assume that the mental symptoms resulted from this effect. However, psychotic reactions with a very similar symptomatology were also observed as a side-effect of isoniazid therapy (Wiedorn and Ervin, 1954; Jackson, 1957). Isoniazid, though a close congener of iproniazid, is only a weak inhibitor of amine oxidase; its biological activity is presumably due to its interaction with pyridoxal phosphate and other B-vitamins.

Finally, a vast amount of data has been collected purporting to show the existence of an abnormal metabolism of aromatic compounds, particularly of indoles, in schizophrenia. At the beginning of the century it was found that psychotics excrete an abnormal amount of "indican" in the urine (Townsend, 1905; Bruce, 1906; Gullotta, 1930 and others). More recently Sano (1954) found a positive reaction for indoxyl sulfate (the principal constituent of indican) in 50% of schizophrenics though only in 0—4.6% of normal controls, psychoneurotics, manic-depressives and epileptics. Others (Folin, 1904; Shoje et al., 1956; Leyton, 1958) found no abnormal amounts of indican or indoxyl sulfate in the urine of schizophrenics. Since indicanuria is largely determined by the degree of constipation, the nature of the diet and the varieties of the intestinal flora, its nosological significance is now discounted except by those who, like Buscaino (1958), still subscribe to the once popular theory that abnormal processes of intestinal putrefaction may result in the absorption of toxic products, presumably amines, with effects very much like those now postulated by the more sophisticated modern theories based on endogenous hallucinogens.

The advent of paper-chromatographic techniques brought about a great refinement in the analysis of urinary excretion patterns. Young et al. (1951) were the first to report that urine from schizophrenic patients contained several diazo-coupling compounds which were absent, or present in smaller amounts, in the controls. Similar studies were carried out by McGeer et al. (1956, 1957) who confirmed the presence of more diazo-coupling compounds in the urine of schizophrenics than in that of non-schizophrenics. In a later paper from the same laboratory (Acheson et al., 1958) three diazo coupling compounds out of over 80 were found to be consistently absent from normal urine but present in schizophrenic urine. Incidentally these diazo compounds, being colorless or pale yellow, could not account for the differences observed earlier by McGeer et al. since these were due to brightly colored spots. None of the compounds characteristic for schizophrenic urine has yet been identified. When schizophrenic patients were kept on a diet devoid of aromatic amino acids, the number and intensity of spots were reduced to the normal range; supplementation with either tryptophan or with phenylalanine and tyrosine led to the conclusion that the greater part of the colored spots were derived from phenylalanine and tyrosine. The patients derived no benefit from the absence of aromatic amino acids in their diet (McGeer, McGeer and Boulding, 1956; Bogoch, 1957).

In other chromatographic studies Ehrlich's reagent was used to develop colored spots. This reagent is more specific for indoles than the diazo reaction. Several authors (Rodnight and Aves, 1958; Leyton, 1958; Riegelhaupt, 1958; Feldstein, Dibner and Hoagland, 1958; Kemali and Buscaino, 1958) described the presence of spots on chromatograms of "schizophrenic" urine which were either absent from control urine or occurred there less frequently and in lower intensity. At least two such spots have now been tentatively identified as indole acetamide, presumably formed from indole acetylglucuronic acid by ammonolysis (Sprince et al., 1961), and as 6-hydroxyskatole sulfate (Sprince et al., 1960; Nakao and Ball, 1960; Acheson and Hands, 1961). The excretion of the latter compound is abolished by gut sterilization (tetracycline) and thus appears to be of intestinal origin.

The capacity of schizophrenics to dispose of a test load of tryptophan has been investigated, with contradictory results. Price, Brown and Peters (1959) found that among 19 schizophrenics 6 had a distinctly abnormal tryptophan metabolism; the following tryptophan metabolites were excreted by them in larger amounts than by normal controls: kynurenine, kynurenic acid, acetylkynurenine, hydroxykynurenine and o-aminohippuric acid. Schizophrenics whose tryptophan metabolism was not distinctly abnormal excreted some of these compounds in smaller amounts than the controls. Changes similar to those observed in the 6 patients with abnormal tryptophan metabolism were also found in patients with porphyria and with psychoses other than schizophrenia. Banerjee and Agarwal (1958) reported that after a test dose of tryptophan schizophrenics excreted less kynurenine and less 3-hydroxy-anthranilic acid than controls, while Zeller et al. (1957) found a larger than normal excretion of xanthurenic acid.

Most of the studies on the urinary excretion patterns of schizophrenics were poorly controlled with respect to a number of factors, such as diet, intake of drugs, physical activity, the possible existence of vitamin deficiencies, of other forms of malnutrition or of previous or active intestinal infections that are so frequent among institutionalized patients. Armstrong et al. (1958) pointed out that abnormal patterns are frequent in institutionalized patients and that administration of antibiotics usually resulted in the disappearance of the abnormal substances from urine. Admittedly, an ideally controlled experiment would be very difficult to organize in a clinical setting, yet it will have to be carried out eventually if present claims are to be substantiated.

Vague and inconsistent though they were, the reports of a disturbance of indole metabolism in schizophrenics appeared to fit in well with the speculations connecting serotonin with schizophrenia. However, since tryptophan is metabolized by several alternative mechanisms a disturbance of tryptophan metabolism need not necessarily involve the pathway of serotonin formation and breakdown. Most authors agree that the urinary excretion of 5-hydroxyindoleacetic acid, the principal metabolite of serotonin, is normal in schizophrenics (ROBINS et al., 1956; SANO et al., 1957; BUSCAINO and STEFANACCHI, 1958; FELDSTEIN, HOAGLAND and FREEMAN, 1958); only LEYTON (1958) reported a decreased excretion in 20% of cases. The excretion of 5-hydroxyindoleacetic acid has also been studied after the administration of a test dose of tryptophan in the expectation that the excretion increment would serve as an indicator of the rate of serotonin synthesis. Results have been conflicting: while ZELLER et al. (1957) found an increased excretion in the control group, but none in schizophrenics, BANERJEE and AGARWAL (1958) found a higher increment in schizophrenics. KOPIN (1959), finally, reported that schizophrenic and control groups responded with similar increments of 5-hydroxyindoleacetic acid excretion to a test dose of tryptophan.

In summary, then, it may be said that the evidence which can be adduced in support of the serotonin theory of schizophrenia is no more conclusive than that discussed in connection with the adrenaline theory. The speculations centered on serotonin are uncertain as to whether schizophrenia is due to a deficiency or an excess of this substance, according to whether LSD is regarded as mainly an antagonist or synergist of serotonin. Experimental evidence of a very inconclusive nature is available in support of either concept. Thus BULLE and KONCHEGUL (1957) claimed that cerebrospinal fluid from schizophrenics in contrast to that from non-schizophrenics, when injected into the carotid of a dog, produced effects similar to those obtained with serotonin; samples from hyperactive schizophrenics produced symptoms indicative of low serotonin concentrations, those from stuporous cases gave reactions indicative of high serotonin concentrations. These results suggest an excess of cerebral serotonin in schizophrenia and an aggravation of symptoms when its level is raised. Yet SHERWOOD (1955) reported great improvement in 3 cases of catatonic schizophrenia and one case of paranoid schizophrenia who received intraventricular injections of serotonin 2—3 times weekly for a period of several weeks. The patients allegedly became tidier, more rational, interested and sociable, thus reacting as if they had been afflicted by a deficiency of cerebral serotonin. Promising therapeutic results have been claimed after the injection of schizophrenics with 5-hydroxytryptophan (WOOLLEY, 1957). Small doses of the latter substance were also found to alleviate the psychological effects of LSD in normal human subjects (BRENGELMANN, PARE and SANDLER, 1958).

G. Biochemistry of the developing nervous system

One of the most conspicuous and extensively investigated aspects of the maturation of the brain and nerve is the large increase of and change in composition of its lipid fractions. Galacto- and phosphosphingosides seem to be added as new components, being present prior to the period of myelination only in minute amounts if at all (JOHNSON et al., 1948; CUMINGS et al., 1958) (cf. FOLCH, 1955). In accordance with these analytical findings, turnover studies in animals show that the fatty acid moiety of lipids of the brain have a high rate of turnover during the period of growth of the brain (WAELSCH et al., 1941).

The metabolic change which triggers the onset of myelination or that which is responsible for its decline is at present unknown. It has been pointed out in the section on lipid metabolism that acetic acid is burned through the citric acid cycle or alternately used for the synthesis of fatty acids depending on the prevalence of a glycolytic or oxidative metabolic milieu. Since, during the development of the brain, glycolysis accounts for a larger portion of glucose metabolism than in the adult central nervous system (HIMWICH, 1951), it could be that these metabolic conditions favor the synthesis of fatty acid. With increasing prevalence of the citric acid cycle more acetic acid would be burned and less would be available for myelination (SPERRY and WAELSCH, 1952). The greater resistance of the newborn brain as compared with the adult brain to respiratory poisons has also been related to larger participation of glycolysis in metabolism at this period of development (HIMWICH, 1951).

Myelination is only one of the aspects of the biochemical concomitants of structural and functional changes occurring in the developing brain. The most extensive correlated studies of enzymatic structural and functional development were carried out by FLEXNER (1955) with the guinea pig. The investigations on the development of the cerebral cortex of rat, guinea pig and pig suggest that the differentiation of the neuroblast into the nerve cell entails a series of inter-related cytological, chemical and functional changes. The period during which these changes occur depends on the maturity of the animal at birth, and therefore falls, in the guinea pig and pig, in the last part of pregnancy and, in the rat, around the 10th day after birth. ATPase (FLEXNER and FLEXNER, 1948), succinic dehydrogenase and cytochrome oxidase (FLEXNER et al., 1953) activities increase in the cerebral cortex of the guinea pig around the 42nd day of gestation, while succinic dehydrogenase and ATPase (POTTER et al., 1945) as well as glutamic decarboxylase (ROBERTS et al., 1951) and carbonic anhydrase (ASHBY and SCHUSTER, 1950) activities increase in the rat cortex between the 6th and 10th day after birth, and glutamine synthetase in the chick brain up to hatching (RUDNICK et al., 1954).

Many studies have concerned themselves with the changes of cholinesterase during development of the brain. Of these, only few have differentiated between pseudo- and true acetylcholinesterase, and therefore most data offer a composite picture of the development of both enzymes, one being located mainly in the neurons (acetylcholinesterase), the other in the non-neuronal elements (pseudo-cholinesterase). The rise in concentration of cholinesterase in the motor cortex of the guinea pig precedes the critical period of cytological differentiation which is characterized by an increase in the activity of ATPase and respiratory enzymes (KAVALER and KIMEL, 1952). The changes of concentration of cholinesterases with cerebral development have also been followed in rabbit, rat, guinea pig, and sheep (NACHMANSOHN, 1939, 1940). A detailed study of cholinesterase of the developing rat brain showed a peak of activity on the 26th day with a decline up to the 32nd day after birth (METZLER and HUMM, 1951), while other studies suggest a peak around the 80th day of life (BENNETT et al., 1958). In the rabbit the maximal activity was obtained in the medulla oblongata at 15 days, in the superior colliculus at 4 months, and in the caudate nucleus and cortical grey at 18 months (HIMWICH and APRISON, 1955a). During maturation in rat brain, a relative increase of acetylcholinesterase in the olfactory bulb and of pseudo-cholinesterase in thalamus has been demonstrated (ELKES and TODRICK, 1955). While most of the enzymes studied increased during development of the nervous system, some showed a higher level in the cortex of the fetal brain than in that of the adult (FLEXNER and FLEXNER, 1948).

There is in the developing brain an increase of the concentration of the metabolites which are the substrates or products of the enzyme activity increasing during the same period (for instance: glutamic acid and glutamine: WAELSCH,

1951; Himwich and Petersen, 1959; aspartic acid and γ-aminobutyric acid: Baxter et al., 1960).

Data from a variety of investigations suggest that the blood-brain barrier is not fully developed in the immature brain and achieves its characteristics in the mature animal (Waelsch, 1955; Himwich and Himwich, 1955b; Lajtha, 1957a; Lajtha, 1958). Just as the blood-brain barrier will affect the rate of entrance of various substances specifically, the rate of uptake of different substances by the immature brain is not modified to the same degree. Not only the rate of metabolism of lipid constituents but also that of protein appears to be increased during the development of the brain (Lajtha et al., 1957b; Lajtha, 1959; Roberts et al., 1959).

H. Inborn errors of metabolism

The inborn errors of metabolism have had a considerable influence on the concepts of the etiology of mental disease aside from their value in studying the biosynthetic and degradative metabolic pathways in the human organism. The finding that some of the "inborn errors" which are inherited as Mendelian characteristics could be explained by the lack of a specific enzyme has led to the hypothesis that some types of schizophrenia, for which inheritance is suggested on the basis of twin and family studies, may also be the result of an abnormal enzymology.

While at present the lack of a specific enzyme has been shown in only a few "errors", an enzymatic lesion may eventually be found also in those inherited abnormalities characterized by a different hemoglobin, by deficiencies in plasma protein fractions or by abnormal renal transport mechanisms (for review and discussion see Hsia, 1959; Harris, 1957).

Inborn errors of metabolism affect all major metabolic systems of the human organism, i.e., lipids, proteins, amino acids and carbohydrates. Many of them affect the nervous system and are accompanied by mental deficiency.

Of particular interest to the biochemist have been those "inborn errors" which have been related to distinct changes in the composition of a body constituent and/ or to changes in the enzymatic makeup of the cells.

Tay-Sachs (infantile amaurotic familial idiocy) and Niemann-Pick diseases are both transmitted as recessive genes and have a number of features in common — a fact which has resulted in the belief by some investigators that these two diseases are either closely linked or actually the same. It could be shown that in infantile amaurotic idiocy the concentration of cerebral gangliosides is increased, while in Niemann-Pick disease the level of sphingomyelin is raised (Klenk and Langerbeins, 1941; Klenk, 1947). Chemical analysis, therefore, could differentiate between these two diseases of the lipid system despite the great similarity in the respective clinical pictures. One might speculate as to whether in these diseases one of the enzyme systems responsible for the synthesis or degradation of the complex sphingosides is lacking.

While the two above-mentioned "errors" are characterized by changes in the concentration or composition of some member of the lipid family, in oligophrenia phenylpyruvica as well as in galactosemia and in some glycogen storage diseases, the metabolic error can be traced to the lack of one specific enzyme.

Phenylpyruvic oligophrenia or phenylketonuria (Foelling, 1934) is transmitted by a recessive gene. The incidence in the British Isles is about 1 in 40,000 of the general population from which it can be calculated that the incidence of heterozygous carriers is about 1%. The mental defect in the afflicted individuals is usually severe, the I. Q. rarely exceeding 30. The appearance of the patients is typical: they are fair-haired, fair-skinned and have light blue eyes, even when other members of the family are dark.

Biochemically, an abnormally high level of phenylalanine in the blood results in increased excretion of the amino acid itself, together with its deaminated derivatives, phenylpyruvic, phenyllactic and phenylacetic acids (the latter conjugated with glutamine), in the urine. Ingestion of phenylalanine produces a rise of the phenylalanine concentration in the blood, followed by a rise of the tyrosine level in normal but not in phenylketonuric subjects. These and other facts suggested a deficiency of the enzyme system, located in the liver, which converts phenylalanine to tyrosine (phenylalanine hydroxylase). The virtual absence of phenylalanine hydroxylase was confirmed by experiments in which the enzymatic activity of autopsy and biopsy specimens removed from the livers of phenylpyruvic oligophrenia patients was examined (JERVIS, 1953; WALLACE et al., 1957; MITOMA et al., 1957 a).

The urine of phenylpyruvic oligophrenia patients frequently contains abnormal amounts of phenolic acids and it has been suggested that the reason for this is a secondary block in the metabolic pathway of tyrosine. However, in addition to p-hydroxyphenyllactic and p-hydroxyphenylacetic acids, which are indeed abnormal metabolites of tyrosine, there occur significant amounts of o-hydroxyphenylacetic acid (BOSCOTT and BICKEL, 1953; ARMSTRONG et al., 1955). This compound is presumably derived from o-tyrosine (ARMSTRONG and SHAW, 1955; MITOMA et al., 1957 b). The formation of o-tyrosine and that of p-hydroxylated phenylic acids may be attributed to an unspecific oxidation of phenylalanine and its deaminated derivatives (UDENFRIEND et al., 1954; BRODIE et al., 1954).

Abnormalities of indole metabolism have also been observed in phenylpyruvic oligophrenia. They consist in an increased excretion of indolelactic and indoleacetic acids (ARMSTRONG and ROBINSON, 1954), a lowered excretion of 5-hydroxyindoleacetic acid (BERENDES et al., 1958; BALDRIDGE et al., 1959) and a decreased concentration of serotonin in serum (PARE et al., 1957). Various explanations have been offered: a deficiency of the enzyme system responsible for the hydroxylation of tryptophan similar to the deficiency of phenylalanine hydroxylase, an inhibition of tryptophan hydroxylase by phenylalanine or one of its metabolites, or an inhibition of 5-hydroxytryptophan decarboxylase by one of these compounds (DAVISON and SANDLER, 1958). No evidence is available so far which would make it possible to decide which of these explanations, if any, is the correct one.

An inhibition of tyrosinase by phenylalanine has been demonstrated in vitro and it has been suggested that this rather than an inadequate supply of tyrosine may be the reason for the defective melanin formation in phenylpyruvic oligophrenia (DANCIS and BALIS, 1955).

The question arises whether the enzymatic block in phenylpyruvic oligophrenia is always complete or whether its severity may vary from case to case. Mild forms of the disease have been observed, with I. Q.'s from 50 to 70 and with a more normal type of pigmentation. Heterozygous carriers of the disease sometimes show a decreased ability to metabolize a test dose of phenylalanine. The degree of mental deficiency does not generally correlate with the phenylalanine levels in the blood since these are dependent on dietary factors and on renal tubular reabsorption much more than on slight residues of phenylalanine hydroxylase activity (BOREK et al., 1950).

It may further be asked whether the mental defect is caused by an excess of metabolites arising above the block or a deficiency of metabolites arising below the block. The hypothesis under investigation today assumes that a metabolic derivative of phenylalanine is responsible for the mental deterioration. This toxic metabolite is assumed to accumulate owing to the excessive phenylalanine concentrations in the tissues. Support for the formation of such a metabolite is seen in the fact that affected infants raised on a phenylalanine-free diet from birth appear to develop normally (BICKEL et al., 1953). On the other hand, when changed to a phenylalanine-free diet at a later stage of development, beneficial effects of this treatment are ambiguous (HSIA et al., 1958a).

Of considerable significance are the findings with children suffering from galactosemia who are fed on a galactose-free diet. In this inborn error of metabolism, transmitted as an autosomal recessive gene, the metabolic error was related to the inability of the organism to convert dietary galactose to glucose, the pathway by which the former sugar is metabolized. This inability is due to a lack of the specific transferase which catalyzes the exchange of galactose with glucose in uridine diphosphate glucose. The enzyme necessary for the succeeding steps, namely for the conversion of uridine diphosphate galactose into the corresponding uridine diphosphate glucose (epimerase), and the phosphorylase liberating glucose-phosphate from the pyrimidine intermediate, are present in galactosemic subjects in normal concentrations (ISSELBACHER et al., 1956). The result of the inability of these infants to convert galactose to glucose leads to the clinical symptoms, among which are the accumulation of galactose-1-phosphate in the erythrocytes, and of galactose in blood, cirrhosis of the liver, cataract and mental deficiency. These symptoms can be ameliorated or prevented by withholding all milk and milk products and thereby lactose or galactose from the diet shortly after birth. The heterozygous carriers of the abnormal gene can be detected with the aid of a galactose tolerance test (HSIA et al., 1958b).

Several other hereditary conditions associated with mental deficiency have been described, but in none of them has it yet been possible to pinpoint the enzyme system which is at fault. In Hartnup disease (BARON et al., 1956) the metabolism of tryptophan seems to be abnormal; indolic acids are found in the urine in increased amounts and the abnormality is exacerbated after the ingestion of tryptophan (MILNE et al., 1959). In "maple sugar urine disease" (WESTALL et al., 1957) early and rapid mental deterioration occurs in infants whose urine has a marked odour resembling maple sugar. The urinary excretion of the branched amino acids and of α-keto acids derived from them is increased; other amino acids have an abnormally low serum level. Finally, a form of mental deficiency has been described in which large amounts of argininosuccinic acid, an intermediary in the transformation of citrulline into arginine, are excreted in the urine (WESTALL, 1958).

In the glycogen storage diseases, a group of congenital and familial disorders, large quantities of normal or abnormal glycogen are deposited in the tissues. Some of these diseases have by now been related to definite lack of specific enzymes necessary for the degradation of glycogen (CORI, 1953).

These few sketchily described examples of inborn errors of metabolism should serve merely to demonstrate the present line of biochemical research and its application to the understanding of, and therapeutic approaches to, the underlying mechanism in these diseases. In their wider context these findings demonstrate that the study of the "biochemical individuality" may hold out hope for finding biochemical abnormalities in hereditary diseases of the nervous system as well as in those occurring sporadically. The concept of inborn errors of metabolism as a working hypothesis stimulated the extensive search in mental disease, and in particular in schizophrenia, for abnormal proteins or abnormal pathways of tryptophan metabolism, dealt with in other sections of this review.

It is also of importance to be aware of the fact that a metabolic deficiency may not have to be interpreted along the classical lines of essential and non-essential nutrients, e. g., vitamins or indispensable amino acids, but that genetically determined or sporadic metabolic abnormalities may produce situations in which a normally dispensable nutrient cannot be synthesized or degraded by the mammalian organism, e. g., tyrosine in oligophrenia phenylpyruvica. Therefore, the search for metabolic abnormalities in mental disease has to encompass a study of metabolic pathways unencumbered by preconceived notions as to the nutritional status of the particular metabolite. The importance of this concept becomes apparent when the possible functional significance of compounds such as glutamic acid, glutamine, or γ-aminobutyric acid for the nervous system is considered where quantitative abnormalities of regulation of metabolism rather than qualitative differences may be decisive.

Bibliography

A. Introduction

BERL, S., A. LAJTHA and H. WAELSCH: Cerebral compartments of glutamic acid metabolism. J. Neurochem. 7, 186 (1961a). — BERL, S., G. TAKAGAKI, D. D. CLARKE and H. WAELSCH: Metabolic compartments in vivo. Ammonia and glutamic acid metabolism in brain and liver. J. biol. Chem. 231, 2562 (1962). — BERL, S., G. TAKAGAKI and D. P. PURPURA: Metabolic and pharmacological effects of injected amino acids and ammonia on cortical epileptogenic lesions. J. Neurochem. 7, 198 (1961).

EDSTRÖM, J. E., and H. HYDEN: Ribonucleotide analysis of individual nerve cells. Nature (Lond.) 174, 128 (1954).

HELLER, I. H., and K. A. C. ELLIOTT: Metabolism of normal brain and human gliomas in relation to cell type and density. Canad. J. Biochem. 33, 395 (1955). — HYDEN, H.: Protein metabolism in the nerve cell during growth and function. Acta physiol. scand. 6, Suppl. 17, 5—136 (1943). — HYDEN, H.: Biochemical changes in glial cells and nerve cells at varying activity. In: Proceedings of the Fourth International Congress of Biochemistry. Volume III, Biochemistry of the central nervous system. pp. 64—89. (F. BRÜCKE, Ed.), Pergamon Press 1959. — HYDEN, H.: The chemistry of single neurons. In: Biochemistry of the developing nervous system; pp. 358—371. (H. WAELSCH, Ed.), New York: Academic Press Inc. 1955.

LOWRY, O. H.: A study of the nervous system with quantitative histochemical methods. In: Biochemistry of the developing nervous system. pp. 350—357. (H. WAELSCH, Ed.). New York: Academic Press Inc. 1955. — LOWRY, O. H.: Quantitative analysis of single nerve cell bodies. In: Ultrastructure and cellular chemistry of neural tissue. 69—76. (H. WAELSCH, Ed.). New York: Hoeber-Harper 1957. — LOWRY, O. H., N. R. ROBERTS, and M. W. CHANG: The analysis of single cells. J. biol. Chem. 222, 97 (1956a). — LOWRY, O. H., N. R. ROBERTS, K. Y. LEINER, M. WU, A. L. FARR, and R. W. ALBERS: The quantitative histochemistry of brain. J. biol. Chem. 207, 39 (1954). — LOWRY, O. H., N. R. ROBERTS, and C. LEWIS: The quantitative histochemistry of the retina. J. biol. Chem. 220, 879 (1956b).

McILWAIN, H.: Substances which support respiration and metabolic response to electrical impulses in human cerebral tissues. J. Neurol. Neurosurg. Psychiat. 16, 257 (1953).

NURNBERGER, J. I., and M. W. GORDON: The cell density of neural tissue. In: Ultrastructure and cellular chemistry of neural tissue. pp. 100—138. (H. WAELSCH. Ed.). New York: Hoeber-Harper 1957.

PALAY, S. L., and G. E. PALADE: The fine structure of neurons. J. biophys. biochem. Cytol. 1, 69—88 (1955). — POPE, A.: Application of quantitative histochemical methods to the study of the nervous system. J. Neuropath. exp. Neurol. 14, 39 (1955). — POPE, A.: The relationship of neurochemistry to the microscopic anatomy of the nervous system. In: The biochemistry of the developing nervous system. pp. 341—349. (H. WAELSCH, Ed.), New York: Academic Press Inc. 1955. — POPE, A., H. H. HESS, and J. N. ALLEN: Quantitative histochemistry of proteolytic and oxidative enzymes in human cerebral cortex and brain tumors. In: Ultrastructure and cellular chemistry of neural tissue. pp. 182—194. (H. WAELSCH, Ed.). New York: Hoeber-Harper 1957. — POPE, A., H. H. HESS, J. R. WARE, and R. H. THOMSON: Intralaminar distribution of cytochrome oxidase and DPN in rat cerebral cortex. J. Neurophysiol. 19, 259 (1956).

WAELSCH, H.: An attempt at integration of structure and metabolism in the nervous system. In: Structure and function of the cerebral cortex. Elsevier Publishing Company, 1960.

WAELSCH, H.: Compartmentalized biosynthetic reactions in the central nervous system. In Regional Neurochemistry (S. S. KETY and J. ELKES, Eds); p. 57. London: Pergamon Press Ltd. 1961. — WAELSCH, H., and A. LAJTHA: Protein metabolism in the nervous system. Physiol. Rev. **41**, 709 (1961).

B. The brain barrier systems

BAKAY, L.: The blood-brain barrier: with special regard to the use of radioactive isotopes. Springfield, Illinois: Charles C. Thomas 1956. — BAKAY, L.: Dynamic aspects of the blood-brain barrier. In: Metabolism of the nervous system. 136—150. (D. RICHTER, Ed.), London: Pergamon Press 1957. — BAKAY, L., T. F. HUETER, H. T. BALLANTINE, JR., and D. SOSA: Ultrasonically produced changes in the blood-brain barrier. A. M. A. Arch. Neurol. Psychiat. **76**, 457—467 (1956). — BERL, S., G. TAKAGAKI and D. P. PURPURA: Metabolic and pharmacological effects of injected amino acids and amoniam on cortical epileptogenic lesions. J. Neurochem. **7**, 198 (1961). — BRIERLEY, J. B.: The blood-brain barrier: structural aspects. In: Metabolism of the nervous system, 121—135. (D. RICHTER, Ed.). London: Pergamon Press Ltd. 1957.

DAVSON, H.: A comparative study of the aqueous humour and cerebrospinal fluid in the rabbit. J. Physiol. (Lond.) **129**, 111—183 (1955).

EDSTROM, R.: An explanation of the blood-brain barrier phenomenon. Acta psychiat. scand. **33**, 403—416 (1958).

GREEN, J. B.: Recent advances in the chemistry of cerebrospinal fluid. J. nerv. ment. Dis. **127**, 359—373 (1958).

QUADBECK, G., and H. HELMCHEN: Steigerung des Phosphat-Übertrittes vom Blut in das Zentralnervensystem nach schweren Gehirnerschütterungen bei der Katze. Z. Naturforsch. **10**b, 328—331 (1955).

SWEET, W. H., G. L. BROWNELL, J. A. SCHOLL, D. R. BOWSHER, P. BENDA, and E. E. STRICKLEY: The formation, flow and absorption of cerebrospinal fluid; newer concepts based on studies with isotopes. In: Neurology and psychiatry in childhood. Res. Publ. Ass. nerv. ment. Dis. **34**, 101—159 (1954). — SWEET, W. H., and H. B. LOCKSLEY: Formation, flow, and reabsorption of cerebrospinal fluid in man. Proc. Soc. exp. Biol. (N. Y.) **84**, 397—402 (1953).

WAELSCH, H.: The turnover of components of the developing brain; the blood-brain barrier. In: Biochemistry of the developing nervous system. 187—201. (H. WAELSCH, Ed.) New York: Academic Press Inc. 1955. — WAKIM, K. G., and G. A. FLEISHER: The effect of experimental cerebral infarction on transaminase activity in serum, cerebrospinal fluid, and infarcted tissue. Proc. Mayo Clin. **31**, 391—399 (1956). — WEIL-MALHERBE, H., J. AXELROD, and R. TOMCHICK: Blood-brain barrier for adrenaline. Science **129**, 1226—1227 (1959). — WISLOCKI, G. B., and E. H. LEDUC: Vital staining of the hematoencephalic barrier by silver nitrate and trypan blue, and cytological comparisons of the neurohypophysis, pineal body, area postrema, intercolumnar tubercle and supra-optic crest. J. comp. Neurol. **96**, 371—414 (1952).

C. Energy metabolism

ABOOD, L. G., E. BRUNNGRABER, and M. TAYLOR: Glycolytic and oxidative phosphorylative studies with intact and disrupted brain mitochondria. J. biol. Chem. **234**, 1307 (1959). — ABOOD, L. G., and A. GEIGER: Breakdown of proteins and lipids during glucose-free perfusion of the cat's brain. Amer J. Physiol. **182**, 557 (1955). — ABOOD, L. G., R. W. GERARD, and S. OCHS: Electrical stimulation of metabolism of homogenates and particulates. Amer. J. Physiol. **171**, 134 (1952). — ÁCS, G., R. BALÁZS, and F. B. STRAUB: Synthesis of adenosinetriphosphate in slices of brain cortex. Chem. Abstr. **48**, 8923 (1954). — ADAMS, J. E., H. A. HARPER, G. S. GORDAN, M. HUTCHIN, and R. C. BENTINCK: Cerebral metabolism of glutamic acid in multiple sclerosis. Neurology (Minnesota). **5**, 100 (1955). — ALLWEIS, C., and J. MAGNES: The uptake and oxidation of glucose by the perfused cat brain. J. Neurochem. **2**, 326 (1958). — ASHFORD, C. A., and K. C. DIXON: The effect of potassium on the glucolysis of brain tissue with reference to the Pasteur effect. Biochem. J. **29**, 157—168 (1935).

BERGER, M.: Metabolic reactivity of brain and liver mitochondria towards chlorpromazine. J. Neurochem. **2**, 30—36 (1957). — BERL, S., D. D. CLARKE, G. TAKAGAKI, D. P. PURPURA and H. WAELSCH: Carbon dioxide fixation in brain in vivo. Fed. Proc. **20**, No. 1 (1961). — BERL, S., G. TAKAGAKI, D. D. CLARKE and H. WAELSCH: Carbon dioxide fixation in the brain. J. biol. Chem. **231**, 2510 (1962). — BLOOM, B.: Catabolism of glucose by mammalian tissues. Proc. Soc. exp. Biol. (N. Y.) **88**, 317 (1955). — BOSZORMENYI-NAGY, I., and F. J. GERTY: Difference between the phosphorus metabolism of erythrocytes of normals and of patients suffering from schizophrenia. J. nerv. ment. Dis. **121**, 53 (1955). — BOSZORMENYI-NAGY, I., F. J. GERTY, and J. KUEBER: Correlation between an anomaly of the intracellular metabolism of adenosine nucleotides and schizophrenia. J. nerv. ment. Dis. **124**, 413

(1956). — BRACELAND, F. J., L. J. MEDUNA, and J. A. VAICHULIS: Delayed action of insulin in schizophrenia. Amer. J. Psychiat. 102, 108 (1945). — BRODY, T. M., and J. A. BAIN: Barbiturates and oxidative phosphorylation. J. Pharmacol. exp. Ther. 110, 148 (1954).

CHENG, S. C., and H. WAELSCH: Carbon dioxide fixation in lobster nerve. Science in press, 1962.

DANZIGER, L.: Anoxia and compounds causing mental disorders in man. Dis. nerv. Syst. 6, 365 (1945). — DAVIES, P. W., and A. RÉMOND: Oxygen consumption of the cerebral cortex of the cat during metrazol convulsions. Res. Publ. Ass. nerv. ment. Dis. 26, 205—217 (1947). — DAWSON, J., R. P. HULLIN, and A. POOL: Variations in the blood levels of acetoin and butane-2:3-diol in normal individuals and mental patients. J. ment. Sci. 100, 536—542 (1954). — DAWSON, J., R. P. HULLIN, and B. M. CROCKETT: Metabolic variations in manic-depressive psychosis. J. ment, Sci. 102, 168—177 (1956). — DICKENS, F.: Metabolism of normal and tumour tissue. XV. The respiratory quotient of brain cortex. Biochem. J. 30, 661—664 (1936).— DIPIETRO, D., and S. WEINHOUSE: Glucose oxidation in rat brain slices and homogenates. Arch. Biochem. Biophys. 80, 268 (1959). — DOLIVO, M., and M. G. LARRABEE: Metabolism of glucose and oxygen in a mammalian sympathetic ganglion at reduced temperature and varied pH. J. Neurochem. 3, 72 (1958). — DOUST, J. W. LOVETT: Spectroscopic and photo-electric oximetry in schizophrenia and other psychiatric states. J. ment. Sci. 98, 143—160 (1952).

ELLIOTT, K. A. C., and I. H. HELLER: Metabolism of neurones and glia. In: The metabolism of the nervous system. p. 286—290. (Ed. D. RICHTER). New York: Pergamon Press 1957. — ELLIOTT, K. A. C., and N. HENDERSON: Metabolism of brain tissue slices and suspensions from various mammals. J. Neurophysiol. 11, 473 (1948).

FINDLAY, M., W. L. MAGEE, and R. J. ROSSITER: Incorporation of radioactive phosphate into lipids and pentosenucleic acid of cat brain slices. The effect of inorganic ions. Biochem. J. 58, 236 (1954). — FREEMAN, H., J. M. LOONEY, R. G. HOSKINS, and C. G. DYER: Results of insulin and epinephrine tests in schizophrenia. Arch. Neurol. Psychiat. (Chicago) 49, 195 (1943). — FREEMAN, H., and R. ZABORENKE: Relation of changes in carbohydrate metabolism to psychotic states. Arch. Neurol. Psychiat. (Chicago) 61, 569 (1949). — FROHMAN, C. E., N. P. CZAJKOWSKI, E. D. LUBY, J. S. GOTTLIEB and R. SENF: Further evidence of a plasma factor in schizophrenia. Arch. gen. Psychiat. 3, 263 (1960). — FROHMAN, C. E., L. K. LATHAM, P. G. S. BECKETT and J. S. GOTTLIEB: Evidence of a plasma factor in schizophrenia. Arch. gen. Psychiat. 3, 255 (1960). — FROHMAN, C. E., E. D. LUBY, G. TOURNEY, P. G. S. BECKETT and J. S. GOTTLIEB: Steps toward the isolation of a serum factor in schizophrenia. Amer. J. Psychiat. 117, 401 (1960). — FROHMAN, C. E., G. TOURNEY, P. G. S. BECKETT, H. LEES, L. K. LATHAM, and J. S. GOTTLIEB: Biochemical identification of schizophrenia. Arch. gen. Psychiat. 4, 405 (1961).

GALLAGHER, C. H., J. D. JUDAH, and K. R. REES: Glucose oxidation by brain mitochondria. Biochem. J. 62, 436 (1956). — GATT, S., and E. RACKER: Regulatory mechanisms in carbohydrate metabolism. II. Pasteur effect in reconstructed systems. J. biol. Chem. 234, 1024 (1959). — GAYET, J.: Physical reactivity of liver and brain cortex mitochondria. Nature (Lond.) 182, 941 (1958). — GEIGER, A.: Correlation of brain metabolism and function by use of a brain perfusion method in situ. Physiol. Rev. 38, 1 (1958). — GEIGER, A., and J. MAGNES: Isolation of cerebral circulation and perfusion of brain in the living cat. Amer. J. Physiol. 149, 517—537 (1947). — GEIGER, A., J. MAGNES, and R. S. GEIGER: Survival of the perfused cat's brain in the absence of glucose. Nature (Lond.) 170, 754 (1952). — GEIGER, A., J. MAGNES, R. M. TAYLOR, and M. VERALLI: Effect of blood constituents on uptake of glucose and on metabolic rate of the brain in perfusion experiments. Amer. J. Physiol. 177, 138—149 (1954). — GEIGER, A., and S. YAMASAKI: Cytidine and uridine requirements of the brain. J. Neurochem. 1, 93 (1956). — GEY, K. F.: The concentration of glucose in rat tissues. Biochem. J. 64, 145—150 (1956). — GEYER, R. P., L. W. MATTHEWS, and F. G. STARE: Metabolism of emulsified trilaurin (—C¹⁴OO—) and octanoic acid (—C¹⁴OO—) by rat tissue slices. J. biol. Chem. 180, 1037—1045 (1949). — GHOSH, J. J., and J. H. QUASTEL: Narcotics and brain respiration. Nature (Lond.) 174, 28 (1954). — GIBBS, E. L., W. G. LENNOX, and F. A. GIBBS: Bilateral internal jugular blood: comparison of A-V differences, oxygen-dextrose ratios, and respiratory quotients. Amer. J. Psychiat. 102, 184—190 (1945). — GOLDFARB, W., and J. WORTIS: Availability of sodium pyruvate for human brain oxidations. Proc. Soc. exp. Biol. (N. Y.) 46, 121—123 (1941). — GORDAN, G. S.: Influence of steroids on cerebral metabolism in man. Recent Progr. Hormone Res. 12, 153—174 (1956). — GORDAN, G. S., F. M. ESTESS, J. E. ADAMS, K. M. BOWMAN, and A. SIMON: Cerebral oxygen uptake in chronic schizophrenic reaction. Arch. Neurol. Psychiat. (Chicago) 73, 544 (1955). — GORE, M. B. R., and H. McILWAIN: Effects of some inorganic salts on the metabolic response of sections of mammalian cerebral cortex to electrical stimulation. J. Physiol. 117, 471 (1952). — GOTTLIEB, J. S., C. E. FROHMAN, P. G. S. BECKETT, G. TOURNEY, and R. SENF: Production of high energy phosphate bonds in schizophrenia. A. M. A. Arch. gen. Psychiat. 1, 243 (1959). — GOTTLIEB, J. S.,

C. E. FROHMAN, G. TOURNEY, and P. G. S. BECKETT: Energy transfer systems in schizophrenia. Arch. Neurol. Psychiat. (Chicago) 81, 505 (1959). — GREENGARD, O., and H. MCILWAIN: Anticonvulsants and the metabolism of separated mammalian cerebral tissues. Biochem. J. 61, 61 (1955). — GRENELL, R. G., J. MENDELSON, and W. D. MCELROY: Neuronal metabolism and ATP synthesis in narcosis. J. cell. comp. Physiol. 46, 143 (1955).

HAAVALDSEN, R., O. LINGJAERDE, and O. WALAAS: Disturbances of carbohydrate metabolism in schizophrenics. The effect of serum fractions from schizophrenics on glucose uptake of rat diaphragm in vitro. Confin. neurol. (Basel) 18, 270—279 (1958). — HEALD, P. J.: Rapid changes in creatine phosphate level in cerebral cortex slices. Biochem. J. 57, 673—679 (1954).— HEALD, P. J.: Effects of electrical pulses on the distribution of radioactive phosphate in cerebral tissues. Biochem. J. 63, 242 (1956). — HEALD, P. J.: The incorporation of phosphate into cerebral phosphoprotein promoted by electrical impulses. Biochem. J. 66, 659 (1957). — HELLER, I. H., and K. A. C. ELLIOTT: The metabolism of normal brain and human gliomas in relation to cell type and density. Canad. J. Biochem. 33, 395—403 (1955). — HENNEMAN, D. H., M. D. ALTSCHULE, and R. M. GONCZ: Carbohydrate metabolism in brain disease. II. Glucose metabolism in schizophrenic, manic-depressive and involutional psychoses. Arch. intern Med. 94, 402—416 (1954). — HESSELBACH, M. L., and H. G. DUBUY: Localization of glycolytic and respiratory enzyme systems on isolated mouse brain mitochondria. Proc. Soc. exp. Biol. (N. Y.) 83, 62—65 (1953). — HIMWICH, H. E.: Brain metabolism and cerebral disorders. Baltimore: The Williams & Wilkins Co. 1951. — HIMWICH, W. A., and H. E. HIMWICH: Pyruvic acid exchange of the brain. J. Neurophysiol. 9, 133—136 (1946). — HOKIN, M. R., and L. E. HOKIN: The synthesis of phosphatidic acid from diglyceride and adenosine triphosphate in extracts of brain microsomes. J. biol. Chem. 234, 1381 (1959a). — HOKIN, L. E., and M. R. HOKIN: Evidence for phosphatidic acid as the sodium carrier. Nature (Lond.) 184, 1068 (1959b). — HOLMGREN, H., and S. WOHLFAHRT: Blutzuckerstudien bei Geisteskranken und psychisch Abnormen. Acta psychiat. (Kbh.) Suppl. 31 (1944). — HOSKIN, F. C. G.: Chemical stimulation and modification of glucose metabolism by brain. Arch. Biochem. Biophys. 91, 43 (1960). — HYDÉN, H.: Biochemical changes in glia cells and nerve cells at varying activity. IVth Internat. Congr. Biochem., Vol. III. Biochemistry of the central nervous system. London: Pergamon Press 1958.

JASPER, H., and T. C. ERICKSON: Cerebral blood flow and pH in excessive cortical discharge induced by metrazol and electrical stimulation. J. Neurophysiol. 4, 333—347 (1941). — JOHNSON, M. K.: The intracellular distribution of glycolytic and other enzymes in rat-brain homogenates and mitochondrial preparations. Biochem. J. 77, 610 (1960).

KENNEDY, C.: The cerebral metabolic rate in children. In: Neurochemistry p. 230—238. (Eds. S. R. KOREY and J. I. NURNBERGER) London: Cassell and Co. Ltd. 1956. — KERR, S. E., and M. GHANTUS: The carbohydrate metabolism of brain. II. The effect of varying the carbohydrate and insulin supply on the glycogen, free sugar and lactic acid in mammalian brain. J. biol. Chem. 116, 9—20 (1936). — KETY, S. S.: Quantitative determination of cerebral blood flow in man. Meth. med. Res. 1, 204—217 (1948). — KETY, S. S.: Discussion in: Metabolic and toxic diseases of the nervous system. Proc. Ass. Res. nerv. ment. Dis. 32, 362—363 (1953). — KETY, S. S.: The general metabolism of the brain in vivo. In: The metabolism of the nervous system. p. 221—237. (Ed. D. RICHTER) New York: Pergamon Press 1957. — KETY, S. S., and C. F. SCHMIDT: The nitrous oxide method for the quantitative determination of cerebral blood flow in man: theory, procedure and normal values. J. clin. Invest. 27, 476—483 (1948). — KETY, S. S., R. B. WOODFORD, M. H. HARMEL, F. A. FREYHAN, K. E. APPEL, and C. F. SCHMIDT: Cerebral blood flow and metabolism in schizophrenia. The effects of barbiturate seminarcosis, insulin coma, and electroshock. Amer. J. Psychiat. 104, 765 (1948). — KIMURA, Y., and K. ITO: Effect of sodium azide on the carbohydrate metabolism of brain tissue in presence and absence of the potassium effect. Sci. Papers Coll. gen. Educ. Univ. Tokyo 4, 57—70 (1954). — KIMURA, Y., and T. NIWA: Inhibitory effect of malonate on the respiration of brain tissue, with special reference to the potassium effect. Nature (Lond.) 171, 881 (1953). — KLEIN, J. R., R. HURWITZ, and N. S. OLSEN: Distribution of intravenously injected fructose and glucose between blood and brain. J. biol. Chem. 164, 509—512 (1946). — KLEIN, J. R., and N. S. OLSEN: Distribution of intravenously injected glutamate, lactate, pyruvate and succinate between blood and brain. J. biol. Chem. 167, 1—5 (1947). — KOREY, S. R., and M. ORCHEN: Relative respiration of neuronal and glial cells. J. Neurochem, 3, 277 (1959). — KREBS, H. A., L. V. EGGLESTON, and C. TERNER: In vitro measurements of the turnover rate of potassium in brain and retina. Biochem. J. 48, 530—537 (1951). — KUNZ, H. A.: Comparative investigations on the oxidation of pyruvate in liver and brain mitochondria. Biochem. biophys. Acta 28, 104 (1958).

LAJTHA, A., S. BERL, and H. WAELSCH: Amino acid and protein metabolism of the brain. IV. The metabolism of glutamic acid. J. Neurochem. 3, 322 (1959). — LANDAU, W. M., W. H. FREYGANG JR., L. P. ROLAND, L. SOKOLOFF, and S. S. KETY: The local circulation of the living brain; values in the unanesthetized and anesthetized cat. Trans. Amer. neurol. Ass. 80,

125 (1955). — LARRABEE, M. G.: Oxygen consumption of excised sympathetic ganglia at rest and in activity. J. Neurochem. **2**, 81 (1958). — LASSEN, N. A., and O. MUNCK: The cerebral blood flow in man determined by the use of radioactive krypton. Acta physiol. scand. **33**, 30 (1955). — LEVY, L., and R. M. FEATHERSTONE: The effect of xenon and nitrous oxide on in vitro guinea pig brain respiration and oxidative phosphorylation. J. Pharmacol. exp. Ther. **110**, 221 (1954). — LEWIS, J. L., and H. MCILWAIN: The action of some ergot derivatives, mescaline and dibenamine on the metabolism of separated mammalian cerebral tissues. Biochem. J. **57**, 680—684 (1954). — LI, C. L., and H. MCILWAIN: Maintenance of resting membrane potentials in slices of mammalian cerebral cortex and other tissues in vitro. J. Physiol. **139**, 178 —190 (1957). — LINGJAERDE, O.: Adrenocortical functions in the insane. Acta psychiat. suppl. **80**, 202 (1953). — LINGJAERDE, O.: Failure in the utilization of carbohydrates in mental disease. Acta psychiat. suppl. **106**, 302 (1956). — LISOVSKAYA. N. P.: Phosphoproteins and the processes of metabolism in the brain. Dokl. Acad. Nauk SSSR **95**, 1033 (1954); Chem. Abstr. **48**, 9509 (1954). — LÖHR, K., and W. O. SCHÜMANN: Presence of a hyperglycaemia-inducing material in the urine. Z. ges. exp. Med. **122**, 374 (1953). — LYNEN, F.: Fatty acid metabolism. In. Metabolism of the nervous system, p. 381—395. (Ed. D. RICHTER). New York: Pergamon Press 1957.

MACFARLANE, M. G., and H. WEIL-MALHERBE: Changes in phosphate distribution during anaerobic glycolysis in brain slices. Biochem. J. **35**, 1—6 (1941). — MADDOCK, S., J. E. HAWKINS, and E. HOLMES: Inadequacy of substances of "glucose cycle" for maintenance of normal cortical potentials during hypoglycaemia produced by hepatectomy with abdominal evisceration. Amer. J. Physiol. **125**, 551—565 (1939). — MAGEE, W. L., J. F. BERRY, and R. J. ROSSITER: Effect of chlorpromazine and azacyclonol on the labelling of phosphatides in brain slices. Biochim. biophys. Acta **21**, 408 (1956). — MANN, F. C., and T. B. MAGATH: Studies on the physiology of the liver. III. The effect of administration of glucose in the condition following total exstirpation of the liver. Arch. intern Med. **30**, 171—181 (1922). — MAYER-GROSS, W.: The diagnostic significance of certain tests of carbohydrate metabolism in psychiatric patients and the question of "oneirophrenia". J. ment. Sci. **98**, 683—686 (1952). — MAYER-GROSS, W., and J. W. WALKER: The effect of L-glutamic acid and other amino-acids in hypoglycaemia. Biochem. J. **44**, 92—97 (1949). — MCFARLAND, R. A., and H. GOLDSTEIN: The biochemistry of manic-depressive psychosis. Amer. J. Psychiat. **96**, 21 (1939). — MCILWAIN, H.: The effect of depressants on the metabolism of stimulated cerebral tissues. Biochem. J. **53**, 403—412 (1953). — MCILWAIN, H.: Biochemistry and the central nervous system. Boston: Little, Brown and Co. 1955. — MCILWAIN, H.: Electrical influences and speed of chemical change in the brain. Physiol. Rev. **36**, 355—375 (1956). — MCILWAIN, H.: Characterization of naturally occurring materials which restore excitability to isolated cerebral tissues. Biochem. J. **78**, 24 (1961). — MCILWAIN, H., L. BUCHEL, and J. D. CHESHIRE: The inorganic phosphate and phosphocreatine of brain especially during metabolism in vitro. Biochem. J. **48**, 12—20 (1951). — MCILWAIN, H., and M. A. TRESIZE: The glucose, glycogen and aerobic glycolysis of isolated cerebral tissues. Biochem. J. **63**, 250 (1956). — MEDUNA, L. J.: Oneirophrenia. Urbana: The University of Illinois Press 1950. — MEDUNA, L. J., F. J. GERTY, and V. G. URSE: Biochemical disturbances in mental disorders. I. Anti-insulin effect of blood in cases of schizophrenia. Arch. Neurol. Psychiat. **47**, 38 (1942) — MEDUNA, L. J., and J. A. VAICHULIS: A hyperglycemic factor in the urine of so-called schizophrenics. Dis. nerv. Syst. **9**, 248 (1948). — MEYERHOF, O.: The rates of glycolysis of glucose and fructose in extracts of brain. Arch. Biochem. **13**, 485—487 (1947). — MORGAN, M. S., and F. J. PILGRIM: Concentration of a hyperglycaemic factor from the urine of schizophrenics. Proc. Soc. exp. Biol. (N. Y.) **79**, 106—111 (1952). — MOYA, F., J. DEWAR, M. MACINTOSH, S. HIRSCH, and R. TOWNSEND: Hyperglycemic action and toxicity of the urine of schizophrenic patients. Canad. J. Biochem. **36**, 505 (1958).

NADEAU, G., and Y. ROULEAU: Insulin tolerance in schizophrenics. J. clin. exp. Psychopath. **14**, 69 (1953). — NARAYANASWAMI, A., and H. MCILWAIN: Electrical pulses and the metabolism of cell-free cerebral preparations. Biochem. J. **57**, 663—666 (1954). — NURNBERGER, J. I., and M. W. GORDON: The cell density of neural tissues: direct counting method and possible applications as a biologic referent. In: Ultrastructure and cellular chemistry of neural tissue. p. 100—138. (Ed. H. WAELSCH). New York: Hoeber-Harper 1957.

OLKON, D. M.: Capillary structure in patients with schizophrenia. Arch. Neurol. Psychiat. (Chicago) **42**, 652—663 (1939). — OPITZ, E.: Energieumsatz des Gehirns in situ unter aeroben und anaeroben Bedingungen. In: Die Chemie und der Stoffwechsel des Nervengewebes. 3.Coll. Ges. physiol. Chem. p. 66—108 (1952). — ORSTROM, A., and O. SKAUG: The isolation from the blood of chronic schizophrenic patients of compounds active in radioactive phosphate turnover. Acta psychiat. scand. **25**, 437 (1950).

PERUTZ, A.: Turnover of the ether soluble plasma phosphatides in schizophrenia. Acta psychiat. scand. **26**, 411 (1951). — PRYCE, I. G.: The relationship between glucose tolerance body weight and clinical state in melancholia. J. ment. Sci. **104**, 1079 (1958).

RAAFLAUB, J.: Die Metallpufferfunktion der Adenosinphosphate. Helv. physiol. pharmacol. Acta **14**, 304 (1956). — REINER, J. M.: Carbohydrate metabolism in tissue homogenates. Arch. Biochem. **12**, 327—338 (1947). — REISS, J. M., M. REISS, and A. WYATT: Action of thyroid hormones on brain metabolism of new born rats. Proc. Soc. exp. Biol. (N. Y.) **93**, 19—22 (1956). — RICHTER, D.: Brain metabolism and cerebral function. Biochem. Soc. Symp. **8**, 62—76 (1952). — RODNIGHT, R., H. McILWAIN, and M. A. TRESIZE: Analysis of arterial and cerebral venous blood from the rabbit. J. Neurochem. **3**, 209 (1959).

SACKS, W.: Cerebral oxidation of fumarate-2-C^{14} in normal human subjects. J. appl. Physiol. **9**, 43 (1956). — SACKS, W.: Cerebral metabolism of butyrate-1-C^{14} in normal human subjects. Fed. Proc. **16**, 240 (1957). — SCHMIDT, C. F., and J. P. HENDRIX: The circulation of the brain and spinal cord. Res. Publ. Ass. nerv, ment. Dis. **18**, 229—276 (1938). — SCHMITT, F. O.: The structure and properties of nerve membranes. In: The metabolism of the nervous system. p. 35—51. (Ed. D. RICHTER). New York: Pergamon Press 1957. — SCHWERIN, P., S. P. BESSMAN, and H. WAELSCH: The uptake of glutamic acid and glutamine by brain and other tissues of the rat and mouse. J. biol. Chem. **184**, 37—44 (1950). — SEBRELL, W. H.: The mental and neurological aspects of vitamin B complex deficiency. Res. Publ. Ass. Res. nerv. ment. Dis. **22**, 113—121 (1943). — SEBRELL, W. H., JR., and K. SCHWARZ: The role of B-vitamins in the metabolism of the nervous system. Res. Publ. Ass. nerv. ment. Dis. **32**, 174—183 (1953). — SELTZER, H. S., S. EISENBERG, and C. W. SENSENBACH: Cerebral and peripheral carbohydrate utilization during amelioration of hypoglycemic symptoms by fructose. J. Lab. clin. Med. **50**, 953 (1957). — SELYE, H.: The physiology and pathology of exposure to stress; a treatise based on the concepts of the general-adaptation syndrome and the diseases of adaptation. Montreal: Acta 1950. — SHATTOCK, F. M.: The somatic manifestations of schizophrenia. A clinical study of their significance. J. ment. Sci. **96**, 32—142 (1950). — SIEBERT, G., K. H. BAESSLER, R. HANNOVER, E. ADLOFF u. R. BEYER: Enzymaktivitäten in isolierten Zellkernen in Abhängigkeit von der mitotischen Aktivität. Biochem. Z. **334**, 388 (1961). — SOKOLOFF, L.: Relation of cerebral circulation and metabolism to mental activity. In: Neurochemistry. p. 216—229. (Eds. S. R. KOREY, and J. I. NURNBERGER). London: Cassell and Co. Ltd. 1956. — SOKOLOFF, L., S. PERLIN, C. KORNETSKY, and S. S. KETY: The effects of D-lysergic acid diethylamide on cerebral circulation and over-all metabolism. Ann. N. Y. Acad. Sci. **66**, 468—477 (1957). — SPILLANE, J. D.: Nutritional disorders of the nervous system. Baltimore: Williams and Wilkins Co. 1947. — SPIRTES, M. A., and E. BRUNNER: Induced fructolysis in normal rat brain cortex slices. Fed. Proc. **18**, 447 (1959). — STREICHER, E.: Effect of anesthetic and convulsant drugs on P^{32} exchange in rat brain. Fed. Proc. **13**, 146 (1954).

TAGNON, R. F., and J. CORVILAIN: Utilization of fructose by the nervous system in man. J. clin. Endocrin. **19**, 509 (1959). — TERNER, C.: The effects of phosphate acceptors, p-nitrophenol and arsenate on respiration, phosphorylation and Pasteur effect in cell-free suspensions. Biochem. J. **64**, 523—532 (1956). — THORN, W.: Über die anaerobe Glykolyse des Warmblütergehirns in situ. Biochem. Z. **321**, 361—367 (1951). — THORN, W., W. ISSELHARD, and B. MULDENER: Glykogen-, Glucose- und Milchsäuregehalt in Warmblüterorganen, bei unterschiedlicher Versuchsanordnung und anoxischer Belastung mit Hilfe optischer Fermentteste ermittelt. Biochem. Z. **331**, 545—562 (1959). — THORN, W., and H. A. RASZKOWSKI: Über den Verlauf der anaeroben Glykolyse in situ bei verschiedenen Körpertemperaturen gemessen am Kaninchenhirn. Biochem. Z. **323**, 21—27 (1952). — TOWER, D. B.: The effects of 2-deoxy-D-glucose on metabolism of slices of cerebral cortex incubated in vitro. J. Neurochem. **3**, 185 (1958). — TSCHIRGI, R. D., R. W. GERARD, H. JENERICK, L. L. BOYARSKY, and J. Z. HEARON: Metabolism of the rat spinal cord functioning in isolation. Fed. Proc. **8**, 166 (1949). — TSUKADA, Y., G. TAKAGAKI, and S. HIRANO: Incorporation of radioactive phosphate into protein-bound phosphorus fractions of brain slices in reference to its relation to the metabolic activity. J. Biochem. (Tokyo) **45**, 489—501 (1958).

UTENA, H., and T. EZOE: Studies on the carbohydrate metabolism in brain tissue of schizophrenic patients. Reports I and II. The aerobic metabolism of glucose. Psychiat. Neurol. jap. **52**, 204—250 (1951). — UTENA, H., T. EZOE, and N. KATO: Biochemical studies on addiction due to β-phenylisopropylmethylamine. I. Tissue distribution and excretion of the amine. II. Effect on glucose metabolism in brain tissue. Psychiat. Neurol. jap. **57**, 1—3 (1955).

VIGNAIS, P. M., C. H. GALLAGHER, and I. ZABIN: Activation and oxidation of long chain fatty acids by rat brain. J. Neurochem. **2**, 283 (1958). — VLADIMIROV, G. E., and J. N. RUBEL: The turnover of hexosemonophosphate in the brain and the effect of stimulation, narcosis and hypothermia. In: Metabolism of the nervous system p. 263—266. (Ed. D. RICHTER). New York: Pergamon Press 1957. — VOLK, M. E., R. H. MILLINGTON, and S. WEINHOUSE: Oxidation of endogenous fatty acids of rat tissues in vitro. J. biol. Chem. **195**, 493 (1952).

WANG, R. I. H., and R. R. SONNENSCHEIN: pH of cerebral cortex during induced convulsions. J. Neurophysiol. **18**, 130 (1955). — WEIL-MALHERBE, H.: The action of glutamic acid in hypoglycaemic coma. J. ment. Sci. **95**, 930—944 (1949). — WEIL-MALHERBE, H.: Der Energiestoffwechsel des Nervengewebes und sein Zusammenhang mit der Funktion. In: Die Chemie und der Stoffwechsel des Nervengewebes. 3. Coll. Ges. physiol. Chem. 1952, p. 41—65. — WEIL-MALHERBE, H., and A. D. BONE: Studies on hexokinase. 1. The hexokinase activity of rat brain extracts. Biochem. J. 49, 339—347 (1951). — WEIL-MALHERBE, H., and A. D. BONE: Activators and inhibitors of hexokinase in human blood. J. ment. Sci. 97, 635—662 (1951). — WEIL-MALHERBE, H., and A. D. BONE: The concentration of adrenaline-like substances in blood during insulin hypoglycaemia. J. ment. Sci. 98, 565—578 (1952). — WILSON, W. P., J. F. SCHIEVE, and P. SCHEINBERG: Effect of series of electric shock treatments on cerebral blood flow and metabolism. Arch. Neurol. Psychiat. (Chicago) 68, 651—654 (1952). — WORTIS, J., K. M. BOWMAN, W. GOLDFARB, J. F. FAZEKAS, and H. E. HIMWICH: Availability of lactic acid for brain oxidations. J. Neurophysiol. 4, 243—249 (1941).

D. Metabolism of nitrogenous compounds

ACS, G., A. NEIDLE, and H. WAELSCH: Brain ribosomes and amino acid incorporation. Biochem. biophys. Acta 50, 403 (1961). — ABOOD, L. G., and A. GEIGER: Breakdown of proteins and lipids during glucose-free perfusion of the cat's brain. Amer. J. Physiol. 182, 557—560 (1955). — ABOOD, L. G., F. A. GIBBS, and E. GIBBS: Comparative study of blood ceruloplasmin in schizophrenia and other disorders. A.M.A. Arch. Neurol. Psychiat. 77, 643—645 (1957). — ACS, G., R. BALÁZS, and F. B. STRAUB: Metabolism in slices of brain cortex. The level of adenosine triphosphate and its changes under the influence of glutamic acid. Ukrain. Biokhim. Zhur. 25, 17—27 (1953). — ADAMS, J. E., H. A. HARPER, G. S. GORDON, M. HUTCHIN, and R. C. BENTINCK: Cerebral metabolism of glutamic acid in multiple sclerosis. Neurology 5, 100—107 (1955). — AJMONE-MARSAN, C., M. G. F. FUORTES, and F. MAROSSERO: Influence of ammonium chloride on the electrical activity of the brain and spinal cord. EEG Clin. Neurophys. 1, 291—298 (1949). — AKERFELDT, S.: Oxidation of N,N-dimethyl-p-phenylenediamine by serum from patients with mental disease. Science 125, 117—119 (1957). — ALBERS, R. W., and R. A. SALVADOR: Succinic semialdehyde oxidation by a soluble dehydrogenase from brain. Science 128, 359—360 (1958). — ALBERT, K., P. HOCH, and H. WAELSCH: Glutamic acid and mental deficiency. J. nerv. ment. Dis. 114, 471—491 (1951). — ANSELL, G. B., and D. RICHTER: A note on the free amino acid content of rat brain. Biochem. J. 57, 70—73 (1954). — AWAPARA, J., A. J. LANDUA, R. FUERST, and B. SEALE: Free γ-aminobutyric acid in brain. J. biol. Chem. 187, 35—39 (1950). — AWAPARA, J., and B. SEALE: Distribution of transaminases in rat organs. J. biol. Chem. 194, 497—502 (1952).

BARGMANN, W., and E. SCHARRER: The site of origin of the hormones of the posterior pituitary. Amer. Sci. 39, 255—259 (1951). — BAZEMORE, A. W., K. A. C. ELLIOTT, and E. FLOREY: Isolation of factor I. J. Neurochem. 1, 334—339 (1957). — BELOFF-CHAIN, A., R. CANTANZARO, E. B. CHAIN, I. MASI, and F. POCCHIARI: Fate of uniformly labeled C^{14}-glucose in brain slices. Proc. roy. Soc. B 144, 22—28 (1955). — BENITEZ, D., G. R. PSCHEIDT, and W. E. STONE: Formation of ammonium ion in the cerebrum in fluoroacetate poisoning. Amer. J. Physiol. 176, 488—492 (1954). — BERL, S., and H. WAELSCH: Determination of glutamic acid, glutamine, glutathione and γ-aminobutyric acid and their distribution in brain tissue. J. Neurochem. 3, 161—169 (1958). — BERL, S., D. P. PURPURA, M. GIRADO, and H. WAELSCH: Amino acid metabolism in epileptogenic and non-epileptogenic lesions of the neocortex (cat). J. Neurochem. 4, 311 (1959). — BERL, S., D. P. PURPURA, O. GONZALEZ-MONTEAGUDO, and H. WAELSCH: Effects of injected amino acids on metabolic changes occurring in epileptogenic and non-epileptogenic lesions of the cerebral cortex. In: Inhibition in the nervous system and γ-aminobutyric acid. (E. ROBERTS, Ed.). London: Pergamon Press 1960b. — BERL, S., G. TAKAGAKI, D. D. CLARKE, and H. WAELSCH: Metabolic compartments in vivo. Ammonia and glutamic acid metabolism in brain and liver. J. biol. Chem. 237, 2562 (1962). — BESSMAN, J. P.: Ammonia and coma. In chemical pathology of the nervous system. p. 370. (J. FOLCH-PI, Ed.) London: Pergamon Press Ltd. 1961. — BESSMAN, S. P., J. ROSSEN, and E. C. LAYNE: γ-Aminobutyric acid — glutamic acid transamination in brain. J. biol. Chem. 201, 385—391 (1953). — BESSMAN, S. P., and A. N. BESSMAN: The cerebral and peripheral uptake of ammonia in liver disease with an hypothesis for the mechanism of hepatic coma. J. clin. Invest. 34, 622—628 (1955). — BESSMAN, S. P.: Ammonia metabolism in animals. In: Inorganic nitrogen metabolism. 408—437. (W. D. MCELROY and B. GLASS, Eds.), Baltimore, Maryland: Johns Hopkins Press 1956. — BLOCK, W.: In-vitro-Versuche zum Einbau von ^{14}C-Mescalin und ^{14}C-β-Phenyl-athylamin in Proteine. Hoppe-Seylers Z. physiol. Chem. 296, 1 (1954). — BLOCK, W., K. BLOCK, and B. PATZIG: Zur Physiologie des ^{14}C-radioaktiven Mescalins im Tierversuch. Hoppe-Seylers Z. physiol. Chem. 290, 160 (1952). — BRAGANCA, B. M., P. FAULKNER, and J. H. QUASTEL: Effects of inhibitors of glutamine synthesis on the inhibition of acetylcholine synthesis in brain slices by ammonia ions. Biochim. biophys. Acta 10, 83—88 (1953). — BRATTGARD, S. O.: The importance of adequate stimulation for the chemical composition of retinal ganglion cells during early post-natal development. Acta radiol. (Stockh.) Suppl. **96**, (1952). — BUSCH, H.: Studies on the metabolism of pyruvate-2-C¹⁴ in tumor-bearing rats. Cancer Res. **15**, Suppl. **3**, 365 (1955). — BUSCH, H., M. H. GOLDBERG, and D. C. ANDERSON: Substrate effects on metabolic patterns of pyruvate-2-C¹⁴ in tissue slices. Cancer Res. **16**, 175 (1956).

CASPERSSON, T.: The relations between nucleic acid and protein synthesis. Symp. Soc. Exp. Biol. 1. Nucleic acid, 127—151 (1947). — CHIRIGOS, M. A., P. GREENGARD, and S. UDENFRIEND: Uptake of tyrosine by rat brain in vivo. J. biol. Chem. **235**, 2075 (1960). — CLARKE, D. D., M. J. MYCEK, A. NEIDLE, and H. WAELSCH: The incorporation of amines into protein. Arch. Biochem. **79**, 338 (1959). — CLARKE, D. D., A. NEIDLE, N. K. SARKAR, and H. WAELSCH: Metabolic activity of protein amide groups. Arch. Biochem. **71**, 277—279 (1957). — CLARK, G. M., and B. EISEMAN: Studies in ammonia metabolism. IV. Biochemical changes in brain tissue of dogs during ammonia induced coma. New Engl. J. Med. **259**, 178—180 (1958). — CLOUET, D. H.: On the apparent fixation of serotonin in mitochondrial proteins. Abstract in: Proceedings of the Fourth International Congress of Biochemistry. p. 184. Pergamon Press 1958. — CLOUET, D. H., and D. RICHTER: The incorporation of (³⁵S) labelled methionine into the proteins of the rat brain. J. Neurochem. **3**, 219—229 (1959). — CLOUET, D. H., and H. WAELSCH: The recovery of cholinesterase in the nervous system of the frog after inhibition. J. Neurochem. **8**, 201 (1961). — CRANE, R. K., and E. G. BALL: Factors affecting the fixation of C¹⁴O₂ by animal tissues. J. biol. Chem. **188**, 819—832 (1951).

DAVISON, A. N.: Metabolically inert proteins of the central and peripherial nervous system, muscle and tendon. Biochem. J. **78**, 272 (1961). — DAWSON, R. M. C.: Studies on the glutamine and glutamic acid content of the rat brain during insulin hypoglycaemia. Biochem. J. **47**, 386—395 (1950). — DAWSON, R. M. C.: The metabolism and glutamic acid content of rat brain in relation to thiopentane anaesthesia. Biochem. J. **49**, 138—144 (1951). — DAWSON, R. M. C., and R. A. PETERS: Observations upon the behaviour of some phosphate esters in brain at the start of convulsions induced by fluorocitrate and fluoroacetate. Biochim. biophys. Acta **16**, 254—257 (1955). — DINGMAN, W., and M. B. SPORN: The penetration of proline and proline derivatives into brain. J. Neurochem. **4**, 148—153 (1959). — DINGMAN, W., and M. B. SPORN: The incorporation of 8-azaguanine into rat brain RNA and its effect on maze-learning by the rat: an inquiry into the biochemical basis of memory. J. Psychiatric. Res. **1**, 1 (1961). — DINGMAN, W., M. B. SPORN, and R. K. DAVIES: The chemical fractionation of rat brain proteins. J. Neurochem. **4**, 154—160 (1959).

EINARSON, L.: Structural changes and functional disturbances in the nervous system. Anatomiske Skrifter 1, 27—51 (1954). — EINARSON, L.: Cytological aspects of nucleic acid metabolism. In: Metabolism of the nervous system. 403—420. (D. RICHTER, Ed.), London: Pergamon Press 1957. — EISEMAN, B., W. BAKEWELL, and G. CLARK: Studies in ammonia metabolism. I. Ammonia metabolism and glutamate therapy in hepatic coma. Amer. J. Med. **20**, 890—895 (1956). — ELLIOT, W. H.: Studies on the enzymic synthesis of glutamine. Biochem. J. **49**, 106—112 (1951). — ELLIOTT, K. A. C.: The relation of ions to metabolism in brain. Canad. J. Biochem. **33**, 466 (1955).

FINDLAY, M., W. L. MAGEE, and R. J. ROSSITER: Incorporation of radioactive phosphate into lipids and pentosenucleic acid of cat brain slices. The effect of inorganic ions. Biochem. J. **58**, 236—243 (1954). — FLOCK, E. V., M. A. BLOCK, J. H. GRINDLAY, F. C. MANN, and J. L. BOLLMAN: Changes in free amino acids of brain and muscle after total hepatectomy. J. biol. Chem. **200**, 529—536 (1953). — FLOREY, E.: Über einen nervösen Hemmungsfaktor in Gehirn und Rückenmark. Naturwissenschaften 40, 295—296 (1953). — FURST, S., A. LAJTHA, and H. WAELSCH: Amino acid and protein metabolism of the brain. III. Incorporation of lysine into the proteins of various brain areas and their cellular fractions. J. Neurochem. **2**, 216—225 (1958).

GAITONDE, M. K.: The rate of (³⁵S) methionine and (³⁵S) cystine into proteolipids and proteins of rat brain. Biochem. J. **80**, 277 (1961). — GAITONDE, M. K., and D. RICHTER: The uptake of ³⁵S into rat tissues after injection of (³⁵S) methionine. Biochem. J. **59**, 690—696 (1955). — GAITONDE, M. K., and D. RICHTER: The metabolic activity of the proteins of the brain. Proc. roy. Soc. **145**, 83—99 (1956). — GEIGER, A., J. MAGNES, and J. DOBKIN: Non-carbohydrate sources of excess energy utilized by the brain during convulsions. Fed. Proc. **13**, 52—53 (1954). — GEIGER, A.: Correlation of brain metabolism and function by the use of a brain perfusion method in situ. Physiol. Rev. **38**, 1—20 (1959). — GJESSING, R.: Disturbances of somatic functions in catatonia with a periodic course, and their compensation. J. ment. Sci. **84**, 608—621 (1938). — GJESSING, R.: Beiträge zur Kenntnis der Pathophysiologie periodisch katatoner Zustände, IV. Mitteilung. Versuch einer Ausgleichung der Funktionsstörungen. Arch. Psychiat. Nervenkr. **109**, 525—595 (1939).— GORE, M. B. R., and H. McILWAIN: Effects of some inorganic salts on the metabolic response of sections of mammalian cerebral cortex to electrical stimulation. J. Physiol. **117**, 471—483 (1952). — GRAY, I., J. M. JOHNSTON, and C. W. SPEARING: Biochemical response to trauma. V. Glutamine, glutamic acid, ammonia in the brain. Fed. Proc. **15**, 265 (1956). — GUHA, S. R., and

J. J. Ghosh: Glutamine transaminase activity in rat brain. Ann. Biochem. exp. Med. 19, 33—36 (1959).

Haber, C., and L. Saidel: Glutamic acid in neural activity. Fed. Proc. 7, 47 (1948). — Hamberger, C. A., and H. Hyden: Cytochemical changes in the cochlear ganglion caused by acoustic stimulation and trauma. Acta oto-laryng. (Stockh.) Suppl. 61, (1945). — Hamberger, C. A., and H. Hyden: Production of nucleoproteins in the vestibular ganglion. Acta oto-laryng. (Stockh.) Suppl. 75, 53—81 (1949a). — Hamberger, C. A., and H. Hyden: Transneuronal chemical changes in Deiters nucleus. Acta oto-laryng. (Stockh.) Suppl. 75, 82—113 (1949b). Heath, R. G., S. Martens, B. E. Leach, M. Cohen, and C. Angel: Effect on behavior in humans with the administration of taraxein. Amer. J. Psychiat. 114, 14—24 (1957). — Heath, R. G., B. E. Leach, L. W. Byers, S. Martens, and C. A. Feigley: Pharmacological and biological psychotherapy. Amer. J. Psychiat. 114, 683—689 (1958). — Heinz, E.: Exchangeability of glycine accumulated by carcinoma cells. J. biol. Chem. 225, 305—315 (1957). — Heinz, E., and P. M. Walsh: Exchange diffusion, transport, and intracellular level of amino acids in Ehrlich carcinoma cells. J. biol. Chem. 233, 1488—1493 (1958).— Himwich, H. E., and W. A. Himwich: The permeability of the blood-brain barrier to glutamic acid in the developing rat. In: Biochemistry of the developing nervous system. 202—206. (H. Waelsch, Ed.), New York: Academic Press 1955. — Hyden, H.: Protein metabolism in the nerve cell during growth and function. Acta Physiol. scand. 6, Suppl. 17, 5—136 (1943)— Hyden, H.: The nucleoproteins in virus reproduction. Cold Spr. Harb. Symp. quant. Biol. 12, 104—114 (1947). — Hyden, H., S. Lovtrup, and A. Pigon: Cytochrome oxidase and succinoxidase activities in spinal ganglion cells and in glial capsula cells. J. Neurochem. 2, 304—311 (1958). — Hyden, H.: Biochemical changes in glial cells and nerve cells at varying activity. In: Proceedings of the Fourth International Congress of Biochemistry. Vol. III: Biochemistry of the central nervous system. 64—89. (F. Brücke, ed.), London: Pergamon Press Ltd. 1959. — Hyden, H., and A. Pigon: A cytophysiological study of the functional relationship between oligodendroglial cells and nerve cells of Deiters' nucleus. J. Neurochem. 6, 57 (1960).

Irreverre, F., and R. L. Evans: Isolation of γ-guanidinobutyric acid from calf brain. J. biol. Chem. 234, 1438—1440 (1959).

Kamin, H., and P. Handler: The metabolism of parenterally administered amino acids. II. Urea synthesis. J. biol. Chem. 188, 193—205 (1951). — Katzman, R., and P. H. Leiderman: Brain potassium exchange in normal adult and immature rats. Amer. J. Physiol. 175, 263—270 (1953). — Kety, S. S.: Biochemical theories of schizophrenia. Science 129, 1528—1532 and 1590—1596 (1959). — Keup, W.: Die „Biochemie der Schizophrenie," Eine kritische Stellungnahme. Mschr. Psychiat. Neurol. 128, 56—90 (1954). — Killam, K. F., and J. A. Bain: Convulsant hydrazides I. In vitro and in vivo inhibition of vitamin B_6 enzymes by convulsant hydrazides. J. Pharmacol. exp. Ther. 119, 255—262 (1957). — Killam, K. F., S. R. Dasgupta, and E. K. Killam: Studies of the action of convulsant hydrazides as Vitamin B_6 antagonists in the central nervous system. In: Inhibition in the nervous system and γ-aminobutyric acid (E. Roberts, Ed.). London: Pergamon Press 1960. — Klingmüller, V.: Biochemie, Physiologie und Klinik der Glutaminsäure. Aulendorf/Württ.: Cantor 1955. — Koechlin, B. A.: On the chemical composition of the axoplasm of squid giant nerve fibers with particular reference to its ion pattern. J. biophys. biochem. Cytol. 1, 511—529 (1955). — Koenig, E., and G. B. Koelle: Mode of regeneration of acetylcholinesterase in cholinergic neurons following irreversible inactivation. J. Neurochem. 8, 169 (1961). — Koransky, W.: Fraktionierte Darstellung von Nucleotiden aus dem Gehirn von Ratten im Ruhezustand und im Krampfanfall. Naunyn-Schmiedebergs Arch. exp. Path. Pharmakol. 228, 140—143 (1956). — Korey, S. R., B. de Braganza, and D. Nachmansohn: Choline acetylase. V. Esterification and transacetylations. J. biol. Chem. 189, 705—715 (1951). — Krebs, H. A.: Metabolism of amino-acids. IV. The synthesis of glutamine from glutamic acid and ammonia, and the enzymic hydrolysis of glutamine in animal tissues. Biochem. J. 29, 1951—1959 (1935). — Krebs, H. A., L. V. Eggleston, and R. Hems: Distribution of glutamine and glutamic acid in animal tissues. Biochem. J. 44, 159—163 (1949).

Lajtha, A.: Amino acid and protein metabolism of the brain. II. The uptake of L-lysine by brain and other organs of the mouse at different ages. J. Neurochem. 2, 209—215 (1958). — Lajtha, A.: Amino acid and protein metabolism of the brain. V. Turnover of leucine in mouse tissues. J. Neurochem. 3, 358—365 (1959). — Lajtha, A.: Protein metabolism in peripheral nerve. In: Chemical pathology of the nervous system. (J. Folch, Ed.). London: Pergamon Press. Ltd. 1960. — Lajtha, A., S. Berl, and H. Waelsch: Amino acid and protein metabolism of the brain. IV. The metabolism of glutamic acid. J. Neurochem. 3, 322—332 (1959). — Lajtha, A., S. Berl, and H. Waelsch: Compartmentalization of glutamic acid metabolism in the central nervous system. In: Inhibition in the central nervous system and γ-aminobutyric acid (E. Roberts, Ed.). London: Pergamon Press Ltd. 1960. — Lajtha, A., S. Furst, A. Gerstein, and H. Waelsch: Amino acid and protein metabolism of the brain. I. Turnover of free and protein bound lysine in brain and other organs. J. Neurochem. 1, 289—300 (1957a). —

LAJTHA, A., S. FURST, and H. WAELSCH: The metabolism of the proteins of the brain. Experientia (Basel) **13**, 168—172 (1957b). — LAJTHA, A., and P. MELA: The exchange of free amino acids between plasma and brain. J. Neurochem. **7**, 210 (1961).— LAJTHA, A., P. MELA, and H. WAELSCH: Manganese dependent glutamotransferase, J. biol. Chem. **205**, 553 (1953). — LAJTHA, A., and J. TOTH: Uptake and transport of amino acids by the brain. J. Neurochem. **8**, 216 (1961). — LEACH, B. E., M. COHEN, R. G. HEATH, and S. MARTENS: Studies of the role of ceruloplasmin and albumin in adrenaline metabolism. A. M. A. Arch. Neurol. Psychiat. **76**, 635—642 (1956).

MAURER, W.: Untersuchungen zur Größe des Eiweißumsatzes von Plasma- und Organeiweiß. Wien. Z. inn. Med. **38**, 28 (1957). — MCILWAIN, H.: Glutamic acid and glucose as substrates for mammalian brain. J. ment. Sci. **97**, 674—680 (1951). — MCILWAIN, H.: Phosphates of brain during in vitro metabolism: Effects of oxygen, glucose, glutamate, and calcium and potassium salts. Biochem. J. **52**, 289—295 (1952). MCILWAIN, H.: Substances which support respiration and metabolic response to electrical impulses in human cerebral tissues. J. Neurol. Neurosurg. Psychiat. **16**, 257—266 (1953). — MCILWAIN, H., P. J. W. AYRES, and O. FORDA: Metabolic response to electrical stimulation in separated portions of human cerebral tissues. J. ment. Sci. **98**, 265—272 (1952). — MCILWAIN, H., and M. B. R. GORE: Induced loss in cerebral tissues of respiratory response to electrical impulses, and its partial restoration by additional substrates. Biochem. J. **54**, 305—312 (1953). — MCKHANN, G. M., R. W. ALBERS, L. SOKOLOFF, O. MICKELSEN, and D. B. TOWER: The quantitative significance of the γ-aminobutyric acid pathway in cerebral oxidative metabolism. In: Inhibition in the nervous system and γ-aminobutyric acid (GABA). (E. ROBERTS, ed.). London: Pergamon Press Ltd. 1959. — MAGEE, W. L., and R. J. ROSSITER: Chemical studies of peripheral nerve during Wallerian degeneration. 6. Incorporation of radioactive phosphate into pentosenucleic acid and phospholipin in vitro. Biochem. J. **58**, 243—249 (1954). — MEISTER, A., and S. V. TICE: Transamination from glutamine to α-keto acids. J. biol. Chem. **187**, 173—187 (1950). — MISANI, F., and L. REINER: Studies on nitrogen trichloride treated prolamines. VIII. Synthesis of the toxic factor. Arch. Biochem. **27**, 234—235 (1950). — MYCEK, M. J., D. D. CLARKE, A. NEIDLE, and H. WAELSCH: Amine incorporation into insulin as catalyzed by transglutaminase. Arch. Biochem. **84**, 528 (1959). — MYCEK, M. J., and H. WAELSCH: Enzymatic hydrolysis of protein amide groups. Fed. Proc. **19**, 336 (1960).

NECHAEVA, G. A., N. V. SADIKOVA, and V. A. SKVORTSEVICH: Renewal of amino acids of protein under different functional states. Vop. Biokhim. Nervnoi Sistemy Sbornik **1957**, 31—39; Chem. Abstr. **53**, 1500b (1959).

OCHS, S., and E. BURGER: Movement of substance proximo-distally in nerve axon as studied with spinal cord injection of radioactive phosphorus. Amer. J. Physiol. **194**, 499—506 (1958).

PALAY, S. L., and G. E. PALADE: The fine structure of neurons, J. biophys. biochem. Cytol. **1**, 69—88 (1955). — PALLADIN, A. V.: Proteins of the nervous system under various conditions. In: Metabolism of the nervous system (D. RICHTER, Ed.), 456—458. London: Pergamon Press Ltd. 1957. — PALLADIN, A. V., V. V. BELIK, N. M. POLYAKOVA, and T. P. SILICH: Proteins of the nervous system. Vop. Biokhim. Nervnoi. Sistemy Sbornik **1959**, 9—30. Chem. Abstr. **53**, 1499h (1959). — PALLADIN, A. V., and N. VERTAIMER: Protein renewal in the central nervous system in different functional states. Dokl. Akad. Nauk SSSR **102**, 319—321 (1955); Chem. Abstr. **49**, 14971g (1955). — PISANO, J. J., C. MITOMA, and S. UDENFRIEND: Biosynthesis of γ-guanidinobutyric acid from γ-aminobutyric acid and arginine. Nature (Lond.) **180**, 1125—1126 (1957). — PISANO, J. J., J. D. WILSON. L. COHNE. D. ABRAHAM, and S. UDENFRIEND: Isolation of γ-aminobutyrylhistidine (homocarnosine) from brain. J. biol. Chem. **236**, 499 (1961). — PRICE, J. C., H. WAELSCH, and T. J. PUTNAM: DL-glutamic acid hydrochloride in treatment of petit mal and psychomotor seizures. J. Amer. med. Ass. **122**, 1153—1156 (1943). — PURPURA, D. P., S. BERL, O. GONZALEZ-MONTEAGUDO, and A. WYATT: Brain amino acid changes during methoxypyridoxine-induced seizures (cat). In: Inhibition in the nervous system and γ-aminobutyric acid (E. ROBERTS, Ed.). London: Pergamon Press 1960. — PURPURA, D. P., M. GIRADO, and H. GRUNDFEST: Selective blockade of excitatory synapses in the cat brain by γ-aminobutyric acid. Science **125**, 1200—1201 (1957). — PURPURA, D. P., M. GIRADO, and H. GRUNDFEST: Central synaptic effects of ω-guanidino acids and amino acid derivatives. Science **127**, 1179—1181 (1958). — PURPURA, D. P., M. GIRADO, T. G. SMITH, D. A. CALLAN and H. GRUNDFEST: Structure-activity determinants of pharmacological effects of amino acids and related compounds on central synapses. J. Neurochem. **3**, 238—268 (1959).

RICHTER, D., and R. M. C. DAWSON: The ammonia and glutamine content of the brain. J. biol. Chem. **176**, 1199—1210 (1948). — ROBERTS, E., and H. M. BREGOFF: Transamination of γ-amino-butyric acid and β-alanine in brain and liver. J. biol. Chem. **201**, 393—398 (1953).— ROBERTS, E., and S. FRANKEL: γ-Aminobutyric acid in brain: its formation from glutamic acid. J. biol. Chem. **187**, 55—63 (1950). — ROBINS, E., K. SMITH, and I. P. LOWE: In: Neuropharmacology, Transactions of the Fourth Conference of the Josiah Macy, Jr. Foundation. New York: 1957. — RUISSEAU, J. P. DU, J. P. GREENSTEIN, M. WINITZ, and S. M. BIRNBAUM: Studies on the metabolism of free amino acids and related compounds in vivo. VI. Free amino acid levels in the tissues of rats protected against ammonia toxicity. Arch. Biochem. **68**, 161—171 (1957).

SACHS, H.: Vasopressin biosynthesis. Biochim. biophys. Acta **34**, 572—573 (1959). — SAMUELS, A. J., L. L. BOYARSKY, and R. W. GERARD: Distribution, exchanges and migration of phosphate compounds in the nervous system. Amer. J. Physiol. **164**, 1—15 (1951). — SARKAR, N. K., D. D. CLARKE, and H. WAELSCH: An enzymically catalyzed incorporation of amines into proteins. Biochim. biophys. Acta **25**, 451 (1957). — SCHEINBERG, I. H., A. G. MORELL, R. S. HARRIS, and A. BERGER: Concentration of ceruloplasmin in plasma of schizophrenic patients. Science **126**, 925—926 (1957). — SCHURR, P. E., H. T. THOMPSON, L. M. HENDERSON, J. N. WILLIAMS JR., and C. A. ELVEHJEM: The determination of free amino acids in rat tissues. J. biol. Chem. **182**, 39—45 (1950). — SCHWERIN, P., S. P. BESSMAN, and H. WAELSCH: The uptake of glutamic acid and glutamine by brain and other tissues of the rat and mouse. J. biol. Chem. **184**, 37—44 (1950). — SHAPOT, V. S.: Brain metabolism in relation to the functional state of the central nervous system. In: Metabolism of the nervous system. 257—262. (D. RICHTER, Ed.). London: Pergamon Press 1957. — SILBER, R. H.: The free amino acids of lobster nerve. J. cell. comp. Physiol. **18**, 21—30 (1941). — SPECK, J. F.: The enzymatic synthesis of glutamine, a reaction utilizing adenosine triphosphate. J. biol. Chem. **179**, 1405—1426 (1949). — SPORN, M. B., W. DINGMAN, and A. DEFALCO: A method for studying metabolic pathways in the brain of the intact animal. The conversion of proline to other amino acids. J. Neurochem. **4**, 141—147 (1959). — STERN, J. R., L. V. EGGLESTON, R. HEMS, and H. A. KREBS: Accumulation of glutamic acid in isolated brain tissue. Biochem. J. **44**, 410—418 (1949). — STRECKER, H. J.: Glutamic dehydrogenase. Arch. Biochem. **46**, 128—140 (1953).

TAKAGAKI, G., S. BERL, D. D. CLARKE, D. P. PURPURA, and H. WAELSCH: Glutamic acid metabolism in brain and liver during infusion with ammonia labelled with nitrogen-15. Nature (Lond.) **189**, 326 (1961). — TAKAGAKI, G., S. HIRANO, and Y. NAGATA: Some observations on the effect of D-glutamate on the glucose metabolism and the accumulation of potassium ions in brain cortex slices. J. Neurochem. **4**, 124 (1959).—TALLAN, H. H., S. MOORE, and W. H. STEIN: Studies on the free amino acids and related compounds in the tissues of the cat. J. biol. Chem. **211**, 927—939 (1954). — TALLAN, H. H., S. MOORE, and W. H. STEIN: L-Cystathionine in human brain. J. biol. Chem. **230**, 707—716 (1958). — TASHIRO, S.: Studies of alkaligenesis in tissues. I. Ammonia production in the nerve fiber during excitation. Amer. J. Physiol. **60**, 519—543 (1922). — TERNER, C., L. V. EGGLESTON, and H. A. KREBS: The role of glutamic acid in the transport of potassium in brain and retina. Biochem. J. **47**, 139—149 (1950). — THORN, W., and J. HEIMANN: The effects of anoxia, ischaemia, asphyxia and reduced temperature on the ammonia level in the brain and other organs. J. Neurochem. **2**, 166—177 (1958). — TORDA, C.: Effect of convulsion-inducing agents on the acetylcholine content and on the electrical activity of the brain. Amer. J. Physiol. **173**, 179—183 (1953). — TOWER, D. B.: Nature and extent of the biochemical lesion in human epileptogenic cerebral cortex. Neurology **5**, 113—130 (1955). — TOWER, D. B.: Glutamic metabolism in the mammalian central nervous system. In: Proceedings of the Fourth International Congress of Biochemistry, Vol. III: Biochemistry of the central nervous system. 213—250. (F. BRÜCKE, Ed.) London: Pergamon Press Ltd. 1959. — TOWER, D. B.: The administration of γ-aminobutyric acid to man: systemic effects and anticonvulsant action. In: Inhibition in the nervous system and γ-aminobutyric acid (E. ROBERTS, Ed.), London: Pergamon Press 1960. — TSUKADA, Y., and G. TAKAGAKI: Ammonia-formation systems in brain tissue, Nature (Lond.) **173**, 1138 (1954). — TSUKADA, Y., G. TAKAGAKI, S. SUGIMOTO, and S. HIRANO: Changes in the ammonia and glutamine content of the rat brain induced by electric shock. J. Neurochem. **2**, 295—303 (1958).

UNGAR, G., E. ASCHHEIM, S. PSYCHOYOS, and D. V. ROMANO: Reversible changes of protein configuration in stimulated nerve structures. J. gen. Physiol. **40**, 635—652 (1957). — UNGAR, G., and D. V. ROMANO: Sulfhydryl groups in resting and stimulated rat brain; their relationship with protein structure. Proc. Soc. exp. Biol. (N. Y.) **97**, 324—326 (1958).

VLADIMIROVA, E. A.: Changes in the content of preformed ammonia in the hemispheres of the cerebrum of rats under conditions of block caused by the action of conditional irritants. Dokl. Akad. Nauk SSSR **95**, 905—908 (1954); Chem. Abstr. **48**, 9509e (1954). — VLADIMIROVA, E. A.: The ammonia and glutamine content of the cerebral hemispheres of rats in conditioned reflex stimulation and inhibition. Akad. Nauk SSSR **1956**, 440—448; Chem. Abstr. **51**, 11526e (1957). — VLADIMIROV, G. E.: Functional biochemistry of the brain. Fiziol. Zhur. SSSR **39**, 3—16 (1953); Chem. Abstr. **47**, 4983e (1953). — VLADIMIROV, G. E., and A. P. URINSON: Glycine metabolism in the cerebral tissue of the rat in normal resting and in amytal-induced sleep. Biochemistry **22**, 665—670 (1957). — VRBA, R.: Beitrag zum Studium des Gehirnmetabolismus im Zusammenhang mit körperlicher Anstrengung. III. Über Ammoniakbildung und strukturale Eiweißveränderungen im Gehirn. Physiol. Bohemoslov. **4**, 397—408 (1955). — VRBA, R., and J. FOLBERGROVA: Observations on endogenous metabolism in brain in vitro and in vivo. J. Neurochem. **4**, 338—349 (1959).

WAELSCH, H.: Glutamic acid and cerebral function. Advanc. Protein Chem. **6**, 301—341 (1951). — WAELSCH, H.: Certain aspects of intermediary metabolism of glutamine, asparagine and glutathione. Advanc. Enzymol. **13**, 237 (1952). — WAELSCH, H.: Metabolism of proteins and amino acids. In: Metabolism of the nervous system. 431—447. (D. RICHTER, Ed.), London: Pergamon Press 1957. — WAELSCH, H.: Some aspects of amino acid and protein-metabolism of the nervous system. J. nerv. ment. Dis. **126**, 33—39 (1958). — WAELSCH, H.: Some problems of metabolism in relation to the structure of the nervous system. In: Proceedings of the Fourth International Congress of Biochemistry. Vol. III; Biochemistry of the central nervous system. 36—45. (F. BRÜCKE, Ed.), London: Pergamon Press Ltd. 1959. — WAELSCH, H.: An attempt at integration of structure and metabolism in the nervous system. In: Structure and function of the cerebral cortex. Elsevier Publishing Company 1960. — WAELSCH, H.: Compartmentalized biosynthetic reactions in the central nervous system. In Regional Neurochemistry (S. S. KETY and J. ELKES, Eds); p. 57. London: Pergamon Press Ltd. 1961. — WAELSCH, H., and A. LAJTHA: Protein metabolism in the nervous system. Physiol. Rev. **41**, 709 (1961). — WAELSCH, H., P. OWADES, H. K. MILLER, and E. BOREK: Glutamic acid antimetabolites: The sulfoxide derived from methionine. J. biol. Chem. **166**, 273—281 (1946). — WEBSTER JR., L. T., and G. J. GABUZDA: Ammonium uptake by the extremities and brain in hepatic coma. J. clin. Invest. **37**, 414—424 (1958). — WEIL-MALHERBE, H.: Studies on brain metabolism. I. The metabolism of glutamic acid in brain. Biochem. J. **30**, 665—676 (1936). — WEIL-MALHERBE, H.: Observations on tissue glycolysis. Biochem. J. **32**, 2257—2275 (1938). — WEIL-MALHERBE, H., and A. C. DRYSDALE: Ammonia formation in brain. III. The role of the protein amide groups and of hexosamines. J. Neurochem. **1**, 250—255 (1957). — WEIL-MALHERBE, H., and R. H. GREEN: Ammonia formation in brain. 1. Studies on slices and suspension. Biochem. J. **61**, 210—218 (1955a). — WEIL-MALHERBE, H., and R. H. GREEN: Ammonia formation in brain. 2. Brain adenylic deaminase. Biochem. J. **61**, 218—224 (1955b). — WEISS, P., and H. B. HISCOE: Experiments in the mechanism of nerve growth. J. exp. Zool. **107**, 315—395 (1948). — WINNICK, T., R. E. WINNICK, R. ACHER, and C. FROMAGEOT: Amino acids and peptides of posterior pituitary and hypothalamus tissues. Biochim. biophys. Acta **18**, 488 (1955). — WINTERSTEIN, H., and E. HIRSCHBERG: Über Ammoniakbildung im Nervensystem. Biochem. Z. **156**, 138 (1925).

E. Lipids

ABOOD, L. G., and A. GEIGER: Breakdown of proteins and lipids during glucose-free perfusion of the cat's brain. Amer. J. Physiol. **182**, 557—560 (1955). — ADAMS, R. D., and E. P. RICHARDSON: The chemistry of demyelination. In: Chemical pathology of the nervous system (J. FOLCH, Ed.), Proceedings of the Third International Neurochemical Symposium. London: Pergamon Press. In press. — ANSELL, G. B., and R. M. C. DAWSON: Ethanolamine O-phosphoric acid in rat brain. Biochem. J. **50**, 241—246 (1951).

BLIX, G.: Zur Kenntnis der schwefelhaltigen Lipoidstoffe des Gehirns. Über Cerebronschwefelsäure. Hoppe-Seylers Z. physiol. Chem. **219**, 82—98 (1933). — BLIX, G.: Über die Kohlenhydratgruppen des Submaxillarismucins. Hoppe-Seylers Z. physiol. Chem. **240**, 43—45 (1936). — BLIX, G.: Einige Beobachtungen über eine hexosaminhaltige Substanz in der Protagon-Fraktion des Gehirns. Skand. Arch. Physiol. **80**, 46—51 (1938). — BLIX, G., L. SVENNERHOLM, and I. WERNER: The isolation of chondrosamine from gangliosides and from submaxillary mucin. Acta chem. scand. **6**, 358—362 (1952). — BODIAN, D., and D. DZIEWIATKOWSKI: The disposition of radioactive phosphorus in normal, as compared with regenerating and degenerating nervous tissue. J. cell. Comp. Physiol. **35**, 155—177 (1950). — BRADY, R. O., and G. J. KOVAL: The enzymatic synthesis of sphingosine. J. biol. Chem. **233**, 26—31 (1958).— BRANTE, G.: Filter paper chromatography in lipid analysis. Upsala Làk.-Foren, Forh. **53**, 301—308 (1948). — BURTON, R. M., M. A. SODD, and R. O. BRADY: The incorporation of galactose into galactolipides. J. biol. Chem. **233**, 1053—1060 (1958).

CARTER, H. E., and F. L. GREENWOOD: Biochemistry of the sphingolipides. VII. Structure of the cerebrosides. J. biol. Chem. **199**, 283—288 (1952). — CHIBNALL, A. C., S. H. PIPER, and E. F. WILLIAMS: The fatty acids of phrenosin and kerasin. Biochem. J. **30**, 100—114 (1936).

DAVISON, A. N., and M. WAJDA: Metabolism of myelin lipids: estimation and separation of brain lipids in the developing rabbit. J. Neurochem. In press. — DAWSON, R. M. C.: Studies on the labelling of brain phospholipids with radioactive phosphorus. Biochem. J. **57**, 237—245 (1954). — DAWSON, R. M. C.: Studies on the phosphorylcholine of rat liver. Biochem. J. **62**, 693—696 (1956). — DAWSON, R. M. C., and D. RICHTER: Phosphorus metabolism of the brain. Proc. roy. Soc. **137** B, 252—267 (1950). — DITTMER, J. C., and R. M. C. DAWSON: The isolation of a new lipid, triphosphoinositide, and monophosphoinositide from ox brain. Biochem. J. 81, 535 (1961). — DONALDSON, H.: The Rat. Memoirs. Wistar Inst. Anat. Biol. 6, 228—233 (1924).

EHRLICH, G., and H. WAELSCH: The position of the higher fatty acid metabolism of rat muscle. J. biol. Chem. 163, 195—202 (1946).

FINDLAY, M., W. L. MAGEE, and R. J. ROSSITER: Incorporation of radioactive phosphate into lipids and pentosenucleic acid of cat-brain slices. The effect of inorganic ions. Biochem. J. 58, 236—242 (1954). — FOLCH, J.: Brain cephalin, a mixture of phosphatides. Separation from it of phosphatidyl serine, phosphatidyl ethanolamine, and a fraction containing an inositol phosphatide. J. biol. Chem. 146, 35—44 (1942). — FOLCH, J.: The chemical structure of phosphatidyl serine. J. biol. Chem. 174, 439—450 (1948). — FOLCH, J., S. ARSOVE, and J. A. MEATH: Isolation of brain strandin. A new type of large molecule tissue component. J. biol. Chem. 191, 819—831 (1951). — FRIES, B. A., G. W. CHANGUS, and I. L. CHAIKOFF: Radioactive phosphorus as an indicator of phospholipoid metabolism. IX. The influence of age on the phospholipid metabolism of various parts of the central nervous system of the rat. The comparative phospholipid activity of various parts of the central nervous system of the rat. J. biol. Chem. 132, 23—34 (1940). — FRIES, B. A., H. SCHACHNER, and I. L. CHAIKOFF: The in vitro formation of phospholipid by brain and nerve with radioactive phosphorus as indicator. J. biol. Chem. 144, 59—66 (1942).

GEIGER, A., S. YAMASAKI, and R. LYONS: Changes in nitrogenous compounds of brain produced by stimulation of short duration. Amer. J. Physiol. 184, 239—243 (1956). — GIBSON, D. M., E. B. TICTCHENER, and S. J. WAKIL: Studies on the mechanism of fatty acid synthesis. V. Bicarbonate requirement for the synthesis of longchain fatty acids. Biochim. biophys. Acta 30, 376—383 (1958). — GOTTSCHALK, A.: Neuraminic acid; the functional group of some biologically active mucoproteins. Yale J. Biol. Med. 28, 525—537 (1956).

HOKIN, M. R., and L. E. HOKIN: Enzyme secretion and the incorporation of P^{32} into phospholipides of pancreas slices. J. biol. Chem. 203, 967—977 (1953). — HOKIN, L. E., and M. R. HOKIN: Effects of acetylcholine on the turnover of phosphoryl units in individual phospholipids of pancreas slices and brain cortex slices. Biochim. biophys. Acta. 18, 102—110 (1955).

KENNEDY, E. P., and S. B. WEISS: The function of cytidine coenzymes in the biosynthesis of phospholipides. J. biol. Chem. 222, 193—214 (1956a). — KENNEDY, E. P., and S. B. WEISS: The enzymatic synthesis of triglycerides. J. Amer. chem. Soc. 78, 3550 (1956b). — KLENK, E.: Über die Cerebroside des Gehirns. Hoppe-Seylers Z. physiol. Chem. 166, 268—286 (1927). — KLENK, E.: Neuraminic acid, the cleavage product of a new brain lipoid. Hoppe-Seylers Z. physiol. Chem. 268, 50—58 (1941). — KLENK, E.: Incorporation of ^{14}C-labelled acetate into some lipids of nervous tissue. In: Metabolism of the nervous system. 369—398. (D. RICHTER, Ed.). London: Pergamon Press 1957. — KLENK, E., and H. FAILLARD: Zur Kenntnis der Fettsäuren der Gehirncerebroside. Die Konstitution der ungesättigten Oxysäuren. Hoppe-Seylers Z. physiol. Chem. 292, 268—275 (1953). — KOREY, S. R., and M. ORCHEN: Plasmologens of the nervous system. Arch. Biochem. 83. In press. — KORNBERG, A., and W. E. PRICER JR.: Enzymatic synthesis of the coenzyme and derivatives of long chain fatty acids. J. biol. Chem. 204, 329—343 (1953a). — KORNBERG, A., and W. E. PRICER JR.: Enzymatic esterification of α-glycerophosphate by long chain fatty acids. J. biol. Chem. 204, 345—357 (1953b).

LEES, M., J. FOLCH, G. H. SLOANE STANLEY, and S. CARR: A simple procedure for the preparation of brain sulphatides. J. Neurochem. 4, 9—18 (1959). — LINDBERG, O., and L. ERNSTER: The turnover of radioactive phosphate injected into the subarachnoid space of the brain of the rat. Biochem. J. 46, 43—47 (1950). — LYNEN, F.: Fatty acid metabolism. In: Metabolism of the nervous system. 381—398. (D. RICHTER, Ed.). London: Pergamon Press 1957. — LYNEN, F., and S. OCHOA: Enzymes of fatty acid metabolism. Biochim. biophys. Acta 12, 299—314 (1953).

McCONNELL, P., and R. G. SINCLAIR: Evidence of selection in the building up of brain lecithins and cephalins. J. biol. Chem. 118, 131—136 (1937). — McMILLAN, P. J., G. W. DOUGLAS, and R. A. MORTENSEN: Incorporation of C^{14} of acetate -1-C^{14} and pyruvate-2-C^{14} into brain cholesterol in the intact rat. Proc. Soc. exp. Biol. (N. Y.) 96, 738—740 (1957). — McMURRAY, W. C., J. F. BERRY, and R. J. ROSSITER: Labelling of phospholipid phosphorus in rat-brain mitochondria. Biochem. J. 66, 629—633 (1957). — MAGEE, W. L., J. F. BERRY, and R. J. ROSSITER: Effect of chlorpromazine and azacyclonol on the labelling of phosphatides in brain slices. Biochim. biophys Acta 21, 408—409 (1956). — MAGEE, W. L., and R. J. ROSSITER: Chemical studies of peripheral nerve during Wallerian degeneration. 6. Incorporation of radioactive phosphate into pentosenucleic acid and phospholipin in vitro. Biochem. J. 58, 243—249 (1954). — MAJNO, G., and M. L. KARNOVSKY: A biochemical and morphologic study of myelination and demyelination. I. Lipide biosynthesis in vitro by normal nervous tissue. J. exp. Med. 107, 475—496 (1958). — MOSER, H., and M. L. KARNOVSKY: Studies on the biosynthesis of cerebroside galactose. Neurology (Minneap.) 8, Suppl. 1, 81—83 (1958).

PRITCHARD, E. T.: Labelling of different portions of phosphoglyceride molecule in rat liver and brain slices. Fed. Proc. 15, 330 (1956).

RAPPORT, M. M., and R. E. FRANZL: The structure of plasmogens. III. The nature and significance of the aldehydogenic linkage. J. Neurochem. 1, 303—310 (1957). — ROSENBERG, A., C. HOWE, and E. CHARGAFF: Inhibition of influenza virus haemagglutination by a brain lipid fraction. Nature (Lond.) 1956, 234—235. — ROSSITER, R. J.: Lipid metabolism. In: Metabolism of the nervous system. 355—380. (D. RICHTER, Ed.) London: Pergamon Press Ltd. 1957.

SCHNEIDER, W. C.: Mitochondrial metabolism. Advanc. Enzymol. 21, 1—72 (1959). — SPERRY, W. M., H. WAELSCH, and V. A. STOYANOFF: Lipid metabolism in brain and other tissues of the rat. J. biol. Chem. 135, 281—290 (1940). STETTEN JR., D.: Biological relationships of choline, ethanolamine and related compounds. J. biol. Chem. 140, 143—152 (1941). — STRICKLAND, K. P.: Factors affecting the incorporation of radioactive phosphate into the phospholipids of slices of cat brain. Canad. J. Biochem. 32, 50—59 (1954).

TAUROG, A., I. L. CHAIKOFF, and I. PERLAMAN: The effects of anaerobic conditions and respiratory inhibitors on the in vitro phospholipid formation in liver and kidney with radioactive phosphorus as indicator. J. biol. Chem. 145, 281—291 (1942). — TOMLINSON, R. V., and C. E. BALLOU: Complete characterization of the myo-inositol polyphosphates from beef brain phosphoinositide. J. biol. Chem. 236, 1902 (1961).

WAELSCH, H.: Myelinization and the synthesis of fatty acids and cholesterol. In: The biology of myelin. 265—270. (S. R. KOREY, Ed.). New York: Hoeber-Harper 1959. — WAELSCH H., W. M. SPERRY, and V. A. STOYANOFF: A study of the synthesis and deposition of lipids in brain and other tissues with deuterium as an indicator. J. biol. Chem. 135, 291—296 (1940). — WAELSCH, H., W. M. SPERRY, and V. A. STOYANOFF: The influence of growth and myelination on the deposition and metabolism in the brain. J. biol. Chem. 140, 885—897 (1941). — WATSON, J. B.: An experimental study on the psychical development of the white rat. Univ. Chicago Contrib. Phil. 4, 5—122 (1903). — WEISS, S. B., and E. P. KENNEDY: Enzymatic conversion of CDP-choline and CDP-ethanolamine to phospholipides. Fed. Proc. 15, 381 (1956). — WITTENBERG, J., and A. KORNBERG: Choline phospholinase. J. biol. Chem. 202, 431—443 1953).

F. Neurohumors

ACHESON, R. M., and A. R. HANDS: 6-Sulphatoxyskatole in human urine. Biochim. biophys. Acta 51, 579 (1961). — ACHESON, R. M.. R. M. PAUL, and R. V. TOMLINSON: Some constituents of the urine of normal and schizophrenic individuals. Canad. J. Biochem. 36. 295 (1958). — ADAM, H. M., R. A. McKAIL, S. OBRADOR, and W. C. WILSON: Acetylcholine in the cerebro-spinal fluid. J. Physiol. (Lond.) 93, 45 P (1938). — AMIN, A. H., T. B. B. CRAWFORD, and J. H. GADDUM: The distribution of substance P and 5-hydroxytryptamine in the central nervous system of the dog. J. Physiol. (Lond.) 126, 596 (1954). — ARMSTRONG, M. D., A. McMILLAN, and K. N. F. SHAW: 3-Methoxy-4-hydroxy-D-mandelic acid, a urinary metabolite of norepinephrine. Biochim. biophys. Acta 25, 422 (1957). — ARMSTRONG, M. D., K. N. F. SHAW, M. J. GORTATOWSKI, and H. SINGER: The indole acids of human urine. Paper chromatography of indole acids. J. biol. Chem. 232, 17 (1958). — AXELROD, J.: The metabolism of catecholamines in vivo and in vitro. Pharmacol. Rev. 11, 402—408 (1959). — AXELROD, J., S. SENOH, and B. WITKOP: O-Methylation of catechol amines in vivo. J. biol. Chem. 233, 697 (1958). — AXELROD, J., and R. TOMCHICK: Enzymatic O-methylation of epinephrine and other catechols. J. biol. Chem. 233, 702—705 (1958). — AXELROD, J., H. WEIL-MALHERBE, and R. TOMCHICK: The physiological disposition of H^3-epinephrine and its metabolite, metanephrine. J. Pharmacol. exp. Ther. 127, 251—256 (1959).

BANERJEE, S., and P. S. AGARWAL: Tryptophane-nicotonic acid metabolism in schizophrenia. Proc. Soc. exp. Biol. (N. Y.) 97, 657 (1958). — BENNETT, E. L., D. KRECH, M. R. ROSENZWEIG, H. KARLSSON, N. DYE, and A. OHLANDER: Cholinesterase and lactic dehydrogenase activity in the rat brain. J. Neurochem. 3, 153—160 (1958). — BENNETT, E. L., M. R. ROSENZWEIG, D. KRECH, H. KARLSSON, N. DYE, and A. OHLANDER: Individual, strain and age differences in cholinesterase activity of the rat brain. J. Neurochem. 3, 144—152 (1958) — BERGSMAN, A.: The urinary excretion of adrenaline and noradrenaline in some mental diseases. Acta psychiat. neurol. scand. 34, suppl. 133 (1959). — BERRY, J. F., and R. J. ROSSITER: Chemical studies of peripheral nerve during Wallerian degeneration. VIII. Acetic thiokinase and choline acetylase. J. Neurochem. 3, 59 (1958). — BERTLER, A., and E. ROSENGREN: Occurrence and distribution of dopamine in brain and other tissues. Experientia (Basel) 15, 10 (1959). — BIEL, J. H., A. E. DRUKKER, P. A. SHORE, S. SPECTOR, and B. B. BRODIE: Effect of 1-phenyl-2-hydrazinopropane, a potent monoamine oxidase inhibitor, on brain levels of norepinephrine and serotonin. J. Amer. chem. Soc. 80, 1519 (1958). — BLASCHKO, H., J. M. HAGEN, and P. HAGEN: Mitochondrial enzymes and chromaffine granules. J. Physiol. (Lond.) 139, 316—322 (1957). — BOGDANSKI, D. F., and S. UDENFRIEND: Serotonin and monoamine oxidase in brain. J. Pharmacol. 116, 7 (1956). — BOGDANSKI, D. F., H. WEISS-

Bach and S. Udenfriend: The distribution of serotonin, 5-hydroxytryptophane decarboxylase and monoamine oxidase in brain. J. Neurochem. 1, 272 (1957). — Bogoch, S.: Effect of synthetic diet low in aromatic amino acids on schizophrenic patients. Arch. Neurol. Psychiat. (Chicago) 78, 539 (1957). — Brengelmann, J. D., C. M. B. Pare, and M. Sandler: Alleviation of the psychological effects of LSD in man by 5-hydroxytryptophan. J. ment. Sci. 104, 1237 (1958). — Brodie, B. B., J. S. Olin, R. G. Kuntzman, and P. A. Shore: Possible interrelationship between release of brain norepinephrine and serotonin by reserpine. Science 125, 1293 (1957). — Brodie, B. B., A. Pletscher, and P. A. Shore: Possible role of serotonin in brain function and in reserpine action. J. Pharmacol. 116, 9 (1956). — Brodie, B. B., A. Pletscher, and P. A. Shore: Evidence that serotonin has a role in brain function. Science 122, 968 (1955). — Brodie, B. B., S. Spector, R. G. Kuntzman, and P. A. Shore: Rapid biosynthesis of brain serotonin before and after reserpine administration. Naturwissenschaften 45, 243 (1958). — Brown, G. L., H. H. Dale, and W. Feldberg: Reactions of the normal mammalian muscle to acetylcholine and eserine. J. Physiol. (Lond.) 87, 394 (1936). — Bruce, L. C.: The clinical significance of indoxyl in the urine. J. ment. Sci. 52, 501—505 (1906). — Bülbring, E., and H. H. Burn: Observations bearing on synaptic transmission by acetylcholine in spinal cord. J. Physiol. (Lond.) 100, 337—368 (1941). — Bulle, P. H., and L. Konchegul: Action of serotonin and cerebral fluid of schizophrenics on the brain of the dog. J. clin. exp. Psychopath. 18, 287 (1957). — Burgen, A. S. V., and L. M. Chipman: Cholinesterase and succinic dehydrogenase in the central nervous system of the dog. J. Physiol. (Lond.) 114, 296—305 (1951). — Burgen, A. S. V., and F. C. MacIntosh: Physiological significance of acetylcholine. In: Neurochemistry p. 311. (K. A. C. Elliott, I. H. Page, and J. H. Quastel, Ed.) Springfield, Ill.: C. C. Thomas 1955. — Buscaino, V. M.: Pathogénèsc et étiologie biologiques de la schizophrénie. Acta Neurol. (Naples) 16, 1—26 (1958). — Buscaino, G. A., and L. Stefanachi: Urinary excretion of 5-hydroxyindoleacetic acid in psychotic and normal subjects. Arch. Neurol. Psychiat. (Chicago) 80, 78 (1958).

Carlsson, A., M. Lindqvist, and T. Magnusson: 3,4-Dihydroxyphenylalanine and 5-hydroxytryptophan as reserpine antagonists. Nature (Lond.) 180, 1200 (1957). — Carlsson, A., M. Lindqvist, T. Magnusson, and B. Waldeck: On the presence of 3-hydroxytyramine in brain. Science 127, 471 (1958). — Cerletti, A., and E. Rothlin: Role of 5-hydroxytryptamine in mental diseases and its antagonism to lysergic acid derivatives. Nature (Lond.) 176, 785 (1955). — Chang, H. C., K. F. Chia, C. H. Hsu, and R. K. S. Lim: Humoral transmission of nerve impulses at central synapses. I. Sinus and vagus afferent nerves. Chin. J. Physiol. 12, 1—36 (1937). — Chang, H. C., W. M. Hsieh, T. H. Li, and R. K. S. Lim: Humoral transmission of nerve impulses at central synapses. IV. Liberation of acetylcholine into the cerebrospinal fluid by the afferent vagus. Chin. J. Physiol. 13, 153—166 (1938). — Chute, A. L., W. Feldberg, and D. H. Smyth: Liberation of acetylcholine from the perfused cat's brain. Quart. J. exp. Physiol. 30, 65—72 (1940). — Cohen, M.: Concentration of choline acetylase in conducting tissue. Arch. Biochem. 60, 284 (1956). — Cohen, G., B. Holland, and M. Goldenberg: The stability of epinephrine and arterenol in plasma and serum. Arch. Neurol. Psychiat. (Chicago) 80, 484 (1958). — Cooper, J. R., and I. Melcer: The enzymic oxidation of tryptophan to 5-hydroxytryptophan in the biosynthesis of serotonin. J. Pharmacol. 132, 265 (1961). — Corne, S. J., and J. D. P. Graham: The effect of inhibition of amine oxidase in vivo on administered adrenaline, noradrenaline, tyramine and serotonin. J. Physiol. (Lond.) 135, 339 (1957). — Costa, E.: Effects of hallucinogenic and tranquilizing drugs on serotonin-evoked uterine contractions. Proc. Soc. exp. Biol. (N. Y.) 91, 39 (1956). — Crane, G. E.: Further studies on iproniazid phosphate. J. nerv. ment. Dis. 124, 322 (1956). — Crossland, J., K. A. C. Elliott, and H. M. Pappius: Acetylcholine content of brain during insulin hypoglycaemia. Amer. J. Physiol. 183, 32 (1955). — Crossland, J., and A. J. Merrick: The effect of anaesthesia on the acetylcholine content of brain. J. Physiol. (Lond.) 125, 56 (1954).

Dale, H. H.: The action of certain esters and ethers of choline and their relation to muscarine. J. Pharmacol. 6, 147 (1914). — Dale, H. H.: Junctional transmission of nervous effects by chemical agents. Proc. Mayo Clin. 30, 5—20 (1955). — Dale, H. H., W. Feldberg, and M. Vogt: Release of acetylcholine at voluntary motor nerve endings. J. Physiol. (Lond.) 86, 353 (1936).

Elliott, T. R.: The action of adrenaline. J. Physiol. (Lond.) 32, 401 (1905). — Elmadjian, F., J. M. Hope, and E. T. Lamson: Excretion of epinephrine and norepinephrine in various emotional states. J. clin. Endocrinol. 17, 608 (1957). — Elmadjian, F., J. M. Hope, and E. T. Lamson: Excretion of epinephrine and norepinephrine under stress. Recent Progr. Hormone Res. 14, 513—553 (1958). — Erspamer, V.: Pharmakologische Studien über Enteramin: II. Mitteilung. über einige Eigenschaften des Enteramins, sowie über die Abgrenzung des Enteramins von den anderen kreislaufwirksamen Gewebsprodukten. Naunyn-Schmiedebergs Arch. exp. Path. Pharmak. 196, 366—390 (1940). — Erspamer, V.: The metabolism of endogenous 5-hydroxytryptamine (enteramine) in the rat. Experientia (Basel) 10, 471 (1954). —

ERSPAMER, V., and B. ASERO: Identity of enteramine, the specific hormone of the entero-chromaffin cell system as 5-hydroxytryptamine. Nature (Lond.) **169**, 800—801 (1952). — EULER, U. S., v.: A specific sympathomimetic ergone in adrenergic nerve fibres (sympathin) and its relation to adrenaline and noradrenaline. Acta physiol. scand. **12**, 73—97 (1946). — EULER, U. S., v.: Identification of the sympathomimetic ergone in adrenergic nerves of cattle (sympathin N) with laevo-noradrenaline. Acta physiol. scand. **16**, 63—74 (1948). — EULER, U. S., v.: Noradrenaline. Springfield, Ill.: Charles C. Thomas 1956. — EULER, U. S. v., and N.-Å. HILLARP: Evidence for the presence of noradrenaline in submicroscopic structures of adrenergic axons. Nature (Lond.) **177**, 45 (1956). — EULER, U. S. v., and F. LISHAJKO: Dopamine in mammalian lung and spleen. Acta physiol. pharmacol. neerl. **6**, 295 (1957). — EULER, U. S. v., and U. LUNDBERG: Effect of flying on the epinephrinexcretion in Air Force personnel. J. Appl. Physiol. **6**, 551 (1954). — EVARTS, E. V.: Some effects of bufotenine and lysergic acid diethylamide on the monkey. Arch. Neurol. Psychiat. (Chicago) **75**, 49—53 (1956).

FALCK, B., N.-Å. HILLARP, and B. HOGBERG: Content and intracellular distribution of adenosine triphosphate in cow adrenal medulla. Acta physiol. scand. **36**, 360—376 (1956). — FELDBERG, W.: Acetylcholine. In: Metabolism of the nervous system. p. 493. (Ed. D. RICHTER) New York: Pergamon Press 1957. — FELDBERG, W., and J. H. GADDUM: The chemical trans-mitter at synapses in a sympathetic ganglion. J. Physiol. **81**, 305 (1934). — FELDBERG, W., and T. MANN: Properties and distribution of the enzyme system which synthesizes acetyl-choline in nervous tissue. J. Physiol. **104**, 411—425 (1946). — FELDBERG, W., and H. SCHRIE-VER: Acetylcholine content of cerebrospinal fluid of dogs. J. Physiol. **86**, 277—284 (1936). — FELDBERG, W., and M. VOGT: Acetylcholine synthesis in different regions of the central nervous system. J. Physiol. **107**, 372—381 (1948). — FELDSTEIN, A., I. M. DIBNER, and H. HOAGLAND: Two-dimensional paper chromatography of urinary indoles in normal subjects and chronic schizophrenic patients. In: Chemical concepts of psychosis. p. 204—218. (Eds. M. RINKEL and H. C. B. DENBER). New York: McDowell-Obolensky 1958. — FELDSTEIN, A., H. HOAGLAND, and H. FREEMAN: On the relationship of serotonin to schizophrenia. Science **128**, 358 (1958). — FREEDLAND, R. A., I. M. WADZINSKI, and A. WAISMAN: The enzymatic hydroxylation of tryptophan. Biochem. biophys. Res. Commun. **5**, 94 (1961a). — FREEDLAND, R. A., I. M. WADZINSKI, and H. A. WAISMAN: The effect of aromatic amino acids on the hydroxylation of tryptophan. Biochem. biophys. Res. Commun. **6**, 227 (1961b). — FOLIN, O.: Some meta-bolism studies, with special reference to mental disorders. Amer. J. Insan. **61**, 299—364 (1904). — FUKUDA, T., and G. B. KOELLE: The cytological localization of intracellular neu-ronal acetylcholinesterase. J. biophys. biochem. Cytol. **5**, 433—440 (1959).

GADDUM, J. H., and K. A. HAMEED: Drugs which antagonize 5-hydroxytryptamine. Brit. J. Pharmacol. **9**, 240 (1954). — GIARMAN, N. J., and S. SCHANBERG: The intracellular distri-bution of 5-hydroxytryptamine in the rat's brain. Biochem. Pharmacol. **1**, 301 (1959). — GODDARD, P. J.: Effect of alcohol on excretion of catechol amines in conditions giving rise to anxiety. J. appl. Physiol. **13**, 118 (1958). — GOLDSTEIN, M., and F. CONTRERA: Inhibi-tion of dopamine β-oxidase by imipramine. Biochem. Pharmacol. **7**, 278 (1961). — GOLDSTEIN, M., A. J. FRIEDHOFF, and C. SIMMONS: Metabolic pathways of 3-hydroxy-tyramine. Biochim. biophys. Acta **33**, 572 (1959). — GOODALL, McC.: Metabolic products of adrenaline and noradrenaline in human urine. Pharmacol. Rev. **11**, 416—425 (1959). — GOODALL, McC., and N. KIRSHNER: Biosynthesis of adrenaline and noradrenaline in vitro. J. biol. Chem. **226**, 213 (1957). — GOODMAN, J. R., L. H. MARRONE, and M. C. SQUIRE: Effect of in vivo inhibition of cholinesterase on potassium diffusion from the human red cell. Amer. J. Physiol. **180**, 118 (1955). — GREEN, D. E.: Enzymes in metabolic sequences. In: Chemical pathways of metabolism. p. 27—65. (Ed. D. M. GREENBERG). New York: Acad. Press Inc. 1954. — GRUNDFEST, H.: Electrical inexcitability of synapses and some consequences in the central nervous system. Physiol. Rev. **37**, 337—361 (1957). — GULLOTTA, S.: Untersuchungen über den Harn von Amentia- und Dementia praecox-Kranken. Zyklische Komplexe (Beitrag zum Studium der Aromaturie). Biochem. Z. **218**, 472 (1930).

HAGEN, P.: Biosynthesis of norepinephrine from 3,4-dihydroxyphenylethylamine (dop-amine). J. Pharmacol. exp. Ther. **116**, 26 (1956). — HAWKINS, R. D., and B. MENDEL: True cholin-esterases with pronounced resistance to eserine. J. cell comp. Physiol. **27**, 69—85 (1946). — HAWKINS, R. D., and B. MENDEL: Selective inhibition of pseudocholinesterase by di-iso-propylfluorophosphonate. Brit. J. Pharmacol. **2**, 173—180 (1947). — HAWKINS, R. D., and B. MENDEL: Cholinesterase. VI. Selective inhibition of true cholinesterase in vivo. Biochem. J. **44**, 260 (1949). — HERKEN, H., and D. NEUBERT: Der Acetylcholingehalt des Gehirns bei verschiedenen Funktionszuständen. Naunyn-Schmiedebergs Arch. exp. Path. Pharmak. **219**, 223 (1953). — HESS, S. M., R. H. CONNAMACHER, M. OZAKI, and S. UDENFRIEND: The effects of α-methyl-dopa and α-methyl-meta-tyrosine on the metabolism of norepinephrine and serotonin in vivo. J. Pharmacol. **134**, 129 (1961). — HILLARP, N.-A., and B. HOKFELT: Evidence of adrenaline and noradrenaline in separate adrenal medullary cells. Acta physiol. scand. **30**, 55—68 (1953). — HILLARP, N.-Å., and B. HOKFELT: Cytological demonstration of noradrenaline in the suprarenal medulla under conditions of varied secretory activity. Endocrinology **55**, 255—260 (1954). — HILLARP, N.-Å., and B. HÓK-FELT: Histochemical demonstration of noradrenaline and adrenaline in the adrenal medulla. J. Histochem. Cytochem. **3**, 1—5 (1955). — HODGKIN, A. L.: The ionic basis of electrical activity in nerve and muscle. Biol. Rev. **26**, 339—409 (1951). — HOFFER, A.: Adrenochrome and adrenolutin and their relationship to mental disease. In: Psychotropic drugs. p. 127—140. (Eds. S. GARATTINI and V. GHETTI). New York: Elsevier 1957. — HOFFER, A.: Adrenochrome in blood plasma. Amer. J. Psychiat. **114**, 752—753 (1958). — HOFFER, A., and H. OSMOND: The adrenochrome model and schizophrenia. J. nerv. ment. Dis. **128**,18-35(1959).—HOFFER, A., H. OSMOND, and J. SMYTHIES: Schizophrenia: a new approach. Part II. Result of a year's research. J. ment. Sci. **100**, 29—45 (1954). — HOKIN, L. E., and M. R. HOKIN: Acetylcholine and the exchange of phosphate in phosphatidic acid in brain microsomes. J. biol. Chem. **233**, 822 (1958). — HOKIN, L. E., and M. R. HOKIN: The mechanism of phosphate exchange in phosphatidic acid in response to acetylcholine. J. biol. Chem. **234**, 1387 (1959). — HOLTZ, P., H. BALZER, and W. WESTERMANN: Die Beeinflussung der Reserpinwirkung auf das Nebennierenmark durch Hemmung der Mono-amino-oxydase. Naunyn-Schmiedebergs Arch. exp. Path. Pharmak. **231**, 361—372 (1957). — HOLTZ, P., H. BALZER, E. WESTERMANN, and E. WEZLER: Beeinflussung der Evipannarkose durch Reserpin, Iproniazid und biogene Amine. Naunyn-Schmiedebergs Arch. exp. Path. Pharmak. **231**, 333 (1957). — HOLTZ, P., and E. WESTERMANN: Über die Dopadecarboxylase und Histidindecarboxylase des Nervengewebes. Naunyn-Schmiedebergs Arch. exp. Path. Pharmak. **227**, 538 (1956). — HOLZBAUER, M., and M. VOGT: Depression by reserpine of the noradrenaline concentration in the hypothalamus of the cat. J. Neurochem. **1**, 8—11 (1956). — HORITA, A.: β-Phenylisopropylhydrazine, a potent and long acting monoamine oxidase inhibitor. J. Pharmacol. **122**, 176 (1958). — HORITA, A., and J. H. GOGERTY: The pyretogenic effect of 5-hydroxytryptophan and its comparison with that of LSD. J. Pharmacol. exp. Ther. **122**, 195 (1958).

IGGO, A., and M. VOGT: The effect of reserpine on the electrical activity in preganglionic sympathetic fibres. J. Physiol. (Lond.) **147**, 14 P (1959).

JACKSON, S. L. O.: Psychosis due to isoniazid. Brit. med. J. **1957**, II 743.

KAMIJO, K., Koelle, G. B., and H. H. WAGNER: Modification of the effects of sympathomimetic amines and of adrenergic nerve stimulation by 1-isonicotinyl-2-isopropylhydrazine (IIH) and isonicotinic acid hydrazide (INH). J. Pharmacol. exp. Ther. **117**, 213 (1956). — KEMALI, D., and V. M. BUSCAINO: Indolic substances in schizophrenic patients. In: Chemical concepts of psychosis. p. 219—222. (Eds. M. RINKEL, and H. C. B. DENBER). New York: McDowell-Obolensky 1958. — KEYNES, R. D.: Electrolytes and nerve activity. In: Metabolism of the nervous system. p. 159—173. (Ed. D. RICHTER) New York: Pergamon Press 1957. — KIBJAKOW, A. W.: Über humorale Übertragung der Erregung von einem Neuron auf das andere. Pflügers Arch. ges. Physiol. **232**, 432 (1933). — KIRSHNER, N., and McC. GOODALL: Formation of adrenaline from noradrenaline. Fed. Proc. **16**, 73 (1957). — KOELLE, G. B.: The localization of acetylcholinesterase in neurons. In: Ultrastructure and cellular chemistry of neural tissue. p. 164—173. (Ed. H. WAELSCH), New York: Hoeber-Harper 1957. — KOELLE, W. A., and G. B. KOELLE: The localization of external or functional acetylcholinesterase at the synapses of autonomic ganglia. J. Pharmacol. exp. Ther. **126**, 1—8 (1959). — KOPIN, I. J.: Tryptophane loading and excretion of 5-hydroxyindoleacetic acid in normal and schizophrenic subjects. Science **129**, 853 (1959).

LEACH, B. E., and R. G. HEATH: The in vitro oxidation of epinephrine in plasma. A. M. A. Arch. Neurol. Psychiat. **76**, 444—450 (1956). — LEVIN, E. Y., B. LEVENBERG, and S. KAUFMAN: The enzymatic conversion of 3,4-dihydroxyphenylethylamine to norepinephrine. J. biol. Chem. **235**, 2080 (1960). — LEWIS, P. R., and A. F. W. HUGHES: The cholinesterase of developing neurones of Xenopus laevis. In: Metabolism of the nervous system. p. 511—514 (Ed. D. RICHTER) New York: Pergamon Press 1957. — LEYTON, G. B.: Indolic compounds in the urine of schizophrenics. Brit. med. J. **1958** II, 1136. — LIPMANN, F., and N. O. KAPLAN: Report on a coenzyme for acetylation. Fed. Proc. **5**, 145 (1946). — LOEWI, O.: Über humorale Übertragbarkeit der Herznervenwirkung. Pflügers Arch. ges. Physiol. **189**, 239—242 (1921).

MacINTOSH, F. C.: Formation, storage and release of acetylcholine at nerve endings. Canad. J. Biochem. **37**, 343—356 (1959). — MacINTOSH, F. C., R. I. BIRKS, and P. B. SASTRY: Pharmacological inhibition of acetylcholine synthesis. Nature (Lond.) **178**, 1181 (1956). — MacINTOSH, F. C., and P. E. OBORIN: Abstr. XIX. Internal. Physiol. Congr. 580 (1953). — MANN, P. J. G., and J. H. QUASTEL: Benzedrine (β-phenylisopropylamine) and brain metabolism. Biochem. J. **34**, 414—431 (1940). — MANN, P. J. G., M. TENNENBAUM, and J. H. QUASTEL: On the mechanism of acetylcholine formation in brain in vitro. Biochem. J. **32**, 243—261 (1938). — MANN, P. J. G., M. TENNENBAUM, and J. H. QUASTEL: Acetylcholine metabolism in the central nervous system. The effects of potassium and other cations on acetylcholine liberation. Biochem. J. **33**, 822—835 (1939). — MARRAZZI, A. S., and E. R. HART:

Relationship of hallucinogens to adrenergic cerebral neurohumors. Science **121**, 365 (1955). — McGEER, E. G., W. T. BROWN, and P. L. McGEER: Aromatic metabolism in schizophrenia, II. Bidimensional urinary chromatograms. J. nerv. ment. Dis. **125**, 176 (1957). — McGEER, P. L., E. G.McGEER, and J. E. BOULDING: Relation of aromatic amino acids to excretory pattern of schizophrenics. Science **123**, 1078—1080 (1956). — McGEER, P. L., F. E. McNAIR, E. G. McGEER, and W. C. GIBSON: Aromatic metabolism in schizophrenia. I. Statistical evidence for aromaturia. J. nerv. ment. Dis. **125**, 166 (1957). — McLENNAN, H., and K. A. C. ELLIOTT: Factors affecting the synthesis of acetylcholine by brain slices. Amer. J. Physiol. **163**, 605—613 (1950). — McLENNAN, H., and K. A. C. ELLIOTT: Effects of convulsant and narcotic drugs on acetylcholine synthesis. J.Pharmacol.exp.Ther.**103**,35(1951).—MONTAGU,K.A.:Catechol compounds in rat tissues and in brains of different animals. Nature (Lond.) **180**, 244—245 (1957). — MUSCHOLL, E., and M. VOGT: The action of reserpine on the peripheral sympathetic system. J. Physiol. (Lond.) **141**, 132 (1958).

NACHMANSOHN, D.: On the role of acetylcholine in the mechanism of nerve activity. In: Recent progress in hormone research vol. I, 1—26. (Ed. G. PINCUS), Academic Press, Inc. 1947. — NACHMANSOHN, D.: Symposium on the physiology of acetylcholine. I. The role of acetylcholine in conduction. Johns Hopk. Hosp. Bull. **83**, 463—493 (1948). — NACHMANSOHN, D.: Metabolism and function of the nerve cell. In: Neurochemistry, p. 390—425. (Ed. K. A. C. ELLIOTT, I. H. PAGE, and J. H. QUASTEL). Springfield, Ill.: Charles C. Thomas 1955. — NACHMANSOHN, D.: Chemical and molecular basis of nerve activity. New York: Academic Press 1959. — NACHMANSOHN, D., and M. BERMAN: Studies on choline acetylase. III. On the preparation of the coenzyme and its effect on the enzyme. J. biol. Chem. **165**, 551—563 (1946).— NACHMANSOHN, D., and A. L. MACHADO: The formation of acetylcholine. A new enzyme: "choline acetylase". J. Neurophysiol. **6**, 397—404 (1943). — NAKAO, A., and M. BALL: The appearance of a skatole derivative in the urine of schizophrenics. J. nerv. ment. Dis. **130**, 417 (1960). — NERI, R., M. HAYANO, D. STONE, R. I. DORFMAN, and F. ELMADJIAN: Conversion of hydroxytyramine to norepinephrine-like material. Arch. Biochem. **60**, 297 (1956). — NOVELLI, G. D.: Metabolic functions of pantothenic acid. Physiol. Rev. **33**, 525—543 (1953).

ORLANS, B. F., F. SULSER, and B. B. BRODIE: Depletion of brain norepinephrine by reserpine without producing sedation. Fed. Proc. **19**, 268 (1960). — OSMOND, H., and J. SMYTHIES: Schizophrenia: A new approach. J. ment. Sci. **98**, 309—315 (1952).

PAASONEN, M. K., and N. J. GIARMAN: Brain levels of 5-hydroxytryptamine after various agents. Arch. int. Pharmacodyn. **114**, 189 (1958). — PAASONEN, M. K., P. D. MacLEAN, and N. J. GIARMAN: 5-Hydroxytryptamine content of structures of the limbic system. J. Neurochem. **1**, 326 (1957). — PAPPIUS, H. M., and K. A. C. ELLIOTT: Acetylcholine metabolism in normal and epileptogenic brain tissues. Failure to repeat previous findings. J. appl. Physiol. **12**, 319 (1958). — PELLERIN, J., and A. D'IORIO: Metabolism of DL-3,4-dihydroxyphenylalanine-α-C^{14} in bovine adrenal homogenate. Canad. J. Biochem. **35**, 151 (1957). — PLEASURE, H.: Psychiatric and neurological side-effects of isoniazid and iproniazid. Arch. Neurol. Psychiat. **72**, 313 (1954). — PLETSCHER, A., P. A. SHORE, and B. B. BRODIE: Release of brain serotonin by reserpine. J. Pharmacol. **116**, 46 (1956). — PLETSCHER, A., P. A. SHORE, and B. B. BRODIE: Serotonin as a mediator of reserpine action in brain. J. Pharmacol. **116**, 84—89 (1956). — POPE, A., W. CAVENESS, and K. E. LIVINGSTON: Architectonic distribution of acetylcholinesterase in the frontal isocortex of psychotic and nonpsychotic patients. Arch. Neurol. Psychiat. **68**, 425 (1952). — PORTER, C. C., J. A. TOTARO, and C. M. LEIBY: Some biochemical effects of α-methyl-3,4-dihydroxyphenylalanine and related compounds in mice. J. Pharmacol. **134**, 139 (1961). — PRICE, J. M., R. R. BROWN, and H. A. PETERS: Tryptophan metabolism in porphyria, schizophrenia and a variety of neurologic and psychiatric diseases. Neurology **9**, 456 (1959).

QUASTEL, J. H., M. TENNENBAUM, and A. H. M. WHEATLEY: Choline ester formation in, and choline esterase activities of, tissues in vitro. Biochem. J. **30**, 1668—1681 (1936).

RAPER, H. S.: The tyrosinase-tyrosine reaction. VI. Production from tyrosine of 5,6-dihydroxyindole and 5:6-dihydroxyindole-2-carboxylic acid - the precursors of melanine. Biochem. J. **21**, 89 (1927). — RAPPORT, M. M., A. A. GREEN, and I. H. PAGE: Serum vasoconstrictor (serotonin): Part IV. Isolation and characterization. J. biol. Chem. **176**, 1243—1251 (1948). — RENSON, J., F. GOODWIN, H. WEISSBACH and S. UDENFRIEND: Conversion of tryptophan to 5-hydroxytryptophan by phenylalanine hydroxylase. Biochem. biophys. Res. Commun. **6**, 20(1961).—RESNICK,O., and F.ELMADJIAN:Excretion and metabolism of DL-epinephrine-7-C^{14} D-bitartrate infused into schizophrenic patients. Amer. J. Physiol. **187**, 626 (1956). — RICHTER, D., and J. CROSSLAND: Variation in acetylcholine content of the brain with physiological state. Amer. J. Physiol. **159**, 247 (1949). — RIEGELHAUPT, L. M.: Investigations of the urinary excretion pattern in psychotic patients. J. nerv. ment. Dis. **127**, 228 (1958). — RINKEL, M., R. W. HYDE, and H. C. SOLOMON: Experimental psychiatry, III. A chemical concept of psychosis. Dis. nerv. Syst. **15**, 259 (1954). — ROBINS, E., I. P. LOWE, and N. M. HAVNER:

The urinary excretion of 5-hydroxy-3-indoleacetic acid in patients with schizophrenia and in control subjects. Clin. Res. Proc. 4, 149 (1956). — RODNIGHT, R., and E. K. AVES: Body fluid indoles of normal and mentally-ill subjects. I. Preliminary survey of the occurrence of some urinary indoles. J. ment Sci. 104, 1149—1159 (1958). — ROSENFELD, F., L. C. LEEPER, and S. UDENFRIEND: Biosynthesis of norepinephrine and epinephrine by the isolated, perfused calf adrenal. Fed. Proc. 16, 331 (1957). — ROSENGREN, E.: Are dihydroxyphenylalanine decarboxylase and 5-hydroxytryptophan decarboxylase individual enzymes? Acta physiol. scand. 49, 364 (1960). — ROSENZWEIG, M. R., D. KRECH, and E. L. BENNETT: Brain chemistry and adaptive behavior. In: Biological and biochemical bases of behavior. p. 367—400. (Ed. H. F. HARLOW and C. N. WOOLSEY,) Univ. of Wisconsin Press 1958.

SALMOIRAGHI, G. C., and I. H. PAGE: Effects of LSD-25, BOL-148, bufotenine, mescaline and ibogaine on the potentiation of hexobarbital hypnosis produced by serotonin and reserpine. J.Pharmacol.exp.Ther.120,20(1957).—SANO,I.: Über die kalte Millon-Reaktion beim schizophrenen Formenkreis und den Träger derselben. Folia psychiat. neurol. jap. 8, 218 (1954). — SANO, I., T.GAMO, Y. KAKIMOTO, K. TANIGUCHI, M. TAKESADA, and K. NISHINUMA,: Distribution of catechol compounds in human brain. Biochim. biophys. Acta 32, 586 (1959). — SANO, I., Y. KAKIMOTO, T. OKAMOTO, H. NAKAJIMA, and Y. KUDO: 5-Hydroxyindoleacetic acid (HIAA) excretion in the urine of schizophrenics with reference to the influence of reserpine and chlorpromazine on serotonin (5-HT) metabolism. Schweiz. med. Wschr. 87, 214 (1957). — SCHAYER, R. W., and R. L. SMILEY: The metabolism of epinephrine containing isotopic carbon. J. biol. Chem. 202, 425—430 (1953). — SCHMITT, H., and P. GONNARD: Action de l'iproniazide sur les effets des sympathicomimétiques sur la membrane nictitante du chat. C. R. Acad. Sci. 240, 2573—2575 (1955). — SCHNECKLOTH, R., I. H. PAGE, F. DEL GRECO, and A. C. CORCORAN: Effects of serotonin antagonists in normal subjects and patients with carcinoid tumors. Circulation 16, 523—532 (1957). — SCHÜMANN, H. J.: The distribution of adrenaline and noradrenaline in chromaffin granules from the chicken. J. Physiol. (Lond.) 137, 318—326 (1957).— SCHÜMANN, H. J.: Über die Verteilung von Noradrenalin und Hydroxytyramin im sympathischen Nerven (Milznerven). Naunyn-Schmiedebergs Arch. exp. Path. Pharmak. 234, 17 (1958). — SHAW, E., and D. W. WOOLLEY: Serotonin-like activities of lysergic acid diethylamide (LSD-25) Science 124, 121 (1956). — SHERWOOD, S. L.: The response of psychotic patients to intraventricular injections. Proc. roy. Soc. Med. 48, 855 (1955). — SHOJE, T., M. OHASHI, and S. TADA: Millon reaction at room temperature on the urine of schizophrenic patients. Jap. J. Neurol. Psychiat. 58, 19 (1956). — SHORE, P. A., J. A. R. MEAD, R. G. KUNTZMAN, S. SPECTOR, and B. B. BRODIE: On the physiologic significance of monoamine oxidase in brain. Science 126, 1063 (1957). — SHORE, P. A., S. L. SILVER, and B. B. BRODIE: Interaction of reserpine, serotonin and lysergic acid diethylamide in brain. Science 122, 284—285 (1955). — SJOERDSMA, A., L. GILLESPIE JR., and S. UDENFRIEND: A simple method for the measurement of monoamine oxidase inhibition in man. Lancet 1958 II, 159. — SPIRO, M. J., and E. G. BALL: Adrenal cytochromes. Fed. Proc. 17, 314 (1958). — SPRINCE, H., E. HOUSER, D. JAMESON, and F. C. DOHAN: Differential extraction of indoles from the urine of schizophrenic and normal subjects. Arch. gen. Psychiat. 3, 268 (1960). — SPRINCE, H., C. M. PARKER, D. JAMESON, J. T. DAWSON, jr., M. KNOWLTON, and F. C. DOHAN: Detection and isolation of indole acetamide from human urine: results with schizophrenic and normal subjects. J. Lab. clin. Med. 57, 763 (1961). — STONE, W. E.: Acetylcholine in the brain. I. "Free", "bound" and total acetylcholine. Arch. Biochem. 59, 181—192 (1955). — STRICKLAND, K. P., and R. H. S. THOMPSON: On the mechanism of the potassium loss from brain slices induced by cholinesterase inhibitors. Biochem. J. 60, 468 (1955). — STRÖM-OLSEN, R., and H. WEIL-MALHERBE: Humoral changes in manic depressive psychosis with particular reference to the excretion of catechol amines in urine. J. ment. Sci. 104, 696—704 (1958). — SZÁRA, S., J. AXELROD, and S. PERLIN: Is adrenochrome present in the blood? Amer. J. Psychiat. 115, 162—163 (1958).

TAUBMANN, G.,v.,and H. JANTZ: Untersuchungen über die dem Adrenochrom zugeschriebenen psychotoxischen Wirkungen. Nervenarzt 20, 485—488 (1957). — TAYLOR, I. M., J. M. WELLER, and A. B. HASTINGS: Effect of cholinesterase and cholinacetylase inhibitors on the potassium concentration gradient and potassium exchange of human erythrocytes. Amer. J. Physiol. 168, 658 (1952). — TOMAN, J. E. P., J. W. WOODBURY, and L. A. WOODBURY: Mechanism of nerve conduction block produced by anticholinesterases. J. Neurophysiol. 10, 429 (1947). — TOSCHI, G.: A biochemical study of brain microsomes. Exp. Cell Res. 16, 232—255 (1959). — TOWNSEND, A. A. D.: Mental depression and melancholia considered in regard to auto-intoxication, with special reference to the presence of indoxyl in the urine and its clinical significance. J. ment. Sci. 51, 51—62 (1905). — TWAROG, B. M., and I. H. PAGE: Serotonin content of some mammalian tissues and urine and a method for its determination. Amer. J. Physiol. 175, 157—161 (1953).

UDENFRIEND, S., D. F. BOGDANSKI, and H. WEISSBACH: Biochemistry and metabolism of serotonin as it relates to the nervous system. In: Metabolism of the nervous system. p. 566—577

(Ed. D. RICHTER), New York: Pergamon Press 1957. — UDENFRIEND, S., and H. WEISSBACH: Turnover of 5-hydroxytryptamine (serotonin) in tissues. Proc. Soc. exp. Biol. (N. Y.) **97**, 748 (1958). — UDENFRIEND, S., H. WEISSBACH, and D. F. BOGDANSKI: Increase in tissue serotonin following administration of its precursor 5-hydroxytryptophan. J. biol. Chem. **224**, 803 (1957). — UDENFRIEND, S., H. WEISSBACH, and D. F. BOGDANSKI: Effect of iproniazid on serotonin metabolism in vivo. J. Pharmacol. exp. Ther. **120**, 255 (1957). — UDENFRIEND, S., and J. B. WYNGAARDEN: Precursors of adrenal epinephrine and norepinephrine in vivo. Biochim. biophys. Acta **20**, 48 (1956).

VOGT, M.: The concentration of sympathin in different parts of the central nervous system under normal conditions and after the administration of drugs. J. Physiol. (Lond.) **123**, 451 (1954).—VOGT, M.: Sympathomimetic amines in the central nervous system. Brit. med. Bull. **13**, 166—171 (1957).

WALASZEK, E., and L. G. ABOOD: Fixation of 5-hydroxytryptamine by brain mitochondria. Proc. Soc. exp. Biol. (N. Y.) **101**, 37 (1959). — WEIL-MALHERBE, H.: The effect of convulsive therapy on plasma adrenaline and noradrenaline. J. ment. Sci. **101**, 156—162 (1955). — WEIL-MALHERBE, H., J. AXELROD, and R. TOMCHICK: Blood-brain barrier for adrenaline. Science **129**, 1226—1227 (1959). — WEIL-MALHERBE, H., and A. D. BONE: Intracellular distribution of catecholamines in the brain. Nature (Lond.) **180**, 1050—1051 (1957). — WEIL-MALHERBE, H. and A. D. BONE: The association of adrenaline and noradrenaline with blood platelets. Biochem. J. **70**, 14—22 (1958). — WEIL-MALHERBE, H., and A. D. BONE: The effect of reserpine on the intracellular distribution of catecholamines in the brain stem of the rabbit. J. Neurochem. **4**, 251—263 (1959). — WEIL-MALHERBE, H., H. S. POSNER, and G. R. BOWLES: Changes in the concentration and intracellular distribution of brain catecholamines: the effects of reserpine, β-phenylisopropylhydrazine, pyrogallol and 3,4-dihydroxyphenylalanine. alone and in combination. J. Pharmacol. **132**, 278 (1961). — WHITTAKER, V. P.: The isolation and characterization of acetylcholine containing particles from brain. Biochem J. **72**, 694 (1959). — WIEDORN, W. S., and F. ERVIN: Schizophrenic-like psychotic reactions with administration of isoniazid. Arch. Neurol. Psychiat. (Chicago) **72**, 321 (1954). — WILSON, I. B.: The mechanism of enzyme hydrolysis studied with acetylcholinesterase. In: The mechanism of enzyme action. p. 642—657 (Ed. W. D. MCELROY and B. GLASS). Baltimore: Johns Hopkins Press 1954. — WILSON, I. B.: Designing of a new drug with antidotal properties against the nerve gas sarin. Biochim. biophys. Acta **27**, 196—199 (1958).

YOUNG, M. K., JR., H. K. BERRY, E. BEERSTECHER JR., and J. S. BERRY: Metabolic patterns of schizophrenic and control groups. Biochemical Institute Studies IV. Austin, the Univ. of Texas Publication No. 5109, 1951.

ZELLER, E. A., J. BERNSOHN, W. M. INSKIP, and J. W. LAUER: On the effect of a monoamine oxidase inhibitor on the behaviour and tryptophan metabolism of schizophrenic patients. Naturwissenschaften **44**, 427 (1957). — ZILE, M., and H. A. LARDY: Monoamine oxidase activity in liver of thyroid-fed rats. Arch. Biochem. **82**, 411—421 (1959).

G. Biochemistry of the developing nervous system

ASHBY, W., and E. M. SCHUSTER: Carbonic anhydrase in the brain of the newborn in relation to functional maturity. J. biol. Chem. **184**, 109—116 (1950).

BAXTER, C. F., J. P. SCHADE, and E. ROBERTS: Maturational changes in cerebral cortex. II. Levels of glutamic acid decarboxylase, γ-aminobutyric acid and some related amino acids. In: Inhibition in the central nervous system and γ-aminobutyric acid. London: Pergamon Press Ltd. 1960. — BENNETT, E. L., M. R. ROSENZWEIG, D. KRECH, H. KARLSSON, N. DYE, and A. OHLANDER: Individual, strain and age differences in cholinesterase activity of the rat brain. J. Neurochem. **3**, 144—152 (1958).

CUMINGS, J. N., H. GOODWIN, E. M. WOODWARD, and G. CURZON: Lipids in the brains of infants and children. J. Neurochem. **2**, 289—294 (1958).

ELKES, J., and A. TODRICK: Development of the cholinesterases in the rat brain. In: Biochemistry of the developing nervous system, 309—314 (H. WAELSCH, Ed.). New York: Academic Press Inc. 1955.

FLEXNER, J. B., and L. B. FLEXNER: Biological and physiological differentiation during morphogenesis. VII. Adenyl-pyrophosphatase and phosphatase activities in the developing cerebral cortex and liver of the fetal guinea pig. J. cell. comp. Physiol. **31**, 311—320 (1948). — FLEXNER, L. B.: Enzymic and functional patterns of the developing mammalian brain. In: Biochemistry of the developing nervous system, 281—300 (H. WAELSCH, Ed.). New York: Academic Press Inc. 1955. — FLEXNER, L. B., E. L. BELKNAP, and J. B. FLEXNER: Biochemical and physiological differentiation during morphogenesis. XVI. Cytochrome oxidase, succinic dehydrogenase and succinoxidase in the developing cerebral cortex and liver of the fetal guinea pig. J. cell. comp. Physiol. Suppl. **42**, 151—161 (1953). — FOLCH-PI, J.: Composition of the brain in relation to maturation. In: Biochemistry of the developing nervous system, 121—136 (H. Waelsch, Ed.). New York: Academic Press Inc. 1955.

Himwich, H. E.: Brain metabolism and cerebral disorders. Baltimore, Maryland: The Williams and Wilkins Company 1951. — Himwich, H. E., and M. H. Aprison: The effect of age on cholinesterase activity of rabbit brain. In: Biochemistry of the developing nervous system, 301—307 (H. Waelsch, Ed.). New York: Academic Press Inc. 1955a. — Himwich, H. E., and W. A. Himwich: The permeability of the blood-brain barrier to glutamic acid in the deloping rat. In: Biochemistry of the developing nervous system, 202—207 (H. Waelsch, Ed.). New York: Academic Press Inc. 1955b. — Himwich, W. A., and J. C. Petersen: Correlation of chemical maturation of the brain in various species with neurologic behavior. In: Biological psychiatry, 2—16 (J. H. Masserman, Ed.). New York: Grune and Stratton, Inc. 1959.

Johnson, A. C., A. R. McNabb, and R. J. Rossiter: Lipids of normal brain. Biochem. J. 43, 573—577 (1948).

Kavaler, F., and V. M. Kimel: Biochemical and physiological differentiation during morphogenesis. XV. Acetylcholinesterase activity of the motor cortex of the fetal guinea pig. J. Comp. Neurol. 96, 113—119 (1952).

Lajtha, A.: The development of the blood-brain barrier. J. Neurochem. 1, 216—277 (1957a). — Lajtha, A.: Amino acid and protein metabolism of the brain. II. The uptake of L-lysine by brain and other organs of the mouse at different ages. J. Neurochem. 2, 209—215 (1958). — Lajtha, A.: Amino acid and protein metabolism of the brain. V. Turnover of leucine in mouse tissues. J. Neurochem. 3, 358—365 (1959). — Lajtha, A., S. Furst, A. Gerstein, and H. Waelsch: Amino acid and protein metabolism of the brain. I. Turnover of free and protein bound lysine in brain and other organs. J. Neurochem. 1, 289—300 (1957b).

Metzler, C. J., and D. G. Humm: The determination of cholinesterase activity in whole brains of developing rats. Science 113, 382—383 (1951).

Nachmansohn, D.: Cholinesterase in the central nervous system. Bull. Soc. Chim. biol. (Paris) 21, 761—796 (1939). — Nachmansohn, D.: Choline esterase in brain and spinal cord of sheep embryos. J. Neurophysiol. 3, 396—402 (1940).

Potter, V. R., W. C. Schneider, and G. J. Lieble: Enzymic changes during growth and differentiation in the tissue of the newborn rat. Cancer Res. 5, 21—24 (1945).

Roberts, E., P. J. Harman, and S. Frankel: γ-Aminobutyric acid content and glutamic decarboxylase activity in developing mouse brain. Proc. Soc. exp. Biol. (N. Y.) 78, 799—803 (1951). — Roberts, R. B., J. B. Flexner, and L. B. Flexner: Biochemical and physiological differentiation during morphogenesis. — XXIII. Further observations relating to the synthesis of amino acids and proteins by the cerebral cortex and liver of the mouse. J. Neurochem 4, 78—90 (1959). — Rudnick, D., P. Mela, and H. Waelsch: Enzymes of glutamine metabolism in the developing chick embryo: a study of glutamotransferase and glutamine synthetase. J. exp. Zool. 126, 297—321 (1954).

Sperry, W. M., and H. Waelsch: The chemistry of myelination and demyelination. Multiple Sclerosis and the Demyelinating Diseases 28, 255—267 (1952).

Waelsch, H.: Glutamic acid and cerebral function. Adv. Protein Chem. 6, 299—341 (1951). — Waelsch, H.: The turnover of components of the developing brain; the blood-brain barrier. In: Biochemistry of the developing nervous system, 187—199 (H. Waelsch, Ed.). New York: Academic Press Inc. 1955. — Waelsch, H., W. M. Sperry, and V. A. Stoyanoff: The influence of growth and myelination on the deposition and metabolism of lipids in the brain. J. biol. Chem. 140, 885—897 (1941).

H. Inborn errors of metabolism

Armstrong, M. D., and K. S. Robinson: On the excretion of indole derivatives in phenylketonuria. Arch. Biochem. 52, 287 (1954). — Armstrong, M. D., and K. N. F. Shaw: Studies on phenylketonuria. III. The metabolism of o-tyrosine. J. biol. Chem. 213, 805 (1955). — Armstrong, M. D., K. N. F. Shaw, and K. S. Robinson: Studies on phenylketonuria. II. The excretion of o-hydroxyphenylacetic acid in phenylketonuria. J. biol. Chem. 213, 797 (1955).

Baldridge, R. C., L. Borofsky, H. Baird, III, F. Reichle, and D. Bullock: Relationship of serum phenylalanine levels and ability of phenylketonurics to hydroxylate tryptophan. Proc. Soc. exp. Biol. (N. Y.) 100, 529 (1959). — Baron, D. N., C. E. Dent, H. Harris, E. W. Hart, and J. B. Jepson: Hereditary pellagra-like skin rash, with temporary cerebellar ataxia, constant renal amino-aciduria, and other bizarre biochemical features. Lancet 1956 II, 421. — Berendes, H., J. A. Anderson, M. R. Ziegler, and D. Ruttenberg: Disturbance in tryptophane metabolism in phenylketonuria. A.M.A. J. Dis. Child. 96, 1 (1958). — Bickel, H., J. Gerrard, and E. M. Hickmans: Influence of phenylalanine intake on phenylketonuria. Lancet 1953 II, 812. — Borek, E., A. Brecher, G. A. Jervis, and H. Waelsch: Oligophrenia phenylpyruvica. II. Constancy of the metabolic error. Proc. Soc. exp. Biol. (N. Y.) 75, 86—89

(1950). — BOSCOTT, R. J., and H. BICKEL: Phenylalanine and tyrosine metabolism in patients with phenylketonuria. Biochem. J. **56**, 1 (1954). — BRODIE, B. B., J. AXELROD, P. A. SHORE, and S. UDENFRIEND: Ascorbic acid in aromatic hydroxylation. II. Products formed by reaction of substrates with ascorbic acid, ferrous ion, and oxygen. J. biol. Chem. **208**, 741—750 (1954).

CORI, G. T.: Glycogen structure and enzyme deficiencies in glycogen storage disease. Harvey Lect. **48**, 145—171 (1953).

DANCIS, J., and M. E. BALIS: A possible mechanism for the disturbance in tyrosine metabolism of phenylpyruvic oligophrenia. Pediatrics **15**, 63 (1955). — DAVISON, A. N., and M. SANDLER: Inhibition of 5-hydroxytryptophan decarboxylase by phenylalanine metabolites. Nature (Lond.) **181**, 186 (1958).

FÖLLING, A.: Über Ausscheidung von Phenylbrenztraubensäure im Harn als Stoffwechselanomalie in Verbindung mit Imbezillität. Hoppe-Seilers Z. physiol. Chem. **227**, 169 (1934).

HARRIS, H.: Human biochemical genetics. Cambridge University Press 1959. — HSIA, D. Y.-Y., K. W. DRISCOLL, W. TROLL, and W. E. KNOX: Detection by phenylalanine tolerance tests of heterozygous carriers of phenylketonuria. Nature (Lond.) **178**, 1239—1240 (1956). — HSIA, D. Y.-Y., W. E. KNOX, K. V. QUINN, and R. S. PAINE: A one-year, controlled study of the effect of low-phenylalanine diet on phenylketonuria. Pediatrics **21**, 178 (1958a). — HSIA, D. Y.-Y., I. HUANG, and S. G. DRISCOLL: The heterozygous carrier in galactosaemia. Nature (Lond.) **182**, 1389—1390 (1958b). — HSIA, D. Y.-Y.: Inborn errors of metabolism. Chicago: The Year Book Publishers 1959.

ISSELBACHER, K. J., E. P. ANDERSON, K. KURAHASHI, and H. M. KALCKAR: Congenital galactosemia, a single enzymatic block in galactose metabolism. Science **123**, 635—636 (1956).

JERVIS, G. A.: Studies on phenylpyruvic oligophrenia. The position of the metabolic error. J. biol. Chem. **169**, 651—656 (1947). — JERVIS, G. A.: Phenylpyruvic oligophrenia: deficiency of phenylalanine oxidizing system. Proc. Soc. exp. Biol. (N. Y.) **82**, 514 (1953). — JERVIS, G. A.: Chemical pathology of the nervous system (J. Folch, Ed.). London: Pergamon Press Ltd. (in press).

KLENK, E.: Über die Verteilung der Neuraminsäure im Gehirn bei der familiären amaurotischen Idiotie und bei der Niemann-Pickschen Krankheit. Hoppe Seylers Z. physiol. Chem. **282**, 84—88 (1947). — KLENK, E., and H. LANGERBEINS: Über die Verteilung der Neuraminsäure im Gehirn. (Mit einer Mikromethode zur quantitativen Bestimmung der Substanz im Nervengewebe). Hoppe-Seylers Z. physiol. Chem. **270**, 185—193 (1941).

MILNE, M. D., M. A. CRAWFORD, C. B. GIRAO, and L. LOUGHRIDGE: The metabolic abnormality of Hartnup disease. Biochem. J. **72**, 30 (1959). — MITOMA, C., R. M. AULD, and S. UDENFRIEND: On the nature of enzymatic defect in phenylpyruvic oligophrenia. Proc. Soc. exp. Biol. (N. Y.) **94**, 634—635 (1957a). — MITOMA, C., H. S. POSNER, D. F. BOGDANSKI, and S. UDENFRIEND: Biochemical and pharmacological studies on o-tyrosine and its meta- and para-analogues. A suggestion concerning phenylketonuria. J. Pharmacol. exp. Ther. **120**, 188 (1957b).

PARE, C. M. B., M. SANDLER, and R. S. STACEY: 5-Hydroxytryptamine deficiency in phenylketonuria. Lancet **1957I**, 551.

UDENFRIEND, S., C. T. CLARK, J. AXELROD, and B. B. BRODIE: Ascorbic acid in aromatic hydroxylation. I. A model system for aromatic hydroxylation. J. biol. Chem. **208**, 731—739 (1954.)

WALLACE, H. W., K. MOLDAVE, and A. MEISTER: Studies on conversion of phenylalanine to tyrosine in phenylpyruvic oligophrenia. Proc. Soc. exp. Biol. (N. Y.) **94**, 632 (1957). — WESTALL, R. G.: Argininosuccinicaciduria. Identification of the metabolic defect in a newly described form of mental deficiency. IVth Int. Congr. Biochem., Abstracts 168 (1958). — WESTALL, R. G., J. DEMIS, and S. MILLER: Maple sugar urine disease. A.M.A. J. Dis. Child. **94**, 571 (1957).

Stoffwechselpathologie der Psychosen

Von

Carl Riebeling†, Hamburg

Inhalt

Historische Einleitung

Als Claus und van-der-Stricht 1895 ihre Monographie über die Pathophysiologie der Epilepsie veröffentlichten, war das wohl der erste Ansatz zu einer somatologischen Forschung innerhalb der Psychiatrie, wenn dieser Angriff auch naturgemäß zunächst auf diejenige Krankheit gerichtet war, bei der noch am ehesten ein organisches Korrelat zu erwarten war. Diese Arbeit hat seinerzeit geradezu revolutionierend gewirkt und hat zweifellos auch für Diagnostik und Therapie Bedeutendes gebracht. Erst Jahrzehnte später erschien das kleine Buch von Justschenko, der mit dem Titel der Schrift bereits einen Anspruch erhob, wie nach ihm niemand mehr: Er glaubte nämlich im Titel „Das Wesen der Psychosen" eine Lösung bereits vorwegnehmen zu dürfen. Seine Arbeit ist so ausgesprochen optimistisch, so fortschrittsgläubig, daß man sie heute nur noch mit

Nach Abschluß des Manuskriptes wurden die Überarbeitung und Korrekturen freundlicherweise von Herrn Professor H. Albrecht und Herrn Dr. G. Zahn durchgeführt.

einem leisen Lächeln lesen kann, insbesondere wenn man die recht spärlichen Ergebnisse der damaligen Zeit als Grundlagen ansieht. Nachdem Wuth im Aschaffenburger Handbuch der Psychiatrie einen ausgezeichneten und von hoher Sachkunde zeugenden Artikel geschrieben hatte, erschien wieder einige Jahre später der Artikel von Georgi und Fischer im Bumkeschen Handbuch, der allein durch den unglaublichen Umfang seines Literaturverzeichnisses von über 1300 Stellen imponierte; dieser enthielt wirklich alles, was damals überhaupt bekannt war. Auch die Liquorliteratur wurde vollständig referiert, und es entstand ein Überblick über die Anschauungen und Ergebnisse der damaligen Zeit, der heute allerdings ganz und gar veraltet ist.

Es wirkte für den Interessierten geradezu wie eine Erlösung, als die ersten Arbeiten von Gjessing erschienen, die neben meisterhafter Darstellung eine Sorgfalt und Sachlichkeit der Arbeit dokumentierten, die bisher nicht übertroffen worden ist. Die fortlaufenden Arbeiten von Gjessing wurden niemals buchmäßig publiziert und waren doch nach einigen Jahren, während derer in Deutschland nach Gjessings eigenen Worten „der Verfasser (R.) der einzige war, der sie gewürdigt hatte", in aller Munde. Einige Jahre nach diesen ersten Arbeiten erschien eine Monographie von K. F. Scheid über die febril-cyanotischen Psychosen, in der eine Anzahl hämatologischer Ergebnisse bei einigen Fällen von sog. akuter Katatonie erörtert wurden, und es war eindrucksvoll, wie diese sehr gründlichen und sauberen Arbeiten die für eine Somatologie der Psychosen allerdings reifgewordene Zeit der Insulin- und Cardiazol-Schocktherapie befruchteten. Erst 1940 erschienen zusammenfassende Darstellungen, beginnend mit den Referaten des Verfassers, die seitdem regelmäßig — in „aperiodischen" Abständen allerdings — publiziert wurden, obwohl sie auch mehr auf Vollständigkeit als auf eine Überschau Wert legen mußten, einfach dem Charakter der Darstellung nach. 1942 schrieb C. Schmidt ein kleines, aber sehr eindrucksvolles Buch über die pathophysiologische Forschung innerhalb der Psychiatrie, im wesentlichen aus der Sicht des Internisten, das er seinem Lehrer Volhard widmete. Es wäre sicher für die Psychiatrie bedeutungsvoll geworden, wenn nicht durch das Kriegsende diese Fragestellungen gewissermaßen beiseitegelegt worden wären. Damals übernahm Amerika, begünstigt durch die ungeheure apparatologische Überlegenheit, die Führung auf dem Gebiet der Pathophysiologie der Psychosen. Aber auch die dortigen Arbeitsmöglichkeiten haben nicht vermocht, entscheidend Neues zu erbringen. Auch in England wurde sehr viel auf dem Gebiet gearbeitet (Crammer, Mayer-Gross, Richter u. Dawson). 1957 veröffentlichte D. Richter mit einigen anderen Autoren zusammen eine Arbeit über die somatologischen Gesichtspunkte der Schizophrenie, wobei allerdings eine Anzahl der Fälle ganz zweifellos nicht als Schizophrenie anzusehen sind, sondern teils als Fälle von Cyclothymie, teils als periodische Katatonie. Das Buch liegt auch in deutscher Übersetzung vor. Bleuler schrieb 1947 sein Buch über endokrinologische Psychiatrie, Stoll ein Buch über die Addison-Psychosen. Beide Bücher haben zweifellos die somatologische Seite der Psychiatrie wesentlich beeinflußt, sind dabei sehr zurückhaltend und, wohltuend für das gesamte Bild, glücklicherweise sehr kritisch. Buscaino, der unermüdliche Nestor der italienischen Psychiatrie, publizierte 1958 noch einmal über die Ätiologie der Schizophrenie, in der er das zur Zeit Bekannte an Beiträgen aus der ganzen Welt zusammentrug. Sehr optimistisch versucht er erneut zu beweisen, daß die Schizophrenie seiner ursprünglichen Theorie entsprechend eine Enterohepatotoxicose darstellt. Das Buch von Lamy über die angeborenen Stoffwechselstörungen im Kindesalter ist insofern von besonderem Interesse, als zum ersten Male die Summe aller „inborn errors of metabolism" monographisch dargestellt wird. Der Verfasser hatte bereits vor vielen Jahren

— wohl als erster — darauf hingewiesen, daß mit den inborn errors fast zwangs-läufig intellektuelle oder psychische Störungen einhergehen.

Zweifellos ergab der Züricher Kongreß im Jahre 1957 eine großartige Übersicht über den Stand der Pathophysiologie der Psychosen überhaupt, er ergab aber auch gleichzeitig nicht nur für die Somatologie, sondern auch für die Psycho-pathologie eine derartige Resignation, daß er paradigmatisch wurde für den Stand der Psychiatrie überhaupt. Aus den teilweise sicher interessanten Ausführungen auf unserem spezielleren Gebiet ging doch immer wieder hervor, daß man vor-läufig bezüglich der Ätiologie und Pathogenese der Psychosen außerordentlich vorsichtig sein muß, wenn man auch nicht völlig zu resignieren braucht. GEORGI und seine zahlreichen Schüler trugen äußerst sorgfältig und gewissenhaft durch-geführte Arbeiten speziell über ihre Isolationsversuche vor, aber sie konnten einen wesentlichen Einwand nicht entkräften, der in der Diskussion gemacht wurde. Es waren aus Sammelurinen von vielen Schizophrenen basische Fraktionen extra-hiert worden, die sich als toxisch gegenüber bestimmten biologischen Objekten erwiesen hatten. Es war aber nicht garantiert, daß die Urine von medikamenten-frei-behandelten Schizophrenen stammten. Mögen nun aber unter den Spendern der Urine Patienten gesesen sein, die irgendwelche Hirngifte bekommen hatten, dann müßten diese selbstverständlich auf die Versuchsobjekte genau so schädi-gend bzw. lähmend wirken wie unter anderen Umständen gewonnene Medikamente. Daß solche ausgesprochenen Hirngifte auch für die Versuchstiere schädigend bzw. lähmend wirken müssen, ist evident und aus der Pharmakologie längst bekannt. Auf die Wirkung beim Tier wird später noch einzugehen sein.

Wir fragen erst ganz unverbindlich nach den Möglichkeiten für den Menschen, überhaupt psychotisch zu reagieren, und wollen dies anhand eines groben Schemas „schematisch" zu beantworten versuchen:

Voraussetzung: körperliche und psychische Erbanlage.

A. Konstitution.

B. Disposition.
  1. frühkindliche Störung,
  2. Sexualentwicklung,
  3. Hunger,
  4. inadäquate Forderung.

C. Wirkung auf diese Disposition durch Toxine:
  a) bakterielle oder virusartige Toxine,
  b) Allergene,
  c) Darmgifte,
  d) hormonelle Gifte,
  e) harnpflichtige Stoffwechselgifte.

  Diese Toxine wirken im Sinne von transitorischen Schäden oder Dauer-wirkungen:
    z. B. Spirochätentoxin,
    Avitaminosen,
    Viruswirkungen,
    Indolderivate,
    andere psychotrope Substanzen,
    Spirochäten,
    Phenylalanin,
    Alkoholsucht,
    Endokrinosen.

D. Periodizität, vorzustellen nach Art der

    1. Liesegangschen Ringe,
    2. senilen Drusen,
    3. konzentrischen Sklerose bzw. Anschoppung im Sinne von GJESSING und RIEBELING und mit Kippschwingungen im Sinne von SELBACH gekoppelt,
    4. Anfall — periodische Psychose.

E. Ferner zu berücksichtigen:

    a) frühkindliche Stoffwechselentgleisung (inborn error of metabolism), z.B.:
        Lipoidosen   (schwer)
        Morbus Fölling   (mittelschwer)
        Phosphaturie   (leicht)
    b) Lebensphasen, körperliche Entwicklung, Reifung usw.
    c) Umwelt und Schicksal.

Man könnte sich vorstellen, daß eine toxische Substanz vielleicht nur sehr früh im ersten Beginn einer Krankheit feststellbar ist, wie das ja z. B. auch für die Poliomyelitis gilt. Die Nachwirkungen aber könnten ähnlich wie bei der Poliomyelitis, nur eben nicht als Ganglienzellenschädigung, sondern z. B. als eine Umwandlung eines Stoffwechselvorganges oder Schädigung eines Ferments des intermediären Stoffwechsels, schädigend bleiben. Man könnte sich z. B. den eigenartigen Geruch, der von manchen Psychotikern ausgeht und der angeblich jetzt sogar objektivierbar geworden sein soll, oder man könnte sich vieles andere, z. B. die vertrackte Gestik, das vertrackte Aussehen vieler alter Psychosen in dem gleichen Sinne erklären. Gerade, daß diese Dinge nicht ausschließlich bei einer bestimmten Gruppe von Psychosen zur Beobachtung kommen, sondern daß sie — wenn auch in geringerem Maße — bei verschiedenen Formen von Psychosen auftreten, spricht noch eher dafür, daß eine gewisse Disposition zur psychotischen Entgleisung bei vielen Menschen vorhanden ist, die Art aber, wie sie entgleisen, mit ihren erblichen Anlagen und mit vielen anderen Phänomenen, die oben im Schema aufgeführt sind, zusammenhängt. Wir können uns z. B. vorstellen, daß gewisse Organminderwertigkeiten zu Herdinfektionen bzw. zur „Focalsepsis" disponieren sowohl im Nasen- oder Rachenraum (PICKWORTH) wie im Darm (REITER, BUSCAINO) oder in der Leber (BUSCAINO, GAUPP, RIEBELING). Wir müssen uns auch vorstellen, daß z. B. ein „Toxin" nur da auf einen Organismus wirken kann, wo es angreifen kann; weder ein Allergen noch irgendein anderer Körper kann chemisch wirken, wenn er auf eine Glasplatte fällt: „Corpora non agunt nisi soluta"; es sei denn, daß er sie aufzu*lösen* vermag. Je nachdem aber, wie der Organismus dieses Toxin — wenn überhaupt — aufnimmt, ob er es nämlich an sich bindet und *inaktiviert* oder ob er es an sich bindet und durch die Bindung *aktiviert* oder ob er mit der Bindung, mit der Aufnahme an den Organismus etwas Neues schafft, was nun im Organismus selbständig wirken kann, wird es seine Wirkung entfalten. Dies sind offene Fragen, die aber für die Theorie nicht nur der Psychosen, sondern der Krankheitsentstehung überhaupt, vielleicht einmal von ausschlaggebender Bedeutung sein können. Es sei nur zum Vergleich daran erinnert, daß die Aufnahme von Bakterien bzw. Bakterien-Toxinen und die Reaktion des Organismus auf solche „Gift"-Wirkungen Gegenstand jahrzehntelanger Arbeit der Serologen waren; daß diese Dinge heute nicht mehr die Rolle zu spielen scheinen, die sie gespielt haben, daß die Bedeutung sich teilweise verlagert auf andere Dinge, besagt nicht, daß sie etwa ihre absolute Bedeutung verloren hätten. Warum wirkt ein Bacterium auf den einen Menschen giftig, auf den anderen nicht, warum wirkt es auf ein Tier giftig, wächst aber auf dem zweiten nur saprophytisch, und auf dem dritten wächst es überhaupt nicht, selbst nicht bei massenhafter Inoculation ? So skeptisch man gegen alles, was damit zusammenhängt, auch sein mag, einfach ablehnen kann man solche Beobachtungen auch nicht. Wenn es FEDOROFF gelungen ist, eine *bestimmte* Gewebekultur zu finden, ganz zufällig — wohlgemerkt —, die für die Wirkung von Psychose-Serum empfindlich ist, dann hat er einfach ein Paradigma gefunden, genauso wie eine chemische Reaktion gefunden worden ist, eine Analysensubstanz; daß eine solche Analysensubstanz fast nie spezifisch ist für eine einzige andere, sondern ganz überwiegend für eine Gruppe von ähnlich gebauten, hätte sie gemeinsam mit dem Menschen und seinen Körperflüssigkeiten als Reagens sowohl wie als Reaktor. Es kommt also darauf an, ständig weiter zu forschen und den Mut nicht zu verlieren. Was aber entscheidend zu sein scheint, ist, daß man gerade nicht gleich mit speziellen Theorien anfangen sollte. Man sollte nicht gleich Serotonin, Indol, Adrenalin bzw. deren Derivate als Erreger, Enterotoxine oder Lebergifte oder ähnliche werten, sondern sollte nur einfach versuchen und suchen, selbst wenn man zur groben Orientierung Versuche wie die von FEDOROFF, RIEDER, RIEBELING, GAUPP, KRAL, FISCHER u. v. a. unternimmt. Natürlich muß man immer versuchen, zu den chemischen Grundlagen vorzustoßen. Bei der heutzutage so weit entwickelten chemischen Analysen-Technik müßte es u. E. möglich sein, das „Toxin" in der Gewebsflüssigkeit oder in dem Körpersaft zu finden und zu analysieren oder einer Analyse näherzubringen, wenn es z. B. die Gewebekulturen von FEDOROFF zerstört hat.

Wir suchen nach einer Stoffwechselpathologie der Psychosen, die wir zweifellos noch nicht haben. Wir haben noch nicht einmal das Umgekehrte, eine Psychopathologie der Stoffwechselkrankheiten. Auch diese müßte noch geschrieben werden. Sie berührt sich eng mit dem, was modernerweise „Psychosomatik" genannt wird. Der Begriff wird nicht immer sehr glücklich angewandt, denn nur ganz spezielle Phänomene können überhaupt mit diesem Ausdruck belegt werden; meistens handelt es sich um Parallelen oder Zuordnungen, die aber nicht den ursprünglich von amerikanischer Seite geschaffenen Terminus wiedergeben.

Was kann man untersuchen und was lohnt sich ? Wir müssen zunächst umschreiben, welche Arten von Psychosen wir erörtern wollen bezüglich der Fragestellungen, die im Titel genannt sind. Wir wollen den Stoffwechsel vorwiegend derjenigen Psychosen kritisch betrachten, die wir als sog. endogene Psychosen auffassen. In den Fällen nämlich, in denen exogene, z. B. durch Krankheiten und Vergiftungen verursachte Psychosen Stoffwechselstörungen aufweisen, bliebe bestenfalls offen, ob die Stoffwechselstörung der Grundkrankheit oder der durch sie verursachten Psychose zuzuschreiben ist. Wahrscheinlich ist es, daß sie der Grundkrankheit zuzuschreiben ist. SCHNEIDER hat körperlich begründbare und körperlich noch nicht begründbare Psychosen voneinander abgegrenzt. Vorläufig müssen wir uns damit abfinden, daß gerade diejenigen Psychosen, die uns interessieren, körperlich noch nicht begründbar sind, daß wir bisher noch vergeblich nach einem körperlichen Substrat der Psychosen suchen und daß wir mit den bisher vorhandenen Mitteln zweifellos noch fast nichts gefunden haben. Diese resignierende Feststellung vorweg. Sie an den Beginn eines Artikels über Stoffwechselpathologie der Psychosen setzen zu müssen, ist sicher deprimierend. Es läßt sich aber nicht umgehen, immer wieder mit aller Schärfe zu trennen, was ist und was nicht ist. Es läßt sich auch nicht vermeiden, daß man mit Schärfe ablehnt, was alles an mehr oder weniger sinnlosen Theorien bereits publiziert ist. Wir wissen aus vielfältiger klinischer Erfahrung, daß die endogenen Psychosen im allgemeinen körperlich erstaunlich gesund sind. Ja, wir sehen alte Schizophrene und alte, jahrelang anstaltspflegebedürftige andere endogene Psychosen, z. B.

auch Fälle aus dem cyclothymen Formenkreis, in erstaunlicher körperlicher Rüstigkeit. Allein das Kausalitätsbedürfnis des Menschen verlangt aber, daß diese Krankheiten doch irgendeine Ursache haben müssen, und mit dem Begriff der Konstitution allein will man sich nicht abfinden; ebensowenig findet sich der moderne Mensch mit dem Begriff einer dämonisch verursachten Krankheit ab.

Was kann man untersuchen?

Wenn wir also von der Vorstellung ausgehen, daß mindestens keine gröberen klinisch faßbaren körperlichen Störungen vorliegen, so schränkt sich der Bereich der Stoffwechseluntersuchungen bereits erheblich ein, nämlich in Richtung auf die besonders empfindlichen Funktionsprüfungen, die bei internen Krankheiten gewissermaßen bereits zugedeckt werden von gröber Faßbarem. Wir brauchen nicht damit zu rechnen, daß die Senkungsgeschwindigkeit der Blutkörperchen oder die Takata-Ara-Reaktion, um zwei relativ grobe Reaktionen zu nennen, bei einer endogenen Psychose positiv sind, es sei denn, daß eine Leberfunktionsstörung oder eine Entzündung vorliegt. Wir könnten aber vielleicht noch mit einer Verschiebung der Elektrophorese rechnen, die immerhin sehr viel empfindlicher und genauer reagiert auf selbst geringfügige Veränderungen an der Leber. Wir brauchen nicht damit zu rechnen, daß grobe innersekretorische Störungen bei endogenen Psychosen zu finden sind. Solche weisen vielmehr — wenn sie vorhanden sind — auf eine exogene, in diesem Falle also endokrin verursachte Psychose hin. Es ist aber durchaus möglich, daß hochempfindliche Erfolgsorgane, wie z. B. der Uterus oder die Ovarien der infantilen Maus, wie die Hypophyse mancher Nagetiere, wie die Hypophyse des Menschen selber, unter Umständen auch auf Ausscheidungsprodukte von endogenen Psychosen reagieren, während Ausscheidungsprodukte von schwerer somatisch Kranken so grobe Veränderungen verursachen, daß sie Feineres zudecken. Es könnte sich als sinnvoll erweisen, neue, ganz ad hoc aufgefundene oder erfundene Untersuchungsverfahren anzuwenden, die von vornherein bei gröberen Störungen gewissermaßen versagen würden, als Beispiel sei verwiesen auf die Stabilitätsreaktion mit Kupfer bei Neurosen (Riebeling). Es kommt auch sicher lange nicht so sehr darauf an, einzelne Phänomene an einer Reihe von Kranken zu prüfen und festzustellen, ob sie dabei deutliche Abweichungen von der Norm erkennen lassen, als vielmehr eine möglichst große Summe von verschiedenen, auch normalerweise vorhandenen Phänomenen untereinander in Korrelation zu setzen, und aus diesen Korrelationen eine quasi-Korrelations-Pathologie zu schaffen, wie sie sich schon bei anderen körperlichen Krankheiten bewährt hat. Sicher glaubt heute niemand mehr daran, daß die Tetanie durch eine Störung des Kalkstoffwechsels allein bedingt wäre. Wohl aber werden wir auch heute noch sinnvoll eine *Verschiebung des Verhältnisses* zwischen Kalium und Calcium in die ätiologischen Betrachtungen über die Tetanie einbeziehen. Ähnlich — nur viel breiter und intensiver — könnte man sich die Erforschung z. B. auch der endogenen Psychosen denken. Es sind mit bemerkenswertem Fleiß und einem großen Aufwand chemischer Methoden Fraktionierungen von Ausscheidungen Geisteskranker vorgenommen worden. Aus der Schule von Buscaino ist jüngst eine Arbeit erschienen, in der eine Fraktionierung von Urinen geschildert wird, wie sie nur in ganz großen Laboratorien überhaupt möglich ist mit einem Stab von chemisch geschultem Hilfspersonal und Chemikern. Die Endprodukte dieser Fraktionen sind zum Teil in ihrer Wirkung verschieden von den gleichen Fraktionen aus Urinen Gesunder. Dabei ist aber doch immer wieder zu erörtern, daß der Gesunde prinzipiell nicht nur deswegen anders ist, weil er eben „nicht krank" ist, sondern auch deswegen anders sein muß, weil er weder einförmige Anstaltskost hat, noch einförmiges Anstaltsleben, noch unter dem psychischen Druck des „Eingesperrtseins" oder unter einer Wahnidee oder unter einer Depression leidet. Das sind eben doch Faktoren, die auch die körperliche Leistungsfähigkeit beeinflussen können. Ob sie es tun, wollen wir ja gerade versuchen zu erfahren. Man sollte demnach auch prinzipiell nicht Geisteskranke mit gesunden Pflegern z. B. vergleichen, sondern mit hospitalisierten Kranken anderer, z. B. chirurgischer Abteilungen, die einigermaßen das gleiche Leben führen wie unsere endogenen Geisteskranken selbst. Ein Beispiel, das sehr viel zu denken gab, ist von PINKUS und HOAGLAND im Jahre 1953 berichtet worden. Die Autoren kontrollierten die damals sehr modernen Ergebnisse der Stressforscher, die SELYE u. Mitarb. publiziert hatten, an einer größeren Gruppe von Schizophrenen und fanden ganz erhebliche Abweichungen von der Norm. Als die gleichen Kranken einige Wochen lang ausreichend zu essen bekamen (sie waren vorher insbesondere bezüglich ihrer Eiweißernährung ungenügend versorgt), verschwanden parallel zur Gewichtszunahme sämtliche bisher beobachteten Anomalien, d. h., diese waren gar nicht durch die Psychose verursacht, sondern sie waren iatrogen, sie beruhten auf einem „Hospitalismus".

Wenn auch der Kranke, der von sich aus freiwillig abstiniert oder sich aus wahnhaften Gründen monate-, ja jahrelang einseitig oder insuffizient ernährt, in irgendeiner Form anders lebt als der Durchschnittsmensch in einer durchschnittlichen Umgebung, dann verändert er seinen Organismus sekundär, und seine primären Veränderungen, die vielleicht diese Haltung erst verursacht haben, verschwinden bzw. werden zugedeckt von den sekundären, gröberen. Auch was er dann an Phänomenen, z. B. des Eiweißdefizits, bietet, sind Ergebnisse eines jahrelangen Hungers, wie man sie häufig auch an nicht-psychotischen Kranken, die jahrelang z. B. einsam gelebt hatten, findet. Das sind aber keine Phänomene, die ursächlich für die Psychose verantwortlich sind. Sie sind nur von der Psychose veranlaßt worden.

Schließlich darf man auch nicht vergessen, daß jedes Lebewesen seinen speziellen Rhythmus hat und eine gewisse Periodizität aller Lebensphänomene offenbar doch ein Prinzip des Lebendigen überhaupt ist.

Will man Vergleiche ziehen, muß man selbstverständlich nicht nur gleiche Altersstufen, sondern nach Möglichkeit außerdem Personen gleichen Geschlechts und gleicher Konstitution von psychiatrischen und anderen Krankenabteilungen untersuchen.

Rhythmus und Periodizität

Wir kommen zur Erörterung der Periodizität, mit der wir innerhalb aller Psychosengruppen außerordentlich viel zu tun haben. Alle Arten von Periodik, auch die langfristige, wirken sich innerhalb der Psychiatrie aus. Wir wissen, daß gerade die endogenen Psychosen in der Menarche, bei den Gestationsprozessen und in der Menopause Auslösungshöhepunkte aufweisen. Auch für Männer gelten ähnliche Phasen. Unabhängig von diesen lebensphasisch ausgelösten Psychosen laufen die phasischen Psychosen überhaupt, die ebenfalls als langfristig periodisch bezeichnet werden können, wie die Phasen der Cyclothymie. Die meisten „rezidivierenden Schizophrenien", ebenso wie viele der Fälle, die als Schizophrenie bezeichnet werden und unter irgendeiner, vielleicht nicht einmal sehr angreifenden Therapie nach zwei bis drei Monaten die Klinik gesund wieder verließen, sind u. E. — damit wissen wir uns in Norddeutschland einig mit der Mehrzahl der skandinavischen Psychiater — keine Schizophrenien, sondern Cyclothymien[1].

---

[1] Wenn im folgenden Schizophrenie, Cyclothymie, endogene Psychose stehen, dann muß vorweg betont werden, daß wir in vielen Fallen anders diagnostiziert hätten. Das kann nicht jedesmal neu gesagt werden. Nur da, wo ausdrücklich betont wird, daß an der Diagnose kein Zweifel bestände, gilt diese reservatio mentalis nicht.

Langfristige Periodizität wirkt sich allerdings nicht nur bei Kranken, sondern auch bei Gesunden vielfältig aus, insbesondere scheinen sich doch auch die jahreszeitlichen Schwankungen des Milieus auszuwirken, wie aus sehr eingehenden Untersuchungen von PETERSEN, aber auch aus den viel moderneren Untersuchungen von DE RUDDER über Wetter- und Krankheitsgeschehen eindeutig hervorgeht.

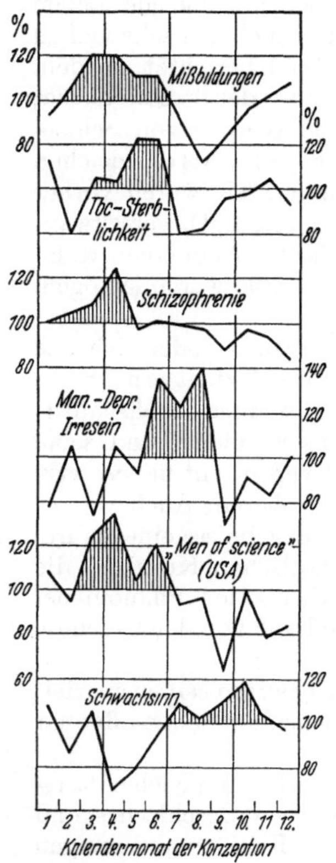

Abb. 1. Jahreszeitliche Schwankungen der Konzeptionsdaten bei einigen charakteristischen Personengruppen (nach PETERSEN)

Aus der Monographie von PETERSEN bringen wir eine Zusammenstellung (Abb. 1), die zeigt, daß zwischen den Jahreszeiten und den Konzeptionsdaten für bedeutende Männer einerseits, bestimmten Psychosen und Schwachsinnsformen andererseits enge Beziehungen bestehen, eine Häufigkeitsverteilung, die sich auch bei genauerem Studium dieser Dinge, wenigstens in Nordamerika, sehr deutlich gezeigt hat. Auf manche anderen bedeutenden Ergebnisse PETERSENs wird hier nicht eingegangen.

Nicht nur langfristige, sondern auch mittelfristige Periodizität spielt innerhalb der Psychiatrie eine nicht zu unterschätzende Rolle. Die meisten klinisch erfahrenen Psychiater kennen Psychosen mit ganz kurzen Phasen, die wenige Tage oder gar nur einige Stunden ausmachen. Gelegentlich finden sich Anomalien wie bei einem Fall von v. STOCKERT, bei dem gelegentlich nicht eine 24-, sondern eine 25 stündige Periodizität aufzudecken war, die für einige Tage mit erstaunlicher Regelmäßigkeit beibehalten wurde. Untersucht man solche Fälle unabhängig vom psychischen Befund, so wird man einmal während einer manischen, einmal während einer depressiven Phase und schließlich während eines Intervalles untersuchen, ohne zu erwarten, daß man nun jeweils die gleichen Abwegigkeiten des Stoffwechsels finden wird. Umgekehrt müßte man fordern, daß eine der Psychose wirklich zu Grunde liegende und ständig wirksame Stoffwechselstörung während aller drei Phasen, nämlich gesund, überantriebig und unterantriebig, gleichmäßig erkennbar wäre. Dann wäre sie ein Konstitutionsmerkmal und als solches eventuell auch verantwortlich für die Psychose. Aber derartige Dinge sind uns eben in keiner Weise bekannt geworden.

PETERSEN berichtet über einen 48-Stunden-Rhythmus in dem Sinne, daß der 68jährige Patient seit fünf Jahren unverändert 24 Std. manisch und 24 Std. depressiv ist. TROLLE hat Untersuchungen gemacht über die Rhodanausscheidung bei Patienten in der depressiven Phase. Die 3,4%ige Lösung wurde per os gegeben, die Ausscheidung untersucht, die während der Depression gegenüber dem Intervall stark verzögert war. Elektroschocks besserten die Ausscheidungsquoten. Die biochemischen Untersuchungen KLEINs in einem Fall von manisch-depressivem Irresein mit kurzen Cyclen sind recht aufschlußreich, wenn sie natürlich auch genauso wenig entscheiden wie alle anderen. Das Körpergewicht stieg bei den depressiven, fiel ab bei den manischen Zuständen. Bei konstanter Diät und konstanter Flüssigkeitszufuhr wurden abnorme Werte des Blutcholesterins und der Ausscheidung von Cortin etwas, aber nicht entscheidend, regularisiert. Während der Depression war regelmäßig eine Salz- und Wasserrentention mit vermehrtem Schlaf zu beobachten, während der Manie Schlaflosigkeit und überschießende Wasser- und Kochsalzausscheidung. Einen interessanten Fall publiziert GREWEL, der bei Jugendlichen über Schlafperioden mit Hunger berichtet, die ebenfalls relativ kurzfristig sind, nur für jeweils 5 Tage anhaltend. Die Jugendlichen scheinen sich überhaupt einer (von außen herangetragenen ?) Periodizität mehr zu fügen als ältere Menschen (s. später auch bei GJESSING).

Pathologische Rhythmen des Zwischenhirns (GROSCH) und periodische Umdämmerungen von 4wöchentlichem Rhythmus sind während der Pubertät beobachtet worden. Auch bei den Fällen von BOCHNIK, der die Tagesschwankungen zentralnervöser und autonomer Funktionen berichtete, handelte es sich überwiegend um junge Menschen. OPPENHEIM beschrieb ein Kind, das nach einem Kopftrauma zu rhythmischen Bewußtseinstrübungen neigte.

Die kurzfristige Periodik von 24 Stunden scheint wohl mehr an organische Zustandsbilder geknüpft zu sein. Immerhin sah BLEULER einen Fall von „Schizophrenie", bei dem manische und depressive Zustandsbilder täglich wechselten. Die Frage der Periodizität von psychischen Störungen ist deswegen so schwer zu beantworten, weil sich endogene Rhythmen, z. B. der Tag-Nacht-Rhythmus zwischen Vagus und Sympathicus, die Schwankungen der Körpertemperatur, die Menses, mit Rhythmen der Psychose überschneiden. Ob diese Rhythmen für das rhythmische oder periodische Auftreten von Psychosen verantwortlich sind, ist keineswegs geklärt. Die Möglichkeit, daß die Periodik des Organismus abhängt von der Periodik der Erdbewegung, von Tag und Nacht bzw. von dem jahreszeitlichen Rhythmus, ist in vieler Beziehung zu belegen, in mancher anderen aber auch eindeutig zu widerlegen. So ist auch ein 25-Stunden-Rhythmus nicht in die Tagesperiodik einzuordnen. Wir wissen schließlich von einer ganzen Anzahl periodisch auftretender Phänomene, daß sie mit den Menses absolut nichts zu tun haben. Das läßt sich z. B. ziemlich klar und eindeutig zeigen an dem epileptischen Anfall, der sicher in der Mehrzahl der Fälle unabhängig von den Menses auftritt. Dagegen verschlägt es gar nichts, daß es auch Fälle gibt, die ihre Anfälle ausgesprochen circum-menstruell haben. Man muß jedenfalls auch erörtern, daß psychische Phänomene, also echte psychogene Verschiebungen des Rhythmus, bei der Entstehung und auch bei der Fixierung solcher rhythmischer Vorgänge interferieren. Es ist gar keine Frage, daß ein mehrfach hintereinander beobachteter Anfall eine mehrfach hintereinander beobachtete Verschiebung der Stimmungslage *auch* im Sinne eines bedingten Reflexes den Betreffenden bestimmt, nun am nächsten Tag und an den folgenden Tagen, wenn nämlich keine Störungen eintreten, in der gleichen Weise weiter seinen Rhythmus aufrechtzuerhalten.

RICHTER, HONEYMAN und HUNTER sahen sogar bei einem Tetaniker echte Schwankungen des charakterlichen und gemütlichen Verhaltens. Sie beobachteten 20 Tage lang depressives und dann wieder 20 Tage fast normales Stimmungsverhalten. Auf regelmäßige Calciumbehandlung verschwanden diese Schwankungen vollkommen. Eine ausgesprochen periodische „diencephale" Störung schildert BETZ bei einem 34jährigen Manne, der in zuletzt einwöchigen Abständen Gehemmtheitszustände von nur 8- bis 12stündiger Dauer erlebte, bei denen eine nennenswerte Blutdrucksteigerung um immerhin 60—80 mm Hg registriert werden konnte. Allerdings waren auch Schlafstörungen und Zwang zu Blickverharren und stärkeres Hervortreten parkinsonistischer Symptome, die auf eine diencephale Genese hinwiesen, festzustellen. Differentialdiagnostisch wird von der Narkolepsie abgetrennt, es ist aber immerhin zu bemerken, daß in der Anamnese echte, offenbar narkoleptische Schlafzustände beobachtet worden waren. Wir dürfen aber auch nicht vergessen, daß sich nicht nur einzelne, sondern viele verschiedene Perioden zu überschneiden vermögen und die eine oder die andere unter Umständen in entscheidender Weise zu beeinflussen vermag. Damit sind wir wieder den psychogenen Beeinflussungen der Periodik, oder richtiger in diesem Falle der Aperiodik, näher-

gekommen. Es besteht zweifellos für sehr viele Menschen die Möglichkeit, willens-
mäßig das Auftreten eines Anfalles, wenn auch nicht gerade eines epileptischen,
aber doch eines Anfalles cerebralen Geschehens, wie z. B. der Migräne, zu beeinflussen. Das Leben in einer modernen Zivilisation wirkt in der Beziehung sicherlich
zerstörend auf eine ganze Anzahl von Rhythmen, die dem einfacheren, unabhängig von der Zivilisation lebenden „Wilden" vielleicht noch zur Verfügung
stehen, obwohl wir uns auf diesem Gebiet auch keinen Illusionen hingeben sollen.
Auch der komplizierte Ritus sehr vieler primitiver Völker vermag deren natürliche
Abläufe entscheidend zu beeinflussen.

Ein für die kurzfristige Periodik sehr bezeichnendes Beispiel gibt Gjessing
(Abb. 2) mit der Wiedergabe von Atemkurven vom Respirationsgerät, die er
anläßlich der Grundumsatzbestimmungen bei seinen periodischen Katatonien erhoben hat. Der Unterschied zwischen dem leichten Wechsel, dem leichten Schwanken der Kurven im Intervall und der stetigen stereotypen Gleichmäßigkeit der
Atemzüge während des Stupors ist evident, d. h. aber, die kurzfristige Periodik
oder Rhythmik der Atmung während der Intervalle wird aufgehoben durch die
stereotypisierende Gleichmäßigkeit des Stuporzustandes. Klein berichtete über
Grundumsatzsteigerungen, Wasser- und Salzausscheidungen bei den manischen,
Senkungen des Grundumsatzes, Wasser- und Salzretentionen bei den depressiven
Phasen. Genau das Gegenteil sah Crammer. Auch die Pulszahlen sind recht
verschieden und in Abhängigkeit von der psychotischen Periodik. Forsgren,
hat bereits 1938 erkannt, daß z. B. die Gallensekretion nicht kontinuierlich,
sondern schubweise oder rhythmisch erfolgt und ihre Maxima und Minima am
Abend bzw. am Morgen hat. Aus seiner Rhythmusvorstellung und aus den
Ergebnissen seiner Gallensekretionsuntersuchungen ergibt sich außerdem, daß
der Mensch während der Vormittagsstunden sich aus dem damit langsam leerer
werdenden Lebervorrat ernährt, während er ab Mittag aus der während des Tages
aufgenommenen Nahrung befriedigt wird. Wenn wir schon eine Intoxikations-
Theorie für möglich oder gar für wahrscheinlich halten, dann würden diese Phänomene ja außerordentlich unterstützend wirken für derartige Vorstellungen, einfach deswegen, weil die Toxine ja wahrscheinlich (?) in der Leber sezerniert werden
und dann in höherem Maße ausgeschieden würden am Vormittag als am Rest
des Tages. Damit wäre aber auch das Schwanken der Stimmung, z. B. bei den
Cyclothymen, die ein schlechtes Befinden an den Vormittagen und langsames
Besserwerden an den Nachmittagen zeigen, immerhin einer Deutung näher-
gebracht. Periodische Depressionszustände hat Lange bereits 1896 beschrieben
und dabei ausdrücklich auf den Zusammenhang mit der harnsauren Diathese
hingewiesen. Diese harnsaure Diathese hat Beziehung zu dem, was in den französischen älteren Konstitutionsbiologien als type digestif auftaucht zum Unterschied vom type cérébral, der nach der Konstitutionslehre von Kretschmer
wiederum bei den Leptosomen (mit schizophreniformen Psychosen) häufiger sein
muß. Häufigkeitsbeziehungen überhaupt zwischen Konstitution, Disposition und
Verhalten sind einfach nicht zu leugnen, man darf sie nur nicht outrieren und als
ausschließliche Phänomene ansehen.

Sicherlich gibt es auch kurzfristige Rhythmusstörungen bei Psychosen wie
auch bei Gesunden. Es hat sich doch herausgestellt, daß sehr viel mehr Kranke
einige — wenn auch uncharakteristische — Veränderungen im EEG aufweisen, als
ursprünglich angenommen werden konnte. Es zeigte sich auch, daß das EEG nicht
nur bei gröberen, auch klinisch schon leicht auffindbaren organischen Störungen
des Zentralnervensystems Abweichungen zeigt, sondern auch bei endogenen
Psychosen, auch bei sog. Neurosen. Diese greifbaren Befunde sprechen dafür, daß
Cerebralfaktoren in den multifaktoriellen Systemen jener klinischen Bilder eine

definierbare Bedeutung haben (Bochnik). Immerhin sind sie im Rahmen des Kapitels über die kurzfristige Periodizität zu erwähnen. Daß früher gelegentlich Pulsanomalien und daneben natürlich auch Blutdruckanomalien sogar ätiologisch mit endogenen Psychosen in Zusammenhang gebracht wurden, sei erwähnt. Wahrscheinlich handelte es sich bei den beobachteten Fällen nicht um der Psychose

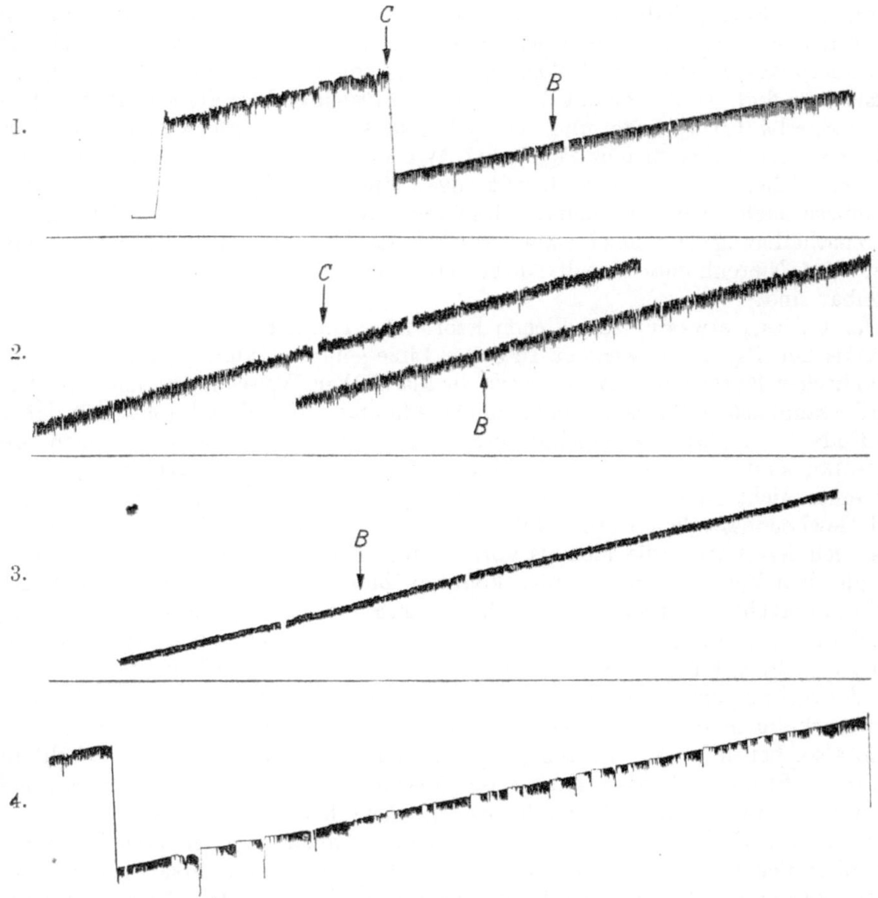

Abb. 2. Änderung kurzfristiger Periodizität unter dem Einfluß von Psychosen. Atemkurven vom Respirationsgerat bei einer Katatonie. 1. Aus der letzten Halfte der wachen Periode. 2. Am ersten Stuportag. 3. Aus der letzten Stuporzeit. 4. Am zweiten Tag nach Erwachen. *B* · Blutentnahme aus dem Ohrlappchen, *C* · Blutentnahme aus der Cubitalvene. (Nach Gjessing)

zuzuschreibende, sondern einfach andersartigen körperlichen Störungen zuzuordnende Kreislaufveränderungen, die sich bei diesen Kranken in den Bereich der Periodizität nur eingeschlichen haben (s. aber weiter unten).

Wenn man bei einem Patienten eine Stoffwechselstörung findet, dann bestehen verschiedene Möglichkeiten, diese Stoffwechselanomalie ätiologisch zu bewerten. Nämlich entweder haben die Psychose oder der Schwachsinn und die Stoffwechselstörung überhaupt nichts miteinander zu tun, sondern sind Zufallsprodukte nebeneinander. Oder wenn sich nun bestätigt hat, daß man öfters diese beiden Krankheiten zusammen beobachtet, dann fragt man sich wieder: Beruht diese Psychose auf der Stoffwechselanomalie oder beruht die Stoffwechselanomalie sekundär auf der Psychose? Bezüglich des Phenylbrenztraubensäure-Schwachsinns ist die Frage u. E. gelöst (s. dort).

Ganz anders gelagert sind aber die Verhältnisse u. E. bei den Fällen, bei denen wir geneigt sind, rein vom klinischen Standpunkt her gesehen, eine endogene Psychose anzunehmen, bei denen wir aber daneben körperliche Veränderungen finden, die wir eben sonst niemals bei diesen Psychosen finden. Da ist die Beantwortung der Frage, ob die beiden Dinge miteinander etwas zu tun haben, deswegen wesentlich schwerer, weil wir ja wissen, daß doch eine ganze Anzahl körperlicher Veränderungen zwar nicht ätiologisch für die endogene Psychose verantwortlich zu machen sind, wohl aber mit der endogenen Psychose korreliert auftreten. Das sind zweierlei Tatbestände, und man sollte sie sorgfältig unterscheiden. Gibt es z. B. eine Niereninsuffizienz-Psychose? Wir möchten es doch annehmen *auch* bei den Fällen, bei denen vielleicht sogar eine Cyclothymie in der Familienanamnese nachweisbar ist, einfach deswegen, weil gerade an der Abstufung der Nierenschädigung vom leichtesten Kopfschmerz bis zum eklamptischen Anfall oder dem Nierenkoma überall Anzeichen *echter* psychischer Einwirkungen erkennbar sind.

Nach dieser etwas umständlichen Erörterung können wir uns zu einigen sog. periodischen Psychosen wenden. In erster Linie gehören dahin die Fälle von sog. periodischer Katatonie, die Gjessing in klassischer Weise dargestellt hat. Die febril-cyanotischen Episoden sind gleichfalls häufig „periodisch". Sie sollen daher am Ende dieses Kapitels ganz kurz besprochen werden. Die Untersuchungen von Gjessing sind schon deshalb vollkommen „außer jeder Konkurrenz", weil sie mit einer nicht zu übertreffenden Akribie, mit einer unvergleichlichen Sorgfalt und Gewissenhaftigkeit, durchgeführt mit einem Stabe von Mitarbeitern, Ergebnisse geliefert haben, die niemals vorher und vielleicht auch niemals wieder in der gleichen Form geliefert werden könnten. Zu dem Stab von Mitarbeitern gehörten nämlich die Kranken selbst, die immerhin so viel Geduld innerhalb ihrer Psychose aufwandten, daß sie sogar im katatonen Stupor noch dafür sorgten, daß sie nicht unter sich ließen, daß Stuhl und Urin gesammelt wurden und daß von der Nahrungsmenge nichts verschüttet wurde. Diese Patienten sind außerdem auch Ausnahmen, da es sich um die sehr seltenen periodischen Katatonien handelt, Fälle also, bei denen in unregelmäßigen Abständen Starrezustände mit echtem katatonen Stupor auftraten, nach deren Abklingen die Kranken wieder traitabel im Anstaltsmilieu waren. Nur sehr wenig, nämlich insgesamt nur 7 Fälle, hat Gjessing innerhalb von 20 Jahren untersuchen können, daneben auch 2 gesunde freiwillige Personen, die mehrere Wochen in gleicher Weise untersucht und beobachtet wurden wie die Kranken. In erster Linie wurde die Stickstoffbilanz geprüft, und Gjessing fand, daß eine positive und eine negative Stickstoffbilanz wechseln. Dieser Wechsel hing zum Teil mit dem Ausbruch des Stupors zusammen. Der Ausbruch des Stupors trat je nach der Art des Falles am Anfang, in der Mitte oder am Ende der Retention ein. Mit dem Beginn der Verminderung der Stickstoffausscheidung im Harn, also mit dem Umschwenken einer negativen in eine positive Stickstoffbilanz, setzte plötzlich der Stupor ein, wie aus der Abb. 3 klar hervorgeht. Daß bei anderen Kranken der Stupor auch an anderen Punkten eintreten kann, ergibt sich aus der Abb. 4. Danach kann die Reaktionsphase, also der katatone Stupor, auf dem Höhepunkt der positiven Stickstoffbilanz eintreten bzw. schon vorher, d. h. auf dem Wege der Anschoppung. Der Stupor kann aber auch während der Wiederausscheidung von Stickstoff auftreten oder sogar am Ende der Mehrausscheidung an der Umschlagstelle, wenn wieder retiniert wird.

Man könnte, wenn immer am Ende einer Anschoppung von Stickstoff der Stupor
einträte, sagen, daß dann dieser die Konsequenz einer bestimmten Höhe von
„Vergiftung" sei. Das ist aber keineswegs der Fall, denn auch im absteigenden
Schenkel der Anschoppung, also wenn bereits wieder viel oder gar alles von dem
retinierten Stickstoff ausgeschieden ist, kann der katatone Stupor eintreten. Auch
beim gleichen Patienten verschoben sich diese Dinge etwas mit zunehmendem

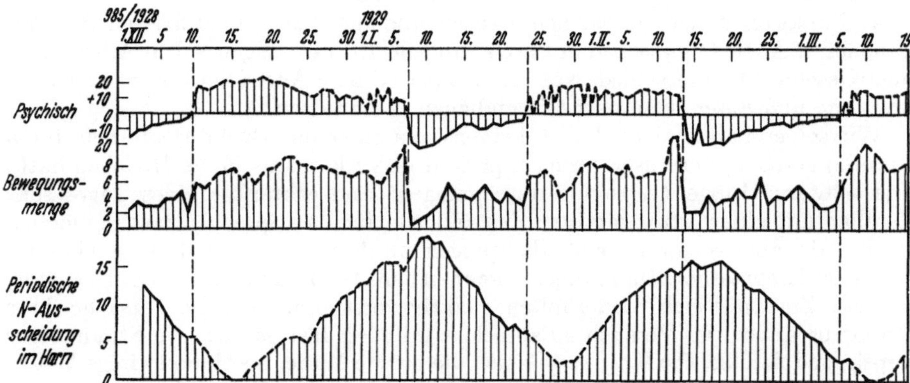

Abb. 3. Periodizität der Stickstoffausscheidung in Beziehung zum psychischen Status und zum Stupor während
zweier wacher und zweier stuporoser Phasen eines Patienten mit periodischer Katatonie. (Nach GJESSING)

Alter. Wir wissen also nicht, was die Retention oder die Ausscheidung von Stickstoff, die auch bei einer völlig gleichmäßigen, bei der absolut gleichmäßigen —
insbesondere auch bezüglich des Stickstoffgehalts absolut gleichmäßigen — Kost
erfolgt, mit der Psyche zu tun hat. Wir könnten allenfalls vermuten, daß die
Stickstoffretention eine Vergiftung darstelle. Warum das Gift aber nicht immer
dann wirkt, wenn es am stärksten im Körper vorhanden ist, sondern unter Umständen auch dann, wenn alles wieder ausgeschwemmt ist, bleibt vollkommen
offen. Ebenso fraglich ist übrigens immer noch, wo eigentlich dieser Stickstoff retiniert wird, der offenbar nach GJESSINGs
Meinung nicht in der Leber retiniert
werden kann, weil die Menge zu groß
ist. Sicherlich ist die Leber geschädigt,
was sich aus der ebenfalls phasisch
schwankenden Ausscheidungshöhe von
Urobilinogen und Harnstoff ergibt.
Welcher Art aber die Schädigung ist,
bleibt unklar. Darüber später noch mehr
im Kapitel über das Leberproblem.

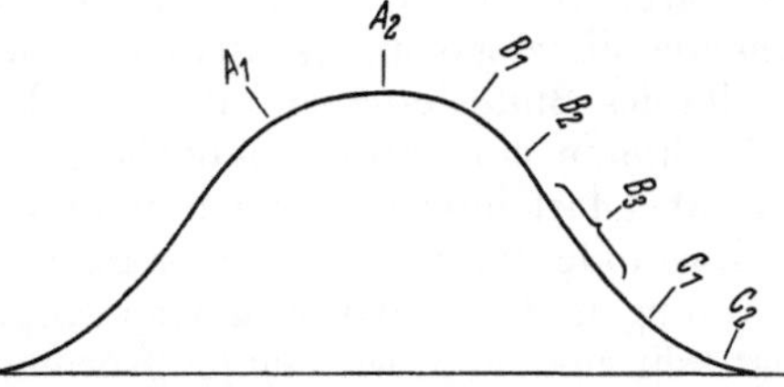

Abb. 4. Beziehungen zwischen der Stickstoffkurve
und dem Beginn eines Stupors bei 7 Patienten mit
periodischer Katatonie. Je nach Eintritt der Reaktionsphase sind sie in A-, B- und C-Typen eingeteilt.
(Nach GJESSING)

Bei den sämtlichen Fällen von
GJESSING ist die Kochsalzausscheidung
durchschnittlich im Intervall größer
als in der Reaktionsphase und richtet
sich nach der psychischen und vegetativen Phase, nicht der Stickstoffbilanz
allein. GJESSING faßt etwa folgendermaßen zusammen:

1. Das zeitlich regelmäßige Eintreten der Reaktionsphase deutet auf eine periodische Speicherung stickstoffhaltiger Substanzen hin, sei es im Zentralnervensystem oder außerhalb des Zentralnervensystems.

2. Die regelmäßig schwankende N-Bilanz hat die gleiche Periodenlänge wie die vegetative Periodik, ist aber beim Reaktionstypus B und C zeitlich gegen diese verschoben und wird durch eine phasisch schwankende Schilddrüsenfunktion mit wechselnder Proteolyse erklärt.

3. Das psychische Zustandsbild (Erregung oder Stupor) scheint durch eine gemeinsame Konstellation der vegetativen Periodik und der N-Bilanz-Phase bzw. ihrer Interferenz auf dem Gebiet des Stoffwechsels bedingt zu sein.

4. Funktionen der endokrinen Drüsen und der Leber modifizieren das Zustandsbild. Auch Organschäden durch exogene Erkrankungen sowie Alters- und auch Geschlechtsunterschiede können das periodische Auftreten von Stupor oder Erregung und deren somatische Grundlagen beeinflussen.

Wir selber haben einen Fall (übrigens aus einer mit Cyclothymie belasteten Familie) gesehen, der ausgesprochen periodisch wirkte. Das junge Mädchen hatte eine schwere Hungerdystrophie durchgemacht und erkrankte eines Tages sehr plötzlich mit einem stuporartigen Zustand, der ihr das Sprechen fast unmöglich machte, der aber — soweit sie überhaupt sich mit ihrer Mutter verständigen konnte — keinerlei depressive Stimmungen erkennen ließ. Die Kranke war lediglich später, als diese Zustände sich wiederholten, reaktiv verstimmt über die Tatsache ihrer Stuporzustände. Der Versuch zu sprechen mißlang fast immer, die Stimme war piepsig und fistelig. Die Kranke gab sich die größte Mühe, überhaupt einige Worte zu bilden. Sie hatte ein ausgesprochen gedunsenes, aufgeschwemmtes Gesicht, war fast anurisch und wirkte ödematös. Dabei bestanden keinerlei Schlafstörung, keine Tagesrhythmusstörung im Sinne von besser oder schlechter im Verlauf des Tages, keine Menstruationsstörung. Gewiß kann man in seltenen Fällen den Ausbruch einer depressiven Verstimmung aus „heiterem Himmel“ auch einmal bei einem Depressiven beobachten. Aber fast immer werden dem depressiven Zustandsbild gewisse Prodrome vorausgehen. In dem genannten Falle war es nun so, daß man innerhalb von Minuten das Entstehen des Ödems im Gesicht und auf der Bauchhaut, der Sprechunfähigkeit sowie des Stupors beobachten konnte. Gelang es ausnahmsweise einmal im ersten Beginn dieser Zustände, starke auf das Gewebe wirkende Diuretica zu geben (wir bedienten uns ganz einfach der „Ableitung auf den Darm“ durch hohe Dosen von Karlsbader Salz), dann konnte der Ausbruch des Stupors mit Sicherheit verhindert werden. War aber erst einmal die Starre für ein oder zwei Tage in Gang gekommen, dann halfen wasserentziehende Mittel gar nichts oder so gut wie gar nichts. Bestimmungen des Wassergehalts des Blutes ergaben in diesem Falle noch mehr als in einigen später noch beobachteten eine ganz erhebliche Hydrämie, die innerhalb der nächsten zwei Tage aber fast immer aufhörte und auch dann beobachtet werden konnte, wenn die Zustände nicht bis zur depressiven Starre, sondern z. B. nur zu einer Mißstimmung und zu migräneartigen Kopfschmerzen führten (Abb. 5). Die Kurve zeigt sehr eindeutig, wie eng die Korrelation zwischen dem Auftreten der Wasserretention und dem Beginn des Stupors ist.

Ähnliche Zustände wurden auch bei anderen Kranken beobachtet, aber es läßt sich auch von diesen ebensowenig wie von den Gjessingschen eine wirklich sichere Korrelation zwischen Schwankungen des Wasserhaushalts oder z. B. des Elektrolythaushaltes oder etwa der Verlaufskurve der Eosinophilen und andererseits der Psyche feststellen (Abb. 6). Man findet immer wieder auch Verschiebungen, so daß zwar beim einzelnen Menschen oft ein hoher Wassergehalt des Serums, hoher Eosinophilengehalt oder niedrige Leukocytenzahl mit dem Beginn der Psychose zusammenliegen, beim nächsten aber die Schwankungen, die ebenfalls beobachtet werden, z. B. in der Mitte der Psychose oder am Ende der Psychose liegen.

Der bemerkenswerte Fall von SPEIJER, bei dem „Phasen" und „Cyclothymien" mit einer Verminderung der Erythrocyten und einer Steigerung des Kalkgehalts des Blutes einhergingen, muß hier ebenfalls erwähnt werden (Abb. 7 u. 8). In diesem Falle hat es sich um einen bereits hospitalisierten Kranken gehandelt, der in unregelmäßigen Abständen immer wieder schwere depressive Zustände bot. Als man zufälligerweise am Beginn eines solchen depressiven Zustandes ein Blutbild anfertigte, fand sich, daß die Zahl der Erythrocyten wesentlich unter der Norm lag. Antianämische Mittel waren erfolglos bezüglich des Stupors. Weitere Untersuchungen ließen aber aufdecken, daß parallel zu der Senkung der Erythrocytenzahl eine nennenswerte Erhöhung des Calciumgehalts des Serums ging. Als nun eine extrem kalkarme Kost gegeben wurde, konnte die Zahl der Stuporen sowohl wie ihre Dauer und ihre Intensität ganz erheblich gesenkt werden. GJESSING schildert bei einigen seiner Fälle plötzliche *Erhöhungen* der Zahlen für die Erythrocyten bei Eintritt der Reaktionsphase. Soll man solche Fälle noch in den cyclothymen Formenkreis hineinnehmen ? Oder sollte man nicht lieber bei solchen Fällen sagen, daß sie in ihrer Symptomatik wohl den endogenen Psychosen sehr

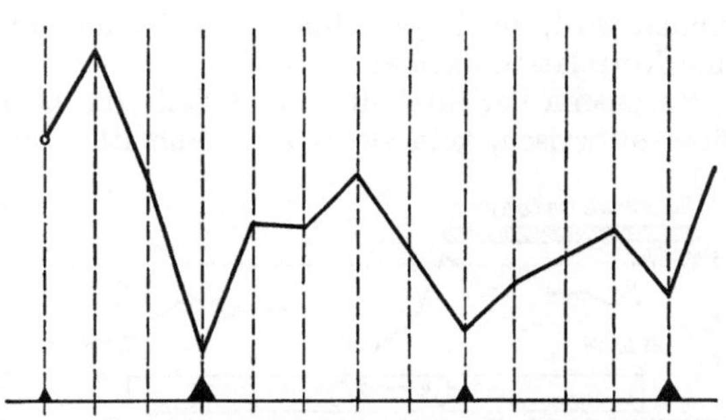

Abb. 5. Wassergehalt des Blutes (ausgezogene Kurve) parallel zu Stuporzustanden (▲). (Nach RIEBELING)

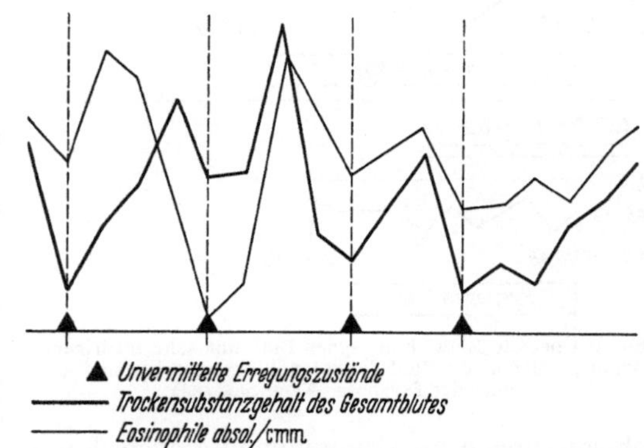

Abb. 6. Beziehungen zwischen Trockensubstanz des Blutes, Eosinophilengehalt pro mm³ und unvermittelten Erregungszustanden bei einer Prozeßpsychose. (Nach RIEBELING)

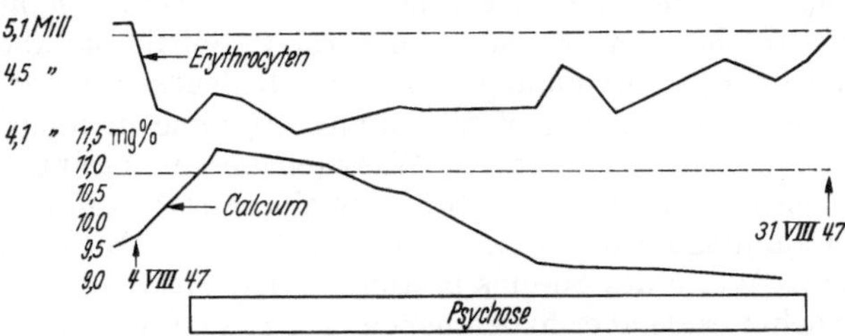

Abb. 7. Beziehung zwischen „Phasen", Calciumgehalt des Blutes und Zahl der Erythrocyten pro mm³. (Nach SPEIJER)

nahestehen, daß sie aber doch gerade diejenigen sind, auf die wir warten, nämlich die einzelnen Ausnahmen, bei denen sich körperliche Symptome nun wirklich erkennen lassen, die einzigen Ausnahmen, die zeigen, daß auch bei körperlichen Veränderungen doch eine endogene Symptomatik möglich ist. Damit sind diese Fälle noch nicht ätiologisch bedeutungsvoll für das Gesamtbild periodischer Psychosen, wenn auch eine Periodizität zweifellos vorliegt. Man kann gerade wegen der Periodizität der körperlichen Phänomene doch hoffen, daß einmal ein Stoff gefunden wird, der in ursächlicher Beziehung zur Psychose steht oder wenigstens eine Korrelation dazu aufweist.

CRAMMER berichtet über zwei Fälle, die beide recht eindrucksvolle Periodizitäten aufweisen, keineswegs aber einheitlich in ihrem Verhalten gegenüber den untersuchten Verhältnissen sind. So war bei dem ersten Fall (48 Jahre), bei dem manische und depressive Zustände abwechselten, das Urinvolumen mit Beginn der Manie erheblich abgesunken, mit dem Beginn von Depressionen steigt es vorläufig wieder an, das Körpergewicht aber sinkt erheblich ab (Abb. 9). Sehr viel klarer ist ein 2. Fall eines 49jährigen Mannes, der mindestens die letzten 5 Jahre seit Beginn der Beobachtung regelmäßige 6- oder 7tägige Cyclen gehabt hat von 2 Tagen Stupor und 4 Tagen manisch-überaktiven Zuständen (Abb. 10). Der Kaliumgehalt des Urins verhielt sich außerordentlich regelmäßig. Der Gewichtsverlust wurde während der Einnahme von etwas Salz wesentlich erheblicher, die

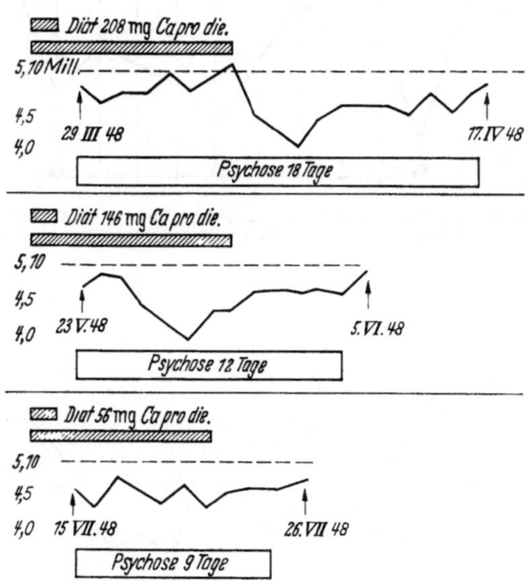

Abb. 8. Über die Einwirkung einer Diät mit sehr niedrigem Calciumgehalt auf die Zahl der roten Blutkorperchen und die Dauer der Psychose. (Nach SPEIJER)

Schwankungen im Urinvolumen gingen damit parallel. Bei dem einen Patienten gingen Gewichtsverlust und Beginn einer Depression zusammen (Abb. 9), bei dem anderen (Abb. 10), begann gerade vor dem Ausklingen des depressiven Substupors und dem Start eines hypomanischen Zustandes der Gewichtsverlust. Wurden Natrium- und Wasserzufuhr wesentlich gesenkt, konnten die Gewichtsschwankungen fast vollkommen aufgehoben, die psychische Symptomatik hingegen kaum auch nur beeinflußt werden. Der Fall ähnelt sehr unserem oben erwähnten (Abb. 5), bei dem allerdings die Psyche noch beeinflußbar ist, *wenn* man zeitig genug die Wasseranschoppung zu bremsen vermag. Sobald sie aber einmal da ist, hat eine Wiederausschwemmung gar keine Bedeutung mehr, dann läuft eine meist über Wochen gehende Verstimmung ab, ohne in irgendeiner Weise weder von Wasseranreicherung noch von Wasserentziehung beeinflußt werden zu können. In meinem Laboratorium hat BÖDIKER eine Anzahl von Psychosen, aber auch einige gesunde junge Studenten, untersucht. Während BÖDIKER hauptsächlich die chemischen Werte des Serums bestimmte, hat MITTRACH hämatologische Faktoren untersucht; beide aber haben neben einigen sehr eindrucksvollen Parallelisierungen zwischen Schwankungen des Blutgehaltes an Wasser, Kalium und Natrium auf der einen Seite, zwischen Eosinophilen und Verhalten der Leukocytenwerte auf der anderen Seite, auch völlig fehlende Parallelen zwischen psychischem Verhalten und körperlichen Zuständen zu beobachten Gelegenheit gehabt. Deswegen haben wir, da diese Ergebnisse eben doch nicht ausreichend klar waren, auf eine Publikation verzichtet. Die Werte von ROWNTREE und KAY zeigen praktisch die gleiche Parallelität wie diejenigen von Bödiker. Uns scheinen auch die Werte von Rowntree und Kay nicht so eindeutig charakteristisch, daß man sie wirklich für eine Somatologie der periodischen Psychosen verwerten könnte. So haben wir den Eindruck, daß die körperlichen Veränderungen bei den periodischen Psychosen Schrittmacher des psychischen Geschehens sein könnten. Daß sie aber miteinander so eng korreliert sind, daß das eine ohne das andere nicht ein-

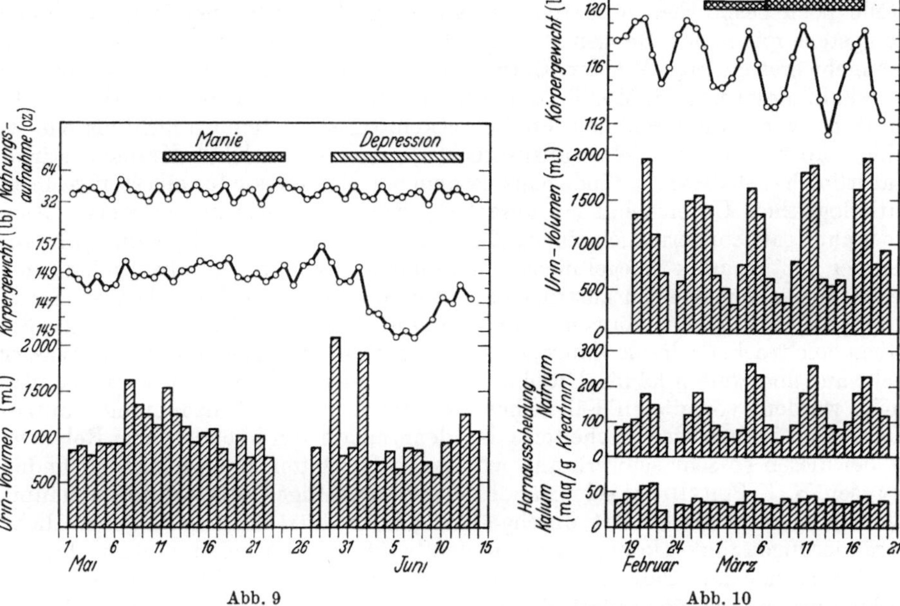

Abb. 9   Abb. 10

Abb. 9. Beziehung zwischen dem Körpergewicht, dem Urinvolumen und dem Verhalten einer periodischen Psychose
Abb. 10. Beziehungen zwischen dem Auftreten kurzfristiger manischer Erregungszustande, dem Körpergewicht und dem Verhalten der Urinmenge mit Kalium- und Natriumausscheidung (Nach Crammer)

treten könnte, kann man u. E. von keinem Fall sagen. Sicherlich sind auch die Fälle von Gjessing zwar häufig oder ganz überwiegend z. B. von der Stickstoffanschoppung begleitet, oder die Stickstoffanschoppung hat irgendeine innere Beziehung zu dem Auftreten der Stuporzustände, aber je älter die Patienten von Gjessing wurden, um so stärker verzögerten sich die Beziehungen zwischen körperlichem und psychischem Befund. Auch bei unseren Kranken, sowie bei den Kranken von Crammer und von Rowntree und Kay scheint es uns so zu liegen, daß der Zusammenhang zwischen psychischem und körperlichem Verhalten nicht immer zwingend ist. Vielleicht spielen da noch andere Dinge, nämlich eine gewisse Gewöhnung oder eine bedingt-reflektorische Auslösung von Verstimmungen eine Rolle. Die bedingt-reflektorische Auslösung wäre auch dann möglich, wenn wirklich die körperlichen Veränderungen unumgänglich mit der psychischen Veränderung verknüpft wären, aber auch die psychischen Veränderungen genau so wie die körperlichen einer entsprechenden Therapie zugänglich wären.

Zustände, wie man sie früher als akute katatone Erregung, später nach Scheid als febril-cyanotische Episode und schließlich unverbindlicher als febrile Hyperkinese bezeichnet hat, kommen prinzipiell bei allen Arten von Psychosen vor, keineswegs ausschließlich bei der Katatonie, wie man das früher angenommen hat. Schon die Fälle von K. F. Scheid sind nach seinen eigenen mündlichen Angaben nicht mit Sicherheit als Schizophrene anzusprechen. Wir selbst haben sie damals, als sie publiziert wurden, im Einverständnis mit Scheid als Zustände innerhalb der Cyclothymie angesehen und aufgefaßt. Aus der Hamburger Klinik sind damals mehrere Untersuchungen veröffentlicht worden, die u. a. zeigten, daß solche Zustände sogar gelegentlich bei Hirntumoren vorkommen!

Diese Zustände waren von jeher äußerst gefährlich, die Kranken waren zweifellos lebensgefährlich krank, und vor Einführung aktiverer Therapie starb die Mehrzahl. Einer der ersten Ansätze zu einer Therapie war der Vorschlag, der an anderer Stelle noch besprochen wird, diese so stark zur Exsikkose neigenden Kranken wenigstens mit hohen Mengen Flüssigkeit zu versorgen, damit die Austrocknung gar nicht erst eintritt. Mit der Einführung der Schocktherapie und insbesondere innerhalb dieser mit der Möglichkeit, Elektroschocks weitgehend gefahrlos durchzuführen, verlor die Krankheit ihre Schrecken. Es ist heute noch nicht als Kunstfehler, aber fast als solcher anzusprechen, wenn ein solcher Kranker stirbt. Natürlich haben diese Zustände ganz besonders viel Interesse für alle stoffwechselpathologischen Untersuchungen ausgelöst, weil man nicht nur schwerste Austrocknung sah, sondern auch regelmäßig den Eindruck hatte, daß bei diesen Kranken der Prothrombin-Spiegel nicht in Ordnung sein könnte. Man beobachtet ausgedehnte flächenhafte Blutaustritte unter der Haut, die z. B. Oberschenkel, Arme, Brustpartien betreffen können, *ohne* daß eine Selbstbeschädigung vorliegt. Sie haben eine trockene, livide Zunge, sind blau im Gesicht, scheiden fast kein Wasser mehr aus und weisen häufig Urobilinogen im Urin auf. Immer wieder ist es versucht worden, von diesen Fällen her die Ätiologie der „Schizophrenie" aufzuklären, und immer wieder scheiterte das, denn nichts von irgendwelcher Relevanz ist bei diesen so sehr schwerkrank wirkenden Patienten nun wirklich zu finden gewesen. K. F. Scheid hat sehr gründliche und sorgfältige Untersuchungen, hauptsächlich hämatologischer Art, durchgeführt und hat tatsächlich einige wesentliche Veränderungen finden können, so u. a. den berühmten Färbeindex-Sturz, der dadurch zustande kam, daß in der akuten Erregung sehr viele rote Blutkörperchen verlorengehen und überstürzt durch neugebildete kleine hyperchrome, häufig sphärocytotisch wirkende Zellen ersetzt werden. Früher hat man auch das bei derartigen Kranken so häufig noch als rot befundene Femurmark, auf das besonders Jahn hingewiesen hat, für pathologisch bedeutungsvoll gehalten. Es hat sich später herausgestellt, daß von jüngeren Menschen weit über 60% rotes Femurmark haben, gerade bei gesunden Verunglückten ließ sich das eindeutig feststellen und beweisen, daß mit dem Auftreten von rotem Femurmark bei jungen Menschen keinerlei pathologische Bedeutung verbunden ist. Ähnlich erging es den Untersuchungen über den Ammoniakgehalt des Blutes. Was Riebeling seinerzeit noch als schizophren erregt bezeichnete *vor* der Arbeit von Scheid, waren im wesentlichen derartige Kranke, bei denen immerhin erheblich mehr Ammoniak im Blut nachgewiesen wurde als in der Norm, obwohl der Ammoniak-Endwert, das, was wir als Ammoniak-Muttersubstanz bezeichnet haben, nicht nennenswert höher war als bei anderen Fällen (s. S. 123).

Conrad und seine Mitarbeiter fanden bei derartigen akuten Katatonien eine deutliche Verkürzung der Prothrombinzeit, die ohne weiteres als Erklärung für die großen Unterhautblutungen dienen könnte. Goldkuhl und Kafka fanden bei Schizophrenen ebenfalls die Prothrombinzeit häufig verkürzt und die Senkung erhöht zum Unterschied von Oezek, der bei Schizophrenen genau das Umgekehrte fand. Das spricht m. E. sehr deutlich dafür, daß die verschiedenen Autoren wahrscheinlich ganz verschiedene Zustandsbilder untersucht haben. Insbesondere hat Oezek seine Untersuchungen an Anstaltsfällen durchgeführt, Conrad an akuten febrilen Episoden. Goldkuhl und Kafka untersuchten wahrscheinlich auch Anstaltsfälle. Daß diese anders gelagert sind als akute frisch Erkrankte, wurde schon verschiedentlich erörtert.

Zur Frage der Hirnschwellung: Wir erwähnten bereits, daß diese Kranken früher sehr gefährdet waren, und wenn sie starben, eine trockene Hirnschwellung aufwiesen. Diese Hirnschwellung hat insbesondere auch RIEBELING sehr interessiert. Er hat in seinen quantitativen Analysen der Gehirne einige bedeutungsvolle Tatsachen gefunden, die sich auch therapeutisch ausgewirkt haben. Sicher ist, daß bei der Hirnschwellung eine Anschoppung von stickstoffhaltigen Substanzen, höchstwahrscheinlich von Serumeiweiß, im Gehirn stattfindet, was sich an einer absoluten Vermehrung des Stickstoffgehalts des Gehirns erkennen läßt und weiterhin an einer nennenswerten, teilweise beträchtlichen Erhöhung der Trockensubstanzgehalte fast sämtlicher Hirnteile (Tab. 1). Daß auch Fälle vorkommen, bei denen nicht alle, sondern nur bestimmte Hirnteile „geschwollen", recte in

Tab. 1. *Trockensubstanz und Stickstoffgehalt bei Fällen, bei denen neben einer Hirnschwellung eine Leberschwellung nachweisbar war. Durchschnittswerte aus 12 Bestimmungen* (Nach RIEBELING)

	Trockensubstanz in g%		Stickstoffgehalt in mg%	
	Durchschnitt	Hirnschwellung	Durchschnitt	Hirnschwellung
Rinde	15,0	16,7	1500	1650
Mark	30,0	32,0	1600	1750
Leber	24	29	2830	3250

ihrer Trockensubstanz vermehrt sind, läßt sich mit pathologisch-anatomischen Untersuchungen ohne weiteres vereinbaren. Insbesondere die Histologen, die sich gerade für die Hirnschwellung interessiert haben, haben immer wieder betont, daß diese keineswegs immer ubiquitär sein müsse. Daß diese Vermehrung von Trockensubstanz nicht, wie das früher üblich war, durch Zufuhr von weiterer hypertonischer Lösung irgendwelcher Art, sei es Traubenzucker, sei es Kochsalz, zu bekämpfen sein konnte, sondern nur durch das Gegenteil, nämlich durch die Zufuhr hypotonischer Lösungen, wurde vom Verfasser verschiedentlich ausgeführt. Alle diese Zustände sind indessen nicht mehr Gegenwart, sondern durch die Einführung der modernen Therapien bereits Vergangenheit.

Über das Körpergewicht

Der unmittelbare Eindruck vermittelt bereits die außerordentlich großen Differenzen im Körpergewicht selbst jahrelang „gleichmäßig" ernährter chronischer Psychosen. Neben dem „gefräßigen" Schizophrenen, unförmig dick und bewegungsarm, steht der dürre ausgemergelte, immer wieder abstinierende und immer wieder nur mit raffinierten Mitteln zum Essen zu zwingende Katatone. Die Schwankungen des Körpergewichts innerhalb einer manischen oder einer depressiven Phase sind dem Pflegepersonal ebenso bekannt wie den Ärzten. Es dürfte ziemlich sicher sein, daß man bei einer phasisch verlaufenden Psychose dann mit einer Besserung der Depression rechnen darf, wenn dieser Mensch an Gewicht wieder zunimmt. Daß das nicht immer der Fall ist, sondern daß auch insbesondere Fettleibige sich dann bessern, wenn sie an Gewicht wieder abnehmen, widerspricht nicht prinzipiell diesen Vorstellungen, daß zwischen den Körpergewichtsschwankungen und den Verhaltensschwankungen bestimmte, wenn auch nur sehr geringe Beziehungen bestehen. Natürlich darf man dabei nicht vergessen, worauf wir an anderer Stelle schon hingewiesen haben, daß unter Umständen die chronischen Psychosen schlecht ernährt werden oder bei ausreichend bereitgestellter Ernährung sich selber nicht genügend versorgen. Geschieht das aber doch, dann sollte man extreme Körpergewichtsschwankungen nur sehr selten finden und immerhin fällt auf, daß PARIN unter 377 Schizophrenen nur 3% mit abnormen Körpergewichten fand, nämlich nur 6 Fettleibige und 5 Magere. Auch bei diesen will er die Gewichtsanomalien durch die Nahrungszufuhr erklären und glaubt, daß endogene Gewichtsschwankungen nicht vorkommen. Wir haben seinerzeit zu dieser Arbeit bemerkt, daß derartige Ergebnisse eindeutig eigenen und z. B. auch denen Gjessings (s. Abb. 11) widersprechen. Auch Post erklärt die meisten Körpergewichtsschwankungen durch Eßgewohnheiten, aber man sollte sich bei jeder Erörterung der Fett- wie auch der Magersucht der alten Tatsache bewußt bleiben, daß *ohne* Essen eben niemand dick werden kann und daß es gute und schlechte Futterverwerter gibt.

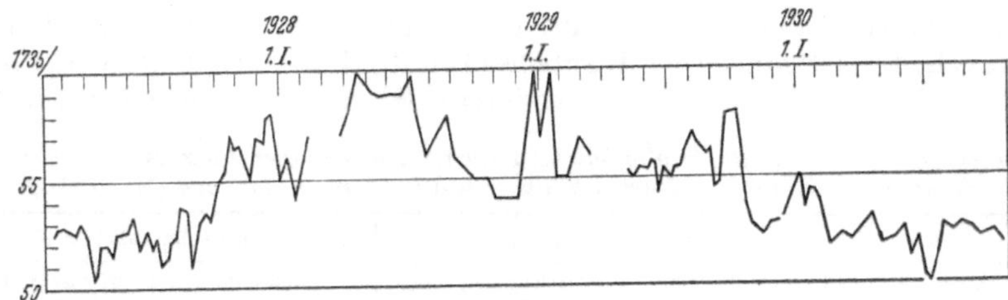

Abb. 11. Körpergewichtsschwankungen eines psychotischen Patienten über mehrere Jahre parallel zur Verhaltensweise (Nach Gjessing)

Am Ende darf man nicht vergessen, daß kurzfristige Körpergewichtsschwankungen, z. B. wie sie Crammer beobachtet hat, nämlich bis zu 4 kg Zu- oder Abnahme innerhalb von 24 Std, meistens auf Wasser- und Salzretention bzw. -verlust beruhen. Die Körpergewichtskurven aber, wie Gjessing sie seinerzeit bei langfristigen Beobachtungen beschrieben hat, geben doch zu denken und wir glauben, daß das Problem so einfach nicht abzutun ist.

Auch Kryspin-Exner hat sich mit den Körpergewichtsschwankungen beschäftigt und glaubt, daß diese sogar ein sehr feines Reagens auf Schwankungen des psychopathologischen Geschehens abgeben. Gar nicht so selten zeige die Gewichtskurve einen Umschwung vor klinisch erkennbaren Änderungen im psychischen Zustand der Kranken. Wir halten seine Meinung, daß nur dann ein Anstieg des Körpergewichtes nach Einsetzen eines akuten psychotischen Zustandes beobachtet wird, wenn eine Depression ohne freies Intervall in eine Manie übergeht, für zu eng gefaßt. Wir selber sahen wenigstens die Gewichtsschwankungen auch durchaus unabhängig vom Verlauf der Psychose ohne sichtbaren Zusammenhang mit irgendwelchen psychischen Schwankungen. Am eindrucksvollsten war in dieser Beziehung ein Mädchen von geradezu grotesken Körpermaßen, eine echte „gefräßige" Schizophrene, die über 120 kg wog und ohne irgendeine erkennbare Änderung weder ihres Regimes noch therapeutischer Art — es war vor der Ära der aktiven Therapie — noch auf Grund irgendwelcher anderer körperlichen Störungen plötzlich an Gewicht abnahm und nach einem Jahr zum Skelet abgemagert genauso inaktiv und genauso „wurstig" im Bett lag wie früher.

Blut und Kreislauf

Von den reichlichen hämatologischen Beobachtungen, die im Laufe der Jahre gemacht worden sind, haben wirkliche Bedeutung für die Ätiologie der Psychosen nur ganz wenige gewonnen. Immerhin ist es eindrucksvoll, daß manche erblichen Anomalien der Erythrocyten oder auch der Leukocyten praktisch nur bei psychotischen bzw. psychopathischen Individuen beobachtet werden. So ist die Pelger-Anomalie eng korreliert mit psychopathischen Persönlichkeitsveränderungen. Man

findet sie nur ausnahmsweise bei psychisch ganz Gesunden. Auch die *Ovalocytose*
findet sich vorzugsweise bei psychopathischen Individuen. Man ist versucht zu
korrelieren, daß diese Veränderungen im gleichen Sinne zu deuten wären wie das,
was man früher einmal als Degenerationszeichen bezeichnet hat. Diese Degenerationszeichen könnten, nunmehr im mikroskopischen Bereich statt wie früher im
makroskopischen Bereich gesucht, auch wieder ein Mehr an Sinter-Phänomenen
oder Domestikationsphänomenen darstellen, was bei den Psychosen, aber vorzugsweise beim Schwachsinn und bei der Epilepsie, eben generell als Sinter-Phänomen
bezeichnet wird. Den ersten Fall von homozygotem Pelger, der überhaupt beim
Menschen beobachtet ist, hat HAVERKAMP beschrieben und bei diesem Patienten
handelte es sich um einen Epileptiker!

Wir beobachteten z. B. in einem Fall ein sehr eigenartiges Verhalten der Färbbarkeit von Blutbildern, das wir bei anderen Psychosen nur sehr selten wieder-
sahen. Um den Schwankungen des „Laborbetriebes" zu entgehen, wurden in allen
seinerzeit durchgeführten Reihenuntersuchungen sämtliche Blutbilder gesammelt
und erst etwa 10 Tage nach dem letzten Blutbild sämtlich auf einmal gefärbt.
Damit entgingen wir den Schwankungen des p_H des destillierten Wassers, eventuellen Schwankungen in der Zusammensetzung der Farbflüssigkeiten, selbst
wenn sie minimal gewesen wären, und außerdem Schwankungen der Färbezeit
usw. Diese Vorsichtsmaßregeln haben aufgedeckt, was wir nicht erwarten konnten, daß nämlich die Blutbilder schon makroskopisch einen ganz wesentlichen
Unterschied aufwiesen, der wenigstens bei dem einen Fall in eindeutiger Beziehung
zu den übrigen Veränderungen, insbesondere des Wassergehalts des Blutes, stand.
Wir waren daher geneigt, die Veränderungen der Färbbarkeit auf Verschiebungen des Wassergehalts der roten Blutkörperchen zurückzuführen. MITTRACH,
die später im Laboratorium des Verfassers eine größere Serie von Fällen untersuchte, konnte diese Resultate nicht bestätigen. Wir haben aber ausdrücklich
bei den beiden Fällen, bei denen wir sowohl verschiedene Färbbarkeit als auch
verschiedene Verteilung der Segmentierung gefunden hatten, einige Monate später
die Duplikate der Ausstriche, die noch vorhanden waren, nachgefärbt und sind
zu genau den gleichen Resultaten gekommen. Erklärt sind sie allerdings nicht.

MITTRACH fand immerhin bei ihren 17 Untersuchungen, daß zwischen dem
hohen Wassergehalt des Blutes und dem psychischen Verhalten eine gewisse
Beziehung bestand. Außerdem fanden sich bei 8 von den gesamt untersuchten
Fällen die gleichen Beziehungen zwischen Wassergehalt und Eosinophilenzahl,
wie wir sie früher auch gefunden hatten.

DEGKWITZ fand eine ganz auffällige Veränderung des Blutvolumens bei bestimmten Psychosen, die zu erklären bisher einfach nicht möglich war (Tab. 2).
Die aktive Blutmenge ist bei manischen Phasen, bei agitierten Depressionen und
bei schizophrenen Erregungszuständen nennenswert verkleinert und wird normalisiert durch die Therapie. Weder mit der Erschöpfung noch mit der Übermüdung
gehetzter Kranker, noch mit dem, was sonst zu einer verminderten aktiven Blutmenge führt, nämlich Schock, Kollaps, Hypotonie, orthostatische Regulationsstörungen, können diese Phänomene etwas zu tun haben. Sie entziehen sich bisher
der Deutung. Gerade bei den Manien, bei denen man insbesondere immer die
geringe Ermüdbarkeit und die hohe Leistungsfähigkeit bewundert, hätte man
am wenigsten — wie DEGKWITZ schreibt — einen Kreislaufbefund erwartet, der
bei anderen einen Kollaps bedeutet. Daß 1937 FINKELMAN und HAFFRON entgegengesetzte Befunde publizierten, dürfte wohl zum großen Teil an der verschiedenen diagnostischen Auffassung der verschiedenen Schulen liegen. Die letzt-
genannten Autoren sind Amerikaner und neigen daher dazu, sehr viel häufiger eine
Schizophrenie zu diagnostizieren, als es in Europa üblich ist. Daraus scheint

Tabelle 2. *Schwankungen von Blutvolumen und von Kochsalz in Blutserum und Harn im Verlauf von Psychosen* (Nach DEGKWITZ)

Fall Nr.	Diagnose	I. Bestimmung					Abstand	II. Bestimmung				
		Blutmenge cm³	Hämatokrit	Spez. Gewicht	NaCl im Ser. mg-%	NaCl im Harn mg-%	Tage	Blutmenge cm³	Hämatokrit	Spez. Gewicht	NaCl i. Serum mg-%	NaCl im Harn mg-%
2	leichte manische Phase	3815	46	1021	595	328	20	4210	42	1022	627	575
3	Manie	4075	44	1008	613	260	14	4453	41	1010	592	457
6	agitierte Depression . .	5085	49,5	1022	611	898	11	5910	47	1025	586	890
10	Depression . .	4785	42,5	1024	572	316						
15	paranoide Schizophrenie.	4925	42	1022	610	678	12	4835	40	1020	610	720

mir aber doch der nur relative Wert auch der so interessanten Feststellungen von
DEGKWITZ hervorzugehen, der nun einmal darin begründet ist, daß Schwankungen
bei den verschiedenen Psychosen ständig vorkommen und daß also diese Zustände
sicherlich keine Specifica für irgendeine besondere Form von Psychosen darstellen
(HODSKINS, GUTHRIE und NAURISON). Signifikant niedriger als normal ist bei
älteren Schizophrenen, die zumindest vier Jahre krank sind, die Sauerstoffauf-
nahme des Gehirns bei im übrigen den Gesunden gleich starker Durchblutung. Die
Messungen ergaben immerhin Werte, die weit außerhalb der Fehlerbreite liegen.
Da sie aber nur bei alten Fällen beobachtet wurden, schließen die Verfasser mit

Tabelle 3. *Blutdruckbestimmungen bei 423 Schizophrenen* (nach LINGJAERDE u. Mitarb.),
verglichen mit einer großen Zahl von Normalen (Nach ROBINSON u. BRUCER)

Alter	Schizophrene		Normalwerte	
	Anzahl	systol. Blutdruck	Anzahl	systol. Blutdruck
20—29	46	$98\pm1{,}4$	833	109
30—39	76	$98\pm1{,}1$	1178	113
40—44	34	$108\pm3{,}0$	495	119
45—49	31	$111\pm3{,}8$	349	125
50—54	23	$118\pm5{,}4$	201	126
55—59	26	$126\pm5{,}3$	141	138
60—64	25	$147\pm7{,}5$	71	143
65—69	24	$147\pm1{,}8$	35	146
70—74	30	$150\pm1{,}4$	8	(137)
75—	18	$175\pm7{,}4$	2	(168)

Recht, daß es sich wahrscheinlich um sekundäre Phänomene handelte, die mit der
eigentlichen Psychose nichts zu tun haben. Die wahrscheinlich ausführlichsten
Blutdruckmessungen an Psychosen haben LINGJAERDE und seine Schüler LAANE
und STROM durchgeführt. Es handelt sich immerhin um 3 000 Blutdruckmessungen
bei 423 Schizophrenen, davon 333 Frauen im Alter zwischen 20 und 85 und 90 Männer im Alter von 50 bis 76 Jahren (Tab. 3). Die Tabelle ist recht aufschlußreich,
insbesondere auch der Vergleich mit den Normalwerten von ROBINSON und
BRUCER. Noch deutlicher zeigen die Werte der Tab. 4, daß bei Schizophrenen
unter 60 Jahren weit mehr Hypotonien vorkommen als im Vergleichsmaterial.
Die Mehrzahl der jüngeren Schizophrenen mit niedrigem Blutdruck befand sich
übrigens in der aktiven Phase der Krankheit. Daß auch diese niedrigen Blut-
drucke nicht ohne weiteres vor einem späteren Hypertonus schützen, fand der

Tabelle 4. *Häufigkeit von systolischem Blutdruck unter 100 mmHg bei Schizophrenen und bei Normalen im Vergleich* (Nach RIEBELING)

Alter	Unter 40 J.	40—49 J.	50—59 J.	60—69 J.	70 J. oder höher
Schizophrene	41%	32,3%	16,3%	6,1%	0
Normale	-19,6%	12,1%	6,1%	4,7%	?

Verfasser 1949, zur Zeit der Nachprüfungen der alten blutdruckuntersuchten Fälle. Bei derartigen Untersuchungen berühren sich vielleicht doch die so heterogenen Begriffe der Psychose überhaupt und der Konstitution. Wenn man sich überlegt, daß ein Pykniker im allgemeinen doch einen höheren Blutdruck hat als der Astheniker und der Leptosome, obwohl diese Beziehungen nicht absolut sind, sondern allenfalls eine Häufigkeitsverteilung darstellen, dann würde das auch wieder unterstreichen, daß die leptosomen und asthenischen Typen unter den Schizophrenen, wenn auch nicht die Norm ausmachen, aber doch überwiegen.

Beziehung zwischen Hormonhaushalt und Psychose

LINGJAERDE hat unter 178 Patientinnen, die er über zwei Jahre lang beobachtet hat, immerhin bei 149 Kranken, das entspricht rund 85%, vor allem in der aktiven Phase, Regelstörungen, meistens sogar Amenorrhoe, beobachtet. Bei einigen Patientinnen setzte das Klimakterium sehr früh ein, gelegentlich sogar schon im Alter von 25 Jahren. REHM hat ausgedehnte Untersuchungen der Menstruation bei Geisteskranken gemacht, ohne indes zu eindeutigen Resultaten zu kommen. Insbesondere ist er sehr viel vorsichtiger als zum Beispiel KNAUS, der apodiktisch erklärt, daß alle jungen schizophrenen Mädchen mit dem Ausbruch der Psychose amenorrhoisch werden, daß alle periodischen Psychosen in ursächlichem und auch in äußerlich zeitlichem Zusammenhang mit Veränderungen der Menstruation stünden. Aus den Untersuchungen von FRÖSHAUG ergibt sich im Gegenteil, daß Stuporphasen gänzlich unabhängig von den Menses auftreten. DALTON hat 276 Frauen mit psychiatrischer Anamnese untersucht. Die Autorin hat in dieser Arbeit sorgfältig zwischen Menstruum, das ist der 1. bis 4. Tag, Ovulation und Prämenstruum, 13. bis 16. bzw. 25. bis 28. Tag, unterschieden. Die Aufnahme ins Krankenhaus erfolgte in weniger als der Hälfte der Fälle in der Menstruationsperiode, aber andererseits fielen sehr viele erfolgreiche Suicide auf die Zeit der Ovulation. Diejenigen Patientinnen, die während des Prämenstruums zur Behandlung kamen, verschlimmerten sich gewöhnlich erst noch bis zum Ende der Menses. Die Zahlen, die die Autorin über die Verhältnisse bringt, sind bei dem niedrigen Prozent der Gesamtzeit (4 bis 8 Tage von 28) relativ hoch. Bei jüngeren Frauen macht sich der Einfluß der Menses wesentlich deutlicher bemerkbar als bei denen über 45 Jahre. GELLER konnte z. B. bei 400 von 500 untersuchten schizophrenen Frauen Regelstörungen der verschiedensten Art feststellen. Dabei handelte es sich aber ausnahmslos um ältere Anstaltsinsassinnen, die vielleicht auch durch das Anstaltsleben bereits verändert worden waren.

So wie man die Manisch-Drepessiven der früheren Psychiatrie insbesondere als ausgeglichene harmonische, auch in ihrem Endokrinium völlig regelmäßige Menschen angesehen hat, so hat man von jeher umgekehrt den Schizophrenen als endokrin-apart, als abwegig, als hypogenital z. B., als hypothyreotisch oder auch hyperthyreotisch angesehen. Immer wieder wurden solche Dinge beobachtet und erwähnt, fast nie aber sind sie sorgfältig untersucht worden. Erst in neuerer Zeit kann man wirklich von einer ernstzunehmenden Endokrinologie der Psychosen sprechen. Mit den endokrinen Psychosen, die BLEULER speziell behandelt, haben diese Erörterungen insofern nichts zu tun, als es sich ja bei den Fällen von Bleuler sicher um echte endokrine Störungen handelt, in deren Gefolge eine Psychose auftritt. Zwar sind mitunter Azoospermien oder Oligospermien bei schizophrenen Männern gefunden worden, zwar hat — wie ja auch an anderer Stelle erwähnt wird — das schizophrene junge Mädchen häufig genug Menstruationsstörungen, aber keineswegs lassen die Organe irgendwelche sicheren Störungen vermuten, und keineswegs bleiben diese Kranken aus endokrinen Gründen außerhalb der Gesellschaft, sondern nur aus psychischen Gründen. Zwar hat Gjessing versucht, und es ist ihm zum Teil auch gelungen, durch sehr langhingezogene regelmäßige Gaben von Thyroxin bzw. Thyreoidin einen Ausgleich der Störungen bei den periodischen Katatonien zu erzielen (Mall hat diese Untersuchungen nachgeahmt, auch er mit teilweisem Erfolg), aber das dürfte wohl mehr eine unmittelbare Beeinflussung eines gesamt-vegetativ veränderten Menschen gewesen sein als eine spezielle Beeinflussung einer endokrinen Störung. Sands drückt sich sehr vorsichtig aus, indem er sagt, daß es unwahrscheinlich sei, daß die „gegenwärtigen großen diagnostischen Gruppen" mit irgendeiner Größe endokriner Veränderungen korreliert werden könnten.

Beziehungen des Wasserhaushaltes zur Psychose

Büssow hat den Wassergehalt bei *Depressiven* durch Tonephin-Wasserstoß beeinflußt und hat dabei genau das gleiche gesehen, was Epileptiker und übrigens Gesunde ebenso zeigen, nämlich eine schnell auftretende Blässe, die wahrscheinlich auf die Wirkung des Tonephins zurückzuführen ist, eine ödematöse Anschwellung des Gesichts und eine Blutdrucksteigerung um 20—30 mm Hg. Der Puls war gespannt. Eine Harnsperre, die beim Gesunden und beim Epileptiker nach einer Tonephin-Injektion im allgemeinen 2 bis 3 Stunden anhält, hielt bei den depressiven Kranken, die er untersuchte, 4 bis 5 Stunden lang an. Etwa 3 bis 4 Stunden nach der Wassergabe wurden die Patienten zunehmend bewegungsarm bis zur Akinese, sie lagen mit geschlossenen Augen zurückgelehnt im Bett, wirkten somnolent, manche schliefen auch ein.

Mit Anfang der Ausscheidung setzte eine Aktivitätssteigerung und eine Besserung des Befindens wie bei Rekonvaleszenz ein. Auch Gesunde, die Karstens untersuchte, denen er 3 bis 4 Liter Flüssigkeit zu trinken gab und von denen übrigens nur einige Studenten überhaupt die gesamte Menge zu trinken vermochten, fühlten sich schläfrig, verlangsamt, die Aufmerksamkeit war gesenkt, die Stimmung allerdings wenig beeinflußt; bei Zugabe von Tonephin war die Stimmung erheblich stärker, bis zu fast depressiven Verhaltensweisen, beeinflußt. Solche Phänomene erinnern doch sehr stark an diejenigen, die wir bei dem Fall von Wasserretention mit Stuporzuständen gesehen haben, der bereits im Rahmen der Periodik ausführlich besprochen wurde. Vielleicht haben die Psychosen doch mehr Beziehungen zu einem gestörten oder labilen Wassergehalt, als wir bisher feststellen konnten. Wissen wir doch, daß z. B. bei den febrilcyanotischen Episoden zu der Zeit, als sie noch überwiegend starben, die wesentliche Todesursache eine Exsiccose war. Heute, wo sie durch Elektroschock mit hoher Sicherheit zu retten sind, kommt nicht mehr zum Zuge, was seinerzeit — als die Schocktherapie noch unbekannt war — in unserer Klinik eine große Rolle spielte, nämlich die Zufuhr hoher Flüssigkeitsmengen, die später auch Lenz unabhängig von mir vorgeschlagen hat.

Verhalten der Elektrolyte bei verschiedenen Formen von Psychosen

Im Verhältnis zu den so einfachen Verfahren, Natrium, Kalium, Calcium zu bestimmen, und der Zahl der Untersuchungen speziell bei Geisteskranken sind die Ergebnisse immer recht mager geblieben. Nur dürfte sicher sein, daß man den

Schwankungen des Calciums mit Recht wenig Bedeutung beizumessen braucht. Wohl kann man mit weitgehender Sicherheit sagen, daß die Ca-Werte im Serum der Depressiven eher etwas höher sind als normal, was wir an zahlreichen Untersuchungen bestätigt haben, und daß die Therapie mit Ca-Ionen, wie sie selbst heute noch mitunter gepflegt wird, allenfalls einen gewissen sedativen Effekt haben kann für einen Moment, niemals aber kausal irgendeine Bedeutung gewonnen hat oder noch gewinnen wird. Bei mir durchgeführte Untersuchungen über den Kochsalzgehalt des Serums von Psychosen ergeben ganz eindeutig in ihrer Verteilung ein Binom, das sich mit dem deckt, das bei Gesunden gefunden wird. Werden aber unter besonderen Belastungen die Vorräte des Organismus an Natrium oder Kalium oder auch an Chlor überbeansprucht, dann können sehr unangenehme Zustände beobachtet werden, wie dies aus einer Arbeit von WELTI hervorgeht, der als Konsiliarius eine Anzahl von Herzoperationen sah. Immerhin zeigte fast ein Drittel der Fälle psychische Symptome, wenn ihr Natriumspiegel einen tiefen Punkt erreicht hatte, der bei der wochenlangen natriumarmen Diät zur Vorbereitung der Operation verständlich geworden war. Drei Fälle sind aber wichtiger als die anderen. Bei diesen fiel der Natriumwert postoperativ ganz bedrohlich ab. Wurden diese Werte — die etwa 113 mäq entsprachen — erreicht, dann brach ein Delir aus, das prompt aufhellte, wenn hypertonische Kochsalzlösungen zugeführt wurden, allerdings abgeschwächt noch blieb. Die Patienten waren besonnen, aber noch desorientiert. Erst bei 135 mäq am 10. Tage war das Delir völlig abgeklungen. Wie aus den Diagrammen — betr. Aufnahme und Ausscheidung von Natrium — hervorgeht, kann es sich z. Z. der Operation nicht darum handeln, daß alles aus dem Serum verschwundene Natrium auch den Körper verlassen hat. Es muß vielmehr ein Teil ins Gewebe abgewandert sein. Die beiden anderen fraglichen Fälle verhielten sich sehr ähnlich. In allen drei Fällen begannen die Symptome bei niedrigem Natriumspiegel und gingen wieder zurück bei etwa 310 mg-% = 135 mäq.

Was den Chlorgehalt des Gewebes angeht, so scheint mir insbesondere wichtig das Ergebnis, das wir beim Liquor der tuberkulös-meningitischen Kinder erheben konnten und im Anschluß an die dort gemachten Beobachtungen an einer Gruppe von Geweben von Tuberkulösen sahen (Tab. 5).

Tabelle 5. *Gewebschlor bei Meningitis tuberculosa und bei anderen Todesfällen*
(Chlorgehalt in mäq) (Nach RIEBELING)

Rinde	Mark	Ges. H.	Leber	Niere	Milz	Herz	Musk.	Pia	
75	69		60	69	67	58	63	96	Carcinome
		75	70	70	71	61	55	125	Meningitis tuberculosa

Wir hatten vor vielen Jahren darauf hingewiesen, daß der Chlorgehalt des Liquors bei der tuberkulösen Meningitis ganz besonders niedrig ist, niedriger als die Chlorgehalte bei anderen Meningitiden, und daß weiterhin die Höhe des Chlorspiegels des Liquors prognostisch bedeutungsvoll sei für die Prognose der tuberkulösen Meningitis, derart nämlich, daß je niedriger der Chlorgehalt am Anfang der Krankheit ist, um so schlechter die Prognose für eine spezifische Therapie moderner Art sei. Der Zuckergehalt des tuberkulösen Liquors spielt in dieser Beziehung überhaupt keine Rolle, ebensowenig der Eiweißgehalt oder der Gehalt an Zellen. Unsere Versuche, den verminderten Chlorgehalt des Liquor cerebrospinalis bei der Meningitis tuberculosa zu erklären, beachteten von vornherein nicht die immer wieder angewandte Theorie vom Donnan-Gleichgewicht, wonach dem niedrigen Eiweißgehalt ein höherer Kochsalzgehalt des Liquors zugehöre, um das Membrangleichgewicht herzustellen. Dieses Membrangleichgewicht wird mit ganz anderen Mechanismen aufrechterhalten. Wir glaubten mit Sicherheit annehmen zu dürfen, daß nicht ein niedriger Chlorgehalt des Serums in Betracht käme, sondern daß die Meningen in irgendeiner Weise dabei beteiligt sein müssen. Deswegen angestellte Untersuchungen des Gehaltes der Meningen an Chlor gegenüber anderen Geweben ergaben die erstaunliche Tatsache, daß die Meningen relativ die chlorreichsten Organe des Körpers sind. Wir sahen allerdings nur einen Fall von Miliartuberkulose, bei dem wir auch die Meningen untersuchen konnten, haben damals aber einen Chlorwert des Gewebes festgestellt, der weit über allem anderen lag, was wir bisher gefunden hatten.

Daraus scheint uns mit Sicherheit hervorzugehen, daß die Meningen ausgesprochen *chlorbedürftig* sind, ebenso wie übrigens auch die Rinde der tuberkulös-meningitischen Kranken ausgesprochen chlorverarmt ist gegenüber normaler Rinde. Auch dieses Gewebschlor wird offenbar verwendet, um die Meningen abzusättigen, und der niedrige Chlorgehalt des Liquors ist maßgebend für den hohen Chlorgehalt der Meningen. Den niedrigen Gehalt des Hirngewebes an Chlor haben bereits Moritz und Kulcsár 1936 beschrieben. Harrison, Finberg und Fleishman untersuchten ebenfalls das Ionengleichgewicht bei tuberkulös-meningitischen Kindern und fanden das gleiche wie wir. Bezüglich des Gehirns konnten wir die Feststellung von Kerpel-Fronius über die Chloropexie der Rinde normaler Gehirne durchaus auch für die Psychosen bestätigen. Wir fanden aber die Unterschiede zwischen verschiedenen Psychosengruppen so auffällig groß, daß es sich lohnt, darauf einzugehen. Bei den akuten katatonen Todesfällen (Tab. 6, erste Rubrik links) war der Gehalt der Rinde fast über 20% höher als bei allen anderen Fällen. Bei Paralyse, Urämie und bei den meisten anderen Psychosen war er ziemlich gleich. Bei einer Reihe von Paralysen war übrigens regelmäßig der Gehalt des Kleinhirns an Chlor am allerhöchsten.

Tabelle 6. *Chlorgehalt des Gehirns bei verschiedenen Todesfällen aus psychiatrischem Material*

Mittelwerte fur den Chlorgehalt, auf Trockensubstanz berechnet, in γ %					
Schizophrenie	Schiz.-ähnliche aber nicht S.	Urämie	Paralyse	andere Falle	Material
2392	1784	1830	1824	1910	Rinde
865	737	854	1357	686	Mark
1396	1117	1108	1560	1111	Stammganglien
1213	1074	1196	2418	1153	Kleinhirn

Ferroni hat den Kochsalzgehalt des Serums bei Epileptikern modifiziert, um dadurch Anfälle auszulösen. Wir selber haben durch Maack mit Schneekloth diese Untersuchungen nachprüfen lassen; es gelang niemals, Anfälle durch Kochsalzbelastung auszulösen. Bei den an anderer Stelle schon erwähnten Fällen von Crammer zeigte sich, daß dem Einsetzen einer Depression ein Gewichtsverlust mit Natriumchlorid-Ausscheidung und dem Abklingen eine Gewichtszunahme durch Oligurie und Natriumretention parallelgeschaltet waren. Wurde die Zufuhr von Wasser und Natrium eingeschränkt, so ließ sich in dem einen Fall die Gewichtsschwankung fast völlig bremsen, die psychische Symptomatik wurde aber nicht wesentlich beeinflußt. Sowohl am Natriumgehalt des Serums als am Hämatokritwert zeigten sich übrigens vor dem Einsetzen jeder polyurischen Phase die relative Hyponatriämie und der große Wassergehalt des Blutes.

Riebeling hat als erster im Liquor Ammoniak nachgewiesen und damals bereits gezeigt, daß der Ammoniakgehalt des Liquors bei einem Status epilepticus wesentlich höher ist als normal. Er hat außerdem eine große Reihe von Ammoniakbestimmungen im Blut von Gesunden und Geisteskranken durchgeführt und damals schon festgestellt, daß innerhalb der ersten Sekunden nach der Blutentnahme bereits der Ammoniakgehalt des Blutes ansteigt, so daß unter Umständen sogar damit gerechnet werden muß, daß freies Ammoniak in vivo überhaupt nicht vorhanden ist.

Tabelle 7. *Ammoniakgehalt des Blutes sofort (A) und nach 2 Std Exposition unter Fermentbedingungen (B)* (in mg-%)

	A-Wert	B-Wert
Normal	0,49	5,71
Nierenschäden . .	0,53	5,58
motor. unruhig . .	0,84	6,21
Schizophr. erregt .	1,20	6,95

Verglichen mit den Befunden von SELIGSON, die mit einer einfacheren Technik als der damals angewandten erhoben wurden, waren die Resultate von RIEBELING durchaus im gleichen Bereich. Angeregt durch den Befund, daß bei der Epilepsie nach Krämpfen Ammoniakvermehrungen zu finden waren, die damals auf Ammoniakaustritt aus der Muskulatur zurückgeführt wurden, wurden auch im Blut und im Gehirn von Psychosen große Mengen von Ammoniakbestimmungen durchgeführt; unabhängig von RIEBELING hatten auch SCHWARZ und DIEBOLD Ammoniakbestimmungen publiziert. Die Autoren hatten die Möglichkeit, mit flüssiger Luft zu arbeiten und lebendfrisches Gehirn anläßlich von Hirnoperationen zu entnehmen. Ihre Werte lagen naturgemäß niedriger als unsere, die an Leichengehirnen erhoben waren, sie lagen aber in der gleichen Größenordnung wie die, die wir bei

Tabelle 8. *Gehalt des Kaninchengehirns an Ammoniak sofort (A) und insgesamt nach 2 Std Exposition (B)*

A-Wert (präf. NH₃)	B-Wert (insgesamt aus Ammoniakmuttersubstanz bildbar)
0,5 mg%	8,0 mg%

unseren Kaninchengehirnen fanden, so daß wir daraus den Schluß ziehen durften, daß unsere Werte durch die Zeitdauer der Entnahme und der Verarbeitung auch ohne die Hilfe von flüssiger Luft nicht nennenswert schlechter waren als die mit möglichst schneller Unterbrechung der Fermentvorgänge.

Tabelle 9. *A- und B-Werte von Rinde und Mark bei verschiedenen Psychosen* Weitere Erklärung s. Text

	Ammoniakgehalt in mg %			
	Rinde		Mark	
	A-Wert	B-Wert	A-Wert	B-Wert
„normal“	4,5	10,0	3,1	12,0
Dem. senilis	4,9	8,9	5,3	9,1
Schizophrenie	5,8	11,3	5,7	13,2
Paralyse	6,4	13,4	7,7	18,4
Urämie	7,7	13,8	9,7	15,7
Status epil.	16	21	15,5	21
Alzheimer	24,7	45,1	28,8	78,1

Aus den Ergebnissen von Expositionsversuchen, bei denen die Gesamtmenge des überhaupt erzielbaren Ammoniaks durch Abspaltung in 2%iger Bicarbonatlösung bei 40° zwei Stunden lang untersucht wurde (sog. B-Wert), konnte der

Schluß gezogen werden, daß eine Abspaltung von Ammoniak aus der Ammoniak-
muttersubstanz nur bis zu einem bestimmten Punkt möglich ist und daß dieser
Punkt schnell erreicht wird, unabhängig von evtl. Eiweißspaltung, denn nach
zwei Stunden bereits war sämtliches abspaltbares Ammoniak gespalten, und ob
man nun länger, bis zu 24 Std. in der gleichen Situation exponierte oder nicht, es
fanden sich keine anderen Werte. Erst nach Tagen weiterer Exposition erfolgte
ein ganz geringfügiger Anstieg, der *dann* vielleicht auf Eiweißfäulnis zurückzuführen war. FISCHLER hatte an Eckfistel-Hunden festgestellt, daß die Tiere nur
dann einigermaßen bei klarem Bewußtsein und einige Tage am Leben bleiben
konnten, wenn sie fleischfrei ernährt wurden, d. h., wenn die Stickstoffzufuhr
von außen minimal blieb. Alle Stoffe, aus denen Ammoniak frei werden konnte,
führten zu schweren Schädigungen der Tiere. Später untersuchten McDERMOTT
einen Fall einer portocavalen Shunt-Operation, bei dem ein Koma aufgetreten
war. Er hielt es für möglich, daß es sich um eine Ammoniakvergiftung handelte,
und konnte das auch durch Ammoniakbestimmungen bestätigen. Auch bei
diesem Menschen blieb der Ammoniakgehalt des Blutes niedrig und er blieb
bewußtseinsklar, wenn möglichst wenig Eiweiß und möglichst wenig stickstoffhaltige Substanzen gegeben wurden. Sobald der Patient Harnstoff, Ammoniumchlorid, Eiweiß oder andere Ammoniak-liefernde Körper einnahm, wurde er wieder
bewußtseinsgetrübt bzw. verwirrt, entwickelte übrigens gegen eiweißreiche Speisen
einen ausgesprochenen Widerwillen, der bis zur völligen Essensverweigerung
führte. Auch REINBOLD sah einen ähnlichen Fall. Er wird aber von SUMMERSKILL
u. Mitarb. widerlegt, die keinerlei Beziehungen zwischen der Höhe des Ammoniak-
spiegels und der Schwere eines Leberkomas fanden. BESSMANN hingegen glaubte,
daß doch eine derartige Beziehung vorliegen müsse. Er nimmt an, daß das Gehirn
dann Ammoniak aus dem Blut aufnimmt, wenn der Blutspiegel über 100 γ liegt.
In den Lebervenen konnte WHITE kein Ammoniak finden. Erst wenn die Nadel
mindestens 3 min gelegen hatte, zeigten sich meßbare Ammoniakwerte. Belastungs-
versuche an Leberkranken zeigten aber, daß bereits nach 3 g Ammoniumchlorid der
Ammoniakspiegel gerade in diesen Venen erheblich ansteigt. Bei seinen Versuchen
fand er etwa in 10% der Fälle neurologische Symptome bei erhöhtem Ammoniakspiegel. SHERLOCK möchte an ihrem Material zeigen, daß die Höhe des Ammoniaks
mit der Bewußtseinstrübung beim Leberkoma doch in enger Korrelation steht.

WEIL-MALHERBE hat an Gehirnschnitten im Warburg-Gerät gefunden, daß die
Ammoniakbildung auf eine von der oxydativen Phosphorylierung unabhängige
Reaktion zurückgeführt werden könnte. Da aber der Gehalt an Ammoniak parallel
zu dem anderen Rest-Stickstoff zunahm, glaubte WEIL-MALHERBE daraus schließen
zu dürfen, daß die Ammoniakbildung doch auf eine Proteolyse zurückzuführen sei.
Wie bereits erwähnt, konnten wir derartiges überhaupt nie finden. Auch VRBA
fand die Ammoniakbildung parallel zu einer Erhöhung des Lipoidstickstoffes und
außerdem, daß eine Erhöhung der Kaliumkonzentration die Bildung von Ammoniak verhindert. Daher meint er, man müsse damit rechnen, daß das Auftreten
von Ammoniak wenigstens teilweise mit einer Wanderung des Kaliums in die
intercellulären Räume verbunden sei. Weiterhin schließt VRBA daraus, daß eine
proteolytische Entstehung des Ammoniaks geradezu ausgeschlossen ist. Hier muß
erwähnt werden, daß RISSEL u. Mitarb. eine Anzahl von Leberkranken mit normalen Versuchspersonen verglichen haben und dabei feststellen konnten, daß die
Hepatitis eine Ammoniakvermehrung häufig erkennen läßt, wie sie bei anderen
schweren Krankheiten im Serum aber auch vorkommt. Cirrhosen haben ebenfalls
hohe Serum-Ammoniak-Werte.

Nachdem EMBDEN sowie RÖSCH und TE KAMP Ammoniak in der Netzhaut nachgewiesen hatte und die Lichtempfindlichkeit der Ammoniakabspaltung zeigen

konnte, später POHLE zusammen mit EMBDEN den Nachweis von Adenylsäure im Gehirn führte, war es für uns naheliegend, Adenylsäure wenigstens als eine Ammoniak-Muttersubstanz anzusehen und die Fermentversuche, die vorher erwähnt wurden, zeigten denn auch Ergebnisse, die einigermaßen denen der quantitativen Verhältnisse, die POHLE mit EMBDEN aufgedeckt hatte, entsprachen. Wir haben seinerzeit so wesentliche Unterschiede im Ammoniakgehalt des Blutes zwischen motorisch unruhigen Kranken, z. B. manischen oder gequälten Depressionen einerseits und katatonen Erregungszuständen, sog. febril-cyanotischen Episoden, andererseits gefunden, daß wir doch annehmen mußten, daß die Erregung der Schizophrenen mit einer Ammoniakvermehrung im Organismus etwas zu tun hätte, was sich auch aus den Ergebnissen der Hirnuntersuchungen mehr oder weniger erschließen ließ. Daß diese Schlüsse seinerzeit nicht endgültig weitergeführt werden konnten aus äußeren Gründen, ist bedauerlich, widerlegt sind aber die Ergebnisse noch nicht, und es scheint uns immer noch wichtig und wünschenswert, darauf einzugehen.

Zur Frage der Abderhalden-Reaktion

Sehr kurz kann das Problem der Abderhaldenschen Reaktion und ihrer Bedeutung für die Psychiatrie abgetan werden, so unendlich viel Mühe und Arbeit auch für diese Reaktion angewandt worden sind. Sicher lag es an der erstaunlichen Persönlichkeit des alten ABDERHALDEN, daß seine Reaktion in dieser Form sich so lange gehalten hat. Wir haben selber mit der Reaktion sowohl mit dem Dialysierverfahren als mit der Reaktion im Urin und im Liquor sehr ausgedehnte Erfahrungen sammeln können und haben uns immer wieder über zweierlei gewundert: Erstens fand sich in erstaunlicher Regelmäßigkeit bei der Epilepsie ein „Abbau" von Schilddrüsensubstanz und Nebennierensubstanz, und zweitens fand sich mit erstaunlicher Regelmäßigkeit ein Abbau von Hirngewebe und Geschlechtsorganen bei den sog. „Schizophrenien". Das sprach dafür, daß der Reaktion eine gewisse Spezifität und eine hohe Empfindlichkeit zuzusprechen war. Auf der anderen Seite konnten wir uns aber niemals davon überzeugen, daß die groben endokrinen Störungen, bei denen man am Ende mit der stärksten Reaktion hätte rechnen müssen, auf der ja ursprünglich (Schwangerschaftsuntersuchung) auch die Reaktion aufgebaut war, überhaupt einen Abbau erkennen ließen. Weder fanden wir bei Schilddrüsenstörungen (Basedow) noch bei schweren ovariellen Störungen oder bei testiculären Störungen irgendwelche sicheren Anhaltspunkte für den Abbau der betreffenden endokrinen Drüsen. Schwere akromegale Zustandsbilder mit schwerer Veränderung oder Degeneration der Hypophyse ergaben ebensowenig einen positiven Abbau von Hypophysensubstanz wie Cushing-Fälle. Wir haben trotzdem jahrelang die Abderhalden-Reaktion weiter angewendet in der Annahme, daß — sorgfältig und sauber genug durchgeführt — die Methode doch ihre Leistungsfähigkeit, wenn auch in sehr beschränktem Maße, bewiese. Nachdem aber durch die moderne Chromatographie viel leichtere Möglichkeiten bestanden, nicht nur überhaupt Aminosäuren, sondern auch sogar die verschiedenen in Frage kommenden Abbauprodukte der Eiweißkörper als Aminosäuren nachzuweisen, war es vollkommen folgerichtig, daß BAHNER und WIES bereits 1951 in Heidelberg papierchromatographische Abbauuntersuchungen durchführten. Und diese ergaben dann eindeutig, daß nichts von den Eiweißkörpern, die dem spezifischen Ferment ausgesetzt waren, abgebaut wurde. Damit entfiel praktisch jede Möglichkeit, die Abderhalden-Reaktion noch weiter zu verwenden, und die berechtigten Zweifel, die sehr viele immer wieder äußerten, insbesondere dadurch gestärkt, daß das Konservierungsverfahren der Substrate durch langes Kochen ja bereits das

Eiweiß weitgehend zerstört und degeneriert haben mußte, müssen als berechtigt
anerkannt werden. Wir halten heute die Abderhalden-Reaktion de facto für vollkommen obsolet und ohne berechtigten Untergrund. Das ist kein Vorwurf gegen
Abderhalden.

Das Leberproblem

Bereits in der antiken Medizin wurde der Zusammenhang zwischen der Leber,
der Milz und auch dem Raum überhaupt, den diese beiden Organe einnehmen,
nämlich dem Hypochondrium, und der Psyche angenommen. Aus dem griechi-
schen Wort Phrene geht ja geradezu hervor, daß man das Gemüt in den Bereich
des Zwerchfells zu lokalisieren versuchte, und Phrene bedeutet sowohl Zwerchfell
wie auch Gehirn. Lag das Gewicht der Forschung oder der Überlegungen einmal
mehr auf der Milz (Spleen!), so andererseits immer häufiger und immer mehr auf
der Leber und auf der Gallenabsonderung (Melan-Cholie). Seit es eine biochemische
Forschung innerhalb der Psychiatrie überhaupt gab, richtete sich das Interesse
auf die Leber, auf ihre Funktion und auf ihre pathologischen Veränderungen.
Und zwar werden sowohl die Wirkung der Psyche auf die Leber als die Wirkung
der Leber auf die Psyche erörtert und in Beziehung gesetzt. Leberfunktionsproben
sind bei allen erdenklichen Psychosen in zahllosen Fällen durchgeführt worden.
Man hat schlechterdings kurzschlüssig die Schizophrenie als eine Leberkrankheit
angesehen, dann hat man wieder mehr die Melancholie, die Cyclothymie als eine
Leberkrankheit angesehen. Es fanden sich allerdings auch zahllose Stützen innerhalb der Literatur für solche Vorstellungen. Angefangen damit, daß — wie an
anderer Stelle schon erörtert — die Abderhalden-Reaktion, als sie innerhalb der
Psychiatrie Interesse fand, für die Schizophrenie einen „Abbau" von Gehirnrinde,
Leber und Geschlechtsdrüsen nachzuweisen versuchte. Man erfuhr sehr frühzeitig
acetonurische und urobilinogenurische Veränderungen, die man mit Leberfunktionsstörungen zusammenbrachte, und V. M. Buscaino, der der mächtige Be-
fruchter der biochemischen Forschung des gesamten 20. Jahrhunderts war und
noch ist, führte das Interesse der Forscher auf die Leber hin, weil er meinte, daß die
Leber mindestens als entgiftendes Organ für die von ihm postulierten enterogenen
Amine von größter Bedeutung sein müßte. Es gibt wohl kaum eine Leberfunktions-
probe, über die nicht in der psychiatrischen Literatur berichtet worden ist, und es
gibt wohl kaum eine Reaktion, die nicht auch als mit Sicherheit beweisend für bestimmte Formen von endogenen Psychosen angesprochen worden ist. Vergleicht
man aber einerseits die Unsumme von Untersuchungen mit den doch sonst immer
so auffällig gesunden und „normalen" klinischen Ergebnissen und überlegt man
sich andererseits, wie wenig eigentlich doch Leberkranke psychisch verändert
sind, dann findet sich kein Zugang zu dieser Diskrepanz. Sicherlich ist die Beobachtung der „Schwarzgalligkeit" völlig richtig, sicherlich ist dieses „Sich-gelb-
oder-grün-Ärgern" richtig, und die Stimmung des Ikterischen, die Stimmung
speziell des Hepatitischen, ist zweifellos auffällig. Sie ist aber eben nicht psychotisch. Trotzdem haben wir alle, die sich für das Thema interessiert haben, unsere
speziellen Untersuchungen durchgeführt und haben alle auch mehr oder
weniger positive und negative Befunde erhoben (Riebeling, Kaps, Rütter,
Strobel). Die meisten dieser Untersuchungen wurden gar nicht publiziert,
weil ihre Ergebnisse nicht beweisend sind. Befunde aber, die zum Teil sehr eindeutig und auch sehr eindrucksvoll erhoben werden konnten, bezogen sich fast
immer auf hochakute Krankheitszustände, nicht auf die chronischen Verläufe,
nicht auf die Endzustände. Eine der empfindlichsten Leberfunktionsproben, die zum
Unterschied von den üblichen Serumlabilitätsproben wiederum eine echte Funktion des Leberparenchyms kontrolliert, ist der sog. Quick-Test, bei dem untersucht

Tabelle 10. *Verhältnis von Körpergewicht zu Lebergewicht und andere Daten bezüglich der Leber*

	Terbrüggen	Riebeling	Roessle
Verhältnis von Körpergewicht zu Lebergewicht	etwa 30	22,4	25—28
Lebergewicht	1800 g	1400 g	1400 g
Lebertrockensubstanz	23,2%	27,1%	24,0%
Wassergehalt	76,8%	72,9%	76,0%
Eiweißgehalt des Lebergesamtgewichtes	15,75%	18,6%[1]	14,9%
Eiweiß in g pro kg Körpergewicht	460	160[2]; 370; 490![3]	

[1] Hoher Durchschnitt, da sämtliche Fälle mit Leberschwellung eingerechnet sind.
[2] Ein Fall von Leberödem.
[3] Durchschnitt der Fälle von Leberschwellung.

wird, wieviel und wie schnell Natriumbenzoat als Hippursäure ausgeschieden wird. Die Bindung der Benzoesäure an Glykokoll ist eine Funktion der intakten Leber. Diesen Test hat GEORGI angewandt, und als er fand, daß verhältnismäßig viel Schizophrene nicht genügend Hippursäure ausschieden, hat er solchen Kranken auch Glykokoll zur Verfügung gestellt in der Annahme, daß vielleicht die Glykokoll-Synthese der Leber dieser Kranken ungenügend sei, so daß einfach mengenmäßig nicht genügend zur Verfügung gestanden hätte. Tatsächlich stellte sich heraus, daß unter der Zugabe von Glykokoll zur Benzoesäure die Bildung von Hippursäure gebessert wurde. PIEPER und FABER haben den „modifizierten Quick-Test" an einer größeren Reihe von Patienten verschiedenster Art untersucht und bestätigen durchaus, daß etwa 40% der Schizophrenen einen pathologischen Quick-Test aufweisen, aber auch 27% von überhaupt nicht psychotischen Kranken wiesen das gleiche Resultat auf, womit der diagnostische Wert dieser Untersuchungen eben wieder stark relativiert wird. Auch der erkenntnistheoretische Wert zur Frage der Ätiologie ist eben doch außerordentlich gering, da es sich ja immer wieder nicht um psychosenspezifische, geschweige denn schizophrenie-spezifische Verhältnisse, sondern um ganz allgemeine Phänomene handelt.

Etwa gleichzeitig, aber völlig unabhängig voneinander, erschienen im Jahre 1930 und 1933 zwei Arbeiten, eine von RIEBELING und eine von GAUPP, die sich beide mit der „Leberschwellung" beschäftigten. Wir hatten Untersuchungen an der Hirnschwellung durchgeführt, und parallel dazu hatten wir festgestellt, daß die Leber auch geschwollen war, und deswegen auch Trockensubstanz-Bestimmungen und Gewichtsbestimmungen der Leber von Psychosen durchgeführt (s. a. weiter oben). Bei diesen Untersuchungen fanden wir eine auffällige Verschiebung sowohl des Eiweißgehalts der Leber (Tab. 10) als auch der Beziehung zwischen Leber und Körpergewicht bei den Fällen von Hirnschwellung, bei denen auch eine Leberschwellung hatte beobachtet werden können. Sehr ähnliche Fälle wie die unseren untersuchte GAUPP, der Hyperämie der Leber unter Bevorzugung der zentralen Läppchen, Auseinanderdrängung der Leberzellbalken, leere Dissésche Räume, in vier von fünf Fällen auch zentrale fettige Degenerationen fand. GAUPP will diese Vorgänge nicht als seröse Entzündungen ansprechen, er nimmt vielmehr an, daß eine Capillarstauung nur sekundäre Bedeutung hat und faßt die degenerative Verfettung als toxisch bedingt auf. Er betont dabei, daß eine Zurückführung der gefundenen Veränderungen auf zusätzliche Schädigung nicht möglich sei. Aber: SCHEIDEGGER hat sehr ähnliche Leberveränderungen wie die von GAUPP *nicht nur* bei akuten Katatonien, sondern auch bei Pneumonie, Herzinsuffizienz und Nierenschäden gefunden!

Lingjaerde zieht den Schluß aus seinen Untersuchungen, daß in der *aktiven Phase* Anzeichen einer Leberkrankheit doch so häufig seien, daß es nicht mehr möglich ist, sie als Zufallsbefund anzusprechen, sondern daß der Zusammenhang zwischen Psychose und Leberstörung evident sei. Aus Ergebnissen von Olaf Bang über Beziehungen zwischen Nahrungsaufnahme, Ketonurie und Urobilinogenurie wurde geschlossen, daß die letzteren pathologischen Urinbefunde auf einem Glykogendefizit der Leber beruhen. Da diese aber relativ häufig bei „aktiven" Schizophrenen gefunden werden, wird der weitere Schluß gezogen, daß bei der Schizophrenie ein Kohlenhydratdefizit, ein innerer Kohlenhydrathunger, vorliege, vielleicht auch die *Verwertung* von Kohlenhydraten schlechter sei, denn nach seinen Beobachtungen konnte die Urobilinogenurie erst nach einer Zufuhr von 6—7 g Kohlenhydrat pro kg Körpergewicht aufgehoben werden, während nach Bang Normale nur 0,7—1,3 g Kohlenhydrate pro kg Körpergewicht brauchen, wenn vorher ein Kohlenhydrathunger oder ein Glykogendefizit der Leber bestanden hatte.

Nachdem Heilmeyer 1941 von einer Vermehrung des Kupfers im Serum der Schizophrenen zum ersten Mal berichtet hatte, wandte sich das Interesse diesem Phänomen zu, das ebenfalls auf eine Leberinsuffizienz zurückgeführt wurde. Zum Teil parallelisierte man zu den absolut pathologischen Kupferverhältnissen beim Morbus Wilson (S. 145). Daß sich die meisten pathologischen Ergebnisse des Kupferstoffwechsels bei sorgfältiger Kontrolle nicht bewahrheitet haben, sei schon vorweg berichtet. Eingehender wird über die Kupferverhältnisse später referiert, hier sollte nur die Beziehung zur Leber erwähnt werden.

Eiweiß

Wenn schon vor Jahrzehnten die Eiweißfraktionen des Serums bei endogenen Psychosen verschiedenster Art untersucht worden sind unter dem Aspekt, daß Verschiebungen des Eiweißquotienten häufig einen Ausdruck für einen Leberschaden darstellen, so bekamen diese Untersuchungen neuen Antrieb, als durch die Papierelektrophorese auch kleineren Laboratorien die Möglichkeit gegeben worden war, Eiweißfraktionierungen mit relativ einfachen Mitteln durchzuführen. Es war bekannt, daß Leberschäden insbesondere mit einer γ-Globulin-Vermehrung einhergehen, und es wurde wiederum bei endogenen Psychosen nach derartigen Veränderungen gefahndet, indes ohne jeden Erfolg. Es läßt sich vielmehr mit Sicherheit sagen, daß — soweit wenigstens keine körperlichen Krankheiten vorliegen — das Pherogramm der endogenen Psychosen völlig regelrecht ist. Daß zahllose Arbeiten erschienen sind, bei denen Abweichungen einzelner Eiweißkörper des Pherogramms um 1% oder weniger als beweisend für eine Veränderung gegenüber der Norm angesehen wurden, sei nebenbei erwähnt. Allerdings geben Consbruch und Faust sehr eindrucksvolle Verschiebungen der Elektropherogramme im Verlaufe der Besserung einer Schizophrenie und einer endogenen Depression an. Es ist keineswegs notwendig, daß ein Pherogramm im Beginn eines schizophrenen Schubes oder einer depressiven Phase etwa pathologisch sein müßte. Viel wichtiger ist, daß es auf Therapie anspricht und eine gewisse Veränderung stattfindet. Sahen die Autoren bei einer posttraumatischen Psychose erst nach vielen Wochen die Albumine zu- und die α-Globuline abnehmen, so zeigte sich umgekehrt im Verlauf der medikamentösen Behandlung einer Manie ein normales Pherogramm im Anfang und eine Verschiebung von Albumin und Globulin bei gleichbleibender Dosierung.

Der Liquor cerebrospinalis

Der Liquor der endogenen Psychose ist praktisch immer völlig „normal". Wenigstens soweit die üblichen Routineuntersuchungen gehen, die ja ganz überwiegend entzündliche und gefäßbedingte Veränderungen degenerativer Art nachzuweisen vermögen, die aber sicherlich nicht in der Lage sind, andersartige Störungen erkennen zu lassen. Derartige Störungen können vorhanden sein.

KRAL und LEHMANN berichteten vor einigen Jahren, daß der Eisengehalt des Liquors bei Gesunden und bei jüngeren Psychosen verschiedenster Art vollkommen gleich sei. Bei chronisch kranken Schizophrenen, die mehrere Jahre krank waren, wenn sie auch ihrem Lebensalter nach noch jung waren, stiegen die Eisenwerte aber erheblich an und erreichten Werte, wie wir sie sonst nur bei alten Menschen, insbesondere bei senilen Psychosen, kennen. Über den Kupfergehalt des Liquors haben meine Schüler KRETH und SCHÖN Untersuchungen angestellt und haben auch gefunden, daß der Liquor bei endogenen Psychosen bezüglich seines Kupfergehaltes normal ist. Frühere Beobachtungen über Kupfervermehrungen bei Schizophrenen im Serum oder im Liquor konnten in keinem Fall bestätigt werden.

Vor wenigen Jahren publizierte BOGOCH einen Befund, der immerhin zum Nachdenken Anlaß gab, der aber — wie gleich vorweg gesagt werden soll — sich bisher nicht überall hat bestätigen lassen. Er bestimmte die Neuraminsäure im Liquor und fand in der Altersstufe von 0—16 Jahren ein Mittel von 42—46 γ im cm³ und bei Erwachsenen etwa 61 γ. Bei den Schizophrenen war das Mittel 36 γ im cm³, und die höchsten Werte lagen nicht über 49 γ, während der Mittelwert bei anderen Patienten 53 γ betrug. Die Schizophrenen waren zwischen 20 und 62 Jahren alt. Der Verfasser schloß aus diesen Befunden, daß die Schizophrenen gewissermaßen „unreifer" oder auf einer „unreiferen Stufe stehen geblieben" seien als andere Patienten und als Gesunde, da er sie eben mit Kindern vergleichen mußte. Wir haben diesen Befund sogleich nachgeprüft und konnten ihn nicht bestätigen. Es wäre ja immerhin sehr wünschenswert, wenn diese Befunde noch weiter nachgeprüft würden, obwohl sie ihrem Wesen nach auch wohl keine entscheidende Bedeutung haben können. BOGOCH bestimmte außerdem die Glucose, das Hexosamin als Galactosamin und fand auch diese beiden Körper bei den Schizophrenen niedriger als bei anderen psychischen Störungen, niedriger insbesondere als bei Manischen, bei denen sie ganz besonders hoch liegen sollen. Leider ist auch in diesen Arbeiten immer wieder die Frage der statistischen und funktionellen Signifikanz nicht genügend getrennt. Sicherlich sind Werte, wie sie BOGOCH angibt, statistisch signifikant. Aber wenn schizophrene Patienten zwischen 4 und 50 mg-% eines bestimmten Körpers ausscheiden, z. B. von Hexose, und chronische Hirnkrankheiten zwischen 11 und 31 mg-%, dann ist das nicht verwertbar.

Sogenannte Focalsepsis

Unter dem Einfluß von HUNTER (London 1910) und FORD-ROBERTSON fanden Theorien von der "oral" oder "focal" infection auch auf die Ätiologie endogener Psychosen Anwendung. Eine zweifellos sehr überlegte, gründliche und sorgfältige Arbeit von PICKWORTH befaßt sich mit diesem Problem sehr ausführlich. Die Arbeit ist seinerzeit auch ins Deutsche übersetzt worden. PICKWORTH ging davon aus, daß die Mehrzahl der damals untersuchten Kranken Hals-Nasen-Ohren-Affektionen verschiedenster Art gehabt hätten und daß diese durch fortgeleitete Schädigungen nicht nur rein toxischer, sondern sogar bakteriämischer Art die

Psychosen verursacht und unterhalten hätten. Er findet denn auch an der Basis des Gehirns sowohl in den Meningen als auch im Parenchym selbst zwischendurch einzelne Bakterien bei Gramfärbung, er findet auch immer wieder Stellen chronisch entzündlicher Veränderungen an der Basis und macht diese verantwortlich für die Psychosen. Insbesondere findet er auch bei auffällig vielen Sektionen chronische Entzündungen der Nebenhöhlen. Daß solche zu erheblichen Störungen führen können, kann nicht geleugnet werden. Ob sie aber ätiologisch in unmittelbaren Zusammenhang mit der Entstehung einer endogenen Psychose zu bringen sind, muß mindestens zweifelhaft bleiben, wenn man es nicht vollkommen ablehnen will. Im Zusammenhang mit diesen Ergebnissen muß aber immer wieder zugegeben werden, daß die Versuche, überhaupt eine Erklärung zu finden, überhaupt eine Beziehung aufzutun zwischen körperlicher Krankheit und psychischer Krankheit, so lange nicht abgetan werden dürfen, so lange wir nichts Besseres haben. Tatsächlich ist es aber doch so, daß dieserlei Veränderungen, insbesondere bakteriämische, bei jedem normalen gesunden Menschen ebenfalls vorkommen und, da sie ubiquitär zu sein scheinen, sicherlich ohne jede Bedeutung für irgendeine Krankheit, geschweige denn für irgendeine Psychose, sind. Im Zusammenhang mit der Arbeit von Pickworth wurde eine ganze Reihe von derartigen Untersuchungen publiziert, insbesondere im Journal of Mental Science, und es wurde selbstverständlich auch über Erfolge nach Herdsanierung berichtet. Daß diese ,,Erfolge'' nach Herdsanierung zweifellos vorlagen und vorliegen, dürfte unter dem Gesichtspunkt keinerlei Besonderheit beanspruchen, daß man sich sagt, daß vorübergehende cyclische Psychosen unter einer eingreifenden Therapie operativer oder auch konservativer Art natürlich Besserungstendenzen zeigen können, natürlich auch Phasenverkürzung zeigen können, die, sowieso kurzfristig ablaufend, durch chronische Schmerzzustände aber scheinbar verlängert worden waren. Anschließend an die Herdsuche in den Zähnen und in den Nebenhöhlen wurden von englischer und dänischer wie auch von italienischer Seite auch vielfach Herde im Magen-Darm-System gesucht und eine Reihe von Arbeiten beschäftigte sich damit, Agglutinationstiter für Coli, Typhus, Paratyphus und andere Erreger von Darmaffektionen zu bestimmen bei Psychosen zum Vergleich bei Gesunden. Auch die Untersuchungen von Reiter spielen da eine große Rolle. Sie sind insofern besonders eindrucksvoll, als der Unterschied gegenüber Gesunden und der Unterschied gegenüber Krankheiten anderer Art mit Sicherheit nachweisbar war und als der Arbeit eine ganze Reihe von histologischen Befunden zugrunde liegt. Es ist nicht zu unterschätzen, daß diese Reiterschen Untersuchungen m. E. niemals genügend widerlegt worden sind bzw. daß man sich einfach nicht genügend damit beschäftigt hat.

Ford-Robertson beschäftigt sich vorzüglich mit den anaeroben Stämmen der Klebs-Löffler-Gruppe und den anaeroben Leptothrix-Bakterien, die er bei ,,insanity'' und ähnlichem so wesentlich häufiger findet als bei allen anderen Kranken, daß er dem eine wesentliche ätiologische Bedeutung zumessen will, und zwar ist bei systematischer Kontrolle sämtlicher Partien des Gastrointestinaltraktes das Colon als der Hauptsitz der Infektion gefunden worden. Von diesen Anaerobiern nun würden Neurotoxine gebildet, die unter Umständen leichte degenerative Veränderungen im Hirnzentrum hervorrufen können, die aber außerdem starke lokale Veränderungen am Auerbachschen Plexus verursachen. Endotoxische Wirkungen sind zusätzlich bedeutungsvoll und Ford-Robertson steht nicht an, diese Ergebnisse in engste ätiologische Beziehung zu den Psychosen überhaupt zu bringen, wohlbemerkt aber nicht zu speziellen Diagnosen. Immer wieder sind derartige Untersuchungen wiederholt worden, und immer wieder haben sich auch pathologische Phänomene am Magen-Darm-Kanal gezeigt, nie aber solche, die man ätiologisch wirklich mit Sicherheit mit den Psychosen in Beziehung setzen könnte.

PLATANIA z. B. fand nicht nur Antikörper gegen verschiedene gastrointestinale Erreger, sondern auch diese selbst wesentlich häufiger bei Schizophrenen als bei Gesunden.

Toxische Wirkung von Körperflüssigkeiten psychotischer Patienten

Toxicitätsbestimmungen mit Körperflüssigkeiten von Psychosen sind in zahllosen Fällen durchgeführt worden. Von der Gewebskultur, von Hefekulturen

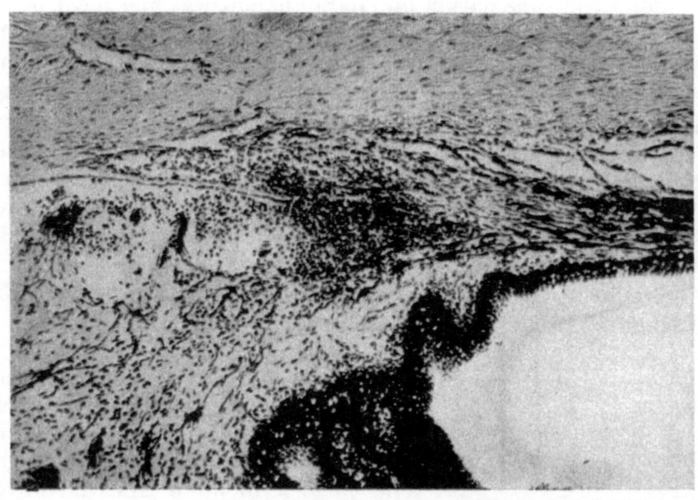

Abb. 12. Entzündliche Infiltrate bzw. Gewebszerstörungen im Kaninchenauge nach Injektion von Liquor von Schizophrenen. (Nach GAMPER, KRAL und STEIN)

bis zum großen Säugetier ist die gesamte Biologie bemüht worden, die Toxicität der Ausscheidungen oder der Körperflüssigkeiten von Psychosen zu beweisen. Nicht immer scheint uns das ganz richtig gewesen zu sein, insbesondere muß man berücksichtigen, daß die Ausscheidungen von Psychosen, die in klinischer Behandlung stehen, unter Umständen doch erhebliche Mengen medikamentöser Gifte bzw. ihrer Abbauprodukte enthalten und daß diese in das Reaktionsgeschehen mit eingreifen können. Sicherlich sind die Versuche von GAMPER, KRAL und STEIN (Abb. 12 u. 13), die schon Jahrzehnte zurückliegen, in der Beziehung sehr viel weniger angreifbar als viele später durchgeführte. RIEDER stellt z. B. die Frage, ob es richtiger sei, höhere oder niedere Tiere als Versuchsobjekte zu benutzen. Er überlegte sich dabei, daß das niedere Tier mit seiner Neigung zu katatonen

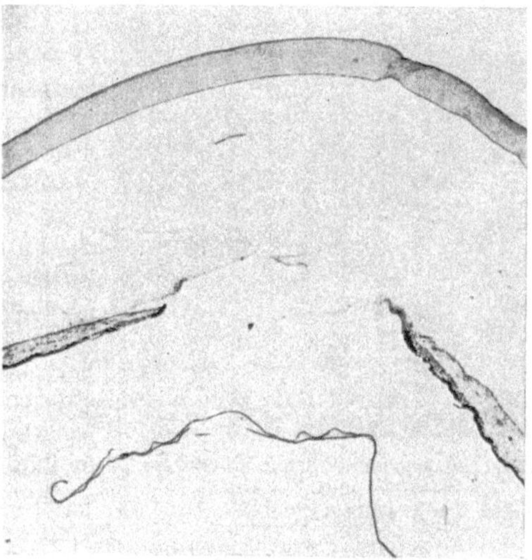

Abb. 13. Vergrößerter entzündeter Iriswinkel. (Nach GAMPER, KRAL und STEIN)

Veränderungen zum Unterschied zum höheren Tier mit seiner Neigung zu epileptiformen Anfällen gleichermaßen geeignet oder ungeeignet sein kann. Es wäre dabei nur daran zu erinnern, daß man keinesfalls Verhaltensweisen oder -änderungen von Tieren untersuchen sollte, sondern nur objektiv nachweisbare Veränderungen. Veränderungen der Verhaltensweisen sind z. B. von WITT mit seinem Spinnennetz-Test oder von WINTER und FLATAKER bezüglich der Reaktionsfreudigkeit von Ratten gegenüber schwer erreichbarem Futter untersucht worden. Dies ist zwar recht eindrucksvoll, die Resultate sind aber andererseits so weitgehend abhängig von medikamentösen Einflüssen anderer Art, vom „Betriebsklima" mit allem, was darum und daran hängt, was hier nicht im einzelnen ausgeführt zu werden braucht, daß solche Untersuchungen sicher weniger Relevanz haben als einfache Absterbeversuche oder Versuche, die zu Entzündungen irgendwelcher Art führen (GAMPER u. Mitarb.). Auch an Hefezellen hat RIEDER die Atmung kontrolliert und konnte feststellen, daß Urin, Liquor und Serum vom Schizophrenen eine wesentlich deutlichere Wirkung haben als die gleichen Stoffe von Normalen oder auch von anderen Psychosen nicht-schizophrener Art.

WADA und GIBSON berichten über Veränderungen, die sie bei Tieren beobachteten nach Injektion von Extrakt aus Urinen Schizophrener. Die Extrakte wurden derart hergestellt, daß nach Absorption an Tierkohle und Wiederauflösung durch physiologische Kochsalzlösung der Urin etwa auf das 500fache angereichert war. Affen reagierten sowohl auf die Extrakte von Gesunden als auch von Schizophrenen, Katzen aber vorzugsweise auf Extrakte von Schizophrenen. Die geringen Mengen wurden prinzipiell intrazisternal gegeben, einige auch in die lateralen Ventrikel. Die Katzen wurden weniger aktiv, blieben aber in ihren Affekten unverändert nach der Injektion eines Extraktes aus normalem Urin. Der Schizophrenen-Extrakt bewirkte eine ausgesprochene Reduktion der Spontanaktivität und insbesondere auch der Affektivität. Bei Affen verursachten beide Extrakte eine deutliche Senkung der emotionellen Färbung. Bei Extrakten aus Schizophrenen-Urinen fanden sich bei den Affen gelegentlich ungewöhnliche Verhaltensweisen, automatismusartige, stuporöse und katalepsie-ähnliche Episoden, während das bei der Injektion normaler Extrakte kein einziges Mal der Fall war. Die Elektrencephalogramme, die durch in die Rinde eingepflanzte Elektroden abgeleitet wurden, waren nach der Injektion normaler Extrakte nicht signifikant verändert, während nach der Injektion von Schizophrenen-Extrakten kleine Wellen mit Hintergrundaktivität beobachtet wurden. Was war in den Urinen alles noch außer dem Unterschied zwischen gesund und krank? Niemals wird das ausdrücklich betont, niemals wird

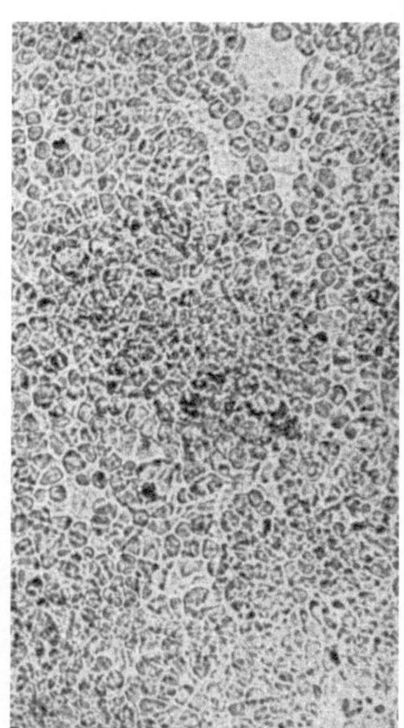

Abb. 14. Gewebskultur nach FEDOROFF mit Serum von Normalen überspult

ausdrücklich unterstrichen, daß die Kranken keinerlei Medikamente bekommen hätten. Es wäre aber nicht verwunderlich, wenn solche Reaktionen z. B. verursacht worden wären durch die Ausscheidung von Medikamenten oder ihren Abbauprodukten. STERN u. Mitarb. hingegen erzielten keinerlei Differenz von Rattenreaktionen auf Seren Normaler bzw. Schizophrener. FISCHER untersuchte Xenopus laevis-Larven, die den Einflüssen der zu untersuchenden Nativflüssigkeiten direkt ausgesetzt wurden. Bezeichnenderweise war der Toxicitätsindex, den FISCHER errechnete, wesentlich geringer als der von LÜHRS aus meinem Laboratorium, obwohl wir gerade nur das Milieu der Kaulquappen verdünnten und die Tiere niemals in konzentrierte Ausscheidungsflüssigkeit gesetzt haben.

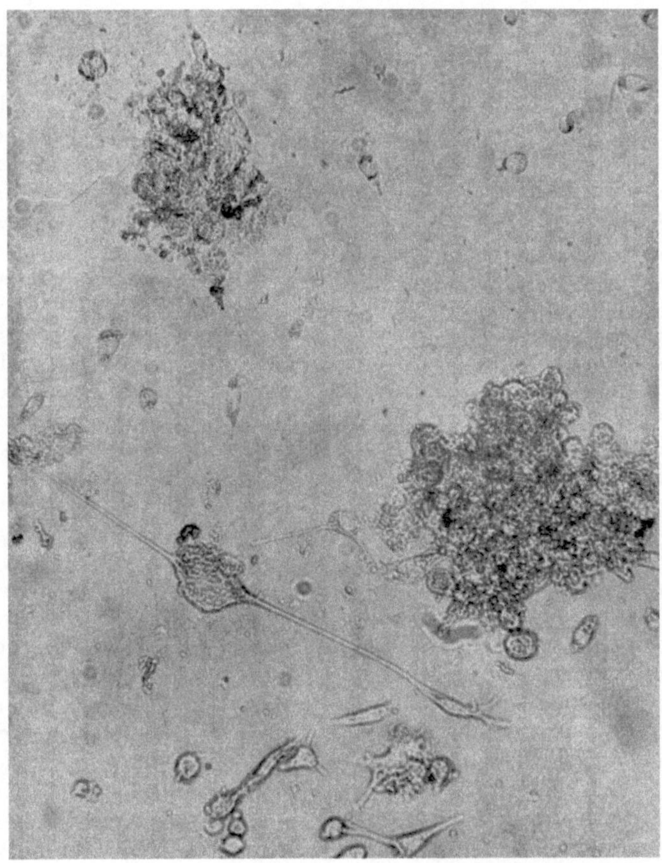

Abb. 15. Gewebskultur nach FEDOROFF mit Serum von Schizophrenen überspult

Uns scheinen Versuche wie die von FEDOROFF deshalb so bedeutungsvoll, weil sie zeigen, daß keineswegs alle Substrate ohne weiteres verwertbar sind (Abb. 14 u. 15), um einen toxischen Effekt eines irgendwie gearteten Körpers nachzuweisen, sondern daß man es teilweise sogar dem Zufall überlassen muß, welches Material nun geeignet ist. So hat FEDOROFF bei der ersten Gewebskultur, die er untersucht hat, keinerlei Effekt durch den Zusatz von schizophrenem Serum erzielt. Als er einen anderen Stamm einer Gewebskultur anwandte, erzielte er Effekte, die immerhin frappierend waren, insbesondere deswegen übrigens, weil sie sich vom gleichen Material des gleichen Patienten — drei Monate später z. B. entnommen — reproduzieren ließen. Sie waren also vom Zufall nicht mehr abhängig. Daß solche Ergebnisse unter Umständen auch mit anderen Seren gefunden werden und daß auch hier keine spezifische Eigenschaft, z. B. des Serums von Schizophrenen, vorliegt, sondern nur wieder ein Mehr/Weniger gegenüber dem Gesunden oder gegenüber anderen Kontrollen, besagt nichts gegen den Wert der Untersuchungen überhaupt, da das Gros der Resultate eben bei den Psychosen liegt. In meinem Laboratorium sind verschiedentlich Untersuchungen durchgeführt worden, um toxische Wirkungen von Ausscheidungen von Psychosen zu kontrollieren gegenüber denen von Gesunden. Die ersten Versuche in dieser Richtung wurden von Franke angestellt, der Paramaecien-Kulturen anlegte. Wir haben uns aber davon überzeugen müssen, daß die Paramaecien von sich aus schon so ungeheuer breit variieren, daß man eine Variation nach Zusatz kaum noch hätte unterscheiden können von der spontanen Variationsbreite. Später hat (wie erwähnt) Lührs Liquoruntersuchungen durchgeführt und hat den Liquor in verschiedenen Mengen dem Lebenselement der Kaulquappen, nämlich dem Frischwasser, in dem wir sie hielten, zugesetzt. Um es mit einigermaßen sicher pathologischen Phänomenen zu tun zu haben, haben wir nicht mit Liquor von Schizophrenen gearbeitet, sondern mit Liquor von Epileptikern, den wir verglichen haben mit dem Liquor von Kontrollen verschiedenster Art, von organischen Nervenkrankheiten, die bestimmt keine Anfälle hatten, die aber zum Teil rein liquorologisch wesentlich pathologischer waren als die Anfallskranken. Bei diesen Untersuchungsreihen hat sich nun ganz eindeutig ein Unterschied ergeben zwischen Anfalls- und anderen Fällen. Jenseits einer bestimmten Zusatzmenge von Liquor starben, gleichgültig, was wir zusetzten, die Mehrzahl aller Kaulquappen. Bei einer Verminderung der Zusatzmenge aber blieben die Unterschiede zwischen den Tieren, die Liquor von Anfallsleidenden bekommen hatten, und den Tieren, die Liquor von anderen Kranken bekommen hatten, erheblich und weit außerhalb jedes Zufallsbereiches.

Während die Wirkung von Körperflüssigkeiten von Psychosen auf die Atmung an sich physiologisch intakter Gewebe oder Kulturen vielfach untersucht worden ist (Lingjaerde), sind Körperzellen von Psychosen weniger untersucht worden. Diese Aufgabe hatte Kosaka übernommen, der die Erythrocyten, die aus einer Arterie entnommen worden waren, in der Warburgapparatur untersuchte und feststellen konnte, daß der Stoffwechsel der Erythrocyten von Schizophrenen doch erheblich anders ist als der von Gesunden. Während die aerobe Glycolyse in der Norm sehr niedrig ist, ist sie bei schweren Schizophrenie-Fällen hoch, selbst bei leichten noch höher als normal. Der Mayerhof-Quotient, d. h. der Quotient aus anaerober minus aerober Glykolyse, dividiert durch den Sauerstoffverbrauch, beträgt bei normalen roten Blutkörperchen etwa 1,1, bei erregten Schizophrenen sinkt er auf 0,5 im Durchschnitt, in Einzelfällen bis auf 0,3 herab! Stuporöse Kranke haben einen sehr niedrigen, die übrigen stationären einen normalen, remittierende Kranke sogar unter Umständen einen erhöhten Wert. Auch der respiratorische Quotient der Erythrocyten ist bei den Schizophrenen dann herabgesetzt, wenn sie erregt sind.

Über den eigenartigen Geruch, den manche Psychiatrische Abteilungen, insbesondere die mit chronischen Patienten, haben, ist schon vielfach gesprochen worden. Wegen der Unmöglichkeit oder außerordentlichen Schwierigkeit, solche Dinge zu objektivieren, ist aber niemals näher darauf eingegangen worden. Das geschah zum ersten Mal von Smith und Sines, die den eigenartigen Geruch auf einer Männerabteilung so penetrant fanden, daß sie versuchten, ihn zu objektivieren, und zwar geschah das damit, daß Ratten auf den Geruch durch bedingte Reflexe trainiert wurden und dann der Schweiß von Schizophrenen, der in einem Gummibett gesammelt wurde, und der Schweiß von Kontrollen nebeneinander den Ratten vorgezeigt wurde. Das, was einzelne Menschen, übrigens bei weitem nicht alle, riechen können, konnten die Ratten in einem hohen Prozentsatz der Fälle mit einem außerordentlich geringen Fehlerresultat bestimmen und auf die Weise doch wenigstens einigermaßen objektivieren. Bezeichnend für das Gesamtresultat ist, daß nicht nur alte Schizophrene, sondern mitunter auch andere

Patienten ganz anderer diagnostischer Kategorien diesen Geruch aufweisen und daß er ganz ausnahmsweise auch bei nicht-hospitalisierten gesunden Menschen vorkommt. Es kann sich nicht um ein Zersetzungsprodukt bakterieller Art handeln, da die Patienten vor der Schweißproduktion mit Septisol oder einer Hexachlorophen-Seife auf das gründlichste abgeseift worden waren. Geklärt ist aber nicht, ob es sich um apokrinen Schweiß oder um Schweißdrüsen-Schweiß handelt. Der Geruch geht beim Schütteln in Äther über, läßt sich bis jetzt aber weder gaschromatographisch noch spektrophotometrisch erfassen.

Kurze Bemerkungen zur Frage der Ausscheidung von Aromaticis und von Serotonin

In dem Artikel von WAELSCH und WEIL-MALHERBE sind bereits die Probleme des Serotonins und seiner Ausscheidungsprodukte so ausführlich wiedergegeben, daß sich eine neuerliche Erörterung erübrigt. Betont werden soll aber doch noch, daß sicherlich nicht die einzige Quelle dessen, was in vielen chromatographischen Untersuchungen als Indol-Derivate gesucht oder großenteils auch gefunden wurde (G. A. BUSCAINO, FERRONI, PLATANIA u. v. a.), aus dem Serotoninstoffwechsel stammen muß, sondern daß auch aus einem gestörten Darmstoffwechsel offenbar noch leichter Oxyphenylgruppen in den Urin abgeschieden werden, als man das früher annahm und als dies in der Norm beobachtet werden kann. SANO hatte mit der Millon-Reaktion in der Kälte bei einer großen Zahl von Schizophrenen, aber nur sehr wenig Gesunden, eine vermehrte Oxyphenyl-Derivat-Ausscheidung schon vor vielen Jahren nachgewiesen. Aus einer Nachprüfung von EDERLE ergab sich indes, daß diese Indolurie keineswegs schizophren-spezifisch war, sondern auch bei anderen psychiatrisch-neurologischen Krankheiten gefunden wurde, bei organischen Erkrankungen des Zentralnervensystems noch häufiger als bei Schizophrenen selbst, und in immerhin nicht geringem Prozentsatz sogar bei Psychopathien zu finden war. Da nun immer wieder darauf hingewiesen wird, wie außerordentlich häufig Darmstörungen, Dysbakterien usw. bei Psychosen vorkommen, war es naheliegend, daß man dieser Dysbakterie und gleichzeitig der Indolurie nachging, um einen eventuellen Zusammenhang zu finden. KANIG und KLUDAS haben sich einer solchen Aufgabe unterzogen, mußten aber feststellen, daß ihre Indolwerte durchaus im Bereich der Norm lagen, obwohl sie eine bemerkenswert hohe Anzahl von dysbakterischen Stuhlbefunden feststellen konnten. Aus der mangelnden quantitativen Parallelisierung schließen die Verfasser, daß eine vermehrte Indol-Ausscheidung, wie sie auch von ihnen gefunden wurde, doch nicht auf Dysbakterie beruht, sondern auf intermediären Störungen des Tryptophanstoffwechsels.

Die Untersuchungen von LEYTON über die Indolverbindungen bei Schizophrenen ergaben selbst bei Anlegen eines sehr kritischen Maßstabes doch Differenzen zwischen („alten"!!) Schizophrenen und Gesunden. Zwei Substanzen, die den Charakter von Indolderivaten haben und als solche nicht zu identifizieren sind, wurden bei Schizophrenen in signifikant höherer Menge ausgeschieden als bei den gesunden Vergleichspersonen. Umgekehrt schieden 20% der Schizophrenen deutlich weniger Hydroxyindolessigsäure aus, also das Abbauprodukt des Serotonins, als die Gesunden. Die Indolausscheidung im Urin vom Schizophrenen ist nicht nennenswert anders als die vom Normalen, wie FORREST erneut nachgewiesen hat.

Die Bedeutung fermentativer Vorgänge

Von einer Fermentschwäche oder Oxydationsschwäche endogener Psychosen ist sehr viel und sehr frühzeitig die Rede gewesen, aber man hat niemals wirklich sichere Anhaltspunkte gefunden, die auch einer Nachprüfung durch objektive

Untersucher wirklich standhielten. Auch die zahlreichen Kupferbestimmungsmetho-
den die angewandt wurden, um die endogenen Psychosen von den anderen Patienten
und von der Norm zu unterscheiden, gingen vielfach entweder davon aus, daß
ein hoher Gehalt des Serums ein Ausdruck für eine Leberschädigung sei, oder,
daß er ein Ausdruck für eine Oxydationsschwäche sei, die eben mit dem normalen
Kupferwert nicht auskomme. Das Kupfer im menschlichen Organismus ist zum
allergrößten Teil an Coeruloplasmin gebunden. Bei diesem Eiweißkörper handelt
es sich um ein α_2-Globulin. Daß das Coeruloplasmin für die Oxydationsvorgänge im
Organismus eine Rolle spielt, dürfte nach Holmberg und Laurell außer Zweifel
stehen. Die Beziehung zwischen diesem Körper und anderen Versuchen, Oxyda-
tionsschwächen oder Reduktionsverstärkungen beim Schizophrenen nachzuweisen,
führten Åkerfeld dazu, eine erhöhte Oxydationsfähigkeit des Serums Schizophrener und anderer Seren gegenüber Dimethylparaphenylendiamin festzustellen.
Dieser Befund, der damals, als er publiziert wurde, geradezu alarmierend wirkte,
konnte sehr bald relativiert werden, denn unabhängig voneinander fanden
Riebeling, Albert, Heath, Martens et al., daß nicht nur keineswegs alle Schizophrenen, sondern umgekehrt auch Gesunde, auch Kranke ganz anderer Art diese
Fähigkeit, das Dimethylparaphenylendiamin schnell zu oxydieren, aufwiesen.
Findet man im gesunden Serum diese Fähigkeit nicht in gleicher Stärke wie im
kranken, dann braucht man es nur gegen physiologische Kochsalzlösung zu dialy-
sieren, um die gleiche Oxydationsgeschwindigkeit wie bei diesem zu finden. Das
sollte nach Åkerfeld darauf beruhen, daß der im gesunden Serum höhere Ascor-
binsäuregehalt zum Teil oder ganz herausdialysiert sei und damit das gesunde
Serum dem krankhaften angeglichen würde. Keineswegs aber ist der Ascorbin-
säuregehalt des schizophrenen Serums immer niedriger als der des gesunden
Serums. Bezüglich des Ascorbinsäuregehaltes und des Glutathiongehaltes verhält
sich vielmehr, wie erst jüngst Abood wieder nachgewiesen hat, das Serum der
Schizophrenen genauso wie das Gesunder. Den Versuch, durch die Bischofschen
und einige andere Ergebnisse, z. B. auch die von Oezek bezüglich des Kupfergehaltes des Serums der Schizophrenen, seine Ergebnisse zu bestätigen, muß man
als mißlungen bezeichnen. Es ist gar keine Frage, daß Oezeks Kupferbestimmungen
gerade ein *normales* Verhalten ergeben haben und nicht eine Veränderung im
Sinne von Åkerfeld. Nun soll die Oxydation von Adrenalin und von Dimethylparaphenylendiamin (DPP) in der gleichen und zueinander proportionalen Weise
vor sich gehen. Diesen beiden Vorgängen proportional ist nun wieder der Coerulo-
plasmingehalt des Serums, den aber Abood u. Mitarb. bei der *Schwangerschaft*
am höchsten, dann beim Carcinom und dann erst bei der Schizophrenie leicht
erhöht fanden. Noch niedriger als bei Normalbefunden zeigte sich die Oxydationsfähigkeit des Serums bei MS-Kranken. Das bestätigt unsere Ergebnisse (Riebeling und Albert), widerspricht aber denen von Åkerfeldt. Martens hat sich
überlegt, daß das Coeruloplasmin des Schizophrenen etwa abnorm zusammengesetzt
sein könnte.

Ljunberg hat vor über 20 Jahren gezeigt, daß das Serum von Schizophrenen
offenbar stärker befähigt ist, Glutathion zu oxydieren, als das Serum von Gesunden. Zum Teil dürfte also die Unfähigkeit oder verminderte Fähigkeit des
Schizophrenen, Glutathion ans Gewebe zu binden, die Barak, Zara und Buondonno, Mariani gefunden haben, darauf beruhen, daß das Glutathion vor
der Bindung oxydiert wird. Riebeling fand aber nun, daß Glutathion im Liquor vieler endogener Psychosen erhöht ist. Nun ist Glutathion ja eigentlich
ein Gewebsferment und kommt frei gar nicht vor. Wenn es im Liquorchromato-
gramm doch gefunden wird, dann könnte das darauf beruhen, daß die Bindungs-
fähigkeit an das Gewebe herabgesetzt ist.

Zur Therapie mit Atmungsgiften

Wieder unter der Vorstellung, daß eine gewisse Oxydationsschwäche vielen endogenen Psychosen zugrunde liegen könnte, versuchten wir bereits 1943 durch eine besonders starke Beeinflussung der Oxydationsfähigkeit des Blutes, diese gewissermaßen anzuregen und zu verbessern. Wir gaben nämlich Natriumcyanid intramusculär, um vorübergehend eine Lähmung der inneren Atmung zu verursachen und nach dieser „Lähmung" eine Aktivierung zu erzielen. Ähnlich wie die Insulintherapie den Kohlenhydratstoffwechsel gewissermaßen trainiert, so sollte sich das Cyanid zum Training der inneren Oxydation eignen. Ähnliches geschah ja einige Jahre später auch mit der Anoxie-Behandlung. Es ließ sich zweifellos erkennen, daß diese Cyanid-Behandlung eine mächtige Anregung der Patienten bedeutete, sie wurde auch nur aus äußeren Gründen aufgegeben. Die Handhabung der Lösungen war schwierig und wegen des Giftcharakters bei oraler Applikation auf den Stationen zu gefährlich. Einige Jahre später wurden von Olsen und Klein Katzenversuche angestellt; mit mäßigen Dosen wurden die Tiere bis zu einem abortiven, mit mittleren Dosen bis zum vollen Krampf und einige Tiere mit hohen Dosen bis zum Tode gereizt. Der Stickstoffgehalt des Gehirns wurde kontrolliert, der regelmäßig gesteigert wurde, während das Phosphokreatin bei Krampfdosis gesteigert war, bei Todesdosen aber wieder absank. Hyden und Hartelius wandten Malononitril an, das im Organismus bekanntlich Cyanid abspaltet. Mit einer noch milderen Therapie (Dinitrilsuccinat) hatte Haries allerdings keine Erfolge bei Depressionen, ebensowenig McKinnon. Diesen Autoren gegenüber wendet aber Hartelius mit Recht ein, daß sie samt und sonders ihre Therapie bereits durch ein Reduktionsmittel unterbrochen hätten, ehe überhaupt eine Wirkung hätte einsetzen können (benutzt wurde meistens Thiosulfat). Noell gab Cyanwasserstoff in 1%iger Lösung subcutan oder intramuskulär, kontrollierte die Wirkung elektrencephalographisch und zeigte, daß sie geringer war als die einer Hypoxämie. Dabei stellte sich aber weiter heraus, daß die Capillarisierung bestimmter Hirnabschnitte durch die Blausäure geradezu günstig beeinflußt werden kann.

Einige Bemerkungen zur Biologie der Epilepsie

Vieles, was über die Chemie oder vielleicht auch die Abnormitäten des Epileptikers zu sagen ist, ist bereits an anderer Stelle gesagt. Auf die Frage des Tonephin-Wasserversuches brauchen wir auch nicht mehr einzugehen.

Es gibt keinen Beweis für Abweichungen von der Norm im Stoffwechsel des Epileptikers. Man wird zwar darauf gedrängt, was Frisch schon früher gefunden hatte, nämlich den relativ hohen Albuminanteil des Gesamteiweißes im Serum, auch elektrophoretisch zu suchen und zu finden, und tatsächlich ist von Fetzner und von italienischen Autoren auch gefunden worden, daß der Albuminanteil relativ hoch ist. Wir glauben diese Befunde aber noch in den Bereich der Norm rechnen zu müssen. Eine gewisse Armut an Elektrolyten und auch an Wasser soll im Serum des Epileptikers festzustellen sein und vorbereitend auf das wirken, was nun für uns interessanter ist, nämlich die *Genese* des epileptischen Anfalls. Mit diesem Thema haben sich unabhängig voneinander u. a. Selbach und Riebeling beschäftigt. Selbach legt besonderen Wert auf die Gültigkeit des Ausgangswertgesetzes oder besser der Ausgangswertregel von Wilder, die dieser 1931 publizierte und die besagt, daß die zusätzliche Erregbarkeit innerhalb der Reichweite überhaupt eines Systems um so geringer ist, je höher die schon vorhandene Erregung war. Umgekehrt also: Da, wo eine Richtung nur *eben* angedeutet ist, wird ein Reiz in dieser um so stärker ausschlagen. Es besteht beim Epileptiker offenbar eine Tendenz zur dekompensierten Alkalose, die sich in einer über die Norm hinausgehenden Labilität des Säure-Basen-Haushalts ausprägt.

Die Anschoppung irgendwelcher Krampfgifte bzw. anfallsauslösender Stoffe hat Selbach am Modell der sog. Kippschwingung zu erklären versucht, eine Vorstellung, die er von Betz übernommen hat. Als Modell der Kippschwingung benutzt er die Glimmlampe, bei der bekanntlich ein Schrittmachersystem und ein Gefolgschaftssystem einen Kondensator aufladen, bis dessen Entladungsschwelle oder eine Grenzwertspannung erreicht ist. Diese Grenzwertspannung ist für die Glimmlampe die Zündspannung. Dadurch, daß die Glimmlampe gezündet wird, sinkt die Spannung des Systems wieder auf die Löschspannung zurück, und die Glimmlampe verlischt wieder. Gewissermaßen ist also die Glimmlampe der Spannungsregler. Ladungen und

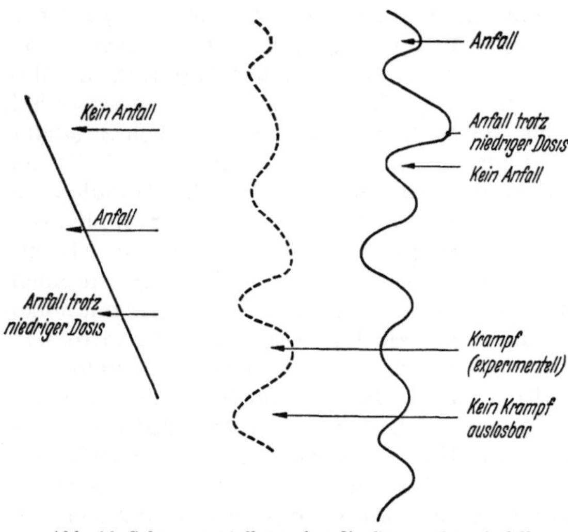

Abb. 16. Schemavorstellung uber die Genese eines Anfalls

Entladungen stehen in dem gleichen Verhältnis zueinander wie assimilatorischer und dissimilatorischer Stoffwechsel.

Riebeling stellt sich eine unregelmäßig schwankende Möglichkeit bei der Disposition zu Anfällen vor, die schematisch dargestellt (Abb. 16) selbstverständlich beim Epileptiker etwas höher liegt als beim Gesunden, höher, also näher bei dem iktogenen Reiz. Die Wellenlinie, die möglichst unregelmäßig und uncharakteristisch willkürlich ausgezogen ist, ebenso wie die gestrichelte, die das Verhalten des Normalmenschen gegenüber Anfallsreizen ausdrücken soll, sollen die Dispositionsmöglichkeiten zeigen. Die Länge der Pfeile soll zeigen, wieviel Anfallsprovokation notwendig ist, um einen Anfall — dabei mag es sich nicht immer um einen epileptischen, sondern es kann sich um einen ganz anderen Anfall handeln — auszulösen. Der erste Anfall wäre ein Spontananfall, und der zweite wäre ein Anfall trotz einer niedrigeren Dosis, weil die Disposition wesentlich höher liegt. Im dritten Fall, bei dem der Reiz genauso groß gedacht ist wie im ersten Fall, erfolgt kein Anfall, weil Reiz und Erfolgsorgan sich nicht erreichen. Beim vierten und fünften Pfeil handelt es sich um die Krämpfe, die auslösbar sind, auch beim gesunden nicht-iktaffinen Menschen, z. B. also Elektroschock, Cardiazol-Schock, Brufaneuxol-Schock etc. Auch der Epileptiker braucht vielleicht die gleiche Dosis eines Krampfgiftes, um einen Anfall auszulösen. Wir haben aber mit den Wellenlinien beim Gesunden anzudeuten versucht, daß auch dabei eine gewisse Disposition vorliegen muß, die zeitlich oder örtlich, lebensaltersmäßig oder irgendwie anders begründet ist, weil sonst auch bei gleich hoher Dosis unter Umständen ein Anfall ausbleibt, ein Phänomen, das von früher her als der Cardiazol- oder Aneuxol-Schock aus therapeutischen Gründen vielfach angewandt wurde, bekannt ist, das nur heute beim reinen Elektroschock unter anderen Verhältnissen, bei dem wesentlich höhere Dosen angewandt werden, nicht mehr beobachtet wird. Die kleine Strecke eines Ansteigens der Prädisposition haben wir noch einmal vergrößert in der unteren Hälfte der Abbildung und haben dabei noch einmal auch während des Anstieges einer Disposition gezeigt, daß auch auf einer so kurzen Strecke noch Differenzen zwischen der den Anfall auslösenden Dosis auftreten können. Am Anfang der Strecke, also in dem Wellental, ist eine Normaldosis eines Anfallsmittels wirkungslos, in der Mitte der Strecke ist sie wirkungsvoll, weil die beiden für den Anfall notwendigen Bestandteile, nämlich die Bereitschaft und der Reiz, sich treffen, und an der Spitze des Wellenberges ist der Anfall trotz einer geringen Dosis ohne weiteres auslösbar. Man könnte den linken Teil der oberen Kurve jenseits des zweiten Anfallspfeiles noch modifizieren, nämlich in dem Sinne, daß man die refraktäre Phase verlängert; nicht nur schwankt die Anfallsbereitschaft spontan, sondern sicherlich auch dadurch, daß unmittelbar nach einem Anfall ein zweiter entweder gar nicht oder nur sehr schwer auslösbar ist. Was aber nun dazu führt, daß die Wellenlinie ansteigt, das dürfte insbesondere bei den Spontananfällen, insbesondere bei allen anfallsartig auftretenden Krankheiten, damit aber auch bei jeder akut auslösbaren phasischen Psychose, eine Anschoppung von irgendwelchen, in keiner Weise näher zu charakterisierenden, Giftsubstanzen sein, eine Anschoppung als Auslöser katatoner Stuporen, wie sie Gjessing bei seinen Patienten sehr schön gezeigt hat. Das Bild zeigt deutlich, was damit gemeint ist, und läßt sich in dieser Form ohne weiteres übertragen auf alle anderen in Betracht kommenden Zustandsbilder. Bei Gjessing handelt es sich um eine Anschoppung von Stickstoffsubstanzen, also um eine negative Stickstoff-Bilanz, bei Rowntree handelt es sich um eine Anschoppung von 17-Ketosteroiden, bei unserem Fall mit der Wasserhaushaltsstörung (s. dort) um eine Anschoppung von Wasser im Gesamtblut. Es dreht sich nicht darum, um welche Substanz es sich handelt, sondern ausschließlich darum, daß dieser Mechanismus ja zwangsläufig zu einem wellenlinienförmigen Verhalten gegenüber einer bestimmten Reizauslösung führen muß. Die Anschoppung, am Boden eines Wellentales beginnend, muß einen Moment erreichen, an dem sie gefährlich wird für den betreffenden Organismus, an dem die Disposition so groß geworden ist, daß nunmehr entweder ein kleiner Reiz von außen oder überhaupt nur noch der Reiz von innen her genügt, um das zu erwartende Phänomen auszulösen. Alle derartigen Modelle sind naturgemäß unglaublich vereinfacht gegenüber der Wirklichkeit, das Selbachsche nicht weniger als meines. Aber sie lassen doch sehr viel mehr von dem verstehen, was im Anfallsgeschehen überhaupt vor sich geht, als die einfache Akkumulation von chemischen Tatsachen; eine derartige Akkumulation kann nur Anhaltspunkte geben, die einfach noch verarbeitet werden müssen, um sinnvoll zu werden.

Albrecht hat in meinem Laboratorium eine Reihe von Epileptikern über längere Zeit regelmäßig untersucht, um einen Zusammenhang zwischen dem Wassergehalt des Blutes sowie dem Chlorgehalt des Serums und den Anfällen zu finden. Sie fand aber regelmäßig, daß die Epileptiker im Prinzip in der Normallage waren und größere Schwankungen zwar gelegentlich, aber keineswegs regelmäßig, vorkamen, weder bezüglich des Wassergehaltes noch der Elektrolyte. Ebenfalls fand sich keinerlei Beziehung zwischen einer besonderen Hydrämie und eventuell einem Anfall. Weinland beobachtete eine Diurese-Hemmung im Anfall. Haury und Hirschfelder fanden den Magnesiumgehalt des Plasmas, und zwar wahrscheinlich den ionisierten Anteil, im Anfall oft herabgesetzt.

Weinland hat auch Untersuchungen des Ammoniakgehalts des Blutes durchgeführt, hat aber keine sicheren Befunde erheben können. Wir selber haben Ammoniak im Liquor bestimmt und beim Status epilepticus einen deutlichen, beim Einzelanfall immerhin meßbaren Anstieg des Ammoniakgehaltes feststellen können. Einen sehr wichtigen Befund teilt Wendt mit, der aber seit 1949 niemals wieder

diskutiert worden ist und dringend nachgeprüft werden sollte, nämlich den auffällig hohen Cholesteringehalt der Nebennieren von Epileptikern, deren Gesamt-
Cholesterin fast das Dreifache des Durchschnitts der Norm ausmacht. Dem steht
allerdings eindeutig entgegen, daß Amantea bei seinen Organuntersuchungen eine
Verminderung des Gewichtes der Nebennieren bei Epileptikern bzw. bei krampfgeneigten Tieren gefunden hat. Amantea hat große Serien von Hunden untersucht und hat eine Gruppe von reflexepilepsiegeneigten Tieren abgetrennt von
solchen, die zu einer Reflexepilepsie offenbar gar nicht fähig sind. Bei den
etwa 50% der gesamten Hundepopulation ausmachenden iktaffinen Hunden
wurden vermehrter Wassergehalt und vermehrter Kochsalzgehalt des Gehirns,
außerdem ein höherer Gehalt des Serums an Phosphor und an Traubenzucker
gefunden als bei nicht-disponierten Tieren. Der Wassergehalt des Serums und
einige andere Eigenschaften, die weniger wichtig sind, waren verändert gegenüber
den nicht-disponierten Tieren. Was aber besonders eindrucksvoll erscheint, sind
die Unterschiede zwischen den Organgewichten. So seien bei disponierten Hunden
die Schilddrüsengewichte durchschnittlich 79% (!!) höher als bei nicht-disponierten. Auch das Pankreas war 61% schwerer auf den Durchschnitt gesehen, während
die Nebennieren, die Nieren und die Lungen 53 bzw. 41 bzw. 30% leichter waren
als bei nicht-disponierten Hunden. Begünstigend für Anfälle wirkt eine Hypoovarie und eine Hyporchie, auch Applikation von Hypophysenhinterlappen-
Hormon. Longo hat beim Epileptiker ein wesentlich geringeres Lebergewicht
als beim normalen Menschen gefunden, und Angrisani hat ausgerechnet, daß
für 100 g Gehirn dem normalen Menschen 117 g Leber, dem Epileptiker aber nur
89 g Leber zur „Entgiftung" zur Verfügung stehen.

Nicht nur die Epilepsie und die Migräne, sondern auch viele Fälle von Allergie
möchte Hoff durch Zwischenhirn-Hypophysen-Regulationsstörungen mindestens
gesteuert wissen. Interessanterweise betont er auch, daß man unter Umständen
eine schwere Allergie durch Herdsanierung heilen könne, was nun wieder Beziehung hat zu weiter oben erörterten Vorstellungen. Bezüglich des epileptischen
Anfalles betont Hoff ausdrücklich die hohe Bedeutung der Regulationen und der
Zwischenhirnsteuerung sowohl für die Epilepsie überhaupt, als insbesondere für die
Genese des epileptischen Anfalles, für die er, ebenso wie Treuheit, ebenfalls eine
vegetative Umschaltung annimmt.

Über die Bedeutung des Wetters für die Auslösung und das Verhalten von Psychosen

Über die Bedeutung des Wetters für die Auslösung von Psychosen hat
am meisten und am genauesten de Rudder gearbeitet, dem wir auch bei
den folgenden Ausführungen folgen werden. Es war schon den älteren Psychiatern
aufgefallen, daß bestimmte „Katastrophen"-Reaktionen wie die akute Katatonie bevorzugt in den ersten warmen Tagen des Frühlings aufzutreten
pflegten. In kalten Sommern und im Herbst brauchte man kaum damit
zu rechnen, daß solche Ergebnisse innerhalb eines Anstaltsbetriebes auftraten.
Auch der Eindruck, daß epileptische Anfälle mit dem Wetter etwas zu tun
haben müßten, ist immer wieder entstanden, hat sich aber oft genug nicht bestätigen lassen, wenn man nämlich anfing zu zählen und objektive Vergleiche
zog. Halbey, Brunner, Lomer bestätigten Zusammenhänge zwischen Wetter
und Epilepsie, Reich leugnete sie. Von einer Arbeit von Bredzina und Schmidt
über das Auftreten von epileptischen Anfällen im Steinhof bei Wien referiert
de Rudder ausdrücklich, daß die Autoren wahrscheinlich eine echte Abhängigkeit des Wetters von den Anfällen gefunden hätten, wenn sie damals

ihre Einzelergebnisse der Wetterqualitäten schon in den modernen Luftkörper-Theorien hätten zusammenfassen können. Aus einer Bearbeitung von 15000 Anfällen in Bethel bei Bielefeld ergab sich keinerlei Anfallshäufung an Fronttagen. Die Ergebnisse waren aber bezüglich der genuinen Epilepsie weder allgemein noch getrennt für Männer oder Frauen ausgerechnet. Ganz anders verhielt sich aber die traumatische Epilepsie, bei der BERG wieder umgekehrt eine eindeutige Frontenabhängigkeit feststellen konnte. Aus der Frontenabhängigkeit ließ sich auch noch erkennen, daß auf Tage mit Gewittern oder Wetterleuchten doppelt soviel Anfälle fielen, wie nach dem Zufall zu erwarten gewesen wäre. Auch eine gehäufte Selbstmordneigung an Fronttagen wird berichtet (THOLUCK). Man darf diesen Dingen nicht zu viel Bedeutung beimessen, ganz ablehnen sollte man sie aber auch nicht, besonders deswegen nicht, weil man hier wenigstens eine greifbare Beziehung zwischen Krankheit und Umwelt hat, die zu verfolgen auf Grund der physikalischen Gesetzmäßigkeiten sachlich gerechtfertigt ist.

Die Rolle der vegetativen Dystonie

WUHRMANN fand bei *vegetativen Dystonien* eine Verbreiterung des Weltmann-bandes, bis zu 0,15⁰/₀₀ Calcium-Chlorid, nur in einem Drittel der Fälle eine Kephalin-Cholesterin-Flockung, aber relativ hohe morgendliche Eisenspiegel im Serum. Die Hälfte davon wies sogar über 200 γ-% auf. Auch eine Neigung zu etwas hoch-normalen Albuminwerten und zu einer geringen Abnahme des γ-Globulins wurde festgestellt. In diesem Zusammenhang muß an die zuerst von HOFFSTEDT beschrie-bene und später von RANGE an recht großem Material bestätigte abnorm niedrige Blutsenkungsgeschwindigkeit der Neurotiker und der vegetativen Dystoniker erinnert werden, die immerhin so auffällig war und ist, daß sie als ganz geläufiger Befund im Laboratorium allgemein bekannt ist. Früher von uns gefundene Serumlabilitätsveränderungen bei der Schizophrenie selber dürften wohl weniger spezifisch für die Schizophrenie sein als einfach Ausdruck einer unspezifischen Labilität. Mit einer Kupferchloridreaktion, die wir nicht weiter ausgebaut haben, weil sie nur bei Psychopathen überhaupt ein „positives" Resultat ergibt, läßt sich das sehr schön demonstrieren. Bei dieser Kupferchloridreaktion handelt es sich darum, daß eine Reihe von $CuCl_2$-Mischungen in sämtlichen Verdünnungen immer Trübungen ergibt, die bei Gesunden etwas geringer sind als bei Kranken, bei den endogenen Psychosen die gleichen Werte ergeben wie bei Gesunden, aber bei Neurotikern überhaupt fast zu keiner Trübung führen. Bei diesen Patien-ten bleibt die Lösung praktisch klar und zeigt damit, daß sie stabiler ist als der Durchschnitt, vielleicht weil die Neurotiker relativ mehr Albumin im Serum haben als der Durchschnitt aller anderen Menschen.

Anorexia nervosa

So wichtig die Anorexia nervosa als Krankheitsbild innerhalb unseres Faches ist, so wenig ist stoffwechselpathologisch dazu zu sagen: Daß extreme Abmagerung zu einer enormen Einsparung von Energieumsatz führt, daß der Grundumsatz folgerichtig um 20—30, ja 40% unter die Norm absinken kann, ergibt sich aus dem Gesamtphänomen, ist aber nicht typisch für die Psychose. Daß die Ver-ursachung dieses Leidens ganz wesentlich psychisch ist und nicht hypophysär, wie man früher annahm, ergibt sich sowohl aus dem nur vorübergehenden Erfolg der Hypophyseneinpflanzung, als auch aus dem mindestens ebenso guten, wenn nicht weit besseren Erfolg einer rein psychiatrischen Therapie. Immerhin kommt STÄUBLI-FRÖHLICH zu dem Schluß, daß mehrere Vorbedingungen zum Zustande-kommen einer Anorexie notwendig sind. Neben der endogenen Schrulligkeit und dem Negativismus auf der einen Seite gehöre dazu die ausgeprägte Leptosomie, oft verbunden mit einem Hypogonadismus auf der anderen Seite. Die Autorin glaubt durchaus an die Möglichkeit, daß das, was sie einmal gesehen hat, nämlich den Ausgang in eine Schizophrenie, mehr als zufällig sei, und fragt, ob die Anorexie etwa eine gutartige Verlaufsform der Schizophrenie darstelle. Alle adaptiven Umstellungen, Amenorrhoe, Grundumsatzsenkung, Lanugobehaarung sind sekundäre Störungen, die als Sparvorgänge aufzufassen sind, um den Körper der Unterernährung anzupassen. Die hochgradige Oligodipsie verhindere die Bildung von Ödemen, das Fehlen von Darminfekten sei ebenfalls ein deutliches Unterscheidungsmerkmal gegenüber der Hungerkrankheit, mit der die Anorexie eben doch nur die Unterernährung und nicht die Konsequenzen gemeinsam hat.

Einiges über sogenannte inborn errors of metabolism

Da praktisch sämtliche Abnormitäten des Stoffwechsels, sog. inborn errors of metabolism (GARROD), mit psychischen Störungen einhergehen, viele mit groben Störungen, manche mit nur eben erkennbaren, scheint es uns notwendig, dieses Thema wenigstens ganz kurz auch zu berühren, zumal mit fortschreitender Untersuchungsmethodik und mit fortschreitender Erhaltungsmöglichkeit auch von offenbar schwer gestörten Neugeborenen eine ganze Anzahl von Kindern am Leben bleibt und zur Untersuchung kommt, die früher offenbar so schnell starben, daß man ihre Abnormitäten gar nicht erkennen konnte. Wir möchten beginnen mit einer leichten und nicht sehr wichtigen Stoffwechselanomalie, der man noch vor 30 Jahren sicher mehr Bedeutung zugemessen hat, als ihr zukommt, die aber immerhin nicht ganz uninteressant ist: die sogenannte Phosphaturie oder besser Calciurie. Ältere Autoren waren geneigt, die Phosphaturie mit der sog. Sexualneurose in unmittelbaren Zusammenhang zu bringen, da sie vorwiegend bei jüngeren Männern auftritt, die einen trüben, schnell zur Ausfällung führenden Urin ausscheiden (sog. Milchpisser). Dieser Urin wird auch nach Zentrifugierung nicht ganz klar, überzieht sich im Gegenteil nach relativ kurzem Stehen mit einem zarten kolloidalen Häutchen, das schillert und das aus einer Eiweißsubstanz besteht, in die Calciumphosphatkristalle in mikroskopischer Größe eingelagert sind. Es ist sehr auffällig, daß Träger dieser Anomalie relativ häufig psychopathische Individuen sind. Es ist weiterhin zu bedenken, daß diese Störung periodisch auftritt und auf Störungen im Säure-Basen-Haushalt beruhen muß. HOFF betont ausdrücklich, daß bei der Phosphaturie eine zentralnervöse oder nervös-humorale Regulationsstörung periodisch und anfallsweise auftritt, während AIGINGER glaubte, einige anstaltsbedürftige Fälle unter seinem Material gefunden zu haben, ohne indes u. E. genügend unterschieden zu haben, ob die Anomalie vielleicht neben echten Psychosen auftrat. So glauben weder HOFF noch KLEINSORGE noch der Verfasser, daß die Phosphaturie eigentlich überhaupt therapiebedürftig ist. Wichtig scheint uns nur, daß man diese Kranken nicht einfach auslachen soll, sondern daß man ihnen zugeben muß, daß sie nicht nur eine Anomalie tragen, sondern auch unter ihr leiden.

Wesentlich wichtiger ist die nächste bedeutende Anomalie, bei der es sich um eine Unfähigkeit des Organismus handelt, Phenylalanin zu Tyrosin zu oxydieren. FÖLLING, PENROSE, RHEIN u. STOEBER, JERVIS haben viele Fälle beschrieben und BOREK u. Mitarb. endgültig die chemische Situation aufgeklärt. Versuche mit C_{14}-markiertem Phenylalanin, die UDENFRIEND und COOPER durchgeführt haben, haben bewiesen, daß etwa $^2/_3$ des aufgenommenen Phenylalanins im Harn als Phenylbrenztraubensäure nachweisbar sind. Normalerweise wird Phenylalanin nicht über Phenylbrenztraubensäure, sondern über Tyrosin abgebaut. KAUFMANN

hat ein kompliziertes System der Leber aufgedeckt, das aus mindestens zwei
Fermenten besteht und das außer hydriertem Triphosphopyridin-Nucleotid und
Sauerstoff auch Pteridin-ähnliche Co-Faktoren zur Verfügung hat. Dieses System
müßte nach JERVIS in der Leber der befallenen Personen fehlen. Aus einem
Schema, das ich einer Arbeit von LANG entnehme (Abb. 17), ergibt sich klar und
eindeutig, worum es sich bei der Anomalie handelt. Warum sie aber auftritt,
dürfte vorläufig noch ungeklärt bleiben.

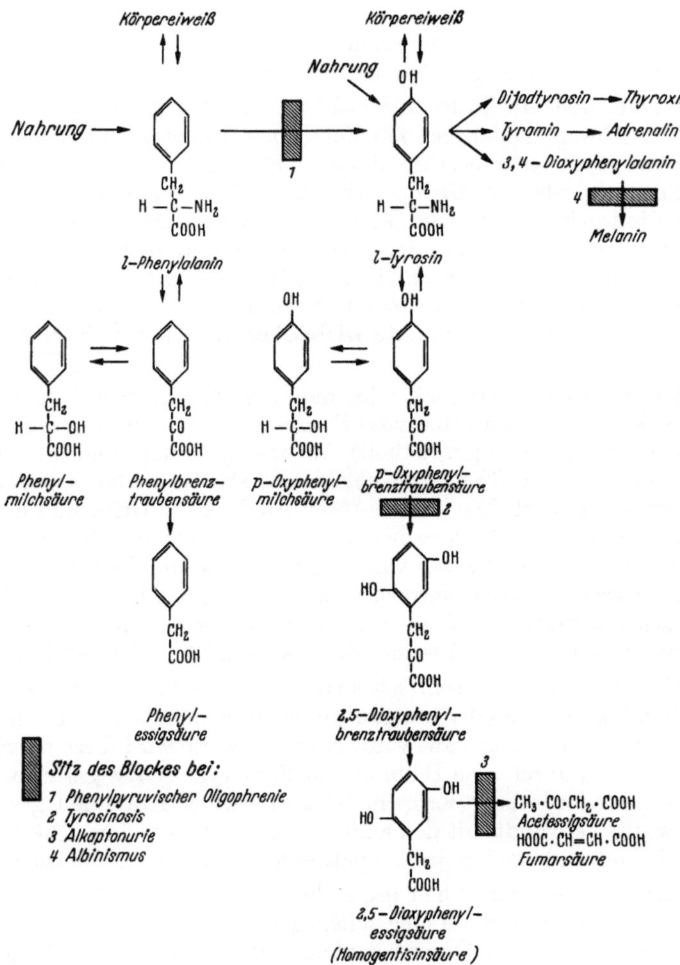

Abb. 17. Stoffwechsel des Phenylalanins und Tyrosins. (Modifiziert nach LANG, Der intermediäre Stoffwechsel)

Bei der Galaktosämie handelt es sich um eine angeborene Unfähigkeit des
Organismus, Galaktose umzubauen. Es fehlt die Galaktose-1-Phosphat-Uridyl-
transferase. Dadurch wird die Umwandlung von Galaktosephosphat in Glucose-
phosphat verhindert, und diese Anreicherung ist für den Körper offenbar giftig oder
mindestens schädlich. Sicher ist, daß unbehandelte Kinder bei weiterer Zufuhr von
Milch eingehen, daß dagegen solche, bei denen beizeiten die Stoffwechselanomalie
erkannt worden ist, bei milchfreier Ernährung tadellos gedeihen und vollkommen

gesund werden, die fettige Infiltration der Leber mit nachfolgender Cirrhose, Kataraktbildung, Aminoacidurie und Schwachsinn also nicht eintreten und man insofern bei dieser Stoffwechselanomalie wirklich einen Schaden vermeiden kann.

Bei der Glykogenose, von der es verschiedene Typen gibt, die sich aber klinisch nicht nennenswert unterscheiden, handelt es sich um eine Störung im Glykogenumbau. Man findet nur einige hundert Fälle in der Literatur beschrieben. Die Folge dieser Störung ist eine Hepatomegalie und ein eigenartig molliger Typ der Kinder, die außerdem psychisch minderwertig sind. Man unterscheidet heute 6 Typen, die durch die Inaktivität einzelner Fermente an verschiedenen Stufen des Abbaus oder durch einen abnormen Glykogenaufbau gekennzeichnet sind. Eine eingehende Beschreibung findet sich bei Stetten und Stetten.

Ältere Berichte über die Fructosurie sowohl wie über die Pentosurie betonen die psychischen Abwegigkeiten bei den Befallenen. Neuerdings hat man weniger darauf geachtet. Mallyoth beschreibt einen Fall eines 7jährigen Knaben, bei dem die Reduktionsproben im Urin positiv waren. Der Knabe macht einen wenig intelligenten Eindruck, was sich im Verlauf der Behandlungen noch stärker betonte. Während Fehling und Nylander positiv waren und die Gärungsprobe ebenfalls, war die Polarisation schwach linksdrehend. Im Urin des Jungen wurde Fructose, Xylose und Mannose gefunden. Nach Belastung fand sich außerdem neben der Glucose der sog. unbekannte Diabetiker-Zucker von Wallenfels und noch ein anderer.

Eine andere familiäre Krankheit wird dadurch charakterisiert, daß der Urin nach Ahornzucker riecht, zentralnervöse Symptome auftreten und der Tod frühzeitig eintritt (sog. Ahornsirupkrankheit). Westall, Dancis und Miller haben ein Kind demonstriert, das 20 Monate gelebt hat. Das ist die längste Überlebenszeit, die bisher bekannt ist. Die Aminosäuren-Analyse des Urins und des Blutes, die während der letzten Lebenswochen möglich war, zeigte sehr auffällige Abweichungen von der Norm. Die drei verzweigten Aminosäureketten Valin, Leucin und Isoleucin waren erheblich vermehrt, während Threonin, Serin, Alanin ungewöhnlich gering auftraten. Es fand sich außerdem eine Erhöhung von Methionin und eine Senkung des Cystins im Plasma. Einen kurzen Überblick gab K. Schreier.

Bei der Alkaptonurie, einer sehr seltenen Stoffwechselanomalie, die höchstens auf 10 Millionen Kinder einmal vorkommt, handelt es sich darum, daß die Homogentisinsäure nicht weiter abgebaut wird. Normalerweise wird diese durch Sprengung des Ringes und durch eine Bildung von Fumarylacet-Essigsäure weiter abgebaut. Das dazu erforderliche Ferment ist aber bei der Krankheit gestört, und sie zeigt sich somit verwandt mit den anderen Fermentanomalien. Die Träger der Anomalie sind samt und sonders psychopathisch, meist auch minderbegabt.

Bei der Hartnupschen Krankheit beobachtet man eine auffällig hohe Indicanausscheidung im Urin. Erst wenn eine solche gesehen wird, lohnt es sich bei verdächtigen Fällen, den Urin auf Aminosäuren zu analysieren. Es liegt nämlich immer eine Aminoacidurie nennenswerten Grades vor. Die Aminosäureausscheidung bei 3 Geschwistern, von denen 2 krank und 1 gesund waren, ergab immerhin bei den kranken etwa das 10fache der Ausscheidung des gesunden Kindes. Auffällig ist besonders eine Ausscheidung von 2—3 g Glutamin täglich und von über 1 g Serin. Auch Tryptophan, Indican, Indolessigsäure und Indolylacetyl-Glutamin werden in abnormen Mengen ausgeschieden. Als Konsequenz der abnorm hohen Ausscheidung von Tryptophan und anderen Indolderivaten ist die Ausscheidung von Kynurensäure und Xanthurensäure, Stoffen, die auf dem Stoffwechselwege zwischen Tryptophan und Nicotinamid liegen, besonders niedrig, wesentlich niedriger als die bei Gesunden.

ALLAN und CUSWORTH beschrieben eine Familie mit Rh-Inkompatibilität. Die beiden Eltern hatten 5 Kinder, eines ist früh gestorben, 2 sind normal, 2 abnorm, geistig schwer zurückgeblieben; davon erkrankte ein 3jähriges an einem epileptischen Status, der aber vollkommen wieder verschwand und einer Ataxie Platz machte, die das Kind zeitweise geradezu unfähig machte, eine Tasse zum Munde zu führen. Es blieb, nachdem dieses verschwunden war, ein schwerer geistiger Defekt, und außer völlig normalen übrigen Befunden fand sich im Chromatogramm eine starke Ausscheidung eines unbekannten Stoffes, der sich nach sorgfältiger Analyse als ein Peptid darstellte, das aber ninhydrin-positiv war. Bei dem zweiten Jungen, der ebenfalls erkrankte (mit dem gleichen eigenartigen Haar übrigens und genau demselben intellektuellen Verhalten), ergab sich genau das gleiche Bild im Chromatogramm. Im Liquor findet sich diese bisher noch unbekannte Substanz wesentlich reichlicher.

Im Mittelpunkt der Stoffwechselschäden beim Morbus Westphal-Strümpell-Wilson oder der hepatolenticulären Degeneration steht die Störung des Kupfer-stoffwechsels. Alle weiteren Stoffwechselstörungen treten hinter seiner Bedeutung sichtlich zurück. Das Coeruloplasmin ist eine unspezifische Oxydase und wurde bereits an anderen Stellen, bei der Erörterung der Oxydationsfähigkeiten des schizophrenen Stoffwechsels, erwähnt (S. 136). Es soll im Gehirn nicht vorkommen, vielmehr sind die an sich kleinen Mengen Kupfer, die im Gehirn überhaupt nach-weisbar sind, offenbar sog. direkt reagierendes, also nicht an α-Globulin gebunde-nes, sondern freies Kupfer, das locker (aus Transportgründen) an Albumin gebun-den ist. Da man nun bei der Lebercirrhose neben verschiedenen anderen Störungen des Kupferstoffwechsels auch eine Oxydationsschwäche gefunden hat, obwohl Coeruloplasmin genügend zur Verfügung steht, hat man den Schluß gezogen, daß hier vielleicht ein abnormes Coeruloplasmin vorliegen könnte. PORTER hat kürzlich vier Gehirne von Wilson-Patienten mit einigen normalen Gehirnen verglichen und dabei festgestellt, daß in den ersteren ein bemerkenswerter Anteil des Kupfers lockerer gebunden ist als bei den Kupfer-Eiweiß-Bindungen im normalen Gehirn. Wäßrige Extrakte aus Gehirn bei pH 4,5 waren der normalen Hirnfraktion ähnlich, während Extrakte bei pH 8,2 nicht direkt mit dem Natriumdiäthyldithiocarbamat, dem klassischen Kupferreagens, reagierten. Die Kupfervermehrungen im Serum, die bei Schwangerschaft und bei Infektionskrankheiten beobachtet werden kön-nen, sind solche des indirekt reagierenden Kupfers, also gewissermaßen Coerul-ämien. Der Gehalt des Serums an Kupfer ist im allgemeinen außerordentlich niedrig, er liegt 30—40% niedriger als bei der Norm. Der Gehalt des Urins schwankt sehr von Hypocuprurien bis zu starken Hypercuprurien, aber ganz regelmäßig ist der Gehalt der Leber und des Gehirns an Kupfer erhöht. Alle Bemühungen, die Kupferstörungen zu beheben, richten sich denn auch darauf, die Kupfer-speicher im Organismus auszuspülen, entweder durch Ionenaustauscher-Harze oder durch BAL. STOKES u. Mitarb. haben sich ganz anders verhalten als GUBLER und viele andere. Sie haben ihrem 22jährigen Kranken, der übrigens auch nicht gerettet werden konnte, Kupfer sogar zugelegt, weil sie sahen, daß unter Kupfer-karenz die Leberschädigung noch deutlicher bemerkbar wurde. Neben der hohen Kupferausscheidung des Kranken war besonders auffällig die enorm hohe Amino-acidurie. Es wird in diesem Zusammenhang auch auf die Beobachtung von UZMAN hingewiesen, der abnorme Oligopeptide, die sich durch Rubeansäure nachweisen ließen, im Urin feststellte. Vielleicht waren die Kupfermengen an diese gebunden. Interessant ist auch, daß GASTAGER und seine Mitarbeiter von der Beobachtung von HOLMBERG und LAURELL noch einmal wieder ausgehen, die ja die oxydativen Eigenschaften des Coeruloplasmins zuerst beschrieben haben. Die beiden genannten Autoren nehmen an, daß die jüngst beschriebene p-Poly-

phenoloxydase vielleicht in Wirklichkeit Coeruloplasmin sei. Sie untersuchten
außer dem Kupfer auch diese Oxydase im Warburg-Gerät, und es stellte sich dabei
heraus, daß nicht nur das Serumkupfer abnorm niedrig war wie erwartet, sondern
daß auch die Oxydaseaktivität wesentlich geringer war als die der Norm. Sie
besserte sich auch auf Kupferbelastung nicht, obwohl der Kupfergehalt des
Serums vorübergehend anstieg. Nun ergaben Untersuchungen von gesunden
Familienangehörigen des Wilson-Falles ebenfalls niedrige Kupferwerte und hohe
Kupferausscheidung im Urin. Daraufhin vorgenommene genauere klinische Untersuchungen deckten übrigens bei zwei von drei Fällen einen Kaiser Fleischerschen
Hornhautring auf.

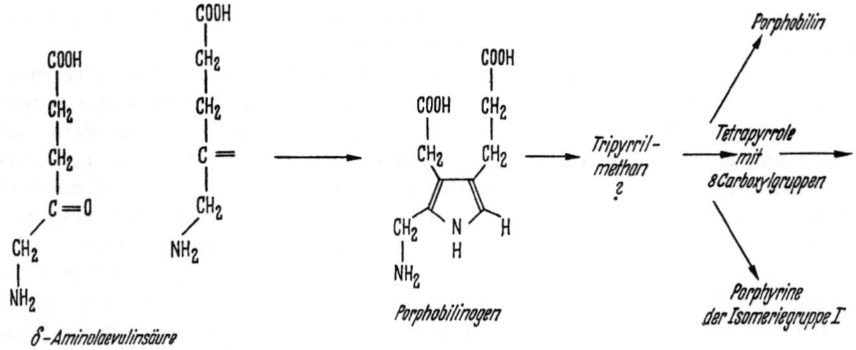

Abb. 18. Entstehung von Porphobilinogen und von Porphyrinen der Isomerie-Gruppe I.

Auch bei den Porphyrien, Krankheiten, die mit der Protoporphyrin-Synthese
im Zusammenhang stehen, kann man wieder mehrere verschiedene Typen unterscheiden, die zum Teil lichtempfindlich und zum Teil völlig lichtunempfindlich
sind. Die congenitale Porphyrie, die auch gelegentlich Günthersche Krankheit genannt wird, ist extrem lichtempfindlich. Es entsteht durch den Einfluß des Lichts
eine Hydroa vacciniformis, die zu erheblichen Störungen führen kann. Psychosen
bei dieser Krankheit sind nicht bekannt (Abb. 18). Die akute Porphyrie des
Erwachsenenalters verhält sich ganz anders. Sie ist im Prinzip ähnlich wie die
symptomatischen Porphyrien, hat aber ihren eigenen Erbverlauf, und insbesondere
sind bei der akuten Porphyrie des Erwachsenenalters, wie MERTENS schon hat
nachweisen können, andere Porphyrine im Urin nachweisbar als bei den symptomatischen Porphyrien. Es handelt sich zweifellos um eine sehr schwere Krankheit,
die der Therapie vorläufig vollkommen unzugänglich ist und die deswegen von
großem Interesse ist, weil die toxische Porphyrie auch heute noch nicht allzu
leicht diagnostiziert wird. Ein Vorschlag, der vor vielen Jahren schon gemacht wurde
und der zweifellos sehr geistreich war, nämlich prinzipiell jeden Urin ganz kurz
unter die Ultraviolett-Analysen-Lampe zu halten und zu finden, ob eine Spur
von Fluorescenz vorhanden ist, die dann weiter auf Porphobilinogen verdächtig
wäre, hat doch viel weniger Erfolg gehabt, als man ursprünglich erwarten
konnte. Wir wenigstens haben den über Monate hindurch geführten Versuch
wieder aufgegeben, weil wir kein einziges Mal eine Porphyrie fanden. Andererseits
wird aber prinzipiell jeder Urin, der beim Stehen nachdunkelt, ultraviolett-
fluorescenzmäßig untersucht, und auf die Weise findet man doch leichter einmal
eine Porphyrie. Bei der akuten Porphyrie werden Uroporphyrin-1, Kopropor-
phyrin und Uroporphyrin III ausgeschieden. Das Schema zeigt ganz gut, worum

es sich handelt (Abb. 19). Andere Anomalien nennenswerter Art sind nicht nachweisbar, insbesondere ist auch keine Störung des Eiweißstoffwechsels erkennbar. Nicht immer dunkelt der Urin sofort nach, sondern das Porphobilinogen kann auch auf dieser Stufe stehenbleiben. Deshalb empfiehlt es sich, das Porphobilinogen in verdächtigen Fällen zu suchen, wozu die Ehrlichsche Aldehydreaktion vollkommen ausreicht.

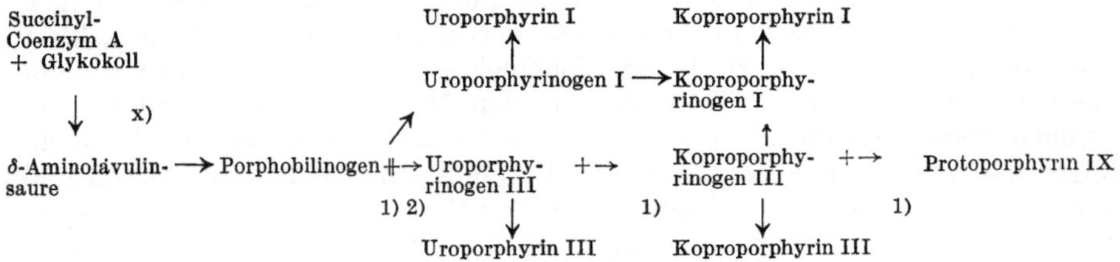

1) Block bei „toxischen" hepatischen Porphyrien und Stimulierung der δ-Aminolävulinsäure-Synthese bei x).
2) Bei herabgesetzter Porphobilinogen-Isomerase-Aktivität (bei erythropoetischer congenitaler Porphyrie) vermehrte Biosynthese von Uroporphyrinogen I usw.

Abb. 19. Fermentblocks, die zu einer Porphyrie führen

Porphobilinogen wird gebildet aus zwei Molekülen δ-Aminolävulinsäure. Der Stoffwechselfaktor, der diese Bildung verursacht, ist wahrscheinlich ererbt, jedenfalls ist er seit Geburt vorhanden. Bei der Porphyrie, bei der das Porphobilinogen einzig auftritt und Vorstufe für Uroporphyrin-1 ist, das gebildet wird auf Grund einer falschen Kondensation, ist diese Störung im Pyrrolstoffwechsel vielleicht auf Grund eines Fehlens der Aladehydrase, die partiell blockt, bezeichnend und spricht außerdem, da sie offenbar nicht regelmäßig auftritt, für das intermittierende Auftreten.

Das von HÜHNERFELD in die Therapie der Depressionen eingeführte Hämatoporphyrin-Nencki kommt in der Natur nicht vor. Sicherlich ist es ein gewisser Zellaktivator und insofern als völlig unspezifisches aktivierendes Mittel, als Hilfsmittel unter Umständen sogar brauchbar. Daß aber die Theorie, von der HÜHNERFELD ausging, als er dieses Material in die Therapie einführte, völlig falsch ist, dürfte ganz sicher sein. HÜHNERFELD glaubte, was damals auch durchaus im Bereich der wissenschaftlichen Vorstellungen seiner Zeit lag, daß das Hämatoporphyrin-Nencki ebenso wie andere Porphyrine, wie das Coproporphyrin-1 zum Beispiel, auf Licht sensibilisiere und glaubte, mit kleinen Dosen die mit dem Material gefütterten Patienten durch ihre Sensibilisierung gegen Licht gewissermaßen zu aktivieren. Keineswegs aber hat Hämatoporphyrin-Nencki überhaupt irgendwelche lichtsensibilisierenden Eigenschaften, weder beim Menschen noch im Tierversuch, andererseits würde auch diese Lichtsensibilisierung, wie wir längst wissen, nicht zu einer Verbesserung der Stimmung oder zu einer größeren Leistungsfähigkeit, sondern im Gegenteil zu einer größeren Schwäche führen. Solche Dinge müssen aber doch noch einmal gesagt werden, weil immer noch wieder in der Literatur Vorstellungen ähnlicher Art auftauchen und auch die Frage der toxischen Porphyrie noch gelegentlich von dieser Seite angegangen wird. Daß häufig auch heute noch die unklaren Abdominalbeschwerden bei der toxischen Porphyrie, die teilweise den neurologischen Symptomen vorhergehen, teilweise ihnen auch folgen (die psychotischen Symptome sind meistens die letzten in der Reihe), chirurgischen Eingriffen unterliegen, geht aus einer Arbeit von WALDENSTRÖM hervor, der immerhin bei weitaus der Mehrzahl der Fälle aus der Weltliteratur der neueren Zeit Operationen wegen abdomineller Beschwerden registriert.

Die Fälle, die wir gesehen haben, sind auch sämtlich mindestens einmal operiert worden, ehe sie neurologischer bzw. psychiatrischer Behandlung zugeführt wurden.

Beim Mongolismus, bei dem es sich nach jüngsten Ergebnissen der erbbiologischen Forschung um eine chromosomale Störung handelt (es treten zwei X-Chromosomen zu dem Y-Chromosom bzw. bei Mädchen sind drei X-Chromosome vorhanden, so, daß die Chromosomen-Gesamtsumme 47 beträgt), finden sich auch Störungen im Stoffwechsel, die insbesondere von amerikanischer Seite geklärt worden sind. Simon u. Mitarb. haben Mongoloide mit Schwachsinnigen anderer Genese und mit Normalen verglichen, bei den Mongoloiden auch Altersgruppierungen vorgenommen, ebenso wie bei den Gesunden und bei den Schwachsinnigen anderer Art, und verglichen ihre Ergebnisse mit denen von Benda und Mader. Von seiten der Schilddrüse vermutete Störungen ließen sich, wenigstens soweit es das eiweißgebundene Jod angeht, nicht bestätigen. Bei der Bestimmung des Jods finden sich keine Unterschiede zwischen mongoloiden Kindern und den Kontrollen. Aber sowohl mongoloide als andere schwachsinnige bzw. idiotische Kinder haben signifikant mehr Serum-Cholesterin als normale Kinder. Die stärksten Unterschiede zwischen Mongolen, normalen und schwachsinnigen Kontrollen zeigen sich bei den großmolekularen Lipoproteiden, die bei Mongolen weitaus am höchsten, bei den schwachsinnigen Kontrollen mittelhoch und bei den normalen am niedrigsten sind.

Bei sämtlichen sog. Speicherkrankheiten ist die Prognose infaust. Es handelt sich mit Ausnahme der Glykogenose, die wir schon besprochen haben, fast nur um Lipoidspeicherungen, und die Speicherung findet keineswegs nur im Gehirn statt, teilweise sind die gespeicherten Lipoide nicht einmal gegenüber der Norm vermehrt, nur ihre Verteilung ist anders als die normale Verteilung. Bei der chronischen Form des Morbus Gaucher handelt es sich um eine cerebrosidartige Verfettung in den Zellen der Milz und des reticuloendothelialen Systems. Sowohl der Fett- als auch der Cholesteringehalt des Blutes sind dabei übrigens normal. Die Diagnose stützt sich also in erster Linie auf die enorm vergrößerte Milz. Im Gehirn findet man keineswegs regelmäßig sog. Gaucher-Zellen.

Die Niemann-Picksche Krankheit, die ebenfalls sehr selten ist, tritt wieder in zwei Formen auf, nämlich einer des kindlichen und einer des Erwachsenen-Alters. Die thesaurierte Substanz bei dieser Krankheit ist ein Sphingomyelin speziell in der Milz, in der Leber und in den Nieren. Im Gehirn haben sowohl Klenk wie Schettler, nicht aber Thannhauser, die Sphingomyeline vermehrt gefunden. Auch die Ganglioside sind zweifellos vermehrt vorhanden.

Bei der Tay-Sachsschen amaurotischen Idiotie handelt es sich um das Auftreten einer Gangliosid-Speicherung, die nach verschiedenen Autoren allerdings sehr verschieden hoch ist. Die Pathogenese der Krankheit ist ebenso unbekannt wie die der vorhergenannten.

Beim *Gargoylismus* liegt offenbar nicht nur eine einzige Stoffwechselstörung vor, sondern es findet sich in der nervösen Substanz ein Glykolipid-Komplex von der üblichen Formel Fettsäure-Sphingosin-Neuraminsäure-Hexose-Hexosamin.

Der chronische Alkoholismus bietet stoffwechselpathologisch keine Besonderheiten. Zwar findet man in vielen Fällen Leberschädigungen, und Yasargil glaubt sogar in allen Fällen chronischen Alkoholmißbrauchs eine Leberfunktionsstörung annehmen zu müssen. Zum Ausbruch eines Delirs hält er eine schwere Alteration der Leber für notwendig, deren Entgiftungsfunktionen lahmgelegt sein sollten, und er glaubt auch mit Neubürger, daß intermediäre toxische Stoffwechselprodukte eine grundlegende Rolle für das Zustandekommen des Delirs spielen. Auch Fournier findet beim chronischen Alkoholismus eine ganze Reihe von körperlichen Veränderungen, die wohl zum größten Teil einfach auf den Vitaminmangel und auf die schlechte Ernährung überhaupt zurückzuführen sind. Man darf nicht vergessen, daß Alkohol ein sehr hochwertiges Nahrungsmittel ist, das aber seinem Wesen nach natürlich völlig frei von Vitaminen ist. Fournier findet eine mäßige Cholesterinämie und eine Störung des Elektrolytgleichgewichts des

Blutes. BINSWANGER hatte vor langer Zeit bereits eine Aufstellung über eine
große Reihe von Leberfunktionsprüfungen durchgeführt, noch wesentlich früher
als die ausgezeichneten Untersuchungen von VÖGTLIN erschienen waren, die nun
sicherlich die gründlichste Erforschung des akuten und des kurzfristig und langfristig chronischen Alkoholismus darstellen. Aus ihnen geht ganz klar hervor,
daß man in der Mehrzahl der Fälle Leberfunktionsstörungen findet, daß sie aber
fast alle vollkommen reversibel sind. Auch MENZI stellt fest, daß das Delir am
häufigsten mit einer Leberfunktionsstörung einhergeht.

Psychosen und Schlafstörungen

Können schon Gesunde nach längerdauerndem Schlafentzug mit erheblichen
subjektiven und meßbaren objektiven Symptomen reagieren — Illusionen, Halluzinationen, Zeitsinnstörungen und Verhaltensstörungen auch anderer Art sind vielfach berichtet worden —, so zeigt sich das noch deutlicher bei einem kontrollierten
Schlafentzug von 72—98 Std, wie ihn MORRIS durchgeführt hat. Während solcher
Schlafentzugsperioden wurden psychologische Tests mehrfach wiederholt, und es
zeigten sich mit der Dauer des Schlafentzugs parallelgehend eine steigende Menge
Fehlleistungen, Fehldeutungen von gezeigten Gegenständen, persönliche und zeitliche Desorientierung, taktile Illusionen und Depersonalisationsphänomene. Die
Fehler gingen bis zu 90%. Wurden ähnliche Experimente bei Psychosen durchgeführt, wie sie KORANYI und LEHMANN in Montreal durchgeführt haben, fanden
sich die Dinge noch wesentlich deutlicher. Bei 6 chronischen Psychosen wurden
nach 100 Stunden Wachsein erhebliche Veränderungen gefunden. 5 der 6 Kranken
boten wieder ihr akut psychotisches Bild, wie es früher bei den ersten Aufnahmen
ins Hospital bestanden hatte. Der 6. Patient zeigte immerhin eine gleichmäßige
Verschlechterung. Sind die bisher berichteten Untersuchungen experimenteller
Natur und zweifellos in der Beziehung anzugreifen, einfach deswegen, weil die
Patienten wohl nicht wußten, was mit ihnen geschehen sollte, aber immerhin
unter allgemeiner Kontrolle standen, so sind die Fälle von STAUDER, der epileptische Anfälle nach Schlafentzug gesehen hat, und diejenigen von KLUGE, der
psychotische Störungen beobachtete und beschrieb, noch klarer und zeigen noch
deutlicher, daß Erschöpfung genauso wie schwere innere Krankheiten zu psychotischen Störungen Anlaß geben können, obwohl sie keineswegs in irgendeiner Form
endogene Psychosen repetieren. Wohl aber können sie das ausgesprochene Bild
einer Manie in den Fällen von KLUGE oder einer Depression zeigen. Nicht immer
sind diese Depressionen vom Typus der reaktiven, sondern sie können auch durchaus wie echte endogene Depressionen aussehen.

Psychotrope Substanzen

Weder gehören die Modellpsychosen zu unserem Thema noch kann die psychische Wirkung der Halluzinogene allgemein in diesem Zusammenhang besprochen werden. Wohl aber ist es ganz unumgänglich, auf die Chemie der Halluzinogene und der sog. psychotropen Substanzen überhaupt etwas einzugehen, und
zwar aus mehreren Gründen. Es ist sehr auffällig und nur spekulativ zu betrachten,
daß eine große Anzahl Stoffe, die zu Psychosen, zu psychotischen Erscheinungen
vorübergehender Art führen, auffällige Ähnlichkeiten untereinander und auffällige
Ähnlichkeiten mit schon lange bekannten Drogen haben, die auf die Psyche
wirken. Außerdem bestehen Ähnlichkeiten mit Stoffen, die im Organismus *vielleicht* etwas mit der Entstehung von Psychosen zu tun haben. Es wurde bereits

früher auf die fraglichen Beziehungen zwischen Adrenalin und Adrenochrom und schließlich Adrenolutin und den sog. endogenen Psychosen eingegangen und an anderer Stelle über die Bedeutung des Serotonins für die Entstehung bzw. auch für die Behandlung von Psychosen gesprochen. Die beiden genannten Körper

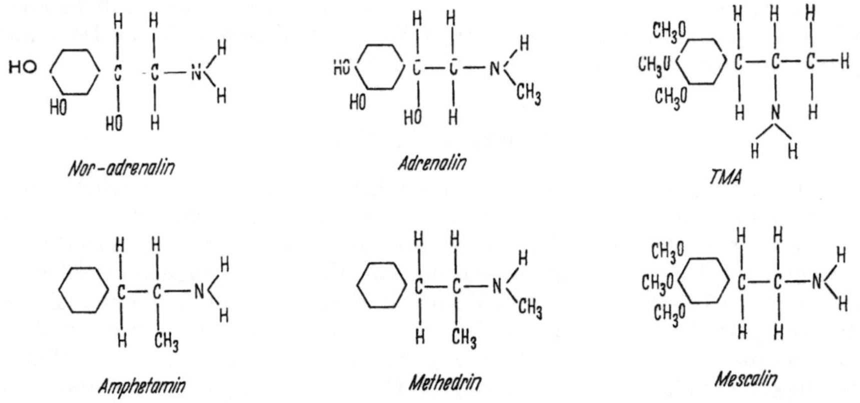

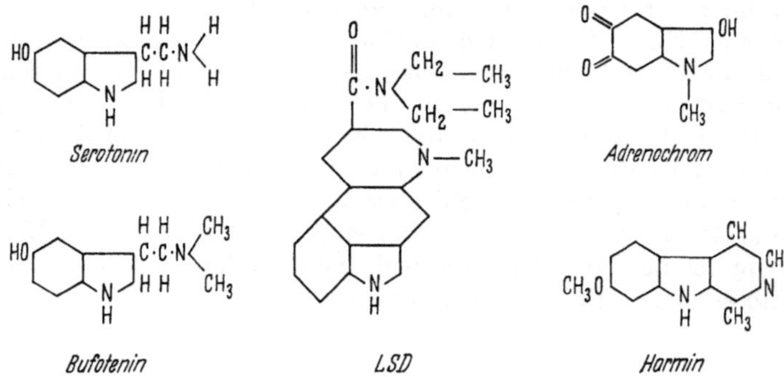

Abb. 20. Beziehungen zwischen Adrenalin und einigen Arzneimitteln

sind aber nun auch Quasi-Modelle oder Standardfiguren für die jetzt zu besprechenden Substanzen. Dem Adrenalin sehr ähnlich sind sowohl das Amphetamin (Abb. 20) als ein Körper, der als Weckmittel schon lange bekannt ist, als auch Metamphetamin, eine relativ neue halluzinogene Substanz, und Mescalin, eine der ältesten. Dem Serotonin, das als 5-Hydroxytryptamin dem Tryptophan in

Abb. 21. Beziehungen zwischen Serotonin und einigen Arzneimitteln

allernächster Nachbarschaft zugehört (Abb. 21), sind nun wieder auffällig ähnlich das Bufotenin, das ist das Gift der Kröte, das Harmin, das früher eine nicht zu unterschätzende Rolle in der Behandlung von Parkinson gespielt hat, das aber auch als Halluzinogen zweifellos eine gewisse Bedeutung hat, und das Adrenochrom, das ebenfalls als für Psychosen-Entstehung von Bedeutung vielfach in den letzten Jahren diskutiert worden ist. Dazwischen steht gewissermaßen ein sicher wesentlich komplizierter aufgebauter, aber doch im ganzen auf dem gleichen Gerüst beruhender Körper, das LSD (Lysergsäurediäthylamid). Dem Bufotenin wieder nahe verwandt sind sowohl das DMT (Dimethyltryptamin) als auch das Diäthyltryptamin, beides synthetische Drogen, die zu den Peptadenia-Alkoloiden gehören.

Die Erörterung der Modellpsychosen kann man vielleicht anfangen mit der Erwähnung der sog. experimentellen Katatonie von DE JONGH, der mit Bufotenin, Harmin und Bulbocapnin Tiere katatonisierte. Da die tierische Katatonie eine allgemeine Reaktion des niederen Wirbeltieres ist, ähnlich etwa dem epileptischen Anfall, der vorzugsweise (aber keineswegs ausschließlich) für höhere Tiere charakteristisch ist, können wir uns von der experimentellen Katatonie schon wieder abwenden, zumal sie weniger Ergebnisse gebracht hat, als ursprünglich angenommen worden war. Es hatte sich herausgestellt, daß sicher eine wesentliche katatonigene Substanz die Nicotinsäure sei.

Viele Rauschgifte der alten und der neuen Welt ähneln — wie gesagt — dem Adrenalin. BERINGER hat zuerst systematisch Rauschgifte zu experimentellen Untersuchungen benutzt, insbesondere um das Erlebnis der Halluzination dem Arzt selber zugänglich zu machen. Er bediente sich dabei des Mescalins, das oben erwähnt wurde, des Alkaloids des Cactus Anhalonium Levinii, der in der Neuen Welt, speziell in Mexiko seit Jahrhunderten als Halluzinogen benutzt wurde. BERINGER betonte immer noch seinerzeit die Ähnlichkeit der Mescalin-Psychose mit der Schizophrenie, insbesondere wegen der reichlichen Halluzinationen und des dereistischen Denkens. Da die Psychose aber fast niemals ohne Bewußtseinsveränderungen, wenn vielleicht auch nur geringfügiger Art, einherging, muß heute eine Ähnlichkeit mit der Schizophrenie bezweifelt oder ganz abgelehnt werden. Dazu kam die interessante Erkenntnis, daß eine Reihe von körperlichen Veränderungen, wie wir sie auch von den akuten Psychosen kannten, die wir aber samt und sonders als unspezifisch haben kennenlernen müssen, auch als Reaktion auf den Mescalinrausch beobachtet werden konnten. Um so näher lag es, den Vergleich zwischen Schizophrenie und der Modellpsychose zu ziehen. Da man u. a. auch einzelne Leberveränderungen unter der Mescalinwirkung beobachten konnte, da man außerdem unter dem Eindruck stand, daß die Leber im Zentrum des Stoffwechselgeschehens auch bei den Psychosen in Betracht kommt, wurden Versuche angestellt, Mescalin zu markieren und den eventuellen Einbau in die Leber bzw. in Lebereiweiße zu kontrollieren. Ehe wir darüber sprechen, aber noch ein Wort über LSD 25, eine halbsynthetische Droge, die HOFMANN 1943 fand, als er die Mutterkorn-Alkaloide untersuchte (STOLL u. HOFMANN). Er stellte fest, daß er nach Arbeiten mit dieser Substanz eigenartig müde und verstimmt wurde, und da er den Schluß zog, daß es sich um das Lysergsäure-Diäthylamid handeln müßte, machte er einen Selbstversuch mit einer winzigen Menge dieser Substanz, und dieser Selbstversuch führte zu zahllosen kontrollierten Versuchen an Gesunden und Kranken, zu zahllosen Publikationen: HOFMANN hatte nämlich Halluzinationen bei sich selber erlebt. Zum ersten Mal war es gelungen, mit winzigen Mengen eines Stoffes, mit solchen, die 1—2 Zehnerpotenzen niedriger lagen als alle bisher angewandten, Halluzinationen zu erzeugen. Es war also ein Stoff in γ-Mengen wirksam, der — zudem nicht ganz leicht zu isolieren und zu finden — vielleicht irgendwelche Parallelen haben könnte zu der Entstehung der sog. endogenen Psychosen. Nun fanden die beiden BLOCK, daß Mescalin in Lebereiweiß nur in winzigen Mengen, nämlich auch etwa in γ-Mengen, eingebaut wurde, während die weitaus größere Menge unverändert durch den Urin ausgeschieden wurde. Man könnte die Parallele ziehen, daß vielleicht auch Muscarin, Ololiuqui, Psilocybin in ähnlich winzigen Mengen eingebaut werden, während die anderen unverändert ausgeschieden werden. Daraus aber nun den Schluß zu ziehen, daß also alle diese Stoffe unmittelbar über die Leber wirkten, weiterhin den Schluß zu ziehen, daß demnach an dieser Stelle das effektive Agens für die Psychosenentstehung zu suchen sei, war sicher voreilig.

Sicherlich sind, wie das auch aus den Ausführungen von Waelsch und Weil-Malherbe hervorgeht, die Akten weder über das Serotonin noch über das Adrenochrom geschlossen. Sehr fragwürdig sind aber die teilweise voreiligen Hypothesen, insbesondere von Hoffer. Auch die Versuche, die chemische Verwandtschaft der Halluzinogene mit dem Serotonin und Adrenalin für eine Theorie der Psychosenentstehung zu verwerten, sind voreilig, unbegründet, und insbesondere erscheinen sie unkritisch. Wissen wir doch, daß wohl eine bestimmte Gruppenwirkung von bestimmten chemischen Strukturen zu erwarten ist, daß sie aber — am Beispiel des LSD und des 2-Brom-LSD läßt sich das zeigen — keineswegs garantiert ist. Es ist natürlich für einen Chemiker heutzutage kein Kunststück mehr, zahllose Derivate z. B. von Serotonin herzustellen, und für den Pharmakologen, die Experimente nachzuprüfen. Es bleibt aber immer nach wie vor das Probieren nötig, es läßt sich niemals voraussagen, wie ein neu synthetisierter Stoff nun wirken wird. Ebensowenig läßt sich voraussagen, daß irgendein solcher Stoff Beziehungen zum Organismus, insbesondere der Psychosen, hätte, die anders gelagert wären als die Beziehungen des gleichen Stoffes zum Gesunden.

Außer dem Lysergsäure-Diäthylamid wurde von Stoll und Hofmann auch das Lysergsäuremonoäthylamid und das Lysergsäureamid ohne Äthylgruppe untersucht. Alle drei Substanzen stellten sich als gleichmäßig psychotrop oder halluzinogen heraus. Die beiden letzteren unterschieden sich aber von dem Diäthylamid durch eine andere wichtige Eigenschaft. Das LSD-Problem erhielt neuen Auftrieb durch die Entdeckung, daß 5-Hydroxytryptamin im Gehirn einen ausgesprochenen Antagonismus gegen LSD ausübt. Es war verständlich, daß man die Hypothese aufkommen ließ, daß psychische Effekte durch LSD auf diesen Antagonismus zurückzuführen seien. Nun wurden aber im Laufe der pharmakologischen Prüfung des LSD auch Nebenprodukte untersucht. LSD und Dibrom-LSD stimmen in gewissen Eigenschaften überein, in anderen zeigen sie aber auch ganz erhebliche Differenzen. So hat z. B. 2-Brom-LSD überhaupt keine Wirkung auf die Psyche, indessen ist 2-Brom-LSD mindestens genauso wirkungsvoll als Antagonist des Hydroxytryptamins wie LSD, sowohl in vitro wie in vivo. Das macht die Hypothese wieder sehr fraglich. Dies nur ein Beispiel von vielen!

Trotz einer Fülle von Befunden moderner und älterer Art, trotz ungeheuren Fleißes und eines ständig noch zunehmenden Interesses an den in Frage stehenden Phänomenen, trotz ganzer Teams von wissenschaftlichen Arbeitern sind die Ergebnisse, die bisher vorliegen, ausgesprochen kümmerlich, insbesondere gibt es für keine Psychose irgendein charakteristisches oder spezifisches Phänomen, nicht einmal ein Phänomen, das nur bei Psychosen, aber überhaupt nicht bei Gesunden, beobachtet wird. Wir haben immer wieder darauf hingewiesen, daß man nicht Gesunde mit Kranken vergleichen kann, sondern vorher die Lebensumstände beider Gruppen prüfen muß. Erst wenn diese in den wesentlichsten Punkten übereinstimmen, hat es überhaupt einen Sinn, Vergleiche zu ziehen. Wir wissen viel zu genau, wie außerordentlich mannigfaltig die — übrigens ephemeren — Veränderungen sind, die durch das tätige Leben, allein schon durch den Unterschied zwischen Liegen und Stehen, verursacht werden. Obwohl wir nun keine verwertbaren Unterschiede zwischen Gesunden und psychiatrisch Kranken — ganz allgemein gesehen — kennen (mit Ausnahme der echten Stoffwechselstörungen), bleibt der Eindruck, daß eine Anzahl von Phänomenen, eine Anzahl von Reaktionsformen insbesondere, bei vielen Kranken anders, empfindlicher, mehr nach oben oder unten ausschlagend ist als bei Gesunden. Man wird den Eindruck nicht los, auch wenn man ihn mit nichts belegen kann, als ob das psychiatrische

Krankengut eben doch seinem Wesen nach korreliert sei mit einer Abnormität, mit einer größeren Variationsbreite seines biochemischen Gesamtverhaltens. Das aber erlaubt immer noch die Hoffnung weiterzusuchen und evtl. doch einmal einen signifikanten Befund zu erheben. Wir sind in keiner Weise optimistisch, aber wir resignieren auch nicht endgültig, sondern wir empfehlen nur immer wieder die größte Kritik und die größte Skepsis.

MASTROGIOVANNI hatte beobachtet, daß im Liquor von Schizophrenen ein pathogenes Agens zu finden sei, das — in der Allantoidflüssigkeit des Hühnchens gezüchtet — dort Virusentwicklung zeige. Die Flüssigkeit wurde weiter verimpft, und die Sterblichkeit bei den nächsten Reihen von Hühnereiern soll anscheinend etwas größer gewesen sein als bei Kontrollen. Die Arbeit selber ist relativ vorsichtig gehalten. Man muß sie aber noch vorsichtiger interpretieren, als die Autoren das getan haben. Leider ergeben Nachprüfungen von solchen Ergebnissen durch Virologen fast niemals eine Bestätigung.

Wir sind uns aber darüber klar, daß auch die Entdeckung der Spirochaeta pallida durch SCHAUDINN auf die größte Skepsis oder auf ironisch-lächelnde Ablehnung gestoßen ist durch sehr kritische Fachkollegen. Erst 1934 ist von FÖLLING der Phenylbrenztraubensäureschwachsinn entdeckt worden. Sind auch die in diesem Beitrag angeführten Phänomene mit größter Skepsis anzusehen, sind für fast alle oder für alle immer wieder auch die gegenteiligen Ergebnisse publiziert worden, so könnte doch das eine oder andere Phänomen einmal einen Baustein zu einer neuen Erkenntnis bilden. Das war der Grund, weshalb sie berichtet wurden.

Literatur

ABOOD, L. G., F. A. GIBBS and E. GIBBS: Comparative study of blood coeruloplasmin in schizophrenia and other disorders. Arch. Neurol. Psychiat. (Chicago) 77, 643—645 (1957). — ABRAMSON, D. I., N. SCHKLOVEN and K. H. KATZENSTEIN: Peripheral blood flow in schizophrenia and other abnormal mental states; plethysmographic study. Arch. Neurol. Psychiat. (Chicago) 45, 973—979 (1941). — AIGINGER, J.: Die Phosphaturie, ein Indikator einer konstitutionellen Komponente von Neurosen. Wien. klin. Wschr. 44, 1397—1401 (1931). — AIVAZIAN, G. H., and J. D. GRIFFITH: Coeruloplasmin reaction in mental disorders. Arch. Gen. Psychiat. 2, 17—21 (1960). — ÅKERFELDT, S.: Oxydation of N,N-Dimethyl-p-phenylenediamine by serum from patients with mental disease. Science 125, 117—119 (1957). — ALBERT, E.: Wechselwirkung zwischen Gehirn und Leber, in „Die Chemie und der Stoffwechsel des Nervengewebes“. Springer 1952. — ALBRECHT, H.: Beitrag zum Wasserhaushalt der Epileptiker. Diss. Hamburg 1938. — ALLAN, D., and W. A. SCHROEDER: A comparison of the phenylalanine content of the hemoglobine of normal and phenylketonuric individuals: determination by Ion Exchange Chromatography. J. clin. Invest. 36, 1343 (1957). — AMANTEA, G.: Sul diverso compartamento dei cani nei riguardi dell'epilessia sperimentale. Boll. Soc. ital. Biol. sper. 1, 1 (1926). — ANGEL, C., B. E. LEACH, S. MARTENS, M. COHEN and R. G. HEATH: Serum oxydation test in schizophrenic and normal subjects. Arch. Neurol. Psychiat. (Chicago) 78, 500—504 (1957). — ANGRISANI, D.: Il magnesia nel sangue di malati di mente. Osped. psychiat. 6, 91—97 (1938).

BAHNER, F., u. H. WIES: Papierchromatographie und Abwehrproteinnasennachweis. Biochem. Z. 321, 410—413 (1951). — BALBI, R.: L'Epilepsie. Act. Neur. Policlinico Napoli 1953. — BANG, O.: Klinische Urobilinstudien. Oslo 1926. — BARAK, A. J., F. L. HUMOLLER and J. D. STEVENS: Blood glutathione levels in the male schizophrenic patient. Arch. Neurol. Psychiat. (Chicago) 80, 237—240 (1958). — BATT, J. C., W. W. KAY, M. REISS and D. E. SANDS: The endocrine concomitants of schizophrenia. J. ment. Sci. 103, 240—256 (1957). — BENDA, P.: Perspectives humorales dans certains types de psychoses. Presse méd. 67, 1818—1821 (1951). — BERINGER, K.: Der Mescalinrausch. Berlin: Springer (1927). — BESSMANN, S. P., and A. N. BESSMANN: The cerebral and peripheral uptake of ammonia in liver disease with an hypothesis for the mechanism of hepatic coma. J. clin. Invest. 34, 622—628 (1955). — BETZ, K.: Periodische diencephale Gehemmtheitszustände mit anfallsweiser Blutdrucksteigerung. Arch. Psychiat. Nervenkr. 183, 664—675 (1950). — BINSWANGER, H.: Leberuntersuchungen bei Alkoholpsychosen, gleichzeitig ein Beitrag zur funktionellen Pathologie der Leber. Arch. Psychiat. Nervenkr. 100, 619—669 (1933). — BISCHOFF, A.: Über die Frage des erhöhten Kupferspiegels im Serum Schizophrener. Mschr. Psychiat. Neurol. 124, 211—222 (1952). — BLEULER, E.: Endokrinologische Psychiatrie. S. 498. Stuttgart: Gg. Thieme 1954. — BLOCK, W., u. K. BLOCK: Synthese von 14-C-radioaktivem Mescalin. Chem. Ber. 11, 1009—1012 (1952). — BOCHNIK, H. J.: Über Tagesschwankungen zentralnervöser und autonomer Funktionen. Acta med. scand. 145, Suppl. 278, 122—128 (1953). — BOCHNIK, H. J.: Sozialfaktoren in vieldimensionalen Strukturen mit Beispielen soziogenetischer Komplettierungen nach

Hirntraumen bei kindlichen Verhaltensstörungen und bei abnormen Persönlichkeiten. Nervenarzt **1962** (im Druck). — BOGOCH, S., K. T. DUSSIK and P. G. LEVER: Clinical status and cerebrospinal fluid „Total Neuraminic Acid". Arch. Gen. Psychiat. **1**, 441—449 (1959). — BOREK, E., A. BRECHER, G. A. JERVIS u. H. WAELSCH: Oligophrenia phenylpyruvica. Constancy of the metabolic error. Proc. Soc. exper. Biol. (N. Y.) **75**, 86 (1950). — BOSZORMENYI-NAGY, I., and F. J. GERTY: Difference between the phosphorus metabolism of erythrocytesm of normals and of patients suffering from schizophrenia. J. nerv. ment. Dis. **121**, 53—59 (1955). — BOVI, A., e A. MASCELLANI: Determinazione del tasso di rame serico negli schizofrenici. G. Psichiat. Neuropat. **86**, 163—173 (1958).   BREDZINA, E., u. W. SCHMIDT. Über Beziehungen zwischen der Witterung und dem Befinden des Menschen, aufgrund statistischer Erhebungen dargestellt. S.-B. Akad. Wiss. Wien, Math.-naturwiss. Kl. **123**, Abt. III 209. Wien 1914. — BROSER, F.: Periodische Bewußtseinsstorungen und paroxysmale Comata bei einem Falle von primärer Oligurie nach Hirntrauma. Arch. Psychiat. Z. Nervenkr.**187**,311—336 (1951). — BROWN, J. A. Liver-brain relationships. Springfield Ill. 1957. — BÜSSOW, H.: Über die Wirkung des Wasser-Tonephin-Versuches auf manisch-depressive Zustandsbilder. Arch. Psychiat. Nervenkr. **184**, 357—376 (1950). — BRUNNER, H.: Gezeitenamplitude und epileptischer Anfall. Dtsch. Arch. klin. Med. **120**, 206 (1916). — BUSCAINO, V. M.: Epilepsie und Epilepsien. Sci. med. ital. (Dtsch. Ausg.) **5**, 46—65 (1965); — Pathogénèse et Etiologie biologique de la Schizophrénie. Acta neurol. belg. **8**, H. 1 (1958). — BUSCAINO, G. A. e L. STEFANACHI: Contributo allo studio del metabolismo delle sostanze indoliche nelle malattie del sistema nervosa. V. Ricerche quantitative sull'eliminazione urinaria del l'ac-5-idrossi-indolacetico in condizioni di base e dopo carico con 5-idrossi-triptamina. Acta neurol. (Napoli) **13**, 156—178 (1958).

CLAUS, A., et O. v. D. STRICHT: Pathogénie et traitement de l'Epilepsie. Brüssel-Paris 1895. — CONRAD, K., K. DOMANOWSKY u. B. OTT: Prothrombinbestimmung bei der akuten Katatonie. Med. Klin. **44**, 673—677 (1954). — CONSBRUCH, U., u. CL. FAUST: Vergleichende Längsschnittbetrachtung der Serumeiweißverhältnisse bei exogenen traumatischen Psychosen und bei endogenen Psychosen unter der Behandlung mit Reserpin, Iminodibenzylderivat und Phenothiazinen. Arch. Psychiat. Nervenkr. **197**, 279—287 (1958). — CORI, G. T.: Biochemical aspects of glycogen deposition diseases. Problèmes actuels de Pédiatrie. Basel: Karger 1957. — CRAMMER, J. L.: Rapid weight-changes in mental patients. Lancet **273**, 259—262 (1957); — Water and sodium in two psychotics. Lancet **1959**, 1122—1126. — CUSWORTH, D. C., C. E. DENT and F. V. FLYNN: The amino-aciduria in galactosamid. Arch. Dis. Childh. **30**, 150—154 (1955).

DALTON, K.: Menstruation und acute Psychiatric Illness. Brit. med. J. **1**, 148—149 (1959). — DAVIDSON, W., W. S. LAWLER and A. H. ACKERLY: The Pelger-Huet anomaly; investigations of family A. Hum. Gen. **19**, 1 (1954). — DEGKWITZ, R.: Kreislaufveränderungen bei endogenen Psychosen. Klin. Wschr. **34**, 732—737 (1956).

EDERLE, W.: Zur Frage der Millon-Reaktion in der Modifikation von SANO und DECKER bei der Schizophrenie. Nervenarzt **28**, 131—132 (1957). — EICHHORN, O.: Über Störungen des Kationengleichgewichtes bei Psychosen. Wien. Z. Nervenheilk. **8**, 261—293 (1954). — ELLIOT, K. A. C.: Biochemical approaches in the study of epil. Electrencephalogr. clin. Neurophysiol. **1**, 29—31 (1949). — EMBDEN, G., M. CARSTENSEN u. H. SCHUMACHER: Über die Bedeutung der Adenylsäure für die Muskelfunktion; 4. Mitteilung: Spaltung und Wiederaufbau der ammoniakbildenden Substanz bei der Muskeltätigkeit. Z. physiol. Chem. **179**, 186—225 (1928).

FAUST D'ANDREA: A proposito delle reazioni agglutinanti sul siero de sangue di soggeti affetti da malattie mentali. Act. neurol. (Napoli) **4**, 663—666 (1949). — FEDOROFF, S.: Toxicity of schizophrenics blood serum in the tissue culture. J. Lab. clin. Med. **48**, 55—62 (1956). — FERRONI, A.: Curva cloremica da carico salino e ondovenoso in epilettici. Act. neurol. (Napoli) **3**, 39 (1947). — FETZNER, H. R.: Zur Stickstoffbilanz des Epileptikers. II. Int. Kongr. Psychiat. Zürich 1957, Congress Report, Vol. IV, S. 90. — FINKELMAN, I., and D. HAFFRON: Observations on the circulating blood volume in schizophrenia, manic-depressive psychosis, epilepsy, involutional psychosis and mental deficiency. Amer. J. Psychiat. **93**, 917—928 (1937). — FISCHER, R.: Schizophrenie, ein regressiver Adaptionsprezeß. Mschr. Psychiat. Neurol. **126**, 315—333 (1953). — FISCHLER, F.: Veränderungen der Leberfunktion als Voraussetzung von Störungen des Zentralnervensystems. Wandervers. d. Neur. u. Psych. Baden-Baden 1937. Arch. Psychiat. Nervenkr. **109**, 311 (1939). — FÖLLING, A.: Über Ausscheidung von Phenylbrenztraubensäure in den Harn als Stoffwechselanomalie in Verbindung mit Imbezillität. Z. physiol. Chem. **227**, 169—176 (1934). — FORD-ROBERTSON, W. M.: The pathogenesis of anaerobic microbic infections in the major and minor psychoses with control cases. J. ment. Sci. **78**, 12—95 (1932). — FORREST, A. D.: Indoluria in schizophrenia. II. Chromatographic study on 40 schizophrenics and 10 normal subjects. J. ment. Sci. **105**, 685—692 (1959). — FORSGREN, E.: Über Methoden, Ergebnisse und Ziele der Rhythmenforschung. Nord. med. Tidskr. **2**, 330—235 (1938). — FOURNIER, E.: Biologie de l'alcoolisme. Vie méd. **38**,

455—459 (1957). — Frank, M., and R. Wurtman: Some sources of error in the Akerfeld test for serum oxydative activity. Society 97, 78 (1958). — Frisch, F.: Das „Vegetative System" der Epileptiker. Monogr. a. d. Gesamtgebiet d. Neur. u. Psychiatr. Hrsg. v. O. Foerster u. K. Wilmans. H. 52. Berlin: J. Springer (1928). — Fröshaug, H.: Periodische Psychosen. II. Int. Kongr. Psychiat. Zürich 1957, Vol. IV, S. 89.

Gamper, E., u. A. Kral: Ergänzender Bericht zur Frage der biologischen Wirksamkeit des Schizophrenenliquors. Z. ges. Neurol. Psychiat. 153, 258—264 (1935). — Gamper, E., A. Kral u. R. Stein: Untersuchungen über die Wirkung von pathologischem Liquor cerebrospinalis bei Einbringung in die Vorderkammer des Kaninchenauges. Z. ges. Neurol. Psychiat. 141, 689—701 (1932). — Garrod, A. E.: The croonian lectures on inborn errors of metabolism. Lancet 1908, 142. — Gastager, H., O. Hornykiewicz u. H. Tschabitscher: Das Verhalten des Serumkupfers und der p-Polyphenoloxidaseaktivität bei klinischen und subklinischen Formen der hepatolentikulären Erkrankungen. Wien Z. Nervenheilk. 9, 312—319 (1954). — Gaupp, R.: Über pathologisch-anatomische Befunde bei akuten Katatonien und ihre Bedeutung für die Pathogenese der Schizophrenie. Z. ges. Neurol. Psychiat. 176, 255—264 (1943). — Geller, W.: Die Bedeutung der Menstruationsstörungen bei der akuten Schizophrenie. Ärztl. Forsch. 7, 14—22 (1953). — Georgi, F., u. H. Fischer in Bumke: Handbuch der Geisteskrankheiten. Berlin: Springer (1928) — Georgi, F., R. Fischer, R. Weber u. P. Weis: Schizophrenie und Leberstoffwechsel. V. Psychophysische Korrelation. Schweiz. med. Wschr. 78, 1194—1200 (1948). — Georgi, F., C. G. Honegger, D. Jordan, H. P. Rieder u. M. Rottenberg: Zur Physiologie und Pathophysiologie körpereigener Amine. Klin. Wschr. 34, 799—801 (1956). — Ghent, L., and A. M. Freedmann: Comparison of effects of normal and schizophrenic serum on motor performance in rats. Amer. J. Psychiat. 115, 465—466 (1958). — Gjessing, R.: Beiträge zur Kenntnis der Pathophysiologie des katatonen Stupors. Arch. Psychiat. Nervenkr. 96, 319—473 (1932); — Beiträge zur Kenntnis der Pathophysiologie der katatonen Erregung. Arch. Psychiat. Nervenkr. 104, 355—416 (1936); — Beiträge zur Kenntnis der Pathophysiologie periodisch katatoner Zustände. IV. Mitteilung: Versuch einer Ausgleichung der Funktionsstörungen. Arch. Psychiat. Nervenkr. 109, 525—595 (1939; — Beiträge zur Somatologie der periodischen Katatonie. V.—VIII. Mitteilung: Arch. Psychiat. Nervenkr. 191, 191—326 (1953); — Beiträge zur Somatologie der periodischen Katatonie. IX. Mitteilung: Die periodische Katatonie in der Literatur. Arch. Psychiat. Nervenkr. 200, 350—365 (1960); — Beiträge zur Somatologie der periodischen Katatonie. X. Mitteilung: Pathogenetische Erwägungen. Arch. Psychiat. Nervenkr. 200, 366—389 (1960). — Goldkuhl, E., V. Kafka u. A. Orström: Zur Biologie der Schizophrenie. Acta. psychiat. scand. Suppl. 4, 118—147 (1947). — Gottlieb, J. S., C. E. Frohmann, G. Tournay and P. G. S. Beckett: Energy transfer system in schizophrenia. Adenosinetriphosphate. Arch. Neurol. Psychiat. (Chicago) 81, 504—508 (1959). — Graves, T. C.: Chronic sepsis and mental disorder. J. ment. Sci. 73, 563—566 (1927). — Grewel, F.: Das Syndrom von Kleine-Lewin: Schlafperioden mit Hunger. Ned. T. Geneesk. 91, 2894—2898 (1947). — Grodzicki, W. D.: Über die Perodizität des epileptischen Krampfanfallgeschehens. Psychiat. Neurol. med. Psychol. 2, 135—138 (1950). — Grosch, H.: Krankheitsbilder mit pathologischen Rhythmen des Zwischenhirns. Dtsch. med. Wschr. 73, 560—562 (1948). — Periodische Umdämmerung von vierwöchentlichem Rhythmus in der Pubertät. Dtsch. Z. Nervenheilk. 160, 105—115 (1949). — Gubler, C. J., H. Brown, H. Markowitz, G. E. Cartwight and M. Wintrobe: Studies on copper metabolism. XXIII. Portal (Laennecs) cirrhosis of the liver. J. clin. Invest. 36, 1208 (1957).

Haavaldsen, R., O. Lingjaerde and O. Walaas: Disturbances of carbohydrate metabolism in schizophrenics. Conf. neurol. (Basel) 18, 270—280 (1958). — Halbey, K.: Einflusse meteorologischer Erscheinungen auf epileptische Kranke. Allg. Z. Psychiat. 67, 252 (1910). — Haries, A.: The treatment of depression by dinitrile succinate. J. ment. Sci. 97, 209—213 (1951). — Harrison, H. E., L. Finberg and E. Fleishman: Disturbances of ionic equilibrium of intracellular and extracellular electrolytes in patients with tuberculos meningitis. J. clin. Inv. 31, 300—308 (1952). — Hartelius, H.: Further experiences in the use of malononitrile in the treatment of mental illnesses. Amer. J. Psychiat. 107, 95—101 (1950). — Haury, V. G., and A. D. Hirschfelder: Variations in magnesium and potassium associated with essential epilepsy. Arch. Neurol. (Chic.) 40, 66—78 (1938). — Haverkamp, Begemann, N., u. A. v. Lookeren, Campagne: Homozygous form of Pelger-Huets nuclear anomaly in man. Acta haemat. (Basel) 7, 295 (1952). — Heath, R. G., S. Martens, B. E. Leach, M. Cohen and C. A. Feigl: Behavioral changes in nonpsychotic volunteers following the administration of Taraxein, the substance obtained from serum of schizophrenic patients. 113 annual meeting of The Amer. Psych. Assoc., May 1957. — Heilmeyer, L., L. Keiderling u. B. Stüwe: Kupfer und Eisen als körpereigene Wirkstoffe. Jena: G. Fischer 1941. — Henry, G. W.: Gastrointestinal motor functions in the manic depressive psychoses. Amer. J. Psychiat. 9, H. 1 (1939). — Hicks, S. P.: Brain metabolism in vivo. Arch. Path. (Chicago) 49, 111—137 (1950).— Hierons, R.: Changes in the nervous system in acute porphyria. Brain 80, 176—192 (1957). — Hodskins, M. B., R. Guthrie u. J. Naurison: Studies on the blood volume of epileptics.

Amer. J. Psychiat. 11, 623—646 (1932). — HOFF, F.: Klinische Physiologie und Pathologie. 5. Aufl. S. 1120. Stuttgart: Gg. Thieme 1957. — HOFFER, A., H. OSMOND and J. SMYTHIES: Schizophrenia: a new approach. II. Result of year's research. J. ment. Sci. 100, 29—45 (1954). — HOFFSTEDT, E.: Die Organneurose im Lichte neuerer Anschauungen. Berl. klin. H. 388, 1—26 (1928). — HOHEISEL, H. P., u. R. WALCH: Über manisch-depressive und verwandte Verstimmungszustände nach Hirnverletzung. Arch. Psychiat. Nervenkr. 188, 1—25 (1952). — HOLMBERG, C. G., and C. B. LAURELL: Oxidase reactions in human plasma caused by coeruloplasmin. Scand. J. clin. Lab. Invest. 3, 103—107 (1951). — HOLMGREN, H.: Studien über 24-stundenrhythmische Variationen des Darm-, Lungen- und Leberfetts. Acta med. scand. Suppl. 74 (1936). — HÜHNERFELD, J.: Über den Einfluß von Porphyrinen auf Resorption und Entfärbung von Methylenblauquaddeln. Klin. Wschr. 24, 433—434 (1947). — HUNTER, W.: Oral or focal infection. London: Cassell u. Co., 1910. — HYDEN, H., and H. HARTELIUS: Stimulation of nucleoprotein production in the nerve cells by malononitrile and its effect on psychic functions in mental disorders. Acta. psychiat. scand. Suppl. 48, 1—117 (1948).

JAHN, D.: Die Somatopathologie der endogenen Psychosen. Arch. Psychiat. Nervenkr. 109, 304—306 (1939). — JAHN, D., u. H. GREVING: Untersuchung über die körperlichen Störungen bei katatonen Stuporen und der tödlichen Katatonie. Arch. Psychiat. Nervenkr. 105, 105—120 (1936). — JAKAB, I., et M. PANCZÉL: Contributions à la pathomorphologie et pathochimie de la maladie de Wilson-Westphal-Strümpell. Acta med. Acad. Sci. hung. 3, 341—346 (1952). — JERVIS, G. A.: Biochemical aspects of certain forms of mental deficiency. Dis. nerv. Syst. 18, Suppl. 93—95 (1957). — JONG, H. DE: Die experimentelle Katatonie als vielfach vorkommende Reaktionsform des Zentralnervensystems. Z. ges. Neurol. Psychiat. 139, 468—499 (1932). — JONXIS, J. H. P.: Oligophrenia phenylpyruvica en de hartnupziekte. Ned. F. Geneesk. 101, 569—574 (1957). — JUSTSCHENKO, A.: Das Wesen der Geisteskrankheiten. Leipzig: Steinkopf, 1914.

KANIG, K., u. M. KLUDAS: Indikanurie und Darmflora bei psychiatrisch-neurologischen Erkrankungen. Psychiat. et Neurol. (Basel) 136, 408—417 (1958). — KAPS, G.: Über die Flockungsreaktion mit Hayemscher Lösung (Grossche Reaktion) und die Salzsäure-Collargol-Reaktion (SCR-RIEBELING) im Blutserum kranker Menschen. Diss. Hamburg 1952; — Über elektrophoretische Untersuchungen an Hirngewebe insbesondere aus der Umgebung von Tumoren. Zugleich ein Beitrag zur Pathogenese von Hirnschwellung und Hirnödem. Arch. Psychiat. Nervenkr. 192, 115—129 (1954). — KARSTENS, P.: Über die Beeinflussung des psychischen Zustandes Normaler durch Aufnahme und Retention unphysiologisch großer Wassermengen. Arch. Psychiat. Nervenkr. 186, 231—237 (1951). — KAUFMANN, S.: Soluble ketoglutaric dehydrogenase from heart muscle and coupled phosphorylation. Phosphorus metabolism. Herausgegeb. v. W. D. McElroy a. B. Glass, Bd. I, 370. Baltimore 1951. — KEMALI, D., L. SORRENTINO e L. SALLUSTRO: Indagini chimiche e biologiche sul metabolismo dei soggetti schizofrenici. I. Ricerche cromatografiche e tossicologiche. Acta neur. (Napoli) 14, 641—664 (1959). — KERPEL-FRONIUS, E.: Hormonal influences on salt and water economy in water deprivation. Z. Vitamin-, Hormon- u. Fermentforsch. 4, 149—161 (1951). — KLEIN, E.: Über den heutigen Stand der Schilddrüsendiagnostik. Ärztl. Forsch. 5, 537—546 (1951); — KLEINSORGE, H.: Phosphaturie und Persönlichkeit. Z. Psychother. 1, 205—214 (1951). — KLENK, E.: Lipoidosen. Hoppe-Seyler Z. physiol. Chem. 229, 151 (1934). — KLINGMÜLLER, V.: Biochemie, Physiologie und Klinik der Glutaminsäure. Aulendorf, Cantor K. G. 1955. — KLOPP, H. W., u. H. SELBACH: Über die Gültigkeit der Ausgangswertregel beim Epileptiker. Dtsch. Z. Nervenheilk. 167, 130—142 (1951). — KLUGE, E.: Klinische und pathologisch-anatomische Befunde bei hyperkinetischen Psychosen. Z. ges. Neurol. Psychiat. 176, 423—433 (1943); — Über psychotische Störungen bei Erschopfung. Psychiat. Neurol. med. Psychol. 3, 10—15 (1951). — KNAUS, H.: Menstrueller Zyklus und Psychosen. Schweiz. Arch. Neurol. Psychiat. 64, 264—281 (1949). — KOSAKA, M.: A study on schizophrenia. I. Respiration and glycolysis of erythrocytes in schizophrenia. Folia psychiat. neurol. jap. 7, 17—29 (1953); — II. On the blood gas in schizophrenia. Folia psychiat. neurol. jap. 7, 30—61 (1953). — KORANYI, E. K., u. H. E. LEHMANN: Experimental sleep deprivation in schizophrenic patients. Arch. of Psychiat., Chicago 2, 534—544 (1960). — KRAL, A., and H. E. LEHMANN: Further studies on the iron content of the cerebrospinal fluid in psychoses. Arch. Neurol. Psychiat. (Chicago) 68, 321—328 (1952). — KRETH, G.: Untersuchung des Kupferspiegels im Serum und Liquor cerebrospinalis bei Psychosen. Diss. Hamburg 1954. — KRETSCHMER, E.: Körperbau und Charakter. Berlin-Göttingen-Heidelberg- Springer-Verlag 1955. — KRYSPIN-EXNER, W.: Beiträge zum Verlauf des Körpergewichts bei Psychosen. Wien. klin. Wschr. 59, 531—534 (1947). — KUPPERS, E.: Puls, Blutdruck, vasomotorische Störungen. Blutverteilung. In: Handbuch der Geisteskrankheiten von O. BUMKE, 3, 130—153. Berlin: Springer-Verlag 1928.

LAMY, M., et R. DU DEBRÉ: Maladies héréditaires du Métabolisme chez l'Enfant. Paris 1959. — LANG, K.: Die phenylpyruvische Oligophrenie. Ergebn. inn. Med. Kinderheilk. 6, 78 (1955). — LANG, K., K. KROPP u. CH. WEBER: Behandlung der phenylpyruvischen

Oligophrenie. Z. Kinderheilk. 80, 311—324 (1957). — LANGE, C.: Periodische Depressionszustände und ihre Pathogenesis auf dem Boden der harnsauren Diathesen. S. 56. Hamburg Leipzig: Leopold Voss 1896. — LENZ, H.: Beitrag zum Mineralstoffwechsel akuter Psychosen. Klin. Wschr. 20, 785—787 (1941). — LEYTON, G. B.: Indolic compounds in the urine of schizophrenics. Brit. med. J. 1136—1139 (1958). — LINGJAERDE, O.: Beiträge zur somatologischen Schizophrenieforschung. Bedeutung des Kohlehydratdefizits. Arch. Psychiat. Nervenkr. 191, 114—133 (1953). — LINGJAERDE, O., C. L. LAANE u. H. STROM: Das Blutdruckverhalten in den verschiedenen Lebensaltern bei Schizophrenen. Zbl. ges. Neurol. Psychiat. 111, 266 (1950). — LJUNGBERG, E.: The glutathione content of the blood in schizophrenia. Acta psychiat. scand. 13, 369, 377 (1932).— LOMER, G.: Über Witterungseinflüsse bei 20 Epileptischen. Arch. Psychiat. Nervenkr. 42, 1061 (1907). — LONGO, V.: Epilessia sperimentale e ghiandole endocrine. I. und II. Boll. Soc. med.-chir. Catania 3, 465 u. 506 (1935). — LÜHRS, E.: Versuche zum Nachweis toxisch wirkender Substanzen im Liquor von organischen Hirnkrankheiten. Diss. Hamburg (1958).

MAACK, U.: Über die Wirkung der intravenösen Kochsalzbelastung bei Psychosen, insbesondere bei Epileptikern. Diss. Hamburg 1951. — MADER, A., u. E. BINGENHEIMER: Die Röntgenbestrahlung des Mongolismus und ihr Einfluß auf den Blutcholesterinspiegel. J. Kinderkrankh. 138, 9 (1933). — MAINTZ, E. (geb. LÜHRS): Versuche zum Nachweis toxisch wirkender Substanzen im Liquor von organischen Hirnkrankheiten. Diss. Hamburg 1958. — MALL, G.: Beitrag zur Gjessingschen Thyroxinbehandlung der periodischen Katatonien. Arch. Psychiat. Nervenkr. 187, 381—403 (1952). — MALLYOTH, G., K. SCHEPPE u. H. W. STEIN: Fructosurie, Pentosurie, Mannosurie. Klin. Wschr. 30, 1018—1020 (1952). — MARIANI, G.: Ricerca della proteina reactiva C nel liquor di ammalati psichici. Neopsichiatria 23, 167—178 (1957). — MASTROGIOVANNI, P. D.: Pathophysiologische Aspekte bei Psychosen. II. Int. Kongr. f. Psychiat., Zürich 1957, Congress Report, S. 96. — MAYER-GROSS, W.: Clinical Psychiatry. London: Cassel u. Co. 1961. — MC DERMOTT, W. V. jr., and R. D. ADAMS: Episodic stupor associated with an Eck fistula in the human with particular reference to the metabolism of ammonia. J. clin. Invest. 33, 1—9 (1954). — MC KINNON, I. H. HOCH, P. H. KAMMER and H. D. WEALSCH: The use of malonitrile in the treatment of mental illness. Amer. J. Psychiat. 105, 686 (1948). — MENDELSOHN, J., D. WEXLER, P. KUBZANSKY, P. LEIDERMAN and P. SALOMON: Serum magnesium in delirium tremens and alcoholic halluzinosis. J. nerv. ment. Dis. 128, 352—357 (1959). — MENZI, W.: Pathogenetische Untersuchungen über das Delirium tremens. Diss. Bern 1955. — MERTENS, R.: Über die bei akuter Porphyrie auftretenden Porphyrine. Z. physiol. Chem. 250, 57—59 (1937). — MEYER, A., and M. MEYER: Nucleoprotein in the nerve cells of mental patients; a critical remark. J. ment. Sci. 95, 180—181 (1949). — MITTRACH, R.: Beitrag zur Hämatologie der endogenen Psychosen. Diss. Hamburg 1953. — MORITZ, D. v., u. M. KULCSÁR: Beiträge zur Pathologie der tuberkulösen Meningitis. Orv. Hetil. 344—345 (1936). — MORRIS, G. O., H. L. WILLIAMS and A. LUBIN: Misperception and disorientation during sleep deprivation. Arch. of Psychiat. Chicago, 2, 247—254 (1960). — MUNCH-PETERSEN, S.: On serum copper in patients with schizophrenia. Acta psychiat. scand. 25, 423—427 (1950). MUNKVAD, I.: Determinations of glutamine and glutamic acid in a material of mental patients. Acta psychiat. scand. 25, 269—274 (1950).

NEUBERGER, M., C. RIMINGTON and J. M. WILSON: Studies on alkaptonuria, 2. Investigations on a case of human alkaptonuria. Biochem. J. 41, 438 (1947). — NEUBURGER, H.: Gehirnveränderung d. Alkoholmißbr. Zblt. Neurol. 135, 159 (1931). — NOELL, W.: Hirnelektr. Untersuchungen über die Blausäurewirkung im Vergleich zur Hypoxämie. Arch. Psychiat. Nervenkr. 181, 1—20 (1948).

OEZEK, M.: Blutgerinnungsphysiologische Untersuchungen bei Psychosen. I. Prothrombinkomplex, Gerinnungs- und Blutungszeitbestimmung im schizophrenen Formenkreis. Arch. Psychiat. Nervenkr. 193, 630—639 (1955); — II. Bestimmung der Blutgerinnungsfaktoren bei Schizophrenen. Arch. Psychiat. Nervenkr. 193, 640—644 (1955); — Untersuchungen über den Kupferstoffwechsel im schizophrenen Formenkreis. Arch. Psychiat. Nervenkr. 195, 408—423 (1957). — OLSEN, N. S., and I. R. KLEIN: Effect of cyanide on the concentration of lactate and phosphates in brain. J. biol. Chem. 167, 739—756 (1947). — OPPENHEIM, H.: Die ersten Zeichen der Nervosität des Kindesalters. Berlin: Karger 1904.

PARIN, P.: Über abnorme Ernährungszustände bei Schizophrenen. Schweiz. Arch. Neurol. Psychiat. 72, 231—243 (1953). — PENROSE, L. S.: Inheritance of phenylpyruvic amentia. Lancet 229, II, 192—194 (1935). — PENTA, P., e G. PARENTE: Alterazioni respiratorie nella depressione malinconica. Ann. Neurophysiol. 4, 210—225 (1957). — PETERSEN, W.: The patient and the weather. Ann. Arbor. Michigan: Eduards bothers Tac. (1934). — PETERSON, J.: Study of a case of cycle affective disorder with forty-eight hour cycle. J. nerv. Dis. 105, 84 (1947). — PICKWORTH, F. A.: Die Beziehungen von Erkrankungen der Nebenhöhlen zu Geisteskrankheiten. Z. Neurol. 141, 420—459 (1932). — PIEPER, J., u. R. FABER: Quick-Test bei Schizophrenie. Klin. Wschr. 31, 157—158 (1953). — PINCUS, G., and H. HOAGLAND: Adrenal cortical responses to stress in normal men and in those with personality disorders. I.

Some stress responses in normal and psychotic subjects. Amer. J. Psychiat. **106**, 641—650 (1950). — PLATANIA, S.: Etiologia dell'amenza e della demenza precoce. Nota 5. Nuovo contributo di ricerche sierodiagnostiche de agglutinazione e primi saggi sul liquor. Osped. psichiat. **9**, 179—200 (1941). — POHLE, K.: Über das Vorkommen von Adenylsäure im Gehirn. Z. physiol. Chem. **185**, 281—283 (1929). — PORTER, H. A., and J. FOLCH: Brain Copper-Protein fractions in the normal and in WILSON's disease. Arch. Neurol. Psychiat. (Chicago) **77**, 8—16 (1957). — POST, F.: Body weight in psychiatric illness. A critical survey of the literature. J. psychosomat. Res. **1**, 219—226 (1957).

RANGE, T.: Über die Erniedrigung der Senkungsgeschwindigkeit der Erythrocyten bei Neurotikern und Psychopathen. Dtsch. Z. Nervenheilk. **131**, 198—204 (1933). — REHM, O.: Über Körpergewicht und Menstruation bei akuten und chronischen Psychosen. Arch. Psychiat. Nervenkr. **61**, 385—420 (1929). — REICH, R.: Über die Beziehung zwischen Epilepsie und meteorologischen Faktoren. Allg. Z. Psychiat. **60**, 493 (1905). — REIMANN, H. A., and C.T. DE BERNADINIS: Periodische (cyclische) Neutropenie, Krankheitsübersicht über 16 Falle. Blood **4**, 1109 (1949). — REINBOLD, A.: Verwirrtheitszustände nach einer portocavalen Shuntoperation. Dtsch. med. Wschr. **81**, 1605—1610 (1956). — REITER, P.: Gastrointestinale Störungen, ihre klinische und ätiologische Bedeutung. Roskilde (Dänemark) 1927. — RHEIN, M., et R. STOE-BER: Conseration des urines conténant de l'acide phenylpyruvique. C. R. Soc. Biol. (Paris) **3**, 807 Paris (1936). — RICHTER, C. P., W. M. HONEYMAN and H. HUNTER: Behavior and mood cycles apparently related to parathyroid deficiency. J. Neurol. Psychiat. **3**, 19—25 (1940). — RICHTER, D.: Schizophrenie. Somatische Gesichtspunkte. Hamburg 1957. — RICHTER, D., and R. M. C. DAWSON: Brain lactate in emotion. J. Amer. med. Ass. **136**, 866 (1948). — RIEBELING, C.: Über das Vorkommen von präformiertem Ammoniak im Liquor cerebrospinalis. Z. ges. Neurol. Psychiat. **128**, 475—477 (1930); — Über Ammoniakbefunde im Gehirn und ihre Bedeutung. Klin. Wschr. **10**, 554 (1931); — Über Psychosen bei Niereninsuffizienz mit Bemerkungen über das Verhalten des Liquors bei diesen Zuständen. Mschr. Psychiat. Neurol. **83**, 39—56 (1932); — Über Ammoniakbestimmung im Blut. Zugleich Bemerkungen zu der Arbeit von HEINZ FULD. Klin. Wschr. **12**, 1572 (1933); — Über Adenylsäure im Zentralnervensystem. Klin. Wschr. **13**, 1422—1424 (1934); — Der Ammoniakgehalt des Blutes, des Liquors und des Gehirns bei Psychosen und seine Bedeutung. Z. ges. Neurol. Psychiat. **157**, 418—448 (1937); — Betrachtungen zum Wesen des Anfalles. Med. Klin. **36**, 1207—1209 (1940); — Chemische Befunde am Hirn und Liquor der Schizophrenen. Wandervers. der Psychiater u. Neurologen Baden-Baden 1937; — Eine chemische Untersuchung der Hirnschwellung. Z. ges. Neurol. Psychiat. **166**, 149—177 (1939). — Das Problem der Hirnschwellung. Dtsch. med. Wschr. **62**, 1440—1442 (1937); — Bemerkungen zur Liquordiagnostik und -prognostik der tuberkulosen Meningitis. Ann. Neurol. **7**, 372 (1951); — Hämatologische Beobachtungen bei Psychosen. Fortschr. Neurol. Psychiat. **20**, 237—246 (1952); — Kupfer als Fällungsreagenz für stickstoffhaltige Bestandteile des Serums und seine Anwendung für eine neuartige Reaktion. Colloquium St. Jans Hospital Brügge 1955; — Methodik zweier Reaktionen zwischen Serum und Kupferchloridlösungen und Bemerkungen zu diesen Reaktionen. Ärztl. Lab. **3**, 197—200 (1957); — Bemerkungen zur Biochemie von Psychosen. Confin. neurol. (Basel) **18**, 205—210 (1958); — Hirnschwellung und Leberschwellung bei Psychosen; — Pathophysiologie der Psychosen. Fortschr. Neurol. Psychiat. **13**, 436—454 (1941); **15**, 86—98 (1943); **18**, 403—437 (1950); **19**, 452—484 (1951); **22**, 181—213 (1954); **25**, 579—623 (1957); **27**, 427—468 (1959). — RIEBELING, C., R. STRÖMME u. W. LEHNHARDT: Studien zur Pathophysiologie der Schizophrenie. Z. ges. Neurol. Psychiat. **147**, 61—72 (1933). — RIEDER, H. P.: Über Gasstoffwechselversuche an Mikroorganismen mit Körperflüssigkeiten Stammhirnaffizierter. Schweiz. Arch. Neurol. Psychiat. **72**, 387—393 (1953); — Biologische Toxizitätsbestimmung in pathologischen Körperflüssigkeiten. Conf. Neurol. (Basel) **14**, 65—87 (1954). — RISSL, E., N. STEFENELLI u. F. WEWALKA: Über den Ammoniakgehalt des Blutes bei Leberkrankheiten. Wien. klin. Wschr. **69**, 172—174 (1957). — ROBINSON, S. C., and M. BRUCER: Range of normal blood pressure. Arch. int. Med. **64**, 409—444 (1939). — RÖSCH, H., u. W. TE KAMP: Über Ammoniakbildung bei der Belichtung der Netzhaut. Z. physiol. Chem. **185**, 281 (1929). — ROESSLE, R.: Maß und Zahl in der Pathologie. Berlin: Springer 1932. — ROWNTREE, D., and W. W. KAY: Clinical biochemical and physiological studies in cases of recurrent schizophrenia. J. ment. Sci. **98**, 100—121 (1952). — RUDDER, B. DE: Grundriß einer Meteorobiologie des Menschen. 3. Aufl. Berlin: Springer 1952.

SANDS, D. E., G. H. A. CHAMBERLAIN: Treatment of inadequate personality in juveniles by dehydroisoandrosterone. Brit. Med. J. 4775, 66—68 (1952). — SANO, I.: Die Bedeutung von Indolderivaten in der Pathogenese-Forschung der endogenen Psychosen. II. Int. Kongr. f. Psychiatrie, Congress Report IV, S. 93. Zürich 1957. — SCHEID, K. F.: Febrile Episoden bei schizophrenen Psychosen. S. 97. Leipzig: Thieme 1937. — SCHEIDEGGER, S.: Liver-tissue changes in schizophrenia. Brief critical note. J. Neuropath. exp. Neurol. **12**, 397—399 (1953).— SCHETTLER, R. G.: Lipoidosen. Handbuch inn. Med. VII, 2, 236. Berlin-Gottingen-Heidelberg: Springer 1955. — SCHMIDT, C.: Pathophysiologische Forschung in ihrer Bedeutung für die Psychiatrische Klinik. Erb- und Konstitutionslehre. Leipzig: Thime 1942. — SCHMIDT, P. R.: Neurologische und psychische Störungen bei Porphyrinkrankheiten. Fortschr. Neurol. Psychiat. 20, H. 9 (1952). — SCHNEIDER, H.: Die Psychopathologie des 5-Hydroxytryptamin-(Serotonin)-Stoffwechsels. Schweiz. Archiv. Neur. 81, 344 (1958). — SCHÖN, H. J.: Über die Beeinflussung des NaCl-Spiegels im Blutserum durch Elektroschock und Anoxie. Diss. Hamburg 1952. — SCHÖN, M. L.: Serumkupferbestimmungen bei Syphilis, Alkoholismus und im Senium. Diss. Hamburg 1955.—SCHREIER, K.: Die nichtdiabetischen Melliturien. Ergebn. inn. Med. N. F. 12, 493—562 (1959). — SCHWARZ, H., u. H. DIEBOLD: Über den Ammoniakgehalt und die Ammoniakbildung des Gehirns. Klin. Wschr. 10, 553—554 (1931). — SCHWARZENBACH, F. H.: Die Reaktion von Körperflüssigkeiten Schizophrener im Sporenkeimungstest. II. Int. Kongr. f. Psychiatrie, Congress Report IV, S. 94 Zürich 1957. — SELBACH, H.: Grundregeln der vegetativen Dynamik. Arch. Ohr-, Nas.- u. Kehlk.-Heilk. 163, 250—253 (1953). — SELIGSON, D., and K. HIRAHARA: The measurement of ammonia in whole blood, Erythrocytes and Plasma. J. Lab. clin. Med. 49, 962—974 (1957). — SELYE, H.: Einführung in die Lehre vom Adaptionssyndrom. Stuttgart: Thieme 1953. — SHERLOCK, S.: Altered consciousness in liver failure (hepatic coma and precoma). I. I. Kongr. Int. Sci., Neurol. 2, 115—133 (1957). — SIMON, A., CH. LUDWIG, J. W. GOFMAN and G. H. CROOK: Metabolic studies in mongolism. Amer. J. Psychiat. 111, 139—145 (1954). — SMITH, H., and J. SINES: Demonstration of a peculiar odor in the sweat of schizophrenic patients. Arch. Gen. Psychiat. 2, 184—188 (1960). — SOLMS, H.: Chemische Struktur und Psychose bei Lysergsäure-Derivaten. Praxis 45, 746—749 (1956). — SPIEGELBERG, U.: Über Beziehungen endogener Psychosen zu körperlichen Krankheiten. Fortschr. Neurol. Psychiat. 23, 221—248 (1955). — SPEIJER, N.: Influencing of a periodical psychosis ("Degenerationspsychose") in connection with haematologic and bio-chemical alterations. Mschr. Psychiat. Neurol. 118, 69—76 (1949). — STÄUBLI-FRÖHLICH, M.: Probleme der Anorexia nervosa. Schweiz. med. Wschr. 83, 811—817 u. 837—841 (1953). — STAUDER, H. K.: Anfall, Schlaf, Periodizität. Nervenarzt 19, 107—119 (1948). — STEGER, J., u. R. STEGER: Die Störungen des Kupfer- und Aminosäuren-Stoffwechsels bei der hepatocerebralen Degeneration und deren Behandlung mit BAL. Dtsch. Z. Nervenheilk. 172, 321—351 (1954). — STERN, J. A. G. A. ULETT and K. SMITH: Effect of blood plasma from psychotic patients upon activity levels of white rats. Arch.Gen. Psychiat. 1, 342—345 (1959).—STETTEN, J. R., u. M. R. STETTEN: Glycogen metabolism. Physiol. Rev. 40, 505—537 (1960). — STICH, W.: Porphyrismus und akute Porphyrie. J. W. Bergmann München (1954). — STOCKERT, F. G. v.: Pathophysiologie einer im 48-Stunden-Rhythmus verlaufenden periodischen Katatonie. Confin. neurol. (Basel) 18, 183—188 (1958). — STÖSSEL, K.: Die Behandlung der Katatonie mit großen Wassergaben, zugleich ein Beitrag zur Theorie der Hirnschwellung. Arch. Psychiat. Nervenkr. 114, 699—759 (1942). — STOKES, I. B., A. B. BECK, D. H. CURNOW, J. G. TOPLISS and E. G. AINT: Aspects of copper metabolism in WILSON's disease. Ann. med. Aust. 4, 36 (1955). — STOLL, W. A.: Wirkung eines Mutterkornstoffes in ungewöhnlich schwacher Dosierung. Schweiz. med. Wschr. 79, 110 (1949); Die Psychiatrie des Morbus Addison. S. 143. Stuttgart: Thieme 1953; Vortrag Südwestdeutscher Neurologenkongreß, Baden-Baden 1956; Lysergsäure-diäthylamid, ein Phantastikum aus der Mutterkorngruppe. Schweiz. Arch. Neurol. Psychiat. 60, 279 (1947). — STOLL, W. A., and A. HOFMANN: Alkaloids of the Ergotoxinegroups. Helvet. Chim. Acta 26, 1570—1601 (1945). — STROBEL, TH.: Über den Trockensubstanzgehalt verschiedener Hirnteile. Z. ges. Neurol. Psychiat. 166, 161—169 (1939). — SUMMERSKILL, W. H. J., ST. J. WOLFE and CH. S. DAVIDSON: The metabolism of ammonia and alpha-keto-acides in liver disease and hepatic koma. J. clin. Invest. 36, 361—372 (1957). — SZARA, S., J. AXELROT and S. PERLIN: Is Adrenochrome present in the blood? Amer. J. Psychiat. 115, 162—163 (1958).

TERBRÜGGEN, A.: Über Einschlußkörperchen in Vacuolen der menschlichen Leberzellen. Virchows Arch. path. Anat. 299, 775—785 (1937). — THANNHAUSER, S. J.: Lehrbuch des Stoffwechsels und der Stoffwechselkrankheiten. S. 1040. 2. Aufl. Stuttgart: Thieme 1957. — THOLUCK, H. J.: Selbstmord und Wetter. Beitr. gerichtl. Med. 16, 121 (1942). — TÖBEL, F.: Beitrag zur Frage der Störungen des Kohlenhydratstoffwechsels bei der Hepatolenticulären Degeneration. Schweiz. Arch. Neurol. Psychiat. 63, 328 (1949). — TREUHEIT, A.: Epileptischer Anfall und Wassereinfluß. Nervenarzt 24, 90—96 (1953). — TROLLE, G.: Investigations into the rhodanide excretion in manic-depressive patients (depr. phase). Acta psychiat. scand. Suppl. 47, 156 (1947).

UDENFRIEND, S., and J. R. COOPER: The encymatic conversion of phenylalanine to tyrosine. J. biol. Chem. 194, 503 (1952). — The chemical estimation of tyrosine and tyramine. J. biol. Chem. 196, 227 (1952). — UZMAN, L., and D. DENNY-BROWN: Amino-aciduria in hepatolenticular degeneration (WILSON's disease). Amer. J. med. Sci. 215, 599—611 (1948).

VÖGTLIN, W. L., W. R. BROZ and M. H. MOSS: Liver function in chronic alkoholic patients. I. The incidence of liver disease as indicated by laboratory methods and suggested screening procedure. Gastroenterology 12, 184—198 (1949). — VRBA, R.: On the participation of ammonia in cerebral metabolism and function. Ref. Zbl. Neurol. 144, 183 (1957).

WADA, J., and W. C. GIBSON: Behavioral and EEG-Changes induced by injections of schizophrenic Extract. Arch Neurol. Psychiat. **81**, 747—764 (1959). — WALDENSTRÖM, J.: The porphyrias as inborn errors of metabolism. Amer. J. med. **22**, 758—773 (1957). — WALLEN-FELS, K.: Über die Anwendung der Papierchromatographie auf Probleme der Klinik. Ärztl. Forsch. **5**, 430 (1951). — WEBER, R.: Ein Weg zur Isolierung basischer Fraktionen. Naturwissenschaften **137**, 397 (1950). — WEIL-MALHERBE, H.: Der Energiestoffwechsel des Nervengewebes und sein Zusammenhang mit der Funktion. Kolloqu. d. Gesellsch. f. physiol. Chem., Mosbach 1952. Berlin-Göttingen-Heidelberg: Springer-Verlag 1952. — WEIL-MALHERBE, H.: L'ammoniaque dans le métabolisme cérébral. Schweiz. med. Wschr **86**. 1223—1227 (1956). — WEINLAND, G., u. W. L. WEINLAND: Zum Verhalten der Blutgerinnung bei Epilepsie. Dtsch. Z. Nervenheilk. **161**, 8—16 (1949). — Über den Einfluß von Acetylcholin und Histamin auf die Blutgerinnung. Dtsch. Z. Nervenheilk. **163**, 125—130 (1949). — WEINLAND, W. L.: Über den Wasserhaushalt bei Epilepsie. Arch. Psychiat. Nervenkr. **183**, 402—417 (1949). — WEINLAND, G.: Zum Verhalten des Kalium und Calcium im Blutserum bei Epilepsie. Arch. Psychiat. Nervenkr. **183**, 731—738 (1950). — WEINLAND, W. L., u. G. WENDTLAND: Zum Verhalten des Blutammoniaks bei Epilepsie. Z. klin. Med. **146**, 155—163 (1950). — WELSH, J. H., and A. C. McCLOY: Actions of d-lysergic acid diethylamide, and its 2-brom derivative on heart of Venus Mercenaria. Science **125**, 348 (1957). — WELTI, W.: Delirium with low serum sodium. Arch. Neurol. Psychiat. Chicago **76**, 559—564 (1956). — WENDT, G. G.: Untersuchungen an den Nebennieren von genuinen Epileptikern unter besonderer Berücksichtigung des Cholesteringehaltes. Arch. Psychiat. Nervenkr. **183**, 418—422 (1949). — WESTALL, R. G., J. DANCIS, and S. MILLER: Maple sugar urine disease. Amer. J. Dis. Child. **94**, 571—572 (1957). — WHITE, L. P., E. A. PHEAR, W. H. SUMMERSKILL and S. SHERLOCK: Ammonium tolerance in liver disease: Observations based on the catheterization of the hepatic veins. J. clin. Invest. **34**, 158—168 (1959). — WINTER, C. A., and L. FLATAKER: Effect of blood plasma from psychotic patients upon performance of trained rats. Arch. Neurol. Psychiat. (Chicago) **80**, 441—449 (1958). — WITT, P. N.: Die Wirkung von Substanzen auf den Netzbau der Spinne als biologischer Test. S. 79. Berlin-Göttingen-Heidelberg: Springer 1956. — WOLF, H., D. ZSCHOCKE, F. W. WEDEMEYER u. H. HÜBNER: Angeborene hereditäre Fructose-Intoleranz. Klin. Wschr. **37**, 693—696 (1959). — WOERMANN, H.: Über das Verhalten der eosinophilen Zellen bei schizophrenen Prozeßpsychosen. Diss. Hamburg 1943. — WUHRMANN, F.: Vegetatives Nervensystem und Bluteiweiße. Fortschr. Med. **72**, 533—534 (1954). — WUTH, O.: Körpergewicht, Endokrines System, Stoffwechsel. in O. BUMKE, Handbuch der Geisteskrankheiten **3**, 154—217, Berlin: Springer 1929.

YASARGIL, M. G.: Zur Pathogenese und Therapie des Delirium tremens und des pathologischen Rauschzustandes. Schweiz. Arch. Neurol. Psychiat. **68**, 342—370 (1952).

ZARA, E., e E. BUONDONNO: Ricerche biologiche in ammalati di mente: fluttuazioni nictemerali della glutationemia. Neuropsichiatria N. S. **11**, 541—558 (1955).

Endokrinologische Psychiatrie*

Von

M. Bleuler, Zürich (Schweiz)

Inhalt

---

* Das Kapitel ist erstmals am 17. Mai 1958 fertiggestellt worden. Da sich die Veröffentlichung unvorgesehenerweise verzögerte, wurde es 1961 neu geschrieben. Seither wurde es durch Anmerkungen und Zusätze den Fortschritten der Forschung angepaßt.

Einleitung

Die endokrinologische Psychiatrie umfaßt die Lehre über die psychischen
Erscheinungen bei veränderten endokrinen Funktionen und umgekehrt über das
Verhalten der endokrinen Funktionen bei Geistesstörungen. Sie soll namentlich
das Wesen des Zusammenspieles endokriner und psychischer Vorgänge klären.
Eines ihrer hohen ärztlichen Ziele liegt in der Nutzbarmachung endokrinologischer
Behandlungsverfahren für Kranke, die in Behandlung des Psychiaters stehen,
und in der Nutzbarmachung psychiatrischer, namentlich psychotherapeutischer
Verfahren für endokrin Kranke.

Hoffnungen, wonach endokrinologische Forschungen unser psychiatrisches
Wissen und Können bereichern würden, sind schon Ende des letzten Jahrhunderts
wach geworden. Laignel-Lavastine sprach bereits 1908 von der «psychiatrie
endocrinienne». Bis vor ein bis zwei Jahrzehnten bestand das junge Fach aber in
der Hauptsache nur aus wenig fundierten spekulativen Behauptungen einerseits,
einer ungeordneten Summe von klinischen Einzel-Erfahrungen andererseits. Erst
in den letzten Jahren ist die endokrinologische Psychiatrie systematisch und vielseitig erforscht worden. Seither erst gelingt es, die Fülle von klinischen, pathologisch-anatomischen, -physiologischen und tierexperimentellen Kenntnissen zu
übersehen und zu ordnen und fruchtbare Hypothesen von allgemeiner Bedeutung
zu entwickeln.

Im Laufe der Jahrzehnte ist die Bedeutung der endokrinologischen Psychiatrie
bald maßlos überschätzt, bald unterschätzt worden. Nach unseren heutigen
Kenntnissen muß es als *Über*schätzung bezeichnet werden, wenn man die Entdeckung einer spezifischen Ursache und einer einfachen spezifischen Therapie für
„die" schizophrene und „die" manisch-depressive Psychose von ihr erwartete oder
wenn man bereits mit Genugtuung von einer „Charakter-Apotheke" sprach, die
in Zukunft für jede Triebstörung ein bestimmtes Hormon vorrätig haben würde.
Wie leichtsinnig glaubte man auch, man könnte bloß durch die psychiatrische
Exploration einiger endokrin Kranker das Wesen der Krankheit erklären! Hatte
man in einigen Fällen festgestellt, daß der Beginn einer endokrinen Erkrankung
in einer belasteten Lebensperiode erfolgte, so wollte man daraus schon schließen,
es handle sich um eine „psychosomatische" Störung im einfachen Sinne einer
somatischen Reaktion auf die Emotionen. Damit hatte man freilich die Vielseitigkeit und die Schwierigkeit der Problematik völlig übersehen. Eine gefährliche
*Unter*schätzung eines wichtigen Wissensgebietes war es hingegen, wenn bis vor
kurzem im Lehrgebäude der Psychiatrie endokrinologische Erkenntnisse überhaupt nicht mehr berücksichtigt wurden, wie es unter dem Eindruck der Enttäuschung der früheren naiven Hoffnungen vorkam. Als ebenso gefährlich hat es
sich erwiesen, wenn sich die endokrinologische Praxis nur nach den Laboratoriums-
Befunden ausrichten würde und die Zusammenhänge der endokrinen Störungen
mit der Persönlichkeit außer acht ließe.

Zur Erforschung der endokrinologischen Psychiatrie ist die Zusammenarbeit
des Psychiaters mit dem Endokrinologen, dem Pädiater, dem Gynäkologen, dem

Vertreter der pathologischen Anatomie und Physiologie und mit manchem anderen Fachmann notwendig. In den Schwierigkeiten einer solchen Zusammenarbeit liegt ein wesentlicher Grund dafür, daß das junge Fach in Forschung und Praxis so oft vernachlässigt wurde. Dasselbe Schicksal teilen ja viele Problemkreise, die in Grenzbereichen zwischen den traditionellen Fachgebieten liegen.

Einfache, aber doch grundlegende Erfahrungen, die es zunächst festzuhalten gilt, betreffen die Häufigkeit der Beziehungen zwischen endokrinologischen und psychischen Erkrankungen: *Psychische Störungen bei endokrinen Krankheiten sind häufig, endokrine Störungen bei jenen psychischen Krankheiten, die das Erfahrungsgut des Nervenarztes bilden, selten.* Der Satz kann noch präzisiert werden, wenn wir den Schweregrad der Störungen berücksichtigen: Schon mittelschwere, langdauernde endokrine Erkrankungen sind meistens von psychischen Veränderungen begleitet, aber in der Mehrzahl der Fälle nur von leichten. Deshalb gelangen diese Kranken meist in die Betreuung des Internisten und Endokrinologen und nicht in diejenige des Psychiaters. Schwere psychische Störungen sind nur bei den seltenen schwersten endokrinen Krankheitszuständen die Regel. Demgegenüber ist festzustellen, daß sogar die schwersten Psychosen, wie sie der Psychiater in der Anstaltspraxis zu betreuen hat, gewöhnlich keine endokrinen Störungen zeigen. Einschränkend zur letzteren Feststellung ist freilich noch hinzuzufügen, daß wir bei ihnen *mit unseren bisherigen Untersuchungsmethoden* keine endokrinen Störungen nachweisen konnten, was noch nicht sicher beweist, daß sie nicht vorhanden wären.

Diese Erfahrungen sind beinahe allgemeines Wissensgut geworden, und ihre Feststellung könnte überflüssig scheinen. Trotzdem finden sich in der Literatur noch oft Vermutungen und Behauptungen, die ihnen widersprechen.

I. Psychopathologische Erscheinungen bei endokrin Kranken. Übersicht

Welchen psychopathologischen Begleiterscheinungen begegnen wir bei endokrinen Erkrankungen?

Heute lassen sich die scheinbar so vielfältigen und unübersichtlichen psychopathologischen Bilder bei endokrinen Krankheiten leicht übersehen und ordnen: Es ist festzustellen, daß sie sich zur großen Hauptsache in Grundformen psychischen Krankseins einreihen[1], nämlich

1. in den akuten exogenen Reaktionstypus nach BONHOEFFER,
2. in das amnestische Syndrom und
3. vor allem in ein Syndrom, das man anschaulich „endokrines Psychosyndrom" nennen kann.

1. Endokrine Störungen, die akute und schwere allgemeine Stoffwechselstörungen mit sich bringen, können zu denselben psychischen Störungen führen wie anders bedingte akute schwere Stoffwechselstörungen und wie akute Hirnkrankheiten. Ihre Symptomatologie hält sich unabhängig von der besonderen Art der Grundkrankheit innerhalb eines großen Rahmens, desjenigen, den BONHOEFFER schon zu Beginn des Jahrhunderts als *akuten exogenen Reaktionstypus* umschrieben hat. BONHOEFFER selbst hat ihm auch Psychosen bei verschiedenen endokrinen Krankheiten eingefügt. Die seitherige Erfahrung zeigt, daß nicht nur einzelne, sondern alle hormonalen Störungen mit akuten schweren körperlichen Folgen auch zu Psychosen des akuten exogenen Reaktionstypus führen können. Beispielsweise sind hier zu erwähnen akute psychische Störungen bei Basedow-Krise (siehe z. B.

---

[1] Eine mehr ins einzelne gehende Übersicht der psychopathologischen Bilder bei endokrinen Erkrankungen findet sich bei BARAHONA FERNANDES.

bei Altman u. Aysenstein), bei akutem Myxödem, bei schwerer operativer Schädigung der Epithelkörperchen, bei schweren Formen von Cushing-Syndrom und von Morbus Addison, bei Überfunktion des Inselapparates, bei akuten Vergiftungen durch Verabreichung von Glucocorticoiden, von Insulin, von Parathormon oder von Schilddrüsenhormonen.

Die Erscheinungsbilder des akuten exogenen Reaktionstypus sind mannigfach; sie finden sich alle auch bei endokrinen Krankheiten; in beginnenden und leichten Fällen sehen wir bloße Verstimmungen oder Erregungen oder Müdigkeit, Apathie und Somnolenz. Diese Zustände können sich zum Koma oder zu Verwirrungen, Delirien oder Dämmerzuständen steigern. Andere Fälle verlaufen als Halluzinosen, wieder andere (seltene) als akute Korsakow-Psychosen. Die Störung des Bewußtseins beherrscht viele schwere Fälle. Bei anderen aber (z. B. den Halluzinosen und den bloßen Erregungen oder apathischen Zuständen) kann man kaum von „Bewußtseinsstörungen" sprechen — es sei denn, man fasse diesen Begriff ungewöhnlich weit. Bewußtseinsstörung im gewöhnlichen Sinne des Begriffes darf man nicht in jedem Falle eines akuten exogenen Reaktionstypus erwarten, sei er durch endokrine oder andere Störungen bedingt.

Die endokrin verursachten psychischen Störungen im Rahmen des akuten exogenen Reaktionstypus zeigen zeitlich und graduell nur eine lose Beziehung zu Verlauf und Grad der körperlichen endokrinen Störungen: Wohl treten sie im allgemeinen während schweren körperlichen Krisen auf, doch scheint es oft, daß sie den schweren körperlichen Erscheinungen zeitlich schon vorangingen oder erst nachhinkten, oder wir stehen in Einzelfällen vor erstaunlichem Mangel an Korrelation zwischen dem Grad des körperlichen und jenem des psychischen Leidens. — Dieselbe Unberechenbarkeit in den Beziehungen zwischen körperlichen und psychischen Störungen fällt ja immer wieder bei der Beobachtung von anderen als endokrinen schweren Krankheiten auf (z. B. zeigen auch Fieberdelirien nicht einfache Beziehungen zu Höhe und Verlauf des Fiebers).

Das Symptomenbild der Geistesstörung innerhalb des weiten Rahmens des akuten exogenen Reaktionstypus wird nicht durch die Art der endokrinen Funktionsstörung bestimmt. Verschiedene, ja gegensätzliche endokrine Störungen können von denselben psychischen Krankheitsbildern begleitet sein. Zum Beispiel läßt sich die Psychopathologie von akuten Begleitpsychosen bei Über- und Unterfunktion der Nebennierenrinde nicht grundsätzlich unterscheiden; umgekehrt kann die Begleitpsychose z. B. eines Cushing-Syndroms als Halluzinose, als Dämmerzustand oder als völlige Apathie und noch andere gekennzeichnet sein. Über die Symptomgestaltung innerhalb des Rahmens des akuten exogenen Reaktionstypus sowie über Schwere und zeitlichen Ablauf dieser Psychosen müssen also noch andere Faktoren mitbestimmen als nur jene endokrinen Veränderungen, die wir mit unserer heutigen Untersuchungstechnik erfassen. Diese anderen, krankheitsauslösenden und krankheitsgestaltenden, Faktoren sind erst mangelhaft und teilweise bekannt. Eine nachgewiesene Rolle spielen Lebensalter und persönliche Konstitution.

2. Chronische schwere endokrine Krankheiten sind oft von ähnlichen Störungen begleitet, wie sie als Ausdruck chronischer cerebraler, besonders diffus-cerebraler Erkrankungen längst bekannt sind: Auffallend ist vor allem die Störung der mnestischen Funktionen, die das Frischgedächtnis mehr betrifft als das Altgedächtnis. Ebenso wichtig sind die organischen Denkstörungen mit Gedankenarmut, Schwierigkeiten, gedanklich über die Berücksichtigung von Einzelheiten oder unbestimmten Allgemeinheiten hinaus zur Erfassung und Gestaltung des Wesentlichen zu gelangen, mit Perseverationstendenz, Kritikschwäche, übertriebener Affektschaltung auf das Denken usw. Dazu kommen affektive Störungen,

Verödung des Gemütslebens(Hand in Hand mit der intellektuellen Verödung) einerseits, emotionelle Unbeherrschbarkeit andrerseits. So bedeutungsvoll dieses ganze Syndrom für die Psychiatrie ist, so fehlt ihm doch immer noch eine einwandfreie und allgemein anerkannte Etiquettierung: Wir wollen es im folgenden mit dem gebräuchlichsten Ausdruck des *amnestischen Psychosyndroms* bezeichnen; dabei müssen wir uns aber bewußt bleiben, daß wir eigentlich die denkerischen und affektiven Störungen neben den bloß mnestischen inbegriffen haben möchten. (Eine andere Bezeichnung wäre diejenige des psychoorganischen Syndroms im engeren Sinne von E. BLEULER oder des hirndiffusen Psychosyndroms; gegen den letzteren Ausdruck ist aber einzuwenden, daß die Annahme einer hirndiffusen Schädigung als hauptsächliche körperliche Grundlage des Syndroms erst wahrscheinlich, aber noch nicht sicher ist.)

Bei chronischen endokrinen Erkrankungen tritt das amnestische Psychosyndrom meistens in leichter Form auf. Dieselben schweren Formen, die wir z. B. vom senilen Irresein, von der einfach-dementen Form der progressiven Paralyse her kennen, d. h. die ausgesprochenen organischen Demenzen, sind bei endokrinen Krankheiten selten. Freilich waren sie früher häufiger, als der Endokrinologie die heutigen Behandlungsmethoden noch nicht zur Verfügung standen. — Bei vielen endokrin Kranken kann man ein beginnendes amnestisches Psychosyndrom erst aus den subjektiven Klagen über den Gedächtnisverlust vermuten, doch sind auch die Fälle nicht selten, bei denen die mnestischen und denkerischen organischen Störungen bei der Untersuchung deutlich werden. Wir stehen dann vor ähnlichen psychischen Veränderungen wie z. B. bei leichten Formen der Hirnarteriosklerose oder bei traumatischen Encephalosen. Bekannt ist auch die Tatsache, daß viele endokrin Kranke „früh altern": Es läßt sich im höheren Alter die Auswirkung einer beginnenden senilen Demenz und diejenige der endokrinen Störung auf Gedächtnis und Denkvermögen nicht auseinanderhalten.

Bekannte Beispiele von schweren Gedächtnisstörungen endokriner Genese bilden das erworbene Myxödem und der erworbene schwere Hypoparathyreoidismus. Leichte Gedächtnisstörungen finden sich z. B. sehr häufig bei Cushing-Syndrom und bei Morbus Addison. Kastraten klagen oft über Gedächtnisstörungen; bei ihnen aber sind sie kaum je bei der Untersuchung nachweisbar, und es bleibt fraglich, ob sich die Klagen auf echte mnestische Störungen leichten Grades beziehen oder ob sie eher nur funktioneller Art sind.

Psychosen vom akuten exogenen Reaktionstypus können vollkommen ausheilen, oder sie können in chronische organische Geistesstörungen, vor allem in ein amnestisches Syndrom (in das psychoorganische Syndrom im engeren Sinne des Wortes) ausgehen. Die *Übergänge* sind fließend. Diese allgemeinen Erfahrungen gelten auch für endokrin bedingte Geistesstörungen im Rahmen des akuten exogenen Reaktionstypus und des chronischen amnestischen Psychosyndroms. In seltenen Fällen können aber auch Symptomenbilder, die gewöhnlich eher dem akuten exogenen Reaktionstypus angehören, chronisch werden. Bekannte Beispiele dafür bilden die chronischen Alkoholhalluzinosen und das sog. Malaria-Paranoid. Endokrin bedingte (oder mitbedingte) ähnliche chronische halluzinatorische oder paranoide Psychosen sind z. B. bei Panhypopituitarismus und beim Cushing-Syndrom beschrieben worden, doch sind sie selten.

3. Endokrines Psychosyndrom. Geistesstörungen im Rahmen des akuten exogenen Reaktionstypus und des amnestischen Psychosyndroms (oder psychoorganischen Syndroms im engeren Sinne) sind nicht alle, ja nicht einmal die häufigsten psychischen Veränderungen bei endokrin Kranken. Die *häufigsten* derselben passen nicht in den Rahmen dieser beiden Grundformen psychischen Krankseins. Es handelt sich bei ihnen nicht um Störungen, die nach Grad und sozialer Bedeutung als Psychosen, als eigentliche Geisteskrankheiten, gekennzeichnet wären. Vielmehr sind es leichtere psychopathologische Erscheinungen, die treffend als *Wesensänderungen* bezeichnet werden. In der Vorstellungswelt des

Laien handelt es sich bei diesen endokrin Kranken demnach nicht um „Verrückte“, wohl aber um „Nervöse“, um Sonderlinge, um Unberechenbare, um Kindische oder umgekehrt um vorzeitig Vergreiste.

Ergriffen sind vor allem *Triebe, gesamte Antriebshaftigkeit und Erregungsniveau* und *Stimmungen*. Die Veränderungen können *dauerhaft* sein oder können *plötzlich von Zeit zu Zeit einschießen und nach kurzer Zeit* (Stunden, Tagen, Wochen) *ebenso plötzlich wieder vergehen*.

Von *einzelnen Trieben*, die oft ergriffen sind, sind bisher vor allem elementare aufgefallen, solche, die Menschen und Tieren gemeinsam zukommen: Nahrungstrieb; Durst; Trieb, Hitze oder Kälte auszuweichen; Schlafbedürfnis; Bewegungstrieb oder Ruhebedürfnis; Trieb zum unruhigen Wandern oder zum Sich-Verkriechen und Stillehalten; Aggressivität oder Schüchternheit; Sexualtrieb; triebhafte Mütterlichkeit u. a. Diese Triebe sind bei endokrin Kranken oft *gesteigert* oder *vermindert*, einzelne davon, namentlich der Sexualtrieb, oft auch *erloschen*. Höhere, rein menschliche Bedürfnisse und Interessen können auch betroffen sein; ihre Störungen sind aber nicht so stark aufgefallen und auch nicht so eingehend studiert worden wie die Störungen der elementaren Triebe. Auch *Veränderungen* einzelner Triebe kommen vor, sind aber weniger auffällig als die Übersteigerungen und die Abschwächungen. Die deutlichsten Veränderungen sind die abnormen Gelüste nach besonderen Speisen, wie sie schon lange bei Schwangeren bekannt sind. Perversionen des Sexualtriebes spielen keine wichtige Rolle; die meisten schweren Sexualperversionen sind nicht von nachweisbaren endokrinen Störungen begleitet, und bei endokrin Kranken sind schwere Sexualperversionen Ausnahmen. — Die Triebsteigerungen treten meistens in vorübergehenden Perioden auf, einer Trieb-Unersättlichkeit folgt oft schließlich doch eine langdauernde Sättigung. Triebabschwächungen sind oft auch dauerhaft.

Die *gesamte Antriebshaftigkeit* und *emotionelle Erregbarkeit* kann gesteigert oder vermindert sein. So kommen einerseits erregte, erethische oder maniforme Zustände, andrerseits apathische, indolente oder somnolente vor. Solche Zustände — namentlich ihre leichteren Formen — sind oft dauerhaft, manchmal aber treten auch sie periodisch auf oder verschlimmern sie sich periodisch.

Stimmungsverschiebungen — andauernde und besonders vorübergehende — sind bei endokrin Kranken ebenfalls überaus häufig. Die Verstimmungen entsprechen selten einer reinen Depression oder einer reinen Manie oder Submanie. Häufig sind dagegen unter anderem: Zustände von Zufriedenheit, ja Glücksgefühlen, verbunden nicht mit Tatendrang, sondern mit Trägheit und Tatenlosigkeit (sog. „Hypophysärstimmung“), dann reizbare, mürrische, verdrossene, satte, weinerliche oder ängstliche Verstimmungen in den verschiedensten Tönungen und Mischungen.

Das *Gesamtbild* dieser endokrin Kranken erinnert, solange sie jung sind, oft an den Infantilismus. Es hat u. a. die Verstimmbarkeit, die Wechselhaftigkeit, die Unberechenbarkeit mit ihm gemein, außerdem oft die unentwickelte oder spielerische Sexualität, die Ängstlichkeit und die Unbeherrschtheit Eß- und Trinkgelüsten gegenüber. Ältere endokrin Kranke machen oft den Eindruck, als ob sie vorzeitig vergreisen würden, auch wenn die mnestischen Funktionen noch intakt sind: In diesem Sinne beeindrucken wieder die Unbeherrschtheit, Verstimmbarkeit und Wechselhaftigkeit, die Abnahme eines zielgerichteten Sexualtriebes, die Einschränkung der differenzierteren Aktivität und der differenzierteren Interessen, eine Karikierung und oft auch Erstarrung der ursprünglichen Persönlichkeit.

Primäre Veränderungen der *intellektuellen Funktionen* gehören nicht in dieses Bild. Selbstverständlich ist aber, daß sich die intellektuellen Funktionen im Zusammenhang mit der Emotionalität ändern. So ist z. B. Denkfaulheit eine Seite von trägen, inaktiven Verstimmungen; sprunghaftes Denken kommt in vielen Erregungen vor; übersteigerte Triebhaftigkeit schaltet kritische Überlegungen aus usw.

Zusammenfassend stehen wir demnach vor der Erfahrung, daß endokrine Störungen ganz gewöhnlich von Wesensänderungen begleitet sind; diese Wesensänderungen bestehen in dauerhaften oder unvermittelt und periodisch auftretenden und wieder zurückgehenden Änderungen von Einzeltrieben, der Triebhaftigkeit, des Erregungsniveaus und von Stimmungen. Die psychopathologische Symptomatik endokriner Krankheiten bildet demnach einen bestimmten Symptomenkomplex. Er kann als *endokrines Psychosyndrom*[1] etiquettiert werden. Daß zwischen den so bezeichneten Persönlichkeitsveränderungen und der endokrinen Störung tatsächlich ein innerer Zusammenhang besteht, ergibt sich nicht nur aus der psychiatrischen Betrachtung endokrin Kranker; vielmehr sind heute auch die Beobachtungen alltäglich geworden, wonach therapeutisch in unphysiologischen Dosen verabreichte Hormone emotionelle Veränderungen im Rahmen des endokrinen Psychosyndroms auslösen.

Nicht zum endokrinen Psychosyndrom zu zahlen sind aber die Störungen im Rahmen des akuten exogenen Reaktionstypus und des amnestischen Psychosyndroms bei endokrin Kranken, wie sie eingangs erwähnt wurden. Diese Störungen hängen viel weniger direkt mit der endokrinen Storung zusammen als das endokrine Psychosyndrom. Der Zusammenhang ist hier aller Wahrscheinlichkeit nach ein mehr indirekter. Er geht das eine Mal über eine allgemeine Stoffwechselkrise, das andere Mal wahrscheinlich über eine allgemeine Hirnschädigung. Akuter exogener Reaktionstypus und amnestisches Psychosyndrom sind also genetisch — und erst recht erscheinungsbildlich — vom endokrinen Psychosyndrom grundsätzlich abzugrenzen. Übergangsformen kommen freilich vor.

Das endokrine Psychosyndrom läßt sich erscheinungsbildlich von jenen Psychosyndromen, die bei umschriebenen chronischen Hirnkrankheiten bekannt sind, nicht abtrennen. Namentlich paßt sowohl das psychopathologische Stirnhirn- wie das Stammhirn-Syndrom erscheinungsbildlich in denselben Rahmen wie das endokrine Psychosyndrom. Kranke mit Folgezuständen von Encephalitis lethargica oder mit gewissen Wesensänderungen bei Schläfenlappenepilepsie z. B. lassen sich psychopathologisch von vielen endokrin Kranken nicht unterscheiden. Wenn man die psychopathologischen Folgen von umschriebenen Hirnkrankheiten verschiedener Lokalisation, die ja untereinander erstaunlich wenig verschieden sind, unter dem Oberbegriff des hirnlokalen Psychosyndroms zusammenfaßt, kommt man zur einprägsamen Formel: *Erscheinungsbildlich sind endokrines und hirnlokales Psychosyndrom in der Hauptsache identisch;* sie unterscheiden sich nur durch die Verschiedenheit der körperlichen Störungen, die sie begleiten. Auf die große theoretische Bedeutung dieser Aussage ist sogleich zurückzukommen.

Während sich das endokrine Psychosyndrom scharf von jenen Zustandsbildern unterscheidet, die Schizophrenie und manisch-depressives Kranksein charakterisieren, und sich auch gegen das amnestische Syndrom (oder das organische Psychosyndrom im engeren Sinne des Wortes) und den akuten exogenen Reaktionstypus deutlich absetzt, sind die Grenzen zu vielen Bildern bei psychopathischen und neurotischen Persönlichkeitsentwicklungen oft verwischt. Immerhin unterscheiden sich Psychopathien und neurotische Persönlichkeitsveränderungen in der Mehrzahl der Fälle doch nicht nur durch ihre andersartige Entstehung von den Zuständen des endokrinen Psychosyndroms, sondern auch durch das vorwiegende Betroffensein anderer psychischer Schichten. Bei den Persönlichkeitsstörungen endokrin Kranker ist mehr das Elementare, im Biologischen Verwurzelte, Urtriebhafte betroffen, wie z. B. Kälte- und Wärme-Empfinden, Hunger, gesamte emotionelle Erregbarkeit und vitale Stimmungen; psychopathische und neurotische Entwicklungen betreffen demgegenüber besonders stark die differenzierteren, rein menschlichen, dem Tiere nicht zukommenden Regungen und Einstellungen; sie betreffen z. B. Gemüt, Gewissen, soziales Verantwortungsgefühl, Selbstbewußtsein, Gesinnung.

---

[1] Ein ähnlicher Begriff ist die Characteropathia endocrinogenes von BILIKIEWICZ.

Setzen bestimmte endokrine Erkrankungen charakteristische, „spezifische" psychische Veränderungen? Im Gegensatz zu den jahrzehntelang vorherrschenden Tendenzen habe ich in der Übersicht über die psychischen Begleiterscheinungen endokriner Krankheiten *das Gemeinsame* hervorgehoben, *das für endokrine Krankheiten verschiedenster Art gilt.* Früher beachtete man die Gemeinsamkeiten der Persönlichkeitsstörungen bei verschiedenen endokrinen Krankheiten kaum; man ging vielmehr von der Überzeugung aus, daß jeder endokrinen Erkrankung ihre spezifische Psychopathologie zukommen würde. Es schien undenkbar, daß somatisch völlig verschiedene oder sogar gegensätzliche endokrine Störungen (wie Hyper- und Hypo-Funktion der Nebennierenrinde) ähnliche oder gleiche psychopathologische Folgen haben könnten.— Heute wissen wir, daß die Gemeinsamkeiten der psychopathologischen Erscheinungen bei verschiedenen endokrinen Funktionsstörungen gegenüber jenen psychischen Folgen überwiegen, welche für bestimmte hormonale Funktionsstörungen typisch sind. Die meisten psychopathologischen Erscheinungen bei allen unter sich so verschiedenen endokrinen Krankheiten konnten wir in einen Rahmen, in den Begriff des endokrinen Psychosyndroms, zusammenfassen. Wenn wir die Psychopathologie einzelner bestimmter endokriner Funktionsstörungen zu beschreiben hätten, so würde der Rahmen oft gleichartig und ungefähr gleich umfangreich wie derjenige des ganzen endokrinen Psychosyndroms. Die Psychopathologie des Cushing-Syndroms oder des Hypoparathyreoidismus z. B. läßt sich in fast denselben Worten darstellen wie die Psychopathologie aller endokriner Erkrankungen. Bei anderen endokrinen Funktionsstörungen gibt es immerhin Einzelzüge, Tönungen und Färbungen, die bei ihnen besonders häufig sind. Man kann solche Eigenarten funktionsspezifisch nennen, aber nur wenn man den Begriff der Spezifität weit faßt. Eine Spezifität im engen Sinne des Wortes, wonach ein psychisches Symptom bei einer bestimmten endokrinen Funktionsstörung immer und sonst niemals vorkäme, gibt es nicht.

Bei den psychopathologischen Erscheinungen einer endokrinen Krankheit haben wir demnach heute zu unterscheiden zwischen *Symptomen, die wir bei verschiedensten anderen endokrinen Funktionsstörungen auch finden, und Symptomen, die einigermaßen funktionsspezifisch sind.*

Die Bedeutung der allen endokrinen Krankheiten gemeinsamen psychopathologischen Erscheinungen kann man sich am besten mit der Vorstellung veranschaulichen, daß jede endokrine Gleichgewichts-Erschütterung dieselbe Prädisposition zu gewissen psychischen Störungen setzt. Wie sich diese psychischen Störungen im einzelnen gestalten, hängt dann weniger von der spezifischen Art der endokrinen Funktionsstörung als von anderen Faktoren ab, unter denen das Lebensalter, der Entwicklungszustand und die persönliche Konstitution bekannt sind. Einmal sind es Störungen im Rahmen des akuten exogenen Reaktionstypus, welche bei jeder endokrinen Krankheit vorkommen, wenn sie schwere akute körperliche Folgen hat. Gerade dabei ist die Symptomgestaltung im einzelnen — soweit wir bis heute wissen — nur selten von der Art der zugrunde liegenden endokrinen Krankheit abhängig. (Ausnahmen von dieser Regel gibt es; die wichtigste liegt wohl im Vorkommen vorübergehender Koma-Zustände ohne auffällige körperliche Verschlimmerungen bei Sheehan-Syndrom.) Auch das amnestische Psychosyndrom kommt bei den verschiedensten schwereren und langdauernden endokrinen Störungen in derselben Weise vor. — Im Rahmen des endokrinen Psychosyndroms ist namentlich die Neigung zu Verstimmungen wenig spezifisch in bezug auf die bestimmte endokrine Funktionsstörung. Die gleichen Verstimmungen können bei jeder endokrinen Krankheit vorkommen, wenn auch in verschiedener Häufigkeit. Schon eher hängen Erregungsniveau und Antriebshaftigkeit und namentlich die einzelnen Triebe mit einzelnen bestimmten hormonalen Störungen zusammen. —

Es sind vor allem psychische Begleiterscheinungen von Über- und Unterfunktionszuständen der Nebennierenrinde und Nebenschilddrüsen, welche innerhalb der großen Rahmen des akuten exogenen Reaktionstypus, des amnestischen Psychosyndroms und des endokrinen Psychosyndroms die verschiedensten Bilder und wenig für sie typische Züge zeigen. (Als eine der Ausnahmen von dieser allgemeinen Regel kann man u. a. das Auftreten von Durst und Appetitlosigkeit beim akuten Hyperparathyreoidismus betrachten.)

Die meisten einigermaßen *funktionsspezifischen psychischen Erscheinungen* bei bestimmten hormonalen Störungen betreffen Einzeltriebe oder — etwas seltener — die Antriebshaftigkeit und das Erregungsniveau als Ganzes. Viele dieser funktionsspezifischen psychischen Erscheinungen lassen sich dem Verständnis von der teleologischen und leistungsphysiologischen Betrachtungsweise aus nahe bringen. Es macht den Anschein, als ob die psychischen Schaltungen den Schaltungen der körperlichen Funktionen gleichgerichtet wären; oft scheinen auch beide gemeinsam danach zu tendieren, eine krankhafte Funktion auszugleichen: Die Drosselung des Stoffwechsels beim Hypothyreoidismus geht mit einer Drosselung der psychischen Aktivität einher; der ungenügenden inneren Wärmeerzeugung kommt die Trägheit mit Einschränkung der Energieausgabe und das gesteigerte Bedürfnis nach äußerer Wärme entgegen; bei Hyperthyreose entspricht die Energieverschleuderung im Stoffwechsel dem erhöhten Energiebedarf, der sich aus Übererregbarkeit und gesteigerter Antriebshaftigkeit ergibt; außerdem macht der gesteigerte Stoffwechsel gegen Kälte unempfindlich, gegen Wärme überempfindlich. Zuckerhunger der Gewebe — sei er durch Hypoglykämie oder durch mangelhafte Verwertung des Blutzuckers bedingt — geht mit Hunger einher, der unter physiologischen Umständen imstande wäre, den Zuckerhunger des Gewebes zu stillen. Exsiccose z. B. bei Hypercalcämie zufolge Hyperparathyreoidismus führt zu Durst. Wenn Sexualhormone körperliche Voraussetzungen für die Fortpflanzung fördern, so fördern sie oft (nicht etwa immer!) auch den Paarungstrieb; umgekehrt ist der Sexualtrieb oft vermindert, wenn mit dem krankhaften Wegfall der Sexualhormonproduktion die körperlichen Voraussetzungen für die Fortpflanzung fehlen. Das laktotrope Hormon fördert gleichzeitig Stillfähigkeit und triebhafte Mütterlichkeit. — Jene Erkrankungen, die funktionsspezifische Veränderungen von Trieben oder der gesamten Antriebshaftigkeit am ehesten erkennen lassen, betreffen besonders die Über- und Unterfunktion von Schilddrüse, die Unterfunktion der Gonaden, den Wegfall des Vasopressins, die Überproduktion von laktotropem Hormon, von Adrenalin und von Insulin: Überfunktion der Schilddrüse ist oft mit Erregung und Kälte-Unterempfindlichkeit verbunden, Unterfunktion umgekehrt mit Apathie und Kälte-Überempfindlichkeit; Unterfunktion der Gonaden führt oft (nicht immer!) zu Verkümmerung der Psychosexualutät; Wegfall des Vasopressins macht durstig; Überproduktion von laktotropem Hormon führt zu Übersteigerung der Mütterlichkeit; Adrenalin bedingt oft Angst; Insulin bedingt (über die Hypoglykämie) Hunger.

II. Die Genese des endokrinen Psychosyndroms; Physiologie und Pathophysiologie der Hormonwirkung auf die Psyche

Auf welchem Wege wirken sich die Hormone auf die Psyche aus? Noch vor wenigen Jahren war die Frage nicht zu beantworten. Im Laufe des letzten Jahrzehnts aber sind Fortschritte erzielt worden, die uns klarer sehen lassen. Sie erlauben uns heute zu antworten: *Aller Wahrscheinlichkeit nach wirken sich Störungen im hormonalen Gleichgewicht vorwiegend über das Hirn auf die psychischen Funktionen aus; sie bewirken lokalisierte oder allgemeine Veränderungen der Hirn funktion, der Hirnchemie und schließlich auch der Hirnstruktur.* Zu diesen Erkenntnissen führen die jüngsten Forschungen auf sehr verschiedenen Gebieten gemeinsam.

Wichtige Teilergebnisse erbrachten klinische Psychiatrie, pathologische Anatomie, Elektroencephalographie und Entwicklungspathologie. Deren Befunde werden durch die Fortschritte der Hirnphysiologie eindrucksvoll ergänzt, namentlich durch diejenigen über die Neurosekretion, über die Verbindungen zwischen Hypophyse und Hypothalamus, über das Vorkommen von Hormonen (im weitesten Sinne des Begriffes) oder doch von neurohumoralen Mediatoren im Hirn und ihre differenzierte Konzentration in verschiedenen Hirnteilen und über die Beziehungen von psychisch aktiven Drogen zu den Hormonkonzentrationen im Hirn. Aufschlußreich sind weiter die Wirkungen von gezielter intracerebraler Hormoninstillation und andere Erfahrungen, welche Beziehungen zwischen bestimmten zentralnervösen Systemen und bestimmten Hormonen und humoralen Mediatoren beweisen. — Aus der Klärung der Zusammenhänge zwischen endokrinen und zentralnervösen Funktionen beginnen sich Erkenntnisse abzuzeichnen, die pathologisch-physiologische Vorgänge mit psychopathologischen in genaueren Zusammenhang bringen. Wenn wir auch noch weit von endgültigem und gesichertem Wissen darüber entfernt sind, so haben doch wichtige Arbeitshypothesen in jüngster Zeit die Forschung mächtig angeregt und vorwärtsgetrieben.

Die *klinische Psychiatrie* hat zu dieser glänzenden wissenschaftlichen Entwicklung vorerst die eine grundlegende Erkenntnis beigetragen: *die psychopathologischen Erscheinungsbilder bei endokrinen Störungen sind denjenigen bei Hirnkrankheiten wesensgleich.* Darauf ist bereits hingewiesen worden. Störungen im Rahmen des akuten exogenen Reaktionstypus bei endokrinen Krankheiten sind erscheinungsbildlich allen anderen akuten psychischen Störungsbildern gleichzusetzen, welche durch allgemeine und damit auch cerebrale Stoffwechselstörungen zur Beobachtung kommen; das amnestische Psychosyndrom bei endokrinen Krankheiten tritt in derselben Art auf, wie es bei diffusen cerebralen Krankheiten alltäglich zur Beobachtung kommt; und vor allem: die häufigsten Störungen bei endokrinen Krankheiten, diejenigen im Rahmen des endokrinen Psychosyndroms, sind wesensgleich mit dem hirnlokalen Psychosyndrom, d. h. den psychopathologischen Erscheinungen bei lokalisierten Hirnkrankheiten.

Diese klinischen Feststellungen müssen schon für sich die Vermutung wachrufen, daß endokrine Funktionsstörungen zentralnervöse Funktionsstörungen nach sich ziehen könnten, weil sich Teile des Endokriniums und Teile des Zentralnervensystems zu Funktionseinheiten zusammenfügten. Die weitere Vermutung liegt ebenfalls nahe, daß schwere funktionelle Veränderungen im Hirn schließlich zu strukturellen Veränderungen führen könnten.

Solche klinische Vermutungen sind nun bereits *pathologisch-anatomisch* unterbaut: Viele, vielleicht die meisten schweren endokrinen Krankheiten sind von Hirnveränderungen begleitet. Bei ihnen erstaunt es nicht, daß die psychischen Symptome denjenigen von Hirnkrankheiten entsprechen. Die Mitteilungen über lokalisierte oder diffuse atrophische Erscheinungen im Hirn bei den verschiedensten endokrinen Erkrankungen sind unübersehbar zahlreich. Sie lassen keinen Zweifel darüber zu, daß strukturelle zentralnervöse Schädigungen bei schweren endokrinen Erkrankungen häufig sind. Im übrigen freilich bedürfen sie in vielerlei Hinsicht der Ordnung und der Ergänzung durch neue Forschungen: Es muß noch bewiesen werden, daß die pathologisch-anatomischen Befunde am Hirn bei endokrinen Erkrankungen regelmäßiger oder schwerer oder anders sind als bei vielen anderen ernsten Körperkrankheiten; der weiteren Klärung bedarf die Frage, ob Schwere, Häufigkeit oder Art der hirnpathologischen Veränderungen endokrin

Kranker sich mit ihren psychopathologischen Veränderungen in Beziehung bringen lassen. Diese und andere Fragen sind in den letzten Jahren vernachlässigt worden, wie überhaupt die Erforschung der genaueren Zusammenhänge zwischen Hirnpathologie und Psychopathologie eine Periode der Stagnation durchmacht.

Um so lebhafter hingegen sind die Forschungen zur *elektrencephalographischen Klärung* hormonaler Einwirkungen auf das Hirn in Gang gekommen. Ihre Ergebnisse lassen sich vorerst dahin zusammenfassen, daß endokrine Störungen tatsächlich oft das Elektrencephalogramm verändern und daß damit ihre Einflußnahme auf die Hirnfunktion in irgendeiner Art erwiesen scheint. Gerade bei jenen Hormonen, die sich psychopathologisch stärker auswirken als andere, ist der deutliche Einfluß auf das Elektrencephalogramm vielfach gezeigt worden: beim adrenocorticotropen Hormon, bei den Glucocorticoiden, bei den Schilddrüsenhormonen[1]. Beim Panhypopituitarismus und bei der Hypothyreose, bei denen besonders schwere psychische Störungen häufig sind, sind Beziehungen zwischen elektroencephalographischen Veränderungen und der Schwere der psychischen Schädigung bereits in einzelnen Fällen wahrscheinlich gemacht (KRUMP, MENTZOS und FISCHER, LANSING und TRUNNELL). Bei einem Teil dieser elektrencephalographischen Befunde ist zu vermuten, daß sie auf thalamische und hypothalamische Funktionsstörungen zu beziehen sind.

Demnach weisen klinische, pathologisch-anatomische und elektrencephalographische Beobachtungen gemeinsam darauf hin, *daß* bei endokrinen Erkrankungen im Hirn lokalisierte und generalisierte, funktionelle und strukturelle Veränderungen vor sich gehen. Es stellt sich die Frage, *wie* sie zustande kommen. Darüber ergeben sich nach den jüngsten Erfolgen der Hirnforschung anschauliche Vermutungen. Sie knüpfen sich vorerst an den Nachweis, daß im Hirn Hormone und hormonähnliche Stoffe in bestimmten Verteilungen und Konzentrationen vorkommen[2]. Sie gewinnen noch an Bedeutung und Wahrscheinlichkeit, nachdem gezeigt worden ist, daß bestimmte Teile des Hirn auf bestimmte Hormone spezifisch empfindlich sind. So drängt sich die Annahme auf, daß endokrine Störungen unphysiologische Schwankungen des Gehaltes von Hormonen und neurohumeralen Mediatoren in bestimmten Hirnteilen verursachen und daß dadurch besonders jene Hirnteile geschädigt werden, die schon physiologischerweise speziell auf Hormone ansprechen. Aus der großen Fülle von Befunden verschiedener Forschergruppen, die im Sinne dieser Annahmen geltend zu machen wären, sollen im folgenden einige der wichtigsten erwähnt werden:

Was zunächst das *Vorkommen von Hormonen* im Hirn betrifft, so ist schon längere Zeit bekannt, daß sich Schilddrüsenhormon (COURRIER et al.; SCHITTENHELM; STURM und SCHNEEBERG; STURM und WERNITZ) und Intermedin im Hirn finden, und zwar in ungleichmäßiger Verteilung. Nach neueren Untersuchungen reichert sich radioaktives Triiodothyronin und Thyroxin im paraventriculären Gebiet des Hypothalamus an (FORD und GROSS)[3]. In den letzten Jahren hat aber vor

---

[1] Literatur zusammengefaßt bei PITT-RIVERS and TATA.

[2] Es bestehen im Hirn große regionale Unterschiede in der Fermentaktivität der Nervenzellen. Der Nachweis, daß die Stoffwechselchemie in bestimmten Hirnregionen anders ist als in andern, läßt zum vornherein spezifische Hormonwirkungen auf spezifische Systeme im Hirn möglich erscheinen.

[3] Thyroxin und besonders Triiodothyronin kommen auch in der Hypophyse, besonders in der Neurohypophyse, vor (Literatur referiert bei PITT-RIVERS and TATA). Ob sie dort eine physiologische Rolle spielen, ist noch fraglich. Vielleicht wirken sie bei der Regulierung der Ausscheidung von thyreotrophem Hormon im Hypophysen-Vorderlappen mit. — Das lebende Hirngewebe kann in vitro Thyroxin und 3:5:3'-Triiodothyronin abbauen. Es erscheint deshalb möglich, daß der Abbau der Schilddrüsenhormone im Hirn für die Hirnfunktion wichtig ist (TATA). Thyroxin ist auch im Liquor nachgewiesen (ALPERS).

allem der Gehalt des Hirns an Noradrenalin, an seinem Vorläufer Dopamin und an 5-Hydroxytryptamin und die Anreicherung des letzteren im Rhinencephalon und Hirnstamm große Beachtung gefunden. Auch Enzyme, die bei der Bildung von neurosekretorischen Substanzen (von 5-Hydroxytryptamin und von Sympathin) entscheidend beteiligt sind, finden sich ungleichmäßig im Hirn verteilt (Blaschko).

Zwischen dem 5-Hydroxytryptamin (Serotonin, 5-HT) und verschiedenen Drogen, die deutliche Wirkung auf die Psyche haben, bestehen enge Beziehungen. Man versuchte daraus den Beweis abzuleiten, daß das 5-HT tatsächlich bei der Genese psychischer Störungen eine wichtige Rolle spiele; wenn auch vieles in diesem Sinne spricht, so ist eine solche Beweisführung bis heute noch nicht endgültig gelungen, und verschiedene gewichtige Gegenargumente bleiben zu widerlegen. Für die Bedeutung des 5-HT für psychische Vorgänge sprechen die Befunde, wonach Reserpin, das psychisch beruhigt und entspannt, 5-HT aus dem Hirn ausschwemmt, während Iproniazid (Marsilid), das ähnliche Psychosen setzen kann wie Cortison und gelegentlich depressiv-stuporöse Zustände bessert, die Konzentration des 5-HT im Hirn steigert. [In der Tat wurde bei anderen ähnlichen Stoffen wie dem Iproniazid eine gewisse Korrelation zwischen psychischer Wirksamkeit und Monoaminooxydase-Hemmung aufgedeckt (Pletscher et al.).] Weiter bestehen chemische Verwandtschaften und pharmakologische Synergismen und Antagonismen zwischen 5-HT und Mescalin, Lysergsäurediäthylamid und anderen Drogen, die toxische Psychosen setzen. — Unter den Argumenten, die eher dagegen sprechen, daß diese Drogen vor allem durch Veränderung des 5-HT-Gehaltes im Hirn auf die Psychose wirksam wären, seien nur erwähnt: Bei Kranken mit Carcinoid, die viel 5-HT im Blute aufweisen, besteht keine Tendenz zu psychischen Veränderungen, soweit die bisherige Beobachtung an den seltenen Fällen ergab (Kind und Schneider; Schneider); ebensowenig hat die Injektion von 5-HT in die Blutbahn deutliche psychische Wirkungen[1]; diese beiden Beobachtungen können freilich dadurch erklärt werden, daß das 5-HT nur in beschränktem Maße aus dem Blut ins Hirn dringt. Gewichtiger ist die Beobachtung von Rothlin, wonach es Stoffe gibt, die gleich wie das Lysergsäurediäthylamid dem 5-HT gegenüber antagonistische Eigenschaften aufweisen, aber ungleich dem Lysergsaurediäthylamid keine Wirkung auf die Psyche haben (d-2-Brom-LSD)[2]. Umgekehrt hat Mescalin ähnliche psychische Wirkungen wie LSD, während Mescalin keine Beziehungen zum 5-HT hat, die dem LSD zukommen. Chlorpromazin hat eine grundsätzlich ähnliche Wirkung auf die Psyche wie Reserpin, schwemmt aber 5-HT nicht in derselben Art aus wie das Reserpin. Kurz: Wenn die psychische Wirkung der in Frage stehenden Drogen durch die Beeinflussung des 5-HT im Hirn zu erklären wäre, müßte man annehmen, daß psychische Wirksamkeit und Wirksamkeit auf den 5-HT-Stoffwechsel bei den verschiedenen Drogen gekoppelt wären — gerade das aber ist nicht immer der Fall. Deshalb können wir aus den zahlreichen Untersuchungen, die über die Beziehungen von psychischer Medikamenten-Wirkung und 5-HT-Stoffwechsel durchgeführt wurden, bis heute noch keine sicheren Schlußfolgerungen auf die Bedeutung des 5-HT-Gehaltes im Hirn für psychopathologische Vorgänge ziehen. Trotzdem erscheint die Hoffnung berechtigt, daß die Fortsetzung dieser Studien zu wichtigen hirnphysiologischen Erkenntnissen fuhren wird.

Das Noradrenalin im Hirn verhält sich unter dem Einfluß von Medikamenten, die auf die Psyche wirken, ähnlich wie das 5-Hydroxytryptamin. Es bleibt noch zu prüfen, ob die dem 5-Hydroxytryptamin in den letzten Jahren zugeschriebene Bedeutung für die physiologischen Grundlagen psychischen Lebens nicht eher dem Noradrenalin zuzusprechen wäre[3]. Für die vorliegenden Überlegungen kommt es

---

[1] Neuerdings wurden auch widersprechende Beobachtungen gemacht, so über erregende Wirkung (Fouks et al.).

[2] Es gibt auch noch andere vom Lysergsäurediäthylamid abgeleitete Stoffe, denen Anti-Serotonin-Eigenschaften in hohem Maße zukommen, ohne daß sie im geringsten auf die Psyche wirken (Deseril) (Fanchamps et al.).

[3] Darüber ist bei der Drucklegung eine lebhafte Diskussion im Gange: Die einen Untersucher finden enge Beziehungen zwischen der beruhigenden Wirkung des Reserpins und ähnlich wirkender Medikamente einerseits und dem Noradrenalin-Gehalt im Hirn andererseits, während sie feststellen, daß die beruhigende Wirkung der Medikamente und ihre Wirkung auf den 5-Hydroxytryptamingehalt im Hirn auseinanderfallen. Andere Untersucher stellen bei anderen Experimenten das Gegenteil fest. Die Differenzen beruhen, soweit bis heute festgestellt ist, zum Teil in Mängeln der angewendeten Meßmethoden, zum Teil aber darin, daß es sich um eine zeitlich rasch ablaufende Reihe von Vorgängen handelt; es kommt mehr, als man beachtet hatte, darauf an, in welchem Zeitpunkt nach der Medikamenten-Applikation Noradrenalin und 5-Hydroxytryptamin bestimmt werden (Karki und Paasonen; Pletscher et al. 1960; Sulser und Brodie).

aber zunächst nur darauf an, daß Verteilungen von hormonähnlichen Stoffen im Hirn für die psychischen Funktionen überhaupt bedeutungsvoll sein könnten, und es ist dann eine weitere Frage, welche Hormone im Spiele sind.

Die Substanz P, ein basisches Polypeptid, ist ein Gewebehormon, das sich im Darm und im Hirn findet. Im Hirn ist es ähnlich verteilt wie das 5-Hydroxytryptamin und das Katecholamin. In Tierversuchen hat es eine erregungsdämpfende Wirkung. Seine Konzentration im Hirn sinkt in der Narkose und steigt in der Erregung. Es wirkt unter gewissen experimentellen Bedingungen antikonvulsiv. Es handelt sich vielleicht um eine Überträgersubstanz im Nervensystem. Wahrscheinlich ist in der Substanz P ein Gewebehormon gefunden, dessen Konzentration in bestimmten Hirnteilen etwas mit dem Funktionszustand des Hirns und der psychischen Aktivität zu tun hat (HAEFELY and HÜRLIMANN; ZETLER 1959 und 1960; ZETLER und OHNESORGE). — Auch die Gamma-Amino-Buttersäure im Hirn hat wahrscheinlich Bedeutung für die Funktion des Nervensystems. Im hypoglykämischen Koma wird ihre Konzentration im Hirn geringer (KNAUFF und BÖCK). Es ist aber noch völlig ungeklärt, ob ihre Abnahme mit dem Versinken ins Koma das Geringste zu tun hat.

Hormone werden nicht nur dem Hirn zugeführt, sondern sogar im Hirn selbst gebildet, und die *Neurosekretion*[1] steht in vielfachen Beziehungen zum Stoffwechsel der bisher bekannten Hormone. Viele Abhängigkeiten der Funktionen der endokrinen Drüsen untereinander sind schon lange bekannt; die Kenntnis darüber ist hingegen neu, daß Verbindungen hinüber und herüber bestehen zwischen

den peripheren endokrinen Drüsen

den offensichtlich endokrin tätigen Teilen des Hirns (Nuclei supraoptici und paraventriculares) und

vielen anderen Hirnteilen (besonders dem Hypothalamus, dem reticulären System und dem limbischen System).

Das Zentralnervensystem beeinflußt die periphere endokrine Sekretion mittels neurosekretorischer Vorgänge; umgekehrt wirken sich die Hormone der peripheren Drüsen steuernd auf zentralnervöse Funktionszentren aus. „Das Hirn ist" (gemäß einem Ausdruck von LUFT) „hormonabhängig".

Damit ist die Frage nach dem „Wie?" der Wirkung endokriner Krankheiten auf das Hirn vorläufig wenigstens summarisch beantwortbar: Hormone wirken auf nervöse Funktionssysteme, die auf spezifische Art hormonempfindlich sind. Krankhafte Störungen im Hormongleichgewicht werden diese Funktionssysteme zuerst funktionell und später strukturell verändern. (Schwere hormonale Gleichgewichtsstörungen können das Hirn darüber hinaus diffus vergiften.)

Die Lehre von der Neurosekretion und den engen funktionellen Beziehungen zwischen nervösem und endokrinem System macht eine andere elementare klinische Tatsache verständlich: Endokrine Erkrankungen führen in der Regel zu psychischen Störungen, psychische Erkrankungen viel seltener zu endokrinen Störungen. Das Zentralnervensystem in seiner Differenziertheit ist auf pathologische Stoffwechselbedingungen empfindlicher als die einfacher gebauten peripheren endokrinen Drüsen auf nervöse Einflüsse.

Um die soeben erwähnten grundsätzlichen Annahmen über die Existenz von funktionellen Systemen, die Teile vom Nervensystem und vom Endokrinium

---

[1] Die Neurosekretion ist bei höheren Tieren vorerst für die Nuclei paraventriculares und supraoptici erwiesen und Neurosekreten sind Verbindungen zwischen Hirnstamm und Hypophyse zuzuschreiben. Vieles spricht aber für eine viel allgemeinere Bedeutung der Neurosekretion, u. a. ihre weite Verbreitung im Nervensystem niedriger Tiere. Die Identität von Hormonen des Nebennierenmarkes mit Mediatoren, die nervöse Erregungen übertragen, bildet einen weiteren Hinweis darauf, wie eng verwandt die Funktion der bisher bekannten endokrinen Drüsen mit Stoffwechselvorgängen im Nervensystem ist. Im selben Sinne sprechen die Vorgänge in den synaptischen Bläschen. — Neuerdings zeigt sich, daß das Hirn wahrscheinlich auch in der Gegend der Epiphyse einen Wirkstoff bildet (Adrenoglomerulotropin), der die Nebennierenrinde zur Sekretion von Aldosteron bringt.

gemeinsam umfassen, näher zu belegen und zu erläutern, erwähne ich die folgenden Reihen von Beobachtungen:

1. über Abhängigkeit der Neurosekretion von Hormonen peripherer Drüsen,

2. über die Steuerung des Hypophysenvorderlappens durch nervöse Zentren, die ihrerseits von peripheren Hormonen gesteuert werden und die gleichzeitig mit anderen Hirnteilen in funktioneller Verbindung stehen,

3. über lokalspezifische Empfindlichkeiten auf Mikroinstillation von Hormonen ins Hirn,

4. über lokalspezifische Empfindlichkeiten auf Hormone, wie sie sich bei der elektrischen Selbstreizung von Tieren ergeben,

5. über Wirkungen auf das endokrine System, die von Hirnläsionen und Hirnreizungen bestimmter Lokalisation ausgehen,

6. über die besonderen Beziehungen zwischen reticulärem System und der endokrinen Funktion,

7. über endokrine Wirkungen auf die Phasenhaftigkeit der Lebensvorgänge, die sich vermutlich über das Hirn auswirken,

8. über entwicklungsphysiologische und -pathologische Beziehungen zwischen einzelnen Teilen des Zentralnervensystems und des Hirns.

1. Abhängigkeit der Neurosekretion von Hormonen peripherer Drüsen. Beispiele für Beziehungen zwischen endokriner Tätigkeit des Zentralnertensystems und peripherer Drüsen liefern u. a. die Arbeiten von Eichner und von Malandra und Corbetta. Sie decken enge Zusammenhänge zwischen Neurosekretion im Hypothalamus und der Nebennierenrinden-Funktion auf. Folgen von Adrenalektomie oder von Cortison-Verabreichung lassen sich am neurosekretorischen Zwischenhirnsystem schon morphologisch nachweisen. Stutinski zeigte, daß auch Sexualhormone die Neurosekretion der Nuclei supraoptici und paraventriculares in sichtbarer Art verändern, und zwar Stilboestrol und Progesteron gegensätzlich. Stutinsky hat aus derartigen Befunden geschlossen, daß der neurosekretorische Anteil des Diencephalons unter direktem Einfluß des Spiegels von Hormonen steht, wie jede endokrine Drüse.

2. Steuerung des Hypophysenvorderlappens durch periphere Hormone, die auf zentralnervöse Systeme wirken. Bard ist schon 1940 zur Ansicht gelangt, daß bereits ein Beispiel entdeckt sei, wonach ein funktionelles Zentrum im Hirn Hormonwirkungen auffange und zur Steuerung des Triebverhaltens verwende. Er zog seine Schlüsse aus den damaligen Arbeiten über die Wirkung von Hirnläsionen auf das sexuelle Verhalten von Versuchstieren. Er stellte fest, daß Funktionszentren im oberen Mittelhirn und hinteren Hypothalamus durch Ovarialhormone aktiviert würden und gleichzeitig das Sexualverhalten steuern hülfen.

Die Erkenntnis der Wechselwirkung zwischen Zentralnervensystem und endokrinen Drüsen wurde erschwert, weil nervöse Verbindungen zwischen endokrinen Drüsen und dem Zentralnervensystem spärlich sind. Es mußten die humoralen Verbindungen vom Zentralnervensystem zur Hypophyse entdeckt werden, bevor man sich die Wechselwirkung vorstellen konnte. Die "feed-back"-Vorgänge, die sich in der Physiologie des Nervensystems immer bedeutungsvoller erweisen, spielen auch zwischen Nervensystem und endokriner Sekretion. Teilweise erfolgen sie dabei humoral. Im Zentralnervensystem dienen die neurosekretorischen Zellen der Integration zwischen nervösem und endokrinem System: Sie erhalten Reize aus anderen Neuronen, aber ihre eigenen Achsencylinder enden gewöhnlich in den Blutgefäßen, in die sie ihre Sekrete entleeren.

BERTA SCHARRER hat das folgende Schema über die Kontrolle der Gonadotropin-Bildung aufgestellt:

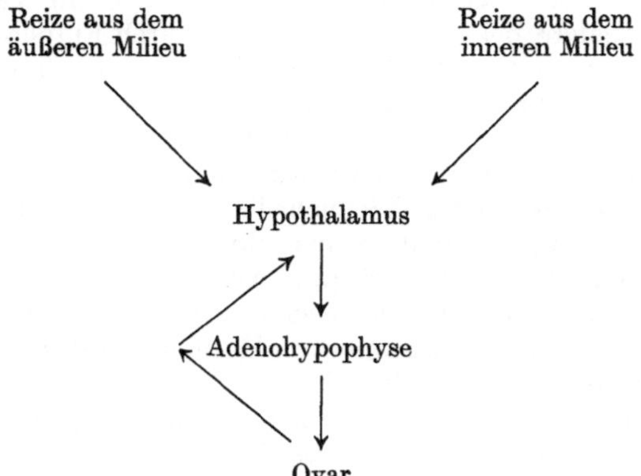

Danach gelangen die Hormone des Ovars in den Hypothalamus. Im Hypothalamus
wird die humoral gemeldete Funktion des Ovars mit der gesamten Lage des Organismus in Beziehung gebracht, wie sie sich aus inneren und äußeren Reizen ergibt.
Gemäß diesem Integrationsprozeß wird auf humoralem Wege die Gonadotropin-
bildung der Hypophyse und damit die endokrine Funktion des Ovars gesteuert.
Wie BERTA SCHARRER — die an der Erforschung der Neurosekretion hervorragend
beteiligt ist — vermutet, gilt ein entsprechendes Schema auch für die "feed-back"-
Kontrolle anderer endokriner Organe als des Ovars[1]. Es wird freilich noch großer
Arbeit bedürfen, um diese Fragen endgültig zu klären.

   3. *Lokalspezifische Empfindlichkeiten im Hirn auf Hormoninstillation.* Eine
wichtige und neuartige Methodik zur Erforschung der Bedeutung von Hormonen im Hirnstoffwechsel ist die *gezielte intracerebrale Hormoninstillation* an
Versuchstieren. Die Methode bezweckt, Hormone an einen bestimmten Ort im
Hirn zu bringen, um sie dort umschrieben einwirken zu lassen. Bisher wurden vor
allem Sexualhormone (HOHLWEG und JUNKMANN 1932, HOHLWEG 1939, HOHLWEG
und JUNKMANN 1946, KENT und LIEBERMANN 1948, HOHLWEG 1952, FISHER 1956,
HARRIS et al. 1958[2]), Gonadotropine (HESS, M., 1951, ENGELHARDT 1957) und
Schilddrüsenhormon (GREER et al. 1950) verwendet. Wirkungen auf Brunst- und
Sexualorgane wurden von bestimmten Stellen des Hirns aus mit viel geringeren
Hormonmengen erzielt, als sie bei subcutaner Injektion zur Erzielung einer Wir-
kung notwendig sind. Die Deutung der bisher mit der Methode erzielten Ergeb-

---

   [1] Wenn die Erhöhung des Spiegels der Hormone der peripheren Drüsen zuerst auf das
Zentralnervensystem und erst von demselben aus bremsend auf die Hypophyse wirkt, so ist
zu erwarten, daß das Zusammenspiel zwischen Hypophyse und peripheren Drüsen durch
Hirnkrankheiten gestört werden kann. Das Gleichgewicht zwischen Cortisol im Blut und
adrenocorticotroper Hypophysenfunktion ist denn auch tatsächlich bei Hirnkranken gestört.
befunden worden (OPPENHEIMER et al.). Aber auch zahlreiche andere endokrine Störungen sind
im Zusammenhang mit Hirnkrankheiten beobachtet worden (siehe z. B. bei WYSS). Naturgemäß
gibt es aber auch Hirnläsionen ohne Folgen am Endokrinium (siehe z. B. ODELL et al.), denn
nur bestimmte Systeme im Hirn haben bestimmte Beziehungen zu endokrinen Drüsen.
   Bereits liegen exakte Experimente vor, welche die Annahme einer Steuerung der Bildung
von thyreotropem Hormon von hypothalamischen Zentren aus sehr wahrscheinlich machen
(CAMPBELL et al.; YAMADA and GREER; Literaturzusammenfassung bei PITT-RIVERS and TATA;
WERNER). Die Überausscheidung einer "Exophthalmus producing substance" mit oder neben
dem Thyreotropin wird vom Diencephalon und vielleicht auch von der Hirnrinde aus gesteuert
(HORST u. ULLERICH).
   [2] Siehe auch S. 185.

nisse ist freilich noch unsicher. Es wird in Zukunft u. a. noch nötig sein, die spezifische Hormonwirkung von unspezifischen Reizwirkungen einwandfrei abzutrennen. Von besonderem Interesse für unsere Thematik sind die Versuchsergebnisse von Harris: Er erzeugte bei kastrierten Katzen durch Einpflanzung von Stilboestrol an bestimmten Stellen des hinteren Hypothalamus (und nur an diesen!) Brunstverhalten. Das Brunstverhalten wurde nicht etwa sekundär ausgelöst, indem sich der hormonale Hirnreiz zuerst auf die Brunstmerkmale an den Sexualorganen ausgewirkt hätte und erst die Brunstveränderungen der Sexualorgane die triebhafte Brunst ausgelöst hätten. Vielmehr löste die Oestrogen-Implantation im Hypothalamus schon Brunstverhalten aus, ohne daß sich die Sexualorgane im Sinne der Brunst verändert hätten. Harris hat so im Tierexperiment bestätigt, was aus der klinischen Erfahrung zu vermuten war: daß hormonal ausgelöstes Triebverhalten durch direkte Einwirkung von Hormonen auf spezifisch reagierende Stellen im Hirn zustande kommen kann[1].

Die Hoffnungen, die sich an die Methode knüpfen, gehen dahin, daß es in Zukunft möglich sein wird, die Wirkwerte der verschiedenen Hormone in verschiedenen Teilen des Hirns zu bestimmen. Vielleicht wird sich dabei feststellen lassen, daß einzelne Hirnteile besondere Empfindsamkeiten auf einzelne Hormone aufweisen und daß diese Empfindsamkeiten nicht nur experimentell, sondern auch biologisch und bei endokrinen Krankheitsvorgängen bedeutungsvoll sind[2].

4. Noch anders nachgewiesene Lokalempfindlichkeiten im Hirn auf Hormone. Im Sinne solcher Erwartungen sprechen Ergebnisse mit einer weiteren neuen Technik, derjenigen der *elektrischen Selbststimulation bestimmter Hirnteile* durch Versuchstiere (Olds). Den Versuchstieren werden Elektroden ins Hirn implantiert; eine raffinierte experimentelle Anlage bewirkt, daß sich diese Tiere bei gewissen Bewegungen selbst elektrisch reizen. Je nachdem, wo die Elektrode ins Hirn implantiert ist, lernen die Tiere die elektrische Reizung vermeiden (vermutlich infolge einer Unlustempfindung), oder aber sie reizen sich immer wieder selbst (vermutlich infolge einer Lustempfindung). Der Androgenspiegel im Blut beeinflußt nun die angelernten Tendenzen zur Selbststimulierung oder ihrer Vermeidung stark, aber nur an ganz bestimmten Hirnstellen und nicht bei jeder Lokalisation der Elektrode. Es läßt sich schließen, daß die Bedeutung des Androgenspiegels für die Hirnfunktion in verschiedenen Hirnteilen verschieden ist. So spricht auch diese Erfahrung dafür, daß Hormone im Zentralnervensystem lokalspezifische Bedeutungen haben können. Erhöhter Androgenspiegel einerseits, Hunger andererseits beeinflussen die Selbststimulation in entgegengesetzter Richtung, wie Hunger und sexueller Drang physiologisch viele Funktionen entgegengesetzt schalten.

5. Lokalisierte Hirnreizung und -Läsion und Endokrinium. Wieder auf eine andere Art zeigten Green *u. Mitarb., daß spezifische Beziehungen zwischen Hormonen und eng begrenzten, kleinen Teilen des Hirns vorkommen:* Läsionen in einem kleinen Teil der piriformen Rinde von Affen führten zu einer Übersteigerung der Sexualität. Nach der Kastration geht der Sexualtrieb bei der-

---

[1] Lisk zeigt neuerdings, daß kleine Mengen Testosteron in bestimmte Stellen des Diencephalons implantiert zu Atrophie der Genitalien führen, aller Wahrscheinlichkeit nach auf dem Wege der Bremsung der gonadotropen Hypophysen-Funktion. Auch Oestradiol-Implantationen in den Hypothalamus lassen Foci erkennen, von denen aus die hypophysäre Gonadotropin-Sekretion gehemmt wird (Davidson and Sawyer 1961 a, b). Nach neuen Versuchen von Grossmann regt Adrenalin und Noradrenalin, als Kristalle ins Hungerzentrum im Nucleus ventrolateralis gebracht, zum Fressen an, während es das Trinken bremst.

[2] Hormonwirkung auf bestimmte Hirnsysteme ergibt sich auch aus neueren von Woolley u. Mitarb. durchgeführten Experimenten: Die Oligodendroglia in Gewebekulturen wird durch Serotonin zu Kontraktionen angeregt.

art verstümmelten Tieren viel langsamer verloren als bei hirngesunden Tieren. Für die endokrinologisch-psychiatrische Grundlagenforschung ist aber wesentlich: Geschlechtshormone haben auf kastrierte Tiere eine stärkere Steigerung der Sexualität zur Folge, wenn eine kleine Stelle in der piriformen Rinde lädiert ist, als beim hirngesunden Tier!

Wie einzelne Hirnteile auf Hormone besonders ansprechen, so bewirkt umgekehrt die *Reizung einzelner Hirnteile Sekretion bestimmter Hormone*, z. B. vom Nucleus amygdalae Ausschüttung von antidiuretischem Hormon (DINGMAN und GAITAN) oder von Teilen des Hypothalamus Ausschüttung von Adrenalin und Noradrenalin und von adrenocorticotropem und gonadotropem Hormon (FOLKOW und VON EULER; HARRIS). Auch das reticuläre System hilft die Gonadotropinbildung zu regulieren (SAWYER). Elektrische Reizung des Hypothalamus führte auch zur Ausschwemmung von thyreotropem Hormon, besonders nach Exstirpation der Nebennierenrinde (HARRIS). In anderen Fällen zeigen sich enge Beziehungen zwischen umschriebenen Hirnteilen und endokrinen Drüsen daran, daß Hirnläsionen zu Drüsenatrophie führen. WOODS erzielte z. B. durch Läsion im Nucleus amygdalae Atrophie der Nebenniere; gleichzeitig wurden seine Versuchstiere (Ratten) zahm.

Mannigfache Reizungen der Peripherie erzeugen bei Tieren spezifische Hormonausschwemmungen, die durch das Hirn vermittelt werden: so bedingt die Paarung der Kaninchen über Erregung des Sexualzentrums im Hypothalamus Ovulation; Saugreize an der Brust können über zentralnervöse Reizung und hormonale Ausschüttung Milchsekretion anregen. Auch die Reaktion auf Stress geht von den Reizungen der Sinnesorgane über das Hirn (reticuläres System und Hypothalamus) und die Hypophyse zu den peripheren Drüsen (Vermehrung von adrenocorticotropem und Verminderung von gonadotropem Hormon) (HARRIS; HAUN und SAWYER u. a.). Zerstörungen in bestimmten Gebieten des Hypothalamus stört die gonadotrope Funktion der Hypophyse (BOGDANOVE, DEY, HILLARP).

Die Tätigkeit der Nebennierenrinde an den Hydroxycorticosteroiden im Blut und Urin gemessen wird dank gewisser Reizungen im Hypothalamus angeregt. Sie wird auch vom limbischen System aus beeinflußt. [Durch die Reizung des Mandelkerns wird sie angeregt; der Reizung des Hippocampus folgt eine Senkung; die Abtragung des Hippocampus stört den Tagesrhythmus im Hydroxycorticosteroid-Spiegel (MASON).]

6. Heute zeigt sich auch, daß *enge Beziehungen zwischen gewissen Hormonen und der Funktion des reticulären Systems* bestehen: Hunger und Hypoglykämie führen zu Adrenalin-Ausschüttung. Adrenalin stimuliert das reticuläre System unter gewissen Umständen und fördert damit die "arousal reaction". Versuchstiere wurden infolge der Adrenalinwirkung auf das reticuläre System lebhafter, sie bewegen sich mit mehr Nachhalt und Aufmerksamkeit, sie werden, wie es genannt wurde, zu einem "exploratory behavior" veranlaßt. Das erhöht ihre Chancen, Nahrung zu wittern, welche Witterung darauf das weitere Hungerverhalten bestimmt[1].— Eine ähnliche stimulierende Wirkung über das reticuläre System auf die allgemeine Aktivität scheint im Tierexperiment weiblichen Sexualhormonen zuzukommen: Zuerst wird das Tier durch Sexualhormone aktiviert und erst wenn es einen Partner gefunden hat sexualisiert. — Es besteht demnach nicht nur ein

---

[1] Nach Untersuchungen von POECK allerdings wirken Acetylcholin und Katecholamin direkt in den cerebralen Kreislauf injiziert, nicht auf das reticuläre System. POECK bestreitet aus diesem und anderen Gründen eine adrenergische und cholinergische Erregungsübertragung im reticulären System. Andererseits fanden SALMOIRAGHI und STEINER, daß viele Neurone im Hirnstamm mit Entladungsfrequenzänderungen auf Acetylcholin reagieren, das in die unmittelbare Nähe dieser Zellen gebracht wurde. — Die unterschiedlichen experimentellen Befunde bedürfen weiterer Abklärung.

Zusammenspiel zwischen Hormonen und lokalisierten Hirnfunktionen in bezug auf die Erfüllung *einzelner* triebhafter Bedürfnisse; vielmehr hilft ein solches Zusammenspiel auch die *allgemeine* Aktivität, den Grad des Wachseins, zu regeln. Wenn Triebbefriedigung zustande kommen soll, so bedarf es zuerst einer allgemeinen Aktivierung und dann erst der Ausrichtung auf ein bestimmtes Triebziel. Die allgemeine Aktivierung schließt es in sich, daß das Territorium durchwandert und durchforscht wird. Wird dann eine Möglichkeit entdeckt, den Hunger zu stillen oder die Sexualspannung zu lösen oder sonst einen Trieb zu befriedigen, bekommt erst die spezielle Getriebenheit in einer bestimmten Richtung Bedeutung. — Mit dem Vorbehalt, daß die Übersetzung tierpsychologischer Beobachtungen in humanpsychologische Begriffe immer nur kritisch erfolgen darf, könnte man anschaulich ausdrücken: Das Streben nach einem bestimmten Ziel setzt vorerst allgemeinen Unternehmungsgeist und allgemeine Regsamkeit voraus (Bonvallet et al.; Zusammenfassung bei P. C. Dell; Einwände bei Domino).

Nervöse Verbindungen vom reticulären System zur Gegend des Nucleus paraventricularis im Hypothalamus und damit zu Regulationszentren des endokrinen Systems sind vorhanden. Demnach erlauben auch die anatomischen Verhältnisse die Erwartung, daß sich unsere Kenntnisse über die funktionellen Beziehungen zwischen Endokrinium und Formatio reticularis noch ausbauen lassen.

Die Erkenntnis, daß Hormone wahrscheinlich auch auf das reticuläre System und damit auf das Wachsein und die Antriebshaftigkeit wirken, ergänzt die bisherigen Kenntnisse über die Physiologie der Hormonwirkung auf die Psyche eindrucksvoll: Das endokrine Psychosyndrom besteht einerseits aus Triebstörungen, andererseits aus Störungen der gesamten Antriebshaftigkeit und der Stimmung. Die Vermutung war schon lange gegeben, daß eine Steuerung einzelner Triebe durch hormonale Einwirkungen auf bestimmte nervöse Zentren erfolgen könnte. — Demgegenüber war es bis vor kurzem kaum möglich, die Wirkung der Hormone auf Antriebshaftigkeit, Aktivität und Stimmung anschaulich zu machen. Heute ist dies möglich: die Hormone haben nicht nur eine Wirkung auf die Regulationszentren für bestimmtes Triebverhalten; vielmehr beeinflussen sie auch jene zentralnervösen Systeme, die die Antriebshaftigkeit, das Wachsein, den Unternehmungsgeist regeln helfen. Es wird damit verständlich, wie sie in das allgemeine Gestimmtsein eingreifen[1].

7. Hormonale Einflüsse über das Zentralnervensystem auf die Phasenhaftigkeit. Das endokrine Psychosyndrom ist gekennzeichnet durch Störungen der Einzeltriebe und der Antriebshaftigkeit, die oft zeitlich unvermittelt und überraschend auftreten und wieder verschwinden. Tierexperimentelle Untersuchungen haben nicht nur das Verständnis für die Genese der Störungen von Einzeltrieben und der Antriebshaftigkeit wesentlich gefördert, vielmehr lassen sie neuerdings sogar die abnormen Aktivitäts-Cyclen besser verstehen. C. P. Richter setzte durch endokrine Eingriffe (im Sinne der Hypothyreose) *abnorme Cyclen der Aktivität*. Er führt sie auf eine Schädigung im Hypothalamus zurück. Dieselben Schädigungen setzt auch schwerer Stress. Sie sind zum Teil irreversibel. Richter vermu-

---

[1] Die Steroide der Nebennierenrinde helfen auch die ganze Hirnerregbarkeit regulieren, soweit sie sich aus der Messung der Reizschwelle bei Auslösung eines Elektroschocks bestimmen läßt. Cortisol erhöht die Reizbarkeit, Desoxycorticosteron setzt sie herab. Die Wirkung dieser Hormone geht wahrscheinlich über eine Verschiebung der intracellulären Natrium-Ionen zu den extracellulären im Hirn. Gleichzeitig verändert sich das Verhältnis von Aminosäuren zu Aminen und damit die unmittelbar greifbaren Energiequellen (Woodbury). Ob dieser Einfluß der Nebennierenrindenhormone auf die Hirnerregbarkeit über das reticuläre System geht, ist noch nicht erforscht. — Auch Thyroxine und 3:5:3'-triiodothyronine erhöhen die Erregbarkeit des Hirns, soweit sie durch die Bestimmung der Reizschwelle für Elektroschock gemessen werden kann (Passouant-Fontaine).

tet, daß Schädigungen des Hypothalamus durch Stress oder endokrine Veränderungen auch beim Menschen cyclisch wiederkehrende Störungen setzen. Sicher ist in der Tat, daß abnorme Aktivitätscyclen bei endokrinen Krankheiten häufig und schwer sind.

8. Von einer weiteren Seite beleuchten *Entwicklungsphysiologie und -pathologie* unsere Problematik. In der Entwicklung und funktionellen Differenzierung der endokrinen Organe und des Nervensystems bestehen gegenseitige Abhängigkeiten. Störungen in der Entwicklung in einem Organsystem können mit Störungen im anderen eng verknüpft sein. In bezug auf den Kretinismus ist dies seit langem bekannt. Für andere Störungen hat MARAÑON dasselbe festgestellt. Seine grundsätzlichen Lehren über den Zusammenhang zwischen der Entwicklung von Hirn und endokrinem System sind heute auch tierexperimentell unterbaut. Zum Beispiel fördert Wuchshormon die Entwicklung des Hirns von Ratten in hohem Maße (ZAMENHOF) und wird die Entwicklung der Nebennierenrinde vom Hirn aus gelenkt (JANIGAN et al.). Diabetes der Mutter führt oft zu Hirnmißbildungen des Fetus (DEKABAN).

KOLLROS und WEISS und ROSETTI haben *Thyroxin in eng umschriebene Teile des Zentralnervensystems von Kaulquappen* eingeführt. An einzelnen Stellen wurde dadurch das Wachstum der Nervenzellen gefördert, an anderen Stellen deren Atrophie. Verschiedene Gruppen von Nervenzellen erwiesen sich auch in diesen Experimenten auf ein Hormon ganz verschieden empfindlich. (Literatur zusammengefaßt bei ERNST SCHARRER.)

Der Mangel an Schilddrüsenhormon wirkt sich hemmend auf die Reifung des Zentralnervensystems aus, und zwar in ähnlicher Weise wie Unterernährung. (Der Grund liegt vielleicht u. a. darin, daß die Grundstoffe zur Eiweiß-Synthese mangelhaft resorbiert werden können.) Überdauert bei Versuchstieren der Schilddrüsenhormon-Mangel eine bestimmte Entwicklungsphase, sind die Schäden irreparabel (Literaturübersicht bei PITT-RIVERS and TATA).

Ganz allgemein weiß man heute um die Bedeutung chemischer Wirkungen auf die organbildenden Vorgänge. Eine Bedeutung von Hormonen auf die Hirnentwicklung kann als Spezialfall allgemeinerer Gesetzlichkeiten betrachtet werden. Die Hormonwirkung am Erwachsenen auf einzelne Hirnteile kann auf dem Hintergrund dieser entwicklungsphysiologischen Annahmen leichter verstanden werden: In beiden Fällen stehen wir vor einem Zusammenspiel zwischen stofflichen Vorgängen im Blut und lokalisierten cerebralen Vorgängen.

Faßt man die Ergebnisse aller dieser Untersuchungen zusammen, so wird gewiß, was früher nur unklar vermutet werden konnte: Nervensystem und Endokrinium sind keineswegs voneinander derart unabhängig, wie es wegen der Verschiedenheit der anatomischen Lage und der Struktur gern angenommen wurde. Teile beider integrieren sich zu Funktionseinheiten. Die gegenseitige Abhängigkeit ist aber nicht nur eine funktionelle, sondern — mindestens unter pathologischen Voraussetzungen — oft auch eine strukturelle. Die Funktion des Nervensystems ist von chemischen Vorgängen begleitet, die der Hormonbildung in den Drüsen mit innerer Sekretion wesensverwandt sind, und die Bildung von Hormonen erfolgt auch im Nervensystem. Allerdings ist die Bildung der Hormone und die Reaktion auf Hormone im Nervensystem ungleich feiner lokalisiert als an der Peripherie.

BLASCHKO hat diese neuen, grundlegenden Vorstellungen kürzlich in folgenden Worten treffend umschrieben: ".... as a first approximation we can say that the brain appears very much like a big gland, the main difference between it and a gland proper being that, in the brain, elaborate precautions are taken to make release localized and effective only over minute distances."

Andere Hirnforscher äußern sich entsprechend darüber: J. H. Welsh: "Developments of the last few decades have made it increasingly clear that the nervous system is, in a sense, itself, a complex endocrine system... The view is now developing rapidly, that neurons are producers and releasers of a variety of active physiological agents."

Berta Scharrer: "...the eminent position of master gland held in the past by the pituitary...., now has to be accorded to, or at least shared with, the neurohumoral center by which it is controlled."

Aus allen diesen Vorstellungen werden die Grundlagen der endokrinologischen Psychiatrie verständlich. Wir verstehen, weshalb die Psychopathologie cerebraler und endokriner Krankheiten dieselbe ist. Wir verstehen, daß Erkrankungen des einen Systems zu funktionellen und strukturellen Schädigungen des anderen führen können. Wir verstehen, daß endokrine Vorgänge die Hirnfunktion beeinflussen. Das große Rätsel über die Art der Hormonwirkung auf die Psyche geht in dem noch größeren Rätsel auf, wie die cerebrale Funktion psychisches Leben ermöglicht.

Älteren Vorstellungen folgend, könnte man erwarten, daß sich bestimmte zentralnervöse Systeme mit bestimmten Funktionen der endokrinen Drüsen in Beziehung setzen ließen. Man wäre versucht, als Ziel der Forschung eine Hirnkarte zu fordern, auf der die Stellen verschiedenster spezifischer Hormonbildungen und -empfindlichkeiten eingetragen werden könnten. Vereinzelte Befunde lassen sich bereits in dieser Hinsicht verwerten. — Vieles aber spricht dafür, daß die Beziehungen des Zentralnervensystems zum Endokrinium von Individuum zu Individuum verschieden sind. Zentralnervöse Lokalisationen, wie sie hier zur Diskussion stehen, könnten nur zum Teil angeboren, weitgehend aber auch durch die Erfahrung erworben sein. In diesem Sinne spricht u. a. die Unregelmäßigkeit der Lokalisation von zentralnervösen Degenerationen bei endokrinen Krankheiten. Auch Erfahrungen von W. R. Hess mit gezielter elektrischer Reizung im Hirn lassen sich in dem Sinne deuten, daß mit erheblichen individuellen Verschiedenheiten der Beziehungen zwischen bestimmten Reizstellen einerseits, vegetativen und emotionellen Reaktionen andererseits zu rechnen ist. Weitere Vermutungen über die individuelle Prägung der Lokalisation von Hirnfunktionen, die mit den endokrinen Funktionen zusammenhängen, können aus den Untersuchungen über die Prägung von cerebralen Lokalisationen bestimmter Funktionen im Laufe der Bildung bedingter Reflexe gezogen werden.

III. Endokrine Funktionen bei schizophrenen und manisch-depressiven Psychosen

Seit Jahrzehnten ist die Frage oft gestellt worden, *ob endokrine Störungen die Genese von Schizophrenien und manisch-depressiven Psychosen erklären könnten.* Die großen Hoffnungen, die man an die Bearbeitung dieser Frage knüpfte, sind bisher zur Hauptsache enttäuscht worden. Es ist keineswegs gelungen, diese Psychosen auf eine endokrine Krankheit zurückzuführen. Immerhin sind die Forschungen darüber noch nicht zu Ende gelangt. Was bisher an positiven Ergebnissen erarbeitet worden ist, liegt aber bloß im Wissen darum, daß endokrine Funktionsstörungen wenigstens bei einem kleinen Teil von schizophrenen Psychosen krankheitsmitgestaltende und -mitauslösende Einflüsse bedeuten.

Zwei wichtige Tatsachen werden bei der Hypothesenbildung über endokrine Genesen von Schizophrenien und manisch-depressivem Kranksein merkwürdigerweise oft übersehen, obschon sie vor voreiligen Schlüssen warnen sollten: Keine der der heutigen Medizin bekannten endokrinen Funktionsstörungen ist für gewöhnlich von schizophrenen oder manisch-depressiven Krankheitsbildern begleitet. Wir haben keinen Grund anzunehmen, daß bei körperlich klar erkennbaren endokrinen Erkrankungen Schizophrenie und manisch-depressives Kranksein viel häufiger vorkommen als in der Durchschnittsbevölkerung. Und umgekehrt: Die große Mehrzahl von Schizophrenen und Manisch-Depressiven läßt mit der bisher üblichen Methodik keine endokrinen Störungen erkennen. Von einer spezifischen endokrinen Störung, die bei der einen oder der anderen dieser Psychosen regelmäßig und nur bei ihr vorkäme, kann schon gar keine Rede sein. Richtig ist allerdings, daß leichte endokrine Funktionsbesonderheiten bei beiden Psychosen etwas häufiger sind als in der Durchschnittsbevölkerung. Sie sind ihrer Natur nach völlig verschiedenartig und manchmal offensichtlich eher Folge als Mitursache der Psychose.

Diese negativen Feststellungen sind nicht bloß darauf zurückzuführen, daß die bisher bekannten endokrinologischen Forschungsmethoden in ungenügendem Maße zur Untersuchung Geisteskranker herangezogen worden wären. Sonderbarerweise sind zwar endokrinologische Untersuchungen an Manisch-Depressiven nicht in wünschbarem Maße mit genügender Technik zur Anwendung gekommen; dafür ist eine ungeheure Arbeit für die Untersuchung Schizophrener mit fast allen, auch den modernsten, Untersuchungsmethoden geleistet worden. Die älteren Arbeiten beziehen sich vor allem auf die Sektionsbefunde an den endokrinen Organen. Es ergab sich nichts Aufschlußreiches[1]. Die Häufigkeit von schizophrenen Psychosen in der Pubertät und im Wochenbett hat die Aufmerksamkeit früh auf die *Sexualhormone* gelenkt. Es hat sich aber nur ergeben, was jeder erfahrene Kliniker ohnehin wußte: Wie bei anderen Psychosen sind Amenorrhoen auch bei diesen in akuten Zuständen häufig; Verspätungen und dauernde Rückstände in der körperlichen sexuellen Reifung sowie die verschiedensten Unregelmäßigkeiten in der Ausprägung der sekundären Geschlechtsmerkmale (z. B. männlicher Behaarungstypus bei Frauen) sind bei Schizophrenen häufiger als in der Durchschnittsbevölkerung (z. B. BERGERON und BENOIT, FERRIER et al., SIVADON et al. u. a.). Eine ähnliche erhöhte Variabilität zeigen Schizophrene aber auch in bezug auf viele andere körperliche Merkmale und nicht nur in bezug auf diejenigen, deren Entstehung durch Sexualhormone gesteuert sein könnte. Auch ist nicht erwiesen, daß sich in bezug auf diese Variabilität Schizophrene etwa von Schwachsinnigen oder Psychopathen wesentlich unterschieden. Bei der Mehrzahl Schizophrener sind keine Störungen feststellbar, die mit den Sexualhormonen in Zusammenhang zu bringen sind.

Besonders eingehend ist seit Jahrzehnten die *Schilddrüsenfunktion* Schizophrener untersucht worden. Diese Untersuchungen litten oft an einseitiger Überbewertung neu eingeführter Untersuchungsmethoden, früher z. B. an derjenigen der Grundumsatzbestimmung, in jüngster Zeit an derjenigen mit Radiojod (s. u. a. CRAMMER und POVER). Es waren keine regelmäßigen Schilddrüsenstörungen bei Schizophrenen zu finden. Abweichungen von der Norm kommen im Sinne einer Über- wie Unterfunktion in einer Minderzahl von Fällen vor, Unterfunktion ist häufiger als Überfunktion (ABÉLY und N. RICHARDEAU, BARUK et al., KIND 1956, REISS 1952, 1955, 1956, STOLL 1956). In diesen Fällen wird aus der Beobachtung der zeitlichen und graduellen Korrelation von körperlich-endokrinen und psychotischen Krankheitserscheinungen manchmal eine krankheitsgestaltende Bedeutung der endokrinen Störung für die Psychose deutlich. In Einzelfällen ist dann auch eine Therapie, die die Schilddrüsenfunktion beeinflußt, auf die Psyche wirksam. Das ist aber lange nicht immer der Fall. — Konstitutionsanalytische Untersuchungen haben ergeben, daß in einzelnen Familien von Schizophrenen, die eine Struma aufweisen, schizophrene und psychopathische Störungen einerseits, Strumen andererseits häufiger zusammen vorkommen, als dem Zufall entsprechen würde. In diesen Familien ist irgendein genetischer Zusammenhang zwischen

---

[1] Eine der wenig zahlreichen neueren Mitteilungen über Sektionsbefunde an endokrinen Organen Schizophrener stellt fest, daß Färbemethoden in den Nebennieren Schizophrener weniger Lipoide erkennen lassen als in denjenigen anderer Geisteskranker. Die Befunde am Sektionsmaterial Schizophrener sind gleich wie an denjenigen von Leberkranken (BEATTIE und HEASMAN).

Psychose und Struma anzunehmen, dessen Natur der Klärung noch wartet. Dagegen spricht nichts dafür, daß beim Gros der Schizophrenen die Genese der Psychose etwas mit der Schilddrüse zu tun hätte.

Neuerdings ist von Flach u. Mitarb. (1959) und Lochner u. Mitarb. versucht worden, das Triiodothyronin bei Sonderformen von Schizophrenie zu verwenden: es käme bei apathischen Schizophrenen in Frage. Eine negative Calcium-Bilanz, wie sie vereinzelte Schizophrene auf Triiodothyronin-Applikation aufwiesen, war mit emotionellem Erwachen verknüpft. — Die Bedeutung der Thyroxin-Behandlung der periodischen Katatonie nach Gjessing steht weiter im Studium (Mall und andere).

Im Zusammenhang mit der glänzenden Entwicklung der Physiologie und Pathologie der *Nebennierenrinde* ist im letzten Jahrzehnt eine mühevolle und groß angelegte Arbeit für die Funktionsprüfung der Nebennierenrinde von Schizophrenen verwendet worden[1]. Heute lassen sich ihre Ergebnisse bereits übersehen. Sie sind leider enttäuschend. Eine Funktionsstörung der Nebennierenrinde als wesentlicher Faktor in der Genese aller oder der meisten schizophrenen Psychosen konnte nicht entdeckt werden. Viele Schizophrene zeigen unveränderte Nebennierenrindenfunktion. In vielen Fällen liegen zwar auch Abweichungen vor, aber sie gehen in verschiedener Richtung und unterscheiden sich nicht deutlich von jenen Veränderungen, wie sie bei zahlreichen anderen psychischen und körperlichen Krankheiten oder unter belastenden und unhygienischen Lebensbedingungen auch gefunden werden. Auch bei den manisch-depressiven Psychosen ergaben Untersuchungen der Nebennierenrindenfunktion widersprüchliche Befunde (Kammerer und Wackenheim; Taban u. a.). — Es hat sich auch die Vermutung nicht bestätigen lassen, daß die Elektroschockbehandlung und andere geläufige körperliche Behandlungsverfahren hauptsächlich durch ihre Einwirkung auf die Nebennierenrinde wirksam wären. Wohl wird ihre Funktion im Schock angeregt, aber nicht in wesentlich stärkerem Maße als durch viele andere Einwirkungen. Die Stress-Reaktion der Nebennierenrinde ist bei schizophrenen und nicht-schizophrenen Psychosen dieselbe (Delay et al. 1953). Bereits ist auch eine erfolgreiche Elektroschock-Behandlung bei einem adrenalektomierten Kranken beschrieben.

In jüngster Zeit hat sich die endokrinologische Schizophrenieforschung mit besonderem Interesse einerseits dem *5-Hydroxytryptamin*, andererseits den *Nebennierenmark-Hormonen* zugewendet. — Es sind bereits auf Seite 172 die wichtigsten Gründe für die Hypothese aufgeführt, wonach das Hormon 5-Hydroxytryptamin (Serotonin oder Enteramin) ganz allgemein für die Hirnphysiologie und elementare psychische Vorgänge, vor allem für den gesamten psychischen Erregungszustand, bedeutungsvoll wäre. Wenn nun darüber hinaus vermutet wird, daß gerade schizophrene Psychosen genetisch eng mit dem 5-Hydroxytryptamin-Stoffwechsel des Hirns verknüpft wären, so auf Grund unzulässiger Annahmen: Man hat nämlich experimentelle, kurzdauernde Psychosen, namentlich diejenige durch Vergiftung mit Lysergsäurediäthylamid, fälschlich Schizophrenien gleichgesetzt; da Lysergsäurediäthylamid pharmakologisch antagonistische Eigenschaften zum 5-Hydroxytryptamin hat, ergab sich dann die Vermutung, der 5-Hydroxytryptamingehalt im Hirn habe Beziehungen zur Genese der Schizophrenie. In Wirklichkeit lassen sich die Lysergsäurediäthylamid-Psychosen zwanglos in den akuten exogenen Reaktionstypus einreihen, und zwar nicht etwa nur wegen ihrer toxischen Genese, sondern gerade wegen ihres Symptomenbildes. Sie sind nicht schizophrene Psychosen. Darauf hat mit Recht schon Stoll in der ersten Publikation, die über die psychischen Wirkungen des Lysergsäurediäthylamids erschienen ist, hingewiesen

---

[1] Literatur bei M. Bleuler: Endokrinologische Psychiatrie. Stuttgart: Thieme 1954.

(1947). Wenn die Lysergsäurediäthylamid-Vergiftungen aber keine Schizophrenien sind, so darf man auch aus den pharmakologischen Beziehungen des Lysergsäurediäthylamids zum 5-Hydroxytryptamin keine Rückschlüsse auf die Genese der Schizophrenie ziehen. Wir wissen heute weiter, daß sich das Lysergsäurediäthylamid nicht über den 5-Hydroxytryptamin-Gehalt des Hirns auf die Psyche auswirkt. — Weiter wurde dahin argumentiert, daß Reserpin die Schizophrenie heile und gleichzeitig 5-Hydroxytryptamin ausschwemme, so daß diese 5-Hydroxytryptamin-Ausschwemmung mit der Heilung schizophrenen Geschehens in Zusammenhang stände. Auch diese Argumentation ist anfechtbar: Reserpin hat beruhigende und inaktivierende Wirkung, ob es bei Schizophrenen, andersartig Psychotischen oder Gesunden (oder sogar bei Versuchstieren) zur Anwendung kommt; es ist kein spezifisches Heilmittel für die Schizophrenie; es wirkt bei Schizophrenen und Nicht-Schizophrenen grundsätzlich ähnlich. Deshalb kann die Ausschwemmung des 5-Hydroxytryptamins durch Reserpin nur zur Vermutung berechtigen, 5-Hydroxytryptamin habe etwas mit dem Erregungs- und Aktivitätszustand der Psyche zu tun, aber nicht mit dem besonderen schizophrenen Krankheitsgeschehen.

Die Frage, ob 5-Hydroxytryptamin mit schizophrenen Erkrankungen genetisch verknüpft sei, kann nur gelöst werden, wenn der 5-Hydroxytryptamin-Haushalt bei Schizophrenen untersucht und in besonderer Art verändert gefunden wird; darüber sind aber noch zu wenig Daten erarbeitet worden, als daß ein Urteil möglich wäre. Die bisherigen Befunde sind widersprechend. Sie deuten darauf hin, daß sich der 5-Hydroxytryptamin-Stoffwechsel nicht bei allen Schizophrenen gleich verhält. Soweit er bei Schizophrenen verändert schien, so waren diese Veränderungen in keiner Weise für die Schizophrenie spezifisch, sondern kamen auch bei andern Krankheiten vor. Unter anderem suchte LJUNGBERG den 5-Hydroxytryptamin-Stoffwechsel Schizophrener an der Ausscheidung der 5-Hydroxyindol-Essigsäure zu messen. Er fand diese Ausscheidung bei Schizophrenen oft herabgesetzt, aber ebenso manchmal bei andern Psychosen. — Übrigens wurden schizophrene Erkrankungen gegensätzlich sowohl mit einer Über- wie Unter-Konzentration von 5-Hydroxytryptamin im Hirn in spekulativen Zusammenhang gebracht.

Wenn es heute den Anschein hat, daß Untersuchungen über das 5-Hydroxytryptamin die Schizophrenie-Forschung nicht fördern können, so besteht hingegen noch gute Hoffnung, daß sie etwas zur Problematik des Schwachsinns beitragen werden: PARE u. Mitarb. fanden die Ausscheidung von 5-Hydroxyindol bei vielen Schwachsinnsformen vermindert (nur bei der Phenylketonurie erhöht und beim Mongolismus normal).

Nach Verabreichung von Abbauprodukten des Adrenalins, nämlich von Adrenochrom und Adrenolutin, wurden psychotische Zustände beobachtet, die in vielen Zügen Ähnlichkeit mit den Lysergsäurediäthylamid-Vergiftungen aufwiesen (HOFFER 1957a—e; HOFFER et al. 1954, 1957). Soweit sich aus den Beschreibungen dieser Psychosen aber schließen läßt, handelt es sich meines Erachtens wieder erscheinungsbildlich deutlich um Störungen des akuten exogenen Reaktionstypus. Wenn man aus der hochinteressanten Beobachtung von Adrenochrom- und Adrenolutin-Psychosen vermutet hat, daß diese toxischen Psychosen Schizophrenien gleich seien, so scheint mir dies anfechtbar. Deshalb kann ich auch nicht der Folgerung zustimmen, daß ein abnormer Abbau der natürlichen Nebennierenmark-Hormone bei der Genese der Schizophrenien beteiligt sein sollte. Berechtigter wäre die Vermutung, daß bei Psychosen des akuten exogenen Reaktionstypus abnormer Adrenalin-Abbau wichtig sein könnte. — Auch der Stoffwechsel der Nebennierenmark-Hormone wird bei schizophrenen Kranken selbst untersucht werden müssen, um deren allfällige Beteiligung an der Genese der Schizophrenie zu klären. Auch darüber liegen noch keine abschließenden Untersuchungen vor. Die Mehrzahl der bisherigen sorgfältig und kritisch durchgeführten Studien spricht entschieden gegen die Annahme, daß wesentliche Zusammenhänge zwischen einem veränderten Auf- oder Abbau des Adrenalins und der Genese schizophrener Psychosen beständen (siehe z. B. Bollard et al.).

Eine umfassende Untersuchung über die Ausscheidung von Adrenalin und Noradrenalin im Urin hat Bergsman angestellt. Bei chronischen Schizophrenen fand er die Ausscheidung von Katecholaminen normal, wenn sie nicht erregt waren. In der Manie war sie im Vergleich zur Depression und zur Norm erhöht. Ob diese Erhöhung nur mit der Erregung im Zusammenhang steht oder tiefere Beziehungen zur Genese des manischen Krankseins hat, bleibt zu prüfen. Bei seniler Demenz war die Ausscheidung von Adrenalin sehr niedrig. Bei Bergsman und bei Almeida findet sich auch eine große Literatur über die neueren Erfahrungen mit Katecholaminen, die in der Psychiatrie Bedeutung haben. Nach Giacobini u. Mitarb. ist die Ausscheidung von Adrenalin und Noradrenalin bei Delirium tremens stark erhöht, nach Prilenski ist Adrenalin im Blut sogar bei toxischen delirienartigen Zuständen bei Tieren erhöht.

Schon in früheren Jahren ist eingehend untersucht worden, ob sich die Wirkung des Elektroschocks und der Insulinschockbehandlung bei endogenen Psychosen endokrinologisch erklären lasse. Die Folgen dieser Behandlungen auf das Endokrinium erwiesen sich aber nicht als derart wesentlich, daß sich die therapeutische Wirkung daraus hätte ableiten können. (Nur wenige Forscher glauben heute das Gegenteil.) In den letzten Jahren sind zahlreiche entsprechende Untersuchungen in bezug auf *die Wirkung der neuen psychisch aktiven Medikamente* vorgenommen worden, ebenfalls ohne daß eine allgemein anerkannte endokrinologische Erklärung für diese Wirkung gefunden worden wäre. Die bedeutungsvollsten Ergebnisse beziehen sich auf die gegenteilige Wirkung von Serpasil einerseits, von Iproniazid und ähnlichen Stoffen anderseits auf den Gehalt an 5-Hydroxytryptamin und Katecholaminen im Stammhirn. Die hemmende Wirkung des Serpasils und die erregende des Iproniazids und anderer Aminooxydasehemmern ist vielleicht mit ihren gegenteiligen Wirkungen auf diese Hirnamine zu erklären. Interessant sind Versuche, die Therapie von Psychosen durch die Bestimmung der Abbauprodukte des 5-Hydroxytryptamins (nämlich der 5-Hydroxy-Essigsäure) im Urin zu lenken (Ljungberg). Je nach den Befunden wären Medikamente zu verabreichen, die auf- oder abbauend auf das 5-Hydroxytryptamin wirkten. Vorläufig liegen aber erst ungenügende Erfahrungen über die klinische Bedeutung einer solchen Verfeinerung der pharmakotherapeutischen Indikationsstellung vor. Sie muß erst vielseitiger erprobt werden, bevor sie endgültig zu beurteilen ist.

Im übrigen wird auf die endokrinologische Bedeutung der neuroleptischen Mittel in einem Sonderabsatz eingegangen (s. S. 234ff.).

Zusammenfassend kann festgestellt werden, daß keineswegs eine spezifische endokrine Wirkung der Neuroleptica bewiesen worden ist, die ihre therapeutische Wirkung auf eine bestimmte Psychose erklären könnte. Wahrscheinlich bleibt nur die Annahme, daß diese Medikamente durch eine allgemeine Beruhigung oder Erregung indirekt auf mannigfaches psychotisches Geschehen einwirken und daß diese allgemeine Beruhigung oder Erregung etwas mit dem Stoffwechsel von 5-Hydroxytryptamin und Katecholaminen im Hirn zu tun hat.

IV. Endokrine Störungen und psychologisch verständliche krankhafte Reaktionen und Entwicklungen

Die häufigsten Wesensänderungen bei schweren endokrinen Krankheiten, wie sie unter dem Überbegriff des *endokrinen Psychosyndroms* bereits zusammengefaßt worden sind, werden von einigen Autoren als einfache psychische Reaktionen auf körperliche Leiden und Entstellungen aufgefaßt: Depressionen beim Cushing-Syndrom z. B. wären nur die Folge der kosmetischen Entstellung; der Verlust der Psychosexualität beim männlichen Kastraten wäre die Folge von Minderwertigkeitsgefühlen; Oestrogene könnten sich höchstens dadurch auf das sexuelle Empfinden auswirken, daß sie die Sekretion der Vaginalschleimhaut sicherten usw. Diese Autoren bestreiten eine direkte Wirkung endokriner Störungen auf die psychischen Lebensvorgänge. In einzelnen Fällen läßt sich gewiß darüber streiten, ob eine Wesensänderung psychogen oder stoffwechselpathologisch zu erklären ist; wenn man aber ein größeres Erfahrungsgut der endokrinologischen Psychiatrie übersieht, wird man direkte Wirkungen des krankhaften Stoffwechsels auf die Psyche nicht übersehen können. Ich möchte hier nur die folgenden unwiderlegten Argumente anführen: Erscheinungen im Rahmen des endokrinen Psychosyndroms lassen sich oft schon bei endokrinen Krankheiten beobachten, die keine kosmetischen Folgen haben und unter denen der Kranke subjektiv kaum leidet; sie gehen z. B. manchmal quälenden körperlichen Erscheinungen voraus[1]. — Das endokrine Psychosyndrom ist den psychischen Erscheinungen bei Hirnkrankheiten wesensähnlich; dagegen sind seine Symptome gewöhnlich elementarer und undifferenzierter als psychische Reaktionen auf körperliches Leiden. Ungünstige reaktive Entwicklungen auf Entstellungen durch Kriegsverletzungen, durch häßliche Naevi oder auf langdauernde schmerzhafte Leiden oder auf uneheliche Mutterschaft z. B. sind, abgesehen von andern Unterschieden, vielfältiger, betreffen mehr persönliche, geistige und rein menschliche Belange. Elementare Störungen wie diejenigen von Hunger, Durst, Wärmebedürfnis usw., die im Rahmen des endokrinen Psychosyndroms so wichtig sind, spielen bei psychogenen Störungen eine geringere Rolle. Die Erscheinungen des endokrinen Psychosyndroms lassen sich wesensähnlich bei Mensch und Tier beobachten. — Bei Verabreichung von Hormonen in unphysiologischen Dosen aus therapeutischen Gründen beobachtet man häufig das Auftreten von psychischen Veränderungen im Rahmen des endokrinen Psychosyndroms, ohne daß sie im geringsten mit körperlichen Leiden in Zusammenhang gebracht werden könnten. Nach Absetzen der Hormontherapie verschwinden sie wieder.

Es läßt sich auch tierexperimentell und nicht nur klinisch beweisen, daß es eine direkte Hormonwirkung auf das Hirn und durch das Hirn auf die Triebe gibt. Die Behauptung, daß Hormone einzig sekundär über ihre Wirkung auf die peripheren Erfolgsorgane und das Erleben dieser Wirkung für die Triebhaftigkeit Bedeutung erhalten könnten, ist angesichts dieser Erfahrungen überholt: Schon ältere Untersuchungen zeigen, daß die Genitalorgane weiblicher Säugetiere für das Brunst-Verhalten nicht notwendig sind. Die Brunst tritt auch ein, wenn die äußeren Genitalien exstirpiert oder anästhesiert sind. — HARRIS und seine Mitarbeiter führten Oestrogene in das Hirn von kastrierten weiblichen Katzen ein. Mit kleinen Dosen wurde Brunstverhalten ausgelöst, wenn das Stilboestrol in den hinteren Teil des Hypothalamus eingelegt wurde. Es ließ sich sicher zeigen, daß das Brunstverhalten direkt von der Einwirkung des Hormons auf diese bestimmten Hirnkerne abhing und nicht etwa (wie früher vermutet worden wäre) von der oestrogenbedingten Veränderung der Genitalien. Brunstverhalten trat nämlich schon dann auf, wenn die in den Hypothalamus eingeführte Oestrogen-Menge zu klein gewesen war, um Veränderungen an Vagina und Uterus zu setzen.

Die Feststellung, daß das endokrine Psychosyndrom seiner Genese nach in der Hauptsache organischer Natur ist, schließt aber nicht aus, daß die endokrin ausgelösten elementaren emotionellen oder triebhaften Erschütterungen und die Verschiebung der nervösen Erregtheit *persönlich verarbeitet werden*. Im Gegenteil, diese persönliche Verarbeitung von emotionellen Erschütterungen ist bedeutsam. Sie ist z. B. offensichtlich bei der Steigerung der Sexualität älterer Frauen während der Behandlung des Mammacarcinoms mit hohen Dosen von Androgenen. Sie reizen elementar die Psychosexualität. Je nachdem, wie sich die Kranke per-

---

[1] Eigene Beobachtungen; BISHOP et al.; LINQUETTE et al. und viele andere.

sönlich dazu einstellt, führt die hormonale Triebaufpeitschung zu Gewissensbissen, zu verstärkten neurotischen Abschirmreaktionen, zu rein körperlich empfundenen genitalen Reizzuständen oder zu glückhaft empfundener Steigerung der erotischen Erlebnisfähigkeit. — Die Kastration des Mannes führt oft zu einem Verlust sexueller Triebhaftigkeit. Dieser Verlust kann als Verlust des Lebensinhaltes oder als Erlösung von einer quälenden Problematik empfunden werden. — Die endokrin bedingte Gleichmut macht den einen zum erbarmungswürdigen Invaliden, der nur noch zu vegetieren scheint und erhalten werden muß, den andern zum großen, verehrungswürdigen Weisen, der sich über die Kleinlichkeit des menschlichen Alltags hinaus zu höherer Geistigkeit erhoben hat[1].

Eine eindrucksvolle experimentelle Illustration zur Formbarkeit chemischer Einflüsse durch die momentanen Emotionen verdanken wir Ploog: Die Blutdruckwirkung des Sympatols hängt stark von der Stimmung ab, während der es verabreicht wird. Schon körperliche Wirkungen von Hormonen werden persönlich gestaltet. Dasselbe gilt für psychische Wirkungen in noch höherem Maße.

Oft hat man den Eindruck, daß die organisch bedingten psychischen Veränderungen in einer Art verarbeitet werden, die dem Kranken sein Leiden erträglich macht. Der Verlust der Sehkraft beim Akromegalen ist nichts Gräßliches mehr, wenn die Lust am Schauen verlorengeht; der Verlust körperlicher Sexualfunktionen ist gleichgültig, wenn die Psychosexualität erlöscht; körperlicher Infantilismus bedeutet dem Kranken keine Entstellung, wenn er sich als Kind erlebt.

Psychische Reaktionen auf die körperlichen Folgen endokriner Erkrankungen sind naturgemäß häufig zu beobachten. Das scheue und anschlußbedürftige Wesen von Kindern mit vorzeitiger Pubertät oder Pseudopubertät scheint z. B. weitgehend durch die grausame Haltung anderer Kinder und Erwachsener bedingt; diese nehmen ja dem Kinde die sexuelle Frühreife oft geradezu übel, als zeigte es damit eine schuldhafte sinnliche Lasterhaftigkeit.

Im Gegensatz zur psychischen Verarbeitung der elementaren, organischen Einflüsse auf die Psyche, im Gegensatz auch zu einfachen psychischen Reaktionen auf die endokrin bedingten körperlichen Leiden sind *neurotische Entwicklungen* von klinischer Bedeutsamkeit bei schweren endokrinen Krankheiten selten. Je schwerer die endokrine Krankheit, um so weniger beobachtet man neurotische Begleiterscheinungen. Dies gilt selbst in bezug auf Körperstörungen, von denen man meinen könnte, sie müßten psychologisch besonders traumatisierend sein und neurotische Entwicklungen fördern. Zum Beispiel zeigen Pseudohermaphroditen und Hermaphroditen, auch wenn gegensätzliche Geschlechtsmerkmale grob auffällig sind, keine Häufung von neurotischen Erkrankungen (und übrigens auch nicht von andern psychischen Störungen).

Viel eher als die großen endokrinen Erkrankungen bilden kleine konstitutionelle und endokrine Besonderheiten Dispositionen zu neurotischen Entwicklungen. Sie können das körperliche Spiegelbild von psychischen Ambitendenzen und Ambivalenzen bilden, in denen Neurosen verwurzelt sind. Hier sind z. B. Infantilismen in der körperlich-sexuellen Entwicklung bei sonst voll entwickelten Frauen zu erwähnen (Wolfgang Kretschmer) oder der Riesenwuchs bei körperlicher Schwäche (J. E. Staehelin). — Die Anorexia nervosa ist, wie man heute sicher weiß, nicht etwa eine Hypophysenerkrankung, sondern ein Symptom einer neurotischen Persönlichkeitsentwicklung. Gerade bei ihr aber findet man häufig körperliche Reifungsverspätungen (schon vor Beginn des Hungerns)[2]. Sie haben

---

[1] Andere Beispiele siehe bei Kind 1963.

[2] Gegenteilige Erfahrungen finden sich in einer Monographie von Thomä, die während der Drucklegung der vorliegenden Arbeit erschien. Der Widerspruch zu den Erfahrungen anderer Autoren bedarf der Klärung.

wahrscheinlich Beziehungen zum übersteigerten Wunsch dieser Kranken, Kind zu bleiben, die elterliche Familie in der alten Art zusammenzuhalten und das Frau-Werden zu verabscheuen. Wenn die Anorexia nervosa keinesfalls eine endokrine Erkrankung ist, so scheinen somit endokrine Besonderheiten, die ihr vorausgehen, doch eine disponierende Rolle zu spielen.

Die *Drang-, Trieb- und Impuls-Krankheiten* stellen Störungen dar, bei denen besonders oft, gleichzeitig und eng miteinander verflochten, endokrine Störungen und neurotische Entwicklungen gemeinsam beteiligt sind (BENEDETTI). Die mitbeteiligten endokrinen Störungen sind meistens leicht, der Art nach äußerst vielfältig (leichte Tetanien, leichte Hyperthyreosen, Pubertas tarda u. a.). Schon im letzten Jahrhundert ist ja der häufige zeitliche Zusammenhang solcher Erkrankungen mit den physiologischen endokrinen Umstellungsphasen aufgefallen (z. B. der Kleptomanie mit Menstruation und mit Schwangerschaft, der Poriomanie mit der Pubertät). Besonders italienische Forscher haben seit Jahrzehnten auf die kriminalistische Bedeutung endokriner Mitursachen bei trieb- und dranghaften Vergehen hingewiesen.

Auch bei *Alkoholikern* findet man häufig (bei etwa 30%) deutliche, aber meist nur leichte endokrine Störungen. Die häufigste derselben, die Hodenatrophie, ist freilich meist schon die Folge des Alkoholismus, wenn sie auch wiederum eine große psychologische Bedeutung bekommt und u. a. bei Eifersuchtszuständen eine Rolle spielt. Andere endokrine Besonderheiten aber, wie leichte Hyperthyreosen, leichte Hypothyreosen (GOLDBERG, ROYER), Diabetes oder Hypogonadismus leichten Grades, haben oft Bedeutung in der neurotischen Charakterentwicklung, die im Alkoholismus gipfelt. Unter anderem wirken viele Verstimmungen im Rahmen des endokrinen Psychosyndroms für den Alkoholismus prädisponierend (M. BLEULER 1955). Bei Alkoholikerinnen spielen oft prämenstruelle Spannungszustände und klimakterische Verstimmungen ursächlich mit.

Sind endokrine Erkrankungen selbst bloße Symptome einer neurotischen Persönlichkeitsentwicklung? Welche von ihnen können als „psychosomatische" Leiden bezeichnet werden, in dem einfachen Sinne, wonach sie emotionell verursacht würden? So vielerlei dogmatische Behauptungen zu dieser Problematik aufgestellt worden sind, so wenig zuverlässige Grundlagen haben wir noch zu ihrer endgültigen Klärung.

Sicher ist bloß, daß viele emotionelle Vorgänge in die endokrinen Funktionen eingreifen. Emotionelle Erregungen mancher Art führen zu einer Steigerung der Nebennierenmark- und -rinden-Funktion, bei gewissen Menschen auch zu einer solchen der Schilddrüsen-Funktion; sie können wahrscheinlich das Wachstum über Bremsung der somatotropen Hypophysenfunktion hindern u. ä. Es ist aber nicht gesichert, daß sich solche Vorgänge zu eigentlichen endokrinen Erkrankungen steigern. — Allbekannt ist die psychogene Amenorrhoe. Viele betrachten sie als ein typisches psychogenes endokrines Krankheitsbild unter der Annahme, daß von der Emotionalität und hirnphysiologischen Grundlagen derselben aus die gonadotrope Hypophysenfunktion (etwa zugunsten der adrenocorticotropen) gebremst würde. Dieser theoretisch naheliegende Zusammenhang ist in vielen Fällen auch erwiesen. (In anderen Fällen von psychogener Amenorrhoe läßt sich keine Verminderung der Gonadotropine nachweisen; sie können durch direkte nervöse Einflüsse auf die Durchblutung des Uterus oder durch beschleunigten Abbau der Oestrogene bedingt sein.)

Unter den großen endokrinen Erkrankungen ist es vor allem der Morbus Basedow, der von alters her oft und mit Überzeugung als emotionell bedingtes Leiden angesprochen wurde. In diesem Sinne spricht die Häufigkeit, mit der sich die Krankheit im Anschluß an Schreckerlebnisse einstellt oder verschlimmert. Die eingehende Psychotherapie bringt oft die Erkrankung wie ein neurotisches Symptom dem Verständnis näher. Und schließlich hat man versucht, die Psychogenese durch den Nachweis einer spezifischen psychotraumatischen Situation wahrscheinlich zu machen. Aus diesen und anderen Beobachtungen läßt sich aber eine einfache Psychogenese nicht beweisen. Wenn Hyperthyreose oft nach Schreck auftritt, so ist dem gegenüberzuhalten, daß die meisten schweren Schreckerlebnisse bei der Mehrzahl der Menschen nicht zum Morbus Basedow führen. Die psychologische Verstehbarkeit eines Symptoms beweist noch nicht seine Psychogenese. Die psychotraumatischen Situationen, die man bei der Entstehung der Krankheit aufgedeckt hat, betreffen eine allgemeine menschliche Problematik und können nicht als für die Krankheit spezifisch gedeutet werden. Schließlich ist zu bedenken, daß psychotherapeutische Beeinflussung des Morbus Basedow sicher in manchen Fällen Gutes leistet, daß aber doch die überwältigende Mehrzahl der Erkrankten mit einer vorwiegend körperlichen Behandlung geheilt werden kann. Sichergestellt sind nur emotionelle Einflüsse auf die Krankheit, eine rein emotionelle Genese der Krankheit ist aber unbewiesen und unwahrscheinlich. Ähnliches gilt für andere Erkrankungen, z. B. den Diabetes.

Ohne genügenden Grund wird die Psychogenese bei den einen endokrinen Erkrankungen immer wieder in den Vordergrund gestellt, bei andern aber überhaupt kaum diskutiert. Mit ähnlichem Recht oder Unrecht wie den Morbus Basedow könnte man z. B. einzelne Formen des Cushing-Syndroms oder der Akromegalie als emotionell bedingte Krankheiten ansprechen. — Es wird für die zukünftige Forschung nötig sein, daß wir Vorurteile und spekulative Annahmen über emotionelle Ursachen oder Mitursachen der endokrinen Krankheiten fallen lassen, daß wir uns der Unzulänglichkeit unseres Wissens bewußt werden und unvoreingenommener als bisher weiter beobachten.

Ein wichtiger Hinweis hat sich immerhin beim sorgfältigen Studium der individuellen Krankheitsverläufe heute schon ergeben: Je genauer wir die Korrelationen zwischen emotioneller und körperlicher Entwicklung bei endokrin Kranken beobachten, um so öfter werden wir vor der Frage kapitulieren müssen, ob die emotionellen Erschütterungen den endokrinen Krankheitsvorgängen vorausgegangen sind oder umgekehrt. Ganz gewöhnlich können wir ebensogut annehmen, die emotionelle Wallung sei die Folge eines abnormen endokrinen Ablaufes wie umgekehrt. In vielen Fällen fehlen uns letzten Endes alle und jede Kriterien, um diese Alternative zu entscheiden. Ist wohl die Frage falsch gestellt? Ist es zu naiv zu fragen, ob die emotionelle Schädigung die körperliche trage oder umgekehrt oder wie beide zusammenwirkten? Tatsächlich scheinen beide vielfach einem und demselben Lebensvorgang zu entsprechen. Der klinische Forscher kommt dabei zu Problemstellungen, die auch von philosophischer Seite nahegelegt und neu formuliert werden.

V. Endokrine Funktion und normales psychisches Leben

Emotionelle Einflüsse auf endokrine Funktionen beim Gesunden sind gesichert; umgekehrt ist nur sicher, daß krankhafte Veränderungen der endokrinen Funktionen das gesunde psychische Leben stören; unbewiesen und fraglich ist es hingegen, ob endokrinen Vorgängen innerhalb der Norm beim Menschen eine steuernde und regulierende Bedeutung auf das gesunde psychische Leben zukommt. — Im folgenden soll zuerst unser Wissen über emotionelle Einflüsse auf die endokrinen Funktionen innerhalb der Norm dargestellt werden; nachher gehe ich auf die wichtigsten Vermutungen über endokrine Steuerung gesunder Emotionen ein.

Unter den *emotionellen Einflüssen auf endokrine Funktionen* beim Gesunden sind in den letzten Jahren vor allem diejenigen auf die *Nebennierenrinde* vielfach untersucht worden. Funktionssteigerungen der Nebennierenrinde unter psychischem „Stress" sind heute sichergestellt. Die älteren Arbeiten hatten sie meist nur am Absinken der Zahl der Eosinophilen im Blut nachzuweisen versucht. Heute ist dieser Nachweis auch mit zuverlässigeren Methoden gelungen, u. a. mit der Bestimmung der 17-Hydroxycorticosteroide im Blut und Urin (BLISS et al., FRANKSSON et al. 1954 und 1955; HETZEL et al. 1954 und 1955; HOWARD et al.; THORN et al. u. a.).

Die allerverschiedensten psychischen Belastungen aktivieren die Nebennierenrinde: Kampferlebnisse von Soldaten (HOWARD et al.), Beängstigung eines Anstaltspsychiaters durch die Selbstgefährlichkeit seines Kranken (HETZEL et al. 1955), Freude eines Forschers über die Fortschritte seiner Arbeiten (HETZEL et al. 1955), Spannung vor dem Absprung mit dem Fallschirm (BASOWITZ et al.), Erregung der Angehörigen von Verunfallten (BLISS et al.), Examens-Anstrengungen von Studenten (BLISS et al.), emotionelle Wallungen während der Psychotherapie beim Patienten und seinem Therapeuten (BLISS et al., ELMADJIAN et al. 1958), Angst vor bevorstehenden Operationen (FRANKSSON et al. 1954 und 1955)[1]. In quantitativer Hinsicht ist die Steigerung des 17-Hydroxysteroid-Spiegels im Blut nach psychischer Stress-Wirkung nicht so stark ausgeprägt wie unter vielen pathologischen Umständen. — Von einem Individuum zum andern ergeben sich erhebliche Unterschiede in der Reaktion der Nebennierenrinde auf Stress.

Unter allen psychischen Stresswirkungen ist die Wirkung der Angst am eingehendsten untersucht worden. Eine Beziehung zwischen gesteigerter Angst und erhöhter Sekretion von Glucocorticoiden, gemessen am Hydrocortison (Cortisol) im Blutplasma, ist erwiesen. Die Angst wirkt sich (ausschließlich oder teilweise) über die Hypophyse, durch Vermehrung der Sekretion von adrenocorticotropem Hormon, auf die Nebennierenrinde aus. Eine genauere Korrelation zwischen dem Grade der Angst und Adrenocorticotropin im Blut findet sich freilich nur bei Zuständen höchster Angst und nicht bei alltäglicher Angst. Auch gibt es Zustände von sehr stark erhöhtem Adrenocorticotropin im Blut, ohne daß sie mit der Angst verbunden wären. (Literaturübersicht bei HAMBURG; PERSKY et al.)

Bereits ist auch versucht worden, verschiedenerlei Emotionen in ihrer Wirkung auf die Nebennierenrindenfunktion zu differenzieren (KORCHIN et al.). Wesentliche Unterschiede in der Reaktion der Nebennierenrinde bei verschiedenen Qualitäten von Gefühlswallungen sind bisher aber nicht aufgedeckt worden.

In einer Untersuchungsreihe von FOX et al. hatten Gesunde mit starken emotionellen Reaktionen (und entsprechend vielen Farb-Antworten im Rorschach-Versuch) eine vermehrte Ausscheidung von 17-Ketosteroiden und 17-Hydroxycorticoiden gegenüber Gesunden mit nivellierteren emotionellen Reaktionen[2].

Neuerdings ergeben viele Untersuchungen, daß in der Angst auch die Mineralocorticoide (d. h. Aldosteron und Desoxycorticosteron) vermehrt ausgeschieden werden können. Während Angstzuständen von Gesunden, Neurotikern und Schizophrenen wurde vermehrte Aldosteron-Ausscheidung gefunden (Literatur bei HOAGLAND). Patienten mit chronischer Asthenie und kampferschöpfte Soldaten (im Korea-Krieg) zeigten auf die Verabreichung von adrenocorticotropem Hormon

---

[1] Allerdings gibt es auch Ausnahmen von der Regel: in vereinzelten Fällen wurde unter psychischem Stress Dämpfung statt Anregung der Nebennieren-Rinden-Funktion festgestellt (SCHWARTZ u. SHIELDS).

[2] Lärmstimulation erhöht beim Gesunden den Spiegel von Hydroxycorticoiden im Blut und die Ausscheidung von 17-Hydroxycorticoiden im Urin. Die Erhöhung ist bei ängstlichen Neurotikern stärker ausgeprät gals bei Gesunden, bei Depressiven weniger ausgeprägt (ARGUEELLES, A. E. et al.).

Zeichen einer Vermehrung der Mineralocorticoide (Albeaux-Fernet et al., Pace et al.). Es ergibt sich die Vermutung, daß die Nebennierenrinde zwar auf kurzdauernde Stress-Wirkung vor allem mit der Mehrausscheidung von Glucocorticoiden (Cortison) antwortet, nach langer Stress-Wirkung hingegen würde sie vor allem Mineralocorticoide erzeugen (Elmadjian noch unpubliziert, Hoagland).

Die Wirkung von psychischem „Stress" auf die Nebennierenrinde ist individuellen Schwankungen unterworfen. Sie ist auch in verschiedenen Altersklassen verschieden.

Psychischer „Stress" kann wahrscheinlich bei bestimmten Menschen auch die *Schilddrüsenfunktion* innerhalb der Norm anregen (Hetzel et al. 1955). Bei vielen Gesunden aber ist keine Veränderung der Schilddrüsenfunktion unter psychischem Stress nachweisbar — wenigstens nicht durch Veränderungen im eiweißgebundenen Serum-Jod und auch nicht bei Untersuchungen mit radioaktivem Jod (Dongier, Volpe).

Dank der Arbeiten von Cannon ist seit 30 Jahren bekannt, daß bei Tieren die *Ausschüttung von Adrenalin* Angst und andere Emotionen begleitet. Bei Menschen liegen entsprechende Befunde vor. Zum Beispiel stieg die Adrenalin-Ausscheidung mit dem Aufkommen von Angst bei Versuchspersonen, die bei beschränkter Bewegungsfreiheit in Dunkelheit in einem Respirator lagen (Mendelson u. Mitarb.). Neuerdings wurde der Gehalt an Adrenalin und Noradrenalin im Blut von Menschen mit verbesserten Methoden gemessen (Weil-Malherbe 1955a und b). Der Gehalt von Adrenalin (und in geringerem Maße von Noradrenalin) kann mit dem Grad des Wachseins und der psychischen Aktivität in quantitative Beziehung gebracht werden. Dazu paßt die Entdeckung, wonach Adrenalin die "arousal reaction" fördert (s. S. 177). Einige Befunde sprechen für die Annahme, daß hilflose Angst vor allem mit Adrenalin-Ausschüttung, Angriffslust, Kampfwut und Zorn hingegen eher mit Noradrenalin-Ausschüttung verbunden wären (Funkenstein; Hawkins et al.; Hoagland; Silverman and Cohen).

O. Diethelm und seine Mitarbeiter (1945, 1950, 1963 und Fleetwood und Diethelm) konnten Stoffe mit ähnlichen physiologischen Eigenschaften wie Noradrenalin, Acetylcholin und Bradykinin in bestimmten Stimmungslagen (ängstlichen, gereizten oder ressentiment-geladenen) im Blutserum erhöht finden.

Untersuchungen von H. G. Wolff u. Mitarb. legen eine neue interessante Hypothese über bisher unbekannte *humorale Vorgänge bei psychischer Erwartungsspannung und Anstrengung* nahe: Bei Gefäßerweiterung wurde in perivasculären Geweben ein Polypeptid (und ein bei seinem Aufbau beteiligtes Enzym) gefunden, das *Neurokinin* genannt wurde. Es läßt das isolierte Duodenum von Ratten erschlaffen, den isolierten Uterus kontrahieren und setzt im Rattenversuch den Blutdruck hinauf. Es ist dem seit längerer Zeit bekannten und als Gewebehormon angesprochenen Bradykinin ähnlich. Nach der Hypothese von Wolff und seinen Mitarbeitern wird Neurokinin zum Zwecke der Steigerung der Durchblutung des Nervensystems bei psychischer Anstrengung gebildet. Es erweitert intra- und extrakraniale Blutgefäße am Kopf und macht gleichzeitig die perivasculären Gewebe schmerzempfindlicher. Seine übermäßige Ausscheidung bei ängstlicher Anspannung würde über Gefäßerweiterung und Sensibilisierung der perivasculären Gewebe Migräne auslösen (Chapman et al.; Chapman und Wolff).

Emotionelle Spannungen können wahrscheinlich das Wachstum verzögern, vermutlich durch Bremsung der Sekretion des Wuchshormons (Binning; Fried et al.; Talbot et al.; Widdowson; u. a.).

Die psychogene Amenorrhoe und andere psychogene Zyklusstörungen zeigen offensichtlich, daß von der Emotionalität aus auch das *menstruelle Zyklusgeschehen* beeinflußt, häufig gebremst, werden kann. Es erfolgt das auf mannigfache Art:

über die verminderte Bildung von Gonadotropinen und Oestrogenen, über Beschleunigung des Oestrogen-Abbaus und über das vegetative Nervensystem. Dementsprechend gibt es psychische Amenorrhoe mit gesteigerter, normaler oder verminderter Gonadotropin-Bildung.

Schwerer und langdauernder „Stress" hemmt ganz allgemein neben dem Sexualtrieb auch die *endokrinen Funktionen der Gonaden*; die psychogene Amenorrhoe ist nur die am leichtesten erkennbare Äußerung dieser allgemeinen Gesetzmäßigkeit. So bremst Terror bei unterdrückten Bevölkerungen und in Gefangenenlagern gewöhnlich zuerst die Psychosexualität, dann auch die endokrinen Sexualfunktionen und führt sogar zu Atrophie der Hoden und Ovarien (VON KRESS, STIEVE u. a.).

Anstrengung, Schmerz und viele Emotionen sind mit vermehrter Ausschüttung von *antidiuretischem Hormon* und Hemmung der Diurese begleitet; Mittel, die den Schmerz bekämpfen, wirken umgekehrt.

Alle diese und noch andere hormonale Vorgänge innerhalb der Norm sind möglicherweise nicht nur die Folge von emotionellen Wallungen, sondern könnten vielleicht umgekehrt auch ihre Rückwirkungen auf die Emotionalität haben. Wahrscheinlich entsprechen emotionelle und endokrine Schwankungen oft auch einem einheitlichen Lebensvorgang, der auf eine bestimmte Leistung gerichtet ist, z. B. einer allgemeinen ergotropen oder trophotropen Schaltung im Sinne von W. R. HESS; es wäre dann nicht der emotionelle Vorgang oder der hormonale die Voraussetzung des andern, sondern beide Zeichen derselben Lebensregung. Darüber wissen wir aber noch nichts Sicheres.

Aus der erwiesenen Wirkung vieler krankhafter endokriner Vorgänge auf das psychische Leben *hat man zu leicht geschlossen, daß auch beim Gesunden hormonale Einflüsse viele psychische Funktionen steuerten.* Diese Annahme ist aber noch unsicher. Es läßt sich auch die Möglichkeit denken, daß es endokriner Veränderungen krankhafter Art bedarf, um irgendwelche endokrine Einflüsse auf die Psyche geltend zu machen, während das psychische Leben des gesunden Menschen aber den endokrinen Schaltungen ganz oder weitgehend entzogen wäre. Gesundes psychisches Leben hätte dann zwar gesunde endokrine Funktionen zur Voraussetzung, beim endokrin gesunden Menschen aber wäre es von physiologischen Schwankungen des Hormon-Spiegels unabhängig.

Man hat vor allem Beobachtungen über die Psychologie der physiologischen großen endokrinen Umstellungsphasen (Pubertät, Schwangerschaft, Wochenbett, Menstruationszyklus, Klimakterium) herangezogen, um hormonale Einflüsse auf die Psyche des Gesunden geltend zu machen. Tatsächlich erlauben unsere Kenntnisse darüber aber erst Vermutungen und nicht sichere Aussagen. Unbestritten ist, daß in zeitlichem Zusammenhang mit diesen Umstellungsphasen eine gesteigerte Verstimmbarkeit, Veränderungen der Grundstimmung und der Aktivität, Steigerungen oder Verminderungen von Schlafbedürfnis, Durst, Hunger, Sexualität und andern Trieben oder sonderbare Gelüste auftreten können[1]. Es lag nahe, ihre Ursache in den gewaltigen Umstellungen des Hormongleichgewichtes während dieser Phasen zu suchen. Das Kausalitätsverhältnis ist jedoch nicht einfach und eindeutig. Bisher fehlt der Nachweis, daß die hormonalen Umstellungen bei Menschen, die emotionelle Änderungen in den Umstellungsphasen zeigen, anders verlaufen als bei solchen, die die Umstellungsphase psychisch unberührt durchleben. Frauen im Klimakterium z. B. zeigen — soweit man bis heute weiß — dieselbe hormonale klimakterische Umstellung, ob sie an psychischen Beschwerden leiden

---

[1] Moderne genaue Untersuchungen über Verhaltensänderungen während der Menstruation sind z. B. diejenigen von KATHARINA DALTON: Schülerinnen ziehen sich disziplinarische Beanstandungen während der Menstruation öfters zu als sonst.

oder nicht. Entsprechend ist bei Frauen mit prämenstruellen Spannungserscheinungen keineswegs immer ein anderer Verlauf des hormonalen Zyklus bewiesen als bei solchen, die prämenstruell beschwerdelos sind. Allerdings kommt bei prämenstrueller Spannung Unterfunktion des Ovars oft vor — doch ist umgekehrt Unterfunktion des Ovars gewöhnlich nicht mit prämenstrueller Spannung verbunden. Bei der Entstehung emotioneller Störungen in den Umstellungsphasen kann es sich demnach kaum um einfache und obligatorische Wirkungen bestimmter physiologischer Hormonkonstellationen auf jede Persönlichkeit handeln. Eher prädisponiert die hormonale Umstellungsphase bloß zu übersteigerten Reaktionen auf innere oder soziale Konfliktsituationen. — Klimakterische und prämenstruelle emotionelle Störungen können zwar durch hormonale Behandlungen oft günstig beeinflußt werden. Damit ist aber nicht bewiesen, daß sie ganz einfach durch einen substituierbaren Hormonmangel bedingt wären. Trotz dieser therapeutischen Erfahrungen können die genetischen Zusammenhänge vielfältiger sein.

Viel diskutiert wird die Frage über den *Zusammenhang psychischer Sexualität mit endokrinen Funktionen*. Zu dieser Diskussion stehen bis heute nur wenig Erfahrungen an Gesunden zur Verfügung. Sie muß sich weitgehend auf Rückschlüsse aus der Pathologie stützen. Die Darstellung der Problematik erfolgt deshalb im Anschluß an die Kapitel über die Psychopathologie der sexuellen Endokrinopathien auf S. 228 ff.

Sicher steht fest, daß die endokrinen Funktionen beim Gesunden eine große *individuelle Variationsbreite* haben. Die „biochemische Individualität" im allgemeinen schließt eine „*endokrine Individualität*" im besonderen in sich (Williams). Soweit man Zusammenhänge zwischen emotionellen und endokrinen Lebensvorgängen innerhalb der Norm gefunden oder vermutet hat, sind diese Zusammenhänge nicht bei allen Menschen gleichartig; sie stehen oft im Zeichen der Einmaligkeit jeder Persönlichkeit.

VI. Konstitution und Endokrinopathie

Vor einigen Jahrzehnten, vor allem in der Zeit zwischen den beiden Weltkriegen, spielte in der Psychiatrie wie in der inneren Medizin die Vorstellung eine Rolle, daß gewisse körperliche und psychische Konstitutionstypen endokrin bedingt seien. Man nahm an, sie entsprächen Über- und Unterfunktionszuständen von endokrinen Drüsen, die denjenigen bei den bekannten endokrinen Krankheiten wesensähnlich wären. Man sprach z. B. viel von hypothyreoter, thyreotoxischer, akromegaloider oder später auch von Morbus Cushing-ähnlicher Konstitution. Vermutungen gingen sogar dahin, daß sich die konstitutionelle Eigenheit eines Menschen in einer Formel über die Verteilung der verschiedenen Hormone ausdrücken ließe.

In den letzten Jahren sind keine wesentlichen Fortschritte in der wissenschaftlichen Untermauerung der meisten dieser Ansichten erzielt worden. Der Zusammenhang vieler der früher als „dyskrin" angesprochenen Konstitutionsbesonderheiten mit endokrinen Funktionen hat sich bisher dem Nachweis mit den modernen Laboratoriumsmethoden entzogen. Dabei ist allerdings zu sagen, daß nicht allzu viel Mühe dazu verwendet worden ist, diese Methoden zur Klärung von Konstitutionsbesonderheiten anzuwenden.

Die heute in der Endokrinologie vorherrschenden Richtungen (ganz besonders die amerikanischen) sind der Annahme von endokrin bedingten Konstitutionstypen gegenüber streng und kritisch geworden. Sie wollen sich kaum mehr mit ihnen beschäftigen und beschränken sich auf Krankheiten, bei denen Laboratoriumsuntersuchungen Störungen im Hormonhaushalt und Stoffwechsel zeigen.

Es ist bemühend festzustellen, wie sich der Sprachgebrauch umgekehrt hat: Eine
Zeitlang galt oft „konstitutionell" und „von Kindheit an endokrin verwurzelt"
als fast gleichbedeutend; viele moderne Endokrinologen hingegen gebrauchen den
Ausdruck „konstitutionell" im Gegenteil dann, wenn sie von einer Eigenart aussagen wollen, sie sei *nicht* endokrin bedingt und gehe sie nichts an. Beide Auffassungen sind dogmatisch und nicht naturwissenschaftlich begründet. Es ist
ebenso falsch anzunehmen, eine Eigenart sei endokrin verwurzelt, weil sie als
konstitutionell betrachtet wird, wie das Umgekehrte: eine Eigenschaft könne
nicht endokrin verwurzelt sein, weil sie einen Aspekt der Konstitution bildete.
Eine konstitutionelle Besonderheit kann eben endokrin verwurzelt sein oder nicht
und umgekehrt. Bei konstitutionellen Besonderheiten, die Veränderungen bei
erworbenen endokrinen Krankheiten ähnlich sehen, ist die Frage der endokrinen
Genese sorgfältig zu überprüfen und diese Genese nicht einfach zu behaupten oder
zu leugnen. Diese Aufgabe wurde sowohl von der alten wie von der modernen
Endokrinologie arg vernachlässigt.

Sicher bedeutet es einen großen Verdienst der modernen Endokrinologie, daß
sie das Verfehlte vieler Vorstellungen der älteren psychiatrischen Konstitutionslehre an den Pranger stellte. Sie hat z. B. mit Recht mit der früher geläufigen Vorstellung aufgeräumt, daß es häufige Formen von Fett- und Magersucht gäbe, die
hypophysär bedingt wären, oder daß man nur die Fettverteilung richtig ins Auge
fassen müsse, um die Diagnose einer „hypophysären Fettsucht" zu stellen. (Eine
hypophysäre Fettsucht gibt es gar nicht.)

Wahrscheinlich ist es aber doch nicht immer richtig, wenn heute bei angeborenen Eigenheiten die Beziehungen zu endokrinen Funktionen zum vornherein abgelehnt werden. Die meisten heutigen Lehrbücher der Endokrinologie betonen
z. B., daß die gewöhnliche Form des Hirsutismus der Frau, der „idiopathische
Hirsutismus", mit endokrinen Funktionen nichts zu tun hätte. Sie gehen dabei
aber an Beobachtungen, die für das Gegenteil sprechen, vorbei, z. B. an derjenigen,
daß bei Inzucht von Familien, in denen sich Hirsutismus bei Frauen häuft, schwere
Formen von Intersexualität beschrieben sind (BOSIA). Die akromegaloide
Körperkonstitution ist bei Tieren in deutliche Beziehung zur Hypophyse gebracht
worden (STOCKARD), so daß entsprechende Vermutungen beim Menschen berechtigt sind.

Wenn wenig Fortschritte darin erzielt worden sind, die Bedeutung endokriner
Besonderheiten für die als „dyskrin" vermuteten Konstitutionstypen wirklich zu
beweisen, so sind wenigstens neue Erfahrungen über den Zusammenhang von
„dyskrinen" Körperbautypen (Akromegaloid, Infantilismus, Maskulinismus) mit
Persönlichkeitseigenarten und der Disposition zu psychischen Erkrankungen gesammelt worden. Sie haben ihre Bedeutung schon unabhängig von der Frage, ob diese
Körperbautypen von den endokrinen Funktionen abhängen.

Die *akromegaloide Körperkonstitution* kennzeichnet sich durch gleichgerichtete
Vergrößerungen peripherer Körperteile wie bei Akromegalie, vor allem durch die
Größe von Nase, Ohren, Händen und Füßen. Sie kann sich in der Pubertät, in der
Schwangerschaft und im Klimakterium verdeutlichen, ist im übrigen aber nicht
progressiv. Im Gegensatz zur Akromegalie tritt die akromegaloide Körperkon-
stitution familiär auf. Bedeutsam ist nun die Feststellung, daß in den Familien
Akromegaloider eigenartige und psychopathische Persönlichkeitsentwicklungen
einerseits und Akromegaloid andrerseits korreliert sind. (Mit anderen Worten: Die
akromegaloiden Verwandten eines akromegaloiden Psychopathen sind häufiger
psychopathisch als seine körperlich unauffälligen Verwandten und umgekehrt.)
Es handelt sich nicht um eine absolute, aber um eine weitgehende Korrelation.
Akromegaloide zeigen oft langdauernde oder bleibende Verstimmungszustände,

besonders im Sinne einer unbeschwerten und verantwortungslosen Heiterkeit, in anderen Fällen aber auch anders gerichtete. Sie neigen weiter zu trieb- und dranghaften Ausnahmezuständen, z. B. zu poriomanen oder dipsomanen Episoden, zu Perioden hemmungslosen sexuellen Auslebens oder zu schlafsüchtigen und apathischen vorübergehenden Zuständen. Es handelt sich demnach um Störungen, die erscheinungsbildlich zum endokrinen Psychosyndrom passen. — Unter den akromegaloiden Verwandten von akromegaloiden Schizophrenen ist die Schizophrenie häufiger als unter ihren nicht-akromegaloiden Verwandten. In den Familien, in denen Akromegaloid und Schizophrenie vorkommen, besteht also irgendeine genetische Beziehung zwischen Konstitutionsbesonderheit und Psychose. Selbstverständlich darf diese Beobachtung in den Familien Schizophrener mit Akromegaloid nicht verallgemeinert werden; nichts spricht dafür, daß Akromegaloid oder das Wuchshormon mit der Genese der Mehrzahl der Schizophrenien das Geringste zu tun haben könnten. Wir stehen vielmehr vor einem Beispiel dafür, daß in einzelnen Familien konstitutionelle Einflüsse auf das schizophrene Geschehen anzunehmen sind, die bei den meisten anderen schizophrenen Erkrankungen nicht in Frage stehen. — Verlauf und Symptomgestaltung schizophrener Psychosen bei Akromegaloiden sind im Durchschnitt von denjenigen bei der Mehrzahl der Schizophrenien verschieden (Bleuler, M., 1948a und c; Fleisch; Hofmann; Knoepfel a und b; Seiler; Sorg; Sulzer; Wander-Voegelin; Wolf 1946; Züblin 1948).

Unter den Verwandten von Menschen mit *infantiler Körperkonstitution* besteht eine deutliche Korrelation zwischen körperlichem Infantilismus einerseits, psychischem Infantilismus und leichtem Schwachsinn andrerseits. — Schizophrenien bei infantilem Körperbau sahen wir manchmal in akuten Episoden verlaufen und günstig ausgehen (Barich; Bleuler, M., 1948b; v. Brunn; Furger, 1963; Jacobs).

Maskuline Stigmatisierung ist bei schizophrenen Frauen häufiger als in der Durchschnittsbevölkerung. Schizophrenien bei maskulinen Frauen neigen zu akuten und schweren Verläufen (Baer; Bleuler, M., 1948c; Bosia; Kaufmann; Pedersen 1947; Stockmann; Wolf 1946 und 1948).

Als „gewöhnlichen“, „genuinen“ oder „idiopathischen“ *Hirsutismus* bezeichnet man eine maskuline Behaarung der Frau, die sich nicht als Symptom einer bestimmten Krankheit deuten läßt. Maskulin behaart ist neben dem Gesicht meist der ganze Körper. Verschiedenartige Menstruationsstörungen können dazu kommen. Andere maskuline Zeichen als der Hirsutismus fehlen. Die Eigenart ist häufig, vor allem bei schwarzhaarigen Frauen. Sie tritt oft familiär auf.

Viele Endokrinologen hielten die Eigenart bisher für eine konstitutionelle Überempfindlichkeit der Haarfollikel auf Androgene und bestritten endokrine Störungen. In den letzten Jahren häufen sich aber doch die Befunde, wonach die Androgenbildung in der Nebennierenrinde (weniger wahrscheinlich im Ovar) vermehrt und verändert ist. Nach den Untersuchungen von A. E. Meyer und seinen Mitarbeitern kann die Ursache der vermehrten Androgenbildung nicht dieselbe sein wie beim adrenogenitalen Syndrom, weil Zeichen einer gestörten Cortisol-Synthese fehlen. (Allerdings gibt es leichte Fälle von adrenogenitalem Syndrom, die sich äußerlich vom gewöhnlichen Hirsutismus nicht unterscheiden.)

Deutliche Zeichen eines endokrinen Psychosyndroms wurden beim gewöhnlichen Hirsutismus nicht gefunden. Homosexualität wird nur ausnahmsweise beobachtet. Dagegen finden sich oft neurotische Entwicklungen, die meist schon vor Beginn des Hirsutismus begonnen haben. Diese neurotischen Entwicklungen verstärken sich unter dem Eindruck des Hirsutismus: die Kranken fürchten sich, nicht anerkannt, verspottet und verachtet zu werden; oft versuchen sie, nicht

nur den abnormen Haarwuchs, sondern sich selbst zu verstecken. Es entsteht leicht
Schüchternheit, depressive Verstimmung und Unsicherheit über die eigene Geschlechtsrolle. Vorbestandene Wünsche nach Vermännlichung können verstärkt
werden (JAYLE et al.; A. E. MEYER und von ZERSSEN, 1960a und b; VON ZERRSEN,
1960; VON ZERSSEN et al.).

A. E. MEYER, der der Besonderheit eine eingehende Studie gewidmet hat, stellte fest, daß
beim Auftreten des Hirsutismus häufig infolge der vorbestehenden neurotischen Entwicklung
und ungünstiger Lebensumstände ein großer „Leidensdruck" besteht. Dies trifft vor allem für
die sporadischen, weniger für die familiär gehäuften Fälle zu. MEYER schließt aus seinen Untersuchungen auf einen „androgen betonten Hypercorticismus". Bei starker Expressivität der
Anlage würde die Depression schon familiär gehäuft und ohne starke emotionelle Stress-
Situation manifest; bei geringer Expressivität der Anlage dagegen käme es erst unter einem
besonders starken Leidensdruck zur Ausbildung des Hirsutismus.

VII. Spezielle Psychiatrie bei einzelnen endokrinen Funktionsstörungen

Es kann sich nicht darum handeln, in dem mir zur Verfügung stehenden Raum
unser gesamtes Wissen über die spezielle Psychiatrie bei allen endokrinen Funktionsstörungen abzuhandeln. Dazu wäre heute ein Band von mindestens 1000
Seiten notwendig. In der vorliegenden Kurzdarstellung, zu der ich beauftragt bin,
habe ich nicht nur alles Unwesentliche auslassen müssen, sondern ich habe auch
darauf verzichtet, neu darzustellen, was schon in der Zeit vor dem letzten Weltkrieg bekannt geworden war. Der Zweck der Darstellung liegt darin, auf jene
wichtigeren Erkenntnisse hinzuweisen, die in den letzten 15 Jahren erworben
worden sind, und die aktuellen Forschungsprobleme kurz zu umschreiben. Auch
auf die Lücken unseres Wissens hinzuweisen, hielt ich für wichtig; sie sind oft
erschreckend. — Vorwiegend altes Wissen, das nicht mehr berücksichtigt wurde,
betrifft u. a. besonders die Schilddrüsen-Über- und -Unterfunktion, die Unterfunktion der Nebenschilddrüse und den Diabetes. Große Fortschritte unserer
Kenntnisse, die zu berücksichtigen waren, betreffen u. a. die Funktionen der
Nebenniere und der Gonaden, die Überfunktion der Nebenschilddrüse, die Akromegalie, den Panhypopituitarismus, die Folgen der therapeutischen Anwendung
von Corticoiden und von Sexualhormonen.

Die Überschriften sind im folgenden abgekürzt: Statt „Psychopathologie der Zustände bei
Überfunktion der Nebennierenrinde" z. B. heißt es bloß: „Überfunktion der Nebennierenrinde".

1. Überfunktion der Adenohypophyse

Akromegalie. Akromegale sind in den letzten Jahren in großer Anzahl psychiatrisch untersucht worden, so daß ihre Psychopathologie heute in der Hauptsache
geklärt ist (BLEULER, M., 1951; BLICKENSTORFER 1949, 1951, 1953, 1953/54;
BLICKENSTORFER et al.; HOHL-SPIESS; KELLER; SORG). Frühere Angaben, wonach
die Krankheit zu schizophrenen oder manisch-depressiven Psychosen führe, sind
höchstens für seltene Ausnahmefälle richtig. Alle untersuchten Akromegalen entwickelten im Laufe der Krankheit eine *Wesensänderung.* Sie kennzeichnet sich
vor allem durch eine veränderte Stimmungslage. Sie geht häufig in der Richtung
stiller und passiver Heiterkeit, doch kann die feinere Tönung verschieden sein,
z. B. im Sinne der Wehmut, der Resignation, der Gehässigkeit u. a. Differenziertere
Interessen und Tätigkeiten werden leicht zugunsten eines ruhigen, trägen Lebens
mit Freude am Essen aufgegeben. Die Sexualität erlischt langsam. Durst und
Hunger sind oft gesteigert. In einzelnen Fällen treten Zeichen einer elementaren
Mütterlichkeit auf, besonders bei Fällen, in denen Milchbildung außerhalb der

physiologischen Lactationsperioden darauf hindeutet, daß neben dem somatotropen auch das lactotrope Hormon im Übermaß gebildet wird. Besonders auffällig und krankhaft wirkte diese Mütterlichkeit bei Männern mit Milchbildung, die plötzlich Säuglinge umhegen, Windeln waschen und Kleinkinder adoptieren wollen. — Das gesamte psychische Tempo ist meist verlangsamt. — Zu diesem Bild treten vielfach vorübergehende Verstimmungen sowie vorübergehende Zustände von Drang- und Triebhaftigkeit.

Ein leichtes amnestisches Psychosyndrom ist in Fällen mit chronischem Hirndruck häufig.

Psychosen vom akuten exogenen Reaktionstypus treten heute viel seltener auf als früher; die radiologische und neurochirurgische Therapie vermag ihnen meist vorzubeugen.

Über die Psychopathologie des *hypophysären Riesenwuchses* wissen wir noch wenig. In einzelnen Fällen wurde eine ähnliche Wesensänderung beobachtet wie bei Akromegalie. Dazu gibt Riesenwuchs leicht zu ungünstigen psychoreaktiven Entwicklungen Anlaß (Staehelin, J. E.).

Gesteigerte Sekretion des lactotropen Hypophysenvorderlappen-Hormons, das zu Milchsekretion selbst bei Männern führt, kommt auch bei anderen Störungen als bei Akromegalie vor (bei Cushing-Syndrom, bei Chorionepitheliom). Mehrfach wurde dabei eine krankhafte Anregung von Mutterinstinkten beobachtet. Sie äußerte sich auch bei Männern in einem unbändigen Triebe, kleine Kinder zu pflegen. Die vorliegenden Beobachtungen zwingen zur Annahme, daß lactotropes Hormon bei Menschen unter pathologischen Voraussetzungen Muttertriebe auslösen kann, wie es beim Tier schon physiologischerweise Instinkte zur Pflege der Jungen wachruft (Bleuler, M., 1954; Blickenstorfer 1949; Blickenstorfer et al.; Schwöbel).

Im übrigen ist von einer *gesteigerten Sekretion der adenotropen Hypophysenvorderlappenhormone* (Gonadotropine, adrenocorticotropes und thyreotropes Hormon) keine psychopathologische Wirkung bekannt, die sich von den Wirkungen der Überfunktion der gesteuerten endokrinen Drüsen abheben ließe. Bei einer der ersten *Behandlungen mit menschlichem Wuchshormon*, die bisher durchgeführt wurden, ergab sich keine Wirkung des Hormons auf die intellektuelle und emotionelle Entwicklung (Escamilla u. Mitarb.)[1].— Auch über das *melanocytenstimulierende Hormon* und über die *Exophthalmus produzierende Substanz* kennen wir noch keine sicheren psychiatrischen Daten. Ihre Erforschung wird besonderes Interesse bieten.

2. Panhypopituitarismus

Der Ausfall des Hypophysenvorderlappens, der Panhypopituitarismus oder die Simmondssche Krankheit, schließt auch die meisten Fälle mit der älteren Krankheitsbezeichnung, der multiplen Blutdrüsensklerose nach Falta, in sich. Hervorgehoben werden muß aber, daß die Anorexia nervosa scharf vom Panhypopituitarismus abzutrennen ist. Es war ein verhängnisvoller Irrtum, die Anorexia nervosa auf eine primäre Hypophysenvorderlappeninsuffizienz zurückzuführen[2].

---

[1] Nach neuen Untersuchungen bewirkte Wuchshormon bei hypophysektomierten Frauen (unter Substitutionstherapie mit Cortison und Schilddrüsenhormon) neben Diabetes einen Vergiftungszustand mit Unwohlgefühl, Müdigkeit, „Nervosität", Schlaflosigkeit, Appetitlosigkeit und Tachykardie. Er heilte auf Erhöhung der Cortison-Dose. Vermutlich bestand die Vergiftung in einer Nebennieren-Insuffizienz (Ikkos und Luft).

[2] Allerdings sind endokrine Veränderungen bei Anorexia nervosa vorhanden, am häufigsten eine endokrine Unterfunktion der Ovarien. Sie ist oft — aber nicht immer — sekundär eine Folge von verminderter Gonadotropin-Ausscheidung, was u. a. daraus hervorgeht, daß die Ovarien auf die Verabreichung von gonadotropem Hormon ansprechbar bleiben (Johannis-

Die Aufklärung dieses Irrtums ist vor allem das Verdienst von SHEEHAN (SCHUEP-BACH; SHEEHAN; SHEEHAN et al.). Während die innere Medizin seit mehreren Jahren die Anorexia nervosa nicht mehr als endokrine Krankheit anerkennt, wirkt sich im psychiatrischen Schrifttum die ältere fehlerhafte Auffassung der Internisten immer noch verwirrend aus.

Unsere Kenntnisse über die Psychopathologie des Panhypopituitarismus verdanken wir vor allem einer monographischen Bearbeitung von HANS KIND (1958).

Die psychiatrische Bedeutung der schweren, progressiven Formen ist groß. Die überwältigende Mehrzahl der Kranken mit Panhypopituitarismus erleidet psychische Veränderungen. Ohne Substitutionsbehandlung werden sie im Laufe der Jahre sehr hochgradig. Ihre Art und ihre Schwere lassen deutliche Beziehungen zur Dauer der Erkrankung und zur prämorbiden Persönlichkeit erkennen.

Die psychische Wesensveränderung, die sich fast regelmäßig geltend macht, ist vor allem durch Antriebsschwäche, Interesselosigkeit und allgemeine Verlangsamung gekennzeichnet. Apathisch-depressive Verstimmungen herrschen vor. Die Psychosexualität erlischt langsam. Die Bedürfnisse nach Schlaf, nach Ruhe und nach Wärme werden übersteigert. Manchmal tritt vorübergehend krankhafter Durst auf. Appetitstörungen spielen nur eine untergeordnete Rolle (Gegensatz zur Anorexia nervosa!). Beginnt der Panhypopituitarismus schon im Kindesalter, verzögert er die charakterliche Reifung (hypophysärer Infantilismus), während er nicht oder nur ausnahmsweise zu Schwachsinn führt. Schon in den Stadien, in denen die intellektuellen Funktionen noch erhalten sind, vernachlässigen viele Kranke ihren Haushalt, ihre Kinder, selbst ihre Körperpflege erschreckend. Früher oder später gesellen sich zur Antriebsschwäche Schwerbesinnlichkeit und ein amnestisches Psychosyndrom. — Nach vielen Jahren können ohne Behandlung Zustände erreicht werden, die der sozialen Bedeutung nach einer schweren chronischen Psychose entsprechen (B. STAEHELIN).

Diese überaus chronische Entwicklung kann in akuten Stoffwechselkrisen und vor dem Tode, aber auch ohne erkennbare Ursache, von akuten Zuständen im Rahmen des exogenen Reaktionstypus kompliziert werden. Aufgefallen sind vor allem komatöse Zustände und paranoid-halluzinatorische Bewußtseinstrübungen. (Vereinzelt kamen auch chronische halluzinatorische Psychosen zur Beobachtung.)

Wie ein Hypothyreoidismus im körperlichen Bilde eingeschlossen ist, so ist das beschriebene psychopathologische Bild des Panhypopituitarismus demjenigen des bloßen Hypothyreoidismus ähnlich. In Einzelheiten ergeben sich aber doch leichte Unterschiede. Zum Beispiel beherrscht die bloße Apathie beim Panhypopituitarismus die Szene eher länger als beim schweren Hypothyreoidismus, bei dem die intellektuelle Demenz sich rascher zur Apathie gesellt.

Entsprechend den schweren psychopathologischen Befunden fanden sich bei Sektionen degenerative Befunde im Hirn und bei der elektrencephalographischen Untersuchung deutlich pathologische Befunde (HUGHES und SUMMERS, KRUMP).

SON et al.). In der Hauptsache ist die Störung der Ovarial-Funktion einfach Folge des Hungerns. Allerdings besteht oft schon eine Amenorrhoe, lange bevor die Patientinnen kachektisch sind. Diese ist in den meisten Fällen als emotionelle Amenorrhoe zu deuten. Wahrscheinlich prädisponiert auch ein leichter Infantilismus mit verzögerter Pubertät zur gefühlsgeladenen Abneigung gegen die weibliche Reifung, die den meisten Kranken zukommt. — Der erniedrigte Grundumsatz ist bei Anorexia nervosa gewöhnlich kein Zeichen einer Hypothyreose (Literaturverzeichnis über endokrinologische Untersuchungen bei Anorexia nervosa z. B. bei BLISS und HARDIN BRANCH; DECOURT 1953; THOMÄ 1961). — Kranke mit Anorexia nervosa bleiben gewöhnlich bis in die Endstadien vor dem Tode geistig regsam und wach, in ihrem Empfinden und Trachten differenziert und kompliziert; die Verstumpfung und Verödung der Kranken mit Panhypopituitarismus kommt ihnen nicht zu.

Die moderne Substitutionstherapie (Cortison spielt dabei die Hauptrolle) kann die psychischen Störungen weitgehend verhindern und, wenn sie schon aufgetreten sind, bessern. Ob sie sie völlig ausschalten kann, bleibt zu erforschen. Eine bedeutsame Aufgabe des Arztes liegt darin, die dauernde Fortführung der Therapie sicherzustellen, was infolge der Gleichgültigkeit der Kranken schwierig sein kann.

Nach *therapeutischer Hypophysektomie* wurden Wesensänderungen ähnlicher Art, aber viel leichteren Grades, beobachtet wie beim Sheehan-Syndrom. Am häufigsten ist die Dämpfung der Psychosexualität. Die Geringgradigkeit der Veränderung hängt offenbar mit der kurzen Beobachtungszeit und dem frühzeitigen Einsatz der Substitutionsbehandlung zusammen. Ob die Substitutionstherapie die Wesensänderung völlig oder nur teilweise verhindert, bleibt noch abzuklären. — Wiederholt sind auch nach Hypophysektomie akute psychotische Phasen beobachtet worden (Lindqvist u. a.). Da diese Psychosen den Psychosen gleichsehen, die unter Cortison auftreten, läßt sich gewöhnlich nicht entscheiden, ob sie eher der Substitutionsbehandlung mit Cortison oder der Hypophysektomie zuzuschreiben sind.

3. Hypothalamus-Neurohypophysen-System

Die Psychopathologie des *Diabetes insipidus* ist durch J. Angst (1953 und 1959) weitgehend geklärt worden.

Vorerst ist festzustellen, daß sich der Diabetes insipidus scharf von *psychogener Übersteigerung des Durstes* unterscheidet. Eine Verwischung der Grenzziehung ist versucht worden, hat sich aber nicht bewährt. Charakteristisch für den echten Diabetes insipidus sind die dramatischen Folgen des Wasserentzuges: Er bedeutet eine vitale Bedrohung. Im Durstversuch kann der Urin nicht über ein spezifisches Gewicht von 1008 hinaus konzentriert werden, und die Urinmenge nimmt nicht der Norm entsprechend ab. Auch wird durch Infusionen von hypertonischer Kochsalzlösung die Diurese nicht verringert.

Der *renale Diabetes insipidus* gehört nicht zu den endokrinen Erkrankungen. Er wird durch ein Nicht-Ansprechen der Nierentubuli auf antidiuretisches Hormon verursacht. Er ist im Gegensatz zu den anderen Formen von hereditärem Diabetes insipidus meist mit Infantilismus und Schwachsinn gekoppelt (Forssman).

Der *symptomatische Diabetes insipidus* bei Hirnkrankheiten zeigt naturgemäß oft psychopathologische Folgen der primären Hirnkrankheit. Unter anderem ist er (im Gegensatz zum echten Diabetes insipidus) oft mit amnestischem Psychosyndrom gekoppelt.

Die folgenden Ausführungen beziehen sich auf den *echten Diabetes insipidus*. Bei ihm wird Antidiuretin in den hypothalamischen Kernen nicht oder ungenügend gebildet oder aus dem Hypophysen-Hinterlappen nicht oder ungenügend ausgeschwemmt. Er setzt sich aus einer familiären und einer „idiopathischen" Form zusammen. Die psychopathologischen Begleitsymptome beider Formen sind gleichartig und können zusammen besprochen werden, wenn sie auch im ganzen bei der idiopathischen Form etwas schwerer und häufiger zu sein scheinen als bei der familiären.

In der Mehrzahl der Fälle von echtem Diabetes insipidus sind (abgesehen vom gesteigerten Durst selbst) Persönlichkeitsstörungen feststellbar, die in den Rahmen des endokrinen Psychosyndroms hineinpassen; innerhalb dieses weiten Rahmens aber kommt der Psychopathologie des Diabetes insipidus eine Sonderstellung zu. An elementaren Trieben ist nicht der Durst allein betroffen. Appetit und Schlafbedürfnis sind oft gesteigert, Geschlechtstrieb und Bewegungsbedürfnis vermindert. Die gesamte Antriebshaftigkeit ist oft leicht gedämpft. Es besteht oft eine erhöhte Verstimmbarkeit und eine Neigung zu dauerhaften dysphorischen oder (seltener) depressiv-apathischen Verstimmungen. — Bei Kindern zeigt sich Konzentrationsschwäche, Ermüdbarkeit und Reizbarkeit.

Psychosen vom akuten exogenen Reaktionstypus drohen bei Wasserentzug.

Das endokrine Psychosyndrom macht den Kranken mit Diabetes insipidus bei weitem nicht zum erwerbsunfähigen Invaliden. Es färbt aber doch oft spürbar seine ganze Lebenshaltung und hemmt seine persönliche Entfaltung. Darüber hinaus bildet der Zwang zum häufigen Trinken und Urinieren (bei Kindern auch die Enuresis) eine ernsthafte Behinderung. Er begünstigt Neigungen zur Zurückgezogenheit und Isolierung.

Die große Mehrzahl der Kranken stillt ihren Durst nicht mit alkoholischen Getränken und wird nicht zu Alkoholikern. Bei einer Minderzahl (z. B. bei 6 der 39 Probanden von ANGST) kommt es aber doch zu Alkoholismus. Interessant ist dabei, daß der Durst selbst offenbar nicht die einzige und nicht die wesentliche Ursache des Alkoholismus ist; bedeutsamer erscheinen persönliche Schwierigkeiten, Vereinsamung und Unbefriedigtsein im Verein mit den sozialen Gegebenheiten, die auch bei anderen Alkoholismus züchten.

Theoretisch gesehen ist die dauernde Substitutionstherapie mit antidiuretischem Hormon von größter Bedeutung. Praktisch wichtig und psychologisch interessant ist aber die Feststellung, daß die Mehrzahl der Kranken auf die Dauer auf eine Behandlung verzichtet. Sie wollen eher Trink- und Miktionszwang als die Unbequemlichkeiten und Kosten der Behandlung auf sich nehmen.

Über psychische Wirkungen des zweiten Hormons des Hypothalamus-Neurohypophysensystems, des *Oxytocins*, wissen wir nichts.

4. Schilddrüse

Die Psychopathologie des Morbus Basedow, der Hypothyreose und des endemischen Kretinismus gehört zum alten psychiatrischen Wissen. Auf eine Beschreibung der bekannten typischen Krankheitsbilder und ihrer Behandlung kann hier verzichtet werden. Die Aufgabe des folgenden Absatzes ist es hingegen, die wichtigsten neuen Erkenntnisse und neuen Fragestellungen über die Psychiatrie der Funktionsstörungen der Schilddrüse darzustellen, nämlich:

das Vorkommen einer atypischen Psychopathologie bei Schilddrüsenstörungen

die Beziehungen zwischen vielen atypischen psychischen Begleiterscheinungen von Schilddrüsenstörungen und endogenen Psychosen

die Frage der Psychosen nach Thyreoidektomie

das heute viel diskutierte, aber wahrscheinlich zu Unrecht konzipierte Krankheitsbild der „metabolischen Insuffizienz"

die Psychogenese von Schilddrüsenstörungen

neuere Erfahrungen mit der Therapie.

Atypische psychopathologische Formen: In den letzten Jahren wurde unsere Kenntnis über sporadischen vererbten Kretinismus erweitert. Einzelne Formen sind auf verschiedene, genau bestimmte Störungen der Synthese des Schilddrüsenhormons zurückzuführen. Neue psychiatrische Erkenntnisse haben sich aus diesen Fortschritten der inneren Medizin nicht ergeben. Die Psychopathologie der vererbten Formen des sporadischen Kretinismus ist nicht atypisch; sie unterscheidet sich von derjenigen des endemischen Kretinismus nicht (PARKER und BEIERWALTES). Frühzeitig einsetzende Substitutionsbehandlung zeitigt hier glänzende Ergebnisse.

Von den atypischen psychopathologischen Bildern bei Hyper- und Hypothyreose, die in den letzten Jahren besser bekannt geworden sind, sind zwei Gruppen hervorzuheben:

1. Die Psychopathologie bei Hypo- oder Hyperthyreose entspricht nicht dem als typisch bekannten Bilde, hält sich aber innerhalb des Rahmens des endokrinen Psychosyndroms.

2. Hypo- oder Hyperthyreose gehen mit psychischen Störungen einher, die sich schwer oder gar nicht von „endogenen" Psychosen unterscheiden lassen.

Zu 1. Ausnahmsweise hält sich das psychopathologische Bild bei Morbus Basedow nicht an den gewöhnlichen Rahmen, sondern entspricht im Gegenteil dem Bilde, das wir gewöhnlich bei Hypothyreose sehen: statt Angst, Erregung und Unruhe herrschen Erstarrung und Apathie vor. Umgekehrt zeigen Psychosen bei Hypothyreose gelegentlich ängstlich-erregten oder maniformen Charakter (M. Bleuler 1954; Reiss 1957; Abely 1949). Diese Beobachtungen entsprechen allgemeineren Ergebnissen der endokrinologischen Psychiatrie: eine bestimmte endokrine Funktionsstörung setzt nie mit vollkommener Regelmäßigkeit nur bestimmte psychopathologische Folgen; ihre Folgen im Rahmen des endokrinen Psychosyndroms sind oft für die einzelne endokrine Funktionsstörung uncharakteristisch. — Insbesondere darf man die klassische Psychopathologie der Hyperthyreose bei Kindern nicht immer erwarten. Hyperthyreose bei Kindern führt auch nicht etwa zu beschleunigter Entwicklung, sondern im Gegenteil ähnlich wie der Hypothyreoidismus zu Entwicklungsrückstand (Corboz).

Zu 2. Bei Hypo- wie bei Hyperthyreosen beobachtet man nicht selten Psychosen, die sich erscheinungsbildlich von manisch-depressiven oder akuten schizophrenen Erkrankungen oder — besonders oft — von manisch-depressiv-schizoprenen Mischpsychosen nicht unterscheiden lassen. Häufig steht dabei die Schwere der endokrinen Funktionsstörung zur Schwere der Psychose in einem Mißverhältnis: Die körperliche Störung ist leicht, die psychische schwer. Während des Krankheitsverlaufes fallen manchmal körperliches und psychisches Befinden auseinander: So kann besonders das körperliche Befinden auf endokrinologische Behandlung sich bessern, ohne daß entsprechende Fortschritte im psychischen Befinden auftreten.

Myxödem kann von epileptischen Anfällen verschiedener Art begleitet sein, die im Laufe der Substitutionsbehandlung verschwinden. Im Verlaufe einer hypothyreotischen Erkrankung können ferner (oft im Zusammenhang mit epileptischen Anfällen) Zustände von Stupor und Koma auftreten. Sie sind lebensgefährlich. Sie erheischen sorgfältig (nicht zu hoch) dosierte Substitutions-Therapie und, wenn sie mit Hypothermie verbunden sind, langsame Erwärmung (Literatur zusammengefaßt bei Jellinek).

Welche Beziehungen bestehen zwischen psychischen Begleiterscheinungen von Schilddrüsenstörungen und endogenen Psychosen? Wie sind insbesondere die oben erwähnten Psychosen zu deuten, die wie „endogene" aussehen, die aber von Schilddrüsenstörungen begleitet sind ?

Vorerst ist daran zu erinnern, daß man auf allen Gebieten der Psychiatrie atypischen psychischen Störungen begegnet. Es gibt keine Noxe, die immer charakteristische Begleitpsychosen setzen würde. So gibt es auch Überschneidungen zwischen den psychopathologischen Erscheinungsbildern der endokrinen Erkrankungen und denen von Schizophrenie und manisch-depressivem Kranksein. Man muß mit der Tatsache rechnen, daß das endokrine Psychosyndrom (oder der akute exogene Reaktionstypus) bei Hyper- und Hypothyreose in Ausnahmefällen erscheinungsbildlich nicht von einer schizophrenen oder manisch-depressiven Psychose zu unterscheiden ist. Wir stehen dann vor endokrin bedingter Psychopathologie, die ohne genetische Beziehung zu endogenen Psychosen das Erscheinungsbild einer endogenen Psychose nachäfft. Ein solcher Sachverhalt läßt sich am ehesten aus dem Erfolg der endokrinologischen Therapie erschließen: heilt die psychische Störung mit der Störung der Schilddrüsenfunktion aus, so ist die ursächliche Bedeutung der Schilddrüsenstörung für die psychische Störung beinahe bewiesen.

Ferner kommen zufällige Kombinationen von Schilddrüsenerkrankung und endogener Psychose vor. Dann verlaufen beide Störungen völlig unabhängig voneinander. Wenn z. B. bei einer chronischen Schizophrenen, die zwanzig Jahre lang psychotisch gewesen war, nach Butazolidin-Behandlung eine Hypothyreose auftrat und nach einigen Monaten zur Heilung gebracht wurde, ohne daß sich die Psychose dabei im geringsten verändert hätte, so ist eine derartige Zufallskombination anzunehmen.

Die Mehrzahl der Fälle von Psychosen mit Schilddrüsenstörungen, die einem schizophrenen oder manisch-depressiven Kranksein ähnlich sehen, rufen aber nach einer anderen Erklärung. Bei ihnen besteht weder eine völlige Übereinstimmung noch ein völliges Auseinanderfallen der Verlaufskurven von endokriner und psychischer Störung. Zeitweise scheint es zu gelingen, mit der Normalisierung der Schilddrüsenfunktion die Psychose zu bessern oder zu heilen, später aber verschlimmert sich die Psychose wieder ohne Verschlimmerung der Schilddrüsenfunktion, oder sie heilt trotz der erneuten Sanierung der Schilddrüsenfunktion nach einem Rückfall nicht mehr völlig aus. Wir beobachteten an unserer Klinik eine größere Anzahl derartiger Verläufe über lange Jahre. Die naheliegende Erklärung liegt darin, daß die endokrinen Störungen einerseits, die schizophrene oder manisch-depressive Psychose andererseits teilweise unabhängig entstanden sind, sich aber teilweise auch gegenseitig fördern und beeinflussen (Beispiele u. a. bei KIND, 1963 und REISNER).

Zugunsten dieser Erklärung können noch andere Gesichtspunkte als die Verlaufskurven geltend gemacht werden: Sie ergeben sich aus der Untersuchung der Verwandten von Kranken, die gleichzeitig Schilddrüsenstörungen und schizophrenieähnliche Psychosen aufweisen. Unter diesen Verwandten besteht eine deutliche Korrelation zwischen Schilddrüsenerkrankung und solchen Psychosen (KIND; WEBER u. a.).

Die Beziehung zwischen atypischer Psychose und Schilddrüsenerkrankung besteht keineswegs nur immer in einer verschlimmernden oder auslösenden Wirkung der Schilddrüsenerkrankung auf die Psychose. Im Gegenteil verlaufen schizophrene Psychosen, die Beziehungen zu Schilddrüsenstörungen haben, im Durchschnitt eher akuter und gutartiger als das Gros der Schizophrenien (eigene Beobachtungen; TOMORUG und TANASESCU). — In anderen Fällen sprechen klinische Verläufe dafür, daß die gewaltige Aufregung, die Psychosen mit sich bringen, bei vorbestehender latenter endokriner Krankheitsbereitschaft Hyper- oder Hypothyreosen zum Ausbruch bringt.

Es wäre völlig falsch, aus den Beziehungen zwischen schizophrenie-ähnlichen Psychosen mit der Schilddrüsenfunktion *in einzelnen Fallen* auf eine *generelle* Beziehung Schizophrenie-Schilddrüse zu schließen. Man findet nur in einem kleinen Teil aller Schizophrener und Manisch-Depressiver wesentlich gestörte Schilddrüsenfunktion. In der Durchschnittsbevölkerung besteht keine Korrelation zwischen Schilddrüsenerkrankungen und endogenen Psychosen. (Sie fehlt z. B. in der großen Untersuchung von DASKALOV.) Eine solche Korrelation ist nur in den Familien von Probanden festzustellen, bei denen sich beide Krankheiten kombinieren.

Psychosen nach Thyreoidektomie sind häufiger als nach anderen Operationen. Darüber sind sich die meisten Untersucher einig. (Frühere Arbeiten zusammengestellt bei M. BLEULER 1954, neuere Arbeiten u. a. von CAHILL, von CARPELAN, von KAMMERER et al., von MANTHEY 1959.) Im Gegensatz zu früher haben sie heute nur noch sehr selten die typische Symptomatologie eines akuten exogenen Reaktionstypus. Viel öfter zeigen sie dasselbe Bild wie akute Schizophrenien und besonders Katatonien oder wie Manien oder Depressionen. Am häufigsten sind schizophrene Symptome mit manischen oder depressiven gemischt. Das Wesen dieser Psychosen kann nicht auf eine einzige Formel gebracht werden. In Frage kommen vor allem die folgenden Deutungen:

a) Es handelte sich um eine falsche Operations-Indikation: Die Thyreoidektomie wurde vorgenommen, weil man fälschlich eine psychische Erregung anderer

Ursache auf eine Hyperthyreose zurückgeführt hatte. Eine Psychose, die sich vor der Operation vorbereitet hat, bricht nun im Anschluß an die Operation aus. (Es kann sich um eine Schizophrenie, ein manisch-depressives Kranksein, einen epileptischen Dämmerzustand, eine hysterische Psychose handeln.) Die Schilddrüsenfunktion hat hier mit der Genese der Psychose nichts zu tun. — Dieser Fall trifft meiner Erfahrung nach am häufigsten zu.

b) Die Psychose ist die Folge des Schocks, des Blutverlustes, einer medikamentösen Vergiftung im Zusammenhang mit der Operation: Dann handelt es sich um einen reinen exogenen Reaktionstypus wie nach vielen anderen Operationen. Beim heutigen Stand der Chirurgie ist diese Genese einer Psychose nur selten gegeben.

c) Es handelt sich um die reine Folge einer Hyperthyreose, einer Hypothyreose (bei ungenügender oder zu weit gehender Exstirpation der Schilddrüse) oder einer Tetanie. Auch dies ist heute selten.

d) Bei der Thyreoidektomie wird Schilddrüsenhormon ins Blut ausgeschwemmt, doch normalisiert sich der Hormonspiegel rasch wieder. Neuerdings ist aber bekannt geworden, daß der Operation auch andere tiefgreifende und länger dauernde Veränderungen des Jod-Stoffwechsels folgen: Die Verkleinerung des Hormonjodraums in der Schilddrüse führt zu einer Veränderung in der Dynamik des Jodstoffwechsels und die Schilddrüse schwemmt noch lange nach der Operation abnorm Triiodothyronin aus (Höfer). Ob diese Veränderungen in extremen Fällen und bei besonderen Dispositionen mit psychischen Störungen etwas zu tun haben, bleibt abzuklären.

e) Es handelt sich um die Kombination einer endokrinen Störung mit einer rein psychiatrischen, die sich gegenseitig verschlimmern. Die endokrine Störung kann eine Hypothyreose, einer Hyperthyreose oder eine Tetanie sein, die psychiatrische eine Schizophrenie, ein manisch-depressives Kranksein oder eine Neigung zu psychogenen Erregungen. Eine solche Annahme ist häufig gegeben.

Im Einzelfall ist die Unterscheidung oft schwierig oder unmöglich, bis ein längerer Verlauf sorgfältig beobachtet worden ist.

Unter dem Namen der *metabolischen Insuffizienz* (metabolic insufficiency, euthyroid hypometabolism, low basal metabolism without myxoedema) wurde seit 1955 ein Krankheitsbegriff lebhaft diskutiert, der schon 1917 geprägt worden ist. Wären die Annahmen, die ihm zugrunde liegen, richtig, so hätte er für die Therapie des Nervenarztes in der ambulanten Praxis große Bedeutung. Leider erwiesen sich diese Annahmen aber bereits größtenteils als unrichtig.

Als „metabolische Insuffizienz" sollte ein Krankheitsbild herausgehoben werden, bei dem psychasthenische Beschwerden und Grundumsatzerniedrigung das Bild beherrschten. Vor allem gehörten Schwächegefühle, Müdigkeit und Mangel an Unternehmungslust zum Bilde, dann aber Reizbarkeit, Verstimmbarkeit und andere ganz uncharakteristische Störungen wie u. a. Impotenz, Menstruationsbeschwerden, Verstopfung und Kopfschmerzen. Die Grundumsatzerniedrigung ist freilich in der veröffentlichten Kasuistik oft so geringgradig, daß man sich fragen muß, ob es sich um einen pathologischen Befund handelt. Typisch für das Krankheitsbild wäre nun gewesen, daß Beschwerden und Grundumsatzerniedrigung zwar auf eine Hypothyreose verdächtig gewesen wären, daß sich aber eine Hypothyreose nicht hätte nachweisen lassen. Es fehlte das Myxödem, es fehlten die anderen klinischen Zeichen des Hypothyreoidismus, es fehlte die Erhöhung des eiweißgebundenen Jods im Blutserum, und die Untersuchungen mit radioaktivem Jod zeigten normale Ergebnisse. Dementsprechend erzielte die Behandlung mit Schilddrüsentrockensubstanz keine Erfolge. Es wurde nun die Annahme gemacht, die Störung liege in der mangelhaften Fähigkeit der Gewebe, Thyroxin in Triiodothyronin umzuwandeln und zu verwenden. Deshalb drängte sich die Verwendung von Triiodothyronin anstelle von Schilddrüsentrockensubstanz auf. Einige Untersucher fanden diese Therapie erfolgreich. — Wenn diese Annahmen richtig gewesen wären, so hätten sie es ermöglicht, einen Teil der sogenannten Psychastheniker und Neurastheniker, die bisher behandlungsresistent gewesen sind, auf einfache Weise wirksam zu behandeln.

Es zeigte sich nun aber, daß Triiodothyronin bei dem in Frage stehenden Symptomenkomplex oft unwirksam ist. Ist es wirksam, so ist meist Schilddrüsentrockensubstanz ebenso wirksam (wenn auch die Wirkung von Triiodothyronin rascher eintritt). Außerdem ergaben stoffwechselpathologische Studien Einwände gegen den Krankheitsbegriff.

Vorläufig ist zu befürchten, daß die Fälle, die als metabolische Insuffizienz gedeutet worden sind, zum Teil psychasthenischen Bildern ohne Stoffwechselstörungen entsprechen. Zum Teil handelt es sich um wenig typische und symptomarme Hypothyreosen.

Wichtige Arbeiten zum Thema der metabolischen Insuffizienz sind u. a. diejenigen von KEATING, von KURLAND et al., von LEVIN und von SIKKEMA.

Zur *Frage der Psychogenese* von Schilddrüsenstörungen ist in den letzten Jahren wieder viel publiziert worden, ohne daß wesentlich neue Gesichtspunkte herausgearbeitet werden konnten. Der grundsätzliche Stand der Frage ist auf Seite 181/182 dargestellt.

HARRIS verdanken wir ein Experiment, das vielleicht ein Modell für die Art der Entstehung von einzelnen Formen emotionell ausgelöster Basedow-Krankheit ist: Durch elektrische Reizung des Hypothalamus erzielte er einen Zustand, bei dem sowohl das Thyreotropin wie das eiweißgebundene Jod im Blut erhöht waren, bei dem also die Bremswirkung des Schilddrüsenhormons auf die Thyreotropinbildung versagt hatte. Dasselbe ist manchmal bei Morbus Basedow der Fall. Man kann sich vorstellen, daß unter emotionellen Wallungen eine wesensgleiche Erregung vom Hypothalamus ausgeht wie im Experiment von HARRIS.

Wenn die klinische Erfahrung schon zeigte, daß nicht jeder Mensch auf Schreck mit Übersteigerung der Schilddrüsenfunktion reagiert, so ergaben dementsprechende Untersuchungen von FRANZ ALEXANDER u. Mitarb., daß eben vorwiegend nur Hyperthyreotiker die Schilddrüsenfunktion auf Schreck stark steigern.

Früher diskutierte man nur die Psychogenese der Hyperthyreose, während neuerdings die Psychogenese bei Hypothyreosen besonders studiert wird (MANTHEY 1960 u. a.). Ähnlich wie bei der Hyperthyreose findet man viele Fälle von Hypothyreosen, die in engem Zusammenhang mit schwerster psychischer Belastung entstehen und sich mit der Entlastung bessern. Aus der Psychotherapie allein müßte man folgern, daß es sich um eine psychogenetische Erkrankung handelt. Gegen eine einfache psychogenetische Erklärung lassen sich aber dieselben Überlegungen geltend machen wie oft: Inwiefern sind die endokrinen emotionellen Störungen die Ursachen (und nicht die Folgen) der psychischen Belastung? Weshalb führt psychische Belastung nur in seltenen Ausnahmefällen zu Hypothyreose? Weshalb läßt sich nur bei einem Teil der Hypothyreosen eine außerordentliche psychische Belastung nachweisen?

Im Tierexperiment hemmt „Stress" die Schilddrüsen-Funktion meist. Von dieser Erfahrung aus wäre Hypothyreose als Folge einer emotionellen Belastung eher verständlich als Hyperthyreose. Solche Erfahrungen am Tier dürfen aber natürlich nicht verbindlich auf den Menschen übertragen werden.

Therapeutische Erfahrungen. Vorerst eine Warnung: Thyreoidektomie oder Behandlung mit radioaktivem Jod ohne endokrinologische Indikation bewährt sich nicht! Bis vor kurzem sind manchmal emotionelle Störungen als Anzeige für eine Thyreoidektomie oder eine Behandlung mit radioaktivem Jod betrachtet worden.

Man hoffte, psychische Störungen, wie sie den Morbus Basedow häufig begleiten, auch dann durch Thyreoidektomie heilen zu können, wenn keine körperlichen Zeichen von Basedow festzustellen waren. Eine „Basedow-Therapie ohne Morbus Basedow" bei Angst-, Spannungs- und Erregungszuständen mannigfaltigster Art ist aber nicht erfolgreich. Häufiger als Besserungen treten bei solchen Versuchen Verschlimmerungen der emotionellen Störung auf. Thyreoidektomie und andere auf die Schilddrüse gerichtete eingreifende Behandlungsverfahren sind nur angezeigt, wenn körperliche Symptome[1] die Diagnose einer Schilddrüsen-Störung stützen; die Betrachtung des psychischen Krankheitsbildes allein erlaubt die Indikation für eine auf die Schilddrüse gerichtete Behandlung nicht.

Antithyreoidale Substanzen, die mit fehlerhafter Indikation (bei Annahme nicht existierender Hyperthyreose) verabreicht werden, können schwere Folgen haben: Sie führen zu Verminderung der Produktion von Schilddrüsenhormon, zur vermehrten Produktion von thyreotropem Hormon und damit zu Kropf und manchmal zu irreversibler endokriner Ophthalmopathie — eine furchtbare Folge falscher Medikation (Klein).

Bei Hyper- und Hypothyreosen heilen die psychischen Begleiterscheinungen mit der Normalisierung der Schilddrüsenfunktion meistens, wenn nicht — wie beim Kretinismus — irreparable Hirnschäden vorhanden sind. Die bloße psychotherapeutische Haltung des behandelnden Arztes während der körperlichen Behandlung ist in der Mehrzahl der Fälle genügend. Immerhin sind bei Hyperthyreose die Fälle nicht selten, bei denen eine eingehende Psychotherapie die körperliche Behandlung wirkungsvoll ergänzt (Bennett und Cambor). Bei thyreogenen Psychosen ist vielfach eine medikamentöse Beruhigung und eine Pflege notwendig, wie sie auch sonst in der klinischen Psychiatrie geübt werden.

Große Anforderungen an die Geduld und die Ausdauer des Psychiaters stellen Psychosen, bei denen nur eine lose genetische Beziehung mit Schilddrüsenerkrankungen besteht. Sie erfordern abwechselungsweise Behandlungen, wie sie bei Schizophrenie oder manisch-depressivem Kranksein angezeigt sind, und endokrinologische, gegen die Schilddrüsen-Störung gerichtete Behandlung. Die Indikation zu letzterer kann nur durch fortlaufende Untersuchung auf die Schilddrüsenfunktion nach den Regeln der inneren Medizin richtig gesteuert werden. Zu manchen Zeiten wird die ärztliche Mühe schlecht belohnt: der psychische Zustand will trotz der Normalisierung der Schilddrüsenfunktion nicht bessern. Zu anderen Zeiten aber gewinnt man doch den Eindruck entscheidender Erfolge, wenn die gewohnte psychiatrische Therapie durch die endokrinologische ergänzt wird.

Im Anschluß an die Diskussion des Begriffs über metabolische Insuffizienz sind mit dem Triiodothyronin so zahlreiche therapeutische Versuche gemacht worden, daß erneut festzustellen ist: wie die getrocknete Schilddrüsensubstanz ist es ein Medikament, bei dessen Anwendung Vorsicht not tut! Überdosierungen sind schwer zu erkennen, weil sie gerade die Symptome, die man behandeln will, verstärken können. Müdigkeit, Schwäche und Überregbarkeit können sich verschlimmern, wenn bei Hyperthyreose unterdosiert wird, aber es kann sich dabei auch um Symptome der Überdosierung von Triiodothyronin oder Schilddrüsensubstanz handeln. Zu beachten ist auch, daß bei der Behandlung mit Triiodothyronin das eiweißgebundene Jod im Blutserum nicht ansteigt, wenn das Optimum der Dosierung erreicht oder überschritten wird. Man darf Triiodothyronin nicht deshalb höher dosieren, weil das eiweißgebundene Jod niedrig befunden worden ist.

---

[1] In einer Minderzahl der Fälle enthüllen nur dieLaboratoriumsuntersuchungen und nicht die klinischen Erscheinungen die Schilddrüsenstörung (s. u. a. Hortling et al.).

5. Nebenschilddrüsen

Unsere Kenntnisse über die Psychopathologie des *Hypoparathyreoidismus* haben seit langem keine entscheidenden Fortschritte mehr gemacht. Das Schrifttum enthält mannigfache und zum Teil widersprechende Schilderungen der Symptomatik.

In leichten Fällen werden oft die verschiedensten Störungen beobachtet, die man ins endokrine Psychosyndrom einreihen kann, ohne daß sie aber besonders charakteristisch sind. In der Literatur figurieren sie oft unter Ausdrücken wie „pseudoneurotisch" oder „nervös". In schweren Fällen tritt ein psychoorganisches Syndrom mit mnestischen Störungen auf. Seltener sind in der Literatur Psychosen beschrieben, die z. T. zum akuten exogenen Reaktionstypus gehören, z. T. aber Ähnlichkeit mit schizophrenen und manisch-depressiven Psychosen zeigen (DELAY, DENKO und KAELBLING; JOYEUX[1]).

Es wurde oft schon die Vermutung laut, daß in psychiatrischen Spitälern undiagnostizierte Hypoparathyreotiker gepflegt und daß sie durch routinemäßige Ausführung der einfachen Sulkowitsch-Probe zu erkennen wären (BERARDINELLI u. a.). Reihenuntersuchungen an unserer Klinik an 1200 Kranken und im Columbus Psychiatric Institute an 2082 Kranken (DENKO und KAELBLING) ließen aber keinen einzigen undiagnostizierten Fall entdecken.

Die alten Erfahrungen über die Beziehungen von Tetanie und Epilepsie sind elektrencephalographisch bestätigt worden: Tetanie führt nicht nur klinisch, sondern auch elektrencephalographisch zu epileptiformen Erscheinungen.

Beim *Pseudo-Hypoparathyreoidismus* besteht gewöhnlich eine Oligophrenie mäßigen Grades; er kann zu Verwechslung mit Epilepsie führen.

Neu sind psychiatrische Kenntnisse über den *Hyperparathyreoidismus*: Gleich wie die Vergiftung durch überdosierte Verabreichung von Parathormon führt Hyperparathyreoidismus mit stark erhöhtem Calcium-Blutspiegel häufig zu Psychosen. Beschrieben worden sind vor allem Depression[2], Benommenheit, hochgradige Lethargie, deliriöse Bilder und Halluzinosen. Nach der erfolgreichen Operation des zugrunde liegenden Adenoms sah man solche Psychosen ausheilen. In anderen Fällen traten Rückfälle in ähnliche Zustände (aber auch in andere Formen des akuten exogenen Reaktionstypus) auf, wenn der Kranke nach der Operation eine tetanische Phase durchmachte. — In einigen wenigen Fällen standen psychotische Bilder im Vordergrund der Symptomatologie, bevor sich Skeleterkrankungen oder Nierensteine geltend gemacht hätten. Es bestand die Gefahr, unter der falschen Diagnose einer Involutionspsychose das Grundleiden zu übersehen.

Immerhin wird nur eine Minderheit der Kranken mit Hyperparathyreoidismus psychotisch. Wie die ersten Untersuchungen an einer Reihe unausgelesener Kranker (KIND 1959) vermuten lassen, ist die Mehrzahl der Kranken nicht oder nur

---

[1] Während der Drucklegung sind in der englischen Zeitschrift „Lancet" neue und besonders genaue Untersuchungen über Insuffizienz der Nebenschilddrüsen nach Thyreoidektomie publiziert worden: DAVIS R. HARVARD, P. FOURMAN and J. W. G. SMITH: Prevalence of parathyroid insufficiency after thyroidectomy (Lancet **1961** II, 7218, 1432—1435) und Leading Article: Parathyroid insufficiency (Lancet **1961** II, 7218, 1440).

Danach sind hypoparathyreotische Erscheinungen nach Thyreoidektomie häufiger als vielfach angenommen wird; oft äußern sie sich in psychischen Symptomen: Lethargie, dysphorische ängstliche oder gespannte Stimmungen, Angstzustände und Reizbarkeit. Oft werden sie prämenstruell verschlimmert und gehen überhaupt fließend in das prämenstruelle Spannungssyndrom über. Eine einmalige Calciumbestimmung im Blut genügt für den Nachweis einer solchen Insuffizienz lange nicht immer; oft sind Belastungsproben notwendig. — Bei „nervösen" Beschwerden von Thyreoidektomierten ist die Behandlung mit Dihydrotachysterin erfolgreich, wobei allerdings streng auf eine Erscheinung der Überdosierung zu achten ist (Sulkowitch-Probe!). — Diese Ausführungen entsprechen auch eigenen Erfahrungen.

[2] Die Depression ließ in einem Fall eine genauere Korrelation zum Calcium im Blute vermissen (REINFRANK).

leicht psychisch verändert. Am regelmäßigsten wird übersteigerter Durst und verminderter Appetit beobachtet. Die Kranken bleiben durstig, auch wenn sie viel trinken, und die Unlöschbarkeit des Durstes ist quälend. Amnestische Störungen treten oft früh auf. Dagegen sind Stimmungsverschiebungen selten auffällig. Wernly und König, ebenso u. a. Arnaud et al., sahen vor allem träges, denkfaules Wesen im Zusammenhang mit der Müdigkeit. — Soweit wir wissen, hängen die psychopathologischen Folgen des Hyperparathyreoidismus von der begleitenden Hypercalcämie ab.

6. Überangebot von Nebennieren-Rinden-Hormonen

Über die Psychopathologie des *Cushing-Syndroms* sind in den letzten 20 Jahren vielfache Erfahrungen gesammelt worden (Furger; Schwöbel; Stoll 1950; Wolf 1946). Sie sind in einer großen Literatur zerstreut. — Unterschiede im psychischen Symptomenbild je nach der Genese des Cushing-Syndroms sind nicht entdeckt worden. Wir können die Psychopathologie des Cushing-Syndroms deshalb für alle die verschiedenen genetischen Formen gemeinsam umschreiben. — Wesensänderungen im Rahmen des endokrinen Psychosyndroms sind bei ausgesprochenem Cushing-Syndrom die Regel. Sie sind noch mannigfacher in ihren Erscheinungsweisen als etwa die Wesensänderungen bei Akromegalie. Sowohl apathische wie erregte Stimmungslagen sind häufig. Manchmal sind die Kranken in einer eher gehobenen Stimmungslage, die es ihnen ermöglicht, alle die schweren Nachteile, die ihre Krankheit mit sich bringt, überlegen und gleichmütig zu ertragen. Aber auch wehleidige, gehässige und depressive Grundstimmungen können vorherrschen. Das emotionelle Erleben von Cushing-Kranken wirkt oft besonders innig und stark. Die Sexualität wird oft gedämpft, seltener und nur vorübergehend gesteigert; Hunger und Durst sind meist gesteigert, manchmal wird auch die elementare Mütterlichkeit angeregt. — Akute episodische Verstimmungen, Drang-, Angstund Triebzustände sind häufig. Sie gehen nicht selten in psychotische Episoden über: Erregungen, apathische Zustände oder Verstimmungen übersteigern sich, und es treten Verwirrung, Halluzinationen, Illusionen, wahnhafte Vorstellungen hinzu. Es entstehen mannigfache Bilder von affektiven Psychosen, Delirien, Dämmerzuständen, Halluzinosen in den verschiedensten Mischungen. Die Dauer dieser Psychosen ist meist kurz. Sie können von epileptiformen Anfällen begleitet sein. — Amnestische Symptome sind bei Cushing-Syndrom häufig. Vor allem sind sie zu beobachten, wenn sich das Syndrom mit einer Hirnarteriosklerose kompliziert. In leichten Formen kommen sie aber auch ohne erkennbare Hirnarteriosklerose zur Beobachtung.

Es ist untersucht worden, ob alle oder einzelne psychopathologische Befunde des Cushing-Syndroms in Zusammenhang mit bestimmten Einzelsymptomen der Krankheit zu bringen wären. Zum Beispiel wurde daran gedacht, ob Hypokaliämie die Gefahr psychotischer Komplikationen in sich schlösse, ob Durst und Appetit nur bei latentem Diabetes verändert wären, ob das amnestische Psychosyndrom besonders bei starker Hypertonie vorkäme, ob Beziehungen zwischen den Veränderungen der Psychosexualität und dem Hirsutismus aufzudecken wären. Bisher wurden trotz sorgfältiger Bemühungen (Furger; Linquette et al. u. a.) keine Zusammenhänge psychischer Veränderungen mit einzelnen körperlichen Symptomen gefunden. Der Grad der psychischen Veränderungen steht lediglich mit Dauer und Schwere der körperlichen Erkrankung als Ganzes in einem losen Zusammenhang. Er ist — soweit sich feststellen ließ — unabhängig davon, welche körperlichen Symptome im Krankheitsbild vorherrschen. (Eine Ausnahme von dieser Regel beschrieben Abely et al. 1956: bei einer Patientin bestand ein paralleler Verlauf zwischen Psychose und Ausscheidung von 11 Oxycorticosteroiden und 17-Ketosteroiden.)

Dagegen lassen sich enge Beziehungen zwischen der Psychopathologie des Cushing-Syndroms und der prämorbiden Persönlichkeit aufdecken. Unausgeglichene Persönlichkeiten zeigen im ganzen schwerere psychische Störungen, wenn sie ein Cushing-Syndrom entwickeln, als gesunde und gut angepaßte. Die Art der psychopathologischen Veränderung läßt sich oft als eine Übertreibung vorbestehender Persönlichkeitseigenarten deuten. In einer erheblichen Zahl der Fälle fallen Ausbruch und Verschlimmerungen der Krankheit (ähnlich wie beim Morbus Basedow) in Zeiten starker psychischer Belastung (HOCHSTAEDT, SCHWÖBEL u. a.). Prämorbid sind viele Kranke mit Cushing-Syndrom pyknisch und synton, oft auch emotionell unausgeglichen und verstimmbar. Dieselben psychischen Besonderheiten sind unter ihren Verwandten häufig.

Nach einer erfolgreichen Behandlung des Cushing-Syndroms (durch Hypophysenbestrahlung, Adrenalektomie oder Hypophysektomie mit dauernder Substitutionsbehandlung) sieht man meist auch die psychischen Störungen wesentlich zurückgehen. (Bestrahlungsschäden des Hirns können psychopathologische Folgen zeitigen.) Einzelne Symptome, besonders Libido-Verlust und amnestisches Psychosyndrom, können freilich persistieren. Libido-Verlust bei Frauen kann mit Androgenen behandelt werden. — Nach der Adrenalektomie findet sich oft eine etwas nivellierte, aber ausgeglichene Persönlichkeit, die wie gereift und den Nöten des Lebens gegenüber widerstandsfähig erscheint. Die Vermutung liegt nahe, daß die Stetigkeit der Hormonzufuhr während der Substitutionstherapie und der Wegfall der emotionell bedingten Schwankungen der Nebennieren-Funktion mit dieser Veränderung etwas zu tun haben. Es handelt sich um gleichartige Gestimmtheiten, wie sie schon bei andern hormonalen Substitutionsbehandlungen, aber auch bei Akromegalie oder bei Leukotomierten vorkommen. Die vitale Abhängigkeit von der Substitutionstherapie nach Adrenalektomie bedeutet ein schweres Problem, mit dem sich aber die Mehrzahl der Kranken abfindet. Nur eine Minderzahl leidet dauernd unter dem Gedanken, daß ihr Leben von der Hormon-Medikation abhängt.

Unter Zürcher Verhältnissen erwies sich der behandelnde Internist gleichzeitig als ausgezeichneter Psychotherapeut der Kranken mit Cushing-Syndrom. Das Vertrauensverhältnis mit ihm, seine Aufklärung über die hormonalen Hintergründe der emotionellen Veränderungen und seine fürsorgerischen Maßnahmen waren von größtem Wert. Eine zusätzliche Psychotherapie durch den Spezialisten wünschten die Kranken nicht, und sie schien auch nicht notwendig.

Eine große Bedeutung haben die *psychopathologischen Folgeerscheinungen der Behandlung mit Glucocorticoiden und adrenocorticotropem Hormon*[1]. Die zahlreichsten Erfahrungen über die ersteren beziehen sich auf das *Cortison*. Wesentliche Unterschiede in den psychischen Folgen von ACTH- und Cortison-Behandlungen bestehen nicht. ACTH- und Cortison-Behandlung in mittleren und höheren Dosen hat in den meisten Fällen einen Einfluß auf die Stimmung. Das erste Störungszeichen ist oft Schlaflosigkeit. Am häufigsten ist eine euphorisierende Wirkung beobachtet worden, doch treten auch depressive, gereizte, gehässige und viele anders gefärbte Verstimmungen auf. Depressive Verstimmungen bei Cortison-Verabreichung können zu Selbstmord führen (s. z. B. KIRSNER et al.,), die euphorischen Verstimmungen in seltenen Fällen zu Sucht (s. z. B. KUEMMERLE et al.). Manchmal ist die Behandlung von einer Reihe aufeinanderfolgender verschieden gerichteter Verstimmungen begleitet. Der Grad der Verstimmungen ist in der Mehrzahl der Fälle so leicht, daß besonders darauf geachtet werden muß, wenn

---

[1] Übersicht über Literatur z. B. bei CECCARELLI, VON ZERSSEN; s. z. B. auch BONDAREV.

man sie erkennen will[1]. Manchmal aber fallen sie bei der Pflege der Kranken unangenehm auf. — In der Mehrzahl der Fälle tritt ferner eine Steigerung des Appetites auf. Die Sexualität wird oft gedämpft, und Impotenz ist eine häufige Behandlungsfolge.

Nicht ganz selten steigern sich die Verstimmungen unter ACTH- oder Cortison-Behandlung aber zu *psychotischen Zuständen*. Sie sind gleicher Art wie beim Cushing-Syndrom (Verstimmungen, Erregungen, Verwirrungen, Delirien, paranoide Zustände, Halluzinosen). Gelegentlich treten epileptiforme Anfälle dazu (s.z.B. Bonham oder McMahon and Gordan). Die Häufigkeit von Phychosen kann nicht genau angegeben werden. Sie hält sich in der Größenordnung von 1% der Behandlungen. Psychosen sind in den ersten Jahren nach der Einführung der Therapie mit Glucocorticoiden häufiger beobachtet worden als heute, oft in 10% einer Behandlungsreihe. Hängt die abnehmende Zahl von psychotischen Komplikationen mit vorsichtigerer Indikationsstellung und Dosierung oder mit der Einführung neuer Präparate zusammen? Wir wissen es nicht. Das Auftreten dieser Psychosen steht nur in ganz losem Zusammenhang mit der Dosierung und der Dauer der Verabreichung von ACTH oder Cortison. Psychosen können schon am Anfang einer Behandlung mit mäßigen Dosen auftreten, in vielen Fällen aber sind langdauernde (viele Monate lange) Behandlungen in hohen Dosen nicht mit Psychosen kompliziert. Gelegentlich treten Psychosen erst beim Entzug einer Cortison-Medikation auf (Amatruda et al.). Paradoxerweise hat man sogar Cortison-Psychosen unter hohen Dosen von Cortison wieder abheilen sehen (Delay et al. 1954). *Konstitutionelle Momente erleichtern das Auftreten* von psychotischen Episoden während der Behandlung, doch sind selbst nach durchgemachten Psychosen Neuerkrankungen während der Cortisonbehandlung bei weitem nicht obligatorisch. Wenn die Behandlung bei Kranken erfolgt, deren Zustand an sich schon leicht zu Psychosen des akuten exogenen Reaktionstypus führt, sind psychotische Behandlungskomplikationen häufiger (Fieber, hochgradige Kachexie, Morbus Addison, disseminierter Lupus erythematodes, multiple Sklerose). In der Hauptsache aber ließ sich bis heute nicht erkennen, warum der eine Kranke bei der ACTH- oder Cortisonbehandlung eine Psychose entwickelt und der andere nicht.

Die Psychosen unter ACTH- und Cortisonbehandlung dauern verschieden lang: mehrere Stunden bis viele Monate. Beruhigend ist das Wissen darum, daß keine Übergänge in unheilbare, chronische Psychosen bekannt geworden sind, wenn wenigstens der Behandelte nicht schon früher schizophren gewesen war. (Bei remittierten Schizophrenen sind im Anschluß an die Behandlung Rückfälle mit ungünstigem Verlauf vorgekommen.) Soweit aus der Literatur hervorgeht, sind die Psychosen unter ACTH- und Cortison-Behandlung (wenn sie nicht schon von selbst oder nach Absetzen des Medikamentes zurückgingen) meistens mit Elektroschock behandelt worden — und zwar mit gutem Erfolg. Mir scheint freilich die Anwendung von Elektroschock bei einer organischen Psychose, besonders wenn sie noch zur Komplikation mit spontanen epileptischen Anfällen neigt, bedenklich. Eine bewährte bessere Therapie ist aber noch nicht bekannt. Versuche mit einer Behandlung durch Wuchshormon sind noch nicht zur Beurteilung reif.

Die Gefahr psychotischer Komplikationen sollte davon abhalten, Behandlungen mit ACTH oder Cortison ohne gewichtige Indikation durchzuführen. Angesichts der Seltenheit der Behandlungspsychosen und ihrer Heilbarkeit wäre es aber unberechtigt, nur wegen psychiatrischer Bedenken auf die Behandlung in den Fällen zu verzichten, in denen sie aus körperlichen Gründen dringend indiziert ist.

In der *psychiatrischen Therapie* haben die Corticosteroide eine viel beschränktere Indikation, als nach ihrer Entdeckung von vielen erhofft wurde. Sie bewährten

---

[1] Siehe z. B. bei Kochmann.

sich vor allem bei Delirium tremens (THIELE und HOHMANN) und allgemein bei akuten Psychosen vom Typus des „Delirium acutum", bei Psychosen also, die früher oft zu „tödlichen Katatonien" wurden (LINGJAERDE). Sie können ferner bei akuter Alkoholvergiftung nützlich sein (Lit. bei THIELE). Zur Schockbekämpfung überhaupt sind sie an psychiatrischen Kranken ebenso zu verwenden wie sonst in der Medizin. Bei Hirnmetastasen von Mamma-Carcinom stellte GERHARTZ eine gute Wirkung hoher Dosen von Cortison auf die neurologische Ausfallserscheinungen fest, wohl durch Verminderung des Hirnödems. — Dagegen ist Cortison kein Heilmittel bei Schizophrenien. Auch bei Depressionen bewährt es sich im allgemeinen nicht: Seine euphorisierende Wirkung ist zu unregelmäßig, zu kurzdauernd und zu leicht und steht in keinem befriedigenden Verhältnis zu den Gefahren der Behandlung. — Viele Psychotische reagieren erstaunlich wenig auf die Verabreichung von Corticosteroiden. — In den letzten Jahren haben sich adrenocorticotropes Hormon, Hydrocortison oder Dexamethason zur Behandlung der Propulsiv-Petit-Mal-Epilepsie kleiner Kinder (Blitz-, Nick- und Salaam-Krämpfe) brauchbar erwiesen. Unerkannt ist, wie die therapeutische Wirkung entsteht (MATTHES et al., PAULI et al.; SOREL et al.). — Cortison ist ferner bei Puerperalpsychosen versucht worden (ABÉLY, P., 1950; ABÉLY, P., et al., 1955; DELAY et al., 1954, u. a.), doch ist diese Indikation noch unsicher und umstritten.

Soweit bisher bekannt ist, wirken *alle anderen Corticosteroid-Präparate*, die in der Therapie gebraucht werden, gleichsinnig auf die Psyche wie das Cortison (Cortisol, Prednison, Prednisolon, Dexamethason u. a.) (z. B. STOLL, B. A.). Ob die Anzahl psychotischer Komplikationen unter den neuen Präparaten geringer ist als unter Cortison, wie oft gehofft wurde, ist noch unsicher. — Eine Ausnahmestellung nimmt die Wirkung von Triamcinolon auf den Appetit ein: Es setzt ihn herab, statt daß es ihn wie andere Corticosteroid-Präparate anregt.

Das *adrenogenitale Syndrom* entsteht durch vermehrte Ausscheidung von Androgenen in der Nebennierenrinde. (Krankhafte Vermehrung der adrenocorticalen Oestrogene, die adrenale Feminisierung, ist sehr selten und psychiatrisch nicht erforscht.) Die häufigste Form des adrenogenitalen Syndroms ist auf *kongenitale Nebennierenrinden-Hyperplasie* zurückzuführen. Sie wird einfach-rezessiv vererbt. Die Krankheit führt zur vorzeitigen Entwicklung aller Pubertätsmerkmale, mit Ausnahme der Reifung der Geschlechtsdrüsen selbst (Pseudopubertas praecox). Bei Mädchen bestehen Anomalien der Genitalien im Sinne eines Pseudohermaphroditismus. Ihre vorzeitige Pubertätsentwicklung verläuft in vermännlichendem Sinne wie bei Knaben.

Die Psychopathologie von *Mädchen mit kongenitaler Nebennierenrinden-Hyperplasie* ist heute in den Hauptzügen erforscht (HAMPSON, JOAN G.; HAMPSON, JOAN G., et al. 1955, 1956; HAMPSON, J. L., et al.; JOLLY; MARZI und TEODORI; MONEY, J., 1955; MONEY, J., and JOAN G. HAMPSON; MONEY, J., et al. 1955 a, b, 1956; SECKEL; STUTTE; WALLIS; ZÜBLIN 1953). Es hat sich gezeigt, daß viele frühere Vermutungen und Verallgemeinerungen seltener Einzelfälle ein falsches Bild geben. Die vorzeitige körperliche sexuelle Reifung führt gewöhnlich nicht zu vorzeitiger psychosexueller Reifung; die Virilisierung während der Pseudopubertät führt nur ausnahmsweise zu Homosexualität. Die schwere körperliche Anomalie ist gewöhnlich nicht mit schweren psychischen Störungen gekoppelt. — Mädchen mit Pseudopubertas praecox und Pseudohermaphroditismus sind in ihrer emotionellen Entwicklung meistens eher etwas zurück; sie wirken (in seltsamem Gegensatz zu ihrer körperlichen Frühreife) in ihrem Wesen kindlich, sind oft eher scheu und abhängig von anderen. Ihr Streben geht dahin, nicht aufzufallen. Manchmal sind sie leicht verstimmbar. Ihre Sexualität erwacht eher spät und bleibt oft schwach und kindlich. Wenn die Patientinnen als Mädchen erzogen worden sind, so teilen sie Interessen und Einstellungen ihrer Kameradinnen, und der Gedanke eines offiziellen Geschlechtswandels im Sinne der körperlichen Maskulinisierung ist ihnen meist fremd und widerwärtig. Sind sie, was seltener ist, als Knaben auferzogen, so wollen sie häufig Knaben bleiben. Homosexuelle Triebrichtung ist selten, wenn die Patientinnen als Mädchen erzogen sind. Wenig differenzierte Sexualität und sexuelle Neigungen zu Mädchen weisen manche Patientinnen auf, die als Knaben auferzogen wurden. Die intellektuelle Entwicklung ist meist dem Alter entsprechend. Ausnahmen von der Regel, Patientinnen mit gesteigertem und vorzeitigen Geschlechtstrieb, hat u. a. NIEKISCH beschrieben.

Die einzig wirksame Behandlung besteht in der Dauerverabreichung von Cortison, die möglichst frühzeitig einsetzen soll. Durch die Behandlung wird die Virilisierung korrigiert, mit Ausnahme der Genitalmißbildungen. Die Behandlung bessert auch das psychische Wohlbefinden, namentlich das Selbstbewußtsein (PRADER 1952, eigene Beobachtung). — Wenn freilich die Patientinnen als Knaben auferzogen und in ihrer Gesinnung und sozialen Einstellung männlich geworden sind, darf eine Umwandlung des offiziellen Geschlechtes und eine Feminisierung nicht mehr erzwungen werden. Geschlechtswechsel entgegen den Lebensgewohnheiten und entgegen der eigenen Einstellung nach den ersten Lebensjahren bedeuten meist ein schweres psychisches Trauma.

Knaben mit kongenitaler Nebennierenrinden-Hyperplasie sind erst in geringerer Zahl psychiatrisch untersucht worden als Mädchen. Unsere Kenntnisse über ihre Psychopathologie müssen an größerem Untersuchungsgut ergänzt werden. Soweit wir bisher wissen, wird auch bei der Mehrzahl von ihnen kein vorzeitiges Erwachen der Psychosexualität festgestellt, so daß körperliche und psychische Reifung weit auseinanderfallen. Auch die männlichen Kranken sind oft eher scheu und zurückgezogen. Der Sexualtrieb kann noch in erwachsenem Alter schwach bleiben. Intellektuelle Vorentwicklung ist nicht die Regel. — Immerhin kommen überraschende und eindrucksvolle Ausnahmen mit starker sexueller Triebhaftigkeit bis zu sexuellen Gewalttätigkeitsdelikten im Kindesalter und partielle Vorentwicklung der Interessen, der Psychomotorik oder der Intelligenz vor.

Das *erworbene adrenogenitale Syndrom* (durch erworbene NebennierenrindenHyperplasie oder -Tumor), das zur Virilisierung von Frauen führt, ist psychopathologisch noch nicht systematisch erforscht. In der Hauptsache sind nur grob auffällige psychopathologische Erscheinungen in Einzelfällen beschrieben worden; nur in wenigen Fällen liegen umfassende psychiatrische Untersuchungsberichte vor. Aus der in der Literatur verstreuten Kasuistik über Einzelfälle ergibt sich, daß die denkbar verschiedensten psychischen Störungen mit der Virilisierung zeitlich zusammenfallen können: Steigerung oder Verminderung der Sexualität in heterosexueller Richtung, Veränderung des Sexualempfindens im Sinne der Homosexualität, Wesensänderungen, Depressionen, verschiedenartige Psychosen. Die Vermutung ist berechtigt, daß solche dramatische Entwicklungen in der Wirklichkeit (im Gegensatz zur Literatur) eher die Ausnahme als die Regel bilden. Systematische Untersuchungen zu dieser Frage sind aber dringend nötig.

In den seltenen Fällen, in denen das adrenogenitale Syndrom zu Hypoglykämie führt, sind auch hypoglykämische Verwirrungen und Koma beobachtet worden.

Die psychischen Veränderungen bei Kranken mit *Conn-Syndrom* sind noch nicht genauer bekannt geworden. In den wenigen publizierten Fällen sind leichtere und uncharakteristische emotionelle Begleiterscheinungen erwähnt wie Reizbarkeit und „Nervosität". Bewußtseinsstörungen sind selten.

Nach der Verabreichung von *Desoxycorticosteron* (Cortexon) kommen leichtere und vorübergehende Stimmungsverschiebungen vor, oft im Sinne der Stimmungsanregung und der Euphorie. Die Wirkung des *Aldosterons* in therapeutischen Dosen auf die Psyche ist noch nicht erprobt.

7. Unterfunktion der Nebennierenrinde

Morbus Addison. Die Psychopathologie der Krankheit ist schon bei ihrer ersten Beschreibung durch THOMAS ADDISON 1855 berücksichtigt und seither oft bearbeitet worden. Sie ist 1953 von STOLL monographisch beschrieben und seither weiter verfolgt worden. Es ist zu unterscheiden zwischen Kranken, die überhaupt nicht wirksam oder nur mit Desoxycorticosteron behandelt wurden, und jenen, die langdauernd mit Cortison behandelt sind.

Vor der Einführung des Cortisons in die Therapie ergab sich folgendes psychiatrisches Bild der Krankheit: Eine Wesensänderung im Sinne des endokrinen Psychosyndroms erlitten so gut wie alle Kranke. Depressive und apathische Verstimmungen standen dabei im Vordergrund, aber nicht mit derselben Ausschließlichkeit, wie es in der Literatur oft angegeben worden war. Es kamen auch euphorische Verstimmungen und Zustände von Hast und innerer Spannung und viele andere vor. Oft litten das soziale Verantwortungsgefühl und die differenziertere Aktivität, während die Kranken gutmütig und warmer Herzlichkeit fähig blieben. — Zum Dauerzustand gesellten sich wie bei den meisten anderen schweren endokrinen Krankheiten auch episodische Verstimmungen in mancherlei Richtung. Die Sexualität wurde meist abgeschwächt. Hunger und Durst nahmen oft ab. Es kam vielfach zu außerordentlichen Gelüsten, z. B. zu Salzhunger oder Abneigung gegen gewisse Speisen. Auch das Schlafbedürfnis veränderte sich oft. — Fast regelmäßig entwickelte sich mit dem endokrinen auch ein amnestisches Psychosyndrom. Es trat häufiger und schwerer in Erscheinung als bei manchen anderen endokrinen Krankheiten, z. B. der Akromegalie und dem Cushing-Syndrom. — Psychosen vom akuten exogenen Reaktionstypus begleiteten häufig schwere körperliche Krisen und die Agonie. Sie waren manchmal mit epileptischen Anfällen kompliziert. Früher wurden auch chronische organische Psychosen oft gemeldet.

Seit Einführung der Cortison-Behandlung sind die psychopathologischen Störungen bei Morbus Addison milder und seltener geworden. Erst die Zukunft kann aber lehren, ob die Cortison-Behandlung die Addison-Kranken auf lange Sicht *völlig* vor psychischen Veränderungen bewahren kann.

Interessant sind neue Beobachtungen, wonach Psychosen bei Addison-Kranken nicht nur dann ausbrechen, wenn die unbehandelte Krankheit einer kritischen Verschlimmerung entgegengeht, sondern im Gegenteil gerade auch dann, wenn sie sich unter Cortison-Therapie rasch bessert. Bei Fortsetzung der Therapie können sie wieder heilen (BRACELAND; CLEGHORN und PATTEE). Auch an diesen Erfahrungen wird deutlich, wie wichtig die rasche Umstellung des endokrinen Gleichgewichtes an sich für die psychopathologischen Folgen ist und wie wenig diese Folgen spezifische Reaktionen auf spezifische endokrine Umstellungen bedeuten.

Addison-Kranke sind körperlich oft schon vor der Krankheit Astheniker und weisen mehr infantile Merkmale auf als die Durchschnittsbevölkerung. Unter ihnen selbst finden sich prämorbid auffallend viele psychopathische Entwicklungen, ebenso wie unter ihren Verwandten.

Im Tierexperiment hemmen Barbiturate das Auftreten der "arousal reaction" an der elektrischen Aktivität der Hirnrinde, wenn das reticuläre System gereizt wird. Bei Tieren ohne Nebenniere braucht es zu dieser medikamentösen Hemmwirkung weniger Barbiturate als bei normalen Tieren. Unter der Behandlung nebennierenloser Tiere mit Desoxycorticosteron und besonders derjenigen mit Cortison nähert sich hingegen die Hemmwirkung der Barbiturate der Norm (COOK et al.). — Man könnte deshalb vermuten, daß die erhöhte Ermüdbarkeit bei

Nebennierenrinden-Insuffizienz und die erhöhte Erregbarkeit bei Nebennierenrinden-Hyperfunktion mit der Bedeutung der Nebennierenrinden-Hormone für die "arousal reaction" zusammenhängt. Das ist aber vorläufig eine bloße Spekulation. Um eine genügende „Erklärung" der veränderten Antriebshaftigkeit bei Nebennierenerkrankungen kann es sich schon deshalb nicht handeln, weil ja Erregungen auch bei deren Hypofunktion und umgekehrt Apathie bei deren Hyperfunktion vorkommen.

Addisonismus. In der Psychiatrie taucht seit Jahrzehnten die Vermutung immer wieder auf, daß Zustände von erhöhter Erschöpfbarkeit, Müdigkeit, leichten Depressionen, d. h. neurasthenieartige Krankheitsbilder, zwar nicht mit einem eigentlichen progressiven Morbus Addison, aber mit einer leichteren, nicht progressiven „Nebennierenschwäche", einem „Addisonismus", in Beziehung zu bringen wären. Auf Grund dieser Vermutungen wurden Substitutionsbehandlungen mit vielerlei hormonalen Präparaten, vor allem auch mit Desoxycorticosteron, empfohlen und als wirksam beschrieben. Die heutige Endokrinologie ist diesen hypothetischen Vorstellungen und den entsprechenden Behandlungsversuchen gegenüber skeptisch. Sie kennt zwar einen latenten Morbus Addison mit relativer Nebennierenrindeninsuffizienz bei besonderen Belastungen. Um diese Krankheit handelte es sich aber bei der überwältigenden Mehrheit der „Neurastheniker", die als nebenniereninsuffizient betrachtet wurden, nicht. Weiter ist bekannt, daß bei schweren Erkrankungen verschiedenster Art die Steroide im Urin vermindert sein können, obschon die Nebennierenrinde gut auf adrenocorticotropes Hormon anspricht und auch sonst keine Zeichen der Insuffizienz erkennen läßt („funktionelle Nebennierenrindeninsuffizienz"). Diese Erscheinung scheint aber klinisch bedeutungslos zu sein und ruft nach keiner Hormonbehandlung.

Es ist bisher nicht erwiesen, daß Zustände von Neurasthenie ursächlich auf eine solche funktionelle Nebennierenrindeninsuffizienz zurückzuführen und mit einer hormonalen Substitutionsbehandlung zu heilen wären. Zwar sind in jüngster Zeit einzelne moderne Methoden zur Prüfung der Nebennierenrindenfunktion bei Kranken mit neurasthenieartigen Klagen zur Anwendung gekommen und ein verschieden hoher Prozentsatz derselben wies verminderte 17-Ketosteroid-Ausscheidung auf (Birket-Smith; Høyrup). Der Zusammenhang zwischen den Urinbefunden und den subjektiven Beschwerden ist aber unbewiesen. Behandlungserfolge mit Hormonen könnten auch durch Suggestivwirkung erklärt werden; jedenfalls wurden sie früher auch mit Präparaten gemeldet, denen nach neueren Kenntnissen Hormonwirkungen abzusprechen sind.

Schon aus wissenschaftlichen Gründen ist es zu begrüßen, wenn Kranke mit neurasthenieartigen Klagen in bezug auf ihre Nebennierenrindenfunktion untersucht werden. Dagegen ist nach unserem heutigen Wissen nicht mehr zu empfehlen, bloß auf Grund subjektiver Klagen, ohne Nachweis einer körperlichen Indikation mit Laboratoriumsmethoden, eine Behandlung mit Nebennierenrindenhormonen durchzuführen.

8. Nebennierenmark

Phäochromocytom. Die Anfälle der paroxysmalen Form sind oft von ängstlicher Erregung begleitet. Sie kann sich bis zu Psychosen des akuten exogenen Reaktionstypus steigern. Eine besondere Psychopathologie der persistierenden Form, die sie von anderen Hypertonieformen unterscheiden würde, ist nicht bekannt.

Adrenalin, in größeren subcutanen oder intravenösen Dosen verabreicht, setzt neben körperlichen Beschwerden (Kopfweh, Herzklopfen, Zittern, Kältegefühl, Druckgefühl in der Brust, Ohnmachtsanwandlungen) auch Unruhe, Konzentrationsschwäche und manchmal Angst. Wenn aber auch die Steigerung der Adrenalinausscheidung bei Angst deutlich ist, so werden durch Adrenalininfusion eher bloß körperliche Symptome der Angst und Angstbereitschaft gesetzt als hell auflodernde Angstgefühle (HAWKINS et al.). *Noradrenalin* intravenös in Einzeldosen oder infundiert wirkt kaum auf die Emotionalität. — Lokalisiertes Vorkommen von Noradrenalin im Hirn und seine Ausschwemmung durch Reserpin s. S. 172. Beim Delirium tremens wurde eine vermehrte Ausscheidung von Katecholaminen festgestellt (WEGMANN und GIACOBINI).

Abbauprodukte des Adrenalins (Adrenochrom und Adrenolutin) können in experimentellen Situationen akute psychotische Episoden setzen (HOFFER 1957 d, HOFFER et al.).

9. Hyperinsulinismus

Die *Symptomatologie* ist vielfach eine psychische. Sie ist dem klinischen Psychiater von den Insulinkuren her wohlvertraut. Typisch ist das Auftreten nach Fasten und körperlicher Anstrengung. Es treten oft zuerst Hunger, Müdigkeit, Schwäche, Reizbarkeit und Stimmungsverschiebungen auf. Intellektuelle erleben die hypoglykämische emotionelle Veränderung am Anfang nicht selten in der Art einer Depersonalisation (BLEULER 1948 c, GAYRAL). Unter Schweißen und den bekannten muskulären Erscheinungen treten später am häufigsten Ohnmachten und dann längerdauerndes Koma auf. Seltener steigert sich die anfängliche Unruhe zu Delirien oder Dämmerzuständen. Für die Diagnose beweisend ist die Untersuchung des Blutzuckers im Anfall, die veränderte Ansprechbarkeit auf Glucose-Verabreichung außerhalb des Anfalls dagegen nur hinweisend. Langdauerndes und wiederholtes Koma kann zum amnestischen Psychosyndrom und zu lange anhaltenden elektrencephalographischen Veränderungen führen.

Unter den *Ursachen* figurieren neben dem Inseladenom, dem Pankreascarcinom, Krankheiten der Leber, der Hypophyse, der Nebenniere u. a. und neben der Überdosierung des Insulins bei der Diabetesbehandlung solche, die die Psychiatrie besonders angehen: die heimliche Selbstinjektion von Insulin zur Simulation, in suicidaler Absicht oder aus verschiedenen krankhaften Einstellungen, z. B. bei geltungssüchtigen Psychopathen. Spontane Regulationsstörungen des Zuckerstoffwechsels kommen bei Hirnkrankheiten, vor allem Stammhirnkrankheiten, vor. Besonders eingehend diskutiert wurden die funktionelle und die „nervöse" Hypoglykämie. Im psychiatrischen Schrifttum werden sie allerdings kaum je auseinandergehalten. Bei der „funktionellen" Form ist die Hypoglykämie die Folge einer starken Insulinmobilisation nach alimentärer Hyperglykämie; bei der „nervösen" Hypoglykämie steigt der Blutzucker auf Zuckerbelastung zu wenig an.

Die Möglichkeit spontaner hypoglykämischer Erkrankungen stellt den Psychiater vor wichtige differentialdiagnostische Aufgaben. Namentlich ist bei epileptiformen Anfällen, ungeklärten rauschartigen Zuständen und bei neurasthenischen Bildern daran zu denken. Die Diagnose eines operablen Tumors des Pankreas kann ja dem Patienten das Leben retten. In mohammedanischen Ländern spielt Hypoglykämie bei den psychischen Schwächezuständen während des Ramadan eine Rolle (KHALEQUE et al.). — Überbewertet worden ist die Häufigkeit der funktionellen und „nervösen" Hypoglykämie als Ursache von neurasthenischen oder depressiven Zuständen. — Der Verdacht auf Hypoglykämie ergibt sich vor allem aus der Beobachtung des zeitlichen Zusammenhangs einer Störung mit Nahrungszufuhr und Fasten. (Bei funktioneller Hypoglykämie meist Auftreten der Störungen 2—4 Std nach kohlenhydratreicher Mahlzeit, bei der „nervösen" Form lange nach Mahlzeiten, Behebung der Beschwerden durch Kohlenhydratzufuhr.) Die Differentialdiagnose der verschiedenen Hypoglykämien erfordert neben der Bestimmung der Glucosetoleranz eine eingehende internistische Allgemeinuntersuchung.

Bei funktionellen und „nervösen" Formen der Hypoglykämie sind enge Zusammenhänge mit emotionellen Spannungen aufgedeckt worden. Sie wurden zum Teil mit gespannt-depressiven Zuständen (Rennie und Howard), zum Teil mit dem resignierten Verlust von Initiative und Schwung (Alexander und Portis) in Beziehung gebracht. — Bei diesen Formen sind auch erfolgreiche Psychotherapien durchgeführt worden (Portis; Rennie und Howard). Ihre diätetische Behandlung besteht in eiweißreicher, zuckerarmer Kost, verteilt auf 5—6 Mahlzeiten. — Emotionelle Einflüsse auf das einzelne hypoglykämische Koma wurden wiederholt beobachtet (z. B. Konkov).

10. Diabetes mellitus

Viele psychiatrische Fragen, die mit dem Diabetes zusammenhängen, sind längst bearbeitet worden. Es genügt deshalb, folgende Problemkreise bloß zu erwähnen: Diabetiker sind häufig tüchtige und intelligente Menschen[1]. Die Persönlichkeit von Diabetikern, die früh erkranken, und solchen, die erst in höherem Alter erkranken, erscheint im Durchschnitt andersartig. [Unter den ersteren viele Sensitive, den letzteren viele Syntone (Constam).] Bei der Mehrzahl der Diabetiker sind außer depressiven und seltener anderen Stimmungsverschiebungen leichter Art, außer dem Durst und der Impotenz wenig psychische Veränderungen auffällig. Zu akuten psychotischen Zuständen kommt es (abgesehen vom diabetischen Koma und von hypoglykämischen Komen nach Insulin-Überdosierung) vor allem bei Komplikationen mit Urämie, diabetischer Encephalopathie, Hirnarteriosklerose und Alkoholismus. — Kombination von Diabetes mit manisch-depressivem Kranksein und Hirnarteriosklerose ist häufiger, als es dem Zufall nach zu erwarten wäre, Kombination mit Schizophrenie, Schwachsinn und Epilepsie hingegen seltener.

Besonders bearbeitet und hervorgehoben worden sind in den beiden letzten Jahrzehnten die folgenden psychiatrischen Aspekte der Lehre vom Diabetes:

Beim Altersdiabetes spielt die Fettsucht ursächlich eine erhebliche Rolle. Die ihr zugrunde liegende Eßsucht entsteht, wie heute anzunehmen ist, weitgehend aus emotionellen Gründen. Sie ist kaum die Folge einer primären Stoffwechselkrankheit. Einmal kann Eßsucht von Kind auf gezüchtet und angewöhnt werden; Traditionen in bezug auf die Zubereitung und die Einnahme von Mahlzeiten werden oft sogar als Zeichen eines bestimmten sozialen Ranges oder als Mittelpunkt der Beziehungen unter den Familienangehörigen und Freunden oder als Zeichen der Anhänglichkeit an die verstorbenen Eltern und die Kindheit besonders gepflegt. Hunger nach Nahrung kann nicht nur einem elementaren Nahrungsbedürfnis entsprechen, sondern auch übertragenen Hunger bedeuten: Es besteht die Tendenz, ungestillten Hunger nach Anerkennung, nach Reizen oder nach Liebe durch übermäßiges Essen zu beschwichtigen. Gerade im reifen Alter, in dem Fettsucht und Diabetes oft auftreten, bestehen Gründe zu einem derartigen Hunger: Die beruflichen Aufgaben sind oft zur Routine geworden, und es greifen Enttäuschung und Resignation in bezug auf die berufliche Zukunft um sich; bei der Frau regt sich im Klimakterium ein Gefühl der eigenen Entwertung durch den Verlust der Fortpflanzungsfähigkeit und der jugendlichen Reize; auch nach Erfüllung der mütterlichen Aufgaben an den nunmehr herangewachsenen Kindern bleibt eine Leere zurück. Die aus der Hungrigkeit resultierende Fettsucht fördert die Entstehung des Diabetes.

---

[1] Soweit wir bis jetzt wissen, hemmt ein Diabetes die intellektuelle Entwicklung nur, wenn er schon vor dem 5. Altersjahr beginnt [Ack, M., I. Miller and W. B. Weil, jr.: Intelligence of children with diabetes mellitus. — Pediatrics 28, 5, 764—770 (1961)].

Eine interessante Frage, die aufgeworfen, aber noch nicht beantwortet worden ist, geht dahin, ob ein solcher übertragener Hunger zur physiologischen Schaltung des Stoffwechsels auf gewöhnlichen Hunger Anlaß geben könnte. Emotionelle Hungrigkeit in irgendeiner Richtung (Reizhunger, Liebeshunger, Machthunger usw.) könnte dann direkt zu Stoffwechselschaltungen führen, die im Verlauf des Diabetes eine Rolle spielen; sie würde sich nicht allein über das übertriebene Essen auswirken. Der Stoffwechsel bei Diabetes entspricht ja zum Teil dem Stoffwechsel bei Hunger.

Mehr Berücksichtigung als früher hat die Beobachtung gefunden, daß emotionelle Erschütterungen verschiedener Art eine Verschlimmerung des Diabetes bedingen können. Namentlich hängt die Kohlenhydrattoleranz und damit der Insulinbedarf u. a. von emotionellen Einflüssen ab[1]. — Zum Wohle des Kranken ist auch viel mehr als früher beachtet worden, daß Diätvorschriften seine soziale Lage in mancherlei Art verändern und auch verschlimmern können. Sie belasten ihn nicht nur finanziell, sondern sie können auch seine Beziehungen zu den Eltern, zu Kameraden, zum Ehepartner auf eine harte Probe stellen. Sie können zu Verstimmungen und zu inneren Konflikten führen, die sich wiederum ungünstig auf die Stoffwechsellage auswirken. Ungenügend begründete Diätvorschriften können also nicht nur unnütz, sondern auch schädlich und gefährlich sein.

Zurückhaltend geworden ist man heute in der Annahme von Hirnläsionen als Ursache des Diabetes. Viele Hirnverletzungen, u. a. der Zuckerstich von CLAUDE BERNARD, führen zwar zu vorübergehender Hyperglykämie, aber nicht zum ganzen Krankheitsbild des Diabetes mellitus.

11. Überangebot von Sexualhormonen

Pubertas und Pseudopubertas praecox. Bei der weitaus häufigsten Form der Pubertas praecox sind die Ursachen bisher unentdeckt geblieben; es tritt die körperliche Pubertät in gleicher Art auf wie bei Gesunden; andere Besonderheiten als ihre Vorzeitigkeit fehlen. Man spricht von „konstitutioneller" Frühreife, wohl in etwas leichtfertiger Anwendung des Konstitutionsbegriffes. Die anderen Formen der echten Pubertas praecox sind seltener (Hirntumoren und andere Hirnkrankheiten oder -verletzungen, Albright-Syndrom, endokrin aktive Tumoren[2]). Von der Pseudopubertas praecox (vorzeitige Pubertätserscheinungen ohne Reifung und ohne normale innere Sekretion der Geschlechtsdrüsen) ist die häufigste auf das adrenogenitale Syndrom bei angeborener Nebennierenrindenhyperplasie zurückzuführen, seltenere Formen auf Tumoren von Hoden, Ovar oder Nebennierenrinde oder auf medikamentöse Sexualhormonverabreichung.

Psychiatrisch nehmen die cerebralen Formen natürlich eine Sonderstellung ein, indem die primäre Hirnkrankheit psychopathologische Folgen setzen kann (am häufigsten Schwachsinn und Epilepsie). — Von den übrigen Formen ist die Psychologie der Pseudopubertas praecox bei adrenogenitalem Syndrom psychiatrisch am genauesten bekannt. Sie ist bereits auf S. 209f. behandelt worden. Alle anderen Formen bedürfen sehr der psychiatrischen

---

[1] Möglicherweise geht die Stoffwechselwirkung von psychischer Anspannung beim Diabetiker über das Hypophysen-Nebennieren-System: Die Nebennieren-Steroide haben Einfluß auf den Kohlenhydrat-Stoffwechsel. Sie verursachen einerseits eine Verminderung der Insulinresistenz (durch Verminderung der Bildung von Insulin-Antikörpern), anderseits eine Gluco-Neogenese. Die erstere Wirkung scheint beim insulinbehandelten Diabetiker zu überwiegen. Die Bildung derselben Steroide (beeinflußt vom Hypothalamus und dem Hypophysenvorderlappen aus) hängt u. a. stark von psychischer Anspannung ab (s. u. a. auch BURKART, F. et al.).

[2] Mit Ausscheidung von Gonadotropin.

Erforschung an größerem Krankengut. Vorläufig ist folgendes über sie festzustellen: Ihre Psychopathologie unterscheidet sich nicht merkbar von derjenigen der adrenalen Pseudopubertas praecox. Schwere psychische Störungen bilden Ausnahmen. Am häufigsten hält die psychosexuelle, die allgemein-emotionelle, die charakterliche und die intellektuelle Entwicklung keineswegs mit der vorzeitigen körperlichen Entwicklung Schritt. Im Gegenteil bleiben viele Kinder trotz der körperlichen Reife im Charakter, der Emotionalität, der Psychosexualität und der Intelligenz ihrem Alter entsprechend kindlich. Es kommt sogar oft vor, daß die charakterliche und emotionelle, ja selbst die intellektuelle Entwicklung hinter derjenigen zurückbleibt, die dem Lebensalter entsprechen würde. Die Kinder sind oft unselbständig, scheu, zurückgezogen, mit Minderwertigkeitsgefühlen belastet, was ja weitgehend als psychische Reaktion auf das Entsetzen ihrer Umgebung auf die körperliche Anomalie verständlich ist. — Diese Angaben treffen nun aber keineswegs für alle Fälle zu. Es gibt im Gegenteil eindrucksvolle Beispiele von psychischen Vorentwicklungen Hand in Hand mit der körperlichen Reifung. Der Sexualtrieb kann sich mit beängstigender Hemmungslosigkeit ausleben. Es kommt auch vor, daß die Kinder sich in ihren Interessen ganz den Erwachsenen anschließen. Intellektuelle Reifungsbeschleunigungen sind in Einzelfällen festzustellen, sind aber meist vorübergehend. Häufiger als totale sind partielle psychische Vorentwicklungen, z. B. mimische oder allgemein-motorische Ausdrucksweise des Erwachsenen, altkluges Benehmen, übersteigerte Aggressivität u. a. (Bishop et al.; Jolly; Hampson, Joan G., and J. Money; Hampson, J. L., et al.; Keizer; Marzi und Teodori; Money, J., and Joan G. Hampson; Seckel; Stutte; Thamdrup; Züblin, 1953[1]).

Die älteren Autoren beobachteten und beschrieben sorgfältig und liebevoll Zeichen der psychischen Vorentwicklung. Es ergab sich so aus der älteren Literatur ein falsches Bild über deren Häufigkeit. Die neuen Untersuchungen haben es mit Recht korrigiert. Jedoch ist in der neuen Zeit die Tendenz entstanden, das Zurückbleiben der psychischen im Vergleich zur körperlichen Entwicklung allzu dogmatisch zu betonen. Zeichen psychischer Vorentwicklung werden oft nicht mehr unvoreingenommen zur Kenntnis genommen, ja es wird geradezu versucht, sie mit gewagten Deutungen wegzudisputieren. — Es ist eine faszinierende Forschungsaufgabe der Zukunft, festzustellen, unter welchen Umständen psychische Vorentwicklungen bei körperlicher Reife vorkommen und unter welchen nicht. Einzelne langdauernde Verlaufsuntersuchungen (Lutz und Meyer) lassen bereits Vermutungen begründen: Es scheint, daß die hormonalen Einflüsse, die die körperliche Reifung bedingen, auch mannigfache Anreize für die psychische Entwicklung setzen. Diese Anreize haben aber — wenn sich ihre Existenz überhaupt bestätigt — sicher nicht obligatorische Wirkungen in allen Fällen. Sie werden vielmehr durch die anderen Faktoren, die die Persönlichkeitsentwicklung ausmachen, gestaltet, abgeschwächt, korrigiert, ja überkompensiert.

Körperliche Frühreife macht sorgfältige Untersuchung auf ihre Ursachen notwendig. Wichtige körperliche Behandlungsindikationen bei einzelnen Formen dürfen nicht übersehen werden (hirnchirurgische Eingriffe bei der cerebralen Form, Exstirpation von malignen Tumoren, Cortisonbehandlung beim adrenogenitalen Syndrom u. a.). Umgekehrt sind die Kinder vor unnützen und schädlichen körperlichen Behandlungen zu schützen, wie namentlich vor einer Hormon-

---

[1] Nach einer Aufstellung von Stutte, die während der Drucklegung erschien, sind unter 300 Fällen von körperlicher Frühentwicklung verschiedener Genese 29% dem chronologischen Alter entsprechend psychisch entwickelt, 31% psychisch retardiert oder schwachsinnig, 36% in irgend einer Art vorentwickelt und 4% massiv psychoorganisch verändert.

behandlung der konstitutionellen Form. Eine verständnisvolle Beratung der Eltern und die erzieherische Führung der Kinder sind von großer Bedeutung.

Von den Tumoren, die Androgene oder Oestrogene ausscheiden, sind jene, die die Nebennierenrinde betreffen, sowie jene, die zu Pseudopubertas praecox führen, bereits berücksichtigt. Andere solche Tumoren sind selten, und ihre Psychopathologie ist nur in einzelnen Fällen bekannt geworden. Es scheint, daß die psychische Wirkung oft fehlt oder gering ist; namentlich regt übermäßige Androgen- und Oestrogensekretion aus Tumoren (z. B. Interstitial-Zell-Tumoren der Hoden oder Arrhenoblastome) die Psychosexualität oft nicht an (z. B. WARD et al.; FAURÉ; FAURÉ et al.), Ausnahmen kommen aber vor (z. B. bei BISHOP et al.).

Besonderes Interesse bieten jene seltenen *Tumoren, welche lactotropes Hormon ausscheiden* (Adenome bei Akromegalie, bei Cushing-Syndrom, Chorionepitheliom) (BLEULER, M., 1954,; BLICKENSTORFER, 1949; BLICKENSTORFER et al., SCHWÖBEL). Zusammen mit dem Einfluß auf die Brustdrüse werden elementare Muttertriebe mächtig angeregt (s. S. 195f). Die krankhaften und übersteigerten Pflegeinstinkte kleinen Kindern gegenüber unter dem Einfluß erhöhter Ausschwemmung von lactotropem Hormon sind besonders auffällig, wenn sie bei Männern beobachtet werden.

Unser Wissen über die *psychischen Folgen der medikamentösen Verabreichung von Androgenen und Oestrogenen* ist noch sehr lückenhaft. Eine wichtige Tatsache ist immerhin sichergestellt: Die Sexualhormone haben keine absolute, eindeutige psychische Wirkung, die sich bei allen Menschen zeigen würde. Ihre Wirkung ist vielmehr abhängig von der körperlichen und psychischen Entwicklung, vom Lebensalter, von der sexuellen Erfahrung, der Lebenseinstellung, der erotischen Erlebnisfähigkeit, der Stimmungslage, der psychischen Gesundheit, der persönlichen Disposition und Konstitution. Gesichert sind weiter die folgenden Erfahrungen:

1. Wenn Androgene bei Männern und Oestrogene bei Frauen erfolgreich zur Anwendung gebracht werden, um eine ausbleibende oder krankhaft verspätete Pubertätsentwicklung in Gang zu setzen, zeigt sich sehr oft Hand in Hand mit der körperlichen eine psychische Wirkung. Sie besteht vor allem in einem Erwachen oder einer Verstärkung der Psychosexualität. Daneben aber beobachtet man auch häufig eine Steigerung der Aggressivität (besonders bei Männern), ein Selbständigerwerden, eine Ausweitung der Interessen, eine Reifung der Persönlichkeit ganz allgemein. Die psychische Wirkung kommt oft lange nach der körperlichen. (Zum Beispiel werden solche psychischen Wandlungen bei der Sexualhormon-Behandlung der kongenitalen Anorchie, des Klinefelter-Syndroms, des idiopathischen Eunuchoidismus und der Gonadendysgenesie beobachtet.) Ob es sich bei diesen psychischen Reifungserscheinungen um psychologische Reaktionen auf die körperliche Entwicklung oder um direktere Hormoneinwirkungen auf die Psyche handelt, ist noch umstritten. Meiner Erfahrung nach spielen beide Vorgänge zusammen. — Wenn die Substitutionsbehandlung von Hypogonadalen mit Sexualhormonen unterbrochen wird, so hat das bei Männern gewöhnlich auch eine Dämpfung der Psychosexualität zur Folge; bei Frauen sind die triebhaften Folgen einer solchen Unterbrechung weniger deutlich.

2. Androgene in hohen Dosen bei Frauen in einem reifen oder höheren Alter regen meist die Psychosexualität mächtig an. Mit hohen Dosen sind solche gemeint, die körperliche Vermännlichungserscheinungen hervorzurufen pflegen (d. h. meist über 300 mg Testosteron parenteral im Monat). Die Steigerung der Psychosexualität wird außerordentlich verschieden erlebt und verarbeitet (siehe S. 185f). In der Mehrzahl der Fälle wird auch eine Wirkung auf die Stimmung

beobachtet, häufiger eine euphorisierende und aktivierende als eine deprimierende und inaktivierende. — Diese Erfahrungen wurden vor allem an Frauen mit Mamma-Carcinom gewonnen, an kleinerem Untersuchungsgut auch bei Depressiven. Bei letzteren waren die psychischen Wirkungen der Androgene geringgradiger als bei ersteren.

3. Oestrogene in großen Dosen bei Männern bewirken Hand in Hand mit ihrer Wirkung im Sinne einer Hodenatrophie („chemische Kastration") meist eine wesentliche Abschwächung oder Aufhebung des Geschlechtstriebes. Gleichzeitig werden Stimmungswirkungen beobachtet, eher im Sinne des Depressiven, Mürrischen und Gleichgültigen als im Sinne der Euphorie. An Stelle des Sexualempfindens kann ein allgemeines Zärtlichkeitsbedürfnis treten. — Diese Veränderungen wurden bei der Behandlung von Kranken mit Prostata-Carcinom, von Akromegalen und von Sexualdelinquenten beobachtet. Bei letzteren können Oestrogene in hoher Dosierung mit derselben Indikation angewendet werden wie die Kastration, doch mit dem Unterschied, daß die Kastration endgültige Folgen hat, während die Oestrogene dauernd verabreicht werden müssen; ihre Wirkung auf die Psychosexualität erlöscht nach dem Absetzen.

4. Die gewöhnliche funktionelle Impotenz bei endokrin gesunden Männern wird durch Androgene nicht beeinflußt. Ebensowenig heilen Oestrogene die Frigidität von endokrin gesunden Frauen. Soweit die üblichen Präparate in diesen Fällen eine Wirkung entfalten, muß sie als suggestiv betrachtet werden. Androgene in hoher Dosierung sind meist ebensowenig geeignet, die gewöhnliche Frigidität zu bekämpfen, obschon sie die Psychosexualität anregen: ihre Verabreichung in genügender Dosierung bringt oft Virilisierungs-Erscheinungen mit sich (von denen die Stimmveränderung irreversivel sein kann); außerdem verarbeiten frigide Frauen die Triebanregung leicht durch vermehrte neurotische Abwehr.

5. Sexualhormone im Klimakterium s. S. 219f.

Ungeklärt sind demgegenüber u. a. folgende wichtige Fragen:

1. Haben Androgene und Oestrogene in kleiner Dosierung auf endokrin Gesunde irgendeinen psychischen Einfluß? Auf Grund von einzelnen Untersuchungen ist eine unregelmäßige und geringgradige Stimmungswirkung zu vermuten; in der Praxis werden diese Hormone aber oft angewendet, ohne daß die geringste psychische Veränderung wahrnehmbar wird.

2. Wie wirken sich Androgene und Oestrogene in den üblichen Dosen auf klimakterische Persönlichkeitsveränderungen aus? Nur indirekt, indem sie die heißen Wallungen unterdrücken und der Wegfall dieser lästigen Beschwerden Frohmut aufkommen läßt? Oder auch durch direkte Stimmungswirkung? Letzteres scheint mir wahrscheinlich.

3. Haben Sexualhormone eine Bedeutung bei der Pflege Altersschwacher? Mehrere sorgfältig und groß angelegte Versuche bejahen die Frage mit Entschiedenheit. Es soll eine Aktivierung, Euphorisierung und allgemeine psychische Kräftigung erzielt werden, sogar die amnestischen Störungen sollen günstig beeinflußt werden. Demgegenüber ist erstaunlich festzustellen, daß sich in der Praxis die Behandlung Altersschwacher mit Sexualhormonen trotz der vielen Empfehlungen seit Jahrzehnten nicht durchgesetzt hat — vermutlich weil sie auf längere Sicht eben doch wirkungslos sind. Auch unsere Erfahrungen sind enttäuschend. — Neuerdings ist von Nowakowski und Schmidt die Untersuchung des Fructose-Gehaltes des Ejaculats empfohlen worden, um eine genaue Indikation der Androgentherapie im Alter zu sichern. Unbestimmte Beschwerden, die den Wechseljahrbeschwerden der Frau gleichen, wären beim Mann dann als Folge der Involution der endokrinen Hodenfunktion zu deuten, wenn die Fructose im

Ejaculat erniedrigt ist. In diesem (und nur in diesem!) Falle wäre dann eine Androgentherapie von Involutionsbeschwerden des Mannes (Verstimmungen, mangelnde Konzentrationsfähigkeit, Müdigkeit usw.) erfolgversprechend. Diese Annahmen rechtfertigen weitere klinische Erforschung.

4. Kommen dem Progesteron psychische Wirkungen zu, wenn ja, welche? Die Frage ist bisher in verschiedenster Art beantwortet worden. Oft scheint Progesteron die Psychosexualität der Frau zu mildern, in selteneren Fällen aber zu steigern. Progesteron kann bei emotionellen Spannungszuständen (z. B. im Prämenstruum) günstig wirken[1], in andern Fällen aber erregen. (Die narkotische Wirkung von Progesteron und ähnlichen Stoffen kommt nur in ganz unphysiologischen Dosen zustande.)

Die *anabolen Steroide* regen oft den Appetit an und haben gelegentlich eine ähnliche Stimmungswirkung wie die Androgene (z. B. BEIGLBÖCK und BRUMMUND[2]). Sie wirken körperlich weniger sexualisierend als die Androgene. Man kann deshalb vermuten, daß auch ihre Wirkungen auf die Psychosexualität der Frau geringer sind, wenn sie auch nicht ganz fehlen (Mosso und PERGOLA; WYNN und LANDON), es bleibt aber zu erforschen, ob diese Erwartung stimmt.

12. Psychopathologie der endokrinen Umstellungsphasen der Frau

Die emotionellen Störungen im Klimakterium und im Prämenstruum und die Wochenbetts-Psychosen konnten bis heute nicht eindeutig auf pathologische endokrine Funktionen zurückgeführt werden. Es ist bisher nicht überzeugend gelungen, bei Patientinnen mit Verstimmungen und anderen psychischen Störungen im Klimakterium, mit prämenstrueller Spannung oder mit Wochenbetts-Psychosen wesentlich andere Hormonbefunde zu erheben, als sie auch oft bei Frauen erhoben werden, die diese endokrinen Umstellungsphasen ohne psychische Störungen durchmachen. Auf Grund unserer heutigen Kenntnisse ist zu vermuten, daß klimakterische, prämenstruelle und puerperale Störungen von Stimmung, Triebhaftigkeit und emotioneller Ansprechbarkeit nicht eindeutig auf endokrine Störungen zurückzuführen sind, sondern daß endokrine Umstellungsphasen lediglich eine allgemeine Prädisposition für emotionelle Gleichgewichtsstörungen schaffen. — Die hormonale Therapie dieser Störungen ist bisher nur empirisch begründbar und fußt im Gegensatz zu dem, was vielfach vorausgesetzt wird, noch nicht auf einer genauen Kenntnis einer hormonalen Genese[3].

Bei *klimakterischen emotionellen Beschwerden* ist, wie die Erfahrung zeigt, ein Versuch mit Sexualhormonen angezeigt. Es kommen sowohl Oestrogene wie Androgene in Frage. Erstere können in hohen Dosen Blutungen, letztere Virilisierung (Stimmbruch, Haarwachstum, Vergrößerung der Klitoris) bewirken. Die Kombination von Androgenen und Oestrogenen erlaubt öfters, die Beschwerden wirksam anzugehen, ohne Nebenerscheinungen erwarten zu müssen. Die Dosierung

---

[1] Therapeutische Erfolge mit Progesteron-Präparaten (besonders „Gestanyn") bei Migräne wurden mit der Entspannung der Gefäße in Zusammenhang gebracht (LUNDBERG); vielleicht wirken sie eher über die emotionelle Entspannung.

[2] Sie haben in einzelnen Versuchsreihen auch die psychomotorischen Reaktionen beschleunigt (KALLIOMÄKI).

[3] Wie wenig Theorie und Wirklichkeit in diesen Belangen übereinstimmen, zeigt sich u. a. an folgendem Beispiel: Nach der Theorie wirken sich die Sexualhormone günstig auf klimakterische Beschwerden aus, weil sie die im Klimakterium stark vermehrte Gonadotropin-Bildung herabsetzen. Es ist aber nicht nachgewiesen, daß die Gonadotropine bei Frauen mit klimakterischen Beschwerden stärker erhöht wären als bei klimakterischen Frauen ohne Beschwerden. Die Heilwirkung der Sexualhormone erfolgt sogar oft, ohne daß die Gonadotropine vermindert würden! (Siehe z. B. ROSEMBERG und ENGEL.)

beider Hormonpräparate ist der individuell sehr verschiedenen Wirkung anzupassen. — Die Therapie von emotionellen klimakterischen Störungen mit Sexualhormonen ist um so eher erfolgreich, je leichter die emotionellen Störungen sind und je enger sie zeitlich mit der Menopause und mit körperlichen klimakterischen Beschwerden korreliert sind. Bei schweren klimakterischen Depressionen oder Katatonie sind sie unwirksam.

Als Ursache des *prämenstruellen Spannungs-Syndroms* wurde früher vor allem der Hyperfollikulinismus angenommen — ohne genügende Gründe. In bunter Reihe wurden später die verschiedensten und gegensätzlichsten hormonalen Gleichgewichts-Störungen als Ursachen angesprochen: ein Zuviel oder Zuwenig an Progesteron, an Androgenen, ein Zuwenig an Oestrogenen, ein Zuviel an antidiuretischem Hormon, Hyperthyreose u. a. Mit modernen Methoden wurde neuerdings am häufigsten ein Mangel an Follikelhormon und vor allem an Progesteron gefunden, in anderen (selteneren) Fällen eine Übersekretion dieser Hormone. Beiden Zuständen könnte eine Überausscheidung von gonadotropen Hormonen gemeinsam sein (entweder eine primäre, die die endokrine Funktion des Ovars anregt, oder — häufiger — eine sekundäre bei primärem Darniederliegen der Bremsung der Hypophyse durch die Follikelhormone) (Geller u. a.). Gleichzeitig spielt in vielen Fällen Wasserretention (und Vermehrung des antidiuretischen Hormons) eine Rolle. Unbewiesen sind Hypothesen, nach denen allergische Vorgänge oder Vitaminmangel oder Vergiftung mit hypothetischen Menstruationstoxinen wesentlich beteiligt wären.

Bisher läßt sich die prämenstruelle Spannung aber bei weitem nicht eindeutig und vollständig mit pathologisch-physiologischen Vorgängen erklären. Solche (und besonders endokrine Insuffizienz des Ovars) sind zwar bei Frauen mit prämenstrueller Spannung wahrscheinlich häufiger als bei solchen ohne prämenstruelle Beschwerden; doch gibt es viele Fälle von prämenstrueller Spannung, bei denen keine abnormen endokrinen Vorgänge aufzudecken sind. Umgekehrt leiden lange nicht alle Frauen mit Gewichtszunahme vor der Menstruation oder mit Hypogonadismus an prämenstrueller Spannung.

Auf Grund eines Überblickes der Literatur und eigener Erfahrung scheint mir vorläufig die folgende Auffassung des prämenstruellen Spannungssyndroms nahezuliegen: Die endokrine Umstellung im Prämenstruum hat einen wesensgleichen dysharmonisierenden Einfluß auf die Emotionalität wie viele andere endokrine Umstellungen. (So z. B. beobachtet man häufig dieselben Symptome wie im prämenstruellen Spannungssyndrom in der Schwangerschaft, im Klimakterium, im Beginn einer Hyperthyreose, bei Cortison-Behandlung usw.) Die Symptome der prämenstruellen Spannung fügen sich zwanglos in den weiteren Begriff eines leichten endokrinen Psychosyndroms ein. Sie unterscheiden sich von rein psychogenen emotionellen Störungen dadurch, daß elementare Triebstörungen (Durst, abnorme Gelüste, Veränderungen des Schlafbedürfnisses u. a.) im Vordergrund stehen. — Gestörte endokrine Cyclus-Vorgänge mögen im Durchschnitt die emotionellen Folgen verschärfen.

Die rein endokrinen Einflüsse des Prämenstruums auf die Emotionalität sind aber offensichtlich gering. Die gesunde Frau, die erfüllt und tätig im Leben steht, braucht sie nicht zu beachten. Man beachtet ja sehr viele leichte körperliche Einflüsse auf das gemütliche Befinden nicht: leichte Hungergefühle, leichte Ermüdung leichte Schmerzen bleiben oft völlig unbemerkt, wenn man tätig und lebensfroh ist. Die prämenstruellen endokrinen Einflüsse werden erst zu bewußt empfundenem Leiden, wenn ein inneres Bedürfnis vorhanden ist, sich leiblich mit den Generationsvorgängen auseinanderzusetzen. Ein solches Bedürfnis ist oft wach. Es kann schon in der Lebensproblematik einer gesunden Frau enthalten sein: Der versagte

Wunsch nach Schwangerschaft kann in Erwartung der Periode lebendig und quälend werden; das Spiel mit den gefühlsgeladenen Gedanken „Wenn die Blutung doch ausbliebe!"kann einen geheimnisvollen Reiz haben, der lustgeladen ist, gleichzeitig aber auch weh tut. Ebenso kann die Angst vor der Schwangerschaft auf die endokrinen Einflüsse im Prämenstruum sensibilisierend wirken. Oft entspringt das Bedürfnis nach einer inneren Auseinandersetzung mit den Generationsvorgängen — und sei sie noch so schmerzhaft — neurotischer oder psychopathischer Entwicklung. Es kann u. a. ein Aspekt eines Infantilismus mit Ablehnung der Rolle einer reifen Frau sein.

Wir sehen deshalb vorläufig die prämenstruelle Spannung *gleichzeitig als Folge einer* (normalen oder gestörten) *hormonalen Umstellungsphase und als psychogene Erscheinung*: Die hormonale Umstimmungsphase bedeutet einen störenden Einfluß auf Stimmung, Antriebshaftigkeit und elementare Triebe. Er ist aber so schwach, daß er unbemerkt bleibt, wenn eine Frau nicht durch das Bedürfnis nach der Auseinandersetzung mit der Problematik der Fortpflanzung sensibilisiert ist.

Die prämenstruelle Spannung gehört zu jenen Störungen, die auf vielerlei Behandlungen vorübergehend ansprechen, bei denen aber keine Behandlung völlig zuverlässig ist und bei der alle Behandlungen auf lange Sicht nur selten befriedigen. Erfolge sieht man von verschiedenen Hormonbehandlungen: Bei Zeichen von Hypofollikulinismus wird man zuerst Oestrogene versuchen, sonst Androgene (z. B. Methyltestosteron oder dann Methylandrostendiol) oder Progesteron in der zweiten Cyclushälfte. Oft sind allein oder in Kombination mit Hormonen entwässernde Mittel wirksam. Sie erscheinen bei Gewichtszunahme im Prämenstruum besonders sinnvoll. Auch mit verschiedensten allgemeinen Beruhigungsmitteln lassen sich Milderungen erreichen. — Oft sind psychotherapeutische Bemühungen erfolgreich. Je nach der Persönlichkeit der Patientin, den äußeren Gegebenheiten und der Ausbildung des Arztes kommen alle psychotherapeutischen Verfahren von einfachen Suggestivtherapien oder bloßen Besprechungen über die Gründe von emotionellen Spannungen bis zur Psychoanalyse in Frage.

Erstaunlich ist, daß die Patientinnen gewöhnlich Medikationen nach einiger Zeit aufgeben und aus der Behandlung ausbleiben — auch dann, wenn sie sehr erfolgreich schienen. Es ist, als ob die innere Auseinandersetzung mit der Problematik der Generationsvorgänge in prämenstruellen Beschwerden einem starken Bedürfnis entsprechen würde, dem die Patientinnen trotz aller Klagen schließlich freien Lauf geben wollen. Die Beschwerden hören dann bei Änderungen der Lebensverhältnisse „von selbst" auf: vor dem Klimakterium, nach Geburten, nach der Verheiratung oder wenn das Leben strenge Anforderungen an die Leistungsfähigkeit der Frau stellt.

In vereinzelten Fällen steigert sich die prämenstruelle Spannung bis zu psychotischen Episoden: u. a. sind solche neuerdings von JANINA KRASOWSKA anschaulich beschrieben worden. Sie prägte den Ausdruck des «*Syndrome psychotique de la tension prémenstruelle*». Es fand sich bei jungen Mädchen nach der Pubertät, aber erst nachdem einige Menstruationscyclen ungestört abgelaufen waren. Die üblichen Beschwerden der prämenstruellen Spannung steigerten sich in diesen Fällen zu psychotischen Verstimmungen (mit ängstlicher oder zorniger Erregung oder mit Stupor) und sogar weiter zu schweren Delirien mit Verwirrtheit, Depersonalisationserlebnissen, Halluzinationen (besonders visuellen) und wahnhaften Einfällen. Die psychotischen Episoden, die JANINA KRASOWSKA beschreibt, hinterließen nie Persönlichkeitsstörungen, vielmehr waren die Patientinnen in der ersten Hälfte des Cyclus völlig gesund. Es fanden sich Zeichen von mangelhafter endokriner Funktion des Ovars, namentlich Hypofollikulinismus gemäß dem Befunde am

Scheidenepithel und fehlender Temperaturanstieg in der Mitte des Cyclus. Trotzdem ist die hormonale Grundlage der Störung nicht geklärt und Vermutungen über Hyper- und Hypo-Follikulinismus stehen sich gegenüber. Die Patientinnen wurden sehr erfolgreich mit Testosteronpropionat behandelt. — Ähnliche Fälle finden sich vereinzelt in der Literatur zerstreut unter den verschiedensten Etiquetten (z. B. J. T. Fischer); sie entsprechen auch einem Teil der „Menstruationspsychosen" alter Autoren. — Die meisten Kliniker sehen derartige Psychosen selten oder gar nie. Es bleibt kritisch zu untersuchen, welche ätiologische Bedeutung Besonderheiten im Stoffwechsel der Sexualhormone dabei haben und ob die Therapie mit Hormonen wirklich für die Heilung entscheidend ist (oder ob die Psychosen auch ohne Behandlung gutartig verlaufen).

Das Problem des «syndrome psychotique de la tension prémenstruelle» wird durch die Studien von Wakoh, 1959; Wakoh et al. 1960, neu beleuchtet und erweitert: Er ging von ähnlichen Psychosen bei Japanerinnen aus wie Krasowska bei Polinnen. (Es handelt sich wieder um akute, episodische Bewußtseinsstörungen mit guter Prognose, die im klassischen nosologischen System keinen eindeutigen Platz gefunden haben und die als schizophreniforme Psychosen nach Langfeldt, als Mischpsychosen, als poussées délirantes und noch anders bezeichnet wurden.) Er sah diese Psychosen aber nicht nur bei jungen Mädchen, sondern in jedem Alter. Sie fielen nicht ausschließlich mit der zweiten Hälfte des Cyclus zusammen, sondern kamen auch im Wochenbett und nach Aborten und in einer kleinen Minderzahl von Fällen während der Menstruation oder in der ersten Hälfte des Cyclus vor. (Hingegen fehlten sie in der Schwangerschaft.) Die Bestimmung der Oestrogen-Ausscheidung im Urin ergab während der Psychose Veränderungen gegenüber der Norm: besonders das Fehlen der normalen beiden Gipfel der Ausscheidung von Oestrogenen während des Cyclus. Vermehrte Oestrogen-Ausscheidung fand sich vor allem bei Erregung und Verwirrung, verminderte bei Depression und Stupor. Das Pregnandiol wird vermindert ausgeschieden, vermutlich wegen Veränderungen im Progesteron-Abbau der Leber. (Bei denselben Fällen fand sich eine Veränderung der Zusammensetzung der 17-Ketosteroide: Verminderung des Anteils von Androsteron und — in geringerem Maße — von Eticholanolon.)

Eine klare Beurteilung solcher prämenstrueller Psychosen mit ihrer Ätiologie und ihrer nosologischen Stellung ist noch nicht möglich. Vorläufig ist sogar noch fraglich, ob die endokrinologischen Befunde Ursachen oder Folgen einer Psychose sind. Mir scheint es unwahrscheinlich, daß sich aus solchen Studien eindeutige Kausalitätsverhältnisse und scharf umschriebene Krankheitseinheiten herausschälen werden. Es scheint vorläufig wahrscheinlicher, daß sich die Befunde in die Annahme multifaktorieller Verursachung von Geistesstörungen einordnen: hormonale Störungen würden die Psychosen nur neben anderen Faktoren mitbedingen und mit beeinflussen.

Psychosen in engem Zusammenhang mit dem Menstruationscyclus scheinen übrigens an verschiedenen Orten und zu verschiedenen Zeiten in verschiedener Häufigkeit aufzutreten. In meinem Erfahrungsgut sind sie außerordentlich selten, obschon ich mich besonders dafür interessiere. Zudem betreffen die wenigen Fälle, die ich behandeln konnte, Kranke, die aus südlichen und östlichen Ländern zu mir in Behandlung kamen.

Bei *Wochenbetts-Psychosen* fehlt bisher der sichere Nachweis, daß die hormonale Umstellung anders erfolgt, als der Norm entspricht. Die Wirksamkeit von hormonalen Bchandlungen ist noch völlig ungesichert. Am ehesten scheinen z. Z. Versuche mit Gelbkörper-Hormonen oder Cortison (s. S. 209) nahezuliegen[1]. Französische Autoren wiesen auf Veränderungen von Vaginalschleimhaut und Endometrium hin, die sich durch Hormonbehandlung nicht beeinflussen ließen. Sie führten in solchen Fällen eine Curettage durch. Sie nahmen an, daß sie sich als „neurohumoraler Reflex" auf das Diencephalon auswirke (DELAY et al. 1951, 1954).

13. Echter Hermaphroditismus und Pseudohermaphroditismus

An psychiatrisch gut oder ordentlich bekannten, genetisch einheitlichen Untergruppen sind die folgenden herauszuheben:

a) Pseudohermaphroditismus femininus bei angeborener Nebennierenrinden-Hyperplasie, auf S. 209f. besprochen.

b) Klinefelter-Syndrom (die Verteilung des Chromatins in den Zellkernen entspricht dem weiblichen Typus; in den meisten Fällen sind 3 Geschlechtschromosomen, 2 weibliche und 1 männliches, vorhanden; männliches äußeres Genitale, evtl. Gynäkomastie, evtl. Eunuchoidismus, kleine Hoden mit Tubulus-Sklerose, Azoospermie, Hypergonadotropismus): Das Syndrom ist oft mit unterdurchschnittlicher Intelligenz oder mit Schwachsinn gekoppelt (CORNWELL und HERRMANN; PASQUALINI et al.; PRADER et al.). Dementsprechend fand es sich unter Hilfsschülern gehäuft (z.B. in Zürich an 8 von 671 Untersuchten!) (PRADER et al.)[2]. Geschlechtstrieb und Liebesfähigkeit können normal sein, sind aber oft schwach und kindlich. Die Potenz, die in jugendlichem Alter meist gegeben ist, geht oft vorzeitig wieder verloren. Auch die ganze Persönlichkeit ist meist unselbständig, ziellos, infantil. Verstimmungen und Trotzreaktionen sind häufig und bedingen oft Schwererziehbarkeit.

In seltenen Fällen von Klinefelter-Syndrom ist nicht nur *ein* überzähliges Geschlechtschromosom festzustellen, sondern es bestehen noch schwerere Anomalien des Chromosomensatzes: So fanden sich u. a. 4 Geschlechtschromosomen in allen oder einem Teil der Zellen, also 2 überzählige, und die Formel XXXY. Interessanterweise erwiesen sich Klinefelter-Patienten mit diesen schwersten Chromosomen-Anomalien in höherem Maße schwachsinnig als die Mehrzahl der Klinefelter-Patienten (ANDERS et al.; BARR et al.; FERGUSON-SMITH et al. a und b; NOWAKOWSKI et al. u. a.).

Während somit eine (grobe) Proportion zwischen dem Grad der Chromosomenanomalie und dem Grad des Schwachsinns besteht, wurde bisher keine Korrelation zwischen dem Grad des Hypogonadismus und dem Grad des Schwachsinns gefunden (RABOCH und SIPOVA). Dies entspricht allgemeineren Erfahrungen: Störungen des Chromosomensatzes sind oft mit Schwachsinn gekoppelt, Mangel an Androgenen gewöhnlich nicht. (Schwachsinn fand sich u. a. auch bei einzelnen — nicht allen! — „Superfemales", d. h. bei Patientinnen mit 3 weiblichen Geschlechtschromosomen.)

In sehr seltenen Ausnahmefällen fand sich bei Klinefelter-Syndrom Transvestitismus (MONEY, J., 1963; OVERZIER 1958a und b; WALTER und BRÄUTIGAM; eigene Beobachtung).

c) Gonadendysgenesie (Keimzellenmangel) oder Turner-Syndrom [die Verteilung des Chromatins in den Zellkernen entspricht meist dem männlichen Typus;

---

[1] Vermutungen darüber, daß Wochenbettpsychosen mit Schwankungen in der Ausscheidung von 17-Hydroxysteroiden nach der Geburt (JACOBIDES) oder mit einem Abfall des eiweißgebundenen Jods im Blute nach der Geburt [und damit mit der Schilddrüsenfunktion (HAMILTON)] etwas zu tun hätten, sind noch unbewiesen.

[2] Demgegenüber liegt die Häufigkeit unter allen männlichen Neugeborenen zwischen $1{,}7^0/_{00}$ und $4{,}6^0/_{00}$.

genauere Untersuchungen des Chromosomensatzes zeigen, daß meist nur ein einziges (weibliches) Geschlechtschromosom vorhanden ist, daß also sowohl ein Y-Chromosom wie bei einem normalen Manne als auch ein zweites X-Chromosom wie bei einer normalen Frau fehlt; es kommen aber auch andere Anomalien des Chromosomensatzes vor; rudimentäre Gonaden, Amenorrhoe, weibliche äußere Genitalien, Fehlen sekundärer Geschlechtsmerkmale bis auf leichte Sexualbehaarung, Hypergonadotropismus, dazu in vielen Fällen Kleinwuchs, Pterygium colli u. a. Besonderheiten im Körperbau[1]. — Der körperliche Infantilismus ist fast immer mit einem psychischen Infantilismus gekoppelt, wenn nicht eine Oestrogenbehandlung die Reifung förderte (DE LA CHAPELLE; HAUSER; KRAUTSCHIK; WALLIS; ZÜBLIN 1960 u.a.). Dieser Infantilismus bezieht sich sowohl auf die mangelnde charakterliche Reifung wie auf das Ausbleiben eines reifen Sexualtriebes. Die Patientinnen sind unselbständig, lenksam und in ihrem Wesen wenig profiliert; ihr intellektuelles Leben ist mehr reproduktiv als persönlich. Mehreren Beobachtern ist aufgefallen, daß die Patientinnen kein Bedürfnis haben, sich nach gewöhnlichem weiblichen Geschmack hübsch zu kleiden und sich zu schmücken. Die Intelligenz hält sich demgegenüber (im Gegensatz zum Klinefelter-Syndrom) meistens noch innerhalb normaler Grenzen, doch ist sie oft unterdurchschnittlich; nur eine Minderzahl der Kranken ist schwachsinnig. Entsprechend dem Bau der Genitalien und der Auferziehung als Mädchen fühlen sich die Kranken als Mädchen, auch dann, wenn das Chromosomengeschlecht männlich ist. Die Interessenrichtung ist auch sonst vorwiegend weiblich. Psychosen sind seltene Ausnahmen. Dagegen kann sich der Infantilismus mit Unbeherrschtheit, Trotz, Haltlosigkeit oder Antriebsstörungen sozial schwer auswirken. — Oestrogene können rasch euphorisieren, und über längere Zeit verabreicht, fördern sie die psychische Reifung Hand in Hand mit der körperlichen.

Turner-Syndrom bei männlichem Körperbau ist sehr selten. In einem der bisher beschriebenen 17 Fälle war die Psychosexualität unentwickelt (FRACCARO et al. 1961).

d) Testiculäre Feminisierung oder „hereditäre Intersexform bei äußerlich weiblichen, gonadal und chromosomal männlichen Individuen ohne Uterus und ohne Sexualbehaarung" (PRADER 1957): Nach übereinstimmenden Berichten fast aller Untersucher unterscheidet sich die Psychologie dieser Pseudohermaphroditen in keiner Weise von derjenigen normaler Frauen (z. B. GAYRAL[2]). Frigidität erschien einzelnen Untersuchern sogar seltener als bei normalen Frauen. Die Intelligenz ist nicht beeinträchtigt, die Häufigkeit guter Begabungen scheint im Gegenteil auffällig.

Nach Ausscheidung dieser Sonderformen und abgesehen von besonderen Seltenheiten bleiben zu berücksichtigen: der *nicht-adrenale Pseudohermaphroditismus femininus und masculinus mit intersexuellen Genitalien* und *der echte Hermaphroditismus:* Keine dieser Formen von Intersexualität ist an genügend großem Krankengut psychiatrisch durchuntersucht worden. Soweit aber bekannt ist, unterscheidet sich ihre Psychopathologie weder untereinander noch vom adrenalen Pseudohermaphroditismus: Schwere psychische Störungen aller Art, insbesondere Psychosen und Neurosen von klinischer Bedeutung, sind selten, kaum häufiger als in der Durchschnittsbevölkerung. Es ist erstaunlich, daß die körperliche Mißgestalt so häufig ohne schwere psychische Schädigung ertragen wird. Scheues

---

[1] Das Turner-Syndrom ist um ein Mehrfaches seltener als das Klinefelter-Syndrom.

[2] Aus der Literatur ist mir eine einzige Ausnahme bekannt geworden: KÖNIG (1960) beschreibt ein 13jähriges Mädchen mit testiculärer Feminisierung, das nie Interesse an Puppen hatte und beim Spiel und Sport männlich eingestellt ist. Aus Projektionstests wurde auf „homosexuelle Tendenzen" geschlossen — Testergebnisse sind freilich in dieser Hinsicht höchst unzuverlässig.

Wesen, Gehemmtsein, Selbstkritik und Ängstlichkeit in leichterem Grade finden sich allerdings oft. Die ganze Persönlichkeit trägt oft ein infantiles Gepräge. Im allgemeinen leben sich die Zwitter in das Geschlecht ein, das ihnen nach der Geburt zugeteilt worden ist und scheuen einen Wechsel des offiziellen Geschlechtes. In der Mehrzahl der Fälle wird auch dann an der angewohnten Geschlechtsrolle festgehalten, wenn sie im Gegensatz zum Chromosomengeschlecht, zur Geschlechtsdrüse oder zur vorherrschenden Sexualhormon-Sekretion steht. Die Psychosexualität ist der Richtung nach ebenfalls meist der angewohnten Geschlechtsrolle angepaßt, aber sie ist häufig schwach, zielunsicher und infantil. Ausnahmen kommen aber nicht selten vor, und Zwitter können sehr bestimmte Wünsche nach Umwandlung der Geschlechtsrolle äußern und eine sexuelle Triebrichtung zeigen, die dem zugeteilten Geschlecht widerspricht.

Ein Wechsel in der sozialen Geschlechtsrolle, der gegen den Widerstand der Patienten erfolgt, setzt ein schweres psychisches Trauma. Er muß vermieden werden, wenn das Kind älter als 1—2 Jahre geworden ist. Zwitter, die äußerlich zum anderen Geschlecht gehören als ihren Chromosomen oder ihren Gonaden entspricht, sollen nicht durch Mitteilung der Untersuchungsbefunde unnötig beunruhigt und gequält werden.

14. Hypogonadismus und Infantilismus

(Angeborene und früherworbene Formen)

Zwei Sonderformen, das *Klinefelter-Syndrom* und die *Gonadendysgenesie*, sind bereits besprochen worden. Die *übrigen Formen* sind psychiatrisch noch wenig systematisch erforscht. Psychische Besonderheiten sind nach einzelnen Beobachtungen nur bei jenen Formen auffällig, bei denen die innere Sekretion mitbetroffen ist (nach anderen aber erstaunlicherweise auch bei selektiver Schädigung des tubulären Teils der Testes). Unterschiede der Psychopathologie in den endokrinologischen Unterformen, z. B. zwischen Anorchie und idiopathischem Eunuchoidismus, sind nicht gesichert. In der großen Mehrzahl der Fälle ist der angeborene oder früh erworbene Hypogonadismus, bei dem die endokrine Sekretion beteiligt ist, mit psychischem Infantilismus gekoppelt. (Zu diesen Schlüssen kommen unter vielen anderen z. B. DICZFALUSY und LAURITZEN; VITEBSKAYA.) Er betrifft Psychosexualität und allgemeine Charakterreifung gleichermaßen, viel seltener aber die intellektuelle Entwicklung. Auf dem Boden des Infantilismus entwickeln sich leicht Primitivreaktionen, Trotzzustände, Angstreaktionen, infantile sexuelle Verhaltensweisen, übertriebene Abhängigkeit von anderen.

Der Psychiater begegnet häufig Formen von *körperlichem Infantilismus, bei denen die endokrinen Funktionen nicht nachweisbar gestört sind.* Sie können sich durch kindliche Gesichtszüge, kindliche Stimme, mangelhaften Bartwuchs, geringe und wenig geschlechtstypische Körperbehaarung, undifferenzierte, kindliche Handformen, geringe Geschlechtsdifferenzierung des Skelets u. a. auszeichnen. Die Ausscheidung von 17-Ketosteroiden und von Gonadotropinen, alle Erscheinungen, die den Menstruationszyklus kennzeichnen, Sperma und Histologie der Gonaden sind dagegen in der Hauptsache normal. Die moderne Endokrinologie spricht hier gerne von „Pseudoeunuchoidismus", verweist die Störungen ins Gebiet des „Konstitutionellen", der mangelhaften Ansprechbarkeit der Erfolgsorgane auf Sexualhormone, und beschäftigt sich wenig mit ihnen. Dabei ist es durchaus möglich, daß doch endokrine Störungen bei der Entstehung dieses Infantilismus mitwirken, z. B. solche, die zeitlich an eine bestimmte, kurzdauernde Entwicklungsphase gebunden sind. In der Mehrzahl der Fälle (nicht etwa in jedem einzelnen) besteht eine Korrelation auch zwischen diesem körperlichen Infantilismus einerseits, psychosexuellem und charakterlichem Infantilismus anderseits. Unterintelligenz und leichter Schwachsinn sind häufig. Diese Infantilismusformen treten hochgradig familiär auf. Interessanterweise häufen sich unter den Verwandten der infantilen Probanden wieder körperlich Infantile, psychisch Infantile und leicht Schwachsinnige. Diese Störungen sind auch in der Verwandtschaft häufiger untereinander korreliert, als dem Zufall entsprechen würde, aber eine absolute Korrelation besteht nicht.

Die Psychopathologie dieser Infantilen ist gut erforscht (Lindberg u. a.). Dringlich geworden ist hingegen das Studium ihrer Genese. Wenn endokrine Störungen in einer bestimmten Kindheitsphase beteiligt wären, käme eine Prophylaxe in Frage. — Substitutionsbehandlung Hypogonadaler s. S. 229.

Kastration. Die Wirkung der Kastration *des Mannes* ist schon seit längerer Zeit gut bekannt. Kastration dämpft meistens Sexualtrieb und Potenz oder hebt sie auf. Ausnahmen kommen vor[1]. Nach einer Periode von leichteren emotionellen Wallungen und von Verstimmbarkeit wie im Klimakterium der Frau erfolgt oft eine Beruhigung des ganzen Wesens, und einzelne Charakterzüge, die als besonders „männlich" imponierten, verwischen und verändern sich. Die Charakterwirkung nach Kastration wird aber stark von Nebenumständen mitbeeinflußt, davon, in welchem Alter sie erfolgte, ob sie zu einer sozialen Verachtung und Verstoßung in eine Sonderklasse von Menschen geführt hat u. a. Bei sorgfältiger Indikationsstellung und im Einverständnis der Kranken wirkt sich die Kastration bei einzelnen Sexualperversen therapeutisch sehr wohltätig aus. Die Perversion muß, wenn die Indikation zur Kastration gestellt werden soll, quälend schwere Folgen haben und ein glückbringendes Sexualleben verunmöglichen; sie muß psychotherapeutisch unbeeinflußbar sein; sie muß sich hauptsächlich auf das Körperlich-Triebhafte, den Orgasmus selbst, und nicht hauptsächlich auf den ganzen Charakter und die ganze Lebensführung beziehen; die zugrundeliegende Persönlichkeit darf nicht schwer krankhaft sein; die Operation darf nur im überzeugten Einverständnis des Kranken durchgeführt werden. (Ist fälschlich ein Druck auf ihn ausgeübt worden, so können Beeinträchtigungsvorstellungen und psychogene Übertreibung der Nebenwirkungen die Folge sein.) Diese längst belegten Erfahrungen sind nur deshalb hier zu wiederholen, weil mehrere neuere Autoren angeben, die Kastration habe kaum eine psychische Wirkung. Solche Behauptungen beruhen auf Verallgemeinerungen von einzelnen Ausnahmefällen und auf der dogmatischen Überzeugung, daß beim Menschen keine endokrinen Einflüsse auf die Psyche wirksam seien. Wer viele Kastraten kennt, zweifelt nicht an der Häufigkeit eines herabgesetzten Trieblebens nach der Kastration.

Gewöhnlich enttäuscht eine „therapeutische" Kastration nur dann, wenn die Indikation falsch war. Sie beeinflußt z. B. die Homosexualität als Triebrichtung nicht und dient keinesfalls Homosexuellen, deren Hauptbedürfnis nach Zärtlichkeit, Freundschaft, Umhegtwerden und eheartigen Verhältnissen mit Männern gerichtet ist. Ebensowenig ist sie bei antisozialen Schwachsinnigen zu empfehlen, auch dann nicht, wenn ihre Verstöße gelegentlich die Sexualität berühren. Am wenigsten kann von der Kastration eine Dämpfung von allgemeiner Aggressivität und Erregtheit bei Schwachsinn, Psychopathie oder Schizophrenie erwartet werden. — Bei richtiger Indikationsstellung kann man in über 90% der therapeutischen Kastration Erfolg erwarten.

Die körperlichen Folgeerscheinungen der Kastration des Mannes (Hitzewallungen, Veränderungen der Gesichtszüge, der Fettverteilung, der Haut, der

---

[1] Geringe oder fehlende Wirkung auf Sexualtrieb und Potenz ist noch am häufigsten, wenn die Kastration schon im 3. Lebensjahrzehnt erfolgt.

Behaarung und der Stimme) sind gewöhnlich so leicht, daß sie keine Behandlung notwendig machen oder sie lassen sich mit einer Hormonbehandlung beeinflussen (auch ohne daß diese Substitutionstherapie den Behandlungserfolg stören würde). Die Fettsucht der Kastraten bedeutet nicht eine direkte Stoffwechselwirkung der hormonalen Insuffizienz, sondern ist die Folge einer psychischen Umstellung auf Vielessen und Trägheit. Dementsprechend tritt sie keineswegs regelmäßig nach der Kastration auf, sondern nur in einer Minderzahl der Fälle.

Das alte Wissen um die Kastrationsfolgen ist in den letzten Jahren durch neue Untersuchungen vielfach bestätigt worden (u. a. von Bowman und Crook, von Bremer, von Langelüddeke, von Ohm, von Theiler und von Yamamoto und Seeman). — Neu hinzugekommen sind endokrinologische Untersuchungen von Kastraten: sie zeigen, daß die Verminderung der 17-Ketosteroide nach der Kastration keineswegs regelmäßig und hochgradig ist. Die 17-Ketosteroid-Ausscheidung hängt ja auch lange nicht ausschließlich von den im Hoden gebildeten Androgenen ab.[1]

In zwei Fällen von testiculärer Feminisierung verminderte die Exstirpation der Hoden die Psychosexualität (Wilkins; Witschi und Mengert). Wenn sich diese Beobachtungen an größerem Erfahrungsgut bestatigen sollten, wären sie von großer Bedeutung.

Die psychischen Folgen der *Kastration der Frau* sind viel schwieriger zu beurteilen als diejenigen beim Manne. Sie sind von Pedersen (1950 und 1956) neu untersucht worden. Aus seiner Monographie, aus sehr zahlreichen (aber unsystematischen) Beschreibungen in der Literatur und aus den eigenen Erfahrungen ergibt sich folgendes Bild: In etwa der Hälfte der Fälle sind keine oder nur unbedeutende psychische Änderungen nach dem Eingriff festzustellen. Am häufigsten sind emotionelle Lockerungen mit Verstimmbarkeit wie im Klimakterium. Das Geschlechtsempfinden wird in fast der Hälfte der Fälle als unverändert beschrieben. In einzelnen Ausnahmefällen ist es gesteigert, am ehesten im Zusammenhang mit dem Fortfall von Schwangerschaftsangst. (In unserem Erfahrungsgut ist diese Steigerung immerhin nach der Kastration seltener als nach der Sterilisation.) In einer beträchtlichen Anzahl von Fällen erfolgt nach und nach eine Dämpfung des Geschlechtsempfindens; es ist dabei kaum zu entscheiden, ob sie Folge der Kastration oder eher natürliche Folge des Alterns ist. In vereinzelten Fällen von schwer krankhafter, vieljähriger, jeder anderen Behandlung gegenüber trotzender Übersteigerung des Sexualtriebes konnte nach der Kastration ein schlagartiges Erlöschen der Nymphomanie festgestellt werden, wobei die Heilung dauernd anhielt; solche Umstimmungen können kaum anders als Kastrationserfolge gedeutet werden. Bei eingehend explorierten Frauen glaubt man die Art der Verarbeitung des hormonalen Ausfalles lebensgeschichtlich verstehen und erklären zu können. — Kastrierte Frauen sind oft stark mütterlich. Die „Kastratenfettsucht" beruht nicht auf einer primären Stoffwechselwirkung des hormonalen Ausfalls, sondern auf einer Steigerung des Hungers. — Viele Kastratinnen klagen über leichte Gedächtnisstörungen, die sich aber kaum objektivieren lassen.

Ganz ähnliche Wirkungen wie die Kastration bei Mann und Frau haben viele Hirnverletzungen (Meyer u. a.) und Hungerzustände.

Grundsätzlich entsprechen sich die Kastrations-Folgen bei Mensch und Tier; bei beiden ist eine Dämpfung des sexuellen Verhaltens häufig, aber nicht regelmäßig. Ein Unterschied ist

---

[1] Der mächtige Rückgang der Psychosexualität nach Kastration des Mannes geht keineswegs proportional dem nur leichten Rückgang der 17-Ketosteroide im Urin nach der Kastration. Dafür entspricht die Rückbildung der Psychosexualität der Rückbildung der sekundären körperlichen Geschlechtsmerkmale des Kastraten. Die 17-Ketosteroide im Urin sind eben nur ein völlig ungenügender Hinweis auf die Menge von ausgeschiedenen Hormonen mit androgener Wirkung. Die 17-Ketosteroide des Kastraten entstammen den Hormonen der Nebennierenrinde, die eine schwächere androgene Wirkung haben als die Hoden-Hormone (Hamilton et al. und andere).

jedoch hervorzuheben: Bei vielen Tieren sind die Kastrationsfolgen auf das Sexualverhalten beim Weibchen stärker und regelmäßiger als beim Menschen; beim Menschen wird umgekehrt die Psychosexualität des Mannes durch die Kastration viel stärker und regelmäßiger gebremst als bei der Frau.

15. Hormone und Psychosexualität

Über die Bedeutung der Hormone für die Psychosexualität wurden völlig falsche Theorien gebildet: Lange Zeit stellte man sich simplizistisch vor, Androgene und Oestrogene seien für das Erwachen, den Grad und die Art der psychosexuellen Entwicklung ebenso entscheidend wie für die Entwicklung der sekundären körperlichen Geschlechtsmerkmale. Fehlen der Sexualhormone würde nach dieser Vorstellung Fehlen der Psychosexualität, ihre übertriebene Sekretion übersteigerte Psychosexualität und Überwiegen der gegengeschlechtlichen Hormone Homosexualität bedingen. Später glaubte man, die Sexualhormone, vor allem die Androgene, bestimmten die Stärke, aber nicht die Richtung des Geschlechtstriebes. Heute leugnen viele die Bedeutung der endokrinen Funktionen für die Psychosexualität völlig.

Solchen zu einfachen oder falschen Ansichten gegenüber ist festzustellen:

1. Krankhaft verminderte oder übersteigerte Bildung von Sexualhormonen übt unter vielen Umständen eine mächtige Störwirkung auf die Psychosexualität aus. Sie wird am deutlichsten und regelmäßigsten sichtbar:

a) wenn bei Hypogonadismus die normale Entfaltung der endokrinen Gonadenfunktion ausbleibt; die Folge ist regelmäßig eine Kümmerentwicklung der Psychosexualität;

b) wenn man den Hypogonadismus mit Sexualhormonen behandelt, dann entwickelt sich die Psychosexualität gewöhnlich Hand in Hand mit der körperlichen Reifung. Setzt man die Behandlung aus, so neigt die Psychosexualität bei Männern wieder zum Erlöschen;

c) wenn der geschlechtsreife Mann kastriert wird: die Folge ist fast regelmäßig eine eindrucksvolle Dämpfung der Psychosexualität;

d) wenn der älteren Frau Androgene in großen Dosen verabreicht werden: die Folge ist meistens eine Anregung der Psychosexualität.

2. Gesundes Endokrinium ist aber nicht die einzige Voraussetzung für gesunde psychosexuelle Entwicklung. Die psychosexuelle Entwicklung ist oft auch bei endokrin Gesunden gestört.

3. Die Stärke des Sexualtriebes wird unter völlig unphysiologischen und krankhaften Verhältnissen vom Über- oder Unterangebot von Sexualhormonen deutlich beeinflußt. Sie ist aber nicht ausschließlich von den Sexualhormonen abhängig. Ihre Schwankungen innerhalb der Norm hängen in der Hauptsache nicht mit erkennbaren Schwankungen des Hormon-Haushaltes zusammen.

4. Für die Richtung des Sexualtriebes (im Sinne der Hetero- oder Homosexualität) sind die Geschlechtshormone sicher nicht allein entscheidend. Vielleicht kommt ihnen aber doch eine gewisse Rolle dabei zu, wenn auch nur eine höchst untergeordnete.

Zu Leitsatz 1. Krankhaft verminderte oder übersteigerte Bildung von Sexualhormonen übt unter vielen Umständen eine mächtige Störwirkung auf die Psychosexualität aus. Heute wird diese Tatsache von vielen völlig übersehen, die behaupten, beim Menschen sei die Psychosexualität — im Gegensatz zu den Verhältnissen beim Tier — vom Endokrinium unabhängig. Und doch sind die klinischen Erfahrungen eindrucksvoll: Fast immer bleibt die Psychosexualität verkümmert, wenn die endokrine Pubertätsentwicklung ausbleibt (s. z. B. Vitebskaya). Allerdings fehlt sie nicht völlig, so wenig wie beim gesunden Kinde. Sie äußert sich aber, wenn sie nachweisbar bleibt, in kindlicher, unentwickelter Art, in Neugierde oder in spielerischem Verhalten. Die körperlich sexuellen Empfindungen und die Bindungen an Menschen können nicht zu einer reifen Liebesfähigkeit zusammenfließen. Gewöhnlich ist die Verkümmerung der Psychosexualität beim Hypogonadismus, der vom Jugendalter an besteht, mit mangelhafter Reifung von Selbstbewußtsein, Selbständigkeit, Durchsetzungswillen, des ganzen Charakters, gekoppelt. Eine Substitutionstherapie mit Sexualhormonen fördert zusammen mit der körperlichen auch die triebhafte und charakterliche Reifung. Es kann deshalb nicht daran gezweifelt werden, daß die persönliche Kümmerentwicklung mit dem Mangel an Sexualhormonen zusammenhängt.

Der Hypogonadismus, der von früh an besteht, wirkt sich bei Mann und Frau ähnlich aus. Er wird zusammen mit seinen Folgen auf die Triebe beim Manne durch Androgene, bei der Frau durch Oestrogene mit ähnlichem Erfolg behandelt.

Wird der Hypogonadismus hingegen erst in reifem Alter, durch Kastration, erworben, so stellt sich die Triebschwäche nur beim Manne mit hoher (nicht absoluter) Regelmäßigkeit ein. Nur schon die Tatsache, daß die Emotionalität der Frau nach der Kastration häufig gesund bleibt, macht die vorsichtige Fassung des Leitsatzes nötig: nur *unter bestimmten Umständen* — und nicht immer! — übt eine Verschiebung des hormonalen Gleichgewichtes eine Störwirkung auf die Psychosexualität aus. Es zeigt sich das besonders klar bei der unphysiologischen Überschwemmung mit Sexualhormonen: zwar steigert die künstliche Überschwemmung des Körpers der älteren Frau mit Androgenen (bei der Behandlung des Brustkrebses) ihre Psychosexualität meistens; zwar gibt es auch Überschwemmungen von Sexualhormonen aus Tumoren, die die Sexualität der Frau steigern; häufiger aber sind Beispiele in umgekehrtem Sinne: bei Pubertas und Pseudopubertas praecox reift die Psychosexualität oft nicht mit dem Körper; massive Überschwemmungen des Körpers mit Sexualhormonen aus Tumorgewebe steigern die Psychosexualität nur ausnahmsweise, meist stören sie sie wenig oder lassen sie sogar verkümmern.

Es lag nahe zu vermuten, daß es bei der Frau auf die Oestrogene, beim Manne auf die Androgene ankomme, wenn hormonale Anomalien die Psychosexualität störten. Die Verhältnisse liegen aber lange nicht so einfach: beim Manne ist nur ein Darniederliegen der Psychosexualität unter Mangel von Androgenen bewiesen, nicht aber das Gegenteil: unphysiologische Überschwemmung mit Androgenen führt — soweit wir wissen — gewöhnlich nicht zur Übersteigerung der Sexualität. Bei der Frau folgt Mangel an Oestrogenen nur dann eine Verkümmerung der Psychosexualität mit Regelmäßigkeit, wenn dieser Mangel vom Jugendalter an dauernd besteht. Sexualisierende Wirkung von Oestrogen-Überschuß ist bei der Frau ebensowenig bekannt wie sexualisierende Wirkung von Androgen-Überschuß beim Manne. Starker Überschuß von gegengeschlechtlichem Geschlechtshormon wirkt beim Manne regelmäßig dämpfend auf die Sexualität, bei der Frau unter einzelnen Umständen erregend, unter anderen gar nicht.

Eine weitere, zu einfache Vermutung ging dahin, daß die krankhaften Veränderungen des Androgenspiegels die Psychosexualität bei Mann und Frau beeinflußten, Veränderungen des Oestrogenspiegels aber weder bei Mann noch Frau[1] einen solchen Einfluß hätten. Aber auch diese Formulierung stimmt nicht: Androgenvermehrung beim Mann hat gewöhnlich keine sexualisierende Wirkung auf die Psyche; Oestrogenmangel von einem frühen Alter an bei der Frau läßt die Entwicklung der Psychosexualität verkümmern. Unsere heutige Erfahrung auf diesem Gebiet läßt sich eben noch nicht in eine einfache und anschauliche Formel zusammenfassen.

---

[1] Die Androgene bei der Frau stammen in der Hauptsache aus der Nebennierenrinde.

Interessant und noch ungelöst ist die Frage, ob sich nur das in den Leydig-Zellen gebildete Testosteron auf die Triebhaftigkeit auswirkt oder ob die *Androgene der Nebennierenrinde* ebenfalls eine Triebwirkung haben und welche. Beim *Manne* fehlt eine eindeutige Beziehung der triebhaften Folgen der Kastration zur Ausscheidung der 17-Ketosteroide. Die Folgen der Kastration auf die 17-Ketosteroid-Ausscheidung sind unbedeutender als diejenigen auf die Triebhaftigkeit (Furman und Howard; Hamilton et al. 1959a und b u. a.). Man muß annehmen, daß die Nebennierenrindenhormone, aus denen 17-Ketosteroide beim Kastraten entstehen, nicht wesentlich auf die Psychosexualität einwirken. (Als 17-Keto-steroide werden allerdings nicht nur Abbauprodukte des Testosterons und von Nebennierenrinden-Androgenen ausgeschieden, sondern auch solche von hormonal inaktiven Substanzen.) Überproduktion von Nebennierenrinden-Androgenen beim Manne erzeugt nicht (oder gewöhnlich nicht) eine Steigerung der sexuellen Trieb-haftigkeit.— Dagegen liegen einzelne Beobachtungen vor, die es möglich erscheinen lassen, daß bei der *Frau* Nebennierenrinden-Androgene etwas mit der sexuellen Triebhaftigkeit zu tun hätten; nach Exstirpation der Nebennierenrinden hat man die Sexualität bei Frauen erlöschen sehen (Waxenberg et al. 1959). Ebenso löscht die Hypophysektomie den Sexualtrieb der Frau, wahrscheinlich ebenfalls durch ihre Bremswirkung auf die Nebennierenrinde (Lindqvist). Bei Überproduktion von Nebennierenrindenhormonen ist sie in seltenen Ausnahmefällen gesteigert.

Zu Leitsatz 2. Daß ein gesundes Endokrinium nicht die einzige Voraussetzung für eine gesunde psychosexuelle Entwicklung ist, ist offensichtlich: Es gibt bei endokrin Gesunden häufige neurotische Verkümmerungen, Übersteigerungen oder Perversionen der Psychosexualität. (Allerdings scheinen manchmal leichte Zu-stände von endokriner Unterfunktion eine Prädisposition zu bilden.) Die über-wältigende Mehrheit der Homosexuellen ist — soweit unsere heutigen Methoden erkennen lassen — endokrin gesund. (Allerdings haben sie, worauf vor allem italienische Autoren hingewiesen haben, häufig kleine Körpermerkmale des anderen Geschlechtes: im Behaarungstypus, in der Fettverteilung, im Knochen-bau u. a. Ob und wie diese gegengeschlechtlichen Merkmale endokrin bedingt sind, ist noch kaum erforscht.) — Völlige Isolierung von menschlichen Kontakten verhindert das Reifen der Psychosexualität.

Entgegen vielfachen Behauptungen läßt sich auch für viele Tiere nachweisen, daß das Sexualverhalten *nicht* ausschließlich hormonal gelenkt ist; sexuelle Erfahrung spielt auch bei vielen Tieren eine große Rolle für die Entwicklung des Sexualtriebes (z. B. Rosenblatt et al; Young, W. C.).

Zu Leitsatz 3. Wie häufig und unter welchen Umständen die *Stärke* des Sexual-triebes von grob krankhaftem Über- oder Unterangebot von Sexualhormonen beeinflußt wird, ist schon erwähnt. Ebenso ist bereits ausgeführt, daß diese Ein-flüsse keineswegs regelmäßig wirksam sind. — Hängt aber der Grad der Psycho-sexualität innerhalb der Norm mit der Quantität der Ausschwemmung von Sexualhormonen innerhalb der Norm zusammen? Sicher ist heute, daß kein enger und zwingender Zusammenhang besteht. Darüber, ob überhaupt ein Zusammen-hang besteht, wissen wir nichts Sicheres. Es sind Argumente für und wider geltend zu machen:

Für einen solchen Zusammenhang sprechen Erfahrungen, wie sie vor allem von französischen Klinikern seit Jahrzehnten immer wieder anschaulich und fein beobachtend beschrieben worden sind (P. Abely 1949, 1951, 1959, Decourt 1954, Rocheblave): danach geht bei Männern und Frauen späte Pubertät, geringe Ausprägung der sekundären Geschlechtsmerkmale und eher kindlicher Körperbau mit geringerem Geschlechtsbedürfnis zusammen; frühe Pubertät, starke Aus-prägung der sekundären Geschlechtsmerkmale, „kraftvolle" Körperkonstitution beim Mann und „üppige Formen" bei der Frau hingegen wären mit starker psychischer Geschlechtlichkeit gekoppelt. Einzelne Untersuchungen deckten auch bei körperlich und psychisch Geschlechtsschwachen unterdurchschnittliche Geschlechtshormonproduktion auf und umgekehrt. Es scheint wahrscheinlich, daß diesen Beobachtungen Gesetzmäßigkeiten zugrunde liegen. Heute ist das aber noch nicht sicher. Schon die häufigen Ausnahmen von dem, was man als Regel bezeichnen möchte, müssen stutzig machen. Sie zeigen zum mindesten, daß die Psychosexualität nicht in eindeutiger Beziehung zur Ausprägung der körperlichen Geschlechtsmerkmale steht, sondern daß die Bedeutung der Körperlichkeit für die Psychosexualität von anderen Einflüssen aus überkompensiert werden kann. Es muß auch zugegeben werden, daß bis heute die Vermutungen über den Zusammenhang zwischen dem Grad endokriner und psychischer Geschlechtlichkeit innerhalb der Norm noch keineswegs durch genügend große statistische und genügend vielseitige endokrinologische Untersuchungen gestützt sind. Selbst der Zusammenhang zwischen Ausprägungsstand körperlicher Geschlechtsmerkmale und endokriner Sekretion innerhalb der Norm ist noch unbewiesen und noch mehr der Zusammenhang beider mit dem Grade psychischer Geschlechtlichkeit.— Großangelegte Untersuchungen über den Verlauf der Psychosexualität während des Menstruationszyklus und seine Abhängigkeit von der Hormonbildung haben vor 25 Jahren Benedek und Rubinstein veröffentlicht: Sie versuchten, in psychoanalytischen Sitzungen die Psychosexualität von Frauen quantitativ zu bestimmen und gleichzeitig die Sexualhormonbildung an Vaginal-Abstrichen zu messen. Sie kamen zur Überzeugung, daß erhöhte sexuelle Bedürftigkeit mit den Perioden maximaler Oestrogenausscheidung zusammenfielen, während die maximale Ausscheidung von Progesteronen das Bedürfnis nach Umhegtwerden förderte. Heute können diese Hypothesen nicht mehr in vollem Maße als richtig anerkannt werden. Die Einwände richten sich schon gegen die Technik: Die psychoanalytische Technik erlaubt nicht, Psychosexualität quantitativ genau zu bestimmen, ohne daß dem subjektiven Ermessen des Therapeuten ein breiter Spielraum gegeben wäre. Ebensowenig liefert die Untersuchung der Vaginalschleimhaut derart genaue quantitative Ergebnisse über die Sexualhormone, wie man früher annahm. Auch widersprechen die Ergebnisse von Benedek und Rubinstein vielen anderen Erfahrungen über die Beziehung zwischen Zyklus, Sexualhormonen und Psychosexualität.

Gegen einen engeren Zusammenhang zwischen Psychosexualität und Oestrogenen bei der Frau sprechen u. a. Untersuchungen von Waxenberg (1960): bei (krebskranken) Frauen vor und nach Adrenalektomie (und z. T. Kastration) fand sich kein Zusammenhang zwischen der noch bestehenden Psychosexualität einerseits und Oestrogenwirkung auf die Vaginalschleimhaut andererseits. (Oestrogene können bei kastrierten und adrenalektomierten Patientinnen aus versprengten Teilen der Nebennierenrinde, aus der Nahrung oder aus Verunreinigungen der therapeutisch verabreichten Glucocorticoide stammen.) — Noch überzeugender sind aber alltägliche Erfahrungen. Mit Oestrogenen läßt sich die Psychosexualität hormongesunder Frauen nicht steigern; ebensowenig sind Androgene ein Heilmittel für darniederliegende Psychosexualität bei hormongesunden Männern. Unter anderem ist hier auch zu bedenken, daß die Kastration der Frau ihre Psychosexualität sehr oft unberührt läßt.

Zu Leitsatz 4. Die Auffassung, welche Rolle den Sexualhormonen für die *Richtung des Sexualtriebes* (auf das eigene oder das andere Geschlecht) zukomme, hat in den letzten Jahrzehnten eine vollkommene Wandlung erfahren: Nach der Entdeckung der Sexualhormone glaubten viele bedenkenlos, die männlichen Sexualhormone seien es, die das Sexualbegehren des Mannes auf die Frau richteten;

umgekehrt würde die weibliche Sexualität von den weiblichen Sexualhormonen getragen. In den letzten Jahren hingegen ist die Behauptung beliebt geworden, die Richtung der Sexualität sei von den Hormonen vollkommen unabhängig; die Sexualität werde einzig allein durch die Erziehung und die gesamte Lebenserfahrung im Sinne des Männlichen oder Weiblichen geprägt.

Heute wissen wir, daß die Mehrheit der Homosexuellen in bezug auf die Geschlechtshormone normal sind. Dasselbe gilt für die Transvestiten. Homosexuelle lassen sich nicht etwa zu Heterosexuellen umstimmen, indem man sie mit gleichgeschlechtlichen Hormonen behandelt: nur schon diese elementaren Tatsachen zeigen, wie falsch die alte Ansicht war, wonach die Richtung der Psychosexualität einzig durch das Verhältnis zwischen männlichen und weiblichen Hormonen bestimmt würde.

Fragen wir uns aber, wie die gegenteilige Ansicht — Hormone hätten mit der Richtung der Geschlechtlichkeit gar nichts zu tun — begründet wird, so zeigt sich, daß auch sie auf eher schwachen Füßen steht. Die Bestimmtheit, mit der heute vielerorts angegeben wird, die Richtung der Sexualität werde gar nicht durch Hormone, sondern ausschließlich durch die Erziehung bestimmt, steht in einem bedenklichen Mißverhältnis zu den tatsächlichen Beobachtungen, die eine solche Angabe stützen könnten. Insbesondere sind die „Beweise", die der endokrinologischen Psychiatrie angehören, keine Beweise, sondern höchstens unbestimmte Hinweise. Sie beziehen sich auf die Geschlechtsrichtung von Hermaphroditen und Pseudohermaphroditen und gehen u. a. vor allem auf eine Literaturübersicht von Ellis zurück. Die meisten dieser Zwitter wünschen diejenige Geschlechtsrolle beizubehalten, die ihnen bei der Geburt zivilrechtlich und gesellschaftlich zugeteilt worden ist. In vielen Fällen halten sie an ihrer gewohnten Geschlechtsrolle fest, auch wenn diese Geschlechtsrolle der Hormonbildung widerspricht. Es ist aber voreilig, wenn man schon daraus auf die absolute Abhängigkeit der Geschlechtsrichtung von der Erziehung geschlossen hat. Diese Zwitter haben nämlich oft eine wenig entwickelte, zielunsichere, kindliche Sexualität. Daß ihnen (wie anderen Menschen) der Gedanke an eine Umwandlung der gesellschaftlichen Geschlechtsrolle und damit der meisten vertrauten Lebensgewohnheiten unheimlich und quälend vorkommt, ist begreiflich. Es zeigt vorerst nur die Bedeutung der Gewohnheit bei wenig differenzierter Psychosexualität. Es beweist noch lange nicht sicher, daß die Richtung reifer Sexualität einzig von der Erziehung bestimmt würde. — Zu beachten ist weiter: es gibt auch Gegenbeispiele, nämlich Pseudohermaphroditen, die unbedingt ihre offizielle Geschlechtsrolle, in der sie aufgewachsen sind, wechseln wollen und die jenes Geschlecht annehmen wollen, das ihrem vorherrschenden Geschlechtshormon entspricht[1]. Daß sie stark in der Minderzahl sind, weist gewiß darauf hin, daß die sozialen Umweltfaktoren bei der Geschlechtsbestimmung wichtiger sein könnten als die hormonalen Verhältnisse. Von dieser Feststellung bis zur Behauptung, einzig die Erziehung bestimme die Geschlechtsrichtung, ist aber noch ein weiter Weg.

Außerdem sind es wieder die Beobachtungen an Homosexuellen und Transvestiten, die der Hypothese von der alleinigen Bedeutung der Erziehung für die Geschlechtsrichtung entgegenstehen; bei sehr vielen von ihnen lassen sich keine

---

[1] Ein summarisches Bild der Häufigkeit zwischen zugeteilter Geschlechtsrolle und psychischer Geschlechtseinteilung ergibt sich z. B. aus einer Tabelle von Overzier (1961): Er stellt die Literatur über 146 echte Hermaphroditen zusammen. Soweit sich aus seiner Tabelle beurteilen läßt, sind rund 10% der Hermaphroditen psychisch dem ihnen sozial zugeteilten Geschlecht widersprüchlich eingestellt. — Ein eindrucksvolles Beispiel von psychischer Feminisierung eines pubertierenden Knaben unter dem Einfluß von Oestrogenen siehe bei A. D. Schwabe et al.

Lebensverhältnisse aufdecken, die die Umprägung des Geschlechtsempfindens überzeugend erklären würde.

So lassen klinische Gegebenheiten die Annahme nicht zu, daß die Erziehung für die Richtung des Geschlechtstriebes allein maßgebend wäre; trotzdem sind klinische Tatsachen nur spärlich, welche dafür sprechen würden, daß neben der Erziehung auch die Sexualhormone richtungsbestimmend wären. Man könnte dafür anführen: der Trieb, die angewohnte offizielle Geschlechtsrolle zu wechseln, wird wahrscheinlich häufiger gesehen, wenn er der vorherrschenden endokrinen Sekretion entspricht, als wenn sich die angewöhnte Geschlechtsrolle und die endokrine Sekretion, wie es normal ist, entsprechen. Androgen-Applikation bei Frauen bewirkt zwar keine Homosexualität, aber doch manchmal ein maskulin getöntes, aggressives und männlich-selbstbewußtes Wesen. Oestrogene in hohen Dosen bei Männern bewirken auch keine Homosexualität, aber den Verlust des männlichen Sexualbedürfnisses, oft verbunden mit einem allgemeinen Bedürfnis nach Zärtlichkeit, wie es weiblichem Empfinden nahe steht.

Wir können demnach der Erziehung eine wichtige, aber nicht allein ausschlaggebende Rolle für die Bestimmung der Geschlechtsrichtung zuweisen, den hormonalen Verhältnissen höchstens eine untergeordnete — von was hängt dann aber die Geschlechtsrichtung ab? Sicher nicht direkt vom *Chromosomengeschlecht*. Der Beispiele gibt es viele, wonach Chromosomengeschlecht und triebhafte Geschlechtsrichtung auseinanderfallen: bei Homosexualität und Transvestitismus ist das fast immer der Fall; bei der testiculären Feminisierung in allen beschriebenen Fällen; beim Klinefelter-Syndrom ist die psychische Einstellung männlich (allerdings bleibt der Sexualtrieb infantil,) trotz zweier weiblicher Chromosomen (neben einem männlichen); in einem Einzelfall von Klinefelter-Syndrom ohne männliches Chromosom, mit einem rein weiblichen Chromosomensatz, war die psychische Geschlechtsrichtung ebenfalls männlich (R. R. GORDON et al.); beim echten Hermaphroditismus kann das Chromosomengeschlecht der Triebrichtung widersprechen (DE ASSIS et al.; FERGUSON-SMITH 1960a; R. R. GORDON et al.); bei den sog. „Superfemales", d. h. bei Frauen mit 3 weiblichen Geschlechtschromosomen, ist keine gesteigerte Weiblichkeit aufgefallen usw.[1]. Ebensowenig ist das Vorhandensein eines Hodens für männliche oder eines Ovars für weibliche Geschlechtsrichtung entscheidend, wie man früher voraussetzte. Das Vorhandensein männlicher oder weiblicher Genitalien und das Erleben ihrer Funktionen mag eine wichtige Rolle spielen, doch zeigen u. a. wieder Homosexuelle und Transvestiten, daß auch dadurch die Geschlechtsrichtung nicht immer und eindeutig bestimmt wird. Unter anderem muß man damit rechnen, daß vererbte „Auslöserschemata" wie bei Tieren im Sinne des Tierpsychologen LORENZ wichtig sind. (Es könnte z. B. eine vererbte sexuelle Ansprechbarkeit auf Anblick weiblicher Formen beim Manne gegeben sein.) So interessant diese Frage ist, so wenig ist sie noch gelöst und so schwierig ist sie zu erforschen.

Zusammenfassend ist demnach festzustellen, daß sich Art, Richtung und Stärke des Geschlechtstriebes beim Menschen keineswegs aus hormonalen Verhältnissen allein ableiten lassen — und doch sind die hormonalen Verhältnisse z. T. Grundlagen, z. T. Beeinflussungsfaktoren der psychischen Geschlechtlichkeit. Allgemeine Lehren der endokrinologischen Psychiatrie sind eben auch auf den Zusammenhang zwischen endokrinem und psychosexuellem Geschehen gültig. Die Psychosexualität

---

[1] Von den Erfahrungen der Biologie aus gesehen besteht auch kein Grund, eine direkte Abhängigkeit der Geschlechtsrichtung (die nicht über die Gonaden ginge) vom Chromosomengeschlecht zu vermuten: soweit wir wissen, erfolgt auch die körperliche sexuelle Geschlechts-Differenzierung bei Wirbeltieren unter dem Einfluß der Gonaden und wirkt sich dabei das genetische Geschlecht nur über die Gonade aus.

entwickelt sich gemeinsam mit der gesamten Persönlichkeit. Viele körperliche Faktoren können Einfluß auf diese Entwicklung nehmen: die körperliche Gesundheit an sich, das ganze hormonale Gleichgewicht, die Sexualhormone im speziellen; vor allem aber gestalten Lebenserfahrungen Persönlichkeit und mit ihr psychische Geschlechtlichkeit: das Erleben der eigenen Körperfunktionen, auch der geschlechtlichen, das Erleben der Beziehungen zu den Mitmenschen, jede Lebenserfahrung. Diese ganze Entwicklung geht von konstitutionellen Bereitschaften aus.

Beim Menschen wird kein Trieb einzig von einem Hormon getragen, auch nicht der Geschlechtstrieb. Jeder Trieb lebt als Teil des ganzen individuellen Lebens und hormonale wie andere Einflüsse, die ihn fördern oder stören, treffen je nach der Persönlichkeit und ihrer Lebenslage auf die verschiedensten Abwehrbereitschaften, Empfindlichkeiten und Gestaltungsmöglichkeiten. Wie Psychologie und Psychiatrie im allgemeinen steht die endokrinologische Psychiatrie meist vor Entwicklungen mit vielfältigen Grundlagen, auf die vielfältige Einflüsse einwirken. Im persönlichen Leben werden sie zusammengefaßt und gestaltet.

Die klinische Erfahrung, wonach das menschliche Sexualverhalten keinesfalls eindeutig und absolut von einer einzigen hormonalen Funktion oder irgendeinem anderen einzigen Vorgang abhängig ist, sondern multifaktoriell bestimmt wird, steht in völliger Übereinstimmung mit biologischen Erfahrungen: nicht einmal die körperlichen sekundaren Geschlechtsmerkmale sind immer von der endokrinen Sekretion abhängig, sondern sind bald endokrin, bald unabhängig vom Endokrinium genetisch bedingt, so z. B. der Federschmuck der Vögel zur Brunstzeit. Dasselbe gilt vom tierischen Sexualverhalten: nur teilweise ist es von den Geschlechtshormonen abhängig, in einzelnen Fällen dagegen von Hypophysenhormonen, oft auch ist es (unabhängig vom ganzen Endokrinium) genetisch verwurzelt und in wieder anderen Fällen wird es durch die Erfahrungen mit den Partnern mitgeprägt. (Kurze Zusammenfassung mit Bibliographie z. B. bei Segal oder bei Goldstein oder Young.)

16. Neuroleptica und endokrine Funktionen

Die Wirkung von Neuroleptica auf den Gehalt von 5-Hydroxytryptamin und Noradrenalin im Hirn ist bereits besprochen worden.

Zahlreiche Untersuchungen — klinische wie tierexperimentelle — zeigen, daß *Neuroleptica die Funktion der endokrinen Drüsen mannigfach beeinflussen.* Man hat sogar erwartet, aus ihrem Einfluß auf das Endokrinium ihre Wirkung auf die Psyche erklären zu können. Wichtige Erwartungen gingen dahin, daß sich je nach dem individuellen Stand des endokrinen Gleichgewichtes individuelle Sonder-Indikationen und Sonder-Gegenindikationen für die therapeutische Anwendung der Neuroleptica ergeben könnten. Namentlich hoffte man, eine differenzierte Therapie von prämenstruellen, puerperalen und klimakterischen Geistesstörungen entwickeln zu können.

Vorläufig haben sich alle diese Hoffnungen nicht erfüllt. *Es ist nicht gelungen, die hauptsächliche psychische Wirkung der Neuroleptica auf ihre Wirkung auf die endokrinen Drüsen zurückzuführen.* Ebensowenig können wir vorläufig die Behandlung mit Neuroleptica durch endokrinologische Untersuchungen lenken. Trotzdem verdienen die vielfachen Feststellungen über gegenseitige Beeinflussurg von Neuroleptica und Hormonen Beachtung. Es sind ihnen dann auch bereits sehr viele Arbeiten gewidmet. In seiner Übersicht darüber zitiert von Brauchitsch allein schon über 100 Publikationen.

Es ist wiederholt versucht worden, ganz einfache Gesetzmäßigkeiten über die Wirkung der Neuroleptica auf das Endokrinium zu formulieren. Eine anregende Arbeitshypothese ging dahin, daß Chlorpromazin u. a. Neuroleptica die Ansprechbarkeit des Hypophysenvorderlappens dämpften. Mit einem anschaulichen Schlagwort konnte man von einer „pharmakologischen Hypophysektomie" sprechen. Diese Annahme war verführerisch; sie legte simplizistische Deutungen der Genese und des Heilvorganges von Psychosen (besonders Schizophrenien) nahe; man war versucht festzustellen, Schizophrenien seien eine unspezifische Reaktion auf übermäßige psychische Belastung, überdosierten „Stress"; Neuroleptica dämpften die Wirkung von Stress und seien deshalb heilsam. Daß solche Vermutungen zu einfach sind, um die wesentliche Wahrheit zu enthalten, und daß ihnen zahlreiche andere als endokrinologische Argumente entgegenzuhalten sind, ist hier nicht auszuführen. Hervorzuheben aber ist, daß sie sich in dieser Einfachheit auch durch endokrinologische Tatsachen widerlegen lassen. Es hat sich nämlich bald gezeigt, daß Neuroleptica die Funktion der Hypophyse keineswegs immer und einheitlich dämpfen. Im Gegenteil wirken sie oft selbst als „Stressor"; sie können über die Anregung der Hypophyse die Nebennierenrinden-Funktion steigern.

Heute ist sicher, daß man die Wirkungen der Neuroleptica keinesfalls auf einfache und generelle endokrinologische Formeln bringen kann. Die klinischen und tierexperimentellen Feststellungen sind vielmehr von verwirrender Widersprüchlichkeit: Neuroleptica beeinflussen das Endikrinium nicht dauernd in derselben Art; sie lösen eine Kette von Veränderungen der endokrinen Funktionen aus. Die endokrinologischen Befunde hängen davon ab, wie lange sie nach der Medikation erhoben wurden. Der Faktor Zeit erheischt gebieterisch Berücksichtigung. Auch die Berücksichtigung der Dose und der Dauer der Medikation ist wichtig. Sodann ist zu beachten, daß die Reaktionen auf Neuroleptica bei verschiedenen Tierarten und bei Tier und Mensch verschieden sind. Man kann die Neuroleptica auch nicht als einheitliche Gruppe in ihrer endokrinologischen Wirkung behandeln; nur schon die beiden Hauptvertreter, Chlorpromazin und Reserpin, haben z. T. unterschiedliche endokrinologische Bedeutung. Schließlich hat es den Anschein, daß die endokrinologische Ausgangslage, wie sie von Individuum zu Individuum und von einem Tag zum anderen wechseln kann, für die endokrine Wirkung der Neuroleptica mit eine Rolle spielt. Zum Beispiel kommt eine verspätende Wirkung des Chlorpromazins auf die Menstruation im Prämenstruum, aber kaum im Postmenstruum zustande. Man kann sich unter diesen Umständen leicht vorstellen, was für schwierige und zeitraubende Aufgaben der Forschung auf diesem Gebiete noch harren.

Am Krankenbett sind die auffälligsten Wirkungen der Neuroleptica, die wahrscheinlich durch Veränderungen endokriner Funktionen zustande kommen, die *Verzögerung der Menstruation* einerseits, die *Anregung der Milchdrüse* andererseits («Syndrome galactorrhée-amenorrhée»). Die Menstruation tritt oft verspätet auf oder wird ganz gehemmt, und genaue Untersuchungen (z. B. der Vaginalabstriche) zeigen manchmal einen Hypofollikulinismus. Die Brüste können schwellen und Colostrum und Milch sezernieren, meist nur bei der Frau im geschlechtsreifen Alter, viel seltener bei Frauen nach dem Klimakterium, sehr selten auch beim Manne. Die Häufigkeit dieser Erscheinungen wird von verschiedenen Klinikern verschieden geschätzt. Darüber, daß sie nicht sehr selten sind, herrscht aber Einigkeit. Mit dem Absetzen des Medikamentes bilden sie sich zurück.[1] Viel seltener als Amenorrhoe treten Menorrhagien auf; besonders wurden sie unter Nitoman beschrieben (STOCKHAUSEN). Einige Kliniker haben ferner eine *dämpfende Wirkung des Reserpins auf die Schilddrüsenfunktion* festgestellt, freilich meist nur bei vorbestehender Hyperthyreose. Andere Untersucher finden hingegen keine

---

[1] BORENSTEIN et al.; COLMEIRO-LAFORET; DESHAIES et al.; DONNADIEU et al.; GAEDE und HEINRICH; GAUNT et al.; KAHANA und KAHANA; KRESSIG; KULCSAR et al.; POLISHUK und KULCSAR; SUZUKI et al.; WHITELAW.

Wirkung von Neuroleptica auf die Schilddrüsenfunktion[1]. Im übrigen fallen dem Kliniker kaum Nebenwirkungen der Neuroleptica auf, die mit den endokrinen Funktionen in einen offensichtlichen Zusammenhang zu bringen wären, abgesehen von seltenen und widersprechenden Einzelbeobachtungen.

Aus der Fülle von *tierexperimentellen Untersuchungen* über Neuroleptica-Wirkungen auf endokrine Funktionen, ergänzt durch eine geringe Anzahl von *quantitativen Hormonuntersuchungen am Menschen*, läßt sich zusammenfassend feststellen:

Die *endokrinen Funktionen von Hoden und Ovarien* unter der Wirkung sowohl von Chlorpromazin wie von Reserpin erweisen sich bei Tieren nach den meisten Untersuchern als herabgesetzt[2]. Einzelne Untersucher stellen fest, daß die Bremsung in bestimmten Tierversuchen noch stärker ist als nach einer Hypophysektomie oder daß die Wirkung an den Erfolgsorganen derjenigen bei Kastration gleich sei. Die meisten Autoren setzen voraus, daß die Wirkung auf die Gonaden durch Bremsung der Gonadotropinbildung im Hypophysenvorderlappen erfolge. Reiss (1959) vermutet, daß darüber hinaus auch eine direkte toxische Wirkung des Chlorpromazins auf die Gonaden vorhanden sei (weil die Gonadenatrophie unter dem Medikament stärker sein kann als nach Hypophysektomie). Direkte Bestimmungen des follikelstimulierenden Hormons haben entgegen der häufigsten Erwartung wiederholt normale Ergebnisse gezeitigt[3]. Deshalb wurde die Vermutung geäußert, die Wirkung von Neuroleptica auf die Gonaden erfolge auf nervösem Wege und nicht über die Funktion des Hypophysenvorderlappens. Reserpin hat im Tierversuch Aborte bewirkt, vermutlich durch Störung der Hypophysenfunktion oder des Serotonin-Stoffwechsels (Poulson et al.; Tuchmann-Duplessis et Mercier-Parot 1956b; Gaunt et. al.). In ganz vereinzelten Fällen wird entgegengesetzt zu den gewöhnlichen Erfahrungen über Oestrogenwirkung von Reserpin (bei einer Greisin von Barnard und Barnard) oder von Anregung der Psychosexualität (bei Frauen von Cohen) oder von Anregung der Gonadotropinbildung (Marinoni et al.) berichtet.

Einzelne Autoren (Reiss 1958 und 1959) glauben, daß die hemmende Wirkung der Neuroleptica auf die Gonadenfunktion bei der Indikationsstellung am Krankenbett berücksichtigt werden sollte: Neuroleptica wären dann kontraindiziert, wenn die Gonadenfunktion von vornherein darniederliegt, z. B. bei Jugendlichen mit sexuellem Infantilismus, bei männlichen Depressiven in höherem Alter mit herabgesetzter Ausscheidung von 17-Ketosteroiden oder bei prämenstrueller Spannung. Umgekehrt wären sie bei Übersteigerung der endokrinen Gonadenfunktion besonders angezeigt, z. B. bei Pubertas praecox. Die tägliche Erfahrung an Kranken hat aber bisher den meisten Klinikern die Bedeutung solcher Überlegungen nicht nahegelegt.

Die *Anregung der Milchsekretion* wird von den meisten Autoren aus theoretischen Überlegungen einer gesteigerten Sekretion von laktotropem Hormon zugeschrieben, ohne daß diese Steigerung noch durch quantitative Hormonbestimmungen bewiesen worden wäre. Es wurde schon lange vermutet, daß neuroleptische Mittel sich über die Beeinflussung des Nervensystems auf den Stoffwechsel des laktotropen Hormons auswirkten (Kulcsar et al.)[4]. Neuerdings wurde an Kaninchen

---

[1] Canary und Schaaf, Darnaud et al.; Klein; Moncke; Newman und Fish; Revol; Saarenmaa; Tuchmann-Duplessis 1956a; Vannotti.

[2] Barraclough und Sawyer; Cohen; Tuchmann-Duplessis 1956b; Tuchmann-Duplessis und Mercier-Parot 1956a und b.

[3] Kulcsar et al.; Polishuk und Kulcsar.

[4] Interessanterweise ist bei Kaninchen die Fähigkeit des Reserpins, Pseudoschwangerschaft, Laktation und Thymus-Rückbildung zu setzen, nur in einem bestimmten Tierstamm vorhanden (Tindal).

bewiesen, daß die Entleerung des laktotropen Hormons aus der Hypophyse durch Reserpin nur zustande kommt, wenn bestimmte Teile des Hypothalamus intakt sind. Das Reserpin wirkt sich also über den Hypothalamus auf die Ausschüttung von laktotropem Hormon aus (KANEMATSU et al.).

Die Untersuchungsbefunde über die Wirkung der Neuroleptica auf die *Schilddrüsenfunktion* sind uneinheitlich. Nach vielen Beobachtungen, namentlich solchen am Krankenbett, besteht keine oder keine wesentliche Schilddrüsenwirkung. Nach anderen hemmt das Reserpin die Schilddrüsenfunktion[1]. Dem Chlorpromazin kommt eine solche Hemmwirkung nicht oder nur in geringerem Maße zu; in einzelnen Versuchsserien steigerte es sogar die Aufnahme von radioaktivem Jod in der Schilddrüse[2]; allerdings spielte bei seiner Einführung in die Chirurgie zur «hibernation artificielle» die Annahme, es setze den Grundumsatz herab, eine führende Rolle (LABORIT und HUGUENARD). KAZANETS sah unter erfolgreicher Behandlung mit Chlorpromazin Anregung der Schilddrüse, unter erfolgloser Behandlung Bremsung.

Vermutlich ist auch hier der Zeitfaktor bedeutsam. Eine Dämpfung der Schilddrüsenfunktion scheint vor allem zu Beginn der Medikation vor sich zu gehen; sie nimmt wahrscheinlich später ab, auch wenn die Medikation fortgesetzt wird. VON BRAUCHITSCH weist darauf hin, daß bei längerer Dauer der Medikation eine Anregung der Hypophysen-Nebennierenrinden-Funktion unter Stress gehemmt bleibt, eine solche der Hypophysen-Schilddrüsenfunktion aber dann vielleicht gesichert bliebe. Unter Neuroleptica würde sich — wenn diese Annahme richtig wäre — die Reaktionsfähigkeit auf Stress von der Nebennierenrinde auf die Schilddrüse übertragen, wie es bei einzelnen Disponierten ohnehin der Fall ist. Einer solchen Annahme widerspricht freilich der Befund von ARVAY et al.: Chlorpromazin hemmte bei Ratten die Erregung der Schilddrüse durch Lärm.

Völlig verschiedenartig sind die Ansichten darüber, *auf welche Art* Neuroleptica die Schilddrüsenfunktion hemmen. Einzelne (besonders Kliniker) vermuten, daß es sich eigentlich gar nicht um eine Hemmung der Schilddrüse, sondern nur um eine solche zentralnervöser Erregung handle, welche Erregung die Auswirkung des Schilddrüsenhormons begleite (GIARRITTA, STRAUSS und HILLER, VANNOTTI, u. a.). Wiederholt wurde vermutet, es werde die Bildung von thyreotropem Hypophysenvorderlappen-Hormon gehemmt (BIERWAGEN und SMITH; MILIN und STERN; YAMAZAKI et al.). Andere fanden das thyreotrope Hormon vermehrt (MARINONI et al.). Weitere Annahmen aus Experimenten: Reserpin verminderte die Empfindlichkeit der Schilddrüse auf thyreotropes Hormon; es beeinträchtige die Thyroxin-Sekretion (MOON und TURNER); es hemme die Dejodierung des Thyroxins und die Bildung von Trijodothyronin (VANNOTTI); es hemme die Wirkung des Thyroxins auf die Gewebe (MILCU et al.) u. a.

Was die *Hypophysen-Nebennierenrinden-Funktion* betrifft, so hoben vor allem frühere Untersucher eine Abschirmung der Hypophyse gegen Stress-Wirkung hervor; ähnlich wie nach einer Hypophysektomie sprach die Hypophyse unter Wirkung von Chlorpromazin oder Reserpin nicht mehr (oder nicht mehr so stark) mit vermehrter Bildung von ACTH auf Stress an, oder die Ansprechbarkeit der Nebennierenrinde auf ACTH war gedämpft, und es waren dadurch die Stress-Wirkungen abgebremst. Schon früh zeigte sich aber im Gegenteil, daß Neuroleptica meist die Hypophyse zur Ausscheidung von ACTH anregen wie ein

---

[1] BIERWAGEN u. SMITH; FREYDBERG-LUCAS; GAUNT et al.; KRÜSKEMPER et al.; MILCU et al.; NEGOESCU et al. 1956 und 1957; TUCHMANN-DUPLESSIS 1956a; YAMAZAKI et al.

[2] BLUMBERG; BOBBIO et al.; CRAMMER and POVER; GIARRITTA; IRMER; JENTZER; MARINONI et al.; MAROCCO and BRENA; MILIN u. STERN; NEGOESCU et al. 1956 und 1957; NEWMAN and FISH; REICHLIN et al.; STEINBEREITHNER et al.

Stressor und damit die Nebennierenrinden-Funktion stimulieren. Im allgemeinen erfolgt zuerst eine Stimulierung der ACTH-Ausscheidung, später erst eine Hemmung. Freilich sind die zeitlichen Grenzen beim Menschen noch nicht festgelegt[1].

Die Beziehungen der Neuroleptica zur *Insulinwirkung* sind uneinheitlich. Es hängt das ja schon damit zusammen, daß sie sich auf die Ausscheidung von Glucocorticoiden verschieden auswirken. Vermutet wurde auch, daß die Leberfunktion verändert wird und daß sich daraus ein Einfluß auf den Blutzucker ergibt. Im ganzen gesehen sind die Wirkungen der Neuroleptica auf den Blutzucker wenig bedeutend. Immerhin kann das Reserpin dem Insulin synergistisch wirken und (in geringem Maße) den Blutzucker herabsetzen. In anderen Fällen freilich steigert es ihn. Eine umgekehrte Wirkung zum Insulin kommt bei einigen Versuchsanordnungen auch dem Chlorpromazin zu. Es kann u. a. das Absinken des Blutzuckers nach Aufnahme von Glucose zum Nüchternwert hemmen (Charatan und Bartlett; Dobkin et al.; Dubansky und Brabec, M. Gordon et al.).

Die Beziehungen der Neuroleptica zur Funktion der *Nebenschilddrüsen* ist noch zu wenig studiert worden. Coirault et al. fanden, daß Tofranil die Calcium-Elimination und die neurale Erregbarkeit erhöht.

Über die Wirkung der Behandlung mit Neuroleptica auf die *Katechol-Amine* liegen erst wenige Untersuchungen vor. Während der Behandlung Schizophrener mit Reserpin verminderte sich die Ausscheidung von Noradrenalin im Urin. Die Ausscheidung von Adrenalin war (bei geringer Dosierung) unverändert, nach anderen Untersuchungen (bei höherer Dosierung) auch vermindert. Eine Korrelation zwischen der Wirkung des Reserpins auf die Katechol-Amine und seiner Heilwirkung auf schizophrene Patienten bestand nicht (Carlsson et al. 1959a). Im Gegensatz zur Erwartung fanden Carlsson u. Mitarb. während Iproniazid-Behandlungen von Depressiven keine Veränderung in der Ausscheidung von Adrenalin und Noradrenalin (Carlsson et al. 1959b).

Das *antidiuretische Hormon* kann unter Serpasil etwas vermehrt ausgeschieden werden (Gaunt et al.).

Früher ist die *endokrinologische Bedeutung des Elektroschocks* ebenso eingehend studiert worden wie in den letzten Jahren diejenige der Neuroleptica. Der Elektroschock bedeutet erwartungsgemäß eine starke Stress-Wirkung[2]. Im übrigen aber haben die Stoffwechseluntersuchungen keine wesentlichen Beiträge zum Verständnis seiner Wirkung gezeitigt. Ich kann deshalb mit Rücksicht auf den Umfang meines Beitrages darauf verzichten, auf die endokrinologischen Untersuchungen über die Elektroschockwirkung näher einzugehen, und mich auf die Neuroleptica beschränken, die heute das Hauptinteresse gefangennehmen.

Literatur

Bis vor kurzem existierten nur wenig zusammenfassende und großangelegte Arbeiten über endokrinologische Psychiatrie. Unser Wissen ergab sich hauptsächlich aus einer Vielzahl von kleinen Arbeiten auf eng beschrankten Gebieten und aus Nebenbemerkungen in Abhandlungen, die einer andern Thematik gewidmet waren. Für meine Darstellung benutzte ich neben eigenen Erfahrungen über 4000 Arbeiten, ohne daß ich Vollständigkeit erreicht hätte.

---

[1] Aron et al. Castaigne; Christy et al.; Egdahl et al.; Endicott and Gralnick; Fraser et al.; Gaunt et al.; Georges und Cahn; Hamburger; Harwood; Holzbauer und Vogt; Kahana und Kahana; Kothari et al.; Kulcsar et al.; Mäkelä et al.; Ohler und Weiner; Olling und de Wied; Reiss 1958 und 1959; Revol; Schaumkell; Sloane et al. 1958a und b; Sulman; Suzuki et al.; Tuchmann-Duplessis 1956a.

[2] Literatur bei Fleming.

Die Annahme aber, daß der Elektroschock durch die Stress-Wirkung auf die Nebennierenrinde wirksam wäre, ist falsch: Auch Adrenalektomierte können auf Elektroschock günstig ansprechen (Crisp et al.; Guze et al.).

Dem Umfang und den Aufgaben dieses Handbuches gemäß konnte es nicht in Frage kommen, ein großes Literatur-Verzeichnis beizugeben. In bezug auf die Literatur bis 1954 muß auf mein Buch „Endokrinologische Psychiatrie" (Thieme, Stuttgart 1954) verwiesen werden. Das folgende Literatur-Verzeichnis enthält deshalb vorwiegend Arbeiten, die nach 1954 erschienen sind. Aus Platzgründen konnten aber die neueren Arbeiten nur zu einem kleinen Teil aufgenommen werden. Bei der Aufnahme ins Literaturverzeichnis leiteten mich folgende Gesichtspunkte: Berücksichtigt wurden vor allem Arbeiten, die im Text besonders besprochen worden sind, dann solche, die umfassende Literaturverzeichnisse über ein Spezialgebiet enthalten. Viele meiner Folgerungen hätten sich gleichermaßen durch eine große Zahl von Publikationen belegen lassen. In dieser Lage wählte ich eine oder wenige Publikationen als Beispiele aus, wobei ebensowohl viele andere hätten zitiert werden können.

In bezug auf die klinische Endokrinologie verweise ich vor allem auf A. LABHART: Klinik der inneren Sekretion. Berlin: Springer 1957. Dieses Werk war auch mir ein beständiger Berater. Biologische Grundlagen der endokrinologischen Psychiatrie finden sich u. a. in reicher Mannigfaltigkeit in: BEACH, F. A.: Hormones and behavior. London and New York: P. B. Hoeber 1949 und GORBMAN, A., edit.: Comparative Endocrinology. New York: John Wiley and Sons, Inc., Publishers 1959.

Ein wichtiger Teil der französischen Literatur der letzten Jahre ist zusammengefaßt bei SCHMIDT-OSER, REGINA: Französische Beiträge der letzten zehn Jahre zur Endokrinopsychiatrie (1950—1960). Diss. Zürich 1962.

ABÉLY, P.: Introduction à l'étude de l'endocrino-psychiatrie. Soc. d'édit. d'enseignement supérieur, Paris 1949; — Les traitements récents des psychoses puerpérales. Feuillet Praticien No. 92; ref. Ann. méd.-psychol. 108 II, 704 (1950); — Hypothalamus et troubles psychiques. Ann. méd.-phsychol. 109 I, 417—434 (1951); — Etude clinique et neuro-endocrino-psychologique de quelques embrasées. Ann. méd.-psychol. 117 I, 395—400 (1959).. — ABÉLY, P., J. COR et J. LEMAIRE: Essais de traitement de la schizophrénie par la cortisone ou l'ACTH. Ann. méd.-psychol. 112 II, 394—398 (1955). — ABÉLY, P., B. JOLIVET, G. DE BAUDOUIN et C. BLANC: Les syndromes délirants de la ménopause en dehors des syndromes mélancoliques. Ann. méd.-psychol. 112 I, 700—763 (1954). — ABÉLY, P., et N. RICHARDEAU: La thérapeutique psychiatrique, son évolution depuis quarantes ans. Ann. méd.-psychol. 117 I, 801—818 (1959). — ABÉLY, X., M. DELAVILLE, P. GUIRAUD, J. BROCHERIOU, A. GREEN et G. ROSOLATO: Parallélisme des troubles psychiques et hormonaux dans un cas d'hypercorticisme surrénale. Ann. méd.-psychol. 114 II, 660—665 (1956). — ABÉLY, X., MENDEL et PERIN: Myxoedème hypophysaire avec excitation psychique. Ann. méd.-psychol. 118 I, 288—291 (1960). — ACK, M., I. MILLER and W. B. WEIL, jr.: Intelligence of children with diabetes mellitus. Pediatrics 28, 5, 764—770 (1961). — ALBEAUX-FERNET, M., P. BUGARD and J. D. ROMANI: Excretion of urinary corticoids in conditions of chronic asthenia. J. clin. Endocr. 17, 519 (1957). — ALEXANDER, F., GLENN W. FLAGG, SUSAN FOSTER, TH. CLEMENS and W. BLAHD: Experimental studies of emotional stress: 1. Hyperthyroidism. Psychosom. Med. 23, 104—114 (1961). — ALEXANDER, F., and S. A. PORTIS: A psychosomatic study of hypoglycemic fatigue. Psychosomat. Med. 6, 191 (1944). — ALMEIDA, M.: Adrenalinstoffwechsel bei einigen psychischen Störungen. Rev. Neuro-psiquiat. 22, No. 1 (1959) (spanisch). — ALPERS, J. B., and J. E. RALL: J. clin. Endocr. 15, 1482 (1955). — ALTMAN, Y. A., et F. A. AYSENSTEIN: Quelques données au sujet des psychoses de la maladie de Basedow. Z. Nevropath. (Korsakow-Z.) 60, 334—342 (1960) (russisch, mit französischer Zusammenfassung). — AMATRUDA, T. T., D. R. HOLLINGSWORTH, N. D. ESOPO, W. UPTUN and P. K. BONDY: A study of the mechanism of the steroid withdrawal syndrome. Evidence for integrity of the hypothalamic-pituitary-adrenal system. J. clin. Endocr. 20, 339 (1960). — ANDERS, G., A. PRADER, E. HAUSCHTECK, R. SCHÄRER, R. I. SIEBENMANN u. R. KELLER: Multiples Sex-Chromatin und komplexes chromosomales Mosaik bei einem Knaben mit Idiotie und multiplen Mißbildungen. Helv. paediat. Acta 15, 515 (1960). — ANGST, J.: Familienuntersuchung zur Frage des Zusammenhanges zwischen Diabetes insipidus und Persönlichkeitsstörung. Diss. Zürich 1953; — Die Psychiatrie des Diabetes insipidus. Arch. Psychiat. Nervenkr. 199, 663—707 (1959). — ARGUELLES, A. E., D. IBEAS, J. P. OTTONE and M. CHEKHERDEMIAN: Pituitary-Adrenal stimulation by sound of different frequencies. J. clin. Endocr. 22, 846—852 (1962). — ARNAUD, C. D., J. A. WALKER and R. W. EWER: Primary hyperparathyroidism associated with a cystic lesion in the neck: probable parathyroid cyst. J. clin. Endocr. 21, 833 (1961). — ARON, E., Y. CHAMBON et A. VOISIN: Bull. Acad. Méd. (Paris) 137, 417 (1953). — ARVAY, A., L. LAMPE, L. KERTESZ and L. MEDVECZKY: Changes of thyroid function in response to severe nervous stimulation. Acta endocr. (Kbh.) 35, 469 (1960).

BAER, H.: Maskulin stigmatisierte schizophrene Frauen unter Einfluß von Sexual- und Hypophysenvorderlappenhormonen. Arch. Psychiat. Nervenkr. 180, 390 (1948). — BARAHONA FERNANDES, H. J. DE: Psychosyndromes et personnalité dans les affections endocriniennes. Schweiz. Arch. Neurol. Psychiat. 91, 216 (1963). — BARD, P.: The hypothalamus and sexual behavior. Res. Publ. Ass. nerv. ment. Dis. 20, 551 (1940). — BARICH, DORIS:

Zur Frage der Beziehungen zwischen dyskrinem und schizophrenem Krankheitsgeschehen. Infantil stigmatisierte Schizophrene und ihre Verwandten. Arch. Klaus-Stift. Vererb.-Forsch. **21**, 1—36 (1945). — Barnard, R. D., and Elizabeth H. Barnard: Hormonal effects of tranquilizers. Lancet **270**, 6923 (1956). — Barr, M. L., Evelin L. Shaver, D. H. Carr and E. R. Plunkett: An unusual sex chromatin pattern in three mentally deficient subjects. J. ment. Defic. Res. **3**, 78 (1959). — Barraclough, C. A., and C. H. Sawyer: Blokkade of the release of pituitary ovulating hormone in the rat by chlorpromazine and reserpine: Possible mechanisms of action. Endocrinology **61**, 341—351 (1957). — Baruk, H., J. Ayme, J. Lunay, R. Melzer et C. D. Veziris: L'épreuve d'hyper- et d'hypoglycémie provoquées chez une série de schizophrènes de sexe feminin. Confrontation des résultats avec ceux de la cytologie vaginale et du métabolisme basal. Ann. méd.-psychol. **108 II**, 627—631 (1950). — Basowitz, H., H. Persky, S. J. Korchin and R. R. Grinker: Anxiety and Stress. An interdisciplinary study of a life situation. The Blakiston Division. New York-Toronto-London. McGraw-Hill Book Company, Inc., 1955. — Beattie, M. K., and M. A. Heasman: Adrenal lipoids as seen post mortem in schizophrenia. J. ment. Sci. **105**, 979—984 (1960). — Beiglböck, W., u. W. Brummund: Zur Frage der anabolen Wirkung von Testosteronderivaten (Bericht über Erfahrungen mit Dianabol). Med. Welt **22**, 1192—1205 (1960). — Benedek, Therese, and B. B. Rubinstein: The correlation between ovarian activity and psychodynamic process. Psychosom. Med. **1**, 244 and 461 (1939). — Benedetti, G.: Untersuchungen zur Genese der Drangkrankheiten. Schweiz. Arch. Neurol. Psychiat. **74**, 113—147 (1955). — Bennett, A. W., and C.G.Cambor: Clinical study of hyperthyroidism.Comparison of male and female characteristics. A.M.A. Arch. Gen. Psychiat. **4**, 160—165 (1961). — Berardinelli, W.: Disturbios mentais di origen paratiroidea. Res. clin.-cient. **21**, 363 (1952).— Bergeron, M., et J. C. Benoit: Recherches biotypologiques sur une groupe de schizophrènes. Évolut. psychiat.1954, 559—570.— Bergsman, A.: The urinary excretion of adrenaline and noradenaline in some mental diseases. Acta psychiat. scand., Suppl. **133**, Vol. **34** (1959). — Bierwagen, M. E., and D. L. Smith: A mechanism of action for antithyroid activity of reserpine. Proc. Soc. exp. Biol. (N. Y.) **100**, 108 (1959). — Binning, G.: The effects of emotional tensions on the development and growth of children, based on a study of 800 Saskatoon School Children. Canad. Nat. Health Magazine, March-April 1948. — Birket-Smith, E.: Excretion of neutral 17-ketosteroids in normal and neurasthenic subjects with special reference to its diurnal variations. Acta psychiat. scand. **29**, 423—440 (1955). — Bishop, P. M. F., D. P. van Meurs, D. R. C. Willcox and D. Arnold: Interstitial cell tumor of the testis in a child, report of a case and a review of the literature. Brit. med. J. **5168**, 238—242 (1960). — Blaschko, H.: Metabolism of mediator substances. In: S. Garattini and V. Ghetti: Psychotropic drugs. Amsterdam: Elsevier 1957. — Bleuler, M.: Untersuchungen aus dem Grenzgebiet zwischen Psychopathologie und Endokrinologie: II. Akromegaloid: Übersicht. Arch. Psychiat. Nervenkr. **180**, 282 (1948a); — Untersuchungen aus dem Grenzgebiet zwischen Psychopathologie und Endokrinologie. VI. Infantilismus: Übersicht der bisherigen Befunde an infantilen Schizophrenen. Arch. Psychiat. Nervenkr. **180**, 457 (1948b); — Untersuchungen aus dem Grenzgebiet zwischen Psychopathologie und Endokrinologie. VIII: Überblick und Diskussion unserer bisherigen Gesamtergebnisse. Arch. Psychiat. Nervenkr. **180**, 492 (1948c); — The Psychopathology of acromegaly. J. nerv. ment. Dis. **113**, 497 (1951); — Endokrinologische Psychiatrie. Stuttgart: Thieme 1954; — Familial and personal background of chronic alcoholics. A comparative study of the constitutions of Swiss and American alcoholic patients. In: O. Diethelm: Etiology of chronic alcoholism. pp. 110—166, 167—178. Springfield, Ill.: Charles C. Thomas, Publisher 1955. — Blickenstorfer, E.: Mutterinstinkte bei einem Manne mit krankhafter Bildung von laktotropem Hypophysenhormon. Arch. Psychiat. Nervenkr. **182**, 536 (1949); — Psychiatrie und Genealogie der Akromegalie. Untersuchungen aus dem Grenzgebiet zwischen Psychopathologie und Endokrinologie. Arch. Psychiat. Nervenkr. **186**, 88—122 (1951); — Genealogie und Psychopathologie bei 51 Akromegalen. Acta endocr. (Kbh.) **13**, 123—137 (1953); — Diskussion des akromegalen Krankheitsgeschehens im Sinne einer psychosomatischen-ganzheitlichen Auffassung des Menschen. Psyche (Stuttgart) **7**, 264—285 (1953/54). — Blickenstorfer, E., P. Isler, M. Marti u. Chr. Hedinger: Vermütterlichung eines erwachsenen Mannes mit Chorionepithelion. Dtsch. Arch. klin. Med. **199**, 462—480 (1952). — Bliss, E. L., and Ch. Hardin Branch: Anorexia nervosa. Paul B. Hoeber Inc. 1960. — Bliss, E. L., C. J. Migeon, C. H. Hardin Branch and L. T. Samuels: Reaction of the adrenal cortex to emotional stress. Psychosom. Med. **18**, 56—76 (1956). — Blumberg, A. G.: Effect of chlorpromazine with procyclidine and imipramine on radioactive iodine uptake. J. clin. Endocr. **23**, 881 (1963). — Bobbio, A., P. Goffrini et E. Bezzi: L'hibernation artificielle selon la méthode de Laborit. Presse méd. **60**, 1708—1712 (1952). — Bogdanove, E. M.: Selectivity of the effects of hypothalamic lesions on pituitary trophic hormone secretion in the rat. Endocrinology **60**, 689—697 (1957). — Bollard, B. M., R. H. Culpan, N. Marks, H. McIlwain and M. Shepherd: Purines in the urine of normal and schizophrenic subjects. J. ment. Sci. **106**, 1250—1272 (1960). — Bondarev, V. N.: Les troubles neuro-psychiques chez les enfants au cours du traitment par lest séroides corticaux. Nevropat. i Psichiat. **63**/7, 1094—1096 (1963). — BONHAM. D. T.: A report on the death of a patient with convulsive seizures during treatment of rheumatoid arthritis with cortisone, ACTH, and postpartum plasma. N. Y. med. J. **53**, 1114 (1953). — BONVALLET, M. P. DELL et G. HIEBEL: Tonus sympathique et activité électrique corticale. EEG and Clin. Neurophysiol. **6**, 119 (1954). — BORENSTEIN, P., M. DABBAH et D. BARE: Contribution à l'étude de la Réserpine en psychiatrie. Ann. méd.-psychol. **114**, 545 (1956). — BOSIA, G.: Zur Frage der Beziehungen zwischen dyskrinem und schizophrenem Krankheitsgeschehen. Eine maskuline schizophrene Frau und ihre Verwandtschaft. Arch. Klaus-Stift. Vererb.-Forsch. **25**, 269—308 (1950). — BOWMAN, K. M., and G. H. CROOK: Emotional changes following castration. In: Explorations in the physiology of emotions, ed. by L. J. WEST and M. GREENBLATT. Psychiat. Res. Rep. Amer. Psychiat. Ass., January 1960. — BRACELAND, F. J.: Hormones and their influence on the emotions. In: R. L. CRAIG: Hormones in health and disease. pp. 331—343. New York: The Macmillan Company 1954. — BRAUCHITSCH, H. VON: Endokrinologische Aspekte des Wirkungsmechanismus neuroplegischer Medikamente. Psychopharmacologia **2**/1, 1—21 (1961). — BREMER, J.: Asexualization, a follow-up study of 244 cases. New York: The Macmillan Company 1959. — BRUNN, RUTH, u. W.L.VON: Infantil stigmatisierte Schizophrene. Arch. Psychiat. Nervenkr. **189**, 324—340 (1952). — BURKART, F., G. HARTMANN, S. FANKHAUSER u. F. KOLLER: Insulinresistenz und Insulinallergie. Schweiz. med. Wschr. **93**, 1247 (1963).

CAHILL, C. A.: Post-Thyroidectomy psychoses treated with imipramine. Amer. J. Psychiat. **117**, 837 (1961). — CAMPBELL, H. J., R. GEORGE and G. W. HARRIS: The acute effects of injection of thyrotrophic hormone, or of electrical stimulation of the hypothalamus, on thyroid activity. J. Physiol. (Lond.) **148**, 5 P — 6 P (1959). — CANARY, J. J., and M. SCHAAF: The effects of reserpine in hyperthyroidism. Clin. Res. Proc. **5**, 12 (1957). — CANNON, W. B.: Bodily changes in pain, hunger, fear and rage. London and New York: Appleton 1929. — CARLSSON, A., E. BOJE RASMUSSEN and P. KRISTJANSEN: The urinary excretion of adrenaline and noradrenaline by schizophrenic patients during reserpine treatment. J. Neurochem. **4**, 318—320 (1959). — The urinary excretion of adrenaline and noradrenaline by depressive patients during iproniazid treatment. J. Neurochem. **4**, 321—324 (1959). — CARPELAN, H.: Mental disorders in thyroidectomized patients. Helsingfors 1957. — CASTAIGNE, A.: Sem. Hôp. Paris **30**, 321 (1954). — CECCARELLI, G.: Disturbi psichici durante trattamento terapeutico con ormone adrenocorticotropo (ACTH). Neuropsichiatria **1956**, 343—364. — CHAPMAN, L. F., A. O. RAMOS, H. GOODELL, G. SILVERMAN and H. G. WOLFF: A humoral agent implicated in vascular headache of the migraine type. A.M.A. Arch. Neurol. **3**, 223—229 (1960). — CHAPMAN, L.F., and H.G.WOLFF: Studies of proteolytic encymes in cerebrospinal fluid: patients with chronic-schizophrenic reactions. A preliminary report. Aus: Biological psychiatry. Grune and Stratton, Inc., 1959; — Studies of proteolytic enzymes in cerebrospinal fluid. A.M.A. Arch. intern. Med. **103**, 86—94 (1959). — CHARATAN, F. B. E., and N. G. BARTLETT: The effect of chlorpromazine ("Largactil") on glucose tolerance. J. ment. Sci. **101**, 351—353 (1955). — CLEGHORN, R. A., and C. J. PATTEE: Psychologic changes in 3 cases of Addisons disease during treatment with cortisone. J. clin. Endocr. **14**, 344—352 (1954). — COHEN, I. M.: Complications of chlorpromazine therapy. Amer. J. Psychiat. **113**, 115—121 (1956). — COIRAULT, R., V. GIRARD, R. JARRET, A. FOURNIER et J. CHAZAUD: Mode d'action du G 22355 en pathologie mentale. I. Internat. Neuro-Psycho-Pharmacol. Coll., Rom 1958. — COLMEIRO-LAFORET, K.: Galaktorrhoe bei Chlorpromazinbehandlung. Zbl. Gynäk. **79**, 1569 (1957). — CONSTAM, G.: Therapie des Diabetes mellitus. Basel: Schwabe 1950. — COOK, ST., H. MAVOR and W. F. CHAMBERS: Effects of reticular stimulation in altered adrenal states. EEG and Clin. Neurophysiol. **12**, 601 (1960). — CORBOZ, R.: Zur Psychiatrie des Morbus Basedow im Kindesalter. Z. Kinderpsychiat. **22**, 23—28 (1955). — CORNWELL, J. G., and W. HERRMANN: Intersexuality in mentally deficient patients. Acta endocr. (Kbh.) **27**, 369 (1958). — COURRIER, R. et al.: Etude quantitative de la pénétration de la radio-thyronine dans les cellules hypophysaires. C. R. Soc. Biol. (Paris) **143**, 935—937 (1949). — CRAMMER, J. L., and W. F. R. POVER: Iodine-132-uptakes by the thyroid in psychotics. J. ment. Sci. **106**, 1371—1376 (1960). — CRISP, A. H., and F. J. ROBERTS: The response of an adrenalectomized patient to ECT. Amer. J. Psychiat. **119**, 784 (1963). — CHRISTY, N. P., D. LONGSON, W. A. HORWITZ and MARY M. KNIGHT: Inhibitory effect of chlorpromazine upon the adrenal cortical response to insulin hypoglycemia in man. J. clin. Invest. **36**, 543—552 (1957).

DALTON, KATHARINA: Schoolgirls' behaviour and menstruation. Brit. med. J. No. **5213**, 1647—1649 (1960). — DARNAUD, CH., Y. DENARD, G. MOREAU, R. VOISIN et Y. GAICHIES: Action de la réserpine sur l'hyperthyroidie. Essai d'interprétation et déductions thérapeutiques. Presse méd. **67**, 457 (1959). — DASKALOV, D., u. A. ATANASOV: Eigentümlichkeiten des Verlaufes der Schizophrenie in den Gebieten mit endemischem Kropf in Bulgarien. Mitteilung I. Erkrankungen an Schizophrenie und Kropfendemie im Gebiet des Rila-Gebirges. Z. Nevropath. **60**, 1183—1186 (1960). — DAVIDSON, J. M., and C. H. SAWYER: Effects of localized intracerebral implantation of oestrogen on reproductive function in the female rabbit. Acta endocr.

(Kbh.) **37**. 385 (1961a); — Evidence for an hypothalamic focus of inhibition of gonadotropin by androgen in the male. Proc. Soc. exp. Biol. (N.Y.) **107**, 4—7 (1961b). — DE ASSIS, L. M., DORINA REICHHARDT EPPS and C. BOTTURA: Chromosomal constitution and nuclear sex of a true hermaphrodite. Lancet **1960** II, No. 7142, 129—130. — DECOURT, J.: Nosologie de l'anorexie mentale. Presse méd. Juin 1951; ref. Ann. méd.-psychol. **111** II, 105 (1953). — DECOURT, J., J. GUILLAUME et J. P. MICHARD: Etude physiopathologique d'une amenorrhée accompagnant un syndrome hypothalamique traumatique. Ann. méd.-psychol. **112** II, 271 (1954). — DE LA CHAPELLE. A.: Cytogenetical and clinical observations in female gonadal dysgenesis. Acta endocr. (Kbh.) Suppl. 65 (zu Vol. 50). — DEKABAN, A. S.. and K. R. MAGEE: Neurology 8, 193 (1958). — DENKO J. D.. and R. KAELBLING: The psychiatric aspects of hypoparathyroidism. Acta psychiat. scand. **38**. Suppl.. 164, 1962. — DELAY, J., L. BERTAGNA et A. LAURAS: ACTH et Cortison en psychiatrie. Ann. méd.-psychol. **112** I, 536—540 (1954). — DELAY, J., A. CORTEEL et B. LAINÉ: Sur une observation de psychose puerpérale guérie après currettage. Bull. Soc. Endocrinol., sé. Nov. 1949; ref. Ann. méd.-psychol. **109** I, 673 (1951); — Traitement des psychoses du postpartum. Bull. Soc. Endocrinol. sé. Mai 1953; ref. Ann. méd.-psychol. **112** II, 815 (1954). — DELAY, J., P. DENIKER et J. GALIBERT: Bouffée délirante avec hypocalcémie. Ann. méd.-psychol. **109** II, 211—214 (1951). — DELAY, J., B. LAINÉ, H. AZIMA et J. PUECH: Contribution à l'étude de l'homéostasie dans la schizophrénie et les autres psychoses. Encéphale **42**, 5, 383—400 (1953). — DELL, P. C.: Some basic mechanisms of the translation of bodily needs into behaviour. In: Ciba Foundation Symposium on the Neurological Basis of Behaviour, pp. 187—203. London: J. and A. Churchill 1958a; — Humoral effects on the brain stem reticular formations. In: Reticular formation of the brain (Henry Ford Hospital, International Symposium). pp. 365—379, edit. by H. H. JASPER, L. D. PROCTOR, R. S. KNIGHTON. W. C. NOSHAY, R. T. COSTELLO. Boston-Toronto: Little, Brown and Company 1958b. — DESHAIES G., Mme. N. RICHARDEAU et Mme. F. DECHOSAL: Chlorpromazine et Réserpine en Psychiatrie. Ann. méd.-psychol. **115** I, 417—476 (1957).— DEY, F. L.: Evidence of hypothalamic control of hypophyseal gonadotropic functions in female guinea pig. Endocrinology **33**, 75—82 (1943). — DICZFALUSY, E.. u. CHR. LAURITZEN: Oestrogene beim Menschen. Berlin-Gottingen-Heidelberg: Springer 1961. — DIETHELM, O., E. J. DOTY and A. T. MILHORAT: Emotions and adrenergic and cholinergic changes in the blood. A.M.A. Arch. Neurol. Psychiat. **54**, 110 (1945). — DIETHELM, O., M. F. FLEETWOOD and A. T. MILHORAT: The predicable association of certain emotions and biochemical changes in the blood. In: Life, Stress and Bodily Disease. Ass. Res. nerv. Dis. Proc. **29** (1950). — DIETHELM, O., and J. F. REILLY: Biochemical changes in plasma components in relation to emotions. Schweiz. Arch. Neurol. Psychiat. **91**/1, 239—244 (1963). — DINGMAN, J. F., and E. GAITAN: Subcortical stimulation of the brain and release of antidiuretic hormone in man. J. clin. Endocr. **19**, 1346 (1959). — DOBKIN, A. G.. R. G. B. GILBERT and L. LAMOUREUX: Anaesthesia 9, 157 (1954). — DOMINO, E. F.: A pharmacologic analysis of some reticular and spinal cord systems. In: Reticular Formation of the Brain (Henry Ford Hospital, International Symposium), pp. 285—318. edit. by H. H. JASPER, L. D. PROCTOR, R. S. KNIGHTON, W. C. NOSHAY, R. T. COSTELLO. Boston-Toronto: Little, Brown and Company 1958. — DONGIER, M.: Quelques acquisitions récentes en pathologie psychosomatique thyroidienne. Évolut. psychiat. **1956** II, 405—429. — DONNADIEU, A., M. FLORENTIN et Mme. FLORENTIN: Les incidents au cours du traitement des troubles mentaux par le Largactil. Ann. méd.-psychol. **113** II, 205 (1955). — DUBANSKY, B., u. J. BRABEC: Zur Frage der Wirkung des Reserpins (Serpasil) auf den Blutzucker. Psychiatr. et Neurol. (Basel) **134**, 284 (1957).

EGDAHL, R. H., J. B. RICHARDS and D. M. HUME: Effect of reserpine on adrenocortical function in unanesthetized dogs. Science **123**, 3191 (1956). — EICHNER, D.: Über den morphologischen Ausdruck funktioneller Beziehungen zwischen Nebennierenrinde und neurosekretorischem Zwischenhirnsystem der Ratte. Z. Zellforsch. **38**, 488 (1953). — ELLIS, A.: The sexual psychology of human hermaphrodites. Psychosom. Med. 7, 108 (1945). — ELMADJIAN, F., J. M. HOPE and E. T. LAMSON: Excretion of epinephrine and norepinephrine under stress. Recent Progr. Hormone Res. **14**, 513—553 (1958). — ELMADJIAN, F., E. T. LAMSON, J. M. HOPE and G. PINCUS: (Aldosterone Excretion in Anxiety States.) im Druck. — ENDICOTT, N. A., and A. GRALNICK: Psychosomatic aspects of hyperadrenocorticism treated with chlorpromazine. Dis. nerv. Syst. **22**. 680—687 (1961). — ENGELHARDT, FR.: Über die Wirkung von Gonadotropinen nach gezielter intracerebraler Instillation bei der Ratte. In: H. NOWAKOWSKI: Die partielle Hypophysenvorderlappeninsuffizienz. Berlin-Göttingen-Heidelberg: Springer 1957. — ESCAMILLA, R. F.. J. J. HUTCHINGS. W. C. DEAMER, HAO LI CHOH and P. H. FORSHAM: Long term effects of human growth hormone (LI) in a pituitary dwarf. J. clin. Endocr. **81**, 721 (1961).

FANCHAMPS, A., W. DOEPFNER, H. WEIDMANN u. A. CERLETTI: Pharmakologische Charakterisierung von Deseril, einem Serotonin-Antagonisten. Schweiz. med. Wschr. **90**, 1040 (1960). — FAURÉ, H., CL. IGERT et PH. RAPPARD: Obésité et dysmorphisme sexuel. Ann.

méd.-psychol. **114** II, 454 (1956). — Ferrier, F., J. J. Rondepierre, Veziris et Lamand: Morphogramme de Decourt et Coumic et schizophrenie. Ann. méd.-psychol. **111** II, 73—75 (1953). — Ferguson-Smith, M. A., A. W. Johnston and S. D. Handmaker: Primary amentia and micro-orchidism associated with an XXXY sex-chromosome constitution. Lancet **1960** II, No. 7143, 184—187, b. — Ferguson-Smith, M. A., A. W. Johnston and A. H. Weinberg: The chromosome complement in true hermaphroditism. Lancet **1960** II, Nr. 7142, 126—128, a. — Fischer, J. T.: Réactions schizophréniques et perturbations de l'axe hypophysogonadal. Ann. méd.-psychol. **117** II, 847—863 (1959). — Fisher, A. E.: Maternal and sexual behavior induced by intracranial chemical stimulation. Science **124**, 228—229 (1956). — Flach, F. F., C. J. Celian and R. W. Rawson: Treatment of psychiatric disorders with triiodothyronine. Amer. J. Psychiat. **114**, 841 (1959a). — Flach, F. F., C. J. Celian, P. E. Stokes and R. W. Rawson: The influence of thyroid hormones on metabolism in psychiatric disorders. I. The effect of 3:5:3-triiodo-thyronine on calcium and phosphorus metabolism in psychiatric patients. J. clin. Endocr. **19**, 454 (1959b). — Fleetwood, M. F., and O. Diethelm: Emotions and biochemical findings in alcoholism. Amer. J. Psychiat. **108**, 433 (1951). — Fleisch, A. O.: Die Persönlichkeit Akromegaloider. Schweiz. med. Wschr. **82**, 230 (1952). — Fleming, T. C.: An inquiry into the mechanism of action of electric shock treatments. J. nerv. ment. Dis. **124**, 440—450 (1956). — Folkow, B., U. S. von Euler: Selective activation of noradrenalin and adrenalin from the suprarenal gland of the cat by hypothalamic stimulation. Circulat. Res. **2**, 191 (1954). — Ford, D. H., and J. Gross: Endocrinology **62**, 416 (1958). — Forssman, H.: On hereditary diabetes insipidus. Acta med. scand. Suppl. **159**, 1—169 (1945). — Fouks, Lainé, Pagaud: Utilisation de la sérotonine en psychiatrie. In: S. Garattini and V. Ghetti: Psychotropic drugs. Amsterdam: Elsevier 1957. — Fox, H. M., B. J. Murawski, A. F. Bartholomay and S. Gifford: Adrenal steroid excretion patterns in 18 healthy subjects. Psychosom. Med. **13**, 33 (1961). — Fraccaro, M., D. Ikkos, J. Lindsten, R. Luft and K. G. Tillinger: Testicular germinal dysgenesis (male Turner's syndrome). Acta endocr. (Kbh.) **36**, 98 (1961). — Franksson, C., and C. A. Gemzell: Adrenocortical activity in the preoperative period. J. clin. Endocr. **15**, 1069—1072 (1955). — Franksson, C., C. A. Gemzell and U. S. von Euler: Cortical and medullary activity in surgical and allied conditions. J. clin. Endocr. **14**, 608 (1954). — Fraser, H. F., Anna J. Eisenman and J. W. Brooks: Urinary excretion of 5 HIAA and corticoids after morphine, meperidine, nalorphine, reserpine and chlorpromazine. Fed. Proc. **16**, Ref. No. 1275 (1957). — Freydberg-Lucas, V.: Die Wirkung von Serpasil auf die Thyreoidea. Acta endocr. (Kbh.) **23**, 419—425 (1956). — Fried, R., and M. F. Mayer: Socio-Emotional factors accounting for growth failure in children living in institutions. J. Pediat. **33**, 444—456 (1948). — Funkenstein, D. H.: Nor-Epinephrine-Like and Epinephrine-Like substances in human behavior. J. nerv. ment. dis. **124**, 58—68 (1956). — Furger, R.: Psychiatrische Untersuchungen beim Cushing-Syndrom. Schweiz. Arch. Neurol. Psychiat. **88**, H. 1 (1961); — Über den familiären Infantilismus als psychiatrisches Problem. Schweiz. Arch. Neurol. Psychiat. **91**, 250 (1963). — Furman, R. H., and R. P. Howard: Urinary 17-Ketosteroid excretion in castrated and intact men. J. clin. Endocr. **19**, 1510—1512 (1959).

Gaede, E. B., u. K. Heinrich: Klinische Beobachtungen bei Megaphen-Behandlung in der Psychiatrie. Nervenarzt **26**, 49—54 (1955). — Gaunt, R., A. A. Renzi, Nancy Antonchak, Gloria J. Miller and Martha Gilman: Endocrine aspects of the pharmacology of reserpine. Ann. N. Y. Acad. Sci. **59**, Art. 1, 22—35 (1954). — Gayral, L.: Crises et paroxysmes catathymiques. Ann. méd.-psychol. **114** II, 25—50 (1956). — Gayral, L., M. Barraud, J. Carrie et L. Candebat: Pseudohermaphroditisme mâle à type de testicule feminisant. 11 cas. Etude hormonale, psychologique et génétique. Ann. méd.-psychol. **118** I, 579 (1960). — Geller, S.: Pathogénie et physiopathologie du syndrome prémenstruel. Marseille: M. Leconte, imprimeur-éditeur 1954. — Georges, G., et J. Cahn: Anesth. et Analg. **10**, 409 (1953). — Gerhartz, H.: Ergebnisse der Cortisontherapie des Mammacarcinoms. In: Die endokrine Behandlung des Mamma- und Prostatacarcinoms. 6. Symp. Dtsch. Ges. Endokr., Homburg (Saar) 21.—23. 4. 1960, S. 14—20, Hrsg. von H. Nowakowsky. Berlin-Göttingen-Heidelberg: Springer 1961. — Giacobini, E., S. Izikowitz and A. Wegmann: Urinary norepinephrine and epinephrine excretion in Delirium tremens. A. M. A. Arch. Gen. Psychiat. **3**, 289 (1960). — Giarritta, N.: Der Einfluß von Reserpin und von Chlorpromazin auf die Funktion der endokrinen Drüsen. Diss. Zürich 1957. — Goldberg, M.: The occurrence and treatment of hypothyroidism among alcoholics. J. clin. Endocr. **20**, 609 (1960). — Goldstein, A. C.: The experimental control of sex behavior in animals. In: Hormones, Brain Function, and Behavior, edit. by H. Hoagland. New York: Academic Press Inc., Publ. 1957. — Gorbman A., Edit.: Comparative Endocrinology. New York: John Wiley & Sons, Inc. 1959. — Gordon, M., W. Zeller and J. Onnelly: A biochemical evaluation of the activity of certain tranquillizers and their relationship to hormonal function. Amer. J. Psychiat. **114**, 201—205 (1957). — Gordon, R. R., F. J. P. O'Gorman, C. J. Dewhurst and C. E. Blank: Chromosome count in a hermaphrodite with some features of Klinefelter's syndrome. Lancet **1960** II, No. 7153, 736—739. — Green, J.: The rhinencephalon and behavior. In: Ciba foundation symposium on the neurological basis of behavior. London: J. and A. Churchill 1958. — Greer Monte, A., T. Yamada and S. Iiono: The participation of the nervous system in the control of Thyroid function. Ann. N. Y. Acad. Sci. **86**, Art. 2, 667—675 (1960). — Grossmann, S. P.: Eating and drinking elicited by direct adrenergic or cholinergic stimulation of hypothalamus. Science **132**, 301 —302 (1960). — Guze, S. B., G. Winokur and M. E. Levin: The effect of electroshock therapy in the absence of both adrenal glands. J. nerv. ment. Dis. **124**, 195—198 (1956).

Haefely, W., and A. Hürlimann: Substance P, a highly active naturally occurring polypeptide. Experientia (Basel) **18**, 297 (1962). — Hamburg, D. A.: Some issues in research on human behavior and adrenocortical function. Psychosom. Med. **21**, 387 (1959). — Hamburger, Chr.: Substitution of hypophysectomy by the administration of chlorpromazine in the assay of corticotrophin. Acta endocr. (Kbh.) **20**, 383—390 (1955). — Hamilton, J. A.: Postpartum psychiatric problems. Saint Louis: C. V. Mosby Company 1962. — Hamilton, J. P., L. D. Bunch and G. E. Mestler: Urinary 17-hydroxycorticosteroids and 17-ketosteroids in castrated versus intact men: Supplementary comparisons in feeble-minded versus mentally normal men. J. clin. Endocr. **19**, 535 (1959a); — Urinary 17-ketosteroids in castrated versus non-castrated men. J. clin. Endocr. **19**, 1680 (1959b); — Chromatographic fractions and estimated androgenic activity of urinary 17-ketosteroids in castrated and intact men. J. clin. Endocr. **22**, 1103 (1962). — Hampson, Joan, G.: Hermpaphroditic genital appearance, rearing and eroticism in hyperadrenocorticism. Bull. Johns Hopk. Hosp. **96**, 265—273 (1955). — Hampson, Joan, G., and J. Money: Idiopathic sexual precocity in the female. Psychosom. Med. **17**, 16—35 (1955). — Hampson, Joan, G., J. Money and J. L. Hampson: Hermaphrodism: Recommandations concerning case management. J. clin. Endocr. **16**, 547—556 (1956). — Hampson, J. L., and Joan G. Hampson: The ontogenesis of sexual behavior in man. In: Sex and Internal Secretions, pp. 1401—1342. Edit. by W. C. Young. Baltimore: Williams & Wilkins Co. 1961. — Hampson, J. L., Joan G. Hampson and J. Money: The syndrome of gonadal agenesis (ovarian agenesis) and male chromosomal pattern in girls and women: Psychologic stud. Bull. Johns Hopk. Hosp. **97**, 207—226 (1955). — Harris, G. W.: The reticular formation, stress, and endocrine activity. In: Reticular formation of the brain (Henry Ford Hospital, International Symposium), pp. 207—221. Edit. by H. H. Jasper, L. D. Proctor, R. S. Knighton, W. C. Noshay, R. T. Costello. Boston-Toronto: Little, Brown and Company 1958. — Harris, G. W., R. P. Michael and P. P. Scott: Neurological site of action of stilboestrol in eliciting sexual behaviour. In: Ciba Foundation Symposium on Neurological Basis of Behaviour. London: J. and A. Churchill 1958. — Harvard, Davis R., P. Fourman and J. W. G. Smith: Prevalence of parathyroid insufficiency after thyroidectomy. Lancet **1961** II, 7218, 1432—1435. — Harwood, C. Terese: Effect of tranquilizing agents on ACTH secretion. J. clin. Endocr. **16**, 938 (1956). — Haun, Ch. K., and Ch. H. Sawyer: The role of the hypothalamus in initiation of milk secretion. Acta endocr. (Kbh.) **38**, 99—106 (1961). — Hauser, G. A.: Testikulare Feminisierung und Gonadendysgenesie. In: Die Intersexualität, S. 261 bis 282 und 304—347. Hrsg. von C. Overzier. Stuttgart: Thieme 1961. — Hawkins, D. R., J. T. Monroe, M. G. Sandifer and C. R. Vernon: Psychological and physiological responses to continuous epinephrine infusion — an approach to the study of the affect, anxiety. In: Explorations in the physiology of emotions. Edit. by L. J. West and M. Greenblatt. Psychiat. Res. Rep. Amer. psychiat. Ass. January 1960. — Hess, M.: Arch. Gynäk. **179**, 653 (1951); zit. v. Fr. Engelhardt. — Hetzel, B. S., W. W. Schottstaedt, W. J. Grace and H. G. Wolff: Changes in urinary 17-hydroxycorticosteroid excretion during stressful life experiences in man. J. clin. Endocr. **14**, 805 (1954); — Changes in urinary 17-hydroxycorticosteroid excretion during stressful life experiences in man. J. clin. Endocr. **15**, 1057—1068 (1955). — Hillarp, N. A.: Studies on localization of hypothalamic centres controlling gonadotrophic function of hypophysis. Acta endocr. (Kbh.) **2**, 11—23 (1949). — Hoagland, H.: Some endocrine stress responses in man. In: Stress and psychiatric disorder. Edit. by J. M. Tanner. Oxford: Blackwell Scientific Publications 1960. — Hochstaedt, B.: Emotionally conditioned endocrine disorders. Acta psychother. (Basel) **8** I, 31—43 (1960). — Höfer, R.: Der Jodstoffwechsel nach Strumektomie. In: Fortschritte der Schilddrüsenforschung, S. 70—80, herausgg. v. K. Oberdisse und E. Klein. Stuttgart: Thieme 1962. — Hoffer, A.: Epinephrine derivatives as potential schizophrenic factors. J. clin. exp. Psychopath. **18**, 27—60 (1957a); — Tranquilizing drugs. Edit. by H. E. Himwich. Publ. Assoc. Advance Sci. No. 46, Washington, D. C. 1957b; — Hormones, brain function and behavior. Edit. by H. Hoagland. New York: Acad. Press Inc. 1957c; — Adrenochrom and adrenolutin and their relationship to mental disease. In: S. Garattini and V. Ghetti: Psychotropic drugs. Amsterdam: Elsevier 1957d; — Meeting Boston Soc. Psychiat. and Neurol. March 21, 1957. Zit in: S. Garattini and V. Ghetti: Psychotropic drugs. Amsterdam: Elsevier 1957e. — Hoffer, A., and M. Kenyon: A.M.A. Arch. Neurol. Psychiat. **77**, 437 (1957). — Hoffer, A., H. Osmond and J. Smithies: Schizophrenia: A new approach. II.

Results of a year's research. J. ment. Sci. **100**, 29 (1954). — HOFMANN, G.: Demonstration eines Falles von Schizophrenie bei einem Akromegaloiden. Wien. Z. Nervenheilk. **7**, 244—251 (1953). — HOHL-SPIESS NELLY: Endokrine und psychische Störungen bei Akromegalen und ihren Familien. Diss. Zürich 1951. — HOHLWEG, W.: Zbl. Gynäk. **1939**, 114; zit. v. FR. ENGELHARDT. — In: Handbuch der Gynäkologie von SEITZ-AMREICH, S. 565, 1952; zit. v. FR. ENGELHARDT. — HOHLWEG, W., u. K. JUNKMANN: Klin. Wschr. **1932**, 321; zit. v. FR. ENGELHARDT; — Z. ges. inn. Med. **1946**, 42; zit. v. FR. ENGELHARDT. — HOLZBAUER, M., and M. VOGT: Brit. J. Pharmacol. **9**, 402 (1954). — HORST, W., u. K. ULLERICH: Die endokrine Ophthalmopathie. In: Fortschritte der Schilddrüsenforschung, S. 131—142, herausgg. v. K. OBERDISSE und E. KLEIN. Stuttgart: Thieme 1962. — HORTLING, H., and L. HIISI-BRUMMER: Basal metabolic rate and serum-protein-bound iodine in thyroid disturbances with special reference to goitre and "hypometabolism". Acta med. scand. **165**, 403 (1959). — HOWARD, J. M., J. M. OLNEY, J. P. FRAWLEY, R. E. PETERSON, L. H. SMITH, J. H. DAVIS, S. GUERRA and W. H. DIBRELL: Studies of adrenal function in combat and wounded soldiers (a study in the Korean Theatre). Ann. Surg. **141**, 3 (1955); An. Cir. (B. Aires) **32**, 3, 314—320 (1955). — HØYRUP, E.: Impaired adrenal function as a contributory factor in constitutional asthenia. Acta psychiat. scand. Suppl. **108**, 185—196 (1956). — HUGHES, R. R., and V. K. SUMMERS: Changes in the electroencephalogram associated with hypopituitarism due to post-partum necrosis. EEG and Clin. Physiol. **8**, 87—96 (1956).

IKKOS, D., and R. LUFT: Effects of short term administration of large doses of human growth hormone on carbohydrate metabolism in adult, non diabetic, hypophysectomized women (studies with 14 C-labelled glucose). Acta endocr. (Kbh.) **39**, 567 (1962). — IRMER, W.: Pharmakologische Blockierung der Überträgerstoffe und des Histamins. Anaesthesist **3**, 79—80 (1954).

JACOBIDES, G. M.: Adrenocortical function in puerperal psychoses. University of Athens thesis, 1957. — JACOBS, D. J.: Weitere infantil stigmatisierte Schizophrene und ihre Verwandten. Arch. Psychiat. Nervenkr. **180**, 432 (1948). — JANIGAN, D. T., O. D. SMITH and J. NICHOLS: Observations of the Central Nervous System, Pituitary and Adrenal in 2 Cases of Microcephaly. J. clin. Endocr. **22**, 683 (1962). — JAYLE, M. F., R. SCHOLLER, P. MAUVAIS-JARVIS et S. MÉTAY: Excrétion des stéroides chez des femmes présentant un virilisme pilaire associé à des troubles du cycle menstruel. Acta endocr. (Kbh.) **36**, 375 (1961). — JELLINEK, E. H.: Fits, faints, coma, and dementia in myxoedema. Lancet **1962**, 7264 (1010—1012). — JENTZER, A.: I 131 avec autographie, hyperglycémie, cholinestérase, métabolisme, thiomidil, choc anaphylactique, immunisation dans l'hibernation. Ann. Endocr. (Paris) **13**, 705 (1952). — JOHANNISSON, ELISABETH, C. A. GEMZELL and E. DICZFALUSY: Effect of a single injection of human pituitary follicle-stimulating hormone on urinary estrogens and the vaginal smears in amenorrhoic women. J. clin. Endocr. **21**, 1069 (1961). — JOLLY, H.: Sexual precocity. Springfield: Charles C. Thomas, Publisher 1955. — JOYEUX, J.: Le syndrome neuro-psychiatrique de la spasmophilie. Ann. méd.-psychol. **116 I**, 472—503 (1958).

KAHANA, T. B., et M. S. KAHANA: Le problème de l'action galactogène de l'aminazine chez les malades mentaux. Z. Nevropath. **60**, 1019 (1960). — KAMMERER, TH., et A. WACKENHEIM: L'évolution de l'éosinophilie sanguine pendent les syndromes maniaques et melancoliques. Ann. méd.-psychol. **113 I**, 295 (1955). — KALLIOMÄKI, L.: A therapeutic trial with ethylestrenol in geriatric patients. In: Acta endocr. (Kbh.) Suppl. 63, p. 124 (1962). — KAMMERER, TH., L. SINGER et A. WACKENHEIM: Troubles mentaux après thyroidectomie. Comptes rendus du Congrès des Médecins aliénistes et neurologistes, Liège, 19—26 juillet 1954. — KÄRKI, N. T., and M. K. PAASONEN: J. Neurochem. **3**, 352 (1959). — KANEMATSU, S., J. HILLIARD and C. H. SAWYER: Effect of reserpine on pituitary prolactin content and its hypothalamic site of action in the rabbit. Acta endocr. (Kbh.) **44**, 467—474 (1963). — KAUFMANN, J.: Zur Frage der Beziehungen zwischen dyskrinem und schizophrenem Krankheitsgeschehen: Maskulin stigmatisierte schizophrene Frauen und ihre nächste Verwandtschaft. Arch. J. Klaus-Stift. Vererb.-Forsch. **18**, 53 (1943). — KAZANETS, E. F.: Les particularités de l'état fonctionnel de la glande thyroide au moment du traitement des malades de schizophrénie par l'insuline et l'aminazine. Z. Nevropath. **60**, 1015—1018 (1960). — KEATING, R. F.: Metabolic insufficiency (Editorial). J. clin. Endocr. **18**, 531 (1958). — KEIZER, D. P. R.: Puberté précoce familiale. Arch. franç. Pédiat. **13**, 986—992 (1956). — KELLER, H. H.: Zur Psychiatrie der Akromegalie. Diss. Zürich 1949. — KENT, A., and C. LIEBERMANN: Anat. Rec. **101**, 677 (1948); zit. von FR. ENGELHARDT. — KHALEQUE, K. A., M. G. MUAZZAM and P. ISPAHANI: J. trop. Med. Hyg. **63**, 10, 241—243 (1960). — KIND, H.: Familienuntersuchung zur Frage des Zusammenhangs von Schilddrüsenfunktionsstörungen, Struma und Psychose. Schweiz. Arch. Neurol. Psychiat. **78**, 138—158 (1956). — Die Psychiatrie der Hypophyseninsuffizienz, speziell der Simmondsschen Krankheit. Fortschr. Neurol. Psychiat. **26**, 501—563 (1958); — Psychische Störungen bei Hyperparathyreoidismus. Arch. Psychiat. Nervenkr. **200**, 1—11 (1959); — Psychische und endokrine Funktionen und ihre Wechselwirkungen in der Pathogenese des Infantilismus beim hypophysären Minderwuchs.

Schweiz. Arch. Neurol. Psychiat. **91**, 245 (1963). — Kind, H., u. H. Schneider: Serotonin (5-Oxytryptamin) und psycho-pathologische Erscheinungen (psychiatrische Befunde beim Dünndarm-Karzinoid). Dtsch. med. Wschr. **82**, 1731—1733 (1957). — Kirsner, J. B., M. Sklar and W. L. Palmer: The use of ACTH, cortisone, hydrocortisone and related compounds in the management of ulcerative colitis. Amer. J. Med. **22**, 264 (1957). — Klein, E.: Iatrogene Storungen im Jodhaushalt. In: Fortschritte der Schilddrusenforschung, S. 81—101, herausgg. v. K. Oberdisse u. E. Klein. Stuttgart: Thieme 1962. — Knauff, H. G., u. F. Bock: Der Einfluß der Insulinhypoglykämie auf die freien Aminosäuren und das Aethanolamin des Gehirns. Klin. Wschr. **38**, 11, 553—554 (1960). — Knoepfel, H. K.: Funf akromegaloide Schizophrene und Psychopathen mit ihren Familien. Arch. Psychiat. Nervenkr. **180**, 332 (1948a); — Statistische Verarbeitung von 23 Fällen bereits beschriebener akromegaloider Schizophrener und Psychopathen und ihrer Familien. Arch. Psychiat. Nervenkr. **180**, 361 (1948b). — Kochmann, R.: Pädiatrie und Psychiatrie. Méd. et Hyg. (Genève) **20**, 187—188 (1962). — Kollros, J. J., and V. M. McMurray: The mesencephalic V nucleus in anurans, II. The influence of thyroid hormone on cell size and cell number. J. exp. Zool. **131**, 1—26 (1956). — Konig, P. A.: Genetische, endokrinologische und psychosexuelle Probleme bei testikularer Feminisierung. Geburtsh. u. Frauenheilk. **20**, 2, 166—180 (1960). — Konkov, A. V.: Hypoglycaemic coma arrested by painful massage (russisch). Klin. Med. (Mosk.) **6**, 144 (1961).— Korchin, S. J., and M. Herz: Differential effects of "shame" and "desintegrative" threats on emotional and adrenocortical functioning. A.M.A. Arch. Gen. Psychiat. **2**, 640 (1960). — Kothari, N. J., T. H. Rindani and M. G. Naik: Effect of reserpine free extract of Rauwolfia serpentina on the action of ACTH and hydrocortisone on man. Arch. int. pharmacodyn. **111**, 293 (1957). — Krasowska, Janina: Les syndromes psychotiques de la tension prémenstruelle à l'âge de puberté. Ann. méd.-psychol. **118**, 56 (1960). — Krautschik, Adelheid: Psychologische Untersuchungen bei 6 Kindern mit Gonadendysgenesie. Prax. Kinderpsychol. **11**, 33 (1962) — Kress, H. Frh. von: Zum Thema Krankheit und Umwelt. Schweiz. med. Wschr. **90**, 1423 (1960). — Kressig, R.: Untersuchungen uber die Largactil-(Megaphen-) Amenorrhoe. Diss. Basel 1959. — Kretschmer, W.: Die Neurose als Reifungsproblem. Sammlg. psychiatr. neurol. Einzeldarstellg. Stuttgart: Thieme 1952. — Krump, J. E.: Die klinische und differentialdiagnostische Bedeutung des Elektroencephalogramms bei Sheehan-Syndrom. In: H. Nowakowski: Die partielle Hypophysenvorderlappen-Insuffizienz. Berlin-Göttingen-Heidelberg: Springer 1957. — Krüskemper, H. L., F. J. Kessler u. E. Steinkrüger: Der Einfluß von Reserpin auf die antithyreoidale Wirkung von Kaliumperchlorat. Acta endocr. (Kbh.) **39**, 423 (1962). — Kulcsar, S., W. Z. Polishuk et L. Rubin: Aspects endocriniens du traitement à la chlorpromazine. Presse méd. **65**, 1288 (1957). — Kuemmerle, H. P., A. Senn, P. Rentchnick u. N. Goossens (Herausgeber): Klinik und Therapie der Nebenwirkungen. Stuttgart: Thieme 1960. — Kurland, G. S., M. W. Hamolsky and A. St. Freedberg: Studies in non-myxedematous hypometabolism. I. The clinical syndrome and the effects of triiodo-thyronine alone or combined with thyroxine. J. clin. Endocr. **15**, 1354—1366 (1955).

Labhart, A.: Klinik der inneren Sekretion. Berlin-Gottingen-Heidelberg: Springer 1957. — Laborit, H., et P. Huguenard: L'hibernation artificielle par moyens pharmacodynamiques et physiques. Presse méd. **59**, 1329 (1951). — Laignel-Lavastine, M.: Des troubles psychiques par perturbations des glandes à sécrétion interne. Congr. Méd. aliénistes et neurologistes de France et des pays de langue française, XVIII session, Dijon, du 3 au 9 août 1908, vol. I (Comptes rendus) et vol. II (Rapports).— Leading Article: Parathyroid insufficiency. Lancet **1961** II, 7218, 1440. — Langelüddeke, A.: Die Entmannung von Sittlichkeitsverbrechern. Berlin: W. de Gruyter & Co. 1963. — Lansing, R. W., and J. B. Trunnell: Electroencephalographic changes accompanying thyroid deficiency in man. J. clin. Endocr. **23**, 470 (1963). — Lenz, W.: Medizinische Genetik. Stuttgart: Thieme 1961. — Levin, M. E.: "Metabolic Insufficiency": A double blind study using triiodothyronine, thyroxine and a placebo: Psychometric evaluation of the hypometabolic patient. J. clin. Endocr. **20**, 106 (1960). — Lindberg, B. J.: Psycho-Infantilism. (A survey and some new experiences.) Nord. Med. **49**, 838—843 (1953) (schwedisch). — Lindqvist, G.: Confusional states, depersonalisation syndromes, and pseudo-hallucinations following hypophysectomy. Acta psychiat. scand. **36**, 601 (1961). — Lingjaerde, O.: Delirium acutum — eine akute Nebenniereninsuffizienz? Mit einigen Bemerkungen über die Rolle der Nebennieren in der Pathogenese gewisser Schizophrenien. Nervenarzt **14**, 97—104 (1941). — Linquette, M., P. Graux et A. Gerard: Les troubles psychiques au cours des hypercorticismes non thérapeutiques. Leur traitement chirurgical. Ann. Endocr. (Paris) **21**, 1, 113—128 (1960). — Lisk, R. D.: Testosterone-sensitive centers in the hypothalamus of the rat. Acta endocr. (Kbh.) **41**, 195—204 (1962). — Ljungberg, E.: Die 5-HIES-Bestimmungen im Urin als wertvolle klinisch-chemische Methode in der modernen psychiatrischen Klinik. (Erscheint demnächst im Schweiz. Arch. Neurol.) — Lochner, K. H., Marilyn R. Scheuing and F. F. Flach: The effect of thyroid hormones on schizophrenic patients: review of literature and double-blind study of the effect of L-triiodothyronine on chronic schizophrenic patients. Manuskript aus Payne Whitney Clinic. New York, August 1962. — LUFT, R.: Die endokrine Behandlung des Mammacarcinoms. In: Die endokrine Behandlung des Mamma- und Prostatacarcinoms. 7. Symp. Dtsch. Ges. Endokr. Homburg (Saar) 21.—23. 4. 1960. S. 1—7. Hrsg. v. H. NOWAKOWSKI. Berlin-Göttingen-Heidelberg: Springer 1961. — LUNDBERG, P. O.: Migraineprophylaxis with progestogens. Acta endocr. (Kbh.) Suppl. 68 (zu Vol. 40). — LUTZ, J., u. A. MEYER: Psychische Entwicklung eines 6¹/₂jährigen Mädchens mit konstitutioneller Pubertas praecox. Z. Kinderpsychiat. 20, 161—166 (1953).

MÄKELÄ, S., E. NÄÄTÄNEN and U. K. RINNE: The response of the adrenal cortex to psychic stress after meprobamate treatment. Acta endocr. (Kbh.) 32, 1 (1959). — MALANDRA, BR., e S. CORBETTA: La sostanca Gomori-positiva della neuroipofisi del ratto dopo surrenectomia e trattamento con corticoidi surrenali e sali. Z. Zellforsch. 39, 318 (1953). — MALL, G.: Katamnestische Ergebnisse nach der Gjessingschen Thyroxinbehandlung periodischer Katatonien. Arch. Psychiatr. Nervenkr. 200, 390—401 (1960). — MANTHEY, G.: Psychische Störungen bei Thyreotoxikosen nach Behandlung mit radioaktivem Jod und Strumektomien. Nervenarzt 30, 15 (1959). — MANTHEY, H. G.: Psychoanalysis of myxoedema. Adv. Psychosom. Med. Vol. I, 280—284, Basel-New York: Karger 1960. — MARAÑON, G.: Personalidad y endocrinologia. Rev. Psicol. gen. Madrid 8, 379—398 (1953). — MARINONI, U., G. PURICELLI, S. HUKOVIC e S. CASENTINI: Azione della cloropromazina a livello delle diverse ghiandole endocrine. Endocr. Sci. Cost. 25, 5, 332—340 (1958). — MAROCCO, F., and S. BRENA: Minerva anest. 19, 332 (1953). — MARZI, A., e U. TEODORI: Primi risultati di una indagine sulla personalità nelle turbe dello sviluppo puberale. Folia endocr. (Pisa) 6, 3, 279 (1953). — MASON, J. W.: The central nervous system regulation of ACTH secretion. In: Reticular Formation of the Brain (Henry Ford Hospital, International Symposium). Edit. by H. H. JASPER, L. D. PROCTOR, R. S. KNIGHTON, W. C. NOSHAY, R. T. COSTELLO. Boston-Toronto: Little, Brown and Company 1958. — MATTHES, A., u. E. MALLMANN-MUEHLBERGER: Die Propulsiv-Petit-Mal-Epilepsie und ihre Behandlung mit Hormonen. Dtsch. med. Wschr. 88, 426 (1963). — MAYER, S. W., F. H. KELLY and M. E. MORTON: J. Pharmacol. exp. Ther. 117, 197 (1956). — McMAHON, F. G., and E. S. GORDAN: Side-effects noted in treatment with Methylprednisolone (Medrol). J. Amer. med. Ass. 168, 1208 (1958). — MENDELSON, J. H., P. E. KUBZANSKY, P. H. LEIDEMAN, D. WEXLER and P. SOLOMON: Physiological and psychological aspects of sensory deprivation — a case analysis. In: Sensory Deprivation, A Symposium at Harvard Medical School edited by P. SOLOMON, P. E. KUBZANSKY, P. H. LEIDEMANN, J. H. MENDELSON, R. TRUMBUKL, D. WEXLER. — MENTZOS, ST., u. P. A. FISCHER: Elektroencephalographische Befunde nach Hypophysektomie. Nervenarzt 34, 234 (1963). — MEYER, A.-E.: Zur Endokrinologie und Psychologie intersexueller Frauen. Stuttgart: Enke 1963. — MEYER, A. E., u. H. FRAHM: Zur Steroidbehandlung des gewöhnlichen Hirsutismus. Schweiz. med. Wschr. 90, 1336 (1960). — MEYER, A. E., u. D. v. ZERSSEN: Psychologische Untersuchungen an Frauen mit sog. idiopathischem Hirsutismus. J. psychosom. Res. 4, 206—235 (1960a); — About methods for an initial psychosomatic investigation of clinical syndromes (exemplified by a research of a socalled idiopathic hirsutism). Advanc. Psychosom. Med. 1, 70 (1960b). — MEYER, J.-E.: Die sexuellen Störungen des Hirnverletzten. Arch. Psychiat. Nervenkr. 193, 449—469 (1955). — MILCU, ST.-M., I. NEGOESCU, A. LUPULESCU and FL. COCU: Inhibition of TSH by Reserpine. Com. Acad. R. P. R. 7, 4, 483—489 (1957). — MILIN, R., and P. STERN: Effect of chlorpromazine on hyperthyroidism in hares. Med. Pregl. (serbisch) 8, 5, 280—285 (1955). — MONCKE, C.: Zum Einfluß von Reserpin auf den Stoffwechsel bei der Hyperthyreose. Med. Mschr. 11, 18 (1957). — MONEY, J.: Hermaphroditism, Gender and Precocity in Hyperadrenocorticism: Psychologic Findings. Bull. Johns Hopk. Hosp. 96, 253—264 (1955); — Components of eroticism in man: I. The hormones in relation to sexual morphology and sexual behavior. J. nerv. ment. Dis. 132, 239 (1961); — Sex hormones and other variables in human eroticism. In: Sex and Internal Secretions, pp. 1383—1400, edit. by W. C. YOUNG. Vol. II. Baltimore: Williams & Wilkins Co. 1961; — Cytogenetic and psychosexual incongruities with a note on space-form blindness. Amer. J. Psychiat. 119, 820 (1963). —, and JOAN G. HAMPSON: Idiopathic sexual precocity in the male. Psychosom. Med. 17, 1—15 (1955). — MONEY, J., JOAN G. HAMPSON and J. L. HAMPSON: Hermaphroditism: Recommandations concerning assignement of sex, change of sex, and psychologic management. Bull.Johns Hopk. Hosp. 97, 284—300 (1955a); — An examination of some basic sexual concepts: The evidence of human hermaphroditism. Bull. Johns Hopk. Hosp. 97, 301—319 (1955b); — Sexual incongruities and psychopathology: The evidence of human hermaphroditism. Bull. Johns Hopk. Hosp. 98, 43—57 (1956). — MOON, R. C., and C. W. TURNER: Effect of reserpine on thyroid activity in rats. Proc. Soc. exp. Biol. (N. Y.) 100, 679—681 (1959). — MOSSO, H. E., y F. PERGOLA: Un nuevo preparado anabólico de síntesis: la metandrostenolona. Dia méd. 33, 11, 208—214 (1961).

NEGOESCU, I., C. PETRESCU, FL. COCU and N. RADIAN: The action of promethazine in hyperthyroidism. Endocrinologia (Bucuresti) 1, 1, 66—69 (1956). — NEGOESCU, I., N. RADIAN, FL. COCU, AL. BOJINESCU and A. LUPULESCU: Contributions to the study of the action of reserpine on the calorigenous effect of thyroxine and on iodine fixation. Endocrinologia (Bucuresti) **2**, 1, 40—46 (1957). — Newman, St., and V. J. Fish: The influence of tranquilizing drugs on results of thyroid function studies. J. clin. Endocr. **18**, 1296 (1958). — Niekisch, H.: Zur Psychopathologie des adreno-genitalen Syndroms. Z. Kinderpsychiat. **27**, 292 (1960). — Nowakowski, H., W. Lenz, S. Bergman u. J. Reitalu: Chromosomenstudien beim Klinefelter-Syndrom. In: Endokrine Regulationen des Kohlenhydratstoffwechsels. 7. Symp. Dtsch. Ges. Endokr., Homburg (Saar) 21.—23. 4. 1960. S. 295—298. Hrsg. v. H. Nowakowski. Berlin-Göttingen-Heidelberg: Springer 1961. — Nowakowski, H., u. H. Schmidt: Die Hodenveränderungen beim alternden Manne und ihre klinische Bedeutung. Schweiz. med. Wschr. **89**, 1204 (1959).

Odell, W. D., J. M. van Buren and R. Hertz: Effect of thalamic surgery on endocrine function. J. clin. Endocr. **22**, 1262 (1962). — Ohler, E. A., and A. Weiner: The effect of chlorpromazine on pituitary-adrenal function. J. clin. Endocr. **16**, 915 (1956). — Ohm, A.: Zur Frage der Entmannung. (Eine Auswertung der Berliner „Akten betr. Entmannung".) Z. psychosom. Med. **7**, 21, 106 (1961). — Olds, J.: Persitive emotional systems studied by techniques of Self-Stimulation. In: Explorations in the physiology of emotions, edited by L. J. West and M. Greenblatt. Psychiatric Res. Rep. Amer. Psychiat. Ass., January 1960. — Olling, Ch. C. J., and D. de Wied: Inhibition of the release of corticotrophin from the hypophysis by chlorpromazine. Acta endocr. (Kbh.) **22**, 283 (1956). — Oppenheimer, J. H., L. V. Fisher and J. W. Jailer: Disturbance of the pituitary-adrenal interrelationship in diseases of the central nervous system. J. clin. Endocr. **21**, 1023 (1961). — Overzier, C.: Transvestitismus und Klinefelter-Syndrom. Arch. Psychiat. Nervenkr. **198**, 198 (1958a); — Das chromosomale Geschlecht bei Transvestitismus. Dtsch. med. Wschr. **83**, 181 (1958b); — Hermaphroditismus verus und sog. echtes Klinefelter-Syndrom. In: Die Intersexualität. S. 188—240. Hrsg. v. C. Overzier. Stuttgart: Thieme 1961; — Die Intersexualität. Stuttgart: Thieme 1961.

Pace, N., F. L. Schaffer, F. Elmadjian, D. Minard, S. W. Davis, J. H. Kilbuck, E. L. Walker, M. E. Johnston, A. Zilinsky, R. W. Gerard, P. H. Forsham and J. G. Taylor: Physiological studies on infantrymen in combat. In: California University Publications in Physiology, Berkely **10**, No. 1, 1—48. — Pare, C. M. B., M. Sandler and R. S. Stacey: 5-hydroxyindoles in mental deficiency. J. Neurol. Neurosurg. Psychiat. **23**, 341 (1960). — Parker, Rose H., and W. H. Beierwaltes: Inheritance of defective Organification of Iodine in Familial Goitrous Cretinism. J. clin. Endocr. **21**, 21—30 (1961). — Pasqualini, R. Q., G. Vidal and G. E. Bur: Psychopathology of Klinefelter's Syndrome. A Review of 31 cases. Lancet **1957**, 164—167. — Passouant-Fontaine, T., C. Flander, and P. Passouant: C. R. Soc. Biol. (Paris) **149**, 791 (1955). — Pauli, Lydia, R. O'Neil, M. Ybanez and S. Livingstone: Minor motor epilepsy: Treatment with corticotropin (ACTH) and steroid therapy. J. Amer. med. Ass. **174**, 1408—1412 (1960). — Pedersen, A. L.: Investigations into the metabolism of androgen in normal-haired and in hypertrichotic, schizophrenic women. Rep. 8. Congr. Scand. Psychiatr. Acta psychiat. scand. Suppl. **47**, 130 (1947); — Psykiske symptomer hos kastrerede kvinder og deres pavirkelighed of ostrogenterapi. Nord. med. **44**, 1895 (1950); — Kirurgisk Klimakterium. Eget Vorlag. Aarhus: Amtstidendes Bogtrykkeri 1956. — Persky, H., J. Maroc, E. Conrad and A. Den Breeijen: Blood corticotropin and adrenal weight-maintenance factor levels of anxious patients and normal subjects. Psychosom. Med. **21**, 379 (1959). — Pitt-Rivers, Rosalind, and J. R. Tata: The thyroid hormones. London: Pergamon Press 1959. — Pletscher, A., H. Besendorf and K. F. Gey: Science **129**, 844 (1959). — Pletscher, A., K. F. Gey and P. Zeller: Monoaminooxydase-Hemmer. Fortschr. Arzneimitt.-Forsch. **2**, 417—590 (1960). — Ploog, D.: Verhaltensforschung und Psychiatrie. (s. S. 291 dieses Bandes). — Poeck, K.: Die Wirkung von Adrenalin, Noradrenalin und Acetylcholin auf das aszendierende retikuläre Aktivierungssystem des Hirnstamms. Fortschr. Med. **80/21**, 815—820 (1962). — Polishuk, W. Z., and S. Kulcsar: Effects of chlorpromazine on pituitary function. J. clin. Endocr. **16**, 292—293 (1956). — Portis, S. A.: Life situations, emotions and hyperinsulinism. J. Amer. med. Ass. **142**, 1281—1286 (1950). — Poulson, Evelyn, M. Botros and J. M. Robson: Effect of 5-hydroxytryptamine and iproniazid on pregnancy. Science **131**, 1101—1102 (1960). — Prader, A.: Die Cortisondauerbehandlung des kongenitalen adrenogenitalen Syndroms. Helv. paediat. Acta **8**, 386—423 (1952); — Intersexualität und Gonadendysgenesie. In: A. Labhart: Klinik der inneren Sekretion. S. 659. Berlin-Göttingen-Heidelberg: Springer 1957. — Prader, A., J. Schneider, J. M. Frances and W. Zublin: Frequency of the true (Chromatin-Positive) Klinefelter's Syndrome. Brief an "Lancet" (London), März 1957, persönlich übermittelt. — Prilenski, F.: Adrenalingehalt im Blut der an Acrichin-„Psychose" leidenden Tieren. In: M. A. Goldenberg: Reproduktion der Syndrome der Acrichin-(Atebrin)-„Psychose" bei Tieren. Arbeiten des staatlichen medizinischen Institutes von Nowosibirsk 1961 (Bd. 37).

Raboch, J., and J. Sipova: The mental level in 47 cases of true Klinefelter's Syndrome. Acta endocr. (Kbh.) **36**, 404 (1961). — Reichlin, S., M. G. Koussa and F. W. Witt: Effect of prolonged sleep therapy and of chlorpromazine on plasma protein-bound jodine concentration and plasma thyroxine turn-over. J. clin. Endocr. **19**, 692 (1959). — REINFRANK, R. F.: Primary hyperparathyroidism with depression. Arch. intern. Med. **108**/4, 606—610 (1961). — REISNER, H.: Melancholie und Morbus Basedow. Schweiz. Arch. Neurol. Psychiat. **91**, 233 (1962). — REISS, M.: Untersuchungen über das endokrine Equilibrium von Geisteskranken. Arch. Psychiat. Nervenkr. **187**, 488 (1952); — Psychoendocrinology. J. ment. Sci. **101**, 683—695 (1955); — Endocrine concomitants of certain physical psychiatric treatments. Int. Rec. Med. **169**, 431 (1956); — Die Laboratoriumsdiagnose der partiellen Hypophysenvorderlappeninsuffizienz. In: NOWAKOWSKI, H.: Die partielle Hypophysenvorderlappen-Insuffizienz. Berlin-Göttingen-Heidelberg: Springer 1957; — Psychoendocrinology. Chapter 15. New York and London: Grune and Stratton 1958; — Drug action and endocrine function in mental disorder. In: Neuro-Psycho-Pharmacology. Ed. by P. B. BRADLEY, P. DENIKER and C. RADOUCO-THOMAS. Amsterdam-London New York-Princeton: Elsevier Publishing Co. 1959. — RENNIE, T. A. C., and J. E. HOWARD: Hypoglycemia and Tension-Depression. Psychosom. Med. **4**, 273 (1942). — REVOL, L.: La thérapeutique par la chlorpromazine en pratique psychiat rique. Paris: Masson 1956. — RICHTER, C. P.: Neurological basis of responses to stress. In: Ciba Foundation Symposium on the neurological basis of behavior. p. 204. London: J. and A. Churchill 1958. — ROCHEBLAVE-SPENLE, A. M.: Rôles masculins et rôles féminins dans les états intersexuels. Évolut. psychiat. **1954**, 281—310. — ROSEMBERG, EUGENIA, and L. ENGEL: The influence of steroids on urinary gonadotropin extraction in a postmenopausal woman. J. clin. Endocr. **20**, 1576 (1960). — ROSENBLATT, J. S., and L. R. ARONSON: The decline of sexual behavior in male cats after castration with special reference to the role of prior sexual experience. Behavior **12**, 4, 286—338 (1958); — The influence of experience in the behavioural effects of androgen in prepuberally castrated male cats. Animal Behaviour **6**, 171—182 (1958). — ROTHLIN, E.: Pharmacology of Lysergic Acid Diethylamid (LSD) and some of its related compounds. In: S. GARATTINI and V. GHETTI: Psychotropic drugs. Amsterdam: Elsevier 1957. — ROYER, P., M. BEIS, VERNET et J. BRIGNON: L'élimination des 17-kétostéroides chez les alcooliques. Ann. méd.-psychol. **111 II**, 87 (1953).

SAARENMAA, E.: On the effect of reserpine on serum Protein-Bound-Iodine (PBI). Acta chir. scand. **112**, 199 (1957). — SALMOIRAGHI, G. C., and F. A. STEINER: Acetylcholine sensitivity of cat's medullary neurons. Erscheint demnächst in J. Neurophysiol. — SAWYER, C. H.: Activation and blockade of the release of pituitary gonadotropin as influenced by the reticular formation. In: Reticular formation of the brain (Henry Ford Hospital, International Symposium), pp. 223—230. Edit. by H. H. JASPER, L. D. PROCTOR, R. S. KNIGHTON, W. C. NOSHAY, R. T. COSTELLO. Boston-Toronto: Little, Brown and Company 1958. — SCHARRER, BERTA: The role of neurosecretion in neuro-endocrine integration. In: AUBREY GORBMAN: Comparative endocrinology. New York: John Wiley and Sons, Inc., publishers 1959. — SCHARRER, E.: General and phylogenetic interpretations of neuroendocrine Interrelations. In: AUBREY GORBMAN: Comparative Endocrinology. New York: John Wiley and Sons 1959. — SCHAUMKELL, K. W.: Über die Morphokinese der Ratten-Nebennierenrinde unter Einwirkung von N-(3-Dimethyl-amino)-Propyl-3-Chlorphenothiazin (Megaphen Bayer). Acta endocr. (Kbh.) **20**, 371—378 (1955). — SCHAUMKELL, K. W., u. H. H. STANGE: Klinische, konstitutionsbiologische, histologische Untersuchungen beim Pseudohermaphroditismus masculinus internus mit totaler Verweiblichung. Zbl. Gynäk. **78**, 1449 (1956). — SCHITTENHELM, A.: Über zentrogene Formen des Morbus Basedowii und verwandter Krankheitsbilder. Klin. Wschr. **1935**, 401. — SCHITTENHELM, A., u. B. EISLER: Über die Resorption des Thyroxins nach oraler Zufuhr. Z. ges. exp. Med. **80**, 569—579 (1932). — SCHMIDT-OSER, REGINA: Französische Beiträge der letzten zehn Jahre zur Endokrinopsychiatrie. Diss. Zürich 1962. — SCHNEEBERG, N. G., W. B. LIKOFF and D. R. MERANZE: An evaluation of the blood test for galactose tolerance in the diagnosis of hyperthyroidism. Arch. Surg. **46**, 581—588 (1943). — SCHNEIDER, H.: Die Psychopathologie des Serotoninstoffwechsels, speziell bei Dünndarmkarzinoid. Diss. Zürich 1957. — SCHUPBACH, A.: Postpartuales Myxödem und Simmondssche Krankheit. Schweiz. med. Wschr. **81**, 610 (1951). — SCHWABE, A. D., D. H. SOLOMON, R. J. STOLLER and J. B. BURNHAM: Pubertal feminization of a genetic male with testicular atrophy and normal urinary gonadotropin. J. clin. Endocr. **22**, 839 (1962). — SCHWARTZ, T. B., and D. R. SHIELDS: Urinary excretion of formaldehydogenic steroids and creatinnine. Psychosom. Med. **18**, 159 (1956). — SCHWÖBEL, G.: Psychopathologie des Morbus Cushing. Schweiz. Arch. Neurol. Psychiat. **71**, 380—384 (1953). — SECKEL, H. P. G.: Six examples of precocious sexual development. II. Studies in growth and maturation. Amer. J. Dis. Child. **79**, 287 (1950). — SEGAL, S. J.: Comparative aspects of gonadal morphology, physiology and antigenicity. In: A. GORBMAN: Comparative Endocrinology. New York: John Wiley and Sons 1959. — SEILER, E.: Ein akromegaloider Schizophrener und seine Verwandtschaft. Diss. Zürich 1953. — SHEEHAN, H. L.: Physiopathologie der Hypophyseninsuffizienz. Helv. med. Acta **22**, 324 (1955). — SHEEHAN, H. L., and V. K. SUMMERS: The syndrome of hypopituitarism. Quart. J. Med. N. S. **18**, 319 (1949). — Sikkema, Stella H.: Triiodothyronine in the diagnosis and treatment of hypothyroidism: Failure to demonstrate the metabolic insufficiency syndrome. J. clin. Endocr. **20**, 546 (1960). — Silverman, A. J., and S. J. Cohen: Affect and vascular correlates to catechol amines. In: Exploration in the physiology of emotions. Edit. by L. J. West and M. Greenblatt. Psychiat. Res. Rep. Amer. Psychiat. Ass., January 1960. — Sivadon, P., S. Pollin et J. Sanson: Essais thérapeutiques par la paraoxy-propiophénone (Corps H-365) frénateur hypophysaire de synthèse. Ann. méd.-psychol. **109 II**, 319—324 (1951). — Sloane, B. R., M. Saffran, R. A. Cleghorn: Steroid response to ACTH and the effect of ataractic drugs. In: M. Reiss: Psychoendocrinology. New York and London: Grune and Stratton 1958a; — The effect of chlorpromazine on steroid response to ACTH in psychiatric patients. The Scient. Papers 114th Ann. Meet. Amer. Psychiatr. Ass., San Francisco, May 12—16, 1958b. — Sorel, L., et A. Dusauca-Bauloye: A propos de 21 cas d'hypsarythmia de Gibbs. Son traitement spectaculaire par l'ACTH. Acta neurol. belg. **58**, 130 (1958). — Sorg, E.: Zur Frage der Beziehungen zwischen dyskrinem und schizophrenem Krankheitsgeschehen. Psychische Storungen in den Familien von nicht-schizophrenen Akromegaloiden. Diss. Zürich 1945. — Staehelin, B.: Die Psychopathologie des Sheehan-Syndroms. Acta endocr. (Kbh.) **14**, 145—152 (1953). — Staehelin, J. E.: Über psychische Storungen bei Riesenwuchs. Mschr. Psychiat. Neurol. **125**, 699 (1953). — Steinbereithner, K., E. Lembeck u. St. Hift: Künstlicher Winterschlaf. Wien-Innsbruck: Urban & Schwarzenberg 1955. — Stieve, H.: Der Einfluß des Nervensystems auf Bau und Tätigkeit der Geschlechtsorgane des Menschen. Stuttgart: Thieme 1952. — Stockard, Ch. R.: The genetic and endocrine basis for differences in form and behavior. The Wister Institute of Anatomy and Biology. Philadelphia 1941. — Stockhausen, F. G.: Clinical studies with tetrabenazine (Ro 1-9569). Dis. nerv. Syst. **21**, 115—117 (1960) (Suppl.). — Stockmann, Maria: Zur Frage der Beziehungen zwischen dyskrinem und schizophrenem Krankheitsgeschehen. Weitere maskulin stigmatisierte schizophrene Frauen und ihre Verwandtschaft. Arch. Klaus-Stift. Vererb.-Forsch. **21**, 171 (1946). — Stoll, W. A.: Dexamethasone in advanced breast cancer. Cancer **13**, 5, 1074—1080 (1960). — Stoll, W.A.: Lysergsäure-diäthylamid, ein Phantasticum aus der Mutterkorngruppe. Schweiz. Arch. Neurol. Psychiat. **60**, H. 1/2 (1947); — Psychopathologische Untersuchungen bei Morbus Cushing. Wien. Z. Nervenheilk. **3**, 315 (1950); — Die Psychiatrie des Morbus Addison, insbesondere seiner chronischen Formen. Sammlg. psychiatr.-neurol. Einzeldarstellungen. Stuttgart: Thieme 1953; — Jodtraceruntersuchungen der Schilddrüse nach Reiss bei chronischer Schizophrenie. Schweiz. Arch. Neurol. Psychiatr. **77**, 310—329 (1956). — Strauss, E., u. J. Hiller: Sympathicolytische Substanzen in der Therapie der Schilddrüsenüberfunktion. Med. Klin. **49 II**, 1073—1075 (1954). — Sturm, A., u. Schneeberg: Zitiert von A. Sturm u. W. Wernitz (1932). — Sturm, A., u. W. Wernitz: Hormonjagd im Gehirn. Acta neuroveg. (Wien) **13**, 50—62 (1956). — Stutinsky, Fr.: Action du diéthylstilboestrol sur la neurosécrétion hypothalamique du rat blanc femelle. Ann. Endocr. (Paris) **14**, 101 (1953). — Stutte, H.: Pubertas praecox. In: Die Sexualität des Menschen. Handbuch der medizinischen Sexualforschung. S. 474—505. Hrsg. v. Dr. med. Dr. phil. Hans Giese. Stuttgart: Ferdinand Enke Verlag 1954; — Zustände psychischer Vorentwicklung im Kindesalter. Nervenarzt **33**, 337 (1962). — Sulman, F. G., and H. Z. Winnik: Hormonal effects of chlorpromazine. Lancet **1956**, 1, 161—162. — Sulser, F., and B. B. Brodie: Is reserpine tranquilization linked to change in brain serotonin or brain norepinephrine? Science **131**, 1440—1441 (1960). — Sulzer, H. J.: Zur Frage der Beziehungen zwischen dyskrinem und schizophrenem Krankheitsgeschehen. Ein akromegaloider Schizophrener und seine Familie. Arch. Klaus-Stift. Vererb.-Forsch. **18**, 461 (1943). — Suzuki, M., K. Kamio, M. Yasuda, S. Akiyama, K. Mitani, T. Oyama, K. Sato and T. Yamashita: Effect of chlorpromazine on the function of the endocrine organs. Endocr. jap. **3**, 67 (1956).

Taban, C.-H.: Mélancolie et fonction cortico-surrénale. Encéphale **46 I**, 52—80 (1957). — Talbot, N. B., E. H. Sobel, B. S. Burke, E. Lindemann and S. B. Kaufmann: Dwarfism in healthy children: Its possible relation to emotional, nutritional and endocrine disturbances. New Engl. J. Med. **236**, 783 (1947). — Tata, J. R.: Metabolism of L-thyroxine and L-3:5:3'-triiodothyronine by brain tissue preparations. In: Hormones, Brain Function, and Behavior, edit. by H. Hoagland. New York: Academic Press Inc., Publ. 1957. — Thamdrup, E.: Precocious sexual development. A clinical study of 100 children. Copenhagen: Munksgaard 1961. — Theiler, H.: Untersuchungen an kastrierten Sexualperversen. Diss. Basel 1959. — Thiele, W. u. R.-M.: Die Anwendung von Corticosteroiden in der Neurologie. Fortschr. Neurol. Psychiat. **28**, 627 (1960). — Thiele, W., u. Hs. Hohman: Corticoid-Behandlung des Delirium tremens. Nervenarzt **32**, 405 (1961). — Thomá, H.: Anorexia nervosa. Geschichte, Klinik und Theorien der Pubertätsmagersucht. Gemeinschaftsverlag Hans Huber, Bern/Ernst Klett, Stuttgart 1961. — Thorn, G. W., D. Jenkins and J. C. Laidlaw: The adrenal response to stress in man. In: Recent progress in hormone research: pp. 171—215. Edit. by G. Pincus. New York: Academic Press Inc. 1953. — Tindal, J. S..

A breed difference in the lactogenic response of the rabbit to reserpine. J. Endocr. **20**, 78 (1960).— TOMORUG, E., and G. TANASESCU: Schizophrenoparanoid and paranoid syndromes in hyperthyroid and hypoparathyroid patients. Neurologia (Bucuresti) **5 I**, 53—58 (1960). — TUCHMANN-DUPLESSIS, H.: Influence de la Réserpine sur les glandes endocrines. Presse méd. **64**, 2189—2192 (1956a); — Action de la réserpine sur le testicule et le tractus génital du rat. C. R. Acad. Sci. (Paris) **242**, 1651—1653 (19 mars 1956) b. — TUCHMANN-DUPLESSIS, H., et Mme. LUCETTE MERCIER-PAROT: Action de la réserpine sur l'appareil génital de la ratte adulte. C. R. Acad. Sci. (Paris) **242**, 1233—1235 (27 février 1956) a; — C. R. Acad. Sci. (Paris) **243**, 410 (1956b).

VANNOTTI, A.: Réserpine et fonction thyroidienne. Schweiz. med. Wschr. **87**, 412 (1957). — VITEBSKAYA, K. S.: Les particularités psychiques des enfants avec un retard du développement sexuel lié à une déficience résiduelle. Z. Nevropath. **61**, 1042—1046 (1961) (russisch, mit französischer Zusammenfassung). — VOLPE, R., J. VALE and M. W. JOHNSTON: The effects of certain physical and emotional tensions and strains on fluctuations in the level of serumprotein-bound iodine. J. clin. Endocr. **20**, 415 (1960).

WAKOH, T.: Endocrinological studies on periodic psychosis. Mie med. J. **9**, 2 (1959). — WAKOH, T., A. TAKEKOSHI, S. YOSHIMOTO, K. YOSHIMOTO, K. HIRAMOTO and K. KUROSAWA: Pathophysiological study of the periodic psychosis (atypical endogeneous psychosis) with special reference to the Comparison with the Chronic Schizophrenia. Mie med. J. **10**, 317 (1960). — WALLIS, HEDWIG: Psychopathologische Studien bei endokrin gestörten Kindern und Jugendlichen. Z. Kinderheilk. **83**, 4, 420—453 (1960). — WALTER, K., u. W. BRÀUTIGAM: Transvestitismus bei Klinefelter-Syndrom. Kasuistischer Beitrag zur Problematik von Geschlechtsrolle und genetischem Geschlecht. Schweiz. med. Wschr. **88**, 357 (1958). — WANDER-VOEGELIN, MARGRIT: Schizophrenes und endokrines Krankheitsgeschehen. Akromegaloide Schizophrene und ihre Familien. Arch. Klaus-Stift. Vererb.-Forsch. **20**, 257 (1945). — WARD, J. A., S. KRANTZ, J. MENDELOFF and E. HALTIWANGER: Interstitial-Cell-Tumor of the Testis: Report of two cases. J. clin. Endocr. **20**, 1622 (1960). — WASER, P. G., u. J. SPENGLER: Pharmakologische Beeinflussung von Hunger und Sàttigung. Schweiz. med. Wschr. **93**, 90 (1963). — WAXENBERG, S. E., M. G. DRELLICH and A. M. SUTHERLAND: The role of hormones in human behavior. I. Change in female sexuality after adrenalectomy. J. clin. Endocr. **19**, 193 (1959). — WAXENBERG, S. E., M. G. DRELLICH, J. A. FINKBEINER and A. M. SUTHERLAND: The role of hormones in human behavior. II. Changes in sexual behavior in relation to vaginal smears of Breast-Cancerpatients after Oophorectomy and Adrenalectomy. Psychosom. Med. **12**, 434 (1960). — WEBER, H. J.: Beispiel einer konstitutionsanalytischen Untersuchung an einem Fall von schizophrenen und manisch-depressiven Mischsymptomen, Struma, Adieschem Syndrom und orthostatischem Kollaps. Arch. Klaus-Stift. Vererb.-Forsch. **25**, 243—268 (1950). — WEGMANN, A. und E. GIACOBINI: Katecholaminausscheidung und Kreislaufregulation bei Delirium tremens. Schweiz. med. Wschr. **91**, 658 (1961). — WEIL-MALHERBE, E.: The effect of convulsive therapy on plasma adrenaline and noradrenaline. J. ment. Sci. **101**, 156—162 (1955a); — The concentration of adrenaline in human plasma and its relation to mental activity. J. ment. sci. **101**, 733—755 (1955b). — WEISS, P., and F. ROSETTI: Differential growth response of nerve cells to thyroid hormone. Science **113**, 476 (1951). — WELSH, J. H.: Neuroendocrine substances. In: A. GORBMAN: Comparative Endocrinology. New York: John Wiley and Sons 1959. — WERNER, S. C.: The thyroid: genetic and psychiatric relations. Dis. nerv. Syst. **22**, 4, 33—38 (1961). — WERNLY, M., u. M. P. KÓNIG: Hypercalcämiesyndrom und Hypercalciurie. Schweiz. med. Wschr. **91**, 769 (1961). — WHITELAW, M. J.: Delay in ovulation and menstruation induced by chlorpromazine. J. clin. Endocr. **16**, 972 (1956). — WIDDOWSON, E. M.: Mental contentment and physical growth. Lancet **1951 I**, 1316—1318. — WILLIAMS, R. J.: Biochemical Individuality. New York: John Wiley and Sons 1958. — WILKINS, L.: The diagnosis and treatment of endocrine disorders in childhood and adolescence, 2nd ed. Springfield: Charles C. Thomas 1957. — WITSCHI, E., and W. F. MENGERT: Endocrine studies on human hermaphrodites and their bearing on the interpretation of homosexuality. J. clin. Endocr. **2**, 279 (1942). — WOLF, DELIA: Zur Frage der Beziehungen zwischen dyskrinem und schizophrenem Krankheitsgeschehen. Überprüfung der bisherigen Untersuchungen an größerem Untersuchungsgut. Arch. Klaus-Stift. Vererb.-Forsch. **21**, 149 (1946); — Statistische Verarbeitung von 32 Fällen bereits beschriebener maskulin stigmatisierter schizophrener Frauen und ihrer Familien. Hinweise auf Literatur. Arch. Psychiat. Nervenkr. **180**, 397—413 (1948). — WOLFF, H. G.: Siehe CHAPMAN et al. und CHAPMAN and WOLFF. — WOODBURY, D. M., PAOLA S. TIMIRAS, and ANTONIA VERNADAKIS: Influence of adrenocortical steroids on brain function and metabolism. In: Hormones, Brain Function, and Behavior, edit. by H. HOAGLAND. New York: Academic Press Inc., Publ. 1957. — WOODS, J. W.: Some observations on adrenal cortical function in wild and domesticated Norway rats. Johns Hopkins University, Ph. D. Thesis, 1954. — WOOLLEY, D. W.: Serotonin in mental disorders. In: Hormones, Brain Function, and Behavior, edit. by H. HOAGLAND. New York: Academic Press

Inc., Publ. 1957. — Wynn, V., and J. Landon: A study of the androgenic and some related effects of methandienone. Brit. med. J. Nr. 5231, 998—1003 (1961 I). — Wyss, F.: Das endokrine Orchester. Schweiz. med. Wschr. 93, 155 (1963).

Yamada, T., and M. A. Greer: Studies on the mechanism of hypothalamic control of thyrotropin secretion: Effect of thyroxine injection into the hypothalamus or the pituitary on thyroid hormone release. Endocrinology 64, 1, 559—566 (1959) — Yamamoto, J., and W. Seeman: A psychological study of castrated males. In: Exploration in the physiology of emotions. Edit. by L. J. West and M. Greenblatt. Psychiat. Res. Rep. Amer. psychiat. Ass. January 1960. — Yamazaki, E., D. W. Slingerland and A. Noguchi: The effect of reserpine on thyroxine degradation and thyreotropic secretion. Acta endocr. (Kbh.) 36, 319 (1961). — Young, W. C.: Genetic and psychological determinants of sexual behavior patterns. In: Hormones, Brain Function, and Behavior, edit. by H. Hoagland. New York: Academic Press Inc., Publ., 1957.

Zamenhof, S.: Stimulation of cortical-cell proliferation by the growth hormone. Physiol. zool. 15, 281 (1942). — Zerssen, D. von: Die psychischen Nebenwirkungen der Pharmakotherapie mit Hormonen des Hypophysen-Nebennierenrinden-Systems. Z. psychosom. Med. 3, 172, 241 (1957); 4, 1 (1957). — Zur Ätiologie und Pathogenese des gewohnlichen Hirsutismus. Schweiz. med. Wschr. 90, 1333 (1960). — Zerssen, D. von, A. E. Meyer u. D. Ahrens: Der gewöhnliche Hirsutismus; endokrine, klinische und psychologische Aspekte. Dtsch. Arch. klin. Med. 206, 334—360 (1960). — Zetler, G.: Versuche zur anticonvulsiven Wirksamkeit des Polypeptids Substanz P. Naunyn-Schmiedeberg's Arch. exp. Path. Pharmak. 237, 11—16 (1959); — Pharmacological actions of substance P on the central nervous system. In: Polypeptides which Affect Smooth Muscles and Blood Vessels. pp. 179—191. London: Pergamon Press 1960. — Zetler, G., u. Gerta Ohnesorge: Die Substanz P-Konzentration im Gehirn bei verschiedenen Funktionszuständen des Zentralnervensystems. Naunyn-Schmiedebergs Arch. exp. Path. Pharmak. 231, 199—210 (1957). — Züblin, W.: Untersuchung eines akromegaloiden Psychopathen und seiner Familie. Arch. Psychiat. Nervenkr. 180, 284 (1948); — Zur Psychiatrie des adrenogenitalen Syndroms bei kongenitaler Nebennierenrinden-hyperplasie. Helv. paediat. Acta 8, 2, 117—135 (1953); — Zur Psychopathologie der endokrinen Storungen des Kindes- und Jugend-Alters. Vortrag vor Dtsch Ges. Kinderpsychiatr., Berlin, Oktober 1959 (nicht publiziert).

Neuroradiologie und Psychiatrie

Von

GERD HUBER, Bonn

Inhalt

A. Einleitung

Aus dem in den vergangenen Jahrzehnten sehr umfangreich gewordenen Gesamtgebiet der Neuroradiologie können hier lediglich die für den engeren Bereich der Psychiatrie relevanten Resultate und Fragestellungen und auch diese nur in einigen Grundzügen behandelt werden. Hinsichtlich der Ergebnisse der Schädelröntgenologie (Kraniographie) und der cerebralen Angiographie ist auf die hier vorliegenden zusammenfassenden Darstellungen zu verweisen (*53, 170, 171, 185; 152, 190, 217*). Das Gesamtgebiet der Röntgendiagnostik des Gehirns und Rückenmarks oder wenigstens beide cerebralen Kontrastverfahren wurden, vorwiegend unter neurologischen und neurochirurgischen Gesichtspunkten, in den letzten 30 Jahren von L. GUTTMANN (1936), F. LÜTHY (1939), H. JANTZ

(1953), E. LINDGREN (1952 und 1954), KAUTZKY und ZÜLCH (1955) sowie K. DECKER (1960), die *Pneumencephalographie* (PEG) und das mit dieser Methode am häufigsten diagnostizierte Syndrom, der sog. Hydrocephalus, in den Monographien von SCHIERSMANN (1942 und 1952) sowie von H. E. KEHRER (1955) bearbeitet. Auch auf die Erörterung spezieller Fragen der pneumencephalographischen Methodik muß weitgehend verzichtet werden.

Zur gezielten, isolierten Darstellung einzelner Liquorraumabschnitte wurden eine Reihe von besonderen Verfahren entwickelt (*5, 46, 170, 226*). Die *technischen und physikalischen Bedingungen* der PEG, die Möglichkeiten, Grenzen und Schwächen des Verfahrens (*49, 51, 92, 95, 111, 113, 117, 169, 195, 196, 221, 222, 234, 240, 272, 278, 284*), die Frage der *formalen Pathogenese* des — vielfach sowohl liquorkinetisch wie ex vacuo entstandenen — Hydrocephalus (*113, 139, 196, 235, 282*), die Ursachen von *Fehlfüllungen* (*57, 137, 144*), die Erscheinungen des *1 bis 14 Tage-PEG* und der Spätfüllung (*27, 32, 33, 104, 134, 175, 206, 285, 295*), Meßmethoden und Planimetrie (*97, 216, 240*) wurden in zahlreichen Beiträgen erörtert; von besonderer Bedeutung ist die Kenntnis der Voraussetzungen und der Fehlerquellen bei der encephalographischen Diagnose einer Hirnatrophie (*35a, 66, 111, 113, 117, 120a, 168, 240, 272*).

In topischer Hinsicht deutet eine Erweiterung der *peripheren Liquorräume*, insbesondere wenn Ventrikelveränderungen zurücktreten oder ganz fehlen, gewöhnlich auf eine corticale Atrophie bzw. Hypoplasie hin, eine allgemeine Erweiterung der *Ventrikel* auf eine Substanzminderung im Bereich der Marklager, basale Ausweitung der Vorderhörner und Verstreichung der Stammganglientaille der Seitenventrikel auf eine Caudatus-Affektion und ein isolierter oder bevorzugter Hydrocephalus des *3. Ventrikels* auf eine Atrophie (Hypoplasie) im Bereich der Basalganglien in erster Linie des Zwischenhirns (*27, 28, 94, 96, 102, 111, 113, 117, 127, 240, 244*). Inwieweit die Hirnvolumenverminderung durch Reduktion von Parenchym, von Stützsubstanz oder durch Dehydratation bedingt ist, läßt sich makroskopisch und vielfach auch histologisch nicht sicher entscheiden; das Problem der sog. Hirnatrophie und des „Hirnschwundes ohne histologisches Substrat" ist in vieler Hinsicht noch keineswegs zureichend geklärt (*22, 113, 117, 209*). Ein Substanzverlust ist auch in jedem Falle eines Hydrocephalus liquordynamischer Genese anzunehmen, sofern dieser längere Zeit besteht (*113, 139*).

Die *Indikation* zur PEG aus diagnostischen, z. T. auch aus prognostischen und therapeutischen Gründen — bei Epilepsien, posttraumatischen und cephalgischen Syndromen (*92, 220*), bei endogenen Psychosen („cerebrale Pneumotherapie" — *205, 111*), kann bei jeder der im folgenden besprochenen, mittelbaren oder unmittelbaren Hirnkrankheiten gegeben sein, doch auch bei endogen-psychotischen Residual- und Defektzuständen und bei manchen hirnorganisch determinierten (pseudo-)psychopathischen und hysteriform-neurotoiden Syndromen (*70, 81, 83, 111*). Das eigentliche Feld der PEG sind die sog. hydrocephalen, nichttumorösen Größen- und Formveränderungen der Liquorräume, der Fragenkomplex der Hirnatrophie, den diese Methode erst für die klinische Psychiatrie zuganglich machte.

Die Frage des „*normalen PEG*" verschiedener Altersstufen war Gegenstand zahlreicher Untersuchungen (*28, 59, 80, 82, 101, 203, 307*). Von der klinischen Diagnose ausgehende Studien, die geeignet sind, dem „PEG der Durchschnittsbevölkerung" nahekommende Vergleichswerte zu liefern (*35, 48, 69, 118, 289*), bezogen meist Syndrome mit ein, bei denen organische Hirnläsionen von vornherein nicht auszuschließen sind. Die bis heute gewonnenen Erfahrungen erlauben die Abgrenzung pathologischer Veränderungen, sofern Grenzbefunde unberücksichtigt bleiben und die Abhängigkeit des PEG vom Lebensalter (*15, 28, 101, 111, 117, 118, 184, 240, 310*), geschlechtsspezifische Unterschiede, die Bedeutung einer konstitutionell abnorm kleinen Liquorraumkapazität, die Relationen der verschiedenen Liquorraumabschnitte zueinander sowie Schädelform und -größe beachtet werden (*117, 118, 203, 215, 293*). Fest steht, daß unterhalb des 45. bis 50. Lebensjahres mit einer physiologischen Altersatrophie noch nicht zu rechnen ist. Der bei der Auswertung des Heidelberger Materials zugrunde gelegte, in Anlehnung an DAVIDOFF und DYKE aufgestellte, gegenüber früheren Angaben (*39, 160, 203, 240, 244*) strengere *Maßstab* läßt ein breites Grenzgebiet fraglicher, möglicherweise in die Variationsbreite des Normalen fallender Befunde unberücksichtigt.

Als pathologisch gelten danach an der Hirnrinde eine Furchenverbreiterung ab 3 mm, an den Seitenventrikeln verplumpte und hydrocephale Hirnkammern mit einem Seitenventrikelindex nach SCHIERSMANN unter 4,0 sowie erhebliche Formveränderungen, am 3. Ventrikel eine Erweiterung ab 8 mm (*111, 117, 118*). Kontrolluntersuchungen an einem einer Durchschnittsbevölkerung sich nähernden Material von Persönlichkeitsvarianten (*118*) konnen die Verläßlichkeit dieser Abgrenzungen bestätigen, andererseits darauf hinweisen, daß Hirnoberflächenbefunde mit einer Furchenbreite zwischen 2 und 2,9 mm im allgemeinen, zumindest bei Fehlen einer abnormen Kleinheit der Ventrikel und nach dem 30. Lebensjahr, noch nicht als pathologisch (s. Abb. 5, 8), Erweiterungen des 3. Ventrikels zwischen 6 und 7,9 mm als Grenzbefunde (die u. U. bei weiblichen Patienten und kleinen Seitenventrikeln schon pathologische Bedeutung erlangen) zu werten sind (vgl. Abb. 11).

Grundsätzlich ist zu unterscheiden zwischen der ausschließlich an Hand des PEG-Befundes ohne Kenntnis der klinischen Daten zu beantwortenden Frage, ob und in welchem Ausmaß *pathologische Liquorraumveränderungen* vorliegen, und der weiteren Frage nach der *Genese*, der Beziehung eines so rein röntgenologisch festgestellten krankhaften Befundes zum jeweiligen klinischen Bild, die nur unter Heranziehung sämtlicher klinischen Daten erörtert und vielfach angesichts der ätiologischen Vieldeutigkeit und Unspezifität jedes im PEG darstellbaren hirnatrophischen Syndromes sowie des Umstandes, daß an sich pathologische morphologische, neuroradiologisch faßbare Veränderungen in funktionaler Hinsicht für lange Zeit oder auch zeitlebens ohne Bedeutung bleiben können, nicht zu entscheiden ist (*74, 111, 118, 223, 238*).

Infolge der von Fall zu Fall in verschiedenem Maße eintretenden Veränderungen von Hirnvolumen und Liquorraumgröße unter agonalen und postmortalen Bedingungen scheint das PEG den intravitalen Verhältnissen eher zu entsprechen als der *Sektionsbefund* (*30, 111, 117, 259*). Besonders am Cortex sind neben korrelierbaren Befunden (*111, 113, 117, 275*) Diskrepanzen nicht selten, wird bei deutlichem Hydrocephalus externus im PEG eine Hirnrindenschrumpfung bei der Sektion vermißt (*30, 43, 113*), während an den inneren Liquorräumen eine weitergehende Übereinstimmung mit vielfach gleichsinnigen, doch durch den Einfluß von Hirnschwellung und -quellung weniger ausgeprägten atrophischen Veränderungen besteht (*25, 43, 49, 111, 194, 227, 297*). Am 3. Ventrikel fand sich eine hervorstechende Erweiterung als Hinweis auf eine Atrophie der Wandstrukturen im Bereich des Zwischenhirnes bei posttraumatischen, postencephalitischen oder vasculären Substanzdefekten (*239, 243, 244*) und bei dementen Epileptikern (*270*) auch bei der Sektion bestätigt.

B. Die neuroradiologischen Befunde bei den einzelnen Krankheitsbildern und Abnormitäten

I. Körperlich begründbare Psychosen und Defektsyndrome

1. Hirnbeteiligende Erkrankungen
(Allgemeinkrankheiten, endokrine Störungen und Intoxikationen)

Allgemein- und Stoffwechselkrankheiten. Endokrinopathien. Die Ansicht (*34, 63, 126, 257, 258, 264*), daß nach schweren *Hungerdystrophien* hirnorganische, im PEG in Form einer meist nur leichten symmetrischen Erweiterung der Seitenventrikel und des 3. Ventrikels sowie einer frontal betonten Oberflächenvergröberung faßbare Dauerschäden mit organischer Wesensänderung auftreten, fanden SCHULTE und STIAWA (*259*) an mittlerweile insgesamt 110 positiven eigenen Fällen bestätigt. Für die Annahme eines Zusammenhanges von Hirnatrophie und Dystrophie sind zumindest 3 Jahre dauernde Mangelernährung mit Dystrophieerscheinungen und Hirndruckkrisen und Ausschluß anderer Schädigungsmöglichkeiten zu fordern. Doch ist eine Überschichtung mehrerer Noxen (Hirntraumen,

Fleckfieber, andere Infektionskrankheiten) in vielen Fällen nicht zu übersehen (*63, 139, 259*) (s. Abb. 1). Im Heidelberger Material boten 7 Dystrophiker mit organischer Wesensänderung sämtlich atrophische Veränderungen, insbesondere am 3. Ventrikel, aber auch an der Hirnrinde und an den Seitenventrikeln; ein encephalographisches Zwischenhirnsyndrom wurde in unserem Gesamtmaterial organischer Defektsyndrome überhaupt am häufigsten nach Hungerdystrophie und bei — oft gleichzeitig vorliegenden — traumatischen und fleckfieberbedingten Hirnschäden beobachtet (s. u.). Daß eine schwere Dystrophie unter bestimmten Bedingungen über ein im akuten Stadium klinisch und autop-

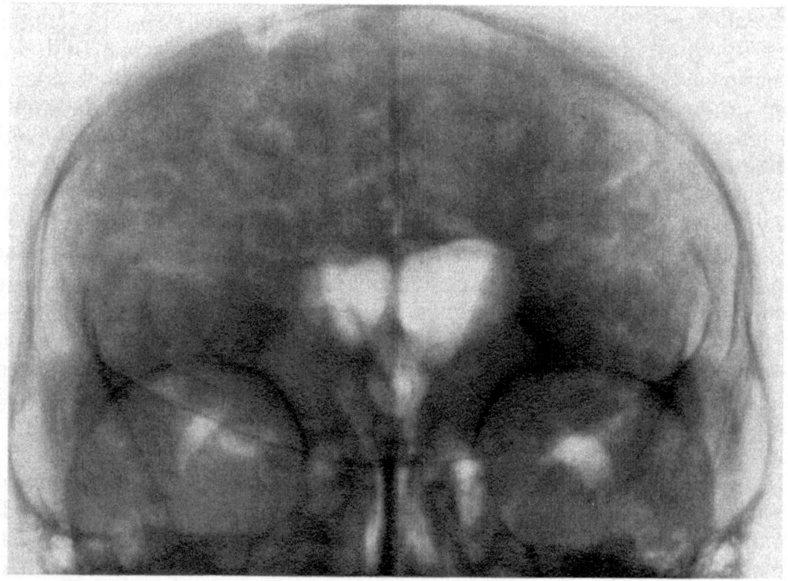

Abb. 1. 54jähriger Mann mit organischer Wesensänderung und episodischer *schizophrenieähnlicher Psychose nach schwerer Dystrophie und Fleckfieber*. A. p.-Aufnahme. Bevorzugte hochgradige Erweiterung des 3. Ventrikels, kombiniert mit erheblichen Formveränderungen der basalen Abschnitte besonders des linken Seitenventrikels. Mäßiggradiger diffuser Hydrocephalus externus

tisch nachgewiesenes (*305*) Hirnödem zu einem hirnatrophischen Defekt führen kann, scheint hinreichend gesichert; ein gleichartiger pathogenetischer Mechanismus liegt bei dystrophiegeschädigten Säuglingen vor, die im Überlebensfall hydrocephale Veränderungen aufweisen.

Die Möglichkeit, daß eine *Ostitis deformans Paget* psychoorganische Störungen zur Folge hat, ist nicht von der Hand zu weisen (*8*). Die gelegentlich von einem Hydrocephalus internus begleitete, häufigste (3 bis 4%) Anomalie der Occipito-Cervical-Region, die *basilare Impression*, kann mit neurologischen und psychopathologischen Störungen, Verstimmungen und Wesensänderung einhergehen (*21, 248, 268, 288*).

Eine angeborene oder durch Strumektomie und andere Ursachen (*279*) erworbene *Nebenschilddrüseninsuffizienz* mit dem klinischen Bild der Tetanie läßt sich nicht selten als Ursache von intracerebralen, besonders in den Stammganglien lokalisierten Verkalkungen nachweisen, die in 60% auf Hypoparathyreoidismus und Pseudohypoparathyreoidismus beruhen sollen (*6*). Ähnliche Kalkablagerungen sieht man bei vermehrter Hormonzufuhr, D-Hypervitaminose und nach langjähriger AT 10-Therapie. Doch tritt das Syndrom der symmetrischen subcorticalen Verkalkung auch ohne Beziehung zur Nebenschilddrüse, u. a. im Rahmen der Fahrschen Erkrankung auf (*37, 231*). Bei *chronischem endokrinem Psychosyndrom* (M. BLEULER) ist mit encephalographisch nachweisbaren Hirnsubstanzschaden zu rechnen, wie eine eigene Beobachtung mit Hydrocephalus externus bei Myxödem und organischer Wesensänderung zeigt.

Die Beziehungen der *Hyperostosis interna frontalis* (MORGAGNI) oder diffusa zu bestimmten Hirnerkrankungen und Psychosen des hoheren Lebensalters sind nicht hinreichend gesichert, die bei Enostosen beobachteten psychischen Störungen weder konstant noch irgendwie charakteristisch; bei Frauen ist die Auffassung als tertiäres, spät sich entwickelndes Geschlechtsmerkmal zu erwagen. Immerhin fanden KNIES und LE FEVER (*147*), die bei 4 Familienmitgliedern typische Frontalhyperostosen sahen und eine hereditäre Basis erörtern, unter 28 Fallen neben intermittierenden Kopfschmerzen bei 12 Patienten psychopathologische, meist psychotische Storungen.

Intoxikationen. Die chronische Intoxikation bei langjährigem *Alkoholismus* kann Ursache einer meist diffusen, auch prognostisch verwertbaren Hirnatrophie

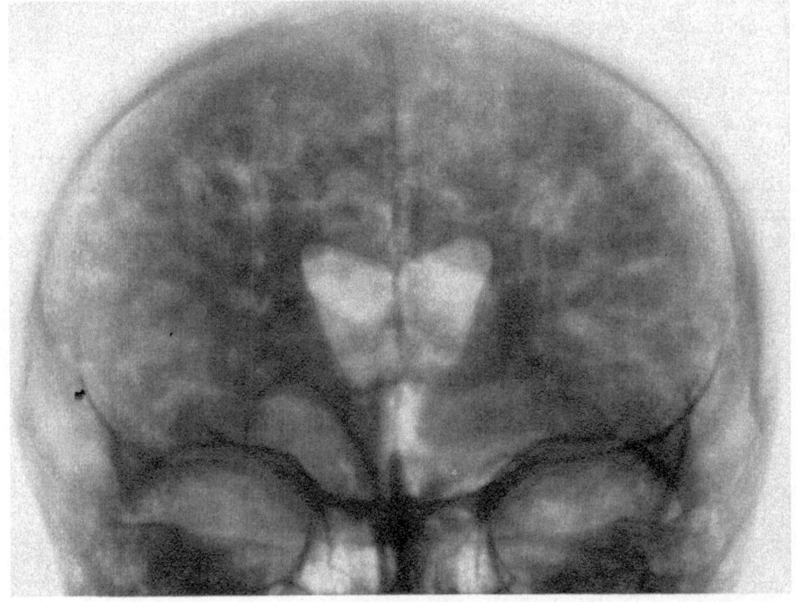

Abb. 2. 54jahriger Patient mit maßiger *Demenz bei chronischem Alkoholismus.* A. p -Bild. Maßiggradiger diffuser Hydrocephalus externus sowie allgemeiner, symmetrischer Hydrocephalus internus

mit organischer Wesensänderung oder dementiellem Abbau vom Typ des *Korsakow* werden (*49, 77, 109, 158, 165, 208, 212*). Die Mitwirkung anderer ätiologischer Momente ist jedoch zu berücksichtigen; vielfach ist eine Hirnatrophie nicht Folge, sondern Ursache des Alkoholismus, indem ein zu Lebzeiten oft nicht erkannter primärer oder sekundärer hirnatrophischer Prozeß über den Persönlichkeitsabbau zum Alkoholmißbrauch führt. Fest steht jedoch, daß die überwiegende Mehrzahl, in einem Material der Münchener Nervenklinik (*165*) 83%, im Heidelberger Krankengut 86%, der klinisch als chronischer Alkoholismus mit Wesensänderung diagnostizierten Fälle eine meist generalisierte und mäßig ausgeprägte Hirnatrophie aufweist. Im Heidelberger Material von 15 fast stets erheblich abgebauten, unkomplizierten Alkoholikern mit einem Durchschnittsalter von 51,6 Jahren waren alle Liquorraumabschnitte betroffen, am regelmäßigsten (73%) jedoch die Hirnrinde (s. Abb. 2).

Spärlich sind die Mitteilungen über andere Suchtfolgen und Intoxikationen. Einen Hydrocephalus als Folge einer *Insulin*-Intoxikation mit mehrwöchiger deliranter Psychose und Ausgang in Demenz beobachteten HEIDRICH und HAMPEL.

Nach *CO-Vergiftung* fand SCHIERSMANN in 2 Fällen mit Demenz und Krampf-
anfällen einen Hydrocephalus externus und internus mit starker Beteiligung
des 3. Ventrikels, Veränderungen, die sich auf autoptisch nachweisbare, gefäßbedingte Läsionen in Stammganglien, Hemisphärenmark und Rinde beziehen
lassen; weitere Beobachtungen mit Hydrocephalus internus erheblichen Grades
stammen von SCHILF sowie von HOPF. Von 8 eigenen Fällen zeigten nur 4 Patienten
nach akuter CO-Intoxikation Veränderungen in Form einer mäßigen Erweiterung
des 3. Ventrikels (2 Fälle), die auf eine Läsion der gegenüber Sauerstoffmangel
vulnerablen Anteile der Basalganglien des Zwischenhirns hindeutet, einer erheblichen Seitenventrikelasymmetrie und eines leichten Hydrocephalus internus;
eine Beobachtung einer chronischen CO-Intoxikation (*250*) bot gleichfalls eine
isolierte erhebliche Erweiterung des 3. Ventrikels.

2. Entzündliche Hirnerkrankungen
(einschließlich Infektionskrankheiten)

Bei der *progressiven Paralyse* zeigt das PEG frontal und temporal betonte
Atrophien an den äußeren und inneren Liquorräumen; je ausgeprägter die Hirn-
substanzeinbuße, um so deutlicher ist für gewöhnlich der nach der Behandlung
zurückbleibende psychoorganische Defekt (*56, 79, 83, 93, 189, 211, 309*). Doch ist

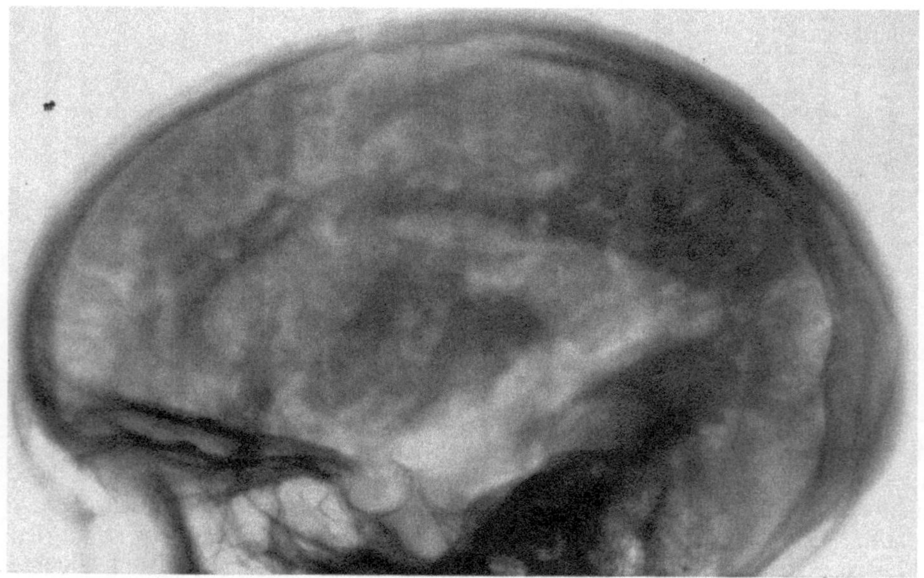

Abb. 3. 34jährige Frau mit *progressiver Paralyse*. Nach 4 Penicillinkuren schwerer dementieller Abbau trotz
weitgehender Sanierung des Liquors. Seitliche Übersichtsaufnahme. Erheblicher Hydrocephalus externus
frontal, parietal und temporal. Mäßiger Hydrocephalus internus

eine Erweiterung des Subarachnoidalraumes, die auch bei meningitischen Vorgängen und Liquorströmungsstörungen zustande kommen oder verstärkt werden
und sich später weitgehend zurückbilden kann (*30, 92, 299*), nicht stets der Ausdruck eines Hirnrindenschwundes; in solchen Fällen wird man daher mit der
Folgerung einer corticalen Atrophie aus dem Hydrocephalus externus zurückhaltend sein. Sicher gibt es auch, entgegen früheren Auffassungen, Paralysen
ohne jede Liquorraumerweiterung, so im Heidelberger Material 2 Fälle mit organischer Persönlichkeitsveränderung; 8 demente Patienten zeigten stets eine

meist erhebliche und cortical betonte allgemeine, in 4 Fällen an den Seitenventrikeln asymmetrische Hirnschrumpfung, wobei der 3. Ventrikel nur in 3 Fällen beteiligt war (s. Abb. 3).

Die markatrophischen, oft mit Füllungsdefekten über der Hirnoberfläche und Erweiterung der Basiszisternen verbundenen Folgezustände nach *Meningitiden* und *Meningoencephalitiden* sind nicht ausschließlich nach dem pathogenetischen Prinzip des aktiven Hydrocephalus — Mißverhältnis zwischen Liquorproduktion und -resorption infolge Hypersekretion, Hyporesorption, partieller oder kompletter Obliteration — zu erklären, primäre Parenchymlasionen sind im wechselnden Ausmaß von Bedeutung (*113, 139, 233*). Eine formalpathogenetische Differenzierung zwischen liquordynamischem und atrophischem Hydrocephalus

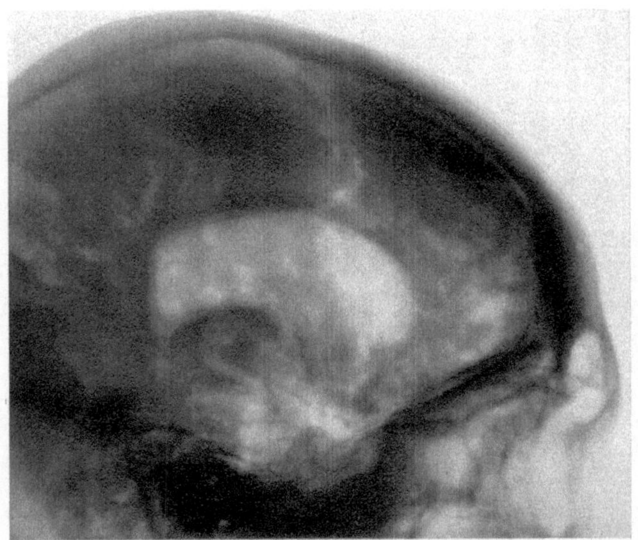

Abb. 4. *Multiple Sklerose* bei jetzt 49jähriger Frau mit schwerer Demenz; seit dem 36. Lebensjahr zunachst schubweise, dann chronisch progredient verlaufend. Im PEG 1953 gegenuber 1947 Progredienz der Atrophie. Horizontales Vorderhornbild (1953). Erheblicher Hydrocephalus externus und internus

ist nach dem morphologischen Ventrikelbild (Kreisbogentyp bzw. Rechteckform—*195*) nicht mit hinreichender Sicherheit moglich (*113*). Bei der *Meningitis tuberculosa* läßt sich die progrediente Erweiterung der inneren und nicht selten auch der äußeren Liquorraume im Krankheitsverlauf verfolgen und gibt Hinweise für die Prognose (*213, 233, 252*). Intrakranielle Verkalkungen werden frühestens 1½ Jahre nach Beginn in 20—40% (*1, 173*) beobachtet.

Primäre, akute oder subakute, vielfach letal endende, (Virus-)*Encephalitiden* zeigen im allgemeinen ein normales PEG, bisweilen die Zeichen der Hirnschwellung, gelegentlich auch — bei umschriebener Ausbreitung des Prozesses — der Verdrängung. Nach abgelaufener und bei chronischer Encephalitis resultieren neben pathologischen Verkalkungen gewöhnlich, im Material von Camblor in 35 von 47, im Heidelberger Untersuchungsgut in 13 von 19 Fällen, atrophische Encephalopathien; man sieht symmetrische, asymmetrische oder umschriebene Erweiterung der Hirnkammern (*78, 119, 187*), ferner diffuse oder partielle Hirnoberflächenatrophien mit oder ohne Hydrocephalus internus (*38, 137*). Auffallende Erweiterungen des 3. Ventrikels wurden beim *postencephalitischen Parkinsonismus* beschrieben (*69, 189, 204*); Flügel hebt wegen der sonstigen Seltenheit in seinem Material diesen Befund besonders hervor. Bei Anwendung unseres Maßstabes fanden wir bei 7 Postencephalitikern mit einem Durchschnittsalter von 44 Jahren nur Grenzbefunde am 3. Ventrikel (5 Fälle) und an den Seitenventrikeln, dagegen 5 Patienten mit pathologischem Hydrocephalus externus.

17*

Bevorzugt cerebrale, mit psychoorganischen Veränderungen einhergehende Formen der *multiplen Sklerose*, die autoptisch nicht nur das Großhirnmark, sondern auch den Cortex betreffen, zeigen im PEG die Zeichen einer allgemeinen, oft an der Rinde überwiegenden Atrophie (Abb. 4), wobei Asymmetrien der Seitenventrikel und eine Beteiligung des Kleinhirnes vorkommen (*9, 69, 137, 290*). Die remittierten und psychisch intakten eigenen Patienten boten dagegen ein normales Hirnluftbild (s. a. *69*). Die Ausweitung der Seitenventrikel bei der konzentrischen Sklerose (*49*) deutet mehr auf ventrikelnahe Veränderungen im Marklager hin.

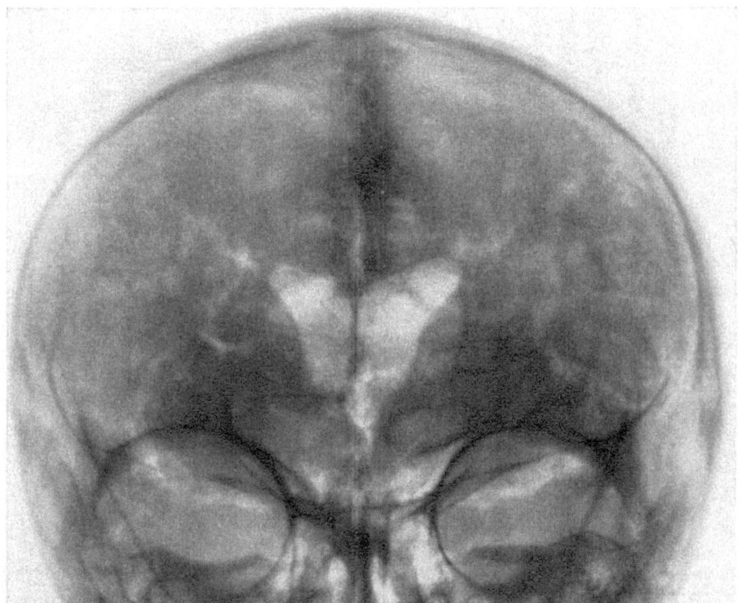

Abb 5. 42jähriger Patient mit nicht progredienter organischer Persönlichkeitsveränderung nach *Fleckfieberence-phalitis*. A. p.-Aufnahme. Leichter linksbetonter Hydrocephalus internus mit Beteiligung des mäßig erweiterten 3 Ventrikels Geringgradige, nicht sicher pathologische Vergroberung der Oberflächenzeichnung über der Hirnkonvexität (Grenzbefund)

Infektionskrankheiten. Der akute, ruckbildungsfähige „toxische Hydrocephalus" nach Infektionen der Nasen-Rachen-Wege (*186*) zeigt die grundsätzliche Reversibilität des „aktiven" Hydrocephalus, sofern innerhalb eines bestimmten Zeitraumes eine Normalisierung der hydrocephalischen Störung (*282*) erfolgt. Wie allgemein beim sog. Druckhydrocephalus und auch beim Hirnödem, die vermutlich bei allen schweren Infektionskrankheiten als mögliche Ursache hirnatrophischer und psychopathologischer Residualsyndrome in Frage kommen, entscheidet neben anderen Bedingungen der Zeitfaktor über Reversibilität oder Irreversibilität und damit über Ausbildung einer Hirnsubstanzschädigung (*113*).

Zum Verständnis von Spätschäden nach epidemischem *Fleckfieber* wurden von SCHMIEDER encephalographische Veränderungen an den inneren Liquorräumen und speziell am 3. Ventrikel herangezogen. Im Heidelberger Material von als Fleckfieberfolgen aufgefaßten Fällen der Jahre 1948 bis 1957 sahen wir bei 6 von 10 Patienten leicht pathologische, die inneren Liquorräume und in 4 Fällen die 3. Hirnkammer betreffende Veränderungen (s. Abb. 5). Auch bei kritischer Einstellung kann man kaum an dem Vorkommen psychischerDauerveränderungen, häufig in Form von uncharakteristischen, mit (auch autoptisch festgestellten— 2) Hirnkammerdilatationen korrelierbaren pseudoneurasthenischen Syndromen zweifeln (s. unten).

3. Traumatische Hirnschäden

Die Entwicklung des posttraumatischen hirnatrophischen Defektsyndromes aus der initialen Ödemphase wird von FAUST im II. Band dieses Werkes dargestellt. Die Hirnschrumpfung mit dem Bild eines symmetrischen oder asymmetrischen Hydrocephalus internus wird bereits in der dritten und vierten Krankheitswoche im PEG sichtbar (*36, 64*). Solche Serienuntersuchungen sind von grundsätzlicher Bedeutung, da sie den zeitlichen Ablauf der Volumenschwankungen des Gehirns und das allgemeine pathogenetische Prinzip der ödembedingten, nach ätiologisch heterogenen cerebralen Affektionen (Trauma, Entzündung, Dystrophie) auftretenden Hirnatrophie auf der Basis von ausgedehnten Marksklerosen (*94, 122*) veranschaulichen. Liquorzirkulationsstörungen und zentral ausgelöste Durchblutungsveränderungen kommen, unabhängig vom Ödem, als Ursachen der Ventrikelerweiterungen in Betracht (*143, 282*). Im Heidelberger, 100 Patienten umfassenden Material von klinisch als Contusio diagnostizierten Hirnschäden, das in etwa $^1/_3$ vegetative Dysregulationen und in $^2/_3$ eine organische Wesensänderung, doch nur in 57% ein pathologisches PEG aufweist, sind der symmetrische, leichte bis mäßige Hydrocephalus der Seitenventrikel (16%) und die isolierte Erweiterung des 3. Ventrikels (24%) relativ häufige, der asymmetrische oder halbseitige Hydrocephalus internus (12%) und umschriebene Rindenveränderungen (2%) seltene Befunde; bei den *offenen Hirnverletzungen* überwogen hingegen örtliche Ausweitungen der Seitenventrikel (29%) sowie halbseitige Kammererweiterungen (22%) (*119*). Doch unterscheiden sich nach TÖNNIS, der unter 375 unkomplizierten Impressionsschüssen 90% diffuse Ventrikeldilatationen fand, die Restzustände nach offenen und gedeckten Hirnschädigungen wenig. Bei den seltenen, in unserem Krankengut nur in 4% beobachteten posttraumatischen Demenzsyndromen sieht man massive Schrumpfungen des Marklagers. Beziehungen zwischen diencephalen Störungen bzw. vegetativem Anteil der Hirnleistungsschwäche und posttraumatischer Erweiterung des 3. Ventrikels wurden von verschiedenen Autoren angenommen (*103, 119, 143, 240*). Obschon ein traumatischer Hydrocephalus sich keineswegs regelmäßig im klinischen Bild äußert, besteht doch, wie Erfahrungen an größerem Material lehren (*113, 119, 143*), eine deutliche Korrelation zwischen hydrocephalen Größen- und Formveränderungen im PEG und psychoorganischen Dauerfolgen.

4. Gefäßerkrankungen des Zentralnervensystems

Die PEG vermag bei der *Hirnarteriosklerose*, als der häufigsten Form der sekundären Hirnatrophie, lediglich über Ausmaß und Lokalisation der Substanzminderung zu orientieren. Man findet bei chronisch psychoorganisch veränderten Patienten ziemlich regelmäßig, im eigenen Krankengut von 115 Fällen in 87%, eine cortical betonte oder sich gleichmäßig auf Rinde, Mark und Stammganglien erstreckende Atrophie. Durch die kraniale Angiographie kann der Gefäßprozeß vielfach direkt nachgewiesen werden; dabei sind abnorme Verplumpung und Ausweitung, andererseits Einengung und Kaliberschwankungen der Gefäße, Unregelmäßigkeiten der Konturen der Carotis, drahtartig starrer oder stark gewundener Gefäßverlauf, Verlängerung der Zirkulationszeit und allgemeine Gefäßarmut besonders der peripheren Arterienverzweigungen nur in ihrer Häufung und Verbindung verwertbare Kriterien (*49, 163, 214*). Auf eine cerebrale Thrombangiitis obliterans können im Angiogramm die schlechte Darstellbarkeit umschriebener peripherer Gefäßgebiete sowie Intimaveränderungen, im PEG eine corticale Atrophie, unter Umständen auch nur strangförmige Verbreiterung einzelner Sulci des Scheitellappens hinweisen (*69, 92, 139, 240*).

Bei der Diagnose des *cerebralen Insultes* sind die Kontrastmethoden, besonders die bei Verdacht auf Subarachnoidalblutung absolut indizierte Angiographie, oft von ausschlaggebender Bedeutung und u. U. die Grundlage einer erfolgversprechenden neurochirurgischen Therapie (*49, 151, 217, 228*). Embolien führen ebenso wie thrombotische Gefäßverschlüsse und Massenblutungen zu umschriebenen, im PEG faßbaren cystischen Substanzverlusten; ähnliche Bilder sieht man nach Aneurysma-Blutungen und bei arteriovenösen Gefäßmißbildungen, die jedoch auch noch nach langjährigem Verlauf ein normales PEG zeigen können. Bei *Carotisthrombosen* verschiedener Ätiologie resultieren homolaterale Ventrikelerweiterungen mit oder ohne Hydrocephalus externus (*237*), nach *Carotisligatur* Schrumpfungen einer

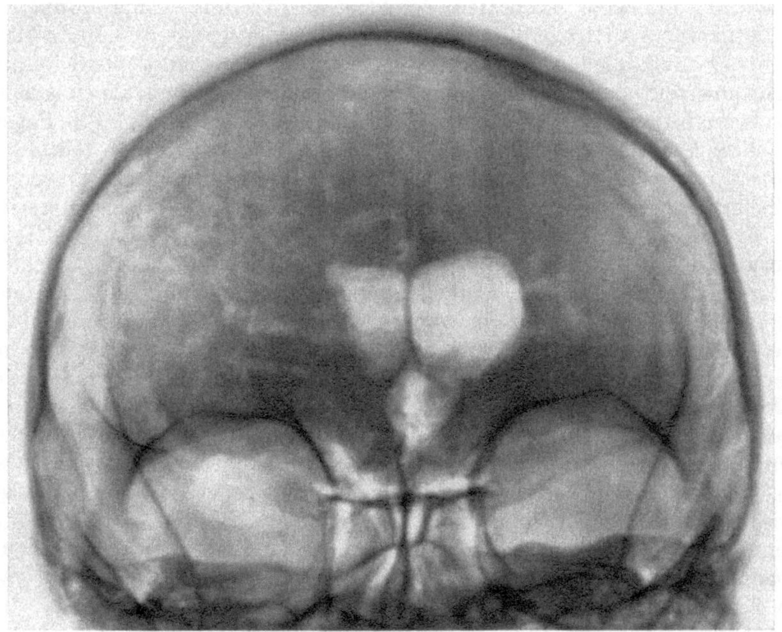

Abb. 6. 28jähriger Gerichtsassessor. Nach *linksseitiger Carotisligatur* (1944) Halbseitenlahmung und Hirnleistungsschwache. 1947 Entwicklung eines schweren, nach PEG weitgehend reversiblen psychoorganischen Syndromes mit schizophrenen Zugen. 1951 voll berufsfähig. A. p.-Aufnahme (1948). Hemiatrophie mit linksseitiger Erweiterung des Ventrikelsystems und Grenzbefund an der Hirnoberfläche

Großhirnhemisphäre mit Hydrocephalus des Seitenventrikels und 3. Ventrikels, Hemiparese und z.T. reversiblem organischem Psychosyndrom (*16, 308*) (Abb. 6). Für die *Sturge-Webersche Erkrankung* sind girlandenförmige Kalkablagerungen, Hypoplasie der Schädelkalotte und eine corticale, oft erheblich über den Verkalkungsbereich hinausreichende Atrophie kennzeichnend.

5. Degenerative Hirnerkrankungen

Diffuse Atrophien. Bei den primären, diffusen oder mehr systemgebundenen hirnatrophischen Prozessen ist das PEG für den Nachweis der Hirnschrumpfung und darüber hinaus für die Differentialdiagnose von Bedeutung. *Senile Demenz* und *Alzheimersche Erkrankung* lassen eine allgemeine, äußere und innere Liquorräume ergreifende, gewöhnlich cortical stärker ausgeprägte Parenchymreduktion erkennen, die an den Ventrikeln nicht das Ausmaß eines Obstruktionshydrocephalus erreicht und an der Hirnoberfläche sich auf alle Regionen annähernd gleichmäßig erstreckt (*72, 139, 262, 294*) (s. Abb. 7). Im eigenen Krankengut von 16 Patienten wurde eine in 7 Fällen deutlich prävalierende Rindenatrophie in keinem Fall, Veränderungen an Seitenventrikeln und 3. Ventrikel nur in je 3 Fällen vermißt.

Die von der allgemeinen Pathoklise der Rinde der Stirn-, Schläfen- und Scheitel-region gegenüber atrophischen Vorgängen (*181*) abweichende fakultative Aus-breitung des Prozesses auch auf den Occipitallappen, der beim Pick und anderen Rindenatrophien verschont bleibt, ist für die Differentialdiagnose verwertbar.

Systematische Atrophien. Für die *Picksche Erkrankung* ist die umschriebene, meist enorme und an der Hirnrinde überwiegende, isolierte oder kombinierte Atrophie des Stirn- und Schläfen-, seltener auch des Scheitellappens mit grob-fleckigen, oft flächenhaften Luftansammlungen über dem Stirnhirn und in der Pro-jektion der mittleren Schädelgrube, sowie oft seitendifferenter Erweiterung vor

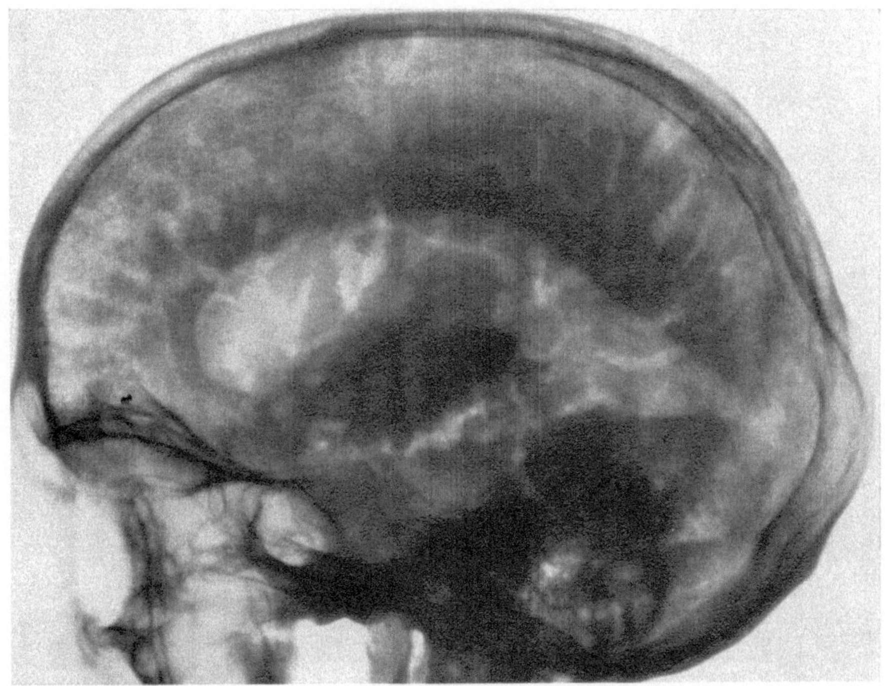

Abb. 7. 60 jahriger Bäckermeister mit seit 3 Jahren progredienter, vorwiegend mnestischer präseniler Demenz. *Alzheimersche Erkrankung*. Seitliche Übersichtsaufnahme. Mäßiger Hydrocephalus externus und internus

allem des Vorder- und Unterhorns der Seitenventrikel charakteristisch (*22, 24, 69, 172, 181, 276*). Die *Chorea Huntington* bietet einen Hydrocephalus der Seiten-ventrikel mit Verbreiterung der Stammganglientaille und basaler Ausweitung des Vorderhorns, entsprechend der Atrophie des Caudatuskopfes (*96*), sowie eine Erweiterung der 3. Hirnkammer und einen weniger ausgeprägten, doch mit fort-schreitender Demenz sich verstärkenden diffusen oder frontal akzentuierten Hydrocephalus externus. Von 6 eigenen Patienten ließen zwei nur stärkere Form-veränderungen an Stammganglientaille und lateraler Umschlagstelle eines Seiten-ventrikels erkennen, während in 4 deutlich dementen Fällen stets ein erheblicher, in 3 Fällen mit Rindenatrophie kombinierter Hydrocephalus internus vorlag. Der *Paralysis agitans* kommt offenbar ein einigermaßen einheitliches hirnatrophi-sches Syndrom nicht zu (*49*).

Klinisch oft nicht eindeutig zu erkennende *Atrophien des Kleinhirnes*, wie sie isoliert oder im Rahmen eines allgemeinen atrophisierenden Hirnprozesses (Morbus Alzheimer) vorkom-men, können mittels der kontrollierten PEG an Hand der Erweiterung des 4. Ventrikels und

der Cisterna magna, abnormer subtentorieller Luftansammlung und verstärkter Furchen-
zeichnung über der Kleinhirnoberfläche sichtbar gemacht werden; Kleinhirnhypoplasien
brauchen klinisch keine Bedeutung zu besitzen (*28, 49, 159, 198, 202*). Patienten mit *Wilson-
scher Krankheit* wurden selten untersucht (*84, 296*); 2 eigene, mit 11 bzw. 18 Jahren sich
manifestierende Fälle zeigten einen Hydrocephalus internus mit Abstumpfung der Stammganglientaille und bevorzugter Erweiterung des 3. Ventrikels (s. Abb. 8). Anomalien des
Skeletsystems werden häufig gefunden (*67*). Normale Hirnluftbilder bei psychisch intakten
Patienten mit *erblichem Tremor*, leichter Hydrocephalus internus mit kontralateraler Abflachung der Caudatuskontur bei *Torticollis spasticus* werden von HASSLER beschrieben.

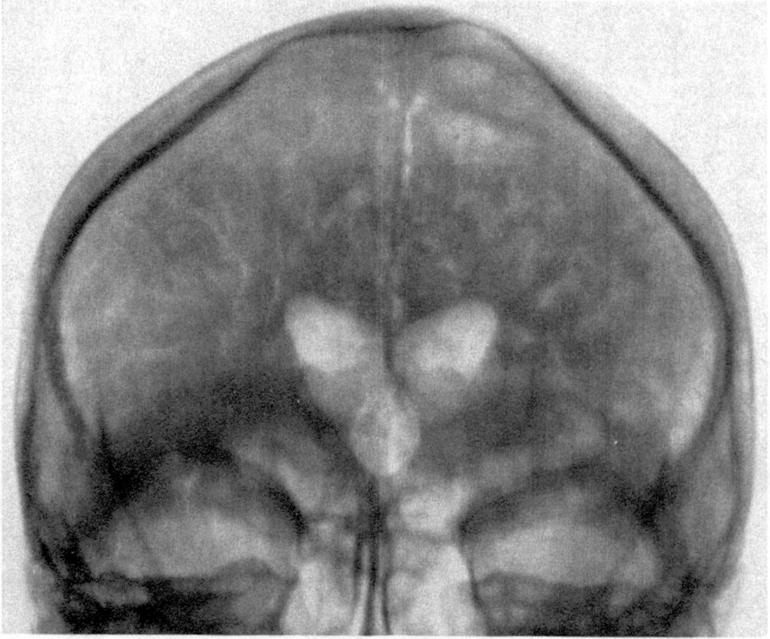

Abb. 8. Im 18. Lebensjahr beginnende *Wilsonsche Krankheit* mit mäßiger Demenz. Annähernd symmetrischer
Hydrocephalus der Seitenventrikel mit Abflachung der Caudatuskontur und bevorzugter hochgradiger
Erweiterung des 3. Ventrikels. Leichte diffuse Oberflachenvergroberung als Grenzbefund

6. Mißbildungen und erbliche Hirnaffektionen im Kindesalter.
Frühkindliche Hirnschäden[1]

Ausgeprägte Formen der gelegentlich mit Hydrocephalus einhergehenden vorzeitigen
Kraniostenosen (*27, 69, 92, 177, 279*) fuhren oft zu einem Zuruckbleiben der geistigen Entwicklung. Von den in den ersten vier Lebensmonaten operativ behandelten Patienten sind
jedoch später nur 11% schwachsinnig. Die haufigste im PEG faßbare Hirnmißbildung (0,6%
im eigenen Material), der sog. *5. Ventrikel*, das erweiterte, geschlossene oder mit dem Ventrikelsystem kommunizierende Cavum septi pellucidi (*3, 29*), besitzt keine sichere Beziehung zu
einem bestimmten Krankheitsbild, ist aber vielfach mit anderen Dysplasien, besonders
Hydrocephalus internus (50% im eigenen Material) kombiniert und kann als Hinweis auf eine
dem Status dysraphicus zuzurechnende Hirnminderwertigkeit angesehen werden; bei Schizophrenen fanden wir einen 5. Ventrikel in 1,3%. Das Cavum Vergae ist anscheinend regelmaßig
mit Ventrikelerweiterung und uberwiegend mit erheblichem Schwachsinn verbunden (*252,
255, 281*). Einen einfachen *Defekt des Septum pellucidum* (*312, 313*) mit mangelnder Trennung
der sonst normal konfigurierten Vorderhörner sahen wir in 4 von 1294 Fallen (0,3%), darunter
bei 2 Patienten mit Schwachsinn und Anfällen bei gleichzeitigem Hydrocephalus internus
und einem Patienten mit dem Bild einer genuinen Epilepsie. Schwere Mißbildungen nach Art
der *Arhinencephalie* gehen klinisch mit Oligophrenie und Epilepsie einher (*3, 252, 312*). Der

---

[1] Vgl. die Beitrage von BENDA und STUTTE im II. Band dieses Werkes.

sehr selten, in unserem Material nur einmal beobachtete *Balkenmangel* ist nach Carpenter in 60% mit fokalen oder generalisierten Anfällen und in 32% mit allgemeiner Retardierung verbunden (*27, 40, 47, 180*) (Abb. 9). Die PEG ist die einzige Methode zur Diagnose der Agenesie des Corpus callosum, die sich auch auf das Splenium beschränken kann und dann in einer Erweiterung des Recessus suprapinealis zum Ausdruck kommt (*223*).

Der neuroradiologische Befund, multiple Ventrikeleinengungen durch ventrikelnahe Tumoren, intracerebrale Verkalkungen und Knochenveränderungen an Schädeldach, Wirbelsäule, Thorax, Becken und Extremitäten kann bei der Diagnose der *tuberosen Sklerose* von Nutzen sein (*65, 105, 130, 148, 189*). Dasselbe gilt für die mannigfachen kraniographischen Befunde (u. a. Usuren und umschriebene Knochendefekte an Felsenbein, Hinterhauptschuppe, Orbita und Keilbeinflügel) bei der *generalisierten Neurofibromatose Recklinghausen* (*13, 49, 62*).

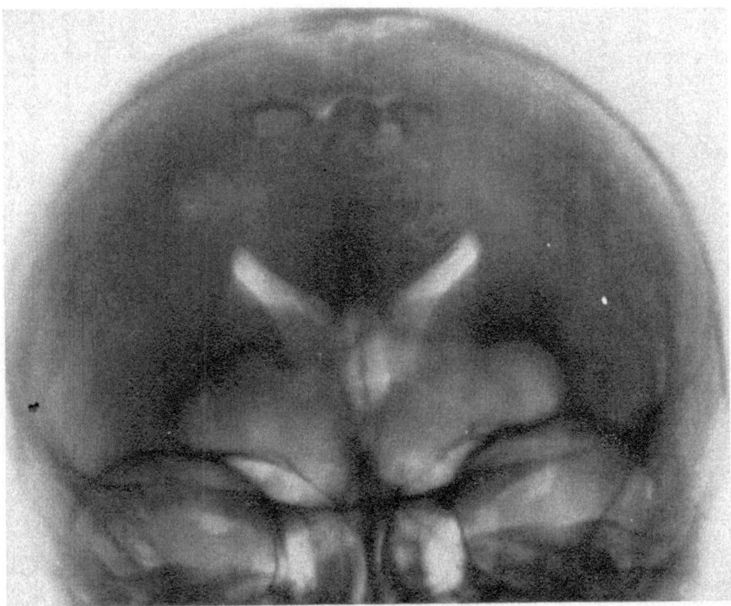

Abb. 9. *Epilepsie*. 23jähriger Patient mit epileptischer Wesensveränderung. Seit dem 6. Lebensjahr generalisierte Anfälle und Absencen bei normalem neurologischem Befund. Im EEG Dysrhythmie sowie Delta- und Krampffocus temporobasal rechts. A. p.-Aufnahme. Balkenmangel mit Verlagerung des stark erweiterten 3. Ventrikels zwischen die Seitenventrikel

Einen Hydrocephalus internus und externus findet man bei den familiaren *diffusen Sklerosen* (*49*) und beim *Laurence-Moon-Bardet-Biedl-Syndrom* (*11, 92, 225*). Für die Existenz eines als primäre Hirnmißbildung aufzufassenden *erblichen Hydrocephalus* beim Menschen sprechen auch die Beziehungen zwischen Status dysraphicus bzw. Meningomyelocele und Ventrikelerweiterung (*207, 230*), die sehr regelmäßige Vergesellschaftung von Spina bifida cystica und Hydrocephalus (*150*) sowie Beobachtungen von konkordantem Auftreten des Hydrocephalus bei eineiigen Zwillingen, die allerdings ohne nur autoptisch möglichen Ausschluß einer exogenen Affektion nicht beweiskräftig sind (*68*). Normale Hirnluftbilder werden beim *Phenylbrenztraubensäureschwachsinn* gefunden (*178*).

Bei Syndromen nach Art der „*cerebralen Kinderlähmung*" und des *früherworbenen Schwachsinns* können neuroröntgenologische Befunde die klinische Diagnose klären oder ergänzen und die exogene Natur einer Epilepsie oder Oligophrenie beweisen; sie ermöglichen ferner prognostische Folgerungen und unter Umständen eine erfolgversprechende operative Behandlung. Das Schädelleerbild erlaubt nicht nur bei stärkeren Hydrocephalien, sondern vielfach auch bei *einseitigen*, atrophischen oder cystischen *Hirnschädigungen* eine Verdachtsdiagnose. Hier sind homolaterale Hypertrophie des Schädeldaches, Volumenverminderung und Abflachung einer Kalottenhälfte, Erweiterung der Neben-, besonders der Stirnhöhlen, Pyramidenhochstand und Schrägstand der Crista galli, des Planum sphenoidale und eines kleinen Keilbeinflügels, seltener einseitige Vorwölbung und Verdünnung der Kalotte (*157*) inkonstante und nicht absolut eindeutige Hinweise auf die klinisch durch Schwachsinn, Hemiplegie und Anfälle, encephalographisch durch halbseitigen Hydrocephalus, umschriebene Ausfälle der Oberflächenzeichnung und Verziehung des Ventrikelsystems gekennzeichneten Syndrome (*54, 71, 188, 210, 224, 303*); Asymmetrien und Skoliosen des Schädels (Plagiocephalie) können aber auch durch extracerebrale Faktoren bedingt sein.

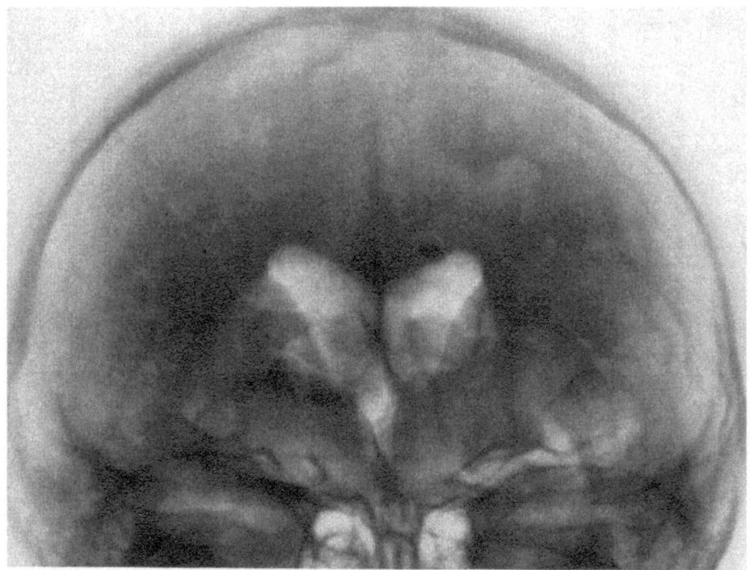

Abb. 10. *Konnatale Toxoplasmose*. Debilitat. Mit 14 Jahren akute Psychose mit schizophrenen Zügen. Arbeitet regelmäßig als Gartner. A. p.-Bild. Hydrocephalus internus mit lokaler Ausweitung des rechten Seitenventrikels im Bereich des Vorderhornes. Hirnrinde o. B. Intracerebrale Verkalkungen

Das PEG zeigt beim frühkindlichen Cerebralschaden, besonders häufig bei Hemi- oder Diplegien, fokalen oder generalisierten Anfällen, mehr umschriebene Veränderungen (innere oder äußere Pori, Cysten und Füllungsdefekte über der Hirnoberfläche, lokale Ausziehungen der Ventrikel) oder mehr diffuse, halb- oder beidseitige Atrophien mit Hydrocephalus internus und — in etwa 50% (*146*) — auch externus (*25, 26, 42, 81, 91, 227, 240, 306*). Starke Hydrocephali interni können durch Druckschädigungen von Hypophyse, Hypothalamus und Epiphyse zu Hypergenitalismus, Nanismus, Fettsucht und konstitutionellen Dysplasien führen (*76, 277*). Im Heidelberger Material von 60, anamnestisch und klinisch gesicherten Fällen, die ausnahmslos psychopathologische, insbesondere psychopathieähnliche (42 Fälle) und leichtere intellektuelle Störungen, doch nur in je etwa $^1/_3$ neurologische Ausfälle und epileptiforme Anfälle boten, zeigten 62% einen pathologischen Befund, darunter 6 Fälle lokale Veränderungen an den Seitenventrikeln, dagegen 12 Patienten eine vorwiegend halbseitige ventrikelnahe Hemisphärenatrophie und 6 Fälle einen symmetrischen Hydrocephalus internus; ein Hydrocephalus externus wurde in 3 und eine hervorstechende Erweiterung des 3. Ventrikels in 9 Fällen beobachtet.

Für eine connatale *Toxoplasmose* sprechen ein meist erheblicher, liquordynamisch und ex vacuo entstandener Hydrocephalus internus und externus, bisweilen auch ein isolierter Hydrocephalus externus in Verbindung mit intracerebralen Verkalkungen (*199, 280*); offen bleibt, ob Plexusverkalkungen öfter als bisher auf eine Toxoplasmose bezogen und nicht einfach als physiologisch angesehen werden dürfen (*174, 256*). Im eigenen Material sahen wir nur 3 sichere Fälle von connataler Toxoplasmose, darunter 2 Patienten mit akuten schizophrenie-ähnlichen Psychosen, die im PEG einen allgemeinen Hydrocephalus internus mit lokalen Ausweitungen der Seitenventrikel bieten (s. Abb. 10). Der *luetische Hydrocephalus* wird bei connataler Syphilis in 10% und auch bei negativem serologischen Befund beobachtet (*229, 274*). Hypoplasien der Nasenbeine und Nebenhöhlen, Häufung von persistierenden Stirnbeinnähten und Schaltknochen, normale und abnorm kleine Ventrikel sowie Erweiterungen der basalen Zisternen wurden beim *Mongolismus* beschrieben (*92, 149, 246, 279, 302*). Beim sporadischen *Kretinismus* bedeuten Erweiterungen der Ventrikel und des Subarachnoidalraumes eine schlechte Prognose für die Hormontherapie (*52*).

7. Epilepsien und andere Anfallserkrankungen

Wie auch sonst, bedingen bei den sog. *genuinen Epilepsien* die Heterogenität des Untersuchungsgutes und des Bewertungsmaßstabes erhebliche Divergenzen hinsichtlich Häufigkeit und Art der im PEG von verschiedenen Autoren beschriebenen Veränderungen (*12, 39, 50, 88, 139, 142, 155, 160, 161*); die Angaben über den Prozentsatz pathologischer Hirnluftbilder schwanken zwischen 6 (*182*) und 80% (*106, 160*). Von den eigenen, in strenger klinischer Auslese als genuin ermittelten, 117 Epileptikern zeigten 32,5% sicher pathologische Veränderungen, am häufigsten (17%) in Form eines leichten, meist symmetrischen, selten asymmetrischen Hydrocephalus der Seitenventrikel, ferner in Gestalt einer isolierten (11%) oder kombinierten (7%) Erweiterung des 3. Ventrikels und einer diffusen corticalen Atrophie (7%). Andere Untersucher (*50, 133, 142*) sahen nur in 5 bis 6,8% eine isolierte Erweiterung des 3. Ventrikels. Die Ansicht (*88, 161, 260*), eine Erweiterung des 3. Ventrikels sei kennzeichnend oder auch nur besonders häufig bei der genuinen Epilepsie, läßt sich in dieser Form nicht aufrecht erhalten. Doch trifft zu (*12, 50, 88, 133, 139, 164*), daß bei Patienten mit langem Verlauf, häufigen generalisierten Anfällen und chronischer psychoorganischer Veränderung Erweiterungen der Seitenventrikel und des 3. Ventrikels häufiger sind als bei frischen, psychisch intakten Fällen mit geringer Anfallsfrequenz; im eigenen Krankengut von 65 wesensveränderten Epileptikern fanden sich 43% pathologische Encephalogramme und 24% mit pathologischen Veränderungen am 3. Ventrikel, gegenüber 19 und 11% in der etwa gleich starken Gruppe psychisch unveränderter Patienten (*120 b*).

Kleine Seitenventrikel mit einem Seitenventrikelindex nach SCHIERSMANN über 4,7, die bei Psychopathien und psychoreaktiven Störungen in 12,7, bei Defektschizophrenen in 23% vorkommen, sahen wir in 15, eine ausgesprochene *Mikroventrikulie* in 5,1%. Umgekehrt konnte BRONISCH (1951) (ferner *254* bei Kindern) das ausschließliche Vorkommen der Mikroventrikulie bei (Spät-)Epilepsien, konstitutioneller Cephalea und Migräne-Epilepsien (*136*) nicht bestätigen; immerhin scheint dieser als Ausdruck einer konstitutionell bedingten, unspezifischen Hirnanomalie angesehene Befund in seiner ausgeprägten, von F. A. KEHRER definierten, im Gesamtmaterial seltenen (3,5%) Form bei Epilepsien haufiger aufzutreten als bei anderen Hirnerkrankungen. Ein sog. *5. Ventrikel* und ein *Septumdefekt* (s. o.), die bei Epilepsien gehauft auftreten sollen (*3, 29, 287, 292*), sind im Heidelberger Epilepsiematerial mit je 0,85% gleichfalls häufiger als im Gesamtmaterial (0,6 bzw. 0,3%, s. o.).

Die Frage nach der Beziehung der atrophischen Befunde zur epileptischen Erkrankung bleibt offen. Ihre Deutung als Ursache der Anfälle hat für das Gros der Fälle wenig für sich, diejenige als Anfallsfolge ist zu erwägen; gegen die Auffassung als konstitutionelle Variante mit besonderer Beziehung zum iktaffinen Typus im Sinne von MAUZ (*155*) läßt sich einwenden, daß das Plump-Amorphe und Dysplastische der äußeren Körperbauform eher in einer anlagemäßigen relativen Volumenvermehrung des Gehirngewebes mit entsprechender Hirnventrikelverkleinerung bis zur Mikroventrikulie zum Ausdruck kommen müßte als in einer hydrocephalen Konfiguration der Ventrikel (*12, 111, 117, 136*). Bei *Temporallappenepilepsien* wurden im Angiogramm eine abnorm enge Schlängelung der Gefäße im Temporalbereich, im PEG Asymmetrien und lokale Erweiterungen der Schläfenhörner beschrieben (*41, 61, 197*), die jedoch nur bei guter Darstellung und Aufnahmen in mehreren Projektionen unter Berücksichtigung des supracornualen Spaltes nachweisbar sind. Ein normales PEG wurde bei *Pyknolepsie* gesehen (*267*, eigene Beobachtungen). Von vier eigenen, ätiologisch unklaren *Narkolepsie*syndromen boten nur ein Patient eine mit einer Verplumpung des rechten Seitenventrikels kombinierte Erweiterung des 3. Ventrikels, die übrigen, abgesehen von einer abnormen Kleinheit und Dysplasie der Ventrikel bzw. einer Brückensella in je einem Fall, einen normalen Befund. Für die Erkennung der progredient oder stationär mit Anfällen verlaufenden meningoencephalen Form der *Hirncysticercose* mit allmählich zunehmender Ventrikelerweiterung (*49*) oder mäßigem Hydrocephalus externus (eigene Beobachtung) sind oft Muskelaufnahmen zum Nachweis der verkalkten Cysticerken entscheidend.

8. Genetisch unklare Demenzen und Versagenszustände

Nicht selten sehen wir in der Psychiatrie ätiologisch unklare, zuerst von Beringer und Mallison (*17*) sowie von Bronisch (*30*) beschriebene Versagenszustände und Demenzen, bei denen wir mittels des PEG eine Hirnatrophie nachweisen, jedoch auch bei Anwendung aller klinischen Verfahren nicht vom „Syndrom“ zu einer speziellen Diagnose vorzudringen vermögen. So berechtigt die Warnung vor einer unkritischen Verwendung der unbestimmten Begriffe „*vorzeitiger organischer Versagenszustand*“ oder „*hirnatrophischer Prozeß im mittleren Lebensalter*“ auch ist (*238*), muß man sich doch häufig mit solchen, auf Anamnese, psychopathologisches Querschnittsbild und neuroradiologischen Befund gegründeten Bezeichnungen begnügen, um so mehr, als auch autoptisch in manchen Fällen ein klar definierbarer Krankheitsprozeß nicht nachweisbar ist, bei makroskopisch sichtbarer Hirnatrophie ein spezifisches histologisches Substrat fehlt, nur abnorm gesteigerte Veränderungen der allgemeinen biologischen Altersinvolution auf vorzeitig einsetzende Alterungsvorgänge hinweisen (*30, 108, 111, 113, 275*). Das röntgenologisch in einem vorwiegend äußeren Hydrocephalus faßbare hirnatrophische Syndrom stellt bei ätiologisch heterogenen, chronischentzündlichen, vasculären oder degenerativen Prozessen das gemeinsame pathogenetische Zwischenglied und ein Korrelat für die psychopathologischen Veränderungen der oft lange Zeit stationären chronischen körperlich begründbaren Psychose dar (Bronisch). Auch bei den bland verlaufenden, zwischen dem 35. und 60. Lebensjahr sich manifestierenden vorzeitigen Versagenszuständen von Beringer und Mallison ist der allen Patienten gemeinsame Befund eines diffusen äußeren und — in 50% — auch inneren Hydrocephalus (s. Abb. 11) nächst dem durch vitale Mißgestimmtheit, Antriebsmangel, emotionale Labilität und leichte intellektuelle und mnestische Störungen gekennzeichneten psychoorganischen Syndrom das für die Zuordnung maßgebliche Kriterium. Autoptisch fanden Peters und Struck bei 3 hierher gerechneten Fällen makroskopisch eine generalisierte Atrophie von Rinde und Mark, feingeweblich jedoch nur die Zeichen des anatomischen Symptomenkomplexes der Rückbildung. Die Annahme eines besonderen vorzeitigen, anlagebedingten Hirnalterungsprozesses (*7*) und einer

„Hirnatrophie ohne charakteristischen histologischen Befund" (*111*) kann durch solche Beobachtungen gestützt werden.

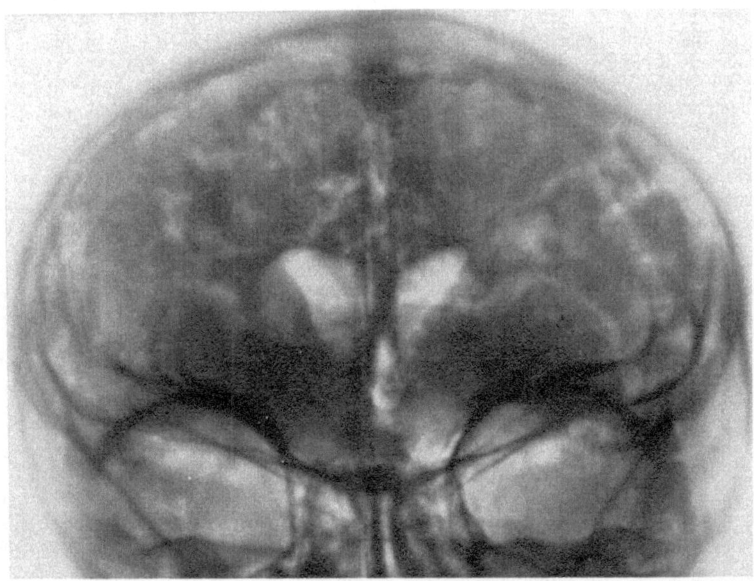

Abb. 11. Im 48. Lebensjahr beginnender *organischer vorzeitiger Versagenszustand* mit Antriebsverarmung, Verlangsamung, emotionaler Labilität und vitaler Mißbefindlichkeit. Mäßiger Hydrocephalus externus. Asymmetrie des Ventrikelsystems mit Formveränderungen am rechten Seitenventrikel, nicht kommunizierendem 5. Ventrikel und Grenzbefund am 3. Ventrikel

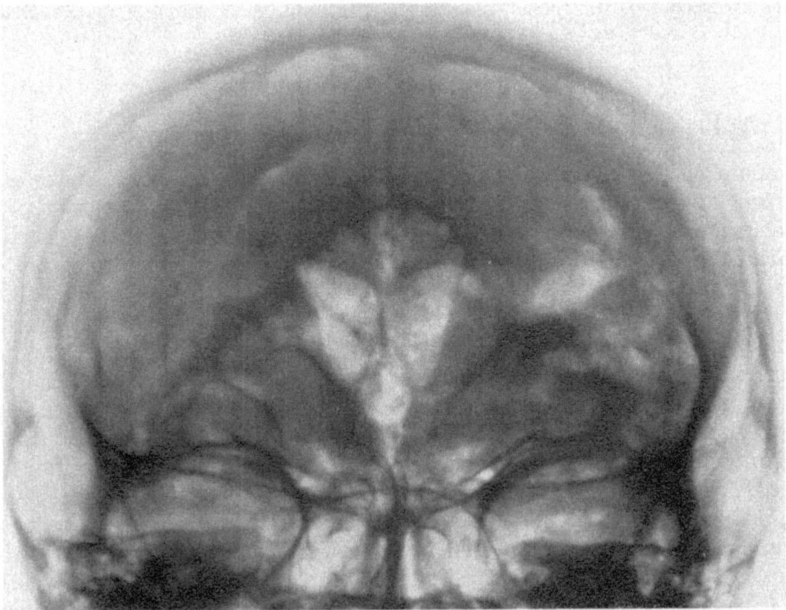

Abb. 12. Syndrom des *Dermatozoenwahnes* bei cerebraler Arteriosklerose. 50jähriger Mann. Seit 49. Lebensjahr chronische taktile Halluzinose mit schwankendem Realitätsurteil. Organische Wesensveränderung mit Verlangsamung, Umständlichkeit und Affektlabilität. Hervorstechende Erweiterung des 3. Ventrikels kombiniert mit leichten Formveränderungen der dysplastischen Seitenventrikel sowie frontal und parietal betontem mäßigem Hydrocephalus externus

Daneben gibt es noch andere diagnostisch vieldeutige *Syndrome vorzeitiger vitaler Erschopfung*, die im PEG, ähnlich wie viele endogen-psychotische Defektzustände, eine vorwiegend subcortical-diencephale Atrophie bei abnorm kleiner und dysplastischer Konfiguration der Seitenventrikel aufweisen, nicht selten bei von Haus aus minderbegabten und schwachsinnigen Individuen (*111, 113*). Manche Versagenssyndrome entwickeln sich vermutlich auf der Grundlage einer unter bestimmten Bedingungen im mittleren oder hoheren Lebensalter eintretenden *Dekompensation fruherworbener Hirnschaden.* Therapieresistente Abbausyndrome, bei denen eine progrediente Horverschlechterung in Verbindung mit Ohrgeräuschen, Akoasmen und — wie in 2 eigenen Fallen — akustischen Halluzinationen im Sinne des Gedankenechos das klinische Bild beherrschen, zeigen gleichfalls eine im PEG darstellbare Hirnatrophie (*87*). Beim sog. *Dermatozoenwahn*, dessen Leibgefuhlalterationen wir mit den coenästhetischen Störungen der Schizophrenen in Parallele setzten und auf eine bestimmte Form eines thalamischen Funktionswandels bezogen, sahen wir im PEG einen symmetrischen leichten Hydrocephalus internus mit bevorzugter Beteiligung des 3. Ventrikels (*111*); ein neuerdings mitgeteilter symptomatischer Fall bei tumorbedingter Läsion des Zwischenhirns scheint die Hypothese einer thalamischen bzw. thalomo-corticalen Genese der „taktilen Halluzinose" (Conrad) stützen zu konnen (*167*) (s. auch Abb. 12). Im *Leerbild* sind regressive Veränderungen am Schädelknochen im 5. und 6. Dezennium oft mit vorzeitiger Alterung des Gehirns vergesellschaftet.

9. Neuroradiologische Befunde bei neurologischen und myopathischen Erkrankungen

Bei der *Syringomyelie* ist, wie allgemein beim Status dysraphicus (s. o.), ein Hydrocephalus internus häufig (*14, 263*). Falle von *amyotrophischer Lateralsklerose* mit den Zeichen eines dementiellen Abbaues bieten im PEG eine maßige, generalisierte und symmetrische Hirnatrophie (eigene Beobachtungen). Kleine Sellen und frontale Hyperostosen, Hydrocephalus internus und z. T. auch externus mit starker Beteiligung des 3. Ventrikels wurden bei *myotonischer Dystrophie* beobachtet (*99, 132*). Die sog. *Trigeminusneuralgie* soll fast immer eine homolaterale und frontal betonte Rindenatrophie vasculärer, fokaltoxisch-allergischer oder arteriosklerotischer Genese zeigen (*139, 166*). Auch bei der *Migrane* kommen gelegentlich neben Mikroventrikulie (*136*) im höheren Lebensalter Hirnoberflächenatrophien in Verbindung mit normalen oder abnorm kleinen Ventrikeln vor (*139*), fur die H. E. Kehrer ahnlich wie bei der Epilepsie eine funktionell-vasculare Genese und eine Beziehung zur Krankheitsdauer annimmt.

II. Endogene Psychosen

1. Cyclothymer (manisch-depressiver) Formenkreis

Dem manisch-depressiven Formenkreis angehörende, phasenhaft vollständig remittierende, psychopathologisch stilrein cyclothym-depressive oder atypische endogene Psychosen zeigen im allgemeinen und unterhalb des 45. Lebensjahres keine pathologischen Befunde im PEG (*18, 111*); dagegen findet man bei den auch schon im 3. und 4. Lebensjahrzehnt nicht allzu seltenen, unter Hinterlassung meist nur leichter Residualsyndrome remittierenden Cyclothymien in vielen Fällen eine bevorzugte, mit Formveränderungen an den Seitenventrikeln kombinierte Erweiterung des 3. Ventrikels (*111*) (s. Abb. 13). Nur das nach Abklingen der grundsätzlich reversiblen, produktiv psychotischen Erscheinungen sichtbare Persönlichkeitsniveau, der Remissionsgrad, läßt bei cyclothymen wie bei schizophrenen endogenen Psychosen Beziehungen zum PEG-Befund erkennen (*111, 117*). Jenseits des 45. und besonders des 50. Lebensjahres sieht man auch bei Endogen-depressiven, bei denen die Ausgangsstruktur der Persönlichkeit nach mehr oder weniger langer Dauer der meist im Rückbildungsalter erstmals sich manifestierenden Psychose wiederhergestellt erscheint, relativ häufig, in unserem Krankengut in 20—25%, neben Ventrikelerweiterungen (*301; 20a*) einen mäßigen Hydrocephalus externus, ein Befund, der überwiegend bei weiblichen Patienten beobachtet wird (s. a. unten) und nicht einfach durch altersgemäßen Abbau (*86*), eher durch vorzeitiges Auftreten der Erscheinungen des anatomischen

Rückbildungskomplexes zu erklären ist, wie es FÜNFGELD bei paranoiden, depressiven und hypochondrischen Involutionspsychosen beschrieb.

Früher von MOORE u. Mitarb. (*192*) beschriebene Hirnrindenbefunde fallen nach dem heutigen Kenntnisstand großteils noch in den Normbereich (*111, 117, 118*). Eine Korrelation zwischen Lebensalter und Haufigkeit pathologischer PEG-Befunde wurde von NAGY (*200*) in einem anscheinend überwiegend aus Rückbildungsdepressionen zusammengesetzten Material beobachtet. Bei den von WEITBRECHT 1953 beschriebenen, zunächst stilrein cyclothym-depressiven, erst nach längerem Verlauf durch hirnorganische Symptombeimengungen im psychopathologischen Bild und durch hirnatrophische, vorwiegend corticale Veränderungen als symptomatisch und körperlich begründbar erkannten Syndromen bedeuten gewöhnlich, wenn auch Fälle mit eindrucksvollen psychopathologischen Remissionen vorkommen, die hirnatrophischen Vorgange eine Trübung der Prognose und Ausgang in psychoorganische Dauerveränderung. Im Heidelberger Material von 24 Fällen *organisch ausmündender cyclothym-depressiver Syndrome*, die stets nach dem 45. und bei 19 Patienten zwischen dem 50. und 68. Lebensjahr sich entwickelten, fanden wir nur 7 Patienten mit Ausgang in Demenz bei eindeutigem Prävalieren des stets nachweisbaren Hydrocephalus externus, während 17 Patienten eine nicht progrediente organische Wesensänderung nach Abklingen der endogen-depressiven Psychose oder eine vollständige Remission (4 Falle) und darunter 14 Fälle im PEG eine Hirnoberfläche und 3. Ventrikel gleich haufig betreffende Atrophie erkennen ließen; bei 8 Patienten waren vollstandig remittierte, nicht organisch gefarbte Phasen vorausgegangen (s. a. *111*).

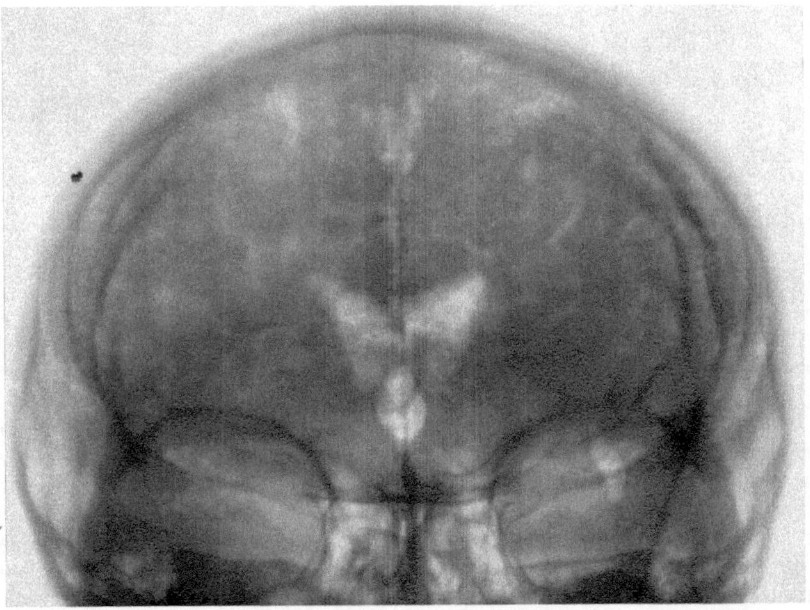

Abb. 13. 46jähriger Landwirt. Mit 31 und 44 Jahren stilrein *cyclothym-depressive, vollstandig geheilte Phasen*. Nach der 3. depressiven Phase bleibt eine deutliche *Wesensanderung* mit sich haufenden, kurzdauernden dysphorisch-leibhypochondrischen Verstimmungszustanden zuruck. Isolierte Erweiterung des 3. Ventrikels kombiniert mit Formveranderungen der basalen Anteile der Seitenventrikel bei nicht pathologischen außeren Liquorraumen

2. Schizophrener Formenkreis

Eine Übersicht über die Resultate encephalographischer Untersuchungen bei Schizophrenen (*111, 117*) ergibt, daß überwiegend normale Befunde von 4 Autoren bei größtenteils akuten Psychosen ohne klinische Defektsymptome erhoben wurden, während bei 17 Untersuchern der Anteil der Fälle mit pathologischen Veränderungen überwog (*117*). Uneinheitlichkeit des Bewertungsmaßstabes und des Untersuchungsgutes, Fehlen einer umfassenden Beziehungsetzung zum klinischen Bild der schizophrenen Psychose und des schizophrenen Defektes erschweren

die Vergleichbarkeit und Beurteilung der Ergebnisse. Eine vom Lebensalter
unabhängige Beziehung zur Krankheitsdauer (*89, 111, 124, 125, 141, 200, 200a,
201, 232, 309*) und zum psychischen Defekt (*162, 191, 309*) wurde mehrfach beobachtet. Von unter Umständen auch therapeutischer Bedeutung ist es, daß eine
Hirnschwellung bei Katatonen im PEG als rückbildungsfähige Mikroventrikulie
in Erscheinung tritt (*98*).

Eigene Untersuchungen an zunächst 195, überwiegend mit nur leichtem Defekt
oder defektfrei remittierten Schizophrenen der Heidelberger Klinik ergaben, daß

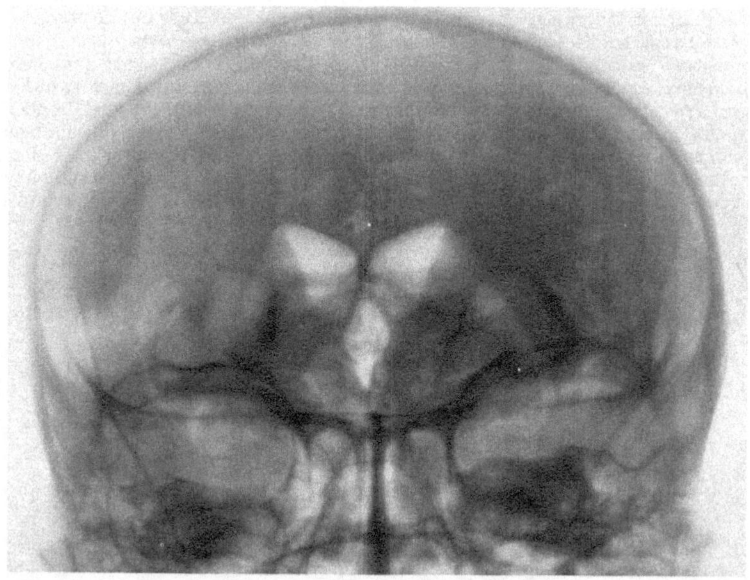

Abb. 14. *Schizophrenie.* 45 jähriger Patient. Seit dem 32. Lebensjahr in Schüben verlaufende Psychose mit jetzt
ausgepragtem, Erwerbsunfähigkeit bedingenden Persönlichkeitsdefekt. Isolierte Erweiterung des 3. Ventrikels.
Formveränderungen der basalen Teile der Seitenventrikel mit breiter Stammganglientaille. Hirnoberfläche o. B.

die bei der Mehrzahl der defektuösen Verläufe nachzuweisenden Atrophien eine
topische Prädilektion im Bereich der Basalganglien insbesondere des Zwischenhirns zeigten, die im Hinblick auf die Korrelationen zwischen Häufigkeit und
Ausmaß der Befunde und psychischem Remissionsgrad eine Inbeziehungsetz-
ung zum klinischen Syndrom und damit eine Hypothese ermöglichte, welche
in den Veränderungen ein Korrelat der bei schizophrenen und cyclothymen Erkrankungen sich entwickelnden post- und parapsychotischen Defektsyndrome
sieht (*108, 110, 111, 114*) (Abb. 14). Von 212 unter 50 Jahre alten, in 68% von
Anfang an einfach progredient verlaufenden defektschizophrenen Anstaltspatienten mit einer durchschnittlichen Prozeßdauer von 12½ Jahren zeigten
81,6% atrophische, an den inneren Liquorräumen überwiegende Veränderungen,
die am häufigsten (71%) den 3. Ventrikel betreffen, seltener die Hirnrinde (25,5%)
und die Seitenventrikel (34%), die in 40,6% eine konstitutionell bedingte, mit
dysplastischer Konfiguration verbundene abnorme Kleinheit aufweisen (*116, 117*).
Die anlagemäßig kleine Ventrikelkapazität, das relativ geringe Ausmaß der Veränderungen an Seitenventrikeln und Rinde und die lokalisatorische Prädilektion
der Atrophie erklären angesichts einer bei Schizophrenen gesteigerten Neigung
zu terminalen und postmortalen Schwellungs- und Quellungsvorgängen die
in der Mehrzahl negativen Autopsiebefunde. Reine und gemischte coenästhetische

Verlaufsformen einschließlich der ausgesprochen psychotischen, paranoid-leib-halluzinatorischen Typen mit vielfach langjährigem leibhypochondrischem Initialverlauf zeigen Veränderungen an den Stammganglien noch häufiger, solche am Cortex dagegen seltener als alle übrigen Unterformen (*111, 112, 115, 117*); den niedrigsten Prozentsatz von Atrophien beobachtet man bei hebephrenen und formal geordneten chronischen paranoiden Krankheitstypen (*117*, s. a. *19*). Die als „alte Katatoniker" bezeichneten, gewöhnlich von Anfang an einfach-progredient verlaufenden Defekttypen unterscheiden sich von den prognostisch

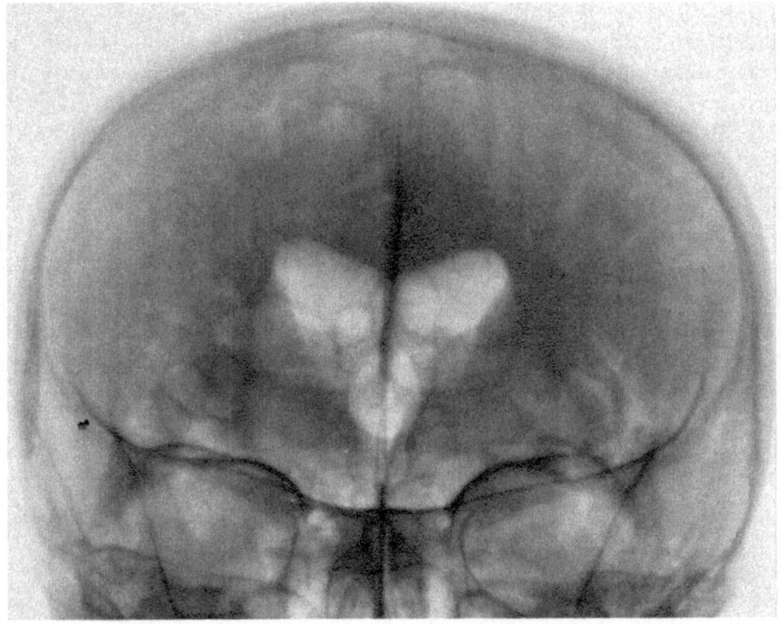

Abb. 15. *Schizophrenie.* 36jähriger Mann. 9jähriger einfach progredienter Verlauf mit raschem Eintritt eines erheblichen Defektes. Bild des „alten Katatonikers". Hydrocephalus der Seitenventrikel mit hochgradiger Erweiterung des 3. Ventrikels bei normaler Hirnoberfläche

relativ günstigen akuten Katatonien mit schubweisem Verlauf auch hinsichtlich der hier geringen, dort hohen Häufigkeit von Hirnatrophien (*117*) (Abb. 15).

Gegen eine Auffassung der Befunde als *konstitutionelle Variante* spricht, daß die Patienten mit psychopathischer Ausgangspersonlichkeit, Unterbegabung, mit ausgepragt asthenischem und dysplastischem Körperbautypus und mit Anomalien am knochernen Hirnschädel eine gegenüber dem Gesamtkrankengut jeweils deutlich geringere Häufigkeit von Veränderungen, insbesondere solcher am 3. Ventrikel, aufweisen. Eine Abhängigkeit der Hirnatrophien vom *Lebensalter*, zumindest unterhalb des 45. Lebensjahres, und von der *Schockbehandlung* läßt sich an unserem Untersuchungsgut nicht nachweisen. Allgemein darf man auf Grund des gesamten, umfangreichen Erfahrungsmaterials annehmen, daß mit dem Vorkommen ence-phalographisch faßbarer Hirnveränderungen als Folge komplikationsloser Schocktherapie in der Regel nicht zu rechnen ist (*111, 117, 139, 266*). Vermutlich infolge *geschlechtsspezifischer Unterschiede* in der Liquorraumkapazitat kommen Veränderungen am 3. Ventrikel und an den Seitenventrikeln bei weiblichen Defektschizophrenen in geringerer, solche am Cortex dagegen in erheblich stärkerer Häufigkeit vor als bei den männlichen Patienten; eine dem weiblichen Geschlecht eigene, bei bestimmten schizophrenen und cyclothym-depressiven (s. o.) Krank-heitstypen besonders ausgeprägte Pathoklise des Cortex allgemein gegenüber atrophischen Vorgängen, möglicherweise auf der Basis einer konstitutionellen Hypoplasie bestimmter Rindenregionen, ist zu erwägen (*22, 117, 273*).

Nach den Erfahrungen an 407 Schizophrenen zeigt die Mehrzahl (80%) ausgeprägter Defektschizophrener atrophische, bevorzugt subcortical-diencephale Veränderungen, dabei 96% eine Erweiterung der 3. Hirnkammer über 6 mm, während das PEG bei den vermutlich 30—50% aller Schizophrenieverläufe umfassenden, ohne deutlichen Defekt remittierenden Schizophrenien in der Regel (84%) im Bereich der Norm liegt. Bei 53 Wiederholungsencephalographien boten 28 Schizophrene eine in erster Linie den 3. Ventrikel betreffende Progredienz der Atrophie, der in 24 Fällen auch ein Fortschreiten der psychischen Veränderungen entsprach (*117*). Unabhängig von der Deutung der Befunde als ätiologisch uneinheitliche, unspezifische Subcorticopathie oder als der Defektpsychose (als immer nur fakultatives Symptom) korrelierte systematische Hirnatrophie im Sinne einer vorzeitigen lokalen Altersinvolution konstitutionell hypoplastischer Systeme (*111, 117*), stellt das an sich unspezifische neuroradiologische Basalganglien-syndrom einen Befund dar, durch den sich ausgeprägte Defektschizophrenien im Durchschnitt nicht nur von nichtpsychotischen Abnormitäten unterscheiden, sondern der bei dieser Kerngruppe auch regelmäßiger vorkommt als bei organischen cerebralen Prozessen und Defektzuständen (*117, 120*, s. unten). Auch bei einer Auffassung als ätiologisch heterogene Diencephalopathie (*117, 128, 129*) wäre diese als prädestinierender und prädisponierender Faktor nicht nur für die Manifestation, sondern auch für Verlauf und Ausgang der Erkrankung von Bedeutung und könnte als Korrelat des sog. schizophrenen, in seiner Essenz mit K. Conrad als „Reduktion des psychischen energetischen Potentials" umschriebenen und erscheinungsbildlich unspezifischen Defektes angesehen werden (*117, 120*).

III. Pseudopsychopathien, Persönlichkeitsvarianten und Konstitutionsanomalien

1. Pseudopsychopathische Syndrome

Auf Grund der Erfahrungen einer Reihe von Autoren (*23, 80, 111, 113, 139, 145, 156, 244, 304*) ist damit zu rechnen, daß sich hinter vielen als Psychopathien und Psychogenien rubrizierten psychiatrischen Syndromen Folgezustände von fetal, paranatal, frühkindlich oder im Erwachsenenalter erworbenen Hirnschäden oder ätiologisch unklare Hirnatrophien verbergen bzw. eine im PEG und durch andere Methoden nachweisbare organische Hirnläsion und die damit verbundene Beeinträchtigung der cerebralen Kompensations- und Anpassungsfähigkeit wenigstens *eine* Bedingung für das Auftreten der psychopathieähnlichen und neurotoiden Störungen darstellt (s. Abb. 16a und b).

Zu beachten ist, daß der frühkindliche, z. Z. noch vorhandener Wachstumsmöglichkeit der Schädelkapsel entstandene Hydrocephalus nicht zu einem wesentlichen Parenchymverlust zu führen braucht und weiter, daß ein — zumal innerer — Hydrocephalus sich weniger im intellektuellen als im affektiven Bereich und hier in völlig uneinheitlicher Form auswirkt; es resultieren als Persönlichkeitsvarianten imponierende Abnormitaten, Verhaltens- und Kontaktstörungen, Mangel an Umweltbezug, an Aktivität und Ausdauer, Gehemmtheit, neurasthenie- und psychopathieähnliche Zustande verschiedenster Art (*108, 113, 277*).

Eine besondere, das höhere Lebensalter bevorzugende Gruppe von oft als Psychopathien und Neurosen verkannten progredienten oder nach Jahren unveränderten *hypochondrischen Zuständen* mit mannigfachen Mißempfindungen und im PEG faßbaren, parietal betonten Erweiterungen der Subarachnoidalräume wie der Ventrikel wurde von H. E. Kehrer (*138*) beschrieben und als hirnorganisches, ätiologisch meist unklares Syndrom aufgefaßt. Wir fanden bei solchen, auch im Heidelberger Untersuchungsgut vorkommenden Patienten die Rindenatrophie gewöhnlich mit einer bevorzugten Erweiterung der 3. Hirnkammer kombiniert. Bei manchen jener unheilbaren „Hypochondrien" dürfte es sich um coenästhetische Verlaufsformen der Schizophrenie handeln, eine Annahme, die durch langjährige Verlaufsbeobachtungen bei solchen im Querschnittsbild uncharakteristischen Fällen, die nur durch passagere psychotische Episoden als Schizophrenien erkennbar werden oder zeitlebens auf der diagnostisch vieldeutigen, dysästhetischen Entwicklungsstufe stehen bleiben, bewiesen werden konntc (*110, 111, 112, 115, 117*). Ausgehend vom morphologischen Befund an der Schädelhirnbasis fand K. H. SCHIFFER (*244, 245*) den Befund einer isolierten Erweiterung des 3. Ventrikels, der bei frühkindlichen Cerebralschäden wie bei anlagebedingten Entwicklungsstörungen und auch familiär und vererbbar vorkommen kann, besonders häufig (17%) bei pseudopsychopathischen Bildern auf der Grundlage früher, vorwiegend basaler meningoencephalitischer Prozesse; während eine Koppelung an bestimmte psychiatrische und neurologische Krankheitsbilder nicht vorlag, ergab die konstitutionsbiologische Auswertung eine deutliche Betonung dysplastischer, dysgenitaler und dyskriner Varianten im Sinne von KRETSCHMER.

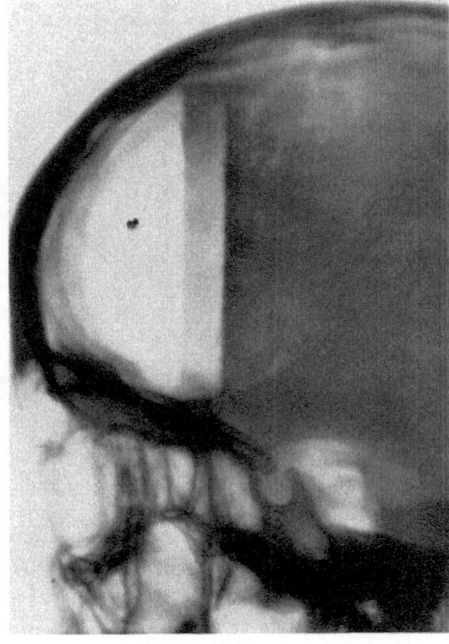
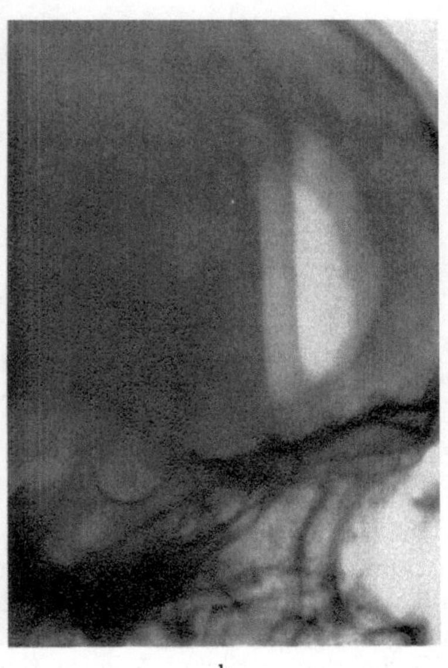

a   b

Abb. 16 a u. b. Horizontales Vorderhornbild. Luftmenge reicht nur zur Darstellung der Vorderhornspitze.
a *Enormer generalisierter Hydrocephalus internus nach frühkindlicher steriler Meningitis.* 15 jähriges Mädchen mit psychomotorischen Anfallen 8 jähriger Volksschulbesuch ohne Sitzenbleiben. Unterbegabung, doch kein Schwachsinn. Vorzeitige Ermüdbarkeit, Konzentrationsschwäche und Verlangsamung. b Hochgradiger *Hydrocephalus internus nach kindlicher Meningitis.* 23 jähriger, überdurchschnittlich intelligenter Student. Psychopathieähnliches Bild mit stimmungslabilen Krisen, sensitiv-selbstunsicheren Zügen und Kontaktstörungen

Manche als stimmungslabile, unstete Persönlichkeiten aufgefaßte Zustände mit *dipso- und poriomanen Krisen* sowie schwere chronische *anankastische Verläufe* zeigen nach eigenen Erfahrungen gleichfalls relativ häufig eine hervorstechende Erweiterung des 3. Ventrikels (Abb. 17). Auch bei diesen Syndromen scheinen exogene hirnorganische Noxen, möglicherweise in Verbindung mit anlagemäßigen Vorbedingungen im Sinne einer Unterwertigkeit bestimmter Hirnsysteme und -zentren, von Bedeutung zu sein (*111, 118*). Wiederholt wurde auf chronisch bestehende, vielfach als Psychopathie oder Psychoneurose verkannte „idiopathische" *Cephalgien* hingewiesen, die im PEG atiologisch aus Anamnese und Befund nicht

18*

zu erklärende Atrophien zeigen (*60, 139, 219, 286*). Die therapeutische Wirkung der Lufteinblasung, deren ausgedehnte Anwendung bei solchen Fällen von genuinen, vermutlich auf frühe Hirnschäden oder Gefäßstorungen zuruckzufuhrenden Kopfschmerzen mit atrophischen Läsionen befürwortet wird (*219*), kann auf Trennung von Adhäsionen und Entleerung von z. T. auch operativ nachgewiesenen (*49*) Arachnoidalcysten beruhen. Im Schadelleerbild sieht man hier häufiger (26%—*218*) als in anderen Krankheitsgruppen eine Vermehrung und Verstärkung der Impressiones digitatae, die bei Fehlen einer aktuellen Hirndrucksteigerung nach Schüller (*256*) eine konstitutionelle Bereitschaft zu Kopfschmerzen anzeigt.

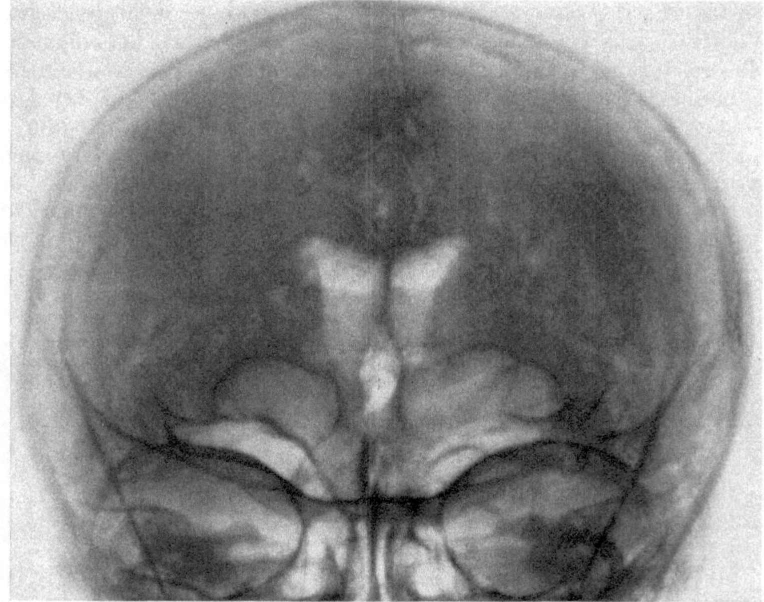

Abb. 17. 23 jähriger Patient, seit dem 14. Lebensjahr bestehendes schweres, therapieresistentes *zwangsneurotisches Syndrom*. Bevorzugte maßige Erweiterung des 3. Ventrikels kombiniert mit frontobasalen Formveranderungen am rechten Seitenventrikel. Verdacht auf fruhkindliche Hirnschadigung

2. Persönlichkeitsvarianten und Konstitutionsanomalien

In einem Material von *Psychopathien und Erlebnisreaktionen* (*118*), die in Anamnese und im klinischen Befund keinerlei Hinweise auf eine (früher durchgemachte oder aktuelle) Hirnaffektion oder eine endogene Psychose boten, fand sich bei Zugrundelegung unseres Maßstabes in über 90% (50 Fälle) ein normales PEG; bei den restlichen 5 Patienten mit pathologischem PEG sind anamnestisch stumme und klinisch unterschwellige hirnorganische Noxen und anlagebedingte Hypoplasien des Hirngewebes zu vermuten. Der Befund doppel- oder auch einseitig abnorm weiter innerer oder äußerer Liquorräume einschließlich der basalen Zisternen kann, z. B. bei manchen erblichen Schwachsinnszuständen, bei Mongolismus (*92, 149, 236*) und bei der Sturge-Weberschen Krankheit (*58*), auch auf einer angeborenen, als Mißbildung anzusehenden *Hypoplasie* des Gehirns oder einzelner Hirnteile beruhen, die dann auf eine anlagemäßige, den Verlauf der Erkrankung ungünstig beeinflussende Unterwertigkeit des Zentralnervensystems hinweist und nicht einfach als morphologische Variante im Bereich der Norm aufzufassen ist (*111, 139, 153, 154*). Die *Formvariante des "Ribbing"* am Dach von Vorderhorn und Cella media der Seitenventrikel (Balkenstrahlung nach Lindgren) ist als ein bei Schizophrenen besonders häufiges dysplastisches Stigma

gewöhnlich mit einer abnormen Kleinheit, nicht selten auch mit einer sog. Ependym-
segelbildung (Verwachsungen zwischen Caudatuskopf und Balken) vergesellschaftet (*111, 113, 117*); davon zu unterscheiden sind ähnliche, jedoch mit Ventrikelerweiterung verbundene Veränderungen, die durch in das Hirnkammerlumen
hineinragende Blutgefäße verursacht und als Hydrocephaluszeichen zu werten
sind (*55, 111, 121*).

Bei den Veränderungen an der Schädelbasis, insbesondere den *Sellaanomalien* (kleine
undifferenzierte Sella, hohes Dorsum oder Dorsum elongatum, sog. Rucksacksella, Einkerbung
am Sellaboden, Brückensella u. a.) ist eine morphologische Differenzierung hinsichtlich einer
endogenen oder exogenen Ätiologie nicht möglich; ähnliche Bilder kommen bei frühen Cerebralschäden bis zum zweiten Lebensjahr, bei anlagebedingten Entwicklungsstörungen wie
auch familiar und vererbbar vor (*243, 244*). Eine Reihe von Sellaformen (ovale, flache, tiefe,
viereckige, verzogene Sella nach MARTIN) sind ebenso wie Verkalkungen des Ligamentum
sellopetrosum als Normvarianten anzusehen (*183, 185, 244*). Zusammenhänge zwischen
Sellabild und Größe und Funktion der Hypophyse, anderen Konstitutionsanomalien und
endokrinen Stigmata, zwischen Sellaverbildung und Hypophysenzwischenhirnschwache,
flacher (oder starker) Schädelbasisknickung und konstitutioneller Retardierung wurden von
zahlreichen Autoren diskutiert (*242, 244, 251, 271*). Besonders ausgeprägte, breite Diploe-
venen sind als ,,Randmerkmal einer konstitutionellen Vasolabilität'' häufig mit vegetativ-
vasomotorischen Syndromen korreliert (*269*).

Die anlagebedingten *Oligophrenien* zeigen in der Regel ein normales PEG
(*179*); in seltenen Fällen lassen sich diffuse oder umschriebene Hypoplasien des
Gehirns feststellen, häufiger aber auf Grund atrophischer, besonders asymmetri-
scher Läsionen, die exogene Natur des Zustandes wahrscheinlich machen (*139*).

C. Die neuroradiologischen Syndrome bei den Grundformen chronischer, irreversibler Psychosyndrome

Die *Unspezifität* aller neuroradiologisch darstellbaren nichttumorösen Liquorraumveränderungen besagt zunächst nichts gegen einen Zusammenhang mit dem
jeweiligen Krankheitsbild (*111, 117*). Alle möglichen cerebralen Affektionen können
zu einem ähnlichen oder gleichartigen hirnatrophischen Syndrom führen, das nur
als das mehr oder weniger identische, grobmorphologisch-encephalographisch
faßbare (End-) Resultat der zugrunde liegenden heterogenen cerebralen Prozesse
und Schäden und möglicherweise als das gemeinsame pathogenetische Zwischenglied und Korrelat für die zugeordneten, gleichfalls erscheinungsbildlich unspezifischen psychopathologischen Dauerveränderungen aufgefaßt werden kann.
Es erhebt sich die Frage, ob verschiedenen Typen neuroradiologisch faßbarer
hirnatrophischer Syndrome auch klinisch unterscheidbare Typen chronischer
irreversibler Psychosyndrome entsprechen.

Ein Zusammenhang zwischen psychoorganischer Dauerveränderung und hirnatrophischem
Befund wurde schon immer vermutet, z. T. jedoch auch in Abrede gestellt (*10, 30, 85, 108,
111, 113, 196*). Diesbezügliche Studien erstreckten sich jedoch allenfalls auf einzelne Krankheitsbilder (*93*); GOSLING fand bei 68 genetisch meist unklaren organischen Demenzen
des höheren Lebensalters in 85% eine cerebrale Atrophie. Untersuchungen mit dem Ziel,
psychoorganische Dauerveränderung und Hirnatrophie in bezug auf das Maß ihrer Zusammen-
gehörigkeit zu prüfen, wurden am Heidelberger, alle Diagnosen umfassenden Material durchgeführt (*120*).

1. Organische Wesensveränderung und Demenz

Unter 535 Patienten mit *psychoorganischer Dauerveränderung* auf der Grundlage von ätiologisch heterogenen Hirnschäden und Hirnprozessen fand sich bei
412 Patienten (77%) eine pathologische, im PEG nachweisbare Hirnatrophie.
Bei einer Aufgliederung des Materials nach dem Typus der psychopathologischen

Veränderung, die zugleich in der Reihenfolge chronisches pseudoneurasthenisches Syndrom bzw. Hirnleistungsschwäche (Gruppe I) — mehr oder weniger isolierte, nicht mit intellektuellem Abbau vergesellschaftete organische Persönlichkeitsveränderung (Gruppe II) — mäßiggradige Demenz (Gruppe III) — schwere Demenz (Gruppe IV) eine solche nach dem Ausmaß der psychischen Defizienz ist, zeigt sich, daß Häufigkeit und Ausmaß der atrophischen Veränderungen insbesondere am Cortex mit dem Grad der psychischen Veränderung eine Zunahme erfahren. Faßt man die Gruppen I und II zusammen und stellt so den isolierten, nicht mit groben intellektuellen und mnestischen Ausfällen verbundenen *organischen Wesensänderungen* (301 Fälle) die ausgesprochenen *Demenzen* (Gruppe III und IV, 228 Fälle) gegenüber, findet man eine Hirnatrophie dort in 66, hier in 91%, eine Atrophie am Cortex bei den Wesensänderungen in 28, den Demenzzuständen dagegen in 73,7% (s. Tab.). Die Demenzprozesse sind gewöhnlich durch Hirnrinde und Hemisphärenmark gleichmäßig betreffende oder aber am Cortex überwiegende, diffuse, meist stärker ausgeprägte Atrophien gekennzeichnet, die Wesensänderungen — auf der Basis von in erster Linie traumatischen, genuin-epileptischen und vasculären Affektionen — durch das Prävalieren von meist geringer ausgeprägten, ventrikelnahen Atrophien im Bereich des Hemisphärenmarks und der Stammganglien.

Tabelle. *Häufigkeit und Lokalisation hirnatrophischer Befunde bei organischer Wesensveranderung, Demenz und schizophrenem Defekt*

| Art der psychopathologischen Dauerveranderung | Zahl der Falle | Pathologische atrophische Veranderungen | | | | Zahl der Falle mit pathologischer Atrophie |
		Seitenventrikel %	3. Ventrikel %	Hirnrinde %	3. Ventrikel isoliert %	%
Organische Wesensveränderung	307	27,0	45,3	28,0	24,2	66,8
Demenz	228	67,9	60,1	73,7	9,6	91,2
Schizophrener Defekt	361	36,3	69,0	22,4	40,1	80,0

Ein Drittel der Syndrome organischer Wesensänderung und selbst 20 von 228 Demenzzustanden (8,8%) besitzen demnach kein pathologisches PEG. Dabei ist zu beachten, daß umschriebene Veränderungen wie Ausweitung und Ausziehung bestimmter Seitenventrikelabschnitte, Cysten- und Porusbildungen an der Hirnoberfläche unberücksichtigt blieben. Man muß damit rechnen, daß darüber hinaus bei einer Anzahl von Fallen mit normalem PEG encephalographisch nicht faßbare *lokale Substanzschaden* vorliegen, die fur manche chronischen psychischen Veränderungen verantwortlich zu machen sind. Man denke z. B. an Charakterveränderungen nach Hirntraumen, die erst autoptisch einen mit den Liquorräumen nicht kommunizierenden und daher dem neuroradiologischen Nachweis sich entziehenden cystischen Defekt im Gebiet der basalen Rinde (H. Spatz) des Orbital- oder Schläfenhirns erkennen lassen. Bemerkenswert ist, daß unter den Demenzen immerhin 17,5% trotz eines Hydrocephalus internus keine Rindenatrophie aufweisen. Es gibt also Ausnahmen von der Regel, daß bei Demenz die durch einen Hydrocephalus externus angezeigte Rindenatrophie überwiegt oder wenigstens in ihrer Ausprägung im Einzelfall nicht hinter dem Hydrocephalus internus zurücksteht (*111*).

Geht man umgekehrt vom PEG-Befund aus, findet man unter insgesamt 285 Fällen mit *Hydrocephalus externus* 236 Patienten, die im klinisch-psychopathologischen Bild die Achsensyndrome der chronischen körperlich begründbaren Psychose (K. Schneider) aufweisen, davon 62% eine ausgeprägte Demenz und 38% eine isolierte organische Persönlichkeitsveränderung. In großer Regelmäßigkeit (82,8%) läßt sich also eine Verbindung von röntgenologisch diagnostizierter Rindenatrophie und organischer psychischer Dauerveränderung aufzeigen. Unter den 49 Patienten ohne chronische psychoorganische Veränderung war kein Fall mit einem Hydrocephalus externus erheblichen Ausmaßes, ein Befund, der demnach ausnahmslos mit den Zeichen einer chronischen körperlich begründbaren Psychose korreliert ist (*120*).

2. Endogen-psychotischer Potentialverlust und neuroradiologisches Basalgangliensyndrom

Wie gezeigt (s. oben), sind die *schizophrenen und cyclothymen Defekt- und Residualsyndrome* in ihrer Mehrzahl durch atrophische Veränderungen im Bereich der Basalganglien ausgezeichnet. Erweiterungen des 3. Ventrikels überhaupt sind bei den schizophrenen Defektsyndromen mehr als dreimal häufiger, bei den Demenzen dagegen seltener als Rindenatrophien. Während mit normalen Befunden an Seitenventrikeln und Hirnrinde kombinierte Veränderungen am 3. Ventrikel bei den Demenzen nahezu vollständig (nur 3,5%) fehlen, werden sie bei den Syndromen organischer Wesensänderung in 18,1 und bei Defektschizophrenen in 30,2% beobachtet (s. Tab.); die isolierte, nicht mit Veränderungen an den übrigen *Ventrikel*abschnitten kombinierte Erweiterung des 3. Ventrikels findet sich bei Demenzen in 9,6, bei Wesensänderungen ohne dementiellen Abbau in 24,2 und bei Defektschizophrenen in 40,1%. Dieses *neuroradiologische Zwischenhirnsyndrom* kommt im Ausgangsmaterial von 1294 Fällen aller Diagnosen in 12,1% und innerhalb der einzelnen Diagnosengruppen am häufigsten bei traumatischen Hirnschäden (22%), Gefäßprozessen (20%), Dystrophie- (28%) und Fleckfieberfolgen (20%), bestimmten vorzeitigen Versagenszuständen (17%) und pseudopsychopathischen Syndromen auf der Grundlage meist früher Hirnschäden vor, also weder im Gesamtmaterial noch in den einzelnen Krankheitsgruppen in gleicher Regelmäßigkeit wie bei Defektschizophrenen (*117, 120*).

Die Frage, ob es für die Fälle mit encephalographischem Basalgangliensyndrom ein gemeinsames, von der jeweiligen Grundkrankheit unabhängiges, als Korrelat der subcorticaldiencephalen Atrophie anzusehendes klinisch-psychopathologisches Syndrom gibt, liegt nahe. Man kann hierfür die „*Reduktion des psychischen energetischen Potentials*" in Anspruch nehmen (*117*), wie wir sie bei endogen-psychotischen Residualsyndromen als deren irreversible Komponente und als mutmaßliches Korrelat der atrophischen Veränderungen angesprochen haben. Die verschiedensten Hirnaffektionen würden also über das *gemeinsame pathogenetische Zwischenglied einer subcorticalen Atrophie* zu einem ähnlichen, psychopathologisch nicht sicher unterscheidbaren, auf die Potentialeinbuße zurückzuführenden, unspezifischen und vielfach nur gering ausgepragten, als „Hirnleistungsschwäche" (s. o.) (*103*) oder asthenisches Versagen imponierenden klinischen Defektsyndrom führen. Solche Beziehungen wurden schon früher, insbesondere von STERTZ (*270*) vermutet.

Die unterschiedliche Häufigkeitsverteilung und Lokalisation der Hirnatrophie bei den drei Grundtypen psychopathologischer Dauerveränderungen veranschaulicht die Tabelle. Es ergibt sich, daß den grob psychopathologisch differenzierbaren, komplexen Grundformen krankheitsbedingter seelischer Dauerveränderungen, die als Leitsyndrome der chronischen, körperlich begründbaren — organische Wesensänderung und Demenz — sowie vieler chronischer endogener und speziell schizophrener Psychosen — Defektsyndrom im Sinne einer Reduktion des psychischen energetischen Potentials (*45, 116, 117*) — gelten, auf der somatischen Seite nach Ausprägungsgrad und Topik in ihren Häufigkeitskorrelationen unterscheidbare Typen neuroradiologisch nachweisbarer hirnatrophischer Syndrome zugeordnet werden können.

3. Inkongruenzen zwischen klinischem und neuroradiologischem Befund

Hirnatrophische Syndrome ohne klinisches Korrelat einerseits, Syndrome chronischer psychoorganischer Veränderung ohne Hirnatrophie andererseits sind bei Auswertung eines genügend großen Untersuchungsgutes (s. oben) relativ selten und kommen nur in 17,2 bzw. 23 % unseres Gesamtmaterials vor (*120*). Diese auf statistischem Wege gewonnenen Ergebnisse besagen für den Einzelfall nichts Zwingendes. Man sieht immer wieder normale PEG-Bilder bei ausgesprochenen psychopathologischen oder neurologischen Symptomen einer schweren Hirnschädigung, andererseits stumme Hydrocephali ohne klinisch faßbare Erscheinungen (*44, 109, 113, 120, 143, 229, 266*). Grundsätzlich gilt, daß ein normales PEG noch keineswegs ein normales Hirngeschehen beweist, ein pathologischer encephalographischer Befund nicht notwendig mit Störungen der Hirnfunktion verbunden zu sein braucht, allgemein eine Beeinträchtigung des Substrates nicht auch eine solche der Funktion bedeutet, besonders wenn es sich nicht um aktuelle Prozesse, sondern um Residuen nach früher durchgemachten Affektionen oder um anlagemäßige Hypoplasien handelt. Die Form- und Größenveränderungen der Liquorräume haben zwar in der Regel eine Beziehung zum Hirngewebe (Atrophie oder Hypoplasie), doch ist eine solche zur Funktion ebensowenig gesetzmäßig vorhanden wie eine konstante Korrelation zwischen Ausprägungsgrad des Hydrocephalus und Schwere des klinischen Bildes (*113*).

Pathologische PEG-Veränderungen ohne oder mit nur geringen klinischen Entsprechungen werden u. a. bei Folgezuständen nach traumatischen (*49, 90, 119, 235*) und entzündlichen (*90, 240*) Hirnläsionen, bei frühkindlichen Cerebralschäden (*91, 240*) und bei Mißbildungen, z. B. beim kommunizierenden, mit Hydrocephalus internus kombinierten 5. Ventrikel gesehen (s. Abb. 16). Unter 213 Encephalographien fanden sich in 11 % hirnatrophische Syndrome ohne klinische Anhaltspunkte (*85*), bei völlig geheilten Fällen von präsenilen Psychosen und Cyclothymien nicht selten Rindenatrophien (*73, 300*, s. oben). Allgemein können Funktionsausfälle besonders bei formalpathogenetisch vorwiegend nach dem Prinzip des aktiven Hydrocephalus entstandenen Liquorraumveränderungen relativ gering sein oder ganz fehlen (*235*). Leichte Hydrocephalien nach frühkindlich durchgemachten oder atypisch verlaufenen Meningitiden, starke Hydrocephali bei Aquäduktstenosen können dauernd symptomlos bleiben (*229*). Im eigenen Material von 285 Fällen mit Hydrocephalus externus fanden sich 17,2 %, darunter am häufigsten Psychopathien, angeborene Schwachsinnszustände, Schädeltraumafolgen sowie Cyclothymien ohne chronische psychoorganische Veränderungen (*120*). Bei einem Teil dieser Fälle ist die Erweiterung der Subarachnoidalräume, die auch bei Tumoren der Medianebene, besonders beim Kraniopharyngiom und als reversibler Befund bei Liquorströmungsstörungen und entzündlichen Prozessen beobachtet wird, vermutlich als Ausdruck einer konstitutionellen Hypoplasie der Hirnrinde anzusehen. Defektfrei remittierte Schizophrenien zeigen in 17 % hirnatrophische Befunde (*111*).

Nichtpathologische Encephalogramme bei schweren klinischen Ausfallserscheinungen wurden u. a. bei traumatischen Epilepsien (*90*), beim Little und sonstigen frühkindlichen Hirnschäden (*90, 91, 240*), bei Halbseitenlähmungen nach cerebralem Insult (*90*), bei organischer Wesensänderung nach Hungerdystrophie (*259*), nach Encephalitis epidemica (*91, 240*) und bei seniler Demenz (*49*) beschrieben, wo histologische Veränderungen im Thalamus bei unauffälligem makroskopischem Befund eine schwere Verblödung verursachen können. Wir selbst sahen chronische, körperlich begründbare Psychosen und Defektsyndrome ohne Hirnatrophie in 123 von insgesamt 535 Fällen (27 %), darunter Syndrome organischer Wesensänderung in 33, Demenzzustände in 8,8 % ohne pathologisches PEG (*120*). Hinsichtlich der Grundkrankheit fanden wir chronische organische Psychosyndrome ohne Hirnatrophie am häufigsten bei genuinen Epilepsien (57 %) und bei gedeckten traumatischen Hirnschäden (39,6 %), bei sämtlichen anderen

Krankheitsbildern dagegen in erheblich geringerer prozentualer Häufigkeit, so bei insgesamt 115 Fällen cerebraler Gefäßprozesse in nur 13%. Bei Hirntraumatikern mit Hirnleistungsschwäche und organischer Persönlichkeitsveränderung ist ein pathologisches PEG in annähernd der Hälfte der Fälle (44,1%) nicht zu erwarten (*120, 120b*, s. auch *4* u. *119*). Unter 361 ausgeprägten schizophrenen Defektzuständen ließen 20% atrophische Veränderungen im PEG vermissen, besonders häufig gerade die psychopathologisch von der organischen Demenz am weitesten entfernten, qualitativ heterogenen, prämorbid psychopathischen und konstitutionell dysplastischen, klassisch schizophrenen Formen (*111, 117*).

4. Verlaufsuntersuchungen bei organischen Abbausyndromen und schizophrenem Defekt

Ergebnisse von encephalographischen Längsschnittuntersuchungen wurden nur selten, so bei traumatischen Hirnschäden (*64, 131, 140*) und bei primären und sekundären hirnatrophischen Prozessen (*30*) mitgeteilt. Bei der von BRONISCH (*30*) beschriebenen ätiologisch heterogenen Gruppe hatte die Hirnatrophie z. Z. der ersten Klinikaufnahme in der Mehrzahl der Fälle und schon voll ausgebildetem psychopathologischem Bild bereits einen Endzustand erreicht und ließ nur in 3 Fällen bei späteren Kontrollen eine wesentliche Progredienz erkennen. Bei neurohistologisch begründbaren hirnatrophischen Prozessen braucht also die Atrophie auch dann nicht fortzuschreiten, wenn klinisch eine Progredienz schon bestehender chronischer psychoorganischer Veränderungen zu verzeichnen ist (*30, 111*). Eine Zunahme der Atrophie, doch auch ein nach Jahren unverändertes PEG wurde bei genuiner Epilepsie beobachtet (*50, 155*). Von grundsätzlicher Bedeutung ist die Unterscheidung zwischen „*hirnatrophischem Prozeß*" und „*hirnatrophischem Defekt*" (*34*), wie er z. B. nach frühkindlich oder im Erwachsenenalter durchgemachten traumatischen, entzündlichen, kreislaufbedingten oder dystrophischen Affektionen vorliegt. Doch besitzen auch manche bland verlaufenden regressiven Prozesse mit irgendwann im Laufe des Lebens allmählich sich entwickelnder Atrophie, z. B. viele vorzeitige Versagenszustände, klinisch wie encephalographisch weitgehend stationären Charakter. Peristatische, zumal psychodynamische Faktoren sind gerade hier, wie grundsätzlich überall im Gebiet chronischer, nur bedingt irreversibler Psychosyndrome, für die soziale Restitution, für Kompensation, Dekompensation und Rekompensation von großer, oft ausschlaggebender Bedeutung (*74, 117*).

Wie bei organischen braucht auch bei *schizophrenen Prozessen* die Hirnatrophie trotz klinischer Progredienz eines schon z. Z. der Erstencephalographie nachweisbaren psychischen Defektes nicht fortzuschreiten (*111, 162*); bei einem Teil chronischer Schizophrenien hat die cerebrale Atrophie offenbar schon z. Z. der Ausbildung eines defektuösen Persönlichkeitswandels einen Endzustand erreicht. Unter 18 von anderen Untersuchern kontrollencephalographierten Schizophrenen zeigten 11 ein zeitliches Parallelgehen des Fortschreitens der psychischen und neuroradiologischen Veränderungen, wobei die Progredienz der Atrophie die Seitenventrikel (*191, 192, 309*) und den 3. Ventrikel (*20*) betraf. Wir selbst sahen bei 24 von 28 Schizophrenen mit Zunahme der Atrophie an den inneren Liquorräumen und in erster Linie am 3. Ventrikel im gleichen Zeitraum ein Fortschreiten des psychischen Defektes, während bei 22 von 23 Patienten mit unverändertem PEG auch das psychopathologische Bild keine Progredienz erkennen ließ (*117*). Die an insgesamt 35 Fällen aufzeigbare Parallelität in der Progredienz der neuroradiologischen und der psychischen Veränderungen einerseits, die verläßliche Konstanz des encephalographischen Befundes bei stationärem klinischen Defektsyndrom andererseits scheint in Verbindung mit anderen Indizien (Korrelationen

zum Remissionsgrad, topische Prädilektion, s. oben) auf eine gleichwie geartete
Beziehung der als systematische Atrophie gedeuteten Befunde zum schizophrenen
Potentialverlust hinzuweisen (*111*, *117*). „Systematische Atrophie", die mit
RAYMOND als vorzeitige lokal betonte Altersinvolution verstanden wird und auch
ohne Schizophrenie vorkommt wie umgekehrt Defektschizophrenie ohne system-
gebundene Atrophie, braucht dabei nicht einen pathologischen Hirnprozeß,
kann vielmehr auch endogene Vorgänge im Grenzgebiet zwischen physiologischer
Altersatrophie und ausgesprochenen Krankheitsprozessen bedeuten (*117*).

Literatur

Die nach Abschluß des Beitrages während der Drucklegung erschienenen einschlägigen
Arbeiten konnten nicht mehr berücksichtigt werden. Hierunter fallen u. a. die Monographien
von J. O. HAUG: "Pneumencephalographic studies in mental disease", Acta Psychiatrica
Scandinavica Supplementum 165, Volume 38 (1962) und von C. SKODA: „Der psychotische
Prozeß und postpsychotische Defekt. Studien zur Frage einer Möglichkeit der objektiven
Unterscheidung besonders bei Schizophrenen". Edition der Abteilung für chemische und biologische Wissenschaften der slowakischen Akademie der Wissenschaften, Bratislava 1963,
sowie die Mitteilung von K. NAGY: Pneumencephalographische Befunde bei endogenen Psychosen. Nervenarzt 34, 543 (1963).

1. ALEKSANDROVA, A. V.: X-ray and differential diagnosis of intracranial calcification in
children who had sustained tuberculous meningitis. Vop. Nejrohir. 22, 21 (1958). — 2. ASCHEN-
BRENNER, R., u. W. V. BAEYER: Das epidemische Fleckfieber. Stuttgart 1944.

3. BANNWARTH, A.: Zur Diagnostik schwerer Gehirnmißbildungen durch die Encephalo-
graphie. Verh. 3. int. neur. Kongr. 549 (1939). — 4. BAY, E.: Die traumatischen Hirnschadi-
gungen. In: Handb. der inn. Med. Hrsg. v. G. V. BERGMANN, W. FREY, H. SCHWIEGK. 4. Aufl.
Redig. v. R. JUNG, Bd. V, 3: Neurologie, S. 373. Berlin-Gottingen-Heidelberg: Springer-
Verlag 1953. — 5. BECKER, H., u. F. RADTKE: Über eine neue encephalographische Methode
Hirnkammern und erweiterte periphere Spalträume isoliert zur Darstellung zu bringen.
Nervenarzt 20, 442 (1949). — 6. BENNETT, J. C., R. H. MAFFLY and H. L. STEINBACH: The
significance of Bilateral Basal Ganglia Calcification. Radiology 72, 368 (1959). — 7. BERIN-
GER, K., u. R. MALLISON: Vorzeitige Versagenszustände. Allg. Z. Psychiat. 124, 100 (1949). —
8. BIASCI, L., e A. JARIA: Malattia ossea di Paget e disturbi psichici (rilievi clinici ed anatomo-
patologici su di un caso a localizazione esclusivement cranica.). Riv. Pat. nerv. mend. 79, 261
(1958). — 9. BINGEL, A.: Encephalographische Erfahrungen. Z. ges. Neurol. Psychiat. 114,
323 (1928). — 10. BLEULER, E.: Lehrbuch der Psychiatrie. 9. Aufl. umgearb. v. M. BLEULER.
Berlin-Gottingen-Heidelberg: Springer-Verlag 1955. — 11. BODECHTEL, G.: Anatomie,
Physiologie, Pathologie und Klinik der zentralen Anteile des vegetativen Nervensystems.
Fortschr. Neurol. Psychiat. 7, 295 (1935). — 12. BOENING, H., u. TH. KONSTANTINU: Encephalographische und erbbiologische Untersuchungen an genuinen Epileptikern. Arch. Psychiat. Nervenkr. 100, 171 (1933). — 13. BÖRLIN, E.: Morbus Recklinghausen (forme fruste mit
Knochendefekt am Hinterkopf). Dermatologica (Basel) 34, 176 (1947). — 14. BOETERS, H.:
Erbleiden des Nervensystems beim Menschen. In: Handbuch der Erbbiologie des Menschen V,
1, S. 187. Berlin: Springer 1938. — 15. BONKALO, A.: The filling of subarachnoid spaces over
the convexity in encephalograms of normal and tumor cases. Acta psychiat. (Kbh.) 25, 323
(1950). — 16. BOOR, W. DE: Psychopathologische Syndrome nach Carotisligaturen. Klin.
Wschr. 1950, 88. — 17. BORENSTEIN, P., M. DABBAH et J. METZGER: L'encéphalographie
fractionnée dans les syndromes schizophréniques. Ann. méd.-psychol. 115, 385 (1957). —
18. BORENSTEIN, P., M. DABBAH et J. METZGER: L'encéphalographie fractionnée et l'électro-
encéphalogramme dans la psychose maniaque dépressive. Ann. méd.-psychol. 116, 417
(1958). — 19. BORENSTEIN, P., et M. DABBAH: L'encéphalographie fractionnée et l'électroence-
phalogramme dans les psychoses délirantes aiguës et chroniques. Ann. méd.-psychol. 117,
793 (1959). — 20. BORREGUERO, A. D.: Estudio encefalográfico seriado de la esquizofrenia
de forma hebefrénica. Arch. Neurobiol. (Madr.) 22, 148 (1959). — 20a. BOVI, A.: Le atrofie
cerebrali nelle psicosi dell' etá media. Ferrara 1961. — 21. BRAILSFORD, J. F.: The
radiology of bones and joints. London 1944. — 22. BRAUNMÜHL, A. V.: Alterserkrankungen des
Zentralnervensystems: Senile Involution. Senile Demenz. Alzheimersche Krankheit. In:
Handbuch der speziellen pathologischen Anatomie und Histologie. Hrsg. v. O. LUBARSCH,
F. HENKE u. R. RÓSSLE. Bd. 13, 1: Nervensystem. Hrsg. v. F. W. SCHOLZ. Bd.-Teil A., S. 337.
Berlin-Gottingen-Heidelberg: Springer-Verlag 1957. — 23. BREDMOSE, G. V., och C. J.
MUNCH-PETERSEN: Encephalographie bei Kranken mit Neurosen und neurotisch gefärbten

Krankheitsbildern. Nord. Med. **1941**, 1367. — 24. BREITENFELD, J.: Beitrag zum klinischen und encephalographischen Bilde der Pickschen Krankheit. Lijecn. Vjesn. **62**, 55 (1940). — 25. BRENNER, W.: Beitrag zur Pathogenese des Hydrocephalus internus. Vergleich von neurologischen, röntgenologischen und anatomischen Befunden. Z. Kinderheilk. **61**, 265 (1939). — 26. BRENNER, W.: Das Encephalogramm bei der cerebralen Kinderlähmung und seine Bedeutung für deren Systematik. Z. Kinderheilk. **62**, 607 (1941). — 27. BRENNER, W.: Die Ergebnisse der Encephalographie im Kindesalter. Ergebn. inn. Med. Kinderheilk. **62**, 1238 (1942). — 28. BRENNER, W.: Die Röntgenologie des Hydrocephalus im Kindesalter unter besonderer Berücksichtigung der Grenzen des Normalen. Fortschr. Neurol. Psychiat. **20**, 445 (1952). — 29. BROBEIL, A.: Die klinische Bedeutung des 5. Ventrikels. Nervenarzt **18**, 180 (1947). — 30. BRONISCH, F. W.: Hirnatrophische Prozesse im mittleren Lebensalter und ihre psychischen Erscheinungsbilder. Stuttgart 1951. — 31. BRONISCH, F. W.: Über die Mikroventrikulie (KEHRER). Nervenarzt **22**, 55 (1951). — 32. BRONISCH, F. W.: Über das 24-Stunden-Encephalogramm. Dtsch. Z. Nervenheilk. **166**, 65 (1951). — 33. BRONISCH, F. W.: Über das 24-Stunden-Encephalogramm. Weitere Ergebnisse. Nervenarzt **23**, 188 (1952). — 34. BRONISCH, F. W.: Gehirnschädigungen nach Dystrophie und Erschöpfung. Dtsch. med. Wschr. **78**, 89 (1953). — 35. BRONISCH, F. W.: Zbl. Neur. Psychiat. **150**, 5 (1959). — 35a. BRUIJN G. W.: Pneumoencephalography in the diagnosis of cerebral atrophy. A quantitative study. Utrecht 1959. — 36. BUES, E.: Zum zeitlichen Ablauf des traumatischen Hirnödems in Serien-Encephalogrammen. Mschr. Unfallheilk. **56**, 151 (1958).

37. CAMBIER, J.: La maladie de Fahr. Calcifications intracérébrales non artério-scléreuses idiopathiques et ses rapports avec la tétanie. Presse méd. **1952**, 765. — 38. CAMBLOR, G. F.: Encefalopatias atróficas en las encefalitis. Su estudio neumoencefalográfico. Neurocirugía **14**, 121 (1956). — 39. CAMPI, L.: Rivievi pneumoencefalografici nell'epilessia (Considerazioni su 99 casi). Radiologia (Roma) **9**, 299 (1953). — 40. CARPENTER, M. B.: Agenesis of the corpus callosum. A study of 18 cases diagnosed during life. Neurology (Minneap.) **4**, 200 (1954). — 41. CASTORINA, G., E. MARCHINI e C. MOROCUTTI: Sui quadri neuroradiologici delle epilessie non tumorali in correlazione alla classificazione clinica ed elettroencefalografica. Osped. psichiat. **25**, 230 (1957). — 42. CHARLES, F., et N. BOINEAU: Enquêtes pneumoencéphalo-graphiques chez l'enfant et le nourrison. Algérie méd. **58**, 427 (1954). — 43. CHODOFF, P., A. SIMON and W. FREEMAN: Pneumoencephalographic diagnosis in the presenile dementias. Amer. J. Roentgenol. **59**, 311 (1948). — 44. CLARKE, E., and J. LAIDLAW: Silent hydrocepha-lus. Neurology (Minneap.) **8**, 382 (1958). — 45. CONRAD, K.: Die beginnende Schizophrenie. Versuch einer Gestaltanalyse des Wahns. Stuttgart 1958.

46. DAVID, M., H. FISCHGOLD, G. RUGGIERO, J. TALAIRACH, J. ABOULKER, P. BENDA et J. CONSTANS: Les explorations radiologiques en neurochirurgie cérébrale. Rev. neurol. **90**, 434 (1954). — 47. DAVIDOFF, L. M., and C. G. DYKE: Agenesis of the Corpus callosum. Its diagnosis by encephalography. Report of three cases. Amer. J. Roentgenol. **32**, 1 (1934). — 48. DAVIDOFF, L. M., and C. G. DYKE: The normal encephalogram. 3rd. ed H. Kimpton. London 1951. — 49. DECKER, K.: Klinische Neuroradiologie. Stuttgart 1960. — 50. DECKER, K., u. J. NAGEL: Rontgenuntersuchung an Anfallskranken. Dtsch. Z. Nervenheilk. **175**, 452 (1956). — 51. DECKER, K., u. O. WIEDEMANN: Mechanismus der cerebralen Luftfüllung nach Beobachtungen bei der kontrollierten Pneumencephalographie. Zbl. Neurochir. **19**, 72 (1959). — 52. DELAY, J., P. DESCLAUX et P. PICHOT: Sur quelques aspects pneumoencé-phalographiques des oligophrénies. Rev. neurol. **79**, 433 (1947). — 53. DIETRICH, H.: Neuro-Rontgenologie des Schädels. Jena 1954. — 54. DYKE, C. G., L. M. DAVIDOFF and C. B. MAS-SON: Cerebral hemiatrophy with homolateral hypertrophy of the skull and sinuses. Surg. Gynec. and Obst. **57**, 588 (1933). — 55. DYKE, C. G., and L. M. DAVIDOFF: An explanation for the ribbing seen in the walls of dilated cerebral ventricles. Yale J. Biol. Med. **11**, 485 (1939).

56. EBAUGH, F. G., H. H. DIXON, H. E. KIENE and K. D. ALLEN: Encephalographic studies in general paresis. Amer. J. Psychiat. **10**, 737 (1931). — 57. ENGELHARDT, H.: Die Ursachen der fehlenden Ventrikelfüllungen im Encephalogramm. Nervenarzt **13**, 490 (1940). — 58. ENGELHARDT, H.: Zur Kenntnis der Sturge-Weberschen Krankheit. Psychiat.-neurol. Wschr. **44**, 313 (1942). — 59. EPSTEIN, B. S., and J. A. EPSTEIN: The normal pneumoence-phalogram. Med. Radiogr. Photogr. **34**, 84 (1959).

60. FALK, B., and B. P. SILFVERSKIÖLD: Pneumoencephalographic changes in the chronic postconcussion syndrome and non-traumatic cephalalgia. Acta psychiat. (Kbh.) **29**, 161 (1954). — 61. FALK, B., L. KIRSTEIN, S. LÓFSTEDT and B. P. SILFVERSKIOLD: Pneumoencephalo-graphic investigations in epilepsy. Acta psychiat. scand. **33**, 440 (1958). — 62. FARBEROW, B. J.: Röntgenologisches Schädelbild bei Neurofibromatosis Recklinghausen. Z. Augenheilk. **89**, 81 (1936). — 63. FAUST, CL.: Hirnatrophie nach Hungerdystrophie. Nervenarzt **23**, 406 (1952). — 64. FAUST, CL.: Die psychischen Störungen nach Hirntraumen: Akute traumatische Psychosen und psychische Spätfolgen nach Hirnverletzungen. In: Psychiatrie der Gegenwart. Hrsg. v. H. W. GRUHLE, R. JUNG, W. MAYER-GROSS, M. MÜLLER. Bd. II: Klinische Psych-

iatrie. S. 552. Berlin-Göttingen-Heidelberg: Springer-Verlag 1960. — 65. Feld, M., B. Duperrat et J. Martinetti: A propos de deux observations de tumeur cérébrale au cours de la sklerose tubéreuse de Bourneville. Rev. neurol. 83, 516 (1950). — 66. Ferey, D., H. Guillerm, Stabert, Javalet, Tuset et Assicot: La pneumatocèle du vertex dans les encéphalographies gazeuses. Les erreurs d'interprétation possibles. Rev. neurol. 92, 148 (1955). — 67. Finby, N., and A. G. Bearn: Roentgenographic abnormalities of the skeletal system in Wilson's disease (hepatolenticular degeneration). Amer. J. Roentgenol. 79, 603 (1958). — 68. Fischer, H.: Ein eineiiges Zwillingspaar mit Hydrocephalus internus communicans und Megalencephalie. Z. ges. Neur. Psychiat. 174, 264 (1942). — 69. Flügel, F. E.: Die Encephalographie als neurologische Untersuchungsmethode. Ergebn. inn. Med. Kinderheilk. 44, 327 (1932). — 70. Flügel, F. E.: Grenzen und Anzeige der Encephalographie. Fortschr. Röntgenstr. 52, 349 (1935). — 71. Friedmann, G., u. E. Schmidt-Wittkamp: Zur Diagnose der einseitigen frühkindlichen Hirnschäden im Übersichtsbild des Schädels. Fortschr. Röntgenstr. 92, 667 (1960). — 72. Di Frisco, S.: Ricerche encefalografiche nella demenza senile e presenile. Rass. Studi psichiat. 27, 395 (1938). — 73. Fromenty, Renault et Salomon: Minimum cérébral vital et pneumoencéphalographie. Rev. neurol. 87, 399 (1952). — 74. Frowein, R.: Zbl. ges. Neur. Psychiat. 150, 5 (1959). — 75. Fünfgeld, E.: Über diffuse Rückbildungs- und Alterserkrankungen des Gehirns. In: Gegenwartsprobleme der psychiatr.-neur. Forsch. Hrsg. v. C. H. Roggenbau. Stuttgart: Enke-Verlag 1939. S. 45.

76. Gelli, G.: Intorno a un caso di macrogenitosomia postidrocefalica. Boll. Soc. ital. Pediat. 3, 170 (1934). — 77. Gelma, E., T. Kammerer, A. Batzenschlager, E. Wolf et J. Forget: Valeur de l'encéphalographie gazeuse dans la maladie de Korsakoff. Chiers Psychiat. 1952, Nr. 2, 21. — 78. Ghersi, J. A., N. E. Piaquadio y A. Fernandez: Imagenes encefalograficas de proceso que ocupa espacio en la encefalitis localizada. Prensa méd. argent. 1952, 355. — 79. Ginzberg, R.: Betrachtungen über das Encephalogramm bei progressiver Paralyse und paralyseverdächtigen syphilitischen Hirnerkrankungen. Arch. Psychiat. u. Nervenkr. 89, 711 (1930). — 80. Göllnitz, G.: Die Bedeutung der frühkindlichen Hirnschadigung für die Kinderpsychiatrie. Leipzig 1954. — 81. Gött, T.: Über die diagnostischen und therapeutischen Indikationen der Encephalographie. Z. Kinderheilk. 53, 411 (1932). — 82. Goette, K.: Über die Darstellung des Encephalogramms und seine Grenzen des Normalen und Pathologischen. Dtsch. Z. Nervenheilk. 110, 9 (1929). — 83. Golant, R.: Die Encephalographie in der psychiatrischen Klinik. Nevropat. Psihiat. 4, Nr. 9/10, 65 (1935). — 84. Goodhart, S. P., B. H. Balser u. I. Bieber: Encephalographic studies in cases of extrapyramidal disease. Arch. Neur. Psychiat. (Chicago) 35, 240 (1936). — 85. Gosling, R. H.: The association of dementia with radiologically demonstrated cerebral atrophy. J. Neur. Neurosurg. Psychiat. N.S. 18, 129 (1955). — 86. Gregoretti, L.: Luftencephalographische Untersuchungen bei depressiven Syndromen. Neuropsichiatria 14, 473 (1958). — 87. Greiner, G., G. Klotz, Wackenheim, M. Champy et Roos: L'atrophie cérébrale et son dépistage par l'encéphalographie fractionnée. Une cause fréquemment méconnue de troubles auditifs et de bourdonnements. Ann. Oto-laryng. (Paris) 76, 58 (1959). — 88. Gross, W.: Die diagnostische Bedeutung der Encephalographie bei der Epilepsie. Arch. Psychiat. Nervenkr. 94, 366 (1931). — 89. Guerner, F., J. Fajardo, M. Yahn e C. P. da Silva: Encephalographische Studien an Schizophrenen. Mem. Hosp. Juquery (Bras.) 11/12, 195 (1935). — 90. Gurdjian, E. S., u. H. A. Jarre: Encephalographic experiences: Medicolegal deductions. Radiology 24, 85 (1935). — 91. Guttmann, L.: Möglichkeiten und Grenzen der Encephalographie bei cerebraler Kinderlahmung. Fortschr. Röntgenstr. 40, 965 (1929). — 92. Guttmann, L.: Róntgendiagnostik des Gehirns und Rückenmarks durch Kontrastverfahren. In: Handb. d. Neurologie. Hrsg. v. O. Bumke u. O. Foerster. Bd. VII, Teil 2: Allgmeine Neurologie. Berlin 1936. — 93. Guttmann, L., u. W. Kirschbaum: Das encephalographische Bild der progressiven Paralyse und seine klinische Bedeutung. Z. Neurol. 121, 590 (1929).

94. Hallervorden, J.: Entwicklungsstörungen und frühkindliche Erkrankungen des Zentralnervensystems. In: Handbuch der inneren Medizin. Hrsg. v. G. v. Bergmann, W. Frey, H. Schwiegk. Bd. V/3: Neurologie. Red. v. R. Jung. S. 905. Berlin-Göttingen-Heidelberg: Springer-Verlag 1953. — 95. Hamne, B., u. S. Jonsell: Wiederholte Encephalogramm-Studien bei ein und demselben Kinde. Z. Kinderheilk. 63, 328 (1942). — 96. Hassler, R.: Extrapyramidal-motorische Syndrome und Erkrankungen. In: Handbuch der inneren Medizin. Hrsg. v. G. v. Bergmann, W. Frey, H. Schwiegk. Bd. V/3: Neurologie. Red. v. R. Jung. S. 676. Berlin-Göttingen-Heidelberg: Springer-Verlag 1953. — 97. Heidrich, R.: Planimetrische Hydrocephalus-Studien. Halle 1955. — 98. Heidrich, R.: Mikroventrikulie bei Psychosen. Arch. Psychiat. Nervenkr. 200, 480 (1960). — 99. Heidrich, R., u. P. Hagemann: Hydrocephalus internus et externus bei Dystrophia myotonica. Psychiat. Neurol. med. Psychol. (Lpz.) 10, 15 (1958). — 100. Heidrich, R., u. R. Hampel: Hydrocephalus internus und externus nach Insulinvergiftung. Nervenarzt 29, 173 (1958). — 101. Heinrich, A.: Alternsvorgänge im Róntgenbild. Leipzig 1941. — 102. Hempel, J.: Über die Bedeutung

eines gewissen Typs des encephalographischen Ventrikelbildes. Z. ges. Neurol. Psychiat. **169**, 522 (1940). — 103. HERTTRICH, P.: Veränderungen an den inneren und äußeren Liquorräumen im Encephalogramm bei Folgezuständen gedeckter Hirnverletzungen. Dtsch. Z. Nervenheilk. **167**, 253 (1952). — 104. HOLUB, K.: Erfahrungen mit der sog. 24-Stunden-Encephalographie. Wien. klin. Wschr. **1958**, 249. — 105. HOLT, J. F., and W. W. DICKERSON: The osseous lesions of tuberous sklerosis. Radiology **58**, 1 (1952). — 106. HOLZMANN, E. M.: Encephalographische Beobachtungen bei Epilepsie. Vestn. Rentgenol. Radiol. **15**, 278 (1935) (Russ.). — 107. HOPF, E. J.: Zur Frage des Hydrocephalus bei CO-Vergiftung. Dtsch. Z. Nervenheilk. **164**, 113 (1952). — 108. HUBER, G.: Zur Frage der mit Hirnatrophie einhergehenden Schizophrenie. Arch. Psychiat. Nervenkr. **190**, 429 (1953). — 109. HUBER, G.: Zur pathologischen Anatomie des Delirium tremens. Arch. Psychiat. Nervenkr. **192**, 356 (1954). — 110. HUBER, G.: Das Pneumencephalogramm am Beginn schizophrener Erkrankungen. Arch. Psychiat. Nervenkr. **193**, 406 (1955). — 111. HUBER, G.: Pneumencephalographische und psychopathologische Bilder bei endogenen Psychosen. Berlin-Göttingen-Heidelberg: Springer-Verlag 1957. — 112. HUBER, G.: Die coenästhetische Schizophrenie. Fortschr. Neurol. Psychiat. **25**, 491 (1957). — 113. HUBER, G.: Zur Frage des sogenannten Hydrocephalus. Nervenarzt **29**, 229 (1958). — 114. HUBER, G.: Endogene Psychosen und hirnatrophischer Befund. Fortschr. Neurol. Psychiat. **26**, 354 (1958). — 115. HUBER, G.: Coenasthetische Schizophrenien. Congress Report Volume II. S. 175. II. Internat. Kongreß f. Psychiatrie Zürich 1957. Zürich 1959. — 116. HUBER, G.: Klinische und neuroradiologische Untersuchungen an chronisch Schizophrenen. Nervenarzt **32**, 7 (1961). — 117. HUBER, G.: Chronische Schizophrenie. Synopsis klinischer und neuroradiologischer Untersuchungen an defektschizophrenen Anstaltspatienten. Heidelberg 1961. — 118. HUBER, G.: Das Pneumencephalogramm bei Psychopathien und psychoreaktiven Storungen. Ein Beitrag zur Frage des „normalen" Encephalogramms. Arch. Psychiat. Nervenkr. **202**, 234 (1961). — 119. HUBER, G.: Zur Frage der pneumencephalographischen Befunde bei traumatischen Hirnschäden. Nervenarzt **33**, 248 (1962). — 120. HUBER, G.: Typen und Korrelate psychoorganischer Abbau-Syndrome. In: Psychopathologie heute. Festschrift zum 75. Geburtstag von KURT SCHNEIDER. Hrsg. H. KRANZ. Stuttgart 1962. — 120a. HUBER, G.: Pacchionische Granulationen im Pneumencephalogramm. Arch. Psychiat. Nervenkr. **203**, 101 (1962). — 120b. HUBER, G.: Zur Frage des pneumencephalographischen Befundes bei idiopathischen Epilepsien. Dtsch. Z. Nervenheilk. **183**, 399 (1962). — 121. HUDOLIN, V., and F. PETROVČIĆ: Irregularities in the contour of the anterior part of the lateral ventricel as shown in air encephalograms. J. Neurol. Neurosurg. Psychiat. N.S. **20**, 136 (1957).

122. JACOB, H.: Über die diffuse Markdestruktion im Gefolge eines Hirnödems. Z. ges. Neurol. Psychiat. **168**, 382 (1940). — 123. JACOB, H.: Pathologisch-anatomisches Substrat und klinisches Bild in der Neurologie und Psychiatrie. Z. ges. Neurol. Psychiat. **171**, 629 (1941). — 124. JACOBI, W., u. H. WINKLER: Encephalographische Studien an chronisch Schizophrenen. Arch. Psychiat. Nervenkr. (D.) **81**, 299 (1927). — 125. JACOBI, W., u. H. WINKLER: Encephalographische Studien an Schizophrenen. Arch. Psychiat. Nervenkr. (D.) **84**, 208 (1928). — 126. JACOBSEN, E.: The air-encephalogram in the concentration camp syndrome. Ugeskr. Laeg. **1955**, 809. — 127. JANTZ, H.: Die Röntgendiagnostik der Hirn- und Rückenmarksräume. In: Handbuch der inneren Medizin. Hrsg. v. G. v. BERGMANN, W. FREY, H. SCHWIEGK. 4. Aufl. Red. v. R. JUNG. Bd. V, 1. Berlin-Göttingen-Heidelberg: Springer-Verlag 1953. — 128. JANZARIK, W.: Ref. über G. HUBER: Pneumencephalographische und psychopathologische Bilder bei endogenen Psychosen. Berlin-Göttingen-Heidelberg: Springer-Verlag 1957. Zbl. ges. Neurol. Psychiat. **142**, 290 (1957). — 129. JANZARIK, W.: Dynamische Grundkonstellationen in endogenen Psychosen. Berlin-Göttingen-Heidelberg: Springer-Verlag 1959. — 130. JONG, R. N. DE: Tuberous sclerosis: Encephalographic interpretation. J. Pediat. **9**, 203 (1936). — 131. JUNGE: Encephalographische Befunde bei Hirnverletzungen. Zbl. ges. Neurol. Psychiat. **113**, 14 (1951). — 132. JUNGMAYR, L.: Myotonische Dystrophie und Sellaveränderung. Klin. Wschr. **1951**, 205.

133. KANAHARA, T., u. Y. TAMURA: Über das Encephalogramm der Epilepsie. Psychiat. Neurol. jap. **40**, 35 (1936). — 134. KASAMATU, HIDEJI, u. K. YOSIKAWA: Die chronologischen Veränderungen der Encephalographie vermittels der serienweisen Aufnahmemethode. Folía psychiat. neurol. jap. **2**, 1 (1938). — 135. KAUTZKY, R., u. K. J. ZÜLCH: Neurologisch neurochirurgische Röntgendiagnostik und andere Methoden zur Erkennung intrakranialer Erkrankungen. Berlin-Göttingen-Heidelberg: Springer-Verlag 1955. — 136. KEHRER, F. A.: Die konstitutionelle Verkleinerung der Hirnventrikel („Mikroventrikulie") und ihre nosologische Bedeutung. Arch. Psychiat. Nervenkr. **179**, 430 (1948). — 137. KEHRER, H. E.: Zur Frage nach den Ursachen des Ausbleibens der Ventrikelfüllung bei der Encephalographie. Nervenarzt **21**, 163 (1950). — 138. KEHRER, H. E.: Zur Anatomie hypochondrischer Zustände. Arch. Psychiat. Nervenkr. **190**, 449 (1953). — 139. KEHRER, H. E.: Der Hydrocephalus internus und externus. Seine klinische Diagnose und Therapie. Basel-New York 1955. —

140. King, G. C.: Encephalography in rapidly progressing cerebral atrophy due to trauma. Amer. J. Dis. Child. **56**, 1330 (1938). — 141. Kisimoto, K.: Beitrage zur Encephalographie der Schizophrenie einschließlich der Resultate der fraktionierten Liquoruntersuchungen und der Einflüsse der Encephalographie auf das vegetative Nervensystem. Psychiat. Neurol. jap. **40**, 1 (1936). — 142. Klar, E.: Die Bedeutung des Rontgenbildes in der Begutachtung von Epilepsien im Erbgesundheitsverfahren. Z. ges. Neurol. Psychiat. **173**, 364 (1941). — 143. Klaue, R.: Zur Beurteilung hirntraumatischer Folgezustande nach stumpfem Schadeltrauma mit besonderer Berucksichtigung encephalographischer Befunde. Dtsch. Z. Nervenheilk. **164**, 259 (1950). — 144. Klausberger, E. M., u. F. Stiegelmayr: Die fehlende Ventrikelfullung bei spinaler Encephalographie. Wien. Z. Nervenheilk. **10**, 127 (1954). — 145. Klein: Psychische Storungen bei encephalographisch nachgewiesenem Hydrocephalus internus. Zbl. ges. Neurol. Nervenkr. **78**, 169 (1936). — 146. Klosovsky, B. N., B. C. Lebedev and Yu I. Barashnev: Open external-internal hydrocephaly in early childhood. Sovetsk. Med. **22**, Nr. 11, 20 (1958). — 147. Knies, P. T., and H. E. Le Fever: Metabolic craniopathy: Hyperostosis frontalis interna. Ann. int. Med. **14**, 1858 (1941). — 148. Koch, G.: Tuberose Sklerose. Zusammenfassender Bericht uber die wichtigsten Forschungsergebnisse des Auslandes. Ärztl. Forsch. **6**, 471 (1952). — 149. Kottgen, H. U.: Encephalographische Befunde bei der mongoloiden Idiotie. Mschr. Kinderheilk. **1942**, 41. — 150. Kottgen, H. U.: Encephalographische Untersuchungen bei der Spina bifida-Cystica. Dtsch. med. Wschr. **1949**, 307. — 151. Krayenbuhl, H.: Neurochirurgische Diagnostik und Therapie der Hemiplegie. Ein Beitrag zur Indikationsstellung der cerebralen Arteriographie. Dtsch. med. Wschr. **1950**, 1177. — 152. Krayenbuhl, H., u. H. R. Richter: Die cerebrale Angiographie. Stuttgart 1952. — 153. Krischek, J.: Über die Bedeutung des gleichmaßig-symmetrischen Hydrocephalus bei psychiatrischen und neurologischen Krankheitsbildern. Dtsch. Z. Nervenheilk. **174**, 61 (1955). — 154. Krischek, J.: Der symmetrische Hydrocephalus internus in der Beurteilung von gedeckten hirntraumatischen Folgezustanden. Psychiat. et Neurol. (Basel) **136**, 129 (1958). — 155. Krischek, J.: Pneumencephalographische Studien bei Epileptikern. Psychiat. et Neurol. (Basel) **138**, 345 (1959).

156. Lafon, R., C. Gros et J.-M. Enjalbert: Les hydrocéphalies latentes en psychiatrie. Rev. neurol. **82**, 435 (1950). — 157. Lafon, R., et R. Labauge: Le syndrome d'expansion cranienne homolatérale au cours des atrophies cérébrales unilatérales de l'enfant. Montpellier méd. **49**, 83 (1956). — 158. Lafon, R., P. Pages, P. Passouant, R. Labauge, J. Minvielle et J. Cadeilhac: Les données de la pneumoencéphalographie et de l'électroencéphalographie au cours de l'alcoolisme chronique. Rev. neurol. **94**, 611 (1956). — 159. Lafon, R., R. Labauge, J. P. Pemple et J. Minvielle: Aspects pneumographiques d'atrophie cérébelleuse. Rev. neurol. **95**, 63 (1956). — 160. Larsby, H., and E. Lindgren: Encephalographic examinations of 125 institutional epileptics. Acta psychiat. (Kbh.) **15**, 337 (1940). — 161. Laubenthal, F.: Encephalographische Erfahrungen bei der erblichen Epilepsie. Zbl. ges. Neurol. Psychiat. **82**, 709 (1936). — 162. Lemke, R.: Untersuchungen uber die soziale Prognose der Schizophrenie unter besonderer Berucksichtigung des encephalographischen Befundes. Arch. Psychiat. Nervenkr. (D.) **104**, 89 (1936). — 163. Lennartz, H., u. U. G. Maass: Cerebrale Gefäßerkrankungen und Hirnangiographie. Med. Klin. **1956**, 44 u. 62. — 164. Leppien, R.: Encephalographische Erfahrungen an klinisch gesichert genuinen Epileptikern (70 sichere und 29 hochstwahrscheinlich genuine Epileptiker, eine Auslese aus den Encephalogrammen von 200 Kranken). Allg. Z. Psychiat. **116**, 119 (1940). — 165. Leuchs, K.: Der cerebrale Alkoholschaden im Pneumencephalogramm. Zbl. ges. Neurol. Psychiat. **148**, 5 (1958). — 166. Lewy, F. H., and F. C. Grant: Physiopathologic and pathoanatomic aspects of major trigeminal neuralgia. Arch. Neurol. Psychiat. (Chicago) **40/2**, 1126 (1938). — 167. Liebaldt, G., u. W. Klages: Morphologische Befunde bei einer „isolierten chronischen taktilen Dermatozoenhalluzinose". Versuch einer Deutung. Nervenarzt **32**, 157 (1961). — 168. Lindgren, E.: Encephalography in cerebral atrophy. Acta radiol. (Stockh.) **35**, 277 (1951). — 169. Lindgren, E.: Pneumographie des Schadels. In: Lehrbuch der Rontgendiagnostik. Hrsg. v. Schinz, Baensch, Friedl, Uehlinger. 5. Aufl. Stuttgart 1952. — 170. Lindgren, E.: Rontgenologie einschließlich Kontrastmethoden. In: Handbuch der Neurochirurgie. Hrsg. v. H. Olivecrona u. W. Tonnis. Bd. II. Berlin-Gottingen-Heidelberg: Springer-Verlag 1954. — 171. Loepp, W., u. R. Lorenz: Rontgendiagnostik des Schadels. Stuttgart 1954. — 172. Lowenberg, K., D. A. Boyd jr. and D. D. Salon: Occurence of Pick's disease in early adult years. Arch. Neurol. Psychiat. (Chicago) **41**, 1004 (1939). — 173. Lorber, J.: Intracranial calcifications following tuberculous meningitis in children. Acta radiol. (Stockh.) **50**, 204 (1958). — 174. Lorenz, K.: Verkalkungen des Plexus chorioideus der Seitenventrikel als Folge kongenitaler Toxoplasmose. Fortschr. Rontgenstr. **73**, 735 (1950). — 175. Lorenz, R.: Die Bedeutung der Luftabsorption nach Encephalographie für Sitz und Art des intrakraniellen Prozesses. Dtsch. Z. Nervenheilk. **152**, 230 (1941). — 176. Lüthy, F.: Liquor cerebrospinalis einschließlich Rontgendiagnostik der Liquorräume. In: Handbuch der inneren

Medizin. Hrsg. v. G. v. BERGMANN u. R. STAEHELIN. Bd. 5: Krankheiten des Nervensystems. S. 403. Berlin 1939. — 177. LUGARESI, E., e R. REGGIANI: Le craniostenosi. Sindromi neurologiche da precoce sinostosi delle suture. Riv. oto-neuro-oftal 33, 247 (1958). — 178. LUZZATTO, A., e A. MASCIOCCHI: A Propotie del quadro pneumoencefalografico e cisternografico nell oligofrenia fenilpiruvica. Neurone (Mantova) 5, 7 (1957).

179. MAURER, H.: Über encephalographische Befunde bei Schwachsinnigen. Med. Welt 13/1, 699 (1939). — 180. MAURER, H.: Zur encephalographischen Diagnose des Balkenmangels. Nervenarzt 13, 454 (1940). — 181. MALLISON, R.: Senile und präsenile Hirnkrankheiten. In: Handbuch der inneren Medizin. Hrsg. v. G. v. BERGMANN, W. FREY, H. SCHWIEGK. Bd. V/3: Neurologie. Red. v. R. JUNG. S. 1031. Berlin-Göttingen-Heidelberg: Springer-Verlag 1953. — 182. MARSHALL, J., and C. W. M. WHITTY: Value of pneumoencephalography in diagnosis of fits. Brit. med. J. 4763, 847 (1952). — 183. MARTIN, H. O.: Sella turcica und Konstitution. Leipzig: G. Thieme 1941. — 184. MATTHIAS, H.: Pneumencephalographische Befunde am alternden Gehirn. Psychiat. Neurol. med. Psychol. (Lpz.) 7, 212 (1955). — 185. MAYER, E. G.: Diagnose und Differentialdiagnose in der Schadelrontgenologie. Wien 1950. — 186. McALPINE, D.: Toxic hydrocephalus. Brain 60, 180 (1937). — 187. McCAUSLAND, A. M., and S. J. McCLENDON: Encephalomyelitis following measles. Case report with encephalogram. Arch. Pediat. 51, 178 (1934). — 188. McRAE, D. L.: Die Krampferkrankungen. In: Klinische Neuroradiologie. Hrsg. v. K. DECKER. S. 181. Stuttgart 1960. — 189. MIURA, N.: Psychiatrische encephalographische Studien. I. Mitt. Tôhoku J. exp. Med. 21, 137 (1933). — 190. MONIZ, E.: Die cerebrale Arteriographie und Phlebographie. In: Handbuch der Neurologie. Erg.-Bd. II. Berlin 1940. — 191. MOORE, M. T., D. NATHAN, A. R. ELLIOT and CH. LAUBACH: Encephalographic studies in schizophrenia (Dementia praecox). Amer. J. Psychiat. 89, 801 (1933). — 192. MOORE, M. T., D. NATHAN, A. R. ELLIOT and CH. LAUBACH: Encephalographic studies in mental disease. Amer. J. Psychiat. 92, 43 (1935). — 193. MOREA, R.: Encephalographie und Ventrikulographie. Übersichtsreferat. Zbl. ges. Neurol. Psychiat. 106, 1 (1949). — 194. MOREL, F., et E. WILDI: Les ventricules cérébraux dans la démence précoce. Mschr. Psychiat. Neurol. 127, 1 (1954). — 195. MULLER, D.: Über die physikalischen Grundlagen der Pneumencephalographie. Dargestellt am Modell und an klinischen Beispielen unter besonderer Berücksichtigung der sogenannten Fehlfullung der Ventrikel. Z. Kinderheilk. 76, 281 (1955). — 196. MÜLLER, D.: Physikalische Faktoren in der Pathogenese des sog. Hydrocephalus. Nervenarzt 29, 1 (1958). — 197. MUNDLER, F.: Recherche sur l'aspect radiologique des ventricules cérébraux dans l'épilepsie temporale. Confin. neurol. (Basel) 19, 415 (1959). — 198. MURPHY, J. P., and R. ARANA: Amer. J. Roentgenol. 57, 545 (1947). — 199. MUTSCHLER, D.: Die Toxoplasmose in ihrer Bedeutung für die Entstehung hirnatrophischer Prozesse. VII. Medizinische 1953, 46.

200. NAGY, K.: Pneumencephalographische Befunde bei akuten und chronischen Psychosen. Arch. Psychiat. Nervenkr. 198, 544 (1959). — 200a. NAGY, K.: Die Ergebnisse wiederholter Pneumencephalographie bei akuten und chronischen Psychosen. Wien. Z. Nervenheilk. 18, 357 (1961). — 201. NOBILE, S., e R. BRIZZI: La pneumoencefalografia negli schizofrenici. Riv. sper. Freniat. 77, 705 (1953). — 202. NOETZEL, H.: Über eine Encephalocele des Kleinhirns und ihr Róntgenbild. Nervenarzt 18, 398 (1947). — 203. NÜRNBERGER, S., u. G. SCHALTENBRAND: Messungen am Encephalogramm. Ein Beitrag zum Begriff des normalen Encephalogramms. Dtsch. Z. Nervenheilk. 174, 1 (1955).

204. OMOROKOW, L., u. A. WISCHNEWSKY: Beitrag zur Pneumencephalographie bei chronischen Formen epidemischer Encephalitis. Fortschr. Rontgenstr. 37, 823 (1928).

205. PAULIAN, D., et M. CHILIMAN: Syndrome schizophrénoide guéri par la pneumo-thérapie cérébrale. Arch. Neurol. (Bukarest) 4, 105 (1940). — 206. PENDERGRASS, E. P., and P. J. HODES: Encephalography: The volue of the second-day examination. Radiology 26, 146 (1936). — 207. PENFIELD, W.: Hydrocephalus and spina bifida. Surg. Gynec. Obstet. 60, 363 (1935). — 208. PÉRON, N., et M. GAYNO: Atrophie cérébrale des ethyliques. Rev. neurol. 94, 621 (1956). — 209. PETERS, G., u. G. STRUCK: Pathomorphologische Befunde bei chronisch verlaufenen hirnorganischen Prozessen. Fortschr. Neurol. Psychiat. 27, 549 (1959). — 210. PETIT-DUTAILLIS, D., et H. FISCHGOLD: Signes radiologiques de l'atrophie cérébrale accompagnée d'épilepsie focale. Rev. neurol. 83, 412 (1950). — 211. PONITZ, K.: Die Encephalographie in ihrer Bedeutung fur die Prognose des Paralyseverlaufs. Dtsch. Z. Nervenheilk. 117—119, 491 (1931). — 212. POSTEL, J., et P. COSSA: L'atrophie cérébrale des alcooliques chroniques, étude pneumoencéphalographique. Rev. neurol. 94, 604 (1956). — 213. PRIESS, H., u. W. BRENNER: Über Veränderungen der liquorführenden Räume bei chronischer tuberkulóser Meningitis. Z. Kinderheilk. 68, 607 (1950).

214. RAUSCH, F., W. SCHIEFER u. G. STRUCK: Über den Wert der cerebralen Angiographie für die Diagnose arteriosklerotischer Gefäßprozesse. Fortschr. Neurol. Psychiat. 24, 512 (1956). — 215. REITMANN, F.: Evaluation of air studies. Dis. nerv. Syst. 12, 44 (1951). — 216. RENNERT, H.: Grundsätzliches zur Planimetrie des Encephalogramms sowie zur einfachen Betrachtung von Schädelröntgenbildern. Arch. Psychiat. Nervenkr. 188, 390 (1952). —

217. RIECHERT, T.: Die Arteriographie der Hirngefäße. 2. Aufl. München 1949. — 218. RIT- TER, F.: Vermehrung der Impressiones digitatae im Rontgenbild. Dtsch. Z. Nervenheilk. **127**, 287 (1932). — 219. RIVES, J.: Encephalography as a therapeutic measure against headaches of nontraumatic origin. Folia neuropath. eston. **15/16**, 298 (1936). — 220. RIVES, J.: Zur Frage über die therapeutische Bedeutung der Encephalo- und Ventrikulographie. Folia neuropath. eston. **17**, 102 (1938). — 221. ROBERTSON, E. G.: Some physical aspects of ence- phalography. Brain **70**, 59 (1947). — 222. ROBERTSON, E. G.: Pneumo-encephalography. Oxford 1957. — 223. ROHMER, F., A. WACKENHEIM et C. VROUSOS: Les agénésies du corps calleux. Rapport de neurologie présenté au congrès de psychiatrie et de neurologie de langue française. LVIIe lession. Tours 1959. — 224. ROSS, A. T.: Cerebral hemiatrophy with compensatory homolateral hypertrophy of the skull and sinuses, and diminution of cranial volume. Amer. J. Roentgenol. **45**, 332 (1941). — 225. RUGGERI, R.: L'encephalografia nella pratica neuropsichiatrica infantile. Arch. ital. Pediat. **6**, 531 (1938). — 226. RUGGIERO, G.: L'encéphalographie fractionnée. Préface de Erik Lindgren. Présentation de Marcel David. Paris 1957. — 227. RUPILIUS, K.: Über cerebrale Storungen im Kindesalter und ihre ence- phalographische Diagnostik. III. Mitt. B. Die rontgenologische Diagnostik durch die Ence- phalographie. II. Pathologische Encephalogramme. Arch. Kinderheilk. **103**, 156 (1934). — 228. RUPRECHT, A., u. E. SCHERZER: Die cerebrale Angiographie in der klinischen Neurologie. Wien. med. Wschr. **1958**, 589. — 229. RUSSELL, D. S.: Observations on the Pathology of Hydrocephalus. Med. Res. Coun. London 1949. — 230. RUSSELL, D. S., and C. DONALD: The mechanism of internal hydrocephalus in spina bifida. Brain **58**, 203 (1935).

231. SAGINARIO, M., V. PELLICCIOLI et G. C. GUAZZI: Les possibilités de diagnostic pendant la vie de la calcinose cérébrale (maladie de Fahr). Etude clinico-radiologique. Rev. Neurol. **97**, 251 (1957). — 232. SANTAGATI, F., e T. DE SANCTIS: Ricerche encefalografiche nella Schizofrenia. Riv. sper. Freniat. **76**, 603 (1952). — 233. SCHALLOCK, G.: Pathologisch-ana- tomische Befunde bei tuberkuloser Meningitis unter Streptomycinbehandlung. Fortschr. Diagn. Therap. 1, Nr. 3 (1949). — 234. SCHALTENBRAND, G.: Die Abhangigkeit des Ence- phalogramms vom äußeren Atmosphärendruck. Zbl. ges. Neurol. Psychiat. **61**, 524 (1932). — 235. SCHALTENBRAND, G., u. W. TONNIS: Traumatischer Hydrocephalus. Zbl. Neurochir. 1, 42 (1936). — 236. SCHEER, W. M. VAN DER: Beiträge zur Kenntnis der mongoloiden Idiotie. Berlin 1927. — 237. SCHEID, W.: Die Zirkulationsstorungen des Gehirns und seiner Haute. In: Handbuch der inneren Medizin. Hrsg. v. G. v. BERGMANN, W. FREY, H. SCHWIEGK. Bd. V/3: Neurologie. Red. v. R. JUNG. S. 1. Berlin-Gottingen-Heidelberg: Springer-Verlag 1953. — 238. SCHEID, W.: Diagnose, Aufbau der Diagnose und Differentialdiagnose in der Neurologie. Nervenarzt **30**, 97 (1959). — 239. SCHEIDEGGER, W.: Katatone Todesfalle in der Psychiatrischen Klinik von Zürich von 1900 bis 1928. Z. ges. Neurol. Psychiat. **120**, 587 (1929). — 240. SCHIERS- MANN, O.: Einführung in die Encephalographie. (Pneumencephalographie). 2. verb. Aufl. Stuttgart 1952. — 241. SCHIFFER, K. H.: Zur Auswertung von Ventrikelbildern am Ence- phalogramm. Fortschr. Rontgenstr. **75**, 50 (1951). — 242. SCHIFFER, K. H.: Cerebrale Früh- schadigung und Schädelbasisdysplasie. Fortschr. Rontgenstr. **75**, 54 (1951). — 243. SCHIFFER, K. H.: Rontgenbefunde an der zentralen Schädel-Hirnbasis als morphologische Indizien in der Konstitutionsbiologie. Fortschr. Rontgenstr. **75**, 59 (1951). — 244. SCHIFFER, K. H.: Konstitutionsbiologische Korrelationen von Schadelbasis- und Encephalogrammbefunden. Z. menschl. Vererb.- u. Konstit.-Lehre **32**, 345 (1954). — 245. SCHIFFER, K. H.: Zur mehr- dimensionalen Betrachtung in der Psychiatrie am Beispiel neuroradiologischer und erb- biologischer Befunde. In: Mehrdimensionale Diagnostik und Therapie. Festschrift zum 70. Ge- burtstag von E. KRETSCHMER. Stuttgart 1958. — 246. SCHIFFER, K. H., u. H. STRUBEL: Über Storungen der Entwicklungsmechanik des Gehirnschädels beim Mongolismus und anderen Konstitutionsanomalien. Nervenarzt **31**, 340 (1960). — 247. SCHILF, E.: Über zwei Zustands- bilder am Nervensystem (Hydroc. internus und Radiculitis) nach Kohlenoxydeinwirkung nebst Erörterung der „Vergiftung" durch Kohlenoxyd. Psychiat. Neurol. med. Psychol. (Lpz.) **3**, 193 (1951). — 248. SCHMIDT, H., u. E. FISCHER: Die occipitale Dysplasie. Stuttgart 1960. — 249. SCHMIEDER, F.: Das Encephalogramm nach Fleckfieber. Klin. Wschr. **1948**, 14. — 250. SCHMITT, W.: Zur Problematik der „chronischen" Kohlenoxydvergiftung. Nervenarzt **31**, 351 (1960). — 251. SCHNEIDER, A.: Sellabrücke und Konstitution. Leipzig: G. Thieme 1939. — 252. SCHÖNENBERG, H.: Klinische und encephalographische Befunde bei Verdacht auf Cavum Vergae. Z. Kinderheilk. **68**, 512 (1950). — 253. SCHONENBERG, H.: Zur Frage des Hydrocepha- lus internus bei der Meningitis tuberculosa vor und im Verlauf der Streptomycinbehandlung. Ärztl. Wschr. **1950**, 106. — 254. SCHONENBERG, H., u. E. J. OTT: Zur Frage der Mikroventri- kulie (KEHRER) im Kindesalter. Z. Kinderheilk. **72**, 258 (1953). — 255. SCHONENBERG, H., u. O. WOLFF: Die klinische Bedeutung der Cisterna interventrikularis. Mschr. Kinderheilk. **104**, 410 (1956). — 256. SCHULLER, A.: Schädelanomalien und psychische Storungen. Wien. klin. Wschr. **40**, Nr. 36 (1927). — 257. SCHULTE, W.: Hirnorganische Dauerschaden nach Dystrophie: Wesensanderung, Epilepsien und Apoplexien. Med. Klin. **46**, 1356 (1951). — 258. SCHULTE, W.: Hirnorganische Dauerschaden nach schwerer Dystrophie. München-

Berlin 1953. — 259. SCHULTE, W., u. R. STIAWA: Organische Hirnschädigungen nach schwerer Hungerdystrophie. Eine Zwischenbilanz über den derzeitigen Stand der Erfahrungen. Fortschr. Neurol. Psychiat. **26**, 66 (1958). — 260. SELBACH, H.: Die cerebralen Anfallsleiden: Genuine Epilepsie, symptomatische Hirnkrämpfe und die Narkolepsie. In: Handbuch der inneren Medizin. Hrsg. v. G. v. BERGMANN, W. FREY, H. SCHWIEGK. Bd. V/3: Neurologie. Red. v. R. JUNG. S. 1082. Berlin-Göttingen-Heidelberg: Springer-Verlag 1953. — 261. SJÖGREN, H.: Neuro-psychiatric studies in presenile and senile diseases, based on a material of 1000 cases. (Introductory lecture.) Acta psychiat. (Kbh.) Suppl. **106**, 9 (1956). — 262. SJÖGREN, T., H. SJÖGREN and A. G. H. LINDGREN: Morbus Alzheimer and Morbus Pick. A genetic, clinical and patho-anatomical study. Copenhagen 1952. — 263. SORNIKOVA, V. A.: Die Beurteilung der Ausdehnung des pathologischen Prozesses bei Syringomyelie nach Befunden der Pneumencephalographie. Z. Nevropath. i. t. d. **55**, 214 (1955). — 264. SOYKA, D.: Hirnatrophische Defektzustände nach Dystrophie und ihre Pathogenese. Nervenarzt **29**, 347 (1948). — 265. SPATZ, H.: Die „systematischen Atrophien". Arch. Psychiat. Nervenkr. **108**, 1 (1938). — 266. STALLWORTHY, K. R., and P. P. E. SAVAGE: Clinical aspects of cerebral atrophy revealed by encephalography. N. Z. med. J. **54**, 457 (1955). — 267. STANKIEWICZ, REMI, et M. KOWALEWSKI: L'encéphalographie et la ventriculographie chez les enfants d'après des observations personnelles. Rev. franç. Pédiat. **14**, 321 (1938). — 268. STENVERS, H. W.: Röntgendiagnostik. In: Handbuch der Neurologie (BUMKE/FOERSTER), VII/2. S. 139. Berlin: Springer 1936. — 269. STENZEL, E.: Bedeutung und Verwertung der Diploëvenen im Röntgenbild des Schädels. Nervenarzt **25**, 11 (1954). — 270. STERTZ, G.: Über den Anteil des Zwischenhirns an der Symptomgestaltung organischer Erkrankungen des Zentralnervensystems: Ein diagnostisch brauchbares Zwischenhirnsyndrom. Dtsch. Z. Nervenheilk. **117/119**, 630 (1931). — 271. STÖCKL, E.: Über Beziehungen zwischen Sellabild, Konstitution und hypophysärer Mangelleistung bei genitalkranken Jugendlichen. Z. Geburtsh. Gynäk. **141**, 65 (1954). — 272. STONE, R. S., and O. W. JONES: Encephalography. A review of 113 cases, and a report of postmortem studies on the injection of air. Radiology **21**, 411 (1933). — 273. STRASSMANN, G. S.: Über die allgemein-medizinische Bedeutung der Altersveränderungen des Gehirns. Medizinische **1956**, 568. — 274. STROHMAYER, W.: Angeborene und im frühen Kindesalter erworbene Schwachsinnzustände. In: Handbuch der Geisteskrankheiten (BUMKE). X. Bd. Berlin: Springer 1928. — 275. STRUCK, G.: Morphologische Untersuchungen bei hirnatrophischen Prozessen des mittleren Lebensalters. Zbl. ges. Neurol. Psychiat. **147**, 13 (1958). — 276. STRUCKE, F.: Zur klinischen Diagnostik beginnender und atypischer hirnatrophischer Prozesse mit Hilfe des Encephalogramms. Allg. Z. Psychiat. **121**, 239 (1942). — 277. STUTTE, H.: Zur Klinik des chronischen Hydrocephalus internus im Kindes- und Jugendalter. Z. ges. Neurol. Psychiat. **173**, 495 (1941).

278. TAMURA, Y., u. T. MATSUMURA: Beiträge zu den encephalographischen Studien. 1. Mitt.: Über die Befunde bei wiederholter Encephalographie. Psychiat. Neurol. jap. **40**, 227 (1936). — 279. TAVERAS, I. M.: Die neuroradiologische Untersuchung im Kindesalter. In: Klinische Neuroradiologie. Hrsg. v. K. DECKER. S. 364. Stuttgart 1960. — 280. THALHAMMER, O.: Die Toxoplasmose bei Mensch und Tier. Wien-Bonn 1957. — 281. THIEFFRY, S., J. LEFÈBVRE, J. LEPINTRE, C. FAURÉ et S. MASSELIN: Contribution à l'étude radiologique des malformations du plan sagittal interhémisphérique à propos de 45 observations. Acta radiol. (Stockh.) **50**, 242 (1958). — 282. TÖNNIS, W.: Hydrocephalus infolge Liquorzirkulationsstörungen. Arch. Kinderheilk. **118**, 65 (1939). — 283. TÖNNIS, W.: Die Behandlung der frischen, gedeckten Hirnverletzung im Hinblick auf die Verhütung der Hirnleistungsschwäche. Nervenarzt **19**, 201 (1948). — 284. TORKILDSON, A., and W. PENFIELD: Ventriculographic interpretation. Arch. Neurol. Psychiat. (Chicago) **30**, 1011 (1933). — 285. TROLAND, C. E., D. H. BAXTER and R. SCHATZKI: J. Neurol. Psychiat. **3**, 390 (1946). — 286. TROLLE, E., and M. FOG: Encephalography in non-surgical neurological diagnostic. Acta psychiat. (Kbh.) Suppl. **74**, 193 (1951).

287. ULRICH: Zur Frage des 5. Ventrikels. Psychiat. Neurol. med. Psychol. (Lpz.) **1**, 158 (1949). — 288. UNGER, H.: Anomalien der Occipito-Cervikal-Region und ihre klinische Symptomatik. Arch. phys. Ther. (Lpz.) **10**, 430 (1958).

289. VASILIU, D. O.: Sur la nécessité de drainer complètement le liquide céphalorachidien et d'injecter une égale quantité d'air, dans l'encéphalo-graphie. Rev. Chir. **41**, 128 (1938). — 290. VERCELLI, G.: Sindromi cliniche di sclerosi a placche con reperto di stato idrocefalico all encefalografia. Forme ipertensive della sclerosi a placche e sindromi da ipertensione. Riv. oto-neuro-oftal. **12**, 658 (1935). — 291. VILLINGER, W.: Abnorme seelische Reaktionen im Kindesalter. (Zum Problem: Psychopathie-Neuropathie-Neurose.) Mschr. Kinderheilk. **99**, 93 (1951). — 292. VINKEN, P. J., and A. STRACKEE-KUJIER: Two cases of absence of the septum pellucidum in the pneumoencephalogram. Folia psychiat. neerl. **60**, 226 (1957). — 293. VINKEN, P. J., F. RODENBOOG and J. HUIZINGA: The ventrikel-index in Epileptics, a pneumencephalographic study. Proceedings, Series C, 61, Nr. 1, 1958.

294. WAGNER, F. F.: Brain atrophy in a psychiatric clinic diagnoses by pneumoencephalography. Acta psychiat. (Kbh.) Suppl. **74**, 212 (1951). — 295. WARTENBERG, R.: Zur Encephalographie. Zbl. ges. Neurol. Psychiat. **61**, 279 (1932). — 296. WEATHERLY, H.: Amer. J. Roentgenol. **45**, 714 (1941). — 297. WEINTRAUB, W.: Étude des variations de la capacité des ventricules cérébraux. Paris 1953. — 298. WEITBRECHT, H. J.: Zur Frage der paranoiden Rückbildungspsychosen. Nervenarzt **12**, 330 (1939). — 299. WEITBRECHT, H. J.: Bemerkungen zu einem wiederholt encephalographierten Fall von progressiver Paralyse. Nervenarzt **13**, 433 (1940). — 300. WEITBRECHT, H. J.: Cyclothymes Syndrom und hirnatrophischer Prozeß. Nervenarzt **24**, 489 (1953). — 301. WEITBRECHT, H. J.: Depressive und manische endogene Psychosen. In: Psychiatrie der Gegenwart. Hrsg. v. H. W. GRUHLE, R. JUNG, W. MAYER-GROSS, M. MÜLLER. Bd. II: Klinische Psychiatrie, S. 73. Berlin-Göttingen-Heidelberg: Springer-Verlag 1960. — 302. WELKER, K.: Das Schädelröntgenbild bei mongoloider Idiotie. Hamburg: Dissertation 1931. — 303. WENDE, S.: Stirnhöhlenhyperplasie bei frühkindlicher Hirnschädigung. Ärztl. Wschr. **14**, 565 (1959). — 304. WIGERT, V.: Encephalographische Befunde bei sogenannten „Psychoneurosen". Acta psychiat. (Kbh.) **13**, 401 (1938). — 305. WILKE, G.: Über den Hirnbefund bei einem Heimkehrer mit schwerer Hungerdystrophie. Dtsch. Z. Nervenheilk. **171**, 388 (1954). — 306. WINKLER, H.: Arbeiten zur Frage des angeborenen Schwachsinns. IV. Mitteilung: Encephalographische Befunde bei angeborenem und früherworbenem Schwachsinn. Arch. Psychiat. Nervenkr. **91**, 495 (1930). — 307. WOLFF, H., u. L. BRINKMANN: Das normale Encephalogramm. Dtsch. Z. Nervenheilk. **151**, 1 (1940). — 308. WORTIS, H.: Ligation of the common carotid artery: Clinical picture and encephalographic study in a case eight years later. Arch. Neurol. Psychiat. (Chicago) **36**, 894 (1936).

309. YAMAMOTO, S.: Über das Encephalogramm der Schizophrenen. Fukuoka Acta med. **33**, Nr. 4 (1940).

310. ZELLWEGER, H.: Die Beurteilung der Subarachnoidalräume im Säuglingsencephalogramm. Ann. paediat. (Basel) **174**, 97 (1950). — 311. ZELLWEGER, H.: Die Cisterna interventricularis und ihre klinische Bedeutung. Helv. paediat. Acta **6**, 484 (1951). — 312. ZELLWEGER, H.: Kasuistischer Beitrag zum Problem der Cyclencephalie und des Congenital single lateral ventricle. Helv. paediat. Acta (Ser. D) **7**, 98 (1952). — 313. ZELLWEGER, H., BEIRUT u. G. v. MURALT: Zur Pathologie des Septum pellucidum im Pneumoencephalogramm (PEG). Helv. paediat. Acta (Ser. D) **7**, 229 (1952).

Verhaltensforschung und Psychiatrie

Von

Detlev Ploog, München

Inhalt

Einleitung

Die Freude der Fische

Tschuang-Tse und Hui-Tse standen auf der Brücke, die über den Hao führt. Tschuang-Tse sagte: „Sieh, wie die Ellritzen umherschnellen! Das ist die Freude der Fische."

„Du bist kein Fisch", sagte Hui-Tse, „wie kannst du wissen, worin die Freude der Fische bestehe ?"

„Du bist nicht ich", antwortete Tschuang-Tse, „wie kannst du wissen, daß ich nicht wisse, worin die Freude der Fische bestehe ?"

„Ich bin nicht du", bestätigte Hui-Tse, „und ich weiß dich nicht. Aber das weiß ich, daß du kein Fisch bist; so kannst du die Fische nicht wissen."

Tschuang-Tse antwortete: „Kehren wir zu deiner Frage zurück. Du fragst mich, ‚wie kannst du wissen, worin die Freude der Fische bestehe‘. Im Grunde wußtest du, daß ich weiß, und fragtest doch. Gleichviel: ich weiß es aus meiner eigenen Freude über dem Wasser."

(Der alte Chinese Tschuang-Tse. Deutsche Auswahl von Martin Buber. Insel-Verlag, Leipzig 1910.)

Dieser Beitrag handelt von *biologischen Grundlagen instinktiven und affektiven Verhaltens*. Unter diesem naturwissenschaftlichen Aspekt nimmt der Mensch seinen Platz als das am höchsten organisierte Säugetier ein. Die Beziehungen zur Psychopathologie und Psychiatrie werden vorwiegend durch die Auswahl des Stoffes — also sozusagen zwischen den Zeilen — hergestellt.

Da das Thema Verhaltensforschung bisher in keinem deutschen psychiatrischen Lehr- oder Handbuch abgehandelt worden ist, schien mir die Aufgabe, eine neue Informationsquelle, Anregung und Diskussionsgrundlage zu geben, vordringlicher zu sein, als das zum Thema gehörige psychiatrische Schrifttum selbst voll zu berücksichtigen. Die Fülle der bisher in der Verhaltensforschung erzielten Ergebnisse ist derart groß, daß eine Beschränkung in der Auswahl des Stoffes notwendig war. So wurden auch nur solche empirisch fundierten Resultate dargestellt, von denen ich hoffe, daß sie für die Psychiatrie wertvoll sind. Der Leser mag dem Inhaltsverzeichnis entnehmen, welche Gebiete berührt werden. Freilich liegt in dieser Auswahl ein subjektives Ermessen, das auch vom eigenen Kenntnis- und Interessenbereich mitbestimmt ist.

Manchmal ist die Darstellung historisch orientiert, nämlich dann, wenn eine Entdeckung entscheidend war und sich die daraus abgeleiteten Folgerungen durch weitere Experimente bestätigen ließen. Meist jedoch wird der nicht-historische Weg unter besonderer Berücksichtigung der Ergebnisse aus den letzten 10 Jahren beschritten.

A. Die vergleichende Erforschung angeborenen Verhaltens (Ethologie)

I. Methoden und Theorien der Ethologie

1. Abgrenzung gegenüber anderen biologischen Verhaltenslehren

Unter dem Titel „Ethologie" inaugurierte JOHN STUART MILL (*147*) in seinem "System of Logic" (1843) die Schaffung einer „exakten Wissenschaft der menschlichen Natur", worunter er eine auf Erfahrungsregeln gründende und zu kausalen Gesetzen vorstoßende Lehre vom Charakter verstanden wissen wollte. MILL sagt: Bevor wir nicht die Erfahrungsregeln in die Gesetze der Ursachen, von denen sie abhängen, aufgelöst haben und uns klar darüber geworden sind, daß diese Ursachen sich auf den Fall, den wir im Auge haben, beziehen, kann man unseren Schlußfolgerungen nicht vertrauen (*2*). Dies entspricht dem Ansatz, den die moderne Ethologie als induktive Naturwissenschaft benutzt, um das *Verhalten* der Lebewesen empirisch zu erfassen und kausal zu erklären. Die Methodik beginnt mit der deskriptiven Erfassung durch Beobachtung und schreitet über ein systematisches Ordnen von Verhaltensweisen zur physiologischen Kausalanalyse des Verhaltens fort. Der Mensch ist in dieser Wissenschaft das im Sinne der Abstammungslehre höchstorganisierte Lebewesen und als solches besonderen Gesetzlichkeiten unterworfen, die durch die speziellen Wissenschaften vom Menschen, also z. B. die Anthropologie, Psychologie, Soziologie und Psychopathologie, untersucht werden. Will man als Naturforscher die speziellen und äußerst komplexen Gesetzlichkeiten, welche menschliches Verhalten und Seelenleben beherrschen, auf die nächst weiteren und allgemeineren Naturgesetze zurückführen, so sind es jene Gesetzlichkeiten, die das Verhalten von Lebewesen schlechthin beherrschen. Alle vom Menschen handelnden Wissenszweige benötigen auch die vergleichende Verhaltensforschung, ähnlich wie die Physiologie der Chemie und die Chemie der Physik bedarf (*134*).

Man wird nun bestürzt fragen: Und wo bleibt das Erleben, das „eigentlich" Seelische in dieser Wissenschaft? Die Antwort ist eindeutig: Da niemals über Erlebnisse von Tieren direkt etwas wird ausgesagt werden können (*74*), ist die subjektive Seite des Verhaltens nicht Gegenstand der Ethologie, sondern gehört in die spezielleren Wissenschaften der Human-Psychologie und -Psychopathologie. Gleichwohl werden wir sehen, daß der Ethologe auf indirekte Weise grundlegende Aussagen über Psychisches machen kann, und erst eine enge und geduldige Zusammenarbeit von Ethologen und Anthropologen verschiedener Disziplinen wird an das Licht bringen, auf welche besondere Weise diese grundlegenden Aussagen für das Seelenleben des Menschen zutreffen (*42, 60, 143, 179, 268, 269, 446*).

Dann wäre also die Ethologie eine Art von *Behaviorismus*, der sich ja radikal auf die objektiv faßbaren Vorgänge des Verhaltens und deren kausale Erklärung zu beschränken versucht? Für den Behavioristen gibt es jedoch den Begriff der angeborenen Verhaltensweisen nicht, obwohl er die Evolution der Organismen bejaht und hinsichtlich morphologischer Merkmale auch durchaus phylogenetisch vergleichend denkt. Das Nervensystem ist in der behavioristischen Lehre eine Art Matrix, die dazu dient, Reflexe auszubilden. Diese gehorchen den Assoziationsgesetzen und bauen als kleinste Elemente das Verhalten auf. So *war* es jedenfalls in starker Vereinfachung gesehen. Daß es heute anders ist, werden wir später lesen (s. S. 395). Immerhin wird auch heute noch von manchen amerikanischen Verhaltensforschern (comparative physiological psychology), die Verhalten ganz unter dem Aspekt des *Lernens* sehen, bestritten, daß es differenzierte angeborene Verhaltensweisen gibt. Angeboren seien lediglich Typen von Nervensystemen bzw. der Bauplan einer Art, während sich Verhaltensweisen allein nach dem Reiz-Reaktions-Modell entwickeln sollen. Die Vererbung reiche bis zur Zygote; alles folgende sei Entwicklung. Über diese Fragen ist in den letzten Jahren eine lebhafte Auseinandersetzung entstanden (*120, 135, 178, 245, 246, 497, 500, 501, 540*), der eine grundsätzliche Bedeutung für die gesamte Verhaltensforschung zukommt (*136*).

Wenn die Ethologen vom „Angeborensein" sprechen, leugnen sie damit keineswegs Umwelteinflüsse, die in das Heranreifen von Verhaltensweisen eingreifen (335). Das Reflex-Modell ist aber auch für dieses Wechselspiel unzulänglich. Für den Ethologen bilden die Reflexe sozusagen einen Mantel um das angeborene Verhalten: sie verändern es im Rahmen seiner erblichen Variationsbreite; sie gehören mit dazu, sind aber gewiß nicht das Ganze (*6, 39, 133, 136*).

Die Behauptung, daß die Vererbung nur bis zur Zygote reicht, ist biologisch unmöglich. Warum sollten sich sonst alle Artangehörigen auf dieselbe Weise artgemäß entwickeln? Freilich mangelt es noch an Untersuchungen über den Erbgang von arteigenen Bewegungsweisen. Immerhin liegen bei Drosophila (*244*) und Vogelbastarden aussichtsreiche Befunde vor. Von Hörmann (*422*) konnte zwei nahverwandte Grillenarten (*639*) kreuzen, die sich in vier Merkmalen ihres Verhaltens deutlich unterschieden. Bei drei Merkmalen war der Erbgang monofaktoriell.

Auch gegen jene Richtung der Verhaltensforschung, die rein final denkt und die *Ziel- und Zweckhaftigkeit* (Directiveness und Purposiveness) *instinktiven Verhaltens* untersucht — wir nennen jetzt nur MacDougall als bekanntesten der älteren Forscher —, grenzt sich die Ethologie ab [s. Diskussion Lorenz—Bierens de Haan (*258, 531*)]. Finale und kausale Naturbetrachtung sind nur *miteinander* von Wert (*177*). Denn die Einsicht in Ziel und Zweck einer Kette von Ereignissen kann zwar das menschliche Bedürfnis nach der Sinnhaftigkeit eines Geschehens befriedigen, verleiht aber keineswegs die Fähigkeit, ein Geschehen zu dem als Ziel erkannten Enderfolg hinzulenken. Diese Macht gibt uns ausschließlich die Einsicht in die kausalen Zusammenhänge (*135*).

Für die *Psychopathologie* spielt diese Auseinandersetzung zwischen teleologischer und kausaler Betrachtungsweise eine große Rolle. Wenn vom Wesen des Menschen, von seinen Daseinsordnungen, aber auch vom Wesen „seiner" Krankheiten, nämlich den Psychosen, gesprochen wird, so mag das für eine philosophisch orientierte Psychopathologie von Wert sein und das Bedürfnis nach Sinnhaftigkeit befriedigen helfen. Dem kranken Menschen dagegen kann nur, wie auch sonst in der Medizin, durch Kausalanalyse der zur Krankheit führenden Vorgänge geholfen werden (*652*).

Die Ethologie legt größten Wert darauf, den Zweck eines Vorganges nicht mit seiner Erklärung zu verwechseln (*236*). Dies sollte man auch in der Human-Psychologie und -Psychopathologie bei der Diskussion der Trieblehren streng beachten. Manche Mißverständnisse ließen sich so vermeiden.

Schließlich haben wir der Ethologie noch die *Umweltlehre* Jacob v. Uexkülls (*200, 201*) gegenüberzustellen. Hier liegt der Unterschied nicht im Methodischen, sondern allein in den von v. Uexküll gezogenen philosophischen Konsequenzen. v. Uexküll leugnet nämlich die Existenz einer außersubjektiven Realität und erkennt nur den Einzel-Umwelten der unzähligen tierischen oder menschlichen Subjekte Wirklichkeitscharakter zu. In seiner Auseinandersetzung mit den Problemen der Phylogenese ist dieser vorzüglich beobachtende und beschreibende Forscher voreingenommen durch seine Lehre vom entelechial gefaßten Begriff des „Bauplanes" und bestreitet die heute von allen maßgebenden Forschern anerkannten Beweise der Evolutionslehre (*66, 70, 71, 83, 135, 167, 170, 171, 173, 333, 613, 614, 695, 696*). Die einzige uns bekannte Ausnahme macht hierin nur der heute häufig zitierte Adolf Portmann (*163*), der sich dann auch wegen seiner naturwissenschaftlich unzulänglichen Beweisführung eine harte Kritik der Ethologen gefallen lassen mußte (*480*).

Die Ethologie hat v. UEXKÜLL Entscheidendes zu verdanken. Er und unabhängig von ihm auch H. S. JENNINGS (*95*) haben die ganzheitsbezogene Analyse in die Verhaltensforschung eingeführt und stets ein Systemganzes untersucht, in dem der Organismus und sein Lebensraum in vielfältiger Wechselwirkung stehen. Die Analyse beginnt mit der Frage: Welche Gegebenheiten der Umgebung sind es, die einerseits reaktionsauslösend auf das Tier wirken, andrerseits aber durch die so ausgelöste Aktivität des Tieres derart verändert werden, daß diese Wirkung ihrerseits wieder vom Organismus rezipierend beantwortet wird? Dieser „Funktionskreis" — eng verwandt dem Gestaltkreis V. v. WEIZSÄCKERs —, diese Doppelbeziehung, die Receptor und Effector zwischen Tier und Umgebung herstellen, ergibt eine Einteilung der tierischen Umwelt in zwei Sektoren, in die „*Merkwelt*", die alle aus der Umgebung rezipierten Reize umfaßt, und

in die „*Wirkwelt*"; diese besteht aus den Angriffsflächen, die den Effectoren des Tieres von der Umgebung geboten werden (siehe Abbildung 1). Bildlich gesprochen, so sagt v. UEXKÜLL, greift jedes Tiersubjekt mit zwei Gliedern einer Zange sein Objekt an — einem Merk- und einem Wirkgliede. Mit dem einen Gliede erteilt es dem Objekt ein Merkmal und mit dem anderen ein Wirkmal. Dadurch werden bestimmte Eigenschaften des Objektes zu Merkmalsträgern und andere zu Wirkmalsträgern. Am recht bekannt gewordenen Beispiel von der Zecke kann man den „Funktionskreis" veranschaulichen:

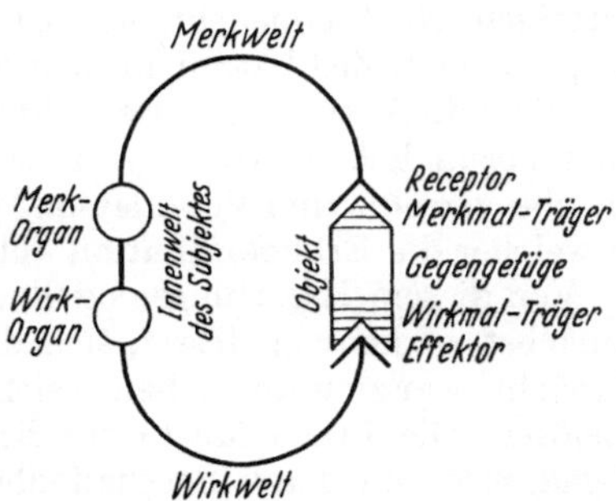

Abb. 1. Der Funktionskreis [J. VON UEXKÜLL (*201*)]

Die Zecke, deren normale Wirtstiere Säuger (Merkmalträger) sind, sticht in alle Objekte, die nach Buttersäure (Merkmal) riechen und eine Temperatur von 37° C (Merkmal) haben, auch wenn diese Objekte keine Angriffsflächen (Wirkmal) für die Effectoren (Bohrrüssel) des Tieres bieten. Am Beispiel der Zecke leitet v. UEXKÜLL die Grundzüge des Aufbaues der Umwelten ab, die für alle Tiere gültig sind.

2. Das Konzept der Ethologie

CHARLES O. WHITMAN (*205*) und OSKAR HEINROTH (*397*) um die Jahrhundertwende und vor diesen schon D. A. SPALDING (*760*) entdeckten unabhängig voneinander, daß es bestimmte Bewegungsweisen gibt, die für Arten, Gattungen, Ordnungen, ja selbst für die größten taxonomischen Kategorien ebenso kennzeichnend sind wie irgendwelche morphologischen Merkmale. Die Kratzbewegung mit dem Hinterbein, die allen Amnioten (Reptilien, Vögeln, Säugern) eigen ist, liefert ein Beispiel dafür, daß solche Bewegungen unter Umständen konservativer durch die Stammesgeschichte gehen als manche morphologische Struktur. WHITMAN und HEINROTH kannten das Verhalten der von ihnen untersuchten Gruppen (Tauben- und Entenvögel) bis in die feinsten Einzelheiten aus jahrelanger, liebevoller Beobachtung und überzeugten davon, daß *der Homologiebegriff*[1] *der morphologischen Phylogenetik (167) auf bestimmte Verhaltensweisen anwendbar* ist (*237*).

---

[1] Homolog sind Strukturen gemeinsamer phylogenetischer Herkunft, auch wenn sie in der Phylogenie heteromorph, heterotop oder heterochron abgewandelt sind (*70, 167*). Lediglich analog sind Organe übereinstimmenden oder ähnlichen Baues, die nicht denselben Bestandteil des Bauplanes verkörpern und somit trotz ihrer Ähnlichkeit einen ganz verschiedenen morphologischen Wert besitzen.

Diese *artgebundenen Bewegungsweisen* sind trotz aller Starrheit oder Gleich-
förmigkeit des Ablaufs nicht Reflexen vergleichbar, sondern durch eine höchst
eigenartige *Spontaneität* ausgezeichnet. Wie Whitmans Schüler Wallace Craig
zeigte, bildet eine starre, artbezeichnende Bewegungskoordination[1] in sehr vielen
Fällen das letzte und konstante Glied einer längeren Kette von solchen Verhaltensweisen, die ihrerseits zweckgerichtet sind. Dieses zweckgerichtete, plastische Verhalten nannte Craig appetitive behavior (*31*) und Lorenz Appetenzverhalten (*131*).
Damit war vorläufig Klarheit in einen alten Streit gebracht: Plastizität und Starrheit von Instinkthandlungen erwiesen sich als zwei voneinander zu trennende Vorgänge. Jede arteigene „Erbkoordination", wie Lorenz die Endhandlung auch
nannte, kann zum Ziel eines Appetenzverhaltens werden. Die Erbkoordination
selbst ist nicht zweckgerichtet. Wer Hunger hat, *strebt nach Nahrung* (Appetenzverhalten) und vollzieht mit der Nahrungsaufnahme die Endhandlung, *ohne* dabei
den biologischen Zweck der Lebenserhaltung, des Größer- oder Dickerwerdens zu
verfolgen. Noch einleuchtender ist es bei der sexuellen Appetenz, die den Begattungsakt zum Ziel hat, nicht aber die arterhaltende Fortpflanzung. Je länger eine
zielbildende Bewegungsweise nicht ausgelöst wird, desto stärker wird sie zum Motiv
im ursprünglichen Wortsinn, indem sie den ganzen Organismus in Bewegungs-
unruhe versetzt und Veranlassung gibt, aktiv nach einer Reizsituation zu suchen,
in welcher die Erbkoordination ablaufen kann.

Von diesem Handlungsmodell, das Lorenz aufstellte, ohne Craigs Ergebnisse
zunächst zu kennen, lassen sich die *Hauptfragestellungen der Ethologie* ableiten.
Zunächst war zu untersuchen, welche Reizsituationen sind es, die eine Endhandlung
auslösen. Die Frage führte zur Entdeckung der sog. *Schlüssel-, Auslöser-* oder
Signalreize und deren Beschaffenheit sowie zu dem für die Verhaltensforschung
zentral wichtigen Begriff des *angeborenen Auslösemechanismus* (AAM), ursprünglich von seinem Entdecker Konrad Lorenz (*531*) „angeborenes Schema" benannt.

Die Beobachtung, daß Erbkoordinationen sich um so leichter auslösen lassen
je länger sie nicht abgelaufen sind, legte die Annahme einer *Schwellenerniedrigung*
für Ablauf und Auslösung der Bewegungen nahe und brachte Lorenz zur *Hypothese
der Kumulierung aktionsspezifischer Energie* infolge einer *endogenen Reizproduktion*
des Nervensystems (*531*). Die zur Stütze dieser Hypothese beigebrachten Beobachtungen trafen mit neurophysiologischen Ergebnissen zusammen, die Erich v.
Holst mit seinen Untersuchungen zur relativen Koordination automatisch-
rhythmischer Vorgänge erzielt hatte (*413, 414*). Diese Versuche dienten als Grundlage für die im Anschluß an Graham Brown entwickelte *Lehre von der Automatie zentralnervöser Elemente*, also der Auffassung, daß viele Neuronensysteme
auf Grund von Stoffwechselprozessen auch dann weiterarbeiten, wenn die peripheren Afferenzen unterbunden sind (*85*). Es lag nahe, eine enge Verwandtschaft
zwischen der endogenen Reizproduktion und der zentralen Automatie anzunehmen[2].

Das sich aus den Arbeiten von Lorenz ergebende *Diagramm einer Handlung*
ist also aus drei verschiedenen Anteilen zusammengesetzt: dem Appetenzverhalten,
dem Ansprechen des angeborenen Auslösemechanismus und dem Ablaufen der
Erbkoordination. Dieses Diagramm entspricht, wie die weitere Forschung zeigte,
einem seltenen, einfachen Spezialfall. Meist aber sind diese Bestandteile zu sehr

---

[1] "consummatory act" (Craig), „triebverzehrende Endhandlung" (Lorenz).
[2] Die Frage, ob es wirklich eine reine Automatie von Ganglienzellen ohne jeglichen afferenten Impulseinstrom gibt, ist noch umstritten. Da es sich letztlich um ein spezifisch neurophysiologisches Problem handelt, gehen wir trotz der Gewichtigkeit dieser Frage auch für die Triebtheorie nicht näher auf sie ein, sondern verweisen auf die entsprechende Literatur (*39, 85, 174,
192, 782, 800*). Wir halten die zentrale Automatie für eine gut gesicherte Tatsache. Auch
Receptoren weisen Automatie auf. Für die Herzphysiologie ist sie seit langem erwiesen.

komplexen Gebilden zusammengefügt, deren Aufbau einer *hierarchischen Organisation* zentralnervöser Leistungen entspricht.

Eine geschlossene und genügend durch Experimente gestützte Theorie der vergleichenden Verhaltensforschung steht noch aus. Fast alle der soeben gedrängt wiedergegebenen Forschungsansätze befinden sich in der Entwicklung. Die verwendeten Begriffe werden von ethologischer Seite selbst noch überprüft und wurden z. B. von BAERENDS eingehend kritisiert (7). Vor allem solche Vergleiche, die auf menschliches Verhalten abzielen, müssen besonders kritisch ausfallen. Fürs erste wollen wir nur bedenken, daß das bisherige *Konzept der Ethologie wesentlich aus Erfahrungen mit Vögeln, Fischen und Insekten entstanden* ist. Der Einwand, daß man so verschiedene Tiergruppen nicht vergleichen dürfe, da die zugrunde liegenden Verhaltensmechanismen nicht identisch sein können (497), hat aber doch kein entscheidendes Gewicht; denn die Physiologie der Säugetiere ist uns letzten Endes auch durch Erfahrungen an Fröschen, Seeigeleiern, Hühnerembryonen und Riesenneuronen von Tintenfischen nähergekommen (23), von den Erfolgen der experimentellen Therapie in der Medizin ganz abzusehen. Dem Mangel an analytischen Beobachtungen bei Säugern (51, 114) bemüht man sich besonders in den letzten Jahren abzuhelfen. Wir werden in unserer Darstellung das *Verhalten der Säuger* besonders berücksichtigen.

II. Kausale Analyse des Instinktverhaltens

Voraussetzung zur Analyse des Instinktverhaltens oder — was für die Ethologie dasselbe bedeutet — des angeborenen Verhaltens ist eine möglichst vollständige *Bestandsaufnahme der Verhaltensweisen* (Ethogramm) einer Tierart (41, 533). Dies kann äußerst mühevoll und langwierig sein, verhindert aber, daß aus der Untersuchung einer speziellen Verhaltensweise unzulässige Verallgemeinerungen entstehen. Die Gefahr der vorzeitigen Verallgemeinerung besteht auch dann, wenn die an einer Verhaltensweise studierten Gesetzmäßigkeiten ohne komplexe Verhaltensanalyse auf andere Arten übertragen werden. Wenn z. B. der Gesang einer Vogelart als angeboren nachgewiesen wurde, so kann er bei einer anderen doch erlernt sein (719).

1. Verhalten als Antwort auf äußere Reize

Um sich eine Vorstellung davon machen zu können, wie ein Tier auf einen Reiz reagiert, müßte man vorher wissen, was es eigentlich wahrnehmen kann. Wie K. v. FRISCH (55, 347) und v. UEXKÜLL (200) so eindrucksvoll gezeigt haben, ist jedes Tier allein durch die Funktionsweise seiner Sinnesorgane, deren Beschaffenheit durch sinnesphysiologische Untersuchungen umrissen werden kann, an eine ganz spezielle Umwelt gekettet. Eine Maus z. B. hört einen anderen Frequenzbereich als der Mensch; von den überhaupt wahrnehmbaren Bereichen sind wiederum nur Teile bestimmter Qualität oder Intensität reaktionsauslösend (724). Erst wenn man weiß, daß der relevante Hörbereich der Maus im Ultraschallfrequenzband liegt, kann man ein systematisches Studium der reaktionsauslösenden Reize beginnen (818).

Um die Beschaffenheit der *Schlüssel-* oder *Auslöserreize* zu studieren, hat man vor allem *Attrappenversuche* angestellt. Zum Beispiel ist das Flugbild der Raubvögel kurznackig und langschwänzig, genau umgekehrt wie das von Enten und Gänsen. Um herauszufinden, welche Schlüsselreize für das Fluchtverhalten von Hühnervögeln wirksam sind, fertigten LORENZ und TINBERGEN 1937 verschieden konfigurierte Flugbilder aus Pappe an und ließen sie an einem waagerecht ausgespannten Draht über ihre Versuchsvögel hinweggleiten. Truthühner schienen

durch jedes kurznackige Modell alarmiert zu werden, dagegen kam es auf sonstige
Formmerkmale wenig an. Die Untersuchungen wurden von anderen mit unterschiedlichen Methoden und Ergebnissen wiederholt. Systematische Versuchsreihen
von Schleidt (725, 726) haben neuerdings ergeben, daß bei *unerfahrenen* Truthühnern allein die relative Größe und Geschwindigkeit von Flugobjekten angeborenermaßen Flugfeind-Reaktionen auslösen, während Gestaltmerkmale gelernt werden.

Abb. 2 soll veranschaulichen, daß bei Schlüsselreizen mehrere Faktoren im
Spiele sein können.

In anderen Fällen sind derartige Beziehungsmerkmale komplizierter: Frisch
geschlüpfte Silbermövenjunge „betteln" um Futter, indem sie nach der Spitze
des Elternschnabels picken (Abb. 3, S. 299). Der Schnabel des Altvogels ist
gelb und hat kurz vor der Unterschnabelspitze einen roten Fleck. Bietet man
dem Jungtier, noch ehe ein Artgenosse es
fütterte, eine Kopfattrappe aus Pappe in
natürlichen Farben mit rotem Fleck und
wahlweise eine andere Attrappe ohne den
roten Fleck, so wird die gefleckte bevorzugt. Die Frage war nun, ob lediglich die
Abhebung des Fleckes von der Grund-
farbe des Schnabels, ob die Farbe von
Schnabel und Fleck selbst oder ob der
Ort des Fleckes am Schnabel reaktionsauslösend sind. Das Ergebnis: Die Abhebung
des Fleckes vom Grunde ist wichtig; die
rote Farbe des Fleckes wirkt stark, dagegen das natürliche Gelb des Schnabels
nicht mehr als andere Farben; die Lage
des Fleckes relativ zu anderen Teilen
des Kopfes ist ausschlaggebend. Das
ganze, optimale Signal heißt also: „Ein

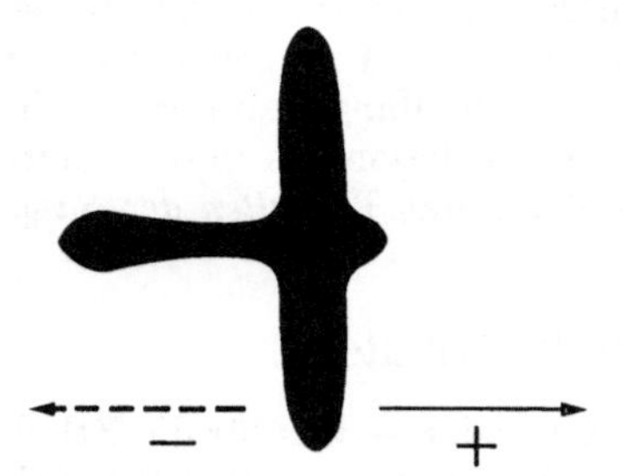

Abb. 2. In der Richtung des ausgezogenen Pfeiles
bewegt, löste die Attrappe Fluchtverhalten bei
Truthuhnern aus, da sie dann einem Raubvogel
ähnelt. In der Gegenrichtung bewegt, blieb sie wirkungslos. [Nach Tinbergen(197)] Durch neue
Untersuchungen von Schleidt (726) wurden diese
vielzitierten und mit unterschiedlichen Ergebnissen
nachgeprüften Versuche richtiggestellt: Relativ-
geschwindigkeit und Größe der Flugobjekte losen
angeborenermaßen Flugfeind-Reaktionen aus;
Gestaltmerkmale müssen gelernt werden

Fleck (am besten ein roter) nahe der Unterschnabelspitze" (*197*). Diese Kombination wirkt, gemessen an der Zahl der Pickbewegungen, am stärksten und gibt
ein gutes Beispiel für einen *figuralen Reiz von Gestaltcharakter* ab (*133*). Es zeigt
aber auch, daß unter Umständen eines oder wenige von mehreren normalerweise
vorkommenden Beziehungsmerkmalen wirksam sein können. Dieses häufig rein
additive Zusammenwirken von Schlüsselreizen hat Seitz (*197*) an Cichliden untersucht und als *Reizsummenregel* zusammengefaßt. Diese Regel besagt, daß in vielen
Fällen qualitativ verschiedene Signalreize gleichsinnig auslösend wirken und sich
quantitativ ersetzen können. Zum Beispiel ist für das Kampfgebaren des drei-
stacheligen Stichlings der rote Bauch des Gegners als Schlüsselreiz maßgebend.
Gerade so kampfauslösend wirkt aber auch ein qualitativ ganz anderer Reiz,
nämlich das Sich-auf-den-Kopf-stellen (Drohstellung) des Nebenbuhlers. Beide
Reize wirken normalerweise zusammen und verstärken einander (*197*). Die Ethologen sprechen in solchen Fällen von einer *Quantifizierung der Schlüsselreize* und
haben die Bedingungen, unter denen Schlüsselreize in verschiedenen Kombinationen reaktionsverstärkend wirken, an mehreren Arten in Attrappenversuchen
gut studiert. (Näheres folgt S. 301 ff., 315 ff.)

Die Tiere reagieren also auf die Attrappe, als sei sie ihresgleichen. Solch ein
„Reinfall" auf Attrappen, die erfahrungsfreien Jungtieren in isolierter Aufzucht
(sog. *Kaspar-Hauser-Versuch*) oder auch erfahrenen erwachsenen Tieren geboten
werden, ist ein Kennzeichen angeborenen Verhaltens. Die Wirksamkeit einzelner

Schlüsselreize oder ihrer Kombinationen kann man auch dadurch untersuchen, daß man die Merkmale der Attrappen übertreibt (Abb. 3). Solche übernormalen Schlüsselreize („Super-Attrappe") fanden zuerst OTTO KOEHLER und ZAGARUS (*197*) beim Sandregenpfeifer, der ein kontrastreicher geflecktes Attrappen-Ei einem natürlichen, arteigenen Ei beim Brüten vorzog. Andere Vögel wählen unter verschieden großen Attrappen-Eiern das größte, obwohl der weitere Fortgang des Brutpflegeverhaltens dadurch erschwert oder unmöglich wird. Mit solchem nicht artgemäßen Riesenei müht sich z. B. die Graugans bei der Ausführung der angeborenen Eirollbewegung vergeblich ab (*197*). In der Abbildung 3 wirkt die übertrieben lange Schnabelspitze in roter Farbe als übernormaler Schlüsselreiz.

Bisher war nur von *auslösenden* Schlüsselreizen die Rede, durch welche eine angeborene Instinktbewegung in Gang gesetzt wird. Man hat aber zwischen *auslösenden* und *richtenden Reizen* zu unterscheiden (*197*) und daher die Instinktbewegung aufgeteilt, und zwar in einen Anteil, der unter Umständen von Anfang bis Ende von Außenreizen unbeeinflußt abrollt, und einen anderen Anteil, der diese Bewegungen im Raum richtet. Diese *Orientierungsreaktionen* sind in vielen Fällen von eigenen, oft differenzierteren Schlüsselreizen abhängig.

Beispiel: Bei noch blinden Drosselnestlingen löst Erschütterung der Unterlage das Sperren des Schnabels aus. Der Reiz hat keinen Einfluß auf die Steuerung der Sperr-Reaktion; die

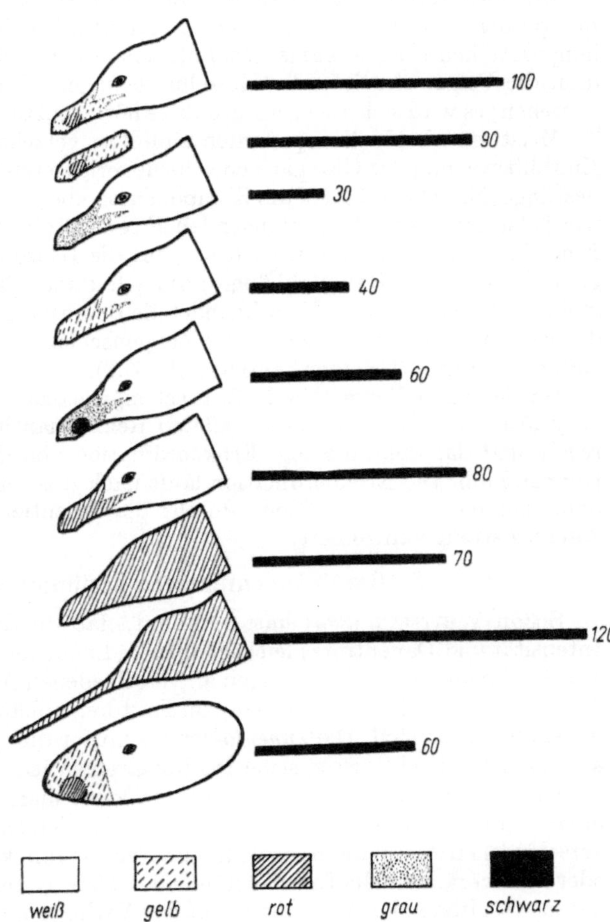

Abb. 3. Zusammenstellung einiger Befunde der Untersuchung von TINBERGEN und PERDECK über die *Auslösung der Bettelbewegung von Silbermöwenjungen.* Das oberste Modell besitzt die normalen Farben. Durch die horizontalen Balken werden die relativen Zahlen der ausgelosten Reaktionen dargestellt. Deutlich kommt der relativ hohe Wert der roten Farbe, des Flecks und der Dünne des Schnabels gegenuber dem relativ geringen Wert des Kopfes und der gelben Schnabelfarbung zum Ausdruck. [Nach BAERENDS (7)]

Nestlinge sperren stets gerade nach oben. Wenn sie nach etwa einer Woche sehen, lassen sich zwei visuelle Auslösemechanismen unterscheiden, ein einfacher, der die Instinktbewegung auslöst, und ein komplizierterer, der sie richtet. Das *auslösende* Objekt muß sich bewegen, muß größer als 3 cm sein und oberhalb der Augenhöhe erscheinen. *Richtende* Signalreize sind Ausbuchtungen an kreisförmigen Attrappen (Schnabel-an-Kopfartigem), von mehreren in gleicher Nähe gebotenen Stäbchen das höchste oder von zwei in gleicher Höhe gebotenen Stäbchen das nächste; von zwei übereinander angebotenen Kreisen richtet der obere optimal dann, wenn sein Durchmesser dreimal kleiner ist als der des unteren. Die erste Komponente, das Sperren, ist relativ starr in ihrer Bewegungskoordination, tritt sofort nach dem Schlüpfen auf und läuft in den ersten Lebenstagen häufig spontan, d. h. ohne Auslöserreize ab. Die zweite Komponente stellt eine erst heranreifende Folge vieler Antworten auf Außenreize dar, welche die Bewegungsrichtung immer erneut und immer genauer gemäß den räumlichen Besonderheiten der Umgebung einstellen und korrigieren. Die erste Bewegungskomponente läuft von selbst weiter, ohne neuer Außenreize zu bedürfen, die zweite ist streng von der afferenten Kontrolle abhängig *(197)*.

Die erste Komponente nannte Lorenz *(531)* die *Erbkoordination* und trennte sie von der *Taxiskomponente (109)* ab. Nicht mehr die ganze Orientierungshandlung wird heute noch Taxis genannt, sondern nur der steuernde Mechanismus, d. h. die Folge orientierender Einzelbewegungen. Diese Trennung mag künstlich aussehen; es wird sich aber zeigen, daß sie nötig und für die Instinktlehre wichtig ist.

Meist sind beide Komponenten simultan verschränkt, wie z. B. bei der Ei-Einrollbewegung der Graugans oder beim gerichteten Sperren der älteren Drosselnestlinge. Manchmal laufen die Komponenten aber auch in strenger Sukzession ab, wie jedermann beim fliegenfangenden Frosch beobachten kann: a) orientierende Einzelbewegungen genau in Richtung auf die Beute und dauernd von der Bewegung der Beute im Raum abhängig; b) nach kurzer Pause Zungenschuß, der nicht mehr ortskorrigierbar ist. Verschwindet die Beute nach dem Einrichten, so schnappt der Frosch gerichtet ins Leere. Der Zungenschlag ist eine echte, verhältnismäßig einfache „starre" Erbkoordination *(109, 731)*.

Wir haben in diesem Abschnitt gesehen, wie das Verhalten durch äußere Reize ausgelöst wird, daß man diese äußeren Reize quantifizieren kann (Reizsummenregel) und daß man die sog. Erbkoordination von den Orientierungsreaktionen trennen muß. Die Erbkoordination läuft nach Auslösung (unter Umständen auch ohne sie) meist bis zum Ende durch; die Orientierungsreaktion wird von der Afferenz streng kontrolliert.

2. Durch Innenfaktoren bestimmtes Verhalten

Schon Whitman *(205)* hatte erkannt, daß die Instinkthandlungen in ihrer Intensität und Dauer trotz gleicher Außenbedingungen schwanken. Das Verhalten, so schloß man aus Beobachtungen an verschiedenen Arten, könne nicht allein von Außenreizen, sondern müsse auch von Faktoren abhängig sein, die im Organismus selbst zu suchen sind. Die *Innenfaktoren* sind für die „Stimmung" des Tieres verantwortlich; sie aktivieren seine Instinkte, einen jeden zu seiner Zeit.

Zur Untersuchung der Innenfaktoren kann man verschiedene Methoden benutzen. Entweder man beobachtet bei gleichbleibenden Außenbedingungen zu verschiedenen Zeiten die Reaktionsstärke und -häufigkeit der Instinkthandlungen, oder man verändert die Innenzustände der Tiere systematisch und beobachtet die daraus resultierenden Wirkungen auf das Verhalten.

Die Erfahrung, daß Erbkoordinationen sich um so leichter auslösen lassen je länger sie nicht abgelaufen sind, hatte, wie schon erwähnt, zu der Arbeitshypothese geführt, eine Schwellenerniedrigung für Auslöserreize infolge Kumulierung aktionsspezifischer Energie anzunehmen. Für Auslösung und Intensität des Ablaufs von Instinktbewegungen nahm man also zwei für sich variable Größen an, nämlich erstens die Intensität der verschiedenen Schlüsselreize, die eine Instinktbewegung auslösen, und zweitens die Menge aktionsspezifischer Erregung im efferenten Zentrum der Instinktbewegung. Dementsprechend wandte man bei Analysen die „*Methode der doppelten Quantifizierung*" an, d. h. Quantifizierung der Innenfaktoren (im Modell vorgestellt als „Ladungsquantum des Instinktzentrums") und der äußeren Reize, wie im vorhergehenden Abschnitt gezeigt. Das Wort Zentrum soll nicht als lokalisatorisch festgelegter, anatomisch definierter Ort, sondern als funktionell zusammengefaßter effectorischer Apparat verstanden werden.

Eine Beobachtung von Lorenz (*531*) trug wesentlich zu der von ihm entwickelten Hypothese von der aktionsspezifischen Erregungskumulierung bei:

Ein junger, zahmer, im Zimmer freifliegender Star, dem eine Beute in Wirklichkeit fehlte, „vollführte mit Augen und Kopf eine Bewegung, als verfolge er ein dahinfliegendes Insekt mit seinen Blicken. Seine Haltung straffte sich, er flog ab, schnappte zu, kehrte auf seine Warte zurück und vollführte die seitlich schlagenden Schleuderbewegungen mit dem Schnabel ... Dann vollführte er mehrmals Schluckbewegungen, worauf sich sein knapp angelegtes Gefieder etwas lockerte und in vielen Fällen der Schüttelreflex eintrat, ganz wie er nach einer wirklichen Sättigung einzutreten pflegt". Der Star produzierte also bei längerem Ausbleiben einer adäquaten Auslösersituation (fliegendes Insekt) den gesamten Handlungsablauf des Insektenfangens mit typischer Totschlage- und Freßbewegung spontan im *Leerlauf*. Solche Leerlaufaktivität ist inzwischen häufiger (*197, 495*) auch bei Säugern (*146, 351*) und bei psychotischen Menschen (*649, 654*) beschrieben worden.

Innere Faktoren, die zur Schwellen-Regulierung führen, sind z. B. innere Sinnesreize, verursacht durch den Füllungszustand von Hohlorganen (Magen, Blase), aber auch alle anderen positiven und negativen Rückmeldungen enterozeptiver Afferenzen, die wiederum von der Tagesperiodik abhängig sind (*5a, 24, 234a—c*), sowie schließlich Faktorenkomplexe aus dem gesamten Stoffwechselgeschehen und darunter vor allem die Hormone. Die Bedeutung endokriner Funktionen für das normale und krankhafte Verhalten des Menschen hat M. Bleuler in diesem Band dargestellt.

Auf welche Weise Hormone spezifischen Einfluß auf das Verhalten nehmen, ist Gegenstand zahlreicher Untersuchungen (*12, 13, 119, 121, 122, 231, 315, 502, 589, 700, 756*).

Sowohl ein direkter Einfluß auf das ZNS (*114, 117*) als auch ein indirekter über die Veränderung peripherer Strukturen (*122, 499, 501*) scheint vorzukommen. Umgekehrt wirken bestimmte Hirnstrukturen auf den Hormonspiegel, u. a. auch auf die Corticosteroid-Produktion zurück (*4, 211, 228, 229, 249, 384, 469, 490, 560, 819*).

Außer inneren Reizen und Hormonen nennen wir noch eine dritte Art von Innenfaktoren. Dafür sprechen die spontan „im Leerlauf" ablaufenden angeborenen Verhaltensweisen, die höchst wahrscheinlich auch ohne innere Sinnesreize, Hormone oder andere Stimuli in Gang kommen können. Diese Innenfaktoren beruhen auf der *Spontanaktivität des Nervensystems* (*192, 234c*) bzw. der Nervenzellen (s. Fußnote S. 296). Wir wollen diesen Vorgang mit einem Ausdruck v. Holsts als *zentrale Automatie* bezeichnen. Wie v. Holst, Aschoff, deren Mitarbeiter und andere Autoren gezeigt haben, sind rhythmische Vorgänge (*5a, 24, 234a—c, 700, 702*) in den Organismen kaum ohne die Annahme einer zentralen Automatie erklärbar. Diese dauernde Produktion nervöser Erregungen trägt entscheidend zur „Stimmung", zur Gestimmtheit des Organismus bei. Darunter ist der aktuelle physiologische Gesamtzustand eines Tieres zu verstehen.

3. Das Zusammenwirken äußerer Reize und innerer Faktoren

Baerends, Brouwer und Waterbolk (*238*) zeigten in einer sorgfältigen Analyse das Zusammenspiel von inneren und äußeren Faktoren bei der Balz des Guppy-Männchens. Der innere Zustand, die physiologische Gestimmtheit des Fischchens, kann an seinem Melanophorenmuster abgelesen werden. Durch charakteristischen Wechsel dieses Musters lassen sich 6 verschiedene Intensitätsstufen der Balzstimmung unterscheiden (s. Abb. 4, S. 302). Setzt man verschieden gezeichnete, d. h. also verschieden gestimmte Männchen zu verschieden großen Weibchen, so entwickelt sich dasselbe Verhalten bei Kombination unterschiedlicher Intensitäten innerer und äußerer Faktoren. Befindet sich z. B. ein Männchen in asexueller Stimmung und bringt man es mit einem sehr großen Weibchen zusammen, so beginnt es dennoch zu balzen. Das großeWeibchen sendet also sehr starke Schlüsselreize aus, welche die an sich unterschwellige Balzstimmung über die Schwelle heben. Umgekehrt beginnt ein Männchen in intensiver Balzstimmung,

erkenntlich am aktuellen Melanophorenmuster, bereits ein sehr kleines Weibchen
anzubalzen. In der Abb. 4 sind 2 Handlungskriterien des Balzverhaltens dargestellt,
nämlich das „Dem-Weibchen-Nachfolgen" und die für die Balz kennzeichnende
Biegung des Männchens in 2 verschiedenen Intensitätsstufen. Die in das Koordi-
natensystem eingetragenen Kurven stellen eine Art „Aequipotentiallinien" des
Verhaltens dar. Verminderung des einen Faktors (Größe des Weibchens) kann

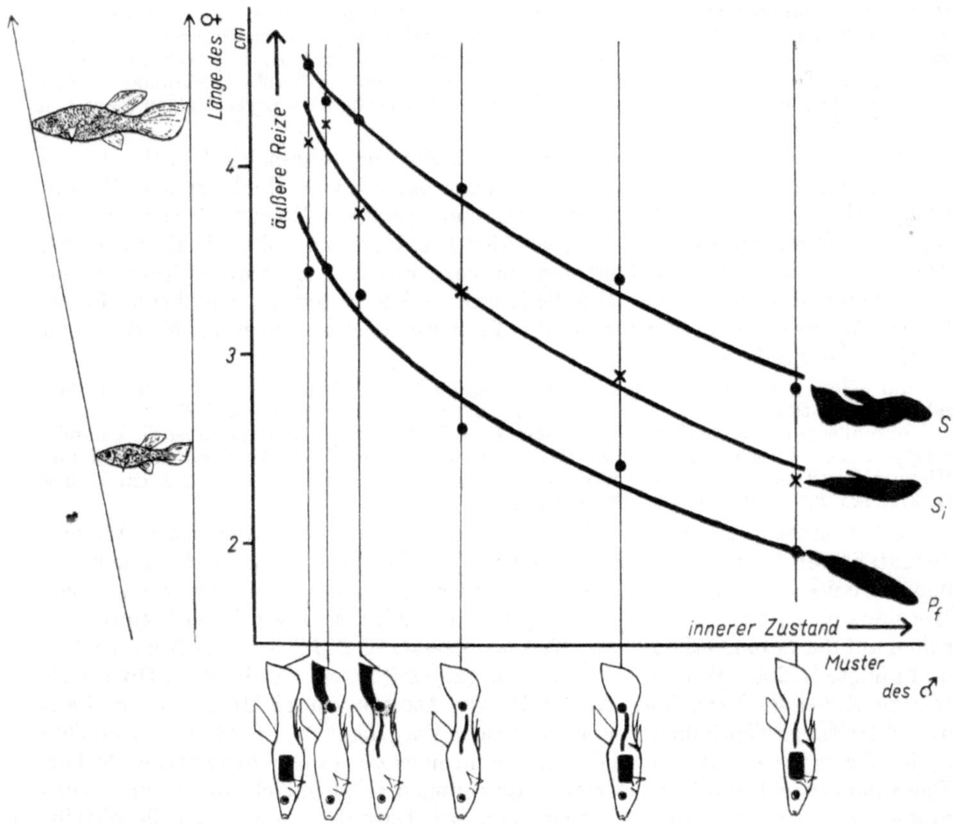

Abb. 4. Der Effekt von Kombinationen verschiedener Quantitäten eines äußeren Reizes mit verschiedenen
Intensitäten des inneren Zustandes eines Tieres. Der Außenreiz kann durch die Wahl der Größe des Weibchens
variiert werden (Ordinate). Der innere Zustand des Männchens ist am Melanophorenmuster ablesbar. Diese
Muster sind in der Abszisse eingetragen. Der Maßstab wurde erhalten durch Messen der Bereitschaft zum Aus-
führen sexueller Handlungen. *Die Kurven geben die Kombinationen an, bei denen das gleiche Verhalten ausgelöst wird.*
Dies ist für zwei verschiedene Verhaltensweisen geschehen: (P_f = Nachfolgen dem Weibchen durch das Männchen
und S = S-Biegung) — sowie für zwei Intensitäten derselben Handlung (S_i und S). (Nach BAERENDS (7)]

durch Zunahme des anderen (Intensität der Stimmung) kompensiert werden und
umgekehrt. Welches Verhalten auftritt, bestimmt die totale Information (716)
durch beide Faktoren zusammen. Je größer diese ausfällt, desto höher ist die Stufe,
auf der das unmittelbar auf die Begegnung von Männchen und Weibchen folgende
Balzverhalten einsetzt. Erhöhung der Information bewirkt also eine entsprechende
Verstärkung der Balzintensität (238). Dies bedeutet bezüglich der Erbkoordination
eine zusätzliche Aktivierung von Muskelelementen in bestimmter, unveränderter
Reihenfolge.

Es gibt genügend Untersuchungen, die zeigen, daß das Zusammenspiel innerer
und äußerer Faktoren bei anderen Tieren und beim Menschen in ähnlicher Weise
funktioniert wie beim Balzverhalten des Guppys (195, 197).

a) Der angeborene Auslösemechanismus (AAM)

Wenden wir uns nochmals den Schlüsselreizen zu. In unserem Guppy-Beispiel war die Größe des Weibchens der Schlüsselreiz für das Balzverhalten. Bei den Drosselnestlingen waren es zuerst taktile, später bestimmte Kombinationen von visuellen Reizen, und ähnlich war es auch bei den jungen Silbermöven. Die Tatsache, daß ein bestimmtes angeborenes Verhalten durch eine bestimmte, für jede Art verschiedene Reizkombination ausgelöst werden kann, bezeichnete LORENZ im Anschluß an ähnliche Gedanken J. v. UEXKÜLLs als „auslösendes angeborenes Schema". Der Ausdruck TINBERGENs (*197*) „angeborener Auslösemechanismus" (AAM) besagt dasselbe und wird jetzt allgemein benutzt. Man stellt sich darunter einen *neuro-sensorischen Mechanismus* vor, der eine spezielle angeborene Verhaltensweise auf passende Außenreize hin freigibt; er bestimmt nach Art eines „Reizfilterapparates" die selektive Empfindlichkeit des Tieres für eben gerade diese Schlüsselreize. Der AAM ist nicht etwa durch die Sinnestüchtigkeit einer Art festgelegt. Denn es gibt bei ein und derselben Art für verschiedene Verhaltensweisen verschiedene AAMs. Beispielsweise reagiert das Samtfaltermännchen nur auf dem Futterflug, nicht aber während des Balzfluges auf Farben (*197*). Ursprünglich stellte man sich vor, daß der AAM eine Hemmung im ZNS aufhebt, daß er einen „Block" beseitigt, so wie der richtige Schlüssel die versperrte Tür freigibt. Dieser Hemmungs- und Enthemmungsmechanismus ordnet nach dieser Vorstellung das richtige Einklinken einer Verhaltensweise im rechten Augenblick. Würde er nicht vorhanden sein, wäre ein chaotisches Durcheinander von angeborenen Reaktionen die Folge.

Gegen diese Vorstellung des „Blocks" und seiner Aufhebung durch den AAM sind inzwischen manche Bedenken aufgetaucht, unter anderem auch der Einwand, daß z. B. die erwähnten Drosselnestlinge die sperrauslösenden Merkmale während des Fütterns *gelernt* haben könnten, wie LEHRMAN (*497*) aus seinen Versuchen an Ringeltauben (*499*) schließt. Mit der Lernhypothese kann jedoch nicht erklärt werden, wie isoliert aufgezogene Drosseln, die nie einen Altvogel gesehen haben, das richtige Verhältnis von Kopf zu Rumpf erlernt haben sollen. Eine Fülle von Tatsachen beweist, daß Lernprozesse den AAM nicht erklären können. Damit ist nun aber keineswegs gesagt, daß nicht auch Lernprozesse in die schließlich reaktionsauslösende Reizkombination eingreifen. LORENZ (*530, 531*) hat auf diese Möglichkeit schon früh aufmerksam gemacht und an Beispielen gezeigt, daß der AAM durch Lernen eingeengt werden kann[1]. Mit dem ganzen Problem der *Instinkt-Dressurverschränkung* (*131*) hat sich THORPE (*195*) auseinandergesetzt und dabei die vor allem von anglo-amerikanischen Forschern bearbeiteten verschiedenen Formen des Lernens berücksichtigt. BAERENDS (*7*) schlägt vor, das Attribut „angeboren" fortzulassen und vorläufig nur vom auslösenden Mechanismus zu sprechen, bis mehr experimentelle Ergebnisse über die Ontogenese des AAM vorliegen.

Die Versuche mit den Guppies werfen die Frage nach den tatsächlichen physiologischen Vorgängen auf, die durch den Begriff des AAM gedeckt werden. Lange Zeit herrschte die Auffassung, daß die Funktion eines AAM wenigstens bei konstanter Stimmung, d. h. bei gleicher spezifischer Handelnsbereitschaft, konstant sei. PRECHTL (*667*) zeigte jedoch für die Sperrbewegung junger Singvögel, daß

---

[1] Auch die Bedingte Reaktion kann man einengen (Diskrimination und Differenzierung, *111, 297, 684*), indem man das Tier z. B. zuerst auf ein breites Ton-Frequenzgemisch dressiert und später nur die Reaktionen auf einen immer schmaler werdenden Ton-Frequenzbereich belohnt. Ähnliches läßt sich im visuellen Bereich erzielen. Es fragt sich, ob der Prozeß der Einengung einer Reaktion bzw. die Selektivität des Ansprechens auf Reizkombinationen beim AAM grundsätzlich verschieden vom Lernprozeß ist.

die Abnahme der Reaktionen nach wiederholten Reizen weder auf einen Refraktärzustand der Sinnesorgane zurückgeführt noch durch Veränderungen im peripheren
oder zentralen motorischen System erklärt werden kann. Es muß sich daher um
Veränderungen im Auslösemechanismus selbst handeln. Wenn nämlich das Sperren
durch fortgesetzte (nachgeahmte) akustische Reize bis zum Verschwinden ausgelöst wird, reagieren die Tiere noch uneingeschränkt auf taktile oder optische
Reize. Wenn der AAM tatsächlich einen „Block" beseitigt hätte, so daß die im
Zentrum „gestaute" aktionsspezifische Erregung sich entladen konnte, wäre es
nach dieser Modellvorstellung schwer erklärbar, daß andere Reize dieselbe Reaktion, deren kumulierte Energie verbraucht sein sollte, doch noch in Gang setzen
können. Prechtl benannte den beobachteten Sachverhalt mit dem mehrfach
präokkupierten Wort „Adaptation" (667, 668). Das gleiche Phänomen wurde inzwischen auch bei anderen Arten gefunden (7, 664, 727). M. Schleidt (723) wählte
bei ihren Untersuchungen an Truthähnen den unseres Erachtens glücklicheren Ausdruck „afferente Drosselung". Soweit wir sehen, nimmt keiner der Autoren Bezug
auf die entsprechenden neurophysiologischen Untersuchungen. Gerade auf akustischem Gebiet ist das Schwinden der zentralen hirnelektrischen Reizantworten auf
auditive Mehrfach-Reize und das Wiedererscheinen der hirnelektrischen Antwort
bei Wechsel der akustischen Reizqualität schon gut untersucht (57). Die „afferente
Drosselung" scheint sich im zentralen Sinnesprojektionsfeld abzuspielen. Auf
psychologischer Ebene findet man Vergleichbares in dem Phänomen der „Sättigung", das bisher von den Ethologen nicht berücksichtigt wurde (445, 651).

b) Übersprung und Leerlauf

Im Zusammenwirken äußerer und innerer Faktoren können, wie wir sahen, diese
oder jene das Übergewicht haben. Die *Leerlaufaktivität* (vgl. S. 360 ff.) gibt ein Beispiel für das wahrscheinlich reine Wirken von Innenfaktoren: Der Drang zur
Triebentladung hat sich so „gestaut", daß die Instinkthandlung ohne erkennbaren
äußeren Anlaß im Leerlauf losgeht, d. h. die Instinkthandlung hat kein Objekt, an
dem sie sich vollzieht. Der Star fängt Fliegen, ohne daß eine Fliege da ist, die Balz
findet ohne den Geschlechtspartner statt.

Anders liegen die Dinge nun, wenn *dieselbe* äußere Reizsituation Handlungen
auslöst, die *verschiedenen* Instinktabläufen angehören. Bei vielen Tieren werden
während der Begegnung zweier Rivalen nicht nur die Angriffshandlungen, sondern
auch zum Fluchtinstinkt gehörige Bewegungen aktiviert (197, 198). In anderen
Fällen können im Beginn der Paarungszeit neben dem Werbespiel Aggression und
Flucht durch den Partner wachgerufen werden. Solange die gleichzeitige Aktivierung verschiedener Instinkte noch ziemlich gering ist, können Handlungen, die
zu verschiedenen Instinkten gehören, gleichzeitig oder abwechselnd nebeneinander
bestehen. Dabei kann die Aktivierung zweier Instinkte gegensätzlich oder gleichgerichtet verlaufen. Im Falle der gegenseitigen Hemmung resultiert im allgemeinen
eine Unvollständigkeit der Handlungen, d. h. es kommt zu *Intentionsbewegungen.*
(Nicht jede Intentionsbewegung beruht jedoch auf gegenseitiger Hemmung.) Im
Falle des gleichgerichteten Verlaufs bei nebeneinander bestehenden Instinktaktivierungen kann zugleich die Zahl der sexuellen und aggressiven Handlungen steigen, wie es bei Stichlingen, Cichliden, Silbermöven (7, 421), Finken (600, 601, 602)
und auch bei einem Säugetier (Hamster) (328) nachgewiesen wurde.

Ist die Aktivierung jedoch stärker, scheint ein Nebeneinanderbestehen nicht
mehr möglich zu sein. Tinbergen und Kortlandt (197, 485) beobachteten in
solchen Situationen Verhaltensweisen, die zu keinem der gerade aktivierten

Instinkte gehörten, und sprachen von *Übersprungbewegungen*[1], TINBERGEN später auch von abgeleiteten Bewegungen. Wird eine Bewegung in dieser Weise abgeleitet, dann spricht KORTLANDT von allochthon aktivierter Instinkthandlung, während er die gleiche, aber situationsgerecht auftretende Instinkthandlung als autochthon aktiviert bezeichnet. Ein Beispiel für solche Übersprunghandlung sind die jedem Beobachter eines Hühnerhofes erkennbaren Pickbewegungen von sich kämpfend oder kampfbereit gegenüberstehenden Haushähnen. Besonders intensiv werden diese allochthon aktivierten Pickbewegungen, wenn die Hähne, wie wir es mehrfach beobachteten, durch einen Drahtzaun getrennt sind. Kämpfende Stare putzen plötzlich ihr Gefieder. Silbermöven in Kampfposition rupfen plötzlich Nestmaterial ab. Andere Vögel nehmen sogar Schlafstellung ein. Auch bei Säugern werden Übersprunghandlungen beobachtet (*113, 126, 146, 149, 158, 354, 608*). Überraschend oft kommt es im unentschiedenen Hin und Her zwischen Angriffs- und Fluchtstimmung an Reviergrenzen zu Übersprunghandlungen.

Außer in den zuletzt genannten Fällen eines Konfliktes (Aggression und Flucht) zwischen sich gegenseitig unterdrückenden Instinkten kann der Übersprung auch dann auftreten, wenn nur ein Instinkt aktiviert ist, der nicht zum Zuge kommen kann, sei es, daß ein Hindernis besteht — eine Versuchsanordnung, die für die experimentellen Tierneurosen häufig benutzt wird (*516*) —, oder sei es, daß die richtige Reizsituation noch nicht eingetreten ist oder plötzlich verschwindet. TINBERGEN und VAN IERSEL (*197*) haben das eindrucksvoll mit ihren Untersuchungen am dreistachligen Stichling gezeigt. Dieser kann nicht ablaichen, solange ihm das Weibchen die hierfür erforderlichen Signalreize vorenthält. Bleibt z. B. ein noch nicht vollbrünstiges Stichlingsweibchen dem stark erregten Männchen die Antwort auf den Zick-Zack-Tanz schuldig, geht das Männchen plötzlich in eine der Balz nebengeordnete und sich im allgemeinen von ihr ausschließende Tätigkeit, zum Nestfächeln, über. Dieses *Übersprungfächeln* gehört an sich „regulär" in die Folge der Brutpflegehandlungen (s. Abb. 5). Die Ausdauer und Stärke eines solchen Übersprungs ist ein zuverlässiges Maß für die nicht zur Abfuhr kommende Trieberregung. Dabei ist aber zu beachten, daß die Übersprungbewegung meist nicht voll in ihrer Bewegungskoordination entfaltet ist.

TINBERGEN deutet den physiologischen Mechanismus der Übersprunghandlung so, „daß die Erregung eines Instinktes, die nicht in die ihm zugeordneten motorischen Mechanismen abfließen kann, sich über das Zentrum eines anderen Instinktes entlädt" (*197*). Die Unvollkommenheit der Übersprunghandlungen zeigt, daß die Entladung über den Umweg auf erheblichen Widerstand stößt (s. die hierfür bestehenden Symbole in der Abb. 5, S. 307).

Drangüberschuß allein genügt für den Übersprung offenbar nicht. Dieser führt zur Leerlaufaktivität, während zum Übersprung sicherlich die Hemmung gehört.

VAN IERSEL und BOLT (*429*) haben kürzlich in einer eingehenden Studie an Seeschwalben die These gut gestützt, daß der *Übersprung tatsächlich allein vom Stärkeverhältnis zweier sich widerstreitender Triebe abhängig* zu sein scheint. Dieses Gleichgewichtsverhältnis von Trieben im Konflikt wird „effektive Gleichheit" genannt. Wenn zwei einander widerstreitende effektiv gleich starke Triebe einander hemmen, so entfällt ihre hemmende Wirkung auf andere Funktionskreise. Im Widerstreit zwischen Brut- und Fluchttrieb z. B. wird das sonst durch Brüten und Flucht gehemmte Sich-Putzen enthemmt. Dies besagt, wie auch BAERENDS und HINDE annehmen, daß allein die *Hemmungs-Enthemmungshypothese genügt*, um das Übersprunggeschehen zu erklären. TINBERGENs umstrittene Vorstellung vom

---

[1] Frühere Beobachter dieses Phänomens sprachen von ''sparking over'' (Überspringen des elektrischen Funkens) und von ''substitute activity'' (Ersatzhandlung). In der britischen Literatur hat sich der Ausdruck ''displacement activity'' eingebürgert.

„Überspringen" aktionsspezifischer Impulse würde damit ebenso hinfällig wie
Kortlandts Unterscheidung von autochthoner und allochthoner Aktivierung der
Instinkthandlungen.

4. Die hierarchische Stufung organisierten Verhaltens

Die bisher geschilderten Ergebnisse machen deutlich, daß wir nur in Ausnahmefällen ein Konkurrieren verschiedener Instinkthandlungen beobachten können.
Gerade diese Ausnahmen zeigen, daß jede Instinktbewegung ihren bestimmten
Stellenwert, ihren bestimmten Platz im Nacheinander von Handlungsfolgen einnimmt. Die Balzhandlungen gehen der Kopulation in fester Reihenfolge voran;
den Nestbauhandlungen folgen die Brutpflegehandlungen (72). Nebenher können
Kampfhandlungen laufen usw. Das klingt selbstverständlich, weil wir als Beobachter einen Sinn in dieser Stufenfolge erblicken. Die Ausnahmen zeigen aber, daß
uns diese Organisation des Verhaltens mehr Fragen aufgibt, als vorläufig kausale
Erklärungen möglich sind. Im Hinblick auf neuropsychiatrische Erfahrungen und
Fragestellungen erscheint die *Modellvorstellung einer hierarchischen Gliederung* im
Aufbau des Verhaltens besonders relevant. Es lassen sich viele Brücken zur Neuro-
logie (*207, 432*), zur Neurophysiologie (*78, 138, 415*), zu den heutigen Vorstellungen
über Hirnorganisation und Verhalten (s. Teil B), zur Psychologie (*486, 510*) und
Psychopathologie (*30, 45, 654*) schlagen.

Die ersten Objekte, an denen diese hierarchische Organisation gründlich studiert wurde, waren die Grabwespe (*7*) und der Stichling (*197*). Andere folgten
(*126, 127, 411*).

Die Grab-Wespe (Ammophila campestris), ein Raupentoter, dem schon Fabre (*46*) besondere Aufmerksamkeit widmete, versorgt ihre Nester in 3 Phasen. In der ersten Phase wird
das Ei ins Nest gelegt, in der zweiten werden einzelne Raupen und in der dritten in der Regel
viele Raupen ins Nest eingetragen. Zwischen diesen Perioden versorgen die Wespen andere
Nester gleichermaßen. Zu Beginn der beiden letzten Phasen steht ein Inspektionsbesuch der
Nester, bei dem keine Raupe ins Nest gebracht wird. Schlüsselreiz fur die Wespe sind Anwesenheit und Größe ihrer Larven und deren Raupen-Futtervorrat. Je nach Phase regen die gleichen
Außenreize verschiedene Instinkthandlungen an (Nestgraben, Raupen-Eintragen, Nest-
verschließen). Durch experimentelle Eingriffe in die strenge Reihenfolge der Kette dieser Brut-
Verproviantierungshandlungen konnte Baerends zeigen, daß der Befund, den die Wespe bei
ihrem ersten Besuch eines Nestes erhebt, fur diesen Tag die Phasen ihres Handelns festlegt,
d. h. sie in eine entsprechende „Stimmung" versetzt, der eine bestimmte Handlungskette
(z. B. Nestgraben, Eintragen usw.) entspricht. Mit „Stimmung" ist also sowohl der physiologische (innere) aktuelle Zustand des Tieres zum Zeitpunkt seiner speziellen Handlungsfolge
gemeint als auch der Integrationsmechanismus, der das Eintreten dieses inneren Zustandes ermöglicht (*7*).

Statt von Stimmungshierarchie sprach Tinbergen von einer Zentren- bzw.
Instinkthierarchie, die am Beispiel des Stichlings erörtert sei (Abb. 5, S. 307):

Im Frühling (Außenfaktor) sind die Männchen, vermutlich durch hormonale
Einflüsse (Innenfaktoren), zunehmend intensiver zur Fortpflanzung gestimmt
(Instinkt I. Ordnung); das treibt sie ins flache, wärmere Süßwasser mit den für das
volle Fortpflanzungsverhalten notwendigen Wasserpflanzen (Außenfaktoren), ihre
Reviere zu suchen und zu besetzen (Instinkt II. Ordnung). Das Männchen bekommt
sein Prachtkleid, den roten Bauch (Innenfaktoren), beginnt sein Nest zu bauen
und fremde, in das Revier eindringende Gegner zu bekämpfen. Einschwimmende
Weibchen werden angebalzt, und wenn deren Eier abgelegt sind, setzen die Brutpflegehandlungen ein. Kampf, Nisten, Balz und Brutpflege gehören zur Instinkthandlung III. Ordnung und setzen die Fortpflanzungs- und Revierstimmung
(Instinkt I. und II. Ordnung) voraus. Was jeweils auf der dritten Stufe geschieht,
hängt wesentlich von Außenreizen ab. Soll das Männchen kämpfen, muß ein anderes, rotbäuchiges ins Revier eindringen. Soll es ein Nest bauen, müssen sich passende Pflanzenteile anbieten. Soll es balzen, muß das erscheinende Weibchen auf

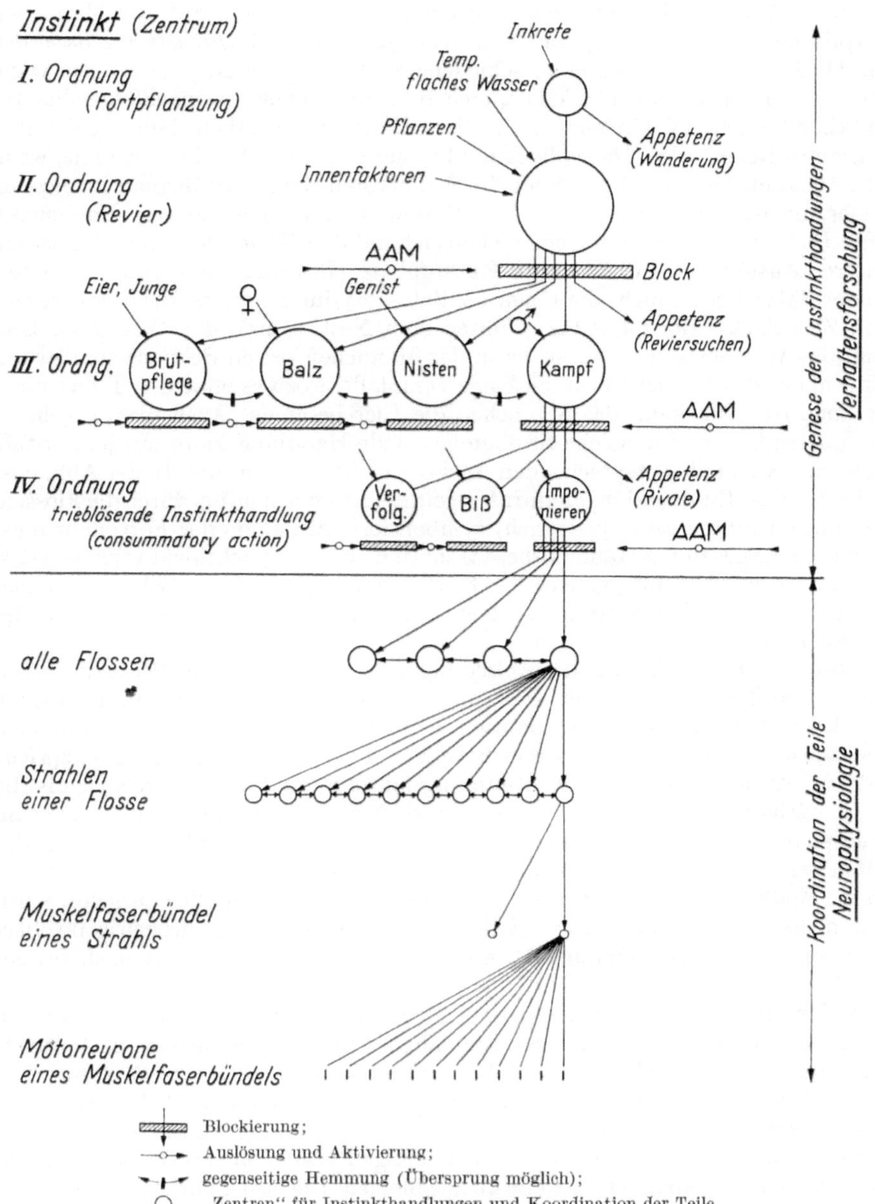

Abb. 5. *Hierarchischer Aufbau der Instinkthandlungen* am Beispiel des Fortpflanzungsverhaltens des Stichlings. [Nach TINBERGEN (*197*), modifiziert]. Die erblich angelegten Instinkthandlungen sind potentiell im Zentralnervensystem vorgebildet, aber blockiert. Erst durch bestimmte Innen- und Außenfaktoren werden sie in Gang gesetzt. Verschiedene Instinkthandlungen auf derselben Ebene schließen sich gegenseitig aus (Hemmungsvorgänge oder intrazentraler Wettstreit), doch ist „Übersprung" vom einen zum anderen möglich. Im speziellen dargestellten Fall des männlichen Stichlings wird ein instinktives Appentenzverhalten mit Wanderung in der Brunstzeit durch endokrine Vorgänge (Sexualhormone) angeregt. Im geeigneten Milieu (warmes Wasser, Pflanzen), das gesucht wird, entwickelt sich ein Instinktkomplex II. Ordnung. Die Manifestierung der einzelnen Handlungen III. Ordnung ist zunächst blockiert, kann aber durch bestimmte angeborene Auslosemechanismen (AAM) ausgeklinkt werden: Balz und Befruchtung beim Erscheinen eines Weibchens, nach Eiablage anschließend die Brutpflegehandlungen. Beim Erscheinen eines anderen Männchens wird der Kampfinstinkt ausgelost, der in der IV. Ordnung als trieblosende Instinkthandlung je nach Verhalten des Gegners wiederum verschieden auftritt: Imponierstellung, Beißen, Verfolgen oder Flucht. Diese einzelnen Handlungen sind neurophysiologisch in der motorischen Koordination der Teile und der diese innervierenden zentralnervosen Strukturen zu analysieren, wie unten schematisch im Anschluß an v. HOLST dargestellt ist.

die erste Phase des Balzens (den Zick-Zack-Tanz) eingehen. Soll das Männchen brutpflegen, muß ein Gelege im Nest sein. Jede dieser 4 *Handelnsbereitschaften* auf III. Stufe wird also durch verschiedene Schlüssel- oder Auslöserreize in Gang gesetzt, d. h. verschiedene AAMs sprechen an und setzen die nachfolgenden Instinkthandlungen IV. Ordnung frei. Diese Handlungen haben dann wieder ihre bestimmte Reihenfolge. Das volle Kampfverhalten z. B. entwickelt sich nur, wenn nach Auslösen der Kampfstimmung durch den roten Bauch des Gegners im eigenen Revier (im fremden überwiegt Fluchtstimmung!) nunmehr das sog. Imponieren folgt: Die kämpfenden Männchen stellen sich auf den Kopf. Diese Stellung ist ein weiterer Auslöser, der die nächste Kampfphase (Biß und Verfolgung) einleitet. Bei der Balz ist es ähnlich; die Folge der Balz wird durch andere Auslöser geregelt. Dem Zick-Zack-Tanz folgt das „Führen zum Nest" durch das Weibchen. Erst wenn das Weibchen im Nest ist, kann das Männchen seinen Schnauzentriller anbringen, der das Weibchen zur Eiablage veranlaßt, wozu es ohne den Triller nicht imstande ist. Nun kann das Männchen die Eier besamen. Auch die Brutpflegehandlungen haben eine solche Stufenfolge. Jede Handlung kann auf jeder Stufe abbrechen, wenn die entsprechenden Auslöser nicht gegeben sind. In der Abb. 5 ist die für jede der Endhandlungen starr festgelegte Erbkoordination durch die Flossenbewegungen (unter dem Querstrich) symbolisiert. Am Ende der Fortpflanzungszeit flauen die gesamten Handelnsbereitschaften ab. Das Prachtkleid verschwindet, die Reviere werden aufgegeben, die Fische vereinigen sich zu Schwärmen und wandern in die Überwinterungsgebiete tieferer Süßwasserschichten oder des Meeres (*197*).

Übersprung entsteht, wie die Abbildung zeigt, nicht auf jeder Stufe der Stimmungs- und Zentrenhierarchie. Das am höchsten integrierte Zentrum hat keinen „Block", d. h. es sind keine bestimmten AAMs bekannt, die enthemmend wirken. Das nächste Zentrum — in unserem Beispiel auf der Stufe II. Ordnung — spricht zwar auf Auslöser an, aber die Stimmungsfaktoren sind viel zahlreicher als die für die nächstfolgenden Stufen. Im ganzen sind die äußeren Reize um so mehr am Auslösen beteiligt, desto tiefer es die „Stimmungstreppe" hinabgeht. Die Anzahl der Stufen kann je nach Art, ja, auch je nach Instinkt verschieden sein, bis es schließlich zur Endhandlung kommt. Wenn die Endhandlung aber endlich ausgelöst wird, werden alle an der motorischen Entladung beteiligten Zentren gleichzeitig aktiviert und koordiniert. Die Handlung ist nicht mehr hemmbar; sie rollt nach festem Muster ab (*197*).

Anders ausgedrückt können wir auch von einem hierarchischen System von Integrationsmechanismen sprechen. Die Zahl der Einzelmechanismen (im Beispiel: alle Flossen, Strahlen einer Flosse, Muskelfaserbündel eines Strahles) ist auf dem tiefsten Niveau, der Erbkoordination, am größten, während sie stufenweise nach oben mehr und mehr abnimmt bis zu einem einzigen an der Spitze. Im gesamten Inventar des Verhaltens kann man viele derartige Pyramiden von Hauptinstinkten unterscheiden, die einander teilweise überschneiden. Die bisher vorliegenden Untersuchungen über die Stimmungshierarchie an Wespen, Spinnen, Vögeln und auch an Säugetieren, wie Mäusen und Hamstern (*7, 328*), den großen Familien der Bären (*146*), der Robben (*149*) und Katzen (*126*), scheinen uns bereits zu zeigen, daß den Säugetieren die höchsten Integrationssysteme eigen sind. *Auf diesen höchsten Stufen wirken sich die jeweiligen Stimmungen vorwiegend als Appetenzverhalten aus.* Ein Appetenzverhalten hat ein nächst spezifischeres Appetenzverhalten zum Ziel und so fort (*411, 510*). Erst tiefer in der Stimmungsleiter werden spezifische Auslöser wirksam oder notwendig. Dennoch kann man bei Säugetieren, analog unserem Stichlingsbeispiel, verschiedene, klar abgrenzbare Stimmungen (zentralnervöse Integrationsmechanismen) unterscheiden. Zum Beispiel versorgen auch Säugetiere ihre Jungen nur dann richtig, solange der Brutfürsorgeinstinkt anhält. Wird dieser Instinkt unterdrückt oder experimentell gestört, werden die Jungen unter Umständen gefressen (*146, 565*), ebenso wie das Ei für die Möve außerhalb der Brutzeit nichts anderes als Futter bedeutet (*198*).

HINDE (*411*) hat auf Grund seiner Untersuchungen an der Kohlmeise manche Abweichungen von TINBERGENs Stichlingsschema aufgezeigt. Nach ihm lassen sich Appetenzverhalten und Endhandlung nicht scharf gegeneinander abgrenzen. Es gibt sehr einfache Appetenzen, zu denen HINDE — verwirrenderweise — auch die Orientierungsreaktionen (vgl. S. 299) zählt, und recht komplizierte Endhandlungen. Die Variationsmöglichkeiten des Appetenzverhaltens sind keineswegs unbeschränkt, sondern werden, je näher dem Ziel, immer eingeengter. Die plastische Zielstrebigkeit, die man als Hauptkriterium für die Appetenz ansieht, reicht oft nicht zur Definition aus (vgl. S. 296). So werden häufig nicht nur die eigentlichen Instinkthandlungen durch Außenfaktoren ausgelöst, sondern auch die Appetenzen, die dann wie die Endhandlungen autonom in sich geordnet sind. Alles greift gleich einem Netzwerk mehr ineinander. Verschiedene Hauptinstinkte und ebenso verschiedene Appetenzen können dieselben Erbkoordinationen benutzen, und die gleichen Stimmungen können an verschiedensten Stellen der Zentrenhierarchie angreifen. Man kann nicht mehr davon sprechen, daß zu jedem Instinkt, gleich welcher Stufe, eindeutig eine Stimmung von derselben Ordnung gehöre. HINDE mochte eine Hierarchie der Instinktzentren von einer Hierarchie der Stimmungen (Appetenzen) unterscheiden, wenn auch beide eng ineinandergreifen. KORTLANDT (*486*) stellt den Appetenzen auf der subjektiven Seite die Bedürfnisse und den Trieben die Affekte gegenüber. Dies ist zwar, wie wir zeigten (*654*), für die Diskussion zwischen Ethologen, Psychologen und Psychopathologen ein ganz entscheidender Fragenkomplex, den man jedoch in der generalisierenden Weise KORTLANDTs kaum klären kann (*478*). KORTLANDT gibt die Hierarchie der Instinkte auf und möchte nur noch die der Bedürfnisse gelten lassen. Abgesehen davon, daß man Bedürfnisse und Appetenzverhalten nicht gleichsetzen kann (*654*), finden sich gerade für die Zentrenhierarchie der Instinkte gute experimentelle Forschungsansätze (s. Teil B).

Weitere Forschungen müssen erweisen, ob das bisher aufgestellte Hierarchie-Modell die zugrunde liegenden physiologischen Vorgänge hinreichend veranschaulicht. Sicher werden noch manche Korrekturen anzubringen sein. Es scheint uns aber vorerst nicht zweckmäßig, anschauliche Modelle mit unanschaulichen neurophysiologischen Hypothesen zu vertauschen (*164*). Die beobachteten Sachverhalte werden dadurch um nichts exakter.

5. Ermüdung und Hemmung angeborener Verhaltensweisen

Wir können dieses Kapitel der kausalen Analyse nicht abschließen, ohne auf weitere Komplikationsgrade des Verhaltens hinzuweisen. Obwohl die folgenden Sachverhalte mit aller Wahrscheinlichkeit auch für Vertebraten, einschließlich Säugetiere, im Prinzip zutreffen und dort auch schon teilweise untersucht worden sind (*146, 158, 331*), wählen wir Untersuchungen an Springspinnen als Modell, weil die Verhältnisse hier noch am übersichtlichsten darzustellen sind.

Wie schon angedeutet, kann das Phänomen der Hemmung von Instinkthandlungen durch die Vorstellung der „Blockierung" im Effectorensystem nicht allein erklärt werden. Das zeigten schon die Versuche von PRECHTL (*667*), SCHLEIDT u. a. (*723, 727*), welche das Prinzip der afferenten Drosselung demonstrierten. Anderes kommt nun hinzu. PRECHT und sein Mitarbeiter FREYTAG (*664*) stellten mit *Springspinnen* Experimente an, die einen bedeutenden Beitrag zum Triebproblem liefern.

Die Beutefanghandlungen der Springspinnen bestehen aus drei selbständigen Teilhandlungen, dem Heranlaufen an die Beute, dem Schleichen und dem Beutesprung. Heranlaufen und Beutesprung wurden unter systematisch variierten Bedingungen mit Beute-Attrappen und im *Hunger-* bzw. partiellen *Sättigungszustand* untersucht. Das Heranlaufen wurde in Zentimetern pro Zeiteinheit, das Springen durch die Zahl der Beutesprünge (auf Attrappen) quantitativ erfaßt.

Die *Erholung* des durch fortgesetzte Wiederholung *ermüdeten* Beutesprunges verlauft zuerst rasch und wird dann immer langsamer. Eine ahnliche Erholungskurve zeigt das Heranlaufen an die Beute. Die Einstellungs- oder Orientierungsreaktionen auf die Beuteattrappen sind sehr viel schwerer ermüdbar als die beiden genannten Instinkthandlungen. Selbst bei der Höchstzahl von 2985 nacheinander ausgelösten Einstellungsreaktionen konnte keine absolute physische Ermattung des Tieres herbeigeführt werden. Als Kriterium der Ermüdung galt das Nichtmehr-Ansprechen auf die Attrappe. Auch hier braucht die Erholung mehr und mehr Zeit, aber verglichen mit der Erholungskurve des Heranlaufens und des Beutesprunges geht es relativ rascher. Somit lassen sich, was Ermüdung und Erholung anbetrifft, die den Reflexen nahestehenden Einstellreaktionen von den Erbkoordinationen (den Instinkthandlungen im engeren Sinne) unterscheiden.

Diesen Unterschied findet man auch, wenn man prüft, welche Handlungen durch die *Ermüdung* anderer in Mitleidenschaft gezogen werden. Der Beutesprung ermüdet das Heranlaufen in meßbarem Grade mit, die Ermüdung des Heranlaufens macht den Beutesprung fast unmöglich. Wird das Heranlaufen gänzlich ermüdet, kann das Tier selbst nach 30 min Erholungzeit nur wenige Beutesprunge machen. Dagegen beeinflußt die Zahl der vorangegangenen Einstellreaktionen die Erholung des ermudeten Heranlaufens nicht. Mit anderen Worten ermüdet also die laufende Auslösung nur einer Teilhandlung den ganzen Funktionskreis der Beutefanghandlungen.

Was nun den Einfluß von *Nahrungsaufnahme* in den Erholungsintervallen auf die Instinkthandlungen betrifft, unterscheiden sich zwar verschiedene Spinnenarten voneinander; die ausgeklugelten Versuche erlauben aber doch die wichtige Feststellung, daß sich nicht der Freßakt (Endhandlung — consummatory action) auf die Triebänderung auswirkt, sondern die Nahrungsaufnahme. Nicht der „Erregungsverbrauch" der Endhandlung, sondern die Nahrungsaufnahme also fuhrt eine langsame Triebanderung herbei. Dabei ist der Fütterungseffekt desto großer, je starker der Hunger ist (gemessen am Intervall des Nahrungsentzuges).

Physische Behinderungen der Tiere (Amputation von Beinen, Aufkleben von Gewichten auf den Cephalothorax) haben weder Einfluß auf den Beutesprung selbst noch auf seine Erholung nach Ermudung. Danach wäre also die Erholung nicht etwa als bemessene Energiebereitstellung fur den Effector zu verstehen.

Ähnlich aufgebaute Untersuchungen betreffen andere Funktionskreise (Fortpflanzungsverhalten, Flucht) und die Beeinflussung der Funktionskreise untereinander bezuglich ihrer Ermudung und Erholung. Auch der *Einfluß der Erfahrungsbildung* auf die Instinkthandlungen wird einbezogen; z. B. beginnt die Balz in einiger Entfernung von der Weibchenattrappe mit einem Zick-Zack-Tanz in zunachst großen, dann kleiner werdenden Amplituden. Die Spinnen mußten nun in einem engen Glaskanal tanzen, dessen Breite variiert werden konnte. Nach „Einfahren" der Bewegungen über eine gewisse Zeit übte die Breite des Kanals einen gesicherten Einfluß auf die Amplitude der Zick-Zack-Bewegungen aus.

PRECHTs Versuche zeigen, daß man *Triebstärke* (z. B. Hungergrad) *von sich ansammelnder Instinkterregung* (z. B. Beutefanghandlung) *trennen* kann und daß eine solche Trennung für die Instinktlehre zweckmäßig ist. Diese Annahme paßt zu einer großen Zahl amerikanischer Untersuchungen (*245, 246, 248*), z. B. auch zum Thema Hunger (als innerem Zustand), Appetit (als Bedürfnisspannung) und Belohnung (als Befriedigung eines Bedürfnisses) (*195, 254, 588, 611*).

Unter den Instinkthandlungen kann man bei dieser engen Fassung des Begriffes „Trieb" *triebabhängige* und *triebunabhängige Instinkthandlungen* unterscheiden. Die Fluchtreaktionen der Spinnen z. B. sind dauernd unabhängig vom Sättigungsgrad auslösbar, insofern nicht deren spezielle Instinkterregung durch fortgesetztes Fluchtauslösen erschöpft ist. Für die Beutefanghandlungen besteht jedoch zugleich Abhängigkeit vom Sättigungszustand. Ähnliche Beispiele lassen sich auch für Säugetiere finden, nur werden die Verhältnisse dort komplizierter, wie z. B. bei der Katze, bei der die Beutefanghandlungen weitgehend unabhängig vom Hungerzustand sind (*126, 127*). Bei jungen Säugetieren drängt die Saugbewegung manchmal im Leerlauf zur Entladung, wenn eine Fütterung unter Umgehung des Saugens erfolgt (*195*).

Wir haben diese Abhängigkeitsverhältnisse von Sättigungsgrad und Saugbewegungen uber Wochen bei zwei Sauglingen im Alter von 4 Wochen bis 6 Monaten untersucht. Eine bestimmte Menge Nahrung führte zu alsbaldigem, befriedigtem Einschlafen, wenn sie mit einer bestimmten Menge von Saugbewegungen — gemessen an der Zeitdauer (20 min) des Saugens — verknüpft war. Dieselbe Menge oder sogar eine um 50% großere Menge Nahrung führte zu keiner Befriedigung, wenn die Saugbewegungen auf ein Minimum (5 min) reduziert wurden (große Öffnung im Sauger). Die Saugbewegungen gingen bei sonst gleichgehaltener äußerer Gesamtsituation im Leerlauf weiter und wurden bald durch intensives Schreien überlagert. Nach Gewinn einer zusätzlichen Saugbewegungsmenge von 10—15 min (mit leerer Flasche und Lutscher) trat befriedigtes Einschlafen ein. Der gleiche Effekt war auch durch reduzierte Nahrungsmenge und vermehrte Saugbewegungen (enges Loch im Sauger) zu erreichen. Die psychoanalytisch interpretierten Beobachtungen von René Spitz (*189*) zeigen ganz ähnliche Abhängigkeitsverhältnisse.

Zeigt sich eine Triebabhängigkeit der Instinkthandlungen, klinkt das Tier durch den aufkommenden Trieb in einen speziellen Funktionskreis ein (Nahrungssuche, Fortpflanzung usw.), wodurch zugehörige AAMs aktiviert werden. Die Zahl der auslösbaren Instinkthandlungen nimmt mit der Triebstärke zu.

Precht versucht unter Einbeziehung dieses Triebbegriffes die beteiligten Mechanismen in einem hydraulischen Modell [modifiziert nach dem alten Lorenzschen (*531*)] zu veranschaulichen und benutzt dabei die Sprache der Reglertechnik. Die Triebänderung kann auf diese Weise als Sollwertverstellung der Stauung von Instinkthandlungen verstanden werden.

III. Angeborene Formen menschlichen Verhaltens im Vergleich zu anderen Säugern

Die vorausgegangenen Kapitel dienen als Basis für die außerordentlich komplex gelagerten Verhältnisse beim Menschen (*37, 38, 132*). Der verläßlichste Anhaltspunkt für den Vergleich angeborenen Verhaltens zwischen Mensch und Tier ist die *Entwicklung des Säuglings* während der ersten Lebensmonate. Darf man doch annehmen, daß in diesem Stadium des Menschseins Erfahrungseinflüsse für das aktuelle Verhalten eine nur untergeordnete Rolle spielen[1]. Zudem befinden sich zu dieser Zeit das Beobachtete und der Beobachter in einer dem Tierexperiment vergleichbaren, nicht sprachlich bestimmten Situation. Reine *Kaspar-Hauser-Versuche* (isolierte Aufzucht) liegen nicht vor; wenn auch gelegentlich Fälle extremer Isolierung von Kindern publiziert wurden (*151*), so sind wegen ihrer Begleitumstände doch keine allgemeineren Aussagen über angeborenes Verhalten zulässig. Vereinzelte Berichte über angeblich unter Wölfen oder anderen Tieren aufgewachsene Menschenkinder (*182, 470, 817*) sind ebenfalls nicht hinreichend sicher auswertbar (*255, 321, 471*). Immerhin darf man aus ihnen schließen, daß bestimmte adäquate äußere Reize notwendig sind, damit sich ein vollkommen menschliches Verhalten entwickeln kann. Dies betrifft besonders die Sprachentwicklung, von der wir hier aber ganz absehen wollen.

1. Über die Motorik des Säuglings

Über die Bewegungs- und Reaktionsweisen des Säuglings und Kleinkindes gibt es eine umfangreiche Literatur. Den besten Überblick bietet das bekannte Buch von Peiper (*156*). Um Fragestellungen und Forschungsabsichten aufzuzeigen, geben wir eine Reihe von Beispielen aus neueren Einzelarbeiten. Ein großer Teil dieser Bewegungsweisen ist spezifisch für die erste Lebenszeit und später unter *normalen* Bedingungen nicht mehr zu beobachten. Es ist ein *charakteristisches Merkmal*

---

[1] Diese Annahme ist bisher von Anhängern verschiedenster Lern- und Milieutheorien zurückgewiesen worden. Der wissenschaftliche Streit entzündet sich, wie auch auf anderen Gebieten der Verhaltensforschung, an dem Begriff „angeboren". Uns erscheint der Streit mit Argumenten wenig förderlich. Interessant ist allein die Frage, welche Verhaltensanteile im wesentlichen vorgebildet sind und welche entscheidend durch Lernvorgänge (Erfahrung) entstehen. Wie die Ethologen bereits an zahlreichen Beispielen belegt haben, ist diese Frage niemals von vornherein dogmatisch zu entscheiden, sondern für jedes isolierbare Verhaltenselement erneut empirisch zu beantworten. Ein gutes Beispiel für solche Fragestellung gibt die Studie von Rheingold und Hess (*697*) an wassertrinkenden Küken: Die erfahrungsfreien Tiere wählten unter 6 verschiedenen Flüssigkeiten Quecksilber statt Wasser (übernormale Schlüsselreize). — Vgl. auch Schiller (*180*) und Eibl-Eibesfeldt (*335*).

dieser Motorik, daß sie *formstarr und stereotyp* ist, d. h. sie bleibt in ihrem Ablauf unveränderlich und ist von der Außensituation weitgehend unabhängig. Dies weist auf vorgebildete zentralnervöse Koordinationsmechanismen im Sinne v. Holsts (*414, 415*) hin. Viele Instinktbewegungen sind funktionslos geworden, wie z. B. der *Handgreif-Reflex* und die *Kletterbewegungen*. Bei den verschiedensten rezenten Affenarten dient der Koordinationsmechanismus zum Festklammern und Hochziehen am Pelz der Mutter. Das entsprechende Instinktverhalten der Säuglinge persistierte in der Stammesgeschichte und ist dem Verhalten der Affenjungen homolog (*156*). Solche stammesgeschichtlichen Bewegungsrudimente, die ihr Wirkmal (s. S. 295) überleben, sind keineswegs selten. Unter diesem Gesichtspunkt sind alternierende Armbewegungen, die mit Öffnung der Hand bei der Aufwärtsbewegung und Schließen der Hand bei der Abwärtsbewegung einhergehen, mit großer Wahrscheinlichkeit als Reste früher in der Phylogenese funktionstüchtig gewesener Kletterbewegungen anzusehen (*666*).

Andererseits muß man annehmen, daß bereits intrauterine Einflüsse eine Rolle für die Entwicklung der postnatalen Motorik spielen. Untersucht man z. B. die Beinmotorik und Fußsohlenreflexe an in Kopf- und in Steißlage gereiften und geborenen Kindern, so läßt sich für die Steißlagen ein Überwiegen der Extensorenaktivität nachweisen, während bei den Kopflagen ein gleichmäßiges Vorkommen von Flexions- und Extensionsbewegungen oder sogar ein Überwiegen von Beugebewegungen zu beobachten ist. Bei Steiß-Fußlagen oder reinen Fußlagen dagegen ist der Beugereflex verstärkt, der Streckreflex vermindert. Man kann daraus schließen, daß Veränderungen der Afferenz modifizierend auf die Reflextätigkeit einwirken (*669*).

In diesem Zusammenhang sei daran erinnert, daß die Entwicklung der Säuglingsmotorik bereits pränatal beginnt (*210*). Die Motoneuronen sind etwas früher reif als die Zellen der Spinalganglien. Die Entwicklungsrichtung verläuft im Rumpfgebiet cervico-caudal, im Kopfgebiet cervico-rostral. Mit der Reifung des neuralen Substrates korrelieren die ersten Bewegungsweisen. Durch einen exterozeptiven Reiz ist zuerst bei einem $9^{1}/_{2}$ Wochen alten Feten ein Öffnen des Mundes nach Berührung im Trigeminusareal auszulösen. 4 Wochen später folgt ein schwaches Schließen der Finger nach taktilem Reiz der Palma. Mit 11—12 Wochen wird der Lidschlagreflex auf Reizung des ersten Trigeminusastes konstant. Die Bewegungsreifung schreitet vom Medullarsystem nach rostral und caudal fort (*165*). Lippenbewegungen, Saugen und Schlucken reifen heran. Schon der Fet trinkt Fruchtwasser, und bei der zeitgerechten Geburt ist der neuronale Integrationsmechanismus für die Nahrungsaufnahme voll aktionsfähig. Normalerweise interferieren Nahrungsaufnahme und ebenfalls koordinierte Atmung nicht miteinander (*37*). Das hungrige Kind dreht den Kopf der Reizquelle zu; wird es aber nach der Nahrungsaufnahme schläfrig, bewirkt der gleiche Reiz ein Wegdrehen des Kopfes (*165*). Bei cerebral geschädigten Kindern scheinen diese frühen, vorgebildeten Bewegungsmuster zu persistieren. Wichtige Hinweise für die motorische Entwicklung primitiver Koordinationsmechanismen liefern auch die „anencephalen" Mißbildungen (*101, 165, 806*).

Besonderes Interesse verdienen die *auslösenden und steuernden Mechanismen des Saugaktes* (*207, 628, 670, 671, 806*). Prechtl und Schleidt (*670, 671*) haben bei neugeborenen Säugetieren eine rhythmische Kopfbewegung beschrieben, die aufhört, wenn die Tiere eine haarlose Stelle im Fell der Mutter berühren. Wie Attrappenversuche beweisen, hängt diese Suchautomatie (vgl. S. 300 f.) mit den Eigenschaften „behaart" und „haarlos" zusammen; das optische System ist zu diesem Zeitpunkt noch funktionsuntüchtig, und Erfahrungseinflüsse sind auszuschließen. Mit dem Bewegungsstop des rhythmischen Brustsuchens setzt gleichzeitig der

Saugakt ein, nämlich das orale Ergreifen der Brustwarze, die dann fest umschlossen wird, so daß durch die Saugbewegungen ein Unterdruck entsteht (Pumpsaugen). Bei besonders kräftigen menschlichen Neugeborenen findet man auch gelegentlich das ontogenetisch jüngere Lecksaugen von Beginn an, was wiederum für eine erfahrungsfreie (angeborene) Reifung dieser beiden Saugformen spricht. Die Suchautomatie gehört zu den gemeinsamen taxonomischen Merkmalen und damit zu den charakterisierenden Verhaltensweisen der Nesthocker einschließlich des Menschen. Es handelt sich um einen orientierenden Vorgang von Instinktcharakter, der die nachfolgenden Greifbewegungen mit dem Mund und das Saugen steuert (805). Wir kommen im nächsten Kapitel auf die oralen Leistungen zurück.

Andere Bewegungsmuster wie die schon bei sehr unreifen Frühgeborenen vorhandenen *Kriechbewegungen*, die *Schreitbewegungen* der Neugeborenen (*191, 627, 629, 778*) und die *Zehenphänomene* wollen wir nur nennen und auf die Bedeutung aller dieser Details für eine vergleichende phylogenetische Betrachtungsweise aufmerksam machen (*156*). Der *Handgreifreflex* ist praktisch bei allen gesunden Neugeborenen nachweisbar. Er verstärkt sich beim Ablaufen der Saugbewegungen und wird mit zunehmender Sättigung schwächer. (Die Mütter erkennen am Schlaffwerden der Hände, daß der Säugling gesättigt ist.) Verständlich wird dies dadurch, daß sich das Affenjunge während der ganzen Zeit des Trinkens im Pelz der Mutter festklammert (*165*). Offenbar ist die muskuläre Grundspannung des Greifens von Haltungsreflexen unabhängig (*811*). Wohl aber kann die Reaktion durch Veränderung der ergriffenen Objekte in ihrer Stärke modifiziert werden. Ein in die Hand gelegter Finger löst schwächere Reaktionen aus als ein erwärmtes, langhaariges Fell, und ein Stückchen Holz wirkt wiederum schwächer als der Finger (*165*).

Seit den Arbeiten von SCHALTENBRAND und H. STRAUSS (*780*) war das *Zusammenschrecken* (Moroscher Reflex, Schreckreflex, Schreckreaktion, startle pattern) mehrfach Gegenstand der Untersuchung. Neuerdings konnte WIESER (*807, 808, 809*) mit Hilfe einer modernen kinematographischen Technik, die eine starke Zeitdehnung (400 bis 600 Bilder pro Sekunde) erlaubt, Licht in die recht verwickelten Zusammenhänge bringen und einen wichtigen Beitrag zur Ontogenese und Phylogenese menschlicher Primitivmotorik liefern.

Meinungsverschiedenheiten bestanden im wesentlichen darin, ob die verschieden bezeichneten Reaktionen mehr den Charakter eines generalisierenden Beuge- oder Streckreflexes tragen, woraus dann divergierende neurophysiologische und phylogenetische Erklärungen abgeleitet wurden (*165, 363, 428*). DUENSING (*325*) stellte bereits bei hirnorganisch Kranken fest, daß das Zusammenschrecken keine einheitliche Latenzzeit hat, und WIESER et al. (*810*) unterschieden ebenfalls auf Grund von Latenzzeitmessungen 2 Phasen des gesamten Bewegungskomplexes.

Der ganze Vorgang des *Schreckverhaltens* gliedert sich in zwei selbständige „motorische Schablonen"[1] (*487*), nämlich die *initiale Beugezuckung* und die mit ihr verkettete, *nachfolgende Spreizphase*. Das Bewegungsbild der Beugezuckung ist durch eine umfassende Flexion gekennzeichnet, an der Wirbelsäule, Hals, Arme, Finger, Beine, Füße und Zehen teilnehmen. Die Schultern werden angehoben. Jede andere Spontan- oder Reaktivbewegung wird unterdrückt, so daß die Beugezuckung, entsprechend einem *Schutzreflex*, die Oberhand behält.

Im Lauf der ersten drei Lebensmonate ist eine Einengung dieser in die Gruppe der Fremdreflexe einzureihenden Verhaltensweise zu beobachten, und zwar sowohl bezüglich der Generalisierung als auch hinsichtlich der Reizqualitäten. Akustische Reize nehmen, wie man auch SPINDLERs Untersuchungen an erwachsenen eineiigen Zwillingen (*764*) entnehmen kann, an Bedeutung zu, während Reize aus der Körperfühlsphäre an Wirksamkeit einbüßen. Diese

---

[1] Diesen Begriff hat KRETSCHMER (*487*) für alle Phänomene geprägt, die sich als genormte Bewegungsabläufe selbständig herausheben, gleichgültig, ob sie in normalen oder pathologischen Zuständen auftreten (*270*).

Entwicklung scheint im wesentlichen schon mit Ende des ersten Lebensjahres abgeschlossen zu sein (*809*). Eine homologe Reaktion zeigen sehr viele Säugetiere auf starke Sinnesreize (*763, 764, 765, 766, 767*).

Die Spreizphase ist durch eine Deflexion des Kopfes mit Strecken der Wirbelsäule und einer symmetrischen Spreizbewegung der Gliedmaßen verbunden, wobei Ellenbogen- und Kniegelenk etwas gebeugt bleiben. Hinzu kommt meist noch eine seitliche Kopfdrehung mit nachfolgender Torquierung des Stammes. Die vergleichende Analyse dieses Bewegungskomplexes erlaubt nicht die früher gern gegebene Deutung als Umklammerungsreflex, sondern stellt vielmehr eine *Homologie zum Bewegungsbild von Säugetieren beim federnden Aufsprung* nach Fallen aus größerer Höhe dar (*808*). Nach dem Schutzreflex folgt also das Relikt einer Fortbewegung. Ohne speziellen Bezug zum Schreckverhalten, sondern allein auf den Sprung abzielend, ist diese Haltungs- und Bewegungshomologie bei Klammeraffen und Schimpansen beschrieben und im Bilde festgehalten worden (*788, 792*). Beim Menschen löst sich diese Reflexsynergie während des ersten Lebensjahres auf, und die verschiedenen an der Reaktion beteiligten Stell- und Haltungsreflexe werden einzeln von den sich allmählich entwickelnden höheren Formationen des Nervensystems überbaut.

Nicht nur beim Säugling können wir erfahrungsfrei sich entwickelnde oder sich wieder zurückbildende Verhaltensweisen studieren. Eine heranreifende Verhaltensweise der Angst und der Flucht scheint z. B. bei Kindern vorzuliegen, wenn sie Schlangen begegnen. Spindler (*765—767*) standen für seine vergleichenden Filmuntersuchungen 75 Kinder im Alter zwischen 8 Monaten und 12 Jahren, erwachsene eineiige und zweieiige Zwillinge, 3 Schimpansen und ein jugendlicher Orang zur Verfügung. Eine Instinktreifung in Form einer spontanen Abwehrreaktion gegenüber einer Schlange tritt bei Kindern, die nie im Leben eine Schlange gesehen haben (Heimkinder), im Laufe des dritten Lebensjahres auf[1]. Die Schlange bekommt in dieser Zeit das spezifische Merkmal des Feindes, das den in diesem Alter gereiften angeborenen Auslösemechanismus anspricht (*665*). Angesichts derartiger Untersuchungen drängt sich die Frage auf, inwieweit phasenspezifische Verhaltensweisen der Kinder, etwa im Fremdel- oder Trotzalter, im ersten Gestaltwandel oder in der Pubertät auf dem Boden angeborenen Verhaltens zu erklären sind. Filmuntersuchungen legen z. B. nahe, daß wie bei Säugetieren auch beim Menschen das Brutpflegeverhalten im Sinne der Ethologie erfahrungsfrei *reift*. Es scheint sich bereits im dritten Lebensjahr auszubilden (*766*). In eine derartige phylogenetische Betrachtungsweise wären dann auch das Fingerlutschen (besser: Fingersaugen), das bei kleinen Kindern beliebte Ins-Haar-des-Erwachsenen-Greifen, das Haarbüscheldrehen und vieles andere einzubeziehen (*567*). Die heute üblichere und oft recht hypothetische psychoanalytische Erklärungsweise (*189*) bekäme ein biologisches Fundament, das gerade Sigmund Freud sicherlich gutgeheißen haben würde. Doch fehlt es in der entwicklungspsychologisch orientierten Triebpsychologie und Psychotherapie nicht an fruchtbaren Ansätzen, Brücken zur Ethologie zu schlagen (s. S. 349 ff.). Über derartige Strömungen kann man sich in den letzten Jahrgängen der Zeitschrift „Psyche" rasch orientieren.

Wie oft bei Einbeziehung neuer Gebiete in eine Wissenschaft besteht allerdings die Gefahr einer allzu raschen und kritiklosen Assimilierung der neuen Erkenntnisquellen. So wird die ethologische Terminologie, die aus jahrelanger induktiver Forschung nach und nach erwächst und noch oft genug wechselt, gerne ohne nähere Prüfung ihres Bedeutungsgehaltes übernommen und umgewertet. Ausdrücke, wie z. B. Leerlaufaktivität oder Übersprunghandlung, werden einfach dort eingesetzt,

---

[1] Vgl. hierzu jedoch Antonius (*232*): Über die Schlangenfurcht der Affen.

wo das zutage liegende (neurotische) Verhalten in Analogie zu diesen Begriffen zu stehen scheint. Aus der Analogie werden dann Erklärungen abgeleitet, ohne daß der Instinktcharakter des in Rede stehenden Verhaltens ' wirklich erhärtet worden ist (s. S. 349 ff.).

2. Über die Motorik im cerebralorganischen Abbau

Ein anderer Weg, die Primitiv-Motorik zu untersuchen und phylogenetisch zu vergleichen, bietet sich beim Studium cerebralorganischer Abbauerscheinungen oder Störungen an. Beginnen wir mit dem Bewegungskomplex der Nahrungsaufnahme.

Bei einer jugendlichen Patientin ließen sich am Verlaufe ihrer Wilson-Krankheit mehrere aufeinanderfolgende Stadien oraler motorischer Schablonen unterscheiden: a) Zuerst wandte sich die Patientin einem etwa 50 cm entfernten Gegenstand mit weit geöffnetem Munde zu, ein Verhalten, das auch durch Berührung der Lippenschleimhaut und der Wangenhaut ausgelöst werden konnte. Nach mehreren einander folgenden Auslöser-Reizen versiegte diese Sperr-Reaktion, erschien aber nach einer gewissen „Erholung" wieder. Ließ die Intensitat der Reaktion auf optische Reize nach, so konnte die Sperr-Reaktion durch andere adaquate Reizqualitäten (Berührungsreize) immer noch voll ausgelost werden (vgl. S. 299). b) Mehrere Wochen später blieb die Orientierungsreaktion (Kopfwendung) aus. Die auslösenden Reize bewirkten jetzt nur noch ein ungerichtetes Sperren des Mundes. c) Das Sperren trat nunmehr mit einer Suchautomatie vergesellschaftet auf (s. S.300). Die rhythmischen seitlichen Kopfbewegungen waren überaus häufig mit spontanem Sperren verbunden, ohne daß Auslöser-Reize gegeben wurden. Während Orientierungs- und Sperr-Reaktion anfangs an bestimmte Auslöser-Reize gebunden waren, wurden diese Reize nun zunehmend unspezifischer. Lichtanknipsen, Erschütterung des Bettes

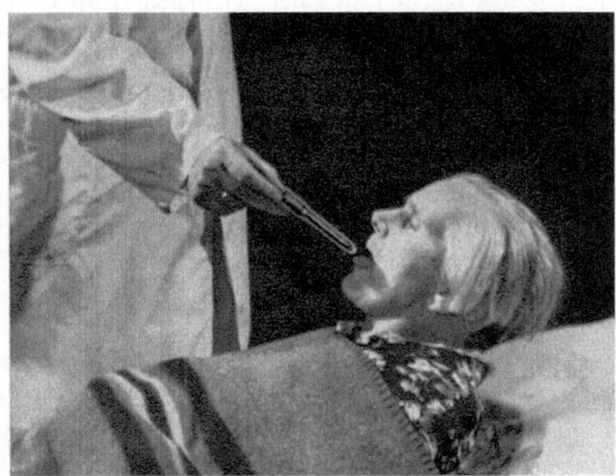

a

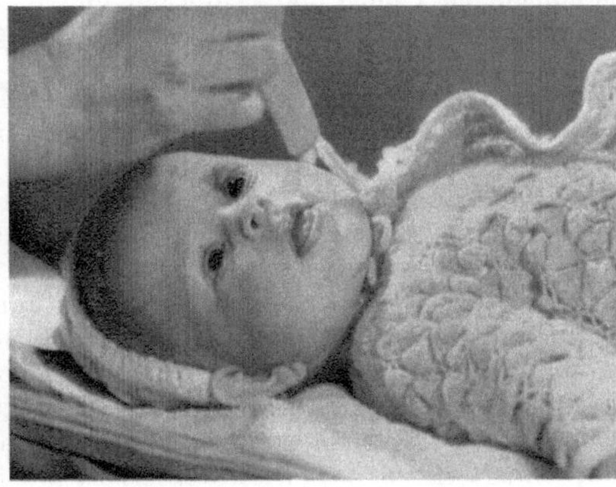

b

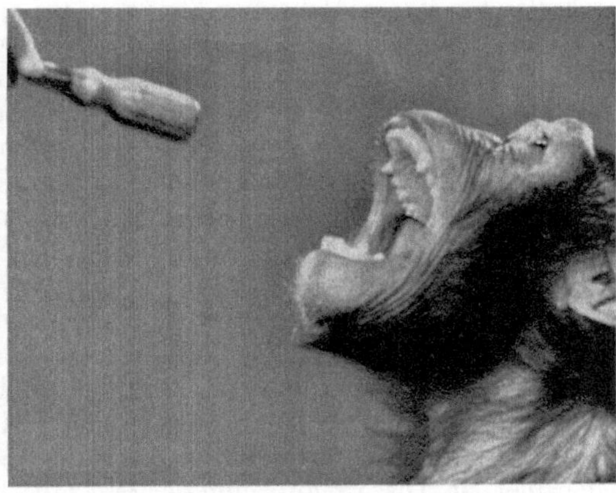

c

Abb. 6a—c. Optisch ausgeloste und optisch orientierte *Sperr-Reaktion* bei einem Kranken mit seniler Demenz, bei einem 6 Monate alten Saugling und bei einem Schimpansen. (Filmaufnahmen von Professor Dr. St. Wieser, Universitatsnervenklinik Gottingen) oder gar das Kneifen an einer beliebigen Körperstelle losten das Sperren und den Such-Automatismus aus (*812*). Pilleri beschreibt einen ähnlichen Fall mit neuro-anatomischem Befund bei Pickscher Krankheit (*642*).

Vergleicht man dieses Beispiel mit dem auf S. 299 geschilderten, so sind hier im Zuge der Desintegration der oralen Leistungen unschwer dieselben Stadien in umgekehrter Reihenfolge wiederzuerkennen, wie sie bei den Drosselnestlingen während der Reifung (Integration) beschrieben wurden.

Abbildung 6 veranschaulicht eine optisch ausgelöste und zugleich auch optisch orientierte Sperr-Reaktion bei einem Kranken mit einer fortgeschrittenen senilen Demenz, bei einem 6 Monate alten Säugling und einem Schimpansen aus dem Frankfurter Zoo. Die drei Reaktionen sind einander homolog. In anderen Fällen folgt dem *Sperren* noch das *Schnappen*: Das dargebotene Objekt wird mit den Lippen oder Zähnen erfaßt. Von diesen beiden Formen oralen Greifens ist das *Ansaugen*, das ebenfalls bei fortgeschrittenem cerebralorganischen Abbau zu finden ist, wohl zu unterscheiden. Es spielt sich im Bereich der Lippen ab und nimmt eine stammesgeschichtliche Sonderstellung ein, da es nur den Säugern eigen ist. Wir übergehen hier weitere Formen motorischer Schablonen des Oralsinnes, wie z. B. das Mundphänomen, das Kauen und Schlucken, und verweisen auf eine Übersicht der umfangreichen, auch älteren Literatur (*207*); bezüglich der oralen epileptischen Phänomene vgl. S. 351 ff.

Allgemein gesagt, ist das Greifen mit dem Mund für alle Wirbeltiere ungemein charakteristisch und als Funktion nicht nur für die Nahrungsaufnahme bereitgestellt (*412*). Die Bewegungen, insbesondere die archaischen Handlungsweisen des Sperrens und Schnappens, können als Drohgeste, bei Angriffs- oder Balzhandlungen und sonstigen arteigenen instinktiven Verhaltensweisen vorkommen. Die Abfolge der Bewegungen ist also als Funktion weitgehend unspezifisch. Auch beim Säugling dient der Mund nicht nur zur Nahrungsaufnahme, sondern auch als Greiforgan. Die Ablösung der Greiffunktion vom Mund und die allmähliche Übertragung auf die Hand beginnt erst mehrere Monate nach der Geburt. Im Zuge des Abbaues der differenzierten zentralnervösen Leistungen erhält der Mund seine frühe Funktion als Greiforgan zurück. Diese oralen motorischen Schablonen können daher mit Recht als *primitive Greifformen* bezeichnet werden (*806*).

Die *Greifphänomene* mit der Hand geben weitere Aufschlüsse über die Entwicklung und den Abbau der Motorik (*208*). Auf Abb. 7 sehen wir den *propriozeptiven Greifreflex* bei einem Alzheimer-Kranken, bei einem 6 Monate alten Säugling und bei einem Schimpansen. Diese tonisch reaktive Beugeantwort der Finger geht regelmäßig mit einer umfassenden Beugekontraktion der Armmuskulatur einher. Daß es sich dabei tatsächlich um eine propriozeptive reflexartige Antwort auf Dehnreize handelt, kann man durch Ausschaltung aller Afferenzen aus der Handfläche mit Hilfe einer Novocainblockade der Nervenstämme am Handgelenk demonstrieren, wie es bei dem Alzheimer-Kranken geschehen ist. (Siehe Markierung der Blockade durch dunkle Flecken am Handgelenk.) Dieser Phase folgt eine exterozeptive Reaktion, das *Nachgreifen* ("instinctive grasp reaction" von Denny-Brown), als Ausdruck einer *Zuwende-Reaktion* im Sinne einer aktiven Hinwendung zu einem Berührungsreiz. Beide Reaktionen können im cerebralorganischen Abbau isoliert vorkommen, sind jedoch gewöhnlich zugleich vorhanden und wirken gegenseitig reaktionsfördernd. Interessant ist dabei, daß jeder Hautzone der Handfläche eine bestimmte, gleichförmige Bewegung eines oder, je nach Reiz, mehrerer Finger zugeordnet ist. Diese Zuordnung der Gliedabschnitte zu den Zonen des receptorischen Feldes geschieht nach dem Prinzip der Bewegungsökonomie (*804*)[1].

---

[1] v. Monakow (*150*), dem ein entscheidendes Verdienst fur die ältere neurologisch und psychopathologisch orientierte Instinktforschung zukommt, entdeckte unseres Wissens als erster das Prinzip der Ökonomie im Rahmen dissolutiver Vorgänge im ZNS. Seine Gedankengänge wurden — auch hinsichtlich der Neurosenlehre — von R. Brun (*21, 22*) weitergeführt.

Die *Zuwende-Reaktionen* sind für die Ethologie deswegen wichtig, weil sich hieran das Grundprinzip von Schlüsselreiz und angeborenem Auslösemechanismus (s. S. 303) auch beim Menschen gut demonstrieren läßt. Zum Beispiel lösen nur ganz bestimmte Schlüsselreize den Mechanismus des Ansaugens, des Sperrens oder des Nachgreifens aus. Für das Ansaugen sind kleinere Objekte mit möglichst glatter, runder oder sphärischer Oberfläche von mittlerer Temperatur optimal, während offene, nicht flächige Objekte (z. B. ein Pinsel) kein Ansaugen hervorrufen. Die Härte oder Weichheit des Materials spielt keine Rolle. So lehrt denn auch die Erfahrung, daß es Säuglingen keine Schwierigkeit bereitet, statt der Mutterbrust den härteren Gummisauger anzunehmen. Für das Sperren und Nachgreifen sind Reizqualitäten der Bewegtheit, des Bewegungstempos, der Bewegungsrichtung, der Entfernung und Größe sowie der Abgehobenheit vom Hintergrund entscheidend. Wir sehen hier also gestalttheoretische Kategorien ins Spiel kommen (*805*). WIESER hat in seinen Experimenten an Patienten mit cerebralorganischen Endzuständen zeigen können, daß bestimmten Reaktionen ein bestimmter Wirkraum zugeordnet ist. In mehr als 57 cm Entfernung vom Kopf folgt der Kranke einem visuellen Reiz mit den Augen oder auch mit dem ganzen Kopf nach. In der nächst näheren Zone löst der optische Schlüsselreiz, unabhängig von der erkannten Bedeutung der Objekte, tastende Handbewegungen mit Erfassen der Objekte aus. Der dritte Raumabschnitt entspricht dem Wirkbereich der oralen Sperr-Reaktion. Die innerste „Raumschale" wird von der Körperoberfläche selbst gebildet, an der sich die taktile

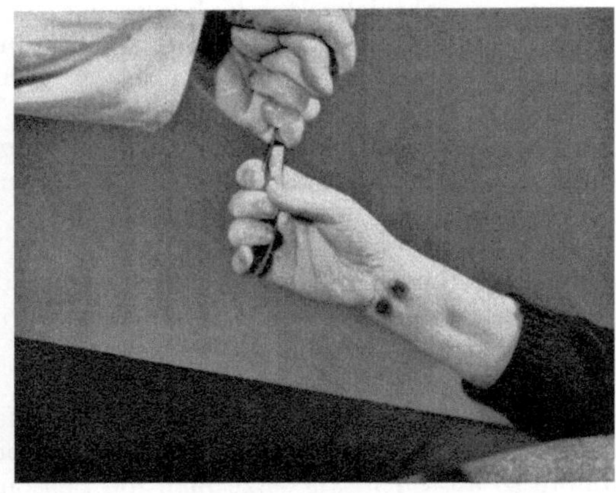

a

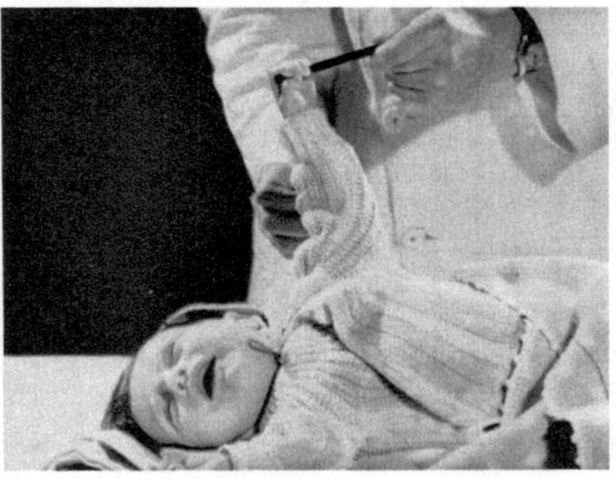

b

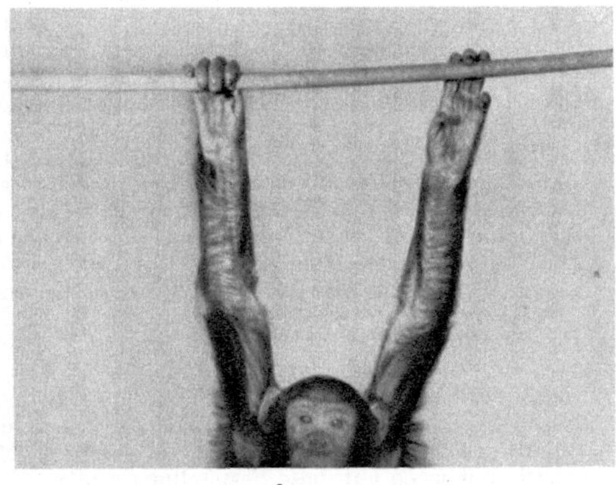

c

Abb. 7 a—c *Proprioceptiver Greifreflex.* Im oberen Bild kommt die reaktive Beugesynergie zum Ausdruck. Der Daumen wird nicht opponiert. Die dunklen Flecken am Handgelenk zeigen die Stelle an, wo eine Blockade der Nn. ulnaris und medianus mit Novocain vorgenommen wurde. Homolog sind die Greifphänomene bei einem etwa 6 Monate alten Säugling (Mitte) und einem erwachsenen Schimpansen (unten). (Filmaufnahmen von Prof. Dr. WIESER)

Orientierung abspielt. Durch Berührung der jeweiligen receptorischen Felder kommt es zu den verschiedenen Greifreaktionen oder zum Ansaugen. Während bei den hirnorganisch Kranken die ehedem differenzierte und reich strukturierte adäquate Reizkonstellation zu einer einfachen taktilen oder optischen Schablone reduziert wird (*805*), sieht man beim Säugling — cum grano salis — den umgekehrten Verlauf: Zwischen dem 3. und 7. Lebensmonat kann man die Ausbildung des Greif- und Seh-Raumes mit zunehmender Differenzierung der Reizkonstellationen beobachten. Auch bei vorübergehenden Zuständen cerebraler Dissolution, wie wir sie in der Klinik beim Erwachen aus dem Insulin-Koma oder nach dem Elektroschock beobachten, können wir schrittweise Restitutionsvorgänge verfolgen, die über motorische Schablonen zur voll integrierten Willkürmotorik führen (*253, 270*).

Um Mißverständnisse zu vermeiden, bedürfen die Beispiele und Vergleiche, die bisher in diesem Kapitel gebracht wurden, noch einiger Erläuterungen. Denn es könnte so aussehen, als setze man die Sensomotorik von Säuglingen, Kranken, Affen und anderen Säugetieren unmittelbar gleich. Die Lehre J. H. JACKSONs (*91*) von der Evolution und Dissolution des Nervensystems muß, obgleich seit langem und häufig angewandt, kurz repetiert werden.

JACKSON fußt auf HERBERT SPENCER (*187*), der die Evolutionslehre CHARLES DARWINs (*32*) abwandelte und als erster von der hierarchischen Ordnung des Nervensystems sprach. JACKSON (*432*) definiert in seinen "Croonian Lectures on the Evolution and Dissolution of the Nervous System" den Terminus Evolution dreifach:

1. "Evolution is a passage from the most to the least organised — that is to say — from the lowest well organised centres to the highest least organised centres." (Dieses „am meisten" und „am wenigsten" Organisiert-Sein bedeutet die Festigkeit des funktionalen Verbandes der jeweiligen Zentren.)

2. "Evolution is a passage from the most simple to the most complex; again from the lowest to the highest centres."

3. "Evolution is a passage from the most automatic to the most voluntary." Diese dreifache Definition bedeutet, so fährt JACKSON fort, daß die hochsten Zentren, welche den Gipfel der nervalen Entwicklung darstellen und das "organ of mind" oder die physische Basis des Bewußtseins bilden, am wenigsten organisiert sind, hochst komplex funktionieren und am meisten dem Willen unterworfen sind. Man beachte, daß es sich hier um eine *rein funktionelle Definition* handelt, in die keine anatomischen Zuordnungen eingeschlossen sind.

Von der Dissolution, einem Terminus SPENCERs, sagt JACKSON zunachst, daß sie die Umkehrung des Evolutionsprozesses bedeute. Daß dies aber nicht im buchstablichen Sinn gemeint ist, wie er oft Anwendung findet, geht aus den weiteren funktionalen Unterscheidungen hervor, die JACKSON für die Dissolutionsprozesse vornimmt. Sie folgen einer „zusammengesetzten Ordnung", und die drei Stadien mögen grob durch die Anfangsbuchstaben der *höchsten*, *mittleren* und *niedrigsten* (*lowest*) Zentren symbolisiert werden: 1. H; 2. $H_2 + M$; 3. $H_3 + M_2 + L$. Diese Unterscheidung bezieht sich auf die allgemeine, d. h. das ganze Hirn betreffende Dissolution.

Die wichtigste Unterscheidung, die JACKSON trifft, scheint uns die zwischen allgemeiner und lokaler Dissolution zu sein: "Obviously disease of a part of the nervous system *could not be a reversal of the evolution of the whole* (vom Verf. kursiv); all that we can expect is a local reversal of evolution, that there should be loss in the order from voluntary towards automatic in what the part diseased represents." JACKSON hebt dann ausdrücklich hervor, daß es auch eine lokale Dissolution der hochsten Zentren gibt, und erwähnt unter den Geisteskrankheiten (insanity) die progressive Paralyse und die Melancholie. "Different kinds of insanity are different local dissolution of the highest centres." Wenn JACKSON dann spater klinische Beispiele gibt, die nach dem damaligen Stande des Wissens mit gewissen anatomischen Systemen korreliert werden — wußte man doch damals z. B. nichts Sicheres über die Neuropathologie der extrapyramidalen Erkrankungen und hielt die neo-motorische Rinde allein verantwortlich für die Willkurbewegungen[1] —, so andert dies nichts an JACKSONs *rein funktional gefaßtem Zentrenbegriff.* Wir legen auf diese Feststellung großen Wert, erstens, weil sich von hier aus fast alle

---

[1] Siehe hierzu die Arbeit von WILDER PENFIELD (*634*): Mechanisms of voluntary movement, in der seine Lehre vom centrencephalen System (*631*) eine wichtige Rolle spielt. Vgl. auch DANDY (*314*) über den „Sitz des Bewußtseins" und ALFORD (*225*) über „Lokalisation von Bewußtsein und Emotion".

Mißverständnisse bezüglich der Lehre von der Evolution und Dissolution beseitigen lassen, und zweitens, weil wir im letzten Kapitel dieses Teiles darauf zurückkommen werden.

Hinsichtlich unserer Beispiele von der Evolution und Dissolution der menschlichen Sensomotorik können wir uns nun kurz fassen und sehen uns in den *Schluß-folgerungen* in Übereinstimmung mit WIESER (*806*): Beim ontogenetischen Vergleichen zwischen dem Aufbau der Sensomotorik des Säuglings und dem Abbau dieser Funktion beim cerebralorganisch Kranken handelt es sich nicht einfach um eine Umkehr des Entwicklungsprozesses. Die Wiederholung der frühen Verhaltensweisen in den Stadien des Abbaues betrifft *nur die erfahrungsfreien, angeborenen Verhaltensweisen*, während die durch Gewöhnung erworbenen, bedingten oder sekundär automatisierten sensomotorischen Vollzüge der Dissolution anheimfallen. Dabei bedenke man, daß sich die ersten bedingten Reaktionen gerade hinsichtlich der Nahrungsaufnahme schon in den ersten Lebenswochen auszubilden beginnen. Der Abbau wiederholt somit nicht die ganze Stufenfolge der früheren Verhaltensweisen, sondern läßt entlang der ontogenetischen Leitlinie die aufeinander folgenden Stadien der artspezifischen und angeborenen Schablonen in umgekehrter Reihenfolge hervortreten. Dies steht im Einklang mit JACKSONs Lehre, da diese „Zentren" von vornherein fester organisiert, einfacher funktionierend, automatischer (formstarr) sind als die erworbenen motorischen Bestände, in denen stets ererbte Teilkoordinationen stecken und die im Sinne JACKSONs einem höheren Zentrum angehören. Wir sehen daraus, daß uns schwere Abbauprozesse vorzüglich dazu verhelfen, Bausteine angeborenen Verhaltens zu erkennen.

Die Beziehungen der Säuglingsmotorik und der pathologisch reduzierten Motorik zu Verhaltensweisen aus der Tierreihe sind anders und vorsichtiger zu beurteilen. Die motorischen Leistungen der Tiere aus der Stammesverwandtschaft des Menschen sind nicht primitiv, schablonenhaft oder unterentwickelt, sondern höchst spezialisiert und in die Umwelt eingepaßt. Beim Säugling hingegen handelt es sich in viel größerem Ausmaß um Durchgangsstufen der Entwicklung, die später umgebaut werden, und im Abbauprozeß schließlich treten nur noch Schablonen hervor, denen die spezifischen Merkmale, die die arterhaltende Leistung garantieren, fehlen. Diesen „motorischen Kernbestand" oder dieses „funktionelle Rohmaterial" (*253, 806*) von Säugling und Hirnkrankem können wir aber nach den Regeln der vergleichenden Morphologie auf homologe Merkmale untersuchen und im Falle hinreichender Übereinstimmung gesicherte Vergleiche zu den Säugetieren ziehen, wie wir an Beispielen zeigten.

3. Das Ausdrucksverhalten des Säuglings

Der Begriff Ausdruck wurde verschieden gefaßt. HEDIGER (*393*) versteht darunter alle am Tier feststellbaren, veränderlichen, nicht pathologischen Erscheinungen, welche zum Verstehen seiner Situation beitragen. Dazu würden dann alle Erscheinungen rechnen, an denen der Beobachter Erregungen eines Tieres erkennt, wie Übersprung und Leerlaufhandlungen (s. S. 304), Lautäußerungen oder Intentionsbewegungen (s. S. 330). Aber auch vegetative Begleitsymptome, die für den Artgenossen zum Signal werden können, wie z. B. Harnen, Koten, Zittern, Drüsensekretionen, wären darunterzuzählen.

Unter den mannigfachen Ausdrucksformen der Säugetiere (*40, 332*) wählen wir eine für den Menschen kennzeichnende Verhaltensweise aus: *das Lächeln.* Wir suchen erstens nach homologem Verhalten bei Säugetieren, und zweitens verfolgen wir die ontogenetische Entwicklung dieses menschlichen Ausdrucksverhaltens. LORENZ (*535*) schlug vor, nur dann von Ausdruck zu sprechen, wenn *ein Verhalten im Dienste der Koordination sozialen Zusammenlebens* eine besondere Differenzierung bekommen hat, da dies beweist, daß die *soziale* Funktion das Wesentliche des betreffenden Phänomens ist. Diese Definition läßt sich gut auf das Lächeln anwenden.

Außer dem Lacheln gibt es freilich noch eine ganze Reihe mimischer Ausdrucksqualitäten, die sich zu phylogenetisch vergleichenden Untersuchungen eignen (*40*), wie LORENZ (*131*) am Beispiel des Hundes gezeigt hat: Durch Superposition von Kampf- und Fluchtintention in der Mimik des Hundes konnen verschiedene Formen des Gesichtsausdrucks entstehen. Fluchtintention wird bei Hundeartigen durch Zuruckziehen der Mundwinkel und Ohren ausgedrückt, Kampfintention durch leichtes Mauloffnen, Emporziehen der Oberlippe und Faltenbildung an Schnauze und Stirn (*721*). Beide Formen überlagern sich häufig, da Kampf- und Fluchtstimmung meist gleichzeitig aktiviert werden (vgl. dazu S. 334 f.). Derartige Überlagerungen von Stimmungen bewirken eine große Variabilität der Ausdrucksbewegungen. Diese sind dem Artgenossen meist primär, d. h. ohne Erfahrung, verstandlich und fungieren als Ausloser (s. S. 330 ff.).

An CHARLES DARWINs beruhmt gewordene Abhandlung „Der Ausdruck der Gemutsbewegungen bei Menschen und Tieren" (*34*) sei erinnert. Über andere Ausdrucksbewegungen wie „Imponieren", „Drohen", Demutsgebarden u. a. lesen wir auf S. 330 ff. weiteres.

a) Das Lächeln

Im Gegensatz zu der üblicherweise herrschenden Meinung ist *das Lächeln des Säuglings eine angeborene Ausdrucksbewegung* und trägt als solche den *Charakter*

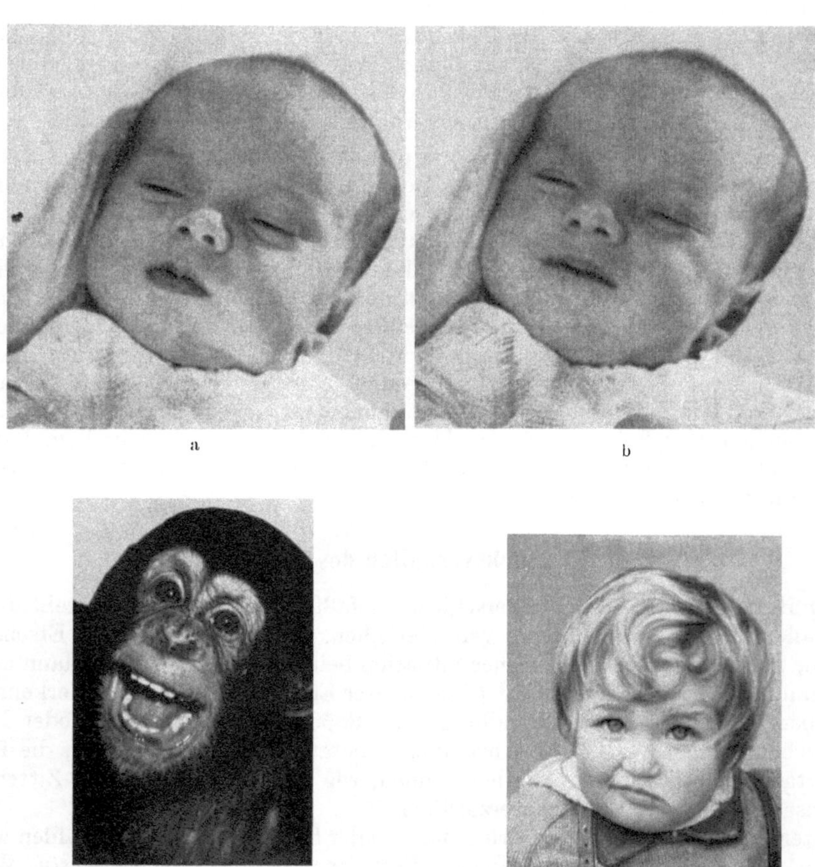

Abb. 8 a—d. *Das Lacheln als angeborene Ausdrucksbewegung.* a 7 Tage altes Madchen, vor dem Lacheln, b wahrend eines etwa 2 sec dauernden Lachelns. c Lacheln der Schimpansin Vicky. d Nach Abdecken der linken Gesichtshalfte des 14 Monate alten Kindes sieht man ein lachelndes, ohne die rechte Halfte ein schmollendes Gesicht. Unmittelbar vor Aufnahme des Bildes schmollte das Kind, gleich danach lachelte es symmetrisch. [Nach KOEHLER (*474*)]

einer echten Instinktbewegung. Das sprach zum ersten Mal Otto Koehler (*475*) aus und stützte sich dabei auf eigene Beobachtungen sowie auf Fotos und Filmstreifen anderer Beobachter (s. Abb. 8). In den ersten Lebenstagen hat der Säugling meist beide Augen geschlossen. Dann sieht man bei seinem Lächeln sich nur Mund und Nasenpartie bewegen. Lächelt er bei offenen Augen, schließt er die Lider etwas, auch können sich am äußeren Augenwinkel „Krähenfüße" bilden.

Der *Zeitpunkt* des ersten Lächelns variiert sehr stark. Kinder, die schon am Tage ihrer Geburt lächeln, hielt man im Altertum für Gotteskinder.

Ein im 6. Schwangerschaftsmonat zur Welt gekommenes Kind lächelte am 2. Tage seiner Geburt drei Stunden vor seinem Tode, und zwar 3mal halbseitig und ungewöhnlich lange, nämlich 2mal 5 sec und einmal 4 sec lang in Abständen von 9 und 15 min. Von 3 Siebenmonatskindern lächelte eines am 9. Lebenstage 4 sec lang halbseitig, das zweite am 4. Tage mehrmals 1—2 sec lang halbseitig und einmal beidseitig, das dritte bereits 7 Std. nach der Geburt mehrmals linksseitig, und zwar nach dem Trinken und Trockenlegen.

Bei den vollausgetragenen und genau auf das Lächeln beobachteten Kindern schwanken die Zeitangaben für halb- und beidseitiges Lächeln zwischen dem ersten und dem 17. Tage. Koehler sah seinen ersten Enkel am Tage der Geburt lächeln (*475*). Meine Frau und ich beobachteten Lachen bei zweien unserer Kinder am 2. Tage, bei den beiden anderen am 5. Tage, und zwar halb- und beidseitig.

Man geht nach allen vorliegenden Angaben nicht fehl, wenn man die erste Woche als durchschnittlichen Zeitpunkt für das Auftreten des ersten Lächelns annimmt, eine Phase der Entwicklung also, wo von einer visuell orientierten Objektbeziehung zur Mutter, von der die Kinder, wie gern geglaubt wird, das Lächeln lernen sollen, nicht die Rede sein kann. Die Erfahrung anderer Beobachter, daß das Lächeln besonders gern nach dem Trinken, Trockenlegen, nach Abgang von Blähungen und sogar im Schlaf auftritt, können wir durchaus auf Grund langer Beobachtung bestätigen. Während einer halben Beobachtungsstunde sah ich Lächeln in der 3. Lebenswoche 5mal beidseitig im Abstand von wenigen Minuten im Schlaf auftreten. Eine Verwechslung mit „Grimassieren", „Stäupchen" oder anderen Gesichtsbewegungen (*156, 628*) halte ich wegen des echten Ausdruckscharakters für ausgeschlossen. Schon dieses frühe Lächeln ist an „Stimmungen" (Sattheit, Schlaf) gebunden und bleibt bei unlustbetonten Zuständen (Hunger, Blähungen) aus. Daß sich solche Stimmungen auch überlagern können, zeigt Bild 4 der Abb. 8: das kurz vorher schmollende, 14 Monate alte Kind beginnt auf der rechten Seite zu lachen, während es auf der linken noch schmollt, um sofort darauf symmetrisch zu lachen (*474*).

Auffälligerweise ist das angeborene Lächeln anfangs häufiger halbseitig als voll, tritt häufig bei geschlossenen Augen auf und währt nur Momente. Es reift also erst zur vollen Erbkoordination heran. Für die Feststellung des erfahrungsfreien Reifens ist die Tatsache, daß blindgeborene Kinder ebenfalls lächeln, von großer Wichtigkeit (*475*). Wie viele Instinkthandlungen zeigt auch das Lächeln mehrere recht verschieden aussehende Intensitätsstufen (vgl. S. 301 f.), was man an 3—5 Monate alten Säuglingen gut beobachten kann. Der Mund wird immer breiter, die Lider nähern sich immer mehr, plötzlich atmet das Kind, zuweilen hörbar, stoßweise aus, ja, es kann sogar zum stimmhaften Lachen kommen. „Und auf dem Gipfel der Freude überrascht uns eines Tages die dritte Stufe, der *Jauchzer*, ein langgezogener Jubelschrei aus weitgeöffnetem Munde" (*474*). Eine der besten Auslösersituationen für die höheren Intensitätsstufen des Lachens ist das Schaukeln. Das Jauchzen hörten wir aber auch bei einem sich allein überlassenen Säugling von knapp 4 Monaten, ohne daß ein äußerer Anlaß zu erkennen war. Sowohl Lachen als auch Jauchzen treten zu einer Zeit auf, wo das Lachen Erwachsener das Baby nicht etwa ansteckt, sondern eher erschreckt und selbst dann noch zum Weinen bringen kann, wenn es selber gerade lacht. Mit der alten Nachahmungsthese ist es nach allem schlecht bestellt.

Schließlich wäre noch nach der *Wirkung* zu fragen, die das Lächeln des Säuglings *auf die Artgenossen,* zumeist die Mutter, ausübt. Nach HERODOT entging Kypselos, der spätere Herrscher von Korinth, als Neugeborener der Tötung, indem er die Schergen anlächelte. Diese Sage zeigt sehr schön den wahren Sachverhalt, daß nämlich für diese angeborene Verhaltensweise keineswegs das Verhalten des

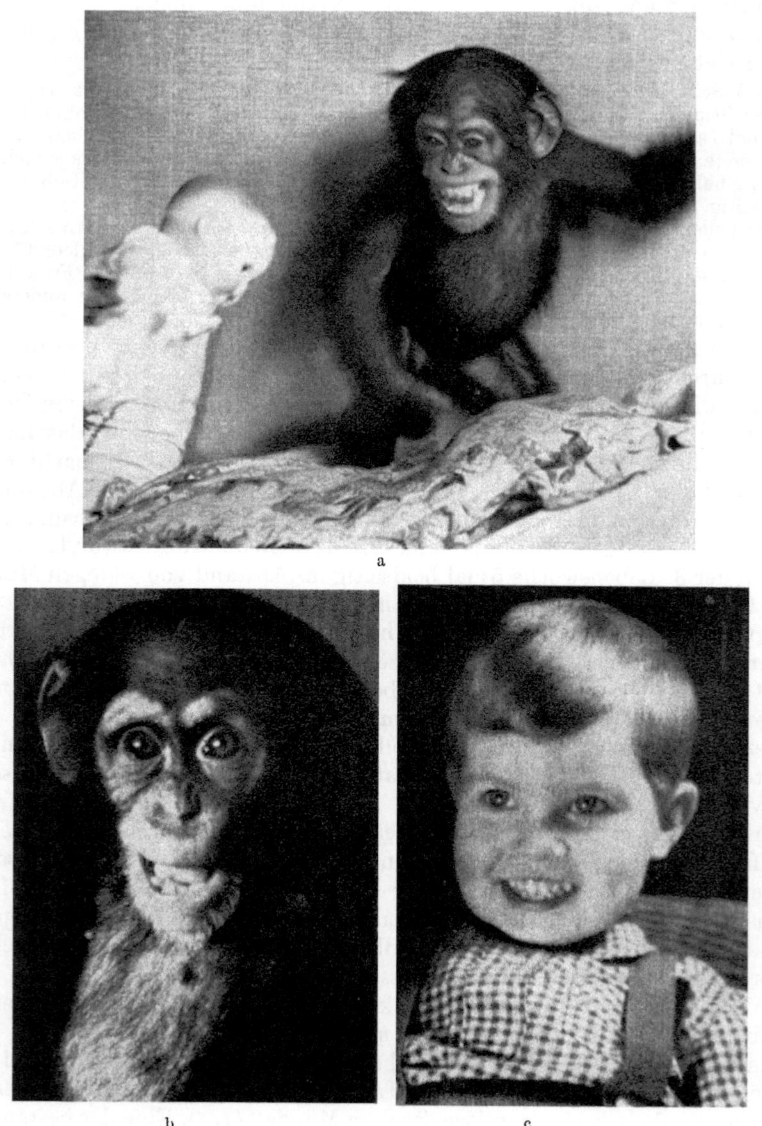

Abb. 9a—c. *Das Lächeln als homologe Instinktbewegung.* a Junge Schimpansin vor einer Puppe. b u. c Erwartungslächeln einer jungen Schimpansin und eines kleinen Jungen. [Aufnahmen von Prof. Dr. B. GRZIMEK (*378*)]

Partners ausschlaggebend ist, daß diese Instinktbewegung aber eine mächtige Kraft auf ihn ausübt und in ihm, wenn nicht den Brutpflegeinstinkt, so doch eine stimmungsbeeinflussende Haltung auslöst. Wie entzückt selbst ganz unbeteiligte

Menschen auf das Lächeln eines Babys reagieren, weiß jedermann aus Erfahrung.
Für die Mutter bedeutet dieser kleine, huschende Ausdruck höchstes Glück. Wir
sehen darin die Verzahnung aller echten Instinktbewegungen mit dem Partner,
ohne daß so etwas wie der Intellekt dabei eine Rolle spielt. Die Instinktbewegung
des Lächelns ist der angeborene Ausdruck der Freude, der seinerseits Freude
auslöst.

Den Vergleich des Lächelns mit der vermutlich homologen Instinktbewegung
junger Schimpansen wollen wir im Bilde demonstrieren (s. Abb. 8 u. 9) und
es dem Betrachter überlassen, ob er diesen Ausdruck als ein Lächeln oder Lachen

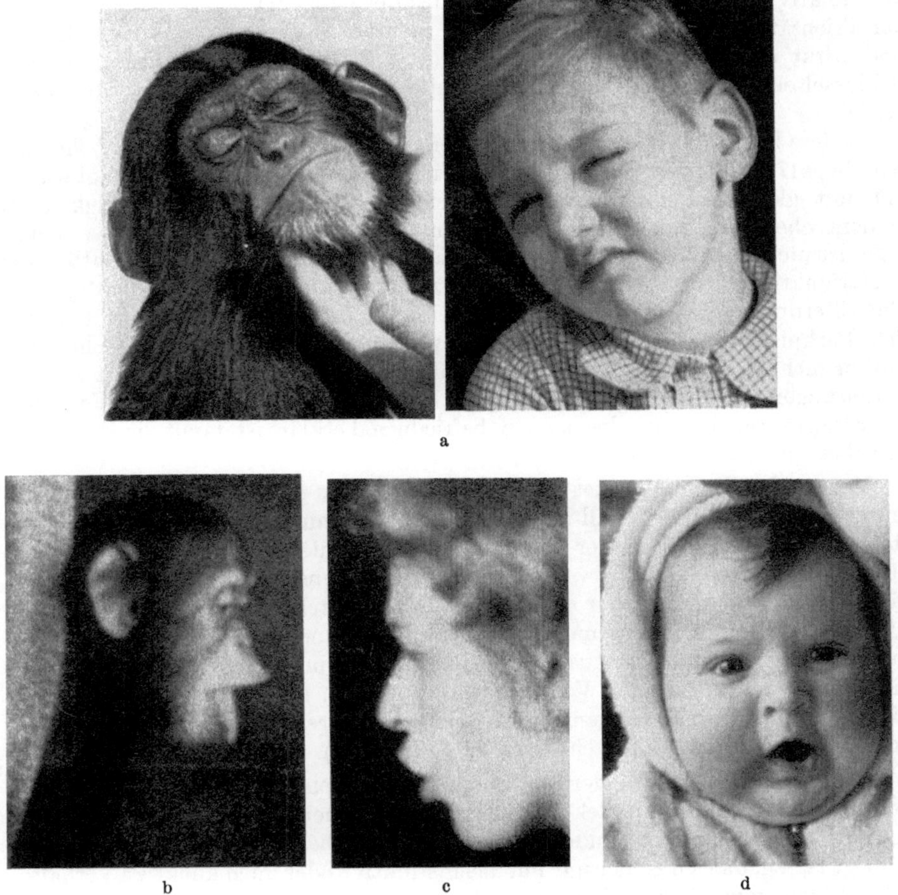

Abb. 10a—d. *Vergleichbare mimische Ausdrucksbewegungen.* a Mißmut; b—d „Schimpfen" eines jungen Schimpansen, eines erwachsenen Menschen und eines 4 Monate alten Mädchens. [Aufnahmen a—c von Prof. Dr. GRZIMEK (*378*), Aufnahme d vom Verfasser]

anerkennen will. Um die Mimik von Schimpansen recht beurteilen zu können,
bedarf es allerdings einiger Erfahrung. Man beachte die Beteiligung der auch beim
Menschen zusammenwirkenden Muskelgruppen. Sicher ist jedenfalls, daß wir eine
derartige Mimik beim jungen Schimpansen nie zu sehen bekommen, wenn er
„ängstlich", „mißtrauisch" oder irgendwie ablehnend gestimmt ist. Einen geradezu komischen Ausdruck des Mißmutes beim Schimpansen und bei einem kleinen
Jungen sehen wir auf Abb. 10, und ebenso das „Schimpfen" im Vergleich zwischen

dem gleichen, noch nicht 1 Jahr alten Schimpansenmädchen, einem 4 Monate alten Menschenmädchen und einem Erwachsenen. Auf Abb. 9 sehen wir ein Lächeln mit dem Unterton: „Ich möchte gern, trau mich aber nicht so recht" (*378*). Bei *erwachsenen Schimpansen* haben wir weder in Wirklichkeit noch auf einem Bilde einen Gesichtsausdruck gesehen, der wie ein Lachen anmutet[1]. Zweifellos lacht ja auch der erwachsene Mensch weit weniger als der jugendliche. So mag denn das Lächeln des Menschen eines der Merkmale persistierender Jugendlichkeit sein (*60*). Auf ein anderes, das Spiel, kommen wir noch zu sprechen.

Halten wir vom Lächeln fest: Es ist angeboren und besteht aus einzelnen Erbkoordinationen, die zunächst noch nicht in vollem Synergismus abzulaufen brauchen, aber relativ rasch reifen. Es ist ein Ausdruck der Gestimmtheit und abhängig von der Triebsättigung (vgl. S. 309). Es zeigt mehrere Intensitätsstufen (vgl. S. 301) und wirkt als starker sozialer Auslöser (s. S. 330), ohne selbst unbedingt von Schlüsselreizen (s. S. 300) abhängig zu sein. Erfahrung spielt nachweisbar keine Rolle.

Andere Formen des Ausdrucksverhaltens, wie z. B. das *Schreien und Lallen* des Säuglings (*785*), können wir nur streifen. Vieles, was über das Lächeln gesagt wurde, gilt mit gleichsam umgekehrten Vorzeichen. Die Stimmungsabhängigkeit ist evident, ebenso die Tatsache des Angeborenseins. „Das Weinen des Verlassenseins" (*740*) ist nicht nur Vögeln, sondern auch vielen Säugetieren eigen. Hinsichtlich der Sozialfunktion (*568*) mag statt vieler Einzelheiten folgender Kurzbericht gelten: Ein Elternpaar geht ins Kino und läßt seinen schlafenden Säugling im Auto auf dem Parkplatz zurück. Der Säugling wird wach und schreit, höchstwahrscheinlich, weil er nichts als Hunger hat. Ein Volksauflauf entsteht, und es kommt zu Ausschreitungen gegen die zurückkehrenden „Raben-Eltern". Man mag das Verhalten der Eltern verantwortungslos nennen, befriedigend erklärt ist damit die Empörung der Masse nicht.

Von großer Wichtigkeit ist das *Lallen*, weil es uns an die Anfänge der Sprachentwicklung führt. Die „Lall-Monologe" (*479*) beginnen im 3. bis 4. Monat und steigern sich hinsichtlich ihrer phonetischen Variabilität bis zum 9. Monat so, daß alle nur denkbaren Laute hervorgebracht werden können (*698*). Mit 1 Jahr nimmt diese Mannigfaltigkeit wieder ab, und gleichzeitig macht sich eine Intentionalisierung der Lautkundgaben bemerkbar (*785*). Man erinnere sich auch in diesem Zusammenhang an Gehlens Ausführungen über die Sprache (*60*). O. Koehler hat mehrfach gezeigt, daß eine Vorstufe des Sprechens, das „unbenannte Denken" (*472*), Menschen und Tieren gemeinsam ist. Auch andere tierische Vorstufen menschlicher Sprache lassen sich nachweisen (*473, 476, 479*).

Die ganze Entwicklung der sog. höheren seelischen Leistungen, alles, was mit der Entwicklung des Intellekts und den zahlreichen Intelligenz-Untersuchungen an Anthropoiden und anderen Affen zusammenhängt, müssen wir unberücksichtigt lassen, da es uns hier nur um das instinktive oder auch affektive Verhalten geht. Einen vorzüglichen Zugang zu diesen Untersuchungen findet man in den älteren Büchern von W. Köhler (*110*) und H. Klüver (*107*) (vgl. S. 346).

b) Das Mimikerkennen

Man mag vom Ausdrucksverhalten des jungen Säuglings und speziell vom Lächeln sagen, es sei nur ein „Grimassieren" und nicht „echt", weil die Gegenseitigkeit der Beziehung fehle. Mit anderen Worten: als „richtiges" Lächeln könne

---

[1] Otto Koehler versichert uns allerdings, man konne bei Schimpanse und Gorilla durch Kitzeln unter der Achsel erst Lächeln und dann dazu stoßweise-phonierte Ausatmung auslösen.

man nur dasjenige bezeichnen, das als Antwort auf das Lächeln eines anderen erscheine (*618*). Eine solche Definition schließt aber die Entwicklung einer Verhaltensweise aus, und so würden denn auch das ungerichtete erste Greifen kein echtes Greifen, die ersten Saugbewegungen im Leerlauf kein richtiges Saugen oder die ersten Laufbewegungen kein echtes Laufen sein.

Gerade für das Antwort-Lächeln läßt sich beweisen, daß es unabhängig von der differenzierten Mimik des Partners reift und keineswegs als persönliche Begrüßung zu verstehen ist. Ohne schon von Schlüsselreizen etwas zu wissen, stellte KAILA (*444*) 1932 die ersten Attrappen-Versuche am Säugling an, und R. SPITZ [zusammen mit K. M. WOLF (*768*)] folgte ihm 1946 nach. SPITZ stellte an 145 Kindern im Alter von 3—6 Monaten fest, daß rohe Gesichtsattrappen, Vogelscheuchen oder eine „sardonisch" verzerrte Fratze das Lächeln geradesogut auslösen wie das menschliche Gesicht. In diesen Untersuchungen blieben viele Fragen offen, die ROLF AHRENS (*221*) mit Hilfe von gründlicheren Attrappen-Versuchen eingehender beantworten konnte. Die Ergebnisse — vorläufig noch auf quantitativ ungesicherter Basis — sind in Abb. 11 veranschaulicht.

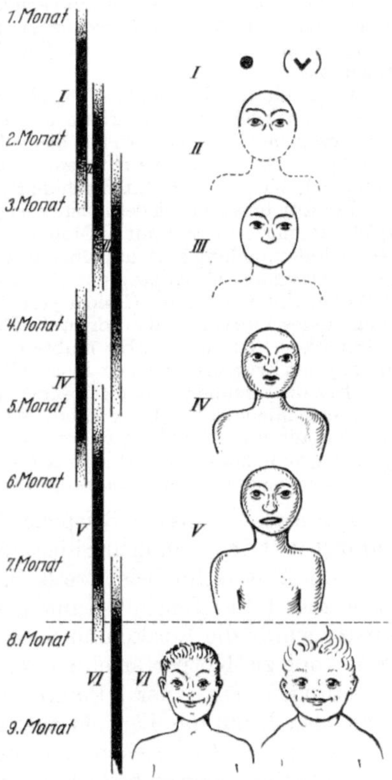

AHRENS ermittelte folgende optische Auslöser, die imstande sind, bei Säuglingen im Alter zwischen 4 und 12 Wochen reaktives Lächeln hervorzurufen: Etwa bis zum Beginn des 2. Monats lösen gut abgegrenzte, etwa augengroße Punkte, die auf einem grob ausgeschnittenen Kopfumriß — gleich, ob oval oder rund — gemalt sind, das Lächeln sicherer aus als ein rechteckiger Balken auf gleichem Grund oder ein gemaltes Gesicht. Die Anordnung der Punkte (ein Paar waagerecht oder senkrecht oder 3 Paare nach Art eines Dominosteines) war dabei gleichgültig. Ein einzelner Punkt hingegen war unwirksam.

Mit Beginn des 2. Monats verlieren diese „Einzelreize" an Wirkung, ohne jedoch die Auslöserwirkung ganz einzubüßen. Die Augenpartie, die Ocula, in welche die Einzelreize gewissermaßen eingebaut sind, entfaltet stärkere Wirksamkeit. Wahrscheinlich steht zwischen diesen beiden Phasen „Einzelreiz" und „Ocula" noch eine Zwischenstufe, in der die Einzelreize (Punkte) in waagerechter Anordnung wirksamer sind als in senkrechter. Man beachte also, daß die Einzelreize der Ocula zeitlich vorangehen und daß diese Entwicklung mit der des optischen Apparates, nämlich der Fähigkeit zum wandernden Fixieren, einhergeht. Die Einzelreize werden zu Relationen. Die untere Gesichtspartie spielt zu diesem Zeitpunkt noch keine Rolle, ebensowenig wie der Blick oder überhaupt der Ausdruck (lachend, indifferent, schreiend) eine Bedeutung hat.

Mit 3 Monaten wird die untere Gesichtshälfte allmählich in das Blickfeld einbezogen, ohne daß deren Infeld (Mundkonfiguration) nennenswerte Beachtung erlangt. Die Augenpartie differenziert sich weiter aus. Die schematische Ocula — und weniger das lebensvolle Bild — verliert im Vergleich zur natürlichen Augenpartie des Erwachsenen an auslösender Wirkung. Plastische Attrappen sind nicht wirksamer als flächige. Mimische Stirnveränderungen stören kaum, und der menschliche Blick spielt noch keine Rolle. Die komplizierte Bedeutung von Bewegungen der Attrappen wollen wir übergehen. Bei Annäherungen können schockartige Reaktionen auftreten, die sich bei Zurückziehen lösen und Lächeln hervorrufen können.

Im Alter von 4 Monaten können Mundbewegungen bereits positiv wirken, ohne daß einzelne Bewegungsformen des Mundes eine Rolle spielen. Obwohl die Durchstrukturierung der Ocula

Abb. 11. *Entwicklung des Mimikerkennens.* (Erläuterung im Text.) [Nach AHRENS (*221*)]

fortschreitet und die schematische Nachbildung nur noch gelegentlich wirksam ist, können manchmal unter besonderen experimentellen Umständen noch Einzelreize in Augenstellung „durchschlagen". Stirnveränderungen können Unmutsreaktionen erzeugen.

Im Laufe des 5. Monats läßt die Ansprechbarkeit auf Attrappen zunehmend nach. Das Kind wendet sich vorwiegend dem Erwachsenen zu; von anderen Säuglingen fühlt es sich bedeutend weniger angesprochen. Das auch von Spitz als charakteristisch hervorgehobene Breitziehen des Mundes entfaltet dieselbe auslösende Wirkung auf das Lachen wie die volle, lachende (bewegte) Mundmimik. Vor die Augen gesetzte Plättchen lösen nachhaltiges Befremden aus.

Beim 6 Monate alten Kind wirken Mundbewegungen, vor allem das Breitziehen, am stärksten. Die Ausdifferenzierung des Erwachsenen-Gesichtes ist im wesentlichen abgeschlossen, wenn auch noch lange kein Mimikverständnis vorhanden ist. Ahrens hat beobachtet, daß bei Heimkindern noch kein Unterschied zwischen fremden und bekannten Personen gemacht wird, räumt jedoch ein, daß die gesamte Entwicklung bei Familienkindern etwas gedrängter vor sich gehen mag.

Im Laufe des 7. Monats schwindet das Interesse für das Erwachsenen-Gesicht, und das Achtmonatskind tritt in die Phase der Gegenstandseroberung ein. Erst jetzt, wo nicht mehr der breitgezogene Mund, sondern nur das volle Lachen wirksam ist, kann man mit einem beginnenden Ausdrucksverständnis rechnen, dessen Entwicklung Ahrens bei Kindern bis zu 2 Jahren untersucht hat. Weitere Untersuchungen beziehen sich auf das Alter zwischen $2^1/_2$ und 6 Jahren.

Ein Ergebnis sei noch besonders hervorgehoben. Die Stirnmimik, die ja zunächst keine Rolle spielt, kommt erst etwa mit 14 Monaten zur vollen Geltung. Dann nämlich dominiert die senkrechte Faltenbildung eindeutig über die waagerechte. Die Heimkinder reagierten darauf prompt mit Wegwenden des Kopfes, mit Fortlaufen, mit Weinen und Schreien; ja, es kam sogar vor, daß dem Untersucher ins Gesicht geschlagen wurde. Mit ziemlicher Sicherheit konnte Erfahrung ausgeschlossen werden; denn die Pflegepersonen waren spontan gar nicht imstande, eine „Drohmiene" zu machen. Sie mußte erst eingeübt werden. Die Erfahrung lehrt zudem, daß kaum je ein Erwachsener einem kleinen Kinde die Drohmiene zeigt. Fast durchwegs werden beim Schelten die Stimme und der Zeigefinger gehoben. Kinder in diesem Alter sind noch nicht in der Lage, eine Miene sinnvoll zu deuten. Selbst in einem Alter, in dem die Übertragung von Gegenständen auf eine Abbildung und ein korrektes Benennen einzelner Teile des Gesichtes sicher gelingen, kann der Gesichtsausdruck keineswegs sinnvoll gedeutet werden. Der zurechtweisende Blick wird nach unseren Erfahrungen frühestens mit 1;6 Jahren wirksam.

Erinnern wir uns der Beispiele, die wir für die Wirksamkeit von Schlüsselreizen anführten. Für die jungen Silbermöven hieß das optimale Signal: Ein roter Fleck nahe der Unterschnabelspitze (s. S. 298f.). Bei den noch blinden Drosselnestlingen löste zuerst die Erschütterung der Unterlage das Sperren des Schnabels aus. Später wurde die Reizkombination zunehmend komplizierter, und das Verhältnis von Kopf zu Körper spielte u. a. eine Rolle (s. S. 299f.). Bei den menschlichen „Nestlingen" sind zuerst Punkte und später 2 Punkte auf einer runden Scheibe ausreichend, um das Lächeln auszulösen. Darauf kann es durch zusätzliche Auslöser-Reize — Breitziehen des Mundes — quantitativ verstärkt werden, und gelegentlich können einfachere, ontogenetisch frühere Auslöser-Reize noch „durchschlagen". Es folgt eine zunehmende Differenzierung des Auslöserschemas, bis schließlich das volle Lächeln des erwachsenen Menschen allein hinreicht, die angeborene, auch spontan im Leerlauf entstehende Ausdrucksbewegung hervorzulocken. Das Erfahrungsmaterial — das voll ausgestaltete menschliche Gesicht — schiebt sich gleichsam über die Grundstruktur, bis die Differenzierung schließlich so weit fortgeschritten ist, daß ein persönliches Erkennen und ein zunehmend nuancierteres Antwortlächeln möglich werden.

Die Untersuchungen geben ein vorzügliches Beispiel für den *fortschreitenden Einbau von Erfahrungen in den angeborenen Auslösemechanismus* ab, und zwar so, daß schließlich die Bausteine des angeborenen Verhaltens nicht mehr erkennbar sind. An diesem „Einbau" haben Gestaltprozesse (im Sinne der Gestaltpsychologie) einen beachtlichen Anteil (*133, 510*). Aber auch hierbei spielt Erfahrung eine Rolle, wie Untersuchungen an Kleinkindern zeigen (*358*). Der Einbau in den AAM ist für den Menschen ganz außerordentlich wichtig und muß besonders hervorgehoben werden. Vergleichbare Entwicklungen finden wir bei anderen „Neugiertieren". Sie sind relativ arm an spezifischen angeborenen Verhaltensweisen, lernen dafür aber *in ihrer Jugend* mit Hilfe fortgesetzter „Anwendung" angeborenen Verhaltens schnell und viel.

Der *Kolkrabe* wendet den Schnabelhieb — eine der wenigen ihm angeborenen Verhaltensweisen — auf alle unbekannten Objekte sozusagen als Testreiz an. Dem Schnabelhieb folgen stets die Flucht und dann die Beobachtung der Reaktion des „explorierten" Objektes. Der Rabe nähert sich von Beginn an lebendigen Objekten stets von hinten; er scheint angeborenermaßen zu „wissen", wo vorn und hinten ist. Schnabelhieb, Fluchtbereitschaft, „Vorn-hinten-Schema" und eine kaum stillbare „Neugier" sind die wenigen Grundelemente des Verhaltens, mit denen der Rabe beginnt, sich *seine* Welt zu erobern. Interessant ist dabei besonders die äußerst labile „Stimmung" von Annäherung und Flucht. Ganz anders dagegen der *Haubentaucher*. Alles, worauf er Bezug nimmt, die Wasserfläche, die Beute, der Nistplatz usw., ist schon beim erfahrungsfreien Jungvogel durch hochspezialisierte AAMs bis in kleinste Einzelheiten festgelegt. Der Vogel braucht außer der Geländetopographie seines eigenen Reviers kaum etwas hinzuzulernen und kann es auch gar nicht. Niemals wird er etwa lernen, einen toten, wenn auch noch so frischen Fisch zu fressen, weil zum Schema des Beutefangens die Bewegung des Fisches gehört.

Unter den Säugetieren ist die *Wanderratte* der Prototyp eines unspezialisierten Neugierwesens. Sie exploriert alle in einem bestimmten Bezirk möglichen Wege und erinnert stets den Rückweg ins Loch. Wege, die „zu nichts führen", läßt sie „dahingestellt" (vgl. S. 344), kann aber bei Bedarf sofort darauf zurückgreifen. Mit dieser Lernfähigkeit hat sich die Ratte den ganzen Erdball erobert. Sie kann sich überall einrichten; selbst auf Inseln, auf denen sie das einzige Landsäugetier ist, verhält sie sich so, als ob sie Spezialist gerade für dieses Milieu wäre (*134*).

Das wesentliche Merkmal des Neugierverhaltens ist seine *Sachbezogenheit*. Nicht etwa Hunger treibt zur „Exploration", wie LORENZ beim Kolkraben (*129, 134*) gezeigt hat, sondern nur gesättigt interessiert sich der Rabe für unbekannte Gegenstände. Durch dieses Erlernen der den Dingen anhaftenden Eigenschaften, unabhängig vom augenblicklichen Bedarf des Organismus, wirkt das Neugierverhalten objektivierend in des Wortes buchstäblicher Bedeutung. Erst durch das *Neugier-Lernen* entstehen „gemeinte" Gegenstände in der Umwelt des Tieres wie des Menschen. Daß das Meinen von Gegenständen beim Menschen dem sprachlichen Ausdruck lange vorangeht, ist wohlbekannt und läßt sich sehr gut mit dem „unbenannten Denken" (*472*) der Tiere vergleichen. So ist denn Sprache Ausdruck und Signal, Meinen und Denken zugleich. Gewiß ist es kein Zufall, daß die Sprachforscher vom stammesgeschichtlichen Ursprung dieser oder jener Wörter sprechen. Es ist höchst unwahrscheinlich, daß z. B. Wörter: Vater, father, pater, padre, pére rein zufällig einen ähnlichen Bau haben. Was ihre Signalfunktion (das Meinen) anbelangt, können sie in nicht stammesverwandten Sprachen auch ganz anders lauten, aber als Ausdruck sind sie eben für einen Völkerstamm charakteristisch.

Die Ausdrucksbewegungen z. B. für die Balz sind bei nicht verwandten Arten außerordentlich verschieden. Je verwandter die Arten sind, desto ähnlicher werden die „Verständigungsbewegungen", so daß sich beispielsweise Stock- und Spießenten noch „verstehen" können, obwohl sie sich im Balzverhalten hinsichtlich ihrer Signale erkennbar unterscheiden. Unter Umständen kann man bei Kreuzungen aber auch „Mißverständnisse" unter den Nachkommen beobachten, eben weil die Signale sich nicht mehr genügend ähnlich sind (*129, 535*). Derartige genetische Untersuchungen an Tieren, die zoologisch nahe genug miteinander verwandt sind, sich aber in wenigen Verhaltensweisen eindeutig unterscheiden, sind zur Untersuchung des Erbganges einzelner Instinktbewegungen von größtem Interesse (*134*; vgl. S. 294).

Was nun die Grundformen menschlicher Ausdrucksbewegungen anbetrifft, dürfen wir mit hinreichender Sicherheit annehmen, daß ihnen primär *phylogenetisch alte Sozialmienen* (*131*) zugrunde liegen, durch welche das Verstehen des Artgenossen gewährleistet ist, ohne daß diesem Verstehen freilich die Bedeutung des sinnvollen Verständnisses — etwa im Sinne des Einfühlens der verstehenden Psychologie — unterlegt werden darf. Vielmehr beruht dieser Vorgang Verstehen auf dem Ansprechen des AAM auf den auslösenden Signalreiz des Artgenossen. Allein auf dieser Basis scheint uns das Lächeln des jungen Säuglings und die gefühlsbetonte Reaktion des Partners (Mutter), dessen AAM auf das Lächeln anspricht, hinreichend erklärt zu sein. Daß solche Sozialmienen nicht vom ersten Lebenstage an fertig geprägt da zu sein brauchen, sondern heranreifen bis zu einer Zeit, wo sie biologisch sinnvoll sind, sehen wir am Beispiel der Drohmiene, die erst als solche wirkt, wenn das Kind ins 2. Lebensjahr eintritt. Wir wollen hier nur hinzufügen, daß auch unter Mantelpavianen Jungtiere nicht angedroht werden, oder, sollte dies einmal vorkommen, nicht darauf reagieren (*113*).

4. Die Prägung

Bei alledem haben wir einen für Mensch und Tier besonders wichtigen Umstand bisher nicht berücksichtigt, nämlich den von O. Heinroth (*397*) erstmals an Graugänsen beobachteten Vorgang der *Prägung*. Der Ausdruck wurde durch Lorenz bekannt (*530*), der ebenfalls an Graugänsen und mehreren Entenarten die Beobachtung machte, daß die Jungen sich ein „erworbenes Eltern-Kumpan-Schema" aneignen, wenn ihnen die rechten Eltern fehlen. Die im Brutschrank geschlüpfte Gans Martina sah Lorenz als erstes Lebewesen nach dem Schlüpfen und behandelte ihn vom ersten Augenblick an wie einen „Führkumpan" (*129*). Sind solche geprägten Tiere erst einmal einem artfremden Adoptivelter gefolgt, so lassen sie sich nicht dazu bringen, Artgenossen zu folgen. Dieser Lernakt geschieht „auf den ersten Blick" und hat eine sehr kurze *sensible Periode*. Diesen Ausdruck entnahm Lorenz der Entwicklungsphysiologie, wo er bedeutet, daß ein Vorgang nur innerhalb eines bestimmten Zeitraumes vonstatten gehen kann; wird der rechte Zeitpunkt verpaßt, so kann er nicht nachgeholt werden. Geschieht aber das Ereignis zur rechten Zeit, eben während der sensiblen Periode, so ist er irreversibel. Ebenso „sitzt" auch die Prägung fest, zumindest solange die betreffende Reaktionsbereitschaft, hier das Sichführenlassen, anhält.

Systematisch untersucht haben die Prägung z. B. E. Fabricius (*341, 342, 343*), A. Ramsay und E. Hess (*401,692*). Weitere Untersuchungen sind am Max-Planck-Institut von Lorenz im Gange. Alle diese Untersucher wählten vor allem Entenarten als Versuchstiere und benutzten neben anderen Methoden verschieden gebaute Attrappen. Die männlichen oder weiblichen Enten ähnelnde Attrappe läuft auf exzentrischen Rädern, gibt arteigene oder auch fremde Locklaute durch einen eingebauten Lautsprecher, spendet Wärme und ist zum Unterschlüpfen geeignet (*692*). Am Lorenzschen Institut versucht man gerade, mit Attrappen auszutesten, wie weit man das „Kumpanschema" vereinfachen kann, ohne daß der Prägungsakt gestört wird. Nach den Untersuchungen von Ramsay und Hess scheint die Zeit zwischen 13 und 16 Lebensstunden die kritische sensible Periode zu sein; bereits nach 28 Std. gelingt die Prägung gewöhnlich nicht mehr. Hess konnte kürzlich (*401*) 2 Faktoren aufdecken, welche die sensible Periode erklären helfen. Sie liegt nämlich gerade im Schnittpunkt der zunehmenden Lokomotionsfähigkeit (Nachfolge-Reaktion!) und der einsetzenden Entwicklung des Fluchtverhaltens. Grad und Dauerhaftigkeit der Prägung hängen von einer Summe von Eigenschaften der Attrappen ab (männlich oder weiblich, lautlos oder „Standard-Ruf", Mutterruf oder „Standard-Ruf", laufend oder bewegungslos usw.). Ist die Prägung erst einmal gelungen, und sei es auch mit einer „schlechten" Attrappe, so wird diese den eigenen Eltern vorgezogen (*692*).

Man kann den Vorgang vielleicht als ungewohnlich raschen Lernprozeß betrachten, durch den ein vorgegebenes Schema (der AAM) ausgefüllt wird. Je merkmalsreicher der AAM ist, desto weniger pragbar ist die Tierart. Je leerer und ärmer an Bestimmungsstücken er ist, desto mehr bleibt der Prägung vorbehalten.

Die Tatsache, daß es auch eine „*unvollstandige Pragung*" gibt, kompliziert das so einfach aussehende Phanomen. Ein Dutzend von 31 durch Fabricius (*341*) untersuchten Reiherentenjungen zeigten zwar das „Nachfolgen", das wichtigste Kriterium fur die gelungene Prägung, bekamen aber, wenn sie gegriffen wurden, eine Schreck-Reaktion, die vollstandig geprägte Entchen nicht zeigten. Die Schreck-Reaktion schwand auch nach langerer Gewohnung nicht. Bei einer anderen, unvollständig auf den Menschen geprägten Gruppe der gleichen Entenart beobachtete Fabricius, daß die Küken zwar auf den Lockruf mit dem „Unterhaltungslaut" grüßten, aber zu Lande nicht nachfolgten. Erst als er mit ihnen ins Wasser ging, folgten sie rasch und dichtaufgeschlossen nach, ließen sich aber trotz aller, sonst erfolgreichen, „komm-komm"-Rufe nicht auf das Land zuruocklocken und verschwanden auf immer im Rohr.

Interessant ist, daß alle Tiere, bei denen eine Prägung auf Artfremde gelang, unabhängig von dieser Tatsache auch sonst die Fähigkeit haben, ein Lebewesen — sei es nun der Artgenosse oder der Mensch — *personlich* zu kennen, d. h. ein Individuum von anderen der gleichen

Art zu unterscheiden und eine persönliche Bindung zu ihm einzugehen. Offenbar wird ein solches Jungtier zunächst auf „den" Menschen geprägt und lernt ihn danach auch persönlich kennen, so wie die Silbermöwe angeborenermaßen jedes artgleiche Junge annimmt, das ebenso alt wie ihre eigenen ist; jedoch nur bis zum 5. Tage, dann kennt sie ein jedes persönlich und lehnt alle fremden ab. FABRICIUS' geprägte Entchen folgten ihm in seiner vollen Größe zu Lande, aber auch im Wasser, wenn gerade nur sein Kopf herausragte. Die Stimme, obwohl ein hervorragendes Unterscheidungsmerkmal, kann für die Prägung nicht allein ausschlaggebend sein. Das Anlegen ungewohnter Kleidung scheint befremdlicher zu wirken als das Ablegen von Kleidung. Aber auch hier gibt es Ausnahmen, wie z. B. die, daß ein Hund den badenden befreundeten Menschen angefallen und getötet hat (379).

Auch bei vollständiger Prägung spielt offenbar der AAM noch eine Rolle und bleibt, wenn auch stark modifiziert und differenziert, wirksam. LORENZ' (129) geprägte Gösselchen ließen sich von ihm jederzeit aus der Luft dadurch herunterholen, daß er schnell lief und sich plötzlich mit ausgebreiteten Armen in die Knie fallen ließ. Auf diese „Landung" reagierten die Gänse angeborenermaßen und „erwarteten" diesen Auslöser auch von ihrem menschlichen „Führ-Kumpan".

Bei Säugetieren ist die empirische Grundlage noch recht schmal (247, 443). GRABOWSKI (368) berichtet kurz über die Prägung eines Jungschafes auf den Menschen. SEITZ (559) sah bei einem am 68. Lebenstage von der Mutter abgesetzten Eisbärenjungen eine bleibende, vollkommene Zahmheit. Junge Eisbären, die erst mit 85 Tagen abgesetzt wurden, waren bereits scheu (146). Isoliert aufgezogene junge Marderhunde (eine Wildform) lassen sich mindestens partiell auf den Menschen prägen. Sie können dann dem Pfleger gegenüber streichelzahm sein und laufen beharrlich nach. Vom Pfleger getrennt, lassen sie das „angeborene Weinen des Verlassenseins" hören (740).

HARLOW u. Mitarb. haben ausgedehnte Isolierungsexperimente an Rhesusaffenbabys vorgenommen, die mit verschieden beschaffenen — teils auch abschreckenden — Mutterattrappen unter extrem unnatürlichen Bedingungen aufgezogen wurden. Im Laufe der Entwicklung zeigten diese Tiere schwere Verhaltensstörungen, vor allem auch hinsichtlich ihres emotionalen und sexuellen Verhaltens. Hingegen scheint regelmäßiger Kontakt mit Spielgefährten, auch wenn er nur auf kurze Tageszeiten beschränkt ist, die natürliche Mutter weitgehend zu ersetzen. HARLOW zieht interessante Parallelen zu psychischen Entwicklungsstörungen des Menschen, z. B. zu solchen, die durch Hospitalisierung von Säuglingen und Kleinkindern auftreten (382, 382a, 383). [Vgl. auch S. 367f. und Nr. (186a).]

Auch von Psychiatern ist der Vorgang der Prägung für den Menschen in Anspruch genommen worden, besonders, was abnorme sexuelle Verhaltensweisen angeht (186a, 511, 512, 513, 820). Hinreichend gesicherte Schlußfolgerungen erscheinen uns verfrüht. Während des ersten Lebenshalbjahres kommt eine Prägung nicht in Frage. Noch das Fünfmonatskind lächelt *jeden* an, der die notwendigen Schlüsselreize aussendet. Man kann die Säuglinge zu dieser Zeit sehr schnell und leicht umgewöhnen, und sie nehmen jeden als Mutter an, der die entsprechende Pflegefunktion erfüllt. Erst um den 8. Monat lernen sie die Mutter persönlich kennen und fremdeln Unbekannten gegenüber. Nun beginnt auch mit der zunehmenden Lokomotionsfähigkeit eine für 1—2jährige Kinder recht typische „Kindestriebhandlung" sich auszubilden, nämlich das speziell Nach-der-Mutter-Verlangen, das der Mutter „Nachfolgen" und „Zulaufen". Wenn also Prägung für den Menschen angenommen werden darf, so kaum vor einem Jahr und auch dann recht unvollständig. Trennt man das Kinde zu diesem Zeitpunkt von seiner Mutter, so erkennt es sie unter Umständen nach 4 Wochen nicht wieder, und nur aus der rascheren Wiedereingewöhnung kann man auf Lernresiduen (169) schließen.

Beim Menschen zieht sich die Prägung also sehr in die Länge, so daß die Charakteristika „früh" und „kurz" gar nicht recht passen und die Abgrenzung zwischen Prägung und anderen Formen des Lernens nicht möglich ist. Man kann dann noch im späteren Leben des Kindes „Prägung auf andere Objekte" außer den Eltern postulieren. So kommt es zwar vor, daß Kinder in sensiblen Perioden von einem Ereignis oder einer Begegnung dauerhaft beeindruckt sind, doch hat dies eigentlich nichts mehr mit der ursprünglichen Bedeutung des Begriffes Prägung zu tun und läßt sich ebenfalls kaum von anderen — unter Affekt ablaufenden — Lernvorgängen abgrenzen. In affektbesetzten Situationen können auch Tiere verblüffende Lern- und Gedächtnisleistungen produzieren. Lorenz' Dohle verlor einen Fuß im Fangeisen und lernte bei dieser Gelegenheit einen ganzen Satz sprechen. *(129)*.

Andererseits — und dies räumt wiederum Prägungsmöglichkeiten auch für den Menschen ein — kann der Prägungsvorgang äußerst stückhaft sein. Lorenz' unter Ornithologen vielberufene Dohle Tschok *(129)* hatte ihn als Elternkumpan. Als sie flügge wurde, brauchte sie Flugkumpane und fand die fliegenden Nebelkrähen. Geschlechtsreif geworden, zeigte sich, trotz aller ihrer Gemeinschaft mit anderen (nicht fliegenden) Dohlen, daß ihre isolierte Aufzucht Spuren hinterlassen hatte: Sie balzte die Hausgehilfin an. Der erwachte Pflegetrieb schließlich fand seine Abfuhr in der Fütterung eines Dohlenjungen.

Analog zu diesem Beispiel darf man auch vom jugendlichen Menschen sagen, daß er den Artgenossen und seine Umgebung je nach gerade vorhandener sensibler Periode stückhaft sieht. Wird ein eben heranreifendes Instinktverhalten vor- oder frühzeitig durch eine abnorme Auslösersituation in Gang gesetzt, so kommt die starre Fixierung an diese Situation einer (abnormen) Prägung sehr nahe. Jedenfalls sollte dieser eigenartige Vorgang bei der auch heute noch offenen Diskussion über das „Psychische Trauma" in Betracht gezogen werden.

Das *Reifen von angeborenen Verhaltensweisen*, von den Ethologen seit langem untersucht *(195, 197)*, ist in der Entwicklungspsychologie und Psychopathologie des Menschen bisher zu wenig beachtet und nie unter vergleichend verhaltensphysiologischen Gesichtspunkten betrachtet worden.

IV. Soziales Verhalten von Mensch und Tier

1. Ausdrucksbewegungen als Verständigungsmittel

Im Grunde haben wir bereits im vorigen Kapitel den Bereich sozialen Verhaltens betreten; bei der Prägung z. B. spielt der Partner die Hauptrolle, und das Ausdrucksverhalten ist auf einen Partner gerichtet.

Definieren wir mit R. Schenkel *(721)* die Ausdrucksbewegung als eine Bewegungsweise, deren arterhaltende Leistung darin liegt, durch Stimmungsübertragung bzw. Reaktionsauslösung an der *Steuerung sozialen Zusammenlebens* mitzuwirken, so stehen die *Auslöser* im Zentrum dieser Definition *(530, 535)*. Diese Auslöser — das sind Instinktbewegungen — sprechen den AAM des Partners an. Im einfachsten Falle verursacht die auslösende Instinktbewegung dieselbe Verhaltensweise beim Artgenossen *(537)*; man nennt das *Stimmungsübertragung*. Ein Beispiel dafür ist das Gähnen, eine unter Wirbeltieren sehr verbreitete, zweifellos als echte Instinktbewegung anzusprechende Verhaltensweise. Ich habe bei den mir gut bekannten Totenkopfäffchen *(657, 659, 661)* (Saimiri sciureus) beobachtet, daß sie sich nicht nur wie z. B. Hunde und Katzen beim Gähnen im Sinne einer Rekelbewegung *(738)* strecken, sondern auch einen oder beide Arme beugen können. Das Gähnen ist zwar noch keine Ausdrucksbewegung im Sinne der Definition. Aber aus solchen Mechanismen der Stimmungsübertragung differenzieren sich häufig echte Ausdrucksbewegungen, das sind Auslöser im eigentlichen Sinne. Nicht mehr die ganze Instinktbewegung tritt in Funktion, sondern nur ein *Teil*, der im Laufe des phyletischen Vorganges eine meist optisch wirksame Übertreibung erfahren hat. Parallel mit dieser reizsendenden Bewegung entwickelt sich der Reizempfangsapparat (AAM), der gerade auf dieses Signal beantwortend anspricht[1]. Dabei richtet sich das Signal nun auch zumeist auf einen Partner, wie man es bei allen Balzhandlungen schön beobachten kann. Es handelt sich jetzt also um eine höchst spezifische Stimmungsübertragung mit dem Erfolg einer Steuerung des sozialen Zusammenlebens von Partnern. Die einstige Funktion der Instinktbewegung kann dabei ganz verlorengegangen sein. So hat die ursprüngliche Drohbewegung primitiver Cerviden (Hirsche), die mit erhobenem Kopf ihre Eckzähne zeigten, das Vorhandensein dieser Waffen um ganze geologische Epochen überdauert (535). Die Eckzähne sind keine Waffe mehr, aber die Drohbewegung ist geblieben [vgl. dazu (34)]. Häufig sind *Intentionsbewegungen* — das sind nach HEINROTH (397) angedeutete, unvollständig ablaufende Instinktbewegungen — der Ursprung von Ausdrucksbewegungen. „Mimisch" übertrieben ist dann also nicht der vollintensive Instinktablauf, sondern die Intentionsbewegung. Die Auffliegebewegungen der Entenvögel bieten reichhaltige Differenzierungsreihen dieser Art, aus denen ein kundiger Beobachter sehen kann, was signalisiert wird. LORENZ verblüffte mich mit Voraussagen über das dem Signal folgende Verhalten, das an Ausführungen nach Kommando auf dem Kasernenhof erinnert.

Auch aus *Übersprungbewegungen* (s. S. 305) können häufig Ausdrucksbewegungen werden (602, 605). Dieser „Auspuff motorischer Erregung", wie TINBERGEN (197) sagt, verwandelt sich in ein Signal. Beim Kranich z. B. entlädt sich gestauter Geschlechtstrieb im Übersprungputzen. Diese Bewegung bedeutet als Auslöser Drohen. Die Verwandlungen der Übersprungbewegungen scheinen besonders gute Aussichten zum Verständnis der Stammesgeschichte angepaßter Instinktbewegungen zu bieten, weil sie sich offenbar weit rascher herauszüchten als andere Instinktbewegungen (s. S. 332ff.).

Wenn sich in einer der beschriebenen Entstehungsweisen der Auslöser eine hochdifferenzierte Ausdrucksbewegung mit neuer Funktion herausbildet, pflegt man von *Ritualisierung*, von *Formalisierung* oder von *Zeremonien* zu sprechen (177, 535, 536, 603, 717). Maßgebend für die Wahl dieser Termini war die Analogie zu entsprechenden Vorgängen im menschlichen Verhalten. Eine Bewegungsfolge verliert ihren ursprünglichen Sinn und gewinnt eine neue Bedeutung. Dabei erstarrt eine Folge von Bewegungsformen zu einer neuen Bewegungsformel. ERWIN STRAUS (779) hat, ohne ethologische Probleme im Sinn gehabt zu haben, einen meisterhaften anthropologischen Beitrag zu diesem Thema gegeben. Es handelt sich, wie gesagt, um Analogien zum menschlichen Verhalten. Die Beweise für Homologien fehlen jedenfalls vorläufig auf diesem Gebiet noch. Auch hier

---

[1] Zwischen solchen angeborenen „Verständigungsmitteln" und den erworbenen Bedingten Reaktionen ließen sich unter Annahme folgender Hypothese manche Brücken schlagen: Einer zunehmend differenzierten Bedingten Reaktion (s. S. 395 ff.) läuft eine fortschreitende Differenzierung der Reizkonstellation parallel, so wie einem sich differenzierenden AAM eine Differenzierung der Auslöser parallel geht. Einem angeborenen Signal wäre also ein erworbenes und einem AAM ein „erworbener Auslösemechanismus" (EAM), eben der der Bedingten Reaktion zugrunde liegende hirnphysiologische Mechanismus, gegenüberzustellen. Die menschliche Sprache z. B. kann man auf diese Weise als ein erworbenes Signalsystem betrachten, durchaus im Sinne des 2. Signalsystems von PAWLOW, wenn auch auf beträchtlich anderer neurophysiologischer Grundlage (s. S. 420), als PAWLOW es sich zur damaligen Zeit vorstellen konnte. „Dieses zweite Signalsystem und sein Organ — (nach PAWLOW das Frontalhirn) — müssen als die allerletzte Errungenschaft des *Evolutionsprozesses* (vom Verf. gesperrt) besonders fein sein" (Bd. 3, S. 451) (155). Sprache ist ohne angeborene Grundlage nicht möglich, wie vor allem OTTO KOEHLER (473) gezeigt hat, sie ist aber auch in ihrer weiteren Ausdifferenzierung ohne erworbene Signale (Lautkombinationen in Syntax) nicht existent. Vielleicht ließen sich heutige Streitfragen (479) auf dieser Basis der Klärung näherbringen. Es ist durchaus möglich, daß *der hirnphysiologische Mechanismus des AAM und des „EAM" im Endeffekt der gleiche, in der Entstehung aber ein verschiedener ist.*

kann uns, wie im cerebralorganischen Abbau, die menschliche Pathologie des
Verhaltens vielleicht weiterhelfen (s. S. 351 ff.). Manche Formeln unserer sozialen
Gepflogenheiten mögen sich als homologisierbare Ausdrucksbewegungen auf-
decken lassen (*34*). Welchen Sinn haben das Händeschütteln, das Auf-die-Schulter-
Schlagen, das Nicken, Kopfschütteln und Verneigen, das höfische Benehmen
beim Verlassen eines Raumes, das Handflächen-Zeigen oder Achselzucken, das
Arme-Ausbreiten, Lippenspitzen, Naserümpfen, Augen-klein-Machen, Beine-
Übereinanderschlagen u. v. a. ursprünglich gehabt? Auf manche dieser Fragen
gibt uns BILZ (*15*), ein Schüler J. v. UEXKÜLLs, vergleichend anthropologische
Antworten. BILZ war es auch, der als erster auf psychiatrischem Felde von einer
vergleichenden Paläophysiologie (*261*) und Paläopsychologie (*262*) gesprochen
hat. Seine anregenden Vergleiche fördern mindestens das biologische Verständnis
für menschliches Verhalten und betonen nicht die Kluft, sondern das Gemeinsame zwischen Mensch und Tier. Bisher hat dieser Blickwinkel die Medizin auf
allen Gebieten weitergeführt und sie zur Hauptdisziplin unter den angewandten
Naturwissenschaften werden lassen. Der Neuropsychiatrie steht das Feld noch
weitgehend offen.

*Für eine Reihe menschlicher Ausdrucksbewegungen ist die stammesgeschichtliche
Parallele evident.*

Drohende Paviane z. B. schlagen mit Steinen gegen den Boden. Wütende Schimpansen
und Gorillas trommeln laut gegen die gewölbte Brust. Schimpansen schlagen im Freien auch
gegen hohle Bäume ihres Reviers, das sie auf diese Weise kennzeichnen. Ein Schimpanse im
Londoner Zoo versetzte sich durch Trommeln gegen eine Blechtür in Kampfstimmung und
bewegte sich dabei in einem komplizierten Rhythmus. Ein anderer Schimpanse tanzte mit zwei
Artgenossen in der Runde und versetzte der Tür einen taktgerechten „Paukenschlag". Auch
Paarungen werden durch Tänze eingeleitet. WOLFGANG KÖHLERs (*483*) Schimpansen schmuck-
ten sich zum Tanz, indem sie sich Tuchfetzen, Schnüre und dgl. umhängten. Das Bedürfnis, zu
imponieren, ist im Tierreich weit verbreitet; es ist je nach Partner meist *Drohen* oder *Werben*.
Sehr viele Kämpfe werden allein durch „Drohduelle" ausgetragen, ja, es gibt kaum Kampfe
zwischen Artgenossen, die nicht durch Drohen eingeleitet werden. Die Auseinandersetzung
vollzieht sich durchaus im Ritus nach Art eines Turniers („Kommentkampf"). Wie beim
Drohen, so ist auch bei der Balz das Imponiergehabe darauf abgestellt, sich in übertriebener
Größe und sozusagen von der besten (stärksten) Seite zu zeigen. Dabei spielen Farbmerkmale,
Abspreizen von Haaren oder Federn, Darbieten der Breitseite, Erheben auf die Hinterbeine,
Ohren-Abwinkeln, Buckel-breitseits-Zeigen, Rüssel-Aufblasen (*149*) u. v. a. eine Rolle.
Geruchliches Drohen ist vor allem bei Makrosmaten zu finden. Nilpferde tragen richtige Stink-
duelle aus, indem sie beim Wutgahnen dem Gegner Verdauungsgase entgegenrülpsen (*40*). Die
neuweltlichen Tylopoden bespucken ihren Gegner mit hochgewürgtem Mageninhalt. Der starke
Geruch löst beim Artgenossen die „*Ekelgebärde*" aus (*158, 644, 645, 646*). Sehr weit verbreitet
sind auch *Drohlaute* wie Zischen, Fauchen oder Brüllen. Beim See-Elefanten genügt allein der
Drohruf, um jüngere Männchen auch außerhalb der Sichtweite eilends in die Flucht zu schlagen (*40, 149*). Aber auch für die Balz sind Lautgebungen ein Teil des Imponiergehabens. An das
Katzen-Konzert brauchen wir kaum zu erinnern. Für die Sattelrobbe gilt der „Gesang" geradezu als Zeichen der Brunst (*149*). Die Beispiele mögen genügen, um den Reichtum der Ausdrucksformen unter den Säugetieren anzudeuten (vgl. Abb. 13 u. 14).

Manches im menschlichen Ausdruck ist klar als *formalisierte Intentionsbewegung*
zu erkennen: So ist z. B. die Gebärde des Hochmutes eine Geste des Sich-Zurück-
ziehens. Der Hochmütige hebt den Kopf in Rückwärtsbewegung hoch, zieht die
Nasenflügel ein und senkt die Augenlider, „beides in symbolisierend übertriebener
Abwehr der vom verachteten Artgenossen kommenden Sinnesreize" (*131*). Dabei
wird, wie DARWIN (*34*) schon beschrieb, kräftig durch die Nase ausgeatmet. Ein
derartiges mimisches Syndrom wird offensichtlich angeborenermaßen vom Artgenossen verstanden. Dieses „Verständnis" ist so unkorrigierbar, daß wir sogar
das Kamel, das alle diese mimischen Auslöser zeigt, für hochmütig halten. Der
Adler mit seinen überdachten Augen und seinem nach vorn gerichteten Blick —
gleich der Mimik des Mutigen — gilt als kühn. Auf ähnliche Weise kommen die

meisten menschlichen Vorurteile über den Charakter von Tieren „instinktiv"
zustande. Das Gefühlsurteil kann nur mit Mühe durch Wissen und Erfahrung
überwunden werden (*131*).

Berühmt geworden ist Lorenz' *Kindchenschema* (*131*) (s. Abb. 12). Der elterliche Pflegeinstinkt antwortet auf Signale, die das Kleinkind aussendet: Kurzes
Gesicht unter hoher Stirn, rundlich vorstehende Backen, relativ große Augen,
großer Kopf und kleiner Körper, runde Formen, kurze Finger, tolpatschige Bewegungen.

Die Abbildung veranschaulicht die morphologischen Schlüsselreize. Puppen-,
Reklame- und Filmindustrie haben von diesem Schema reichlich und mit Erfolg
Gebrauch gemacht. Dem Schema ähnelnde
Lebewesen oder Objekte werden als „her-
zig" oder „niedlich" empfunden und gern
als Ersatzobjekte angenommen. In seiner
Arbeit über „angeborene Instinktformeln
beim Menschen" hat Lorenz (*132*) viele
andere Beispiele ähnlicher Art, u. a.
das Pin-up girl (Anhäufung übernormaler
Schlüsselreize, s. S. 299), angeführt.

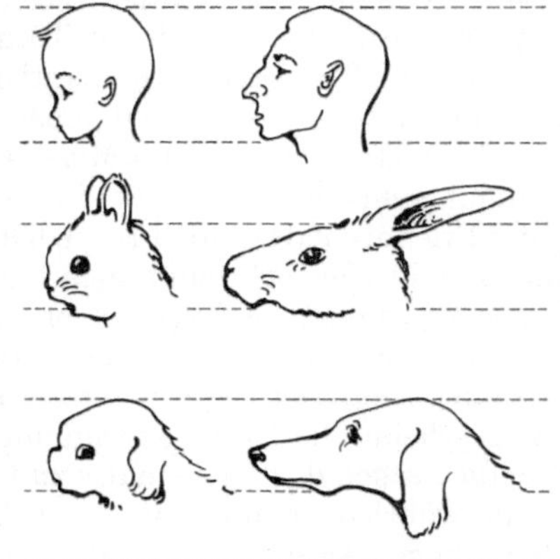

Abb. 12. *Das „Kindchenschema"*. Links: Kleinkind und drei Ersatzobjekte, die durch ihre
Schlüsselreize den menschlichen Pflegetrieb auslösen. Rechts: Erwachsener und drei Tiere, auf
die unser Pflegetrieb weniger anspricht. [Nach
Lorenz (*131*)]

Grußzeremonien und Stimmfühlungslaute sind
im Tierreich weit verbreitet. Viele Säugerweib-
chen kündigen sich ihren Jungen durch Rufe an.
Katzenartige Raubtiere begrüßen sich durch
„Köpfchen-Geben" (*126, 127*). Seelöwen und andere Ohrenrobben berühren sich zum Gruße mit
den Schnauzen und blöken (*149*). Viele Säuger, vor
allem Affen, stellen den sozialen Kontakt — das
eben bedeutet der Gruß — durch „soziale Hautpflege" her. Wo Gefahr besteht, daß sich die Tiere
eines sozialen Verbandes verlieren könnten, sorgen
meist besondere Stimmfühlungslaute für den
Kontakt. Gibbons, Kapuziner (*619*) und andere
Affen rufen unentwegt beim Wandern in den
Wipfeln und ziehen so auch die Nachzügler heran
(*40*). Das zu einem Zwillingspärchen gehörende,
von der Mutter verlassene und dem Untergang
geweihte Seehundbaby schreit kläglich, als ob ein kleines Kind weinend „Mama" ruft (*149*).

Kommen wir auf die oben über den Schimpansen gemachten Bemerkungen
zurück. Das Trommeln ist möglicherweise eine formalisierte Intentionsbewegung
des Zuschlagens. Der hocherregte Mitteleuropäer schlägt nur noch mit der Faust
auf den Tisch, wobei er sich in deutlicher Angriffsintention erhebt, sich „empört".
Das Schmücken als Imponiergehabe ist evident (*267*). Helmbüsche, Stiergehörn
und bunte Tracht machen den Träger größer und auffälliger (*447*). In Drohstellung
werden, wie beim Schimpansen, die Arme leicht vom vorgebeugten Körper
abgehoben und einwärtsgedreht. Ja, die Haare können sich sträuben wie beim
Schimpansen das Fell an der Außenseite der Arme und am Oberrücken. „Der
Mensch sträubt also im Affekt kämpferischer Begeisterung einen Pelz, den er gar
nicht mehr hat!" (*131*). Das wütende Kleinkind zeigt noch das Aufstampfen mit
dem Fuß als Intentionsbewegung des aggressiven Entgegenschreitens. Demuts-
gebärden kennen wir in zahlreichen Variationen bei Mensch und Tier (*40*). Sie
verhindern bei Tieren den Mord des Artgenossen. Wölfe und Haushunde (*50*), die
im Kampf unterliegen, bieten dem Gegner gleichsam zum tödlichen Biß den Hals.
Der Partner steht dann knurrend mit Beißintention davor, *kann* aber nicht
zupacken; die *Aggression* wird durch dieses Signal *gehemmt*. Homer berichtet, daß
die Schutz- und Hilfesuchenden mit ihrer Hand das Kinn des Partners berühren.

Odysseus umfaßt flehend Aretes Knie, und Priamos fällt auf gleiche Weise vor Achill nieder, womit der Beispiele genug sein müssen. Alle „alten Sozialgebärden" und „Sozialmienen" lösen zwingend eine von Emotion begleitete Antwort aus, und mag sie auch nur wiederum als Intentionsbewegung erscheinen.

Zweifellos sind auch dem Menschen *Tötungshemmungen* angeboren, und zwar besonders den Schwachen und Wehrlosen, den Frauen, Kindern und Alten, ja, auch Tieren gegenüber. Kindermord wird als das verabscheuungswürdigste aller Verbrechen empfunden. Vater- oder Muttermörder, Mörder überhaupt hatten seit altersher die scheußlichsten Qualen durch personifizierte Gewissensbisse, die Erinnyen, auszustehen. — Die Tötung eines Tieres in der Jagdsituation ist von ganz andersartigen Emotionen begleitet als das Schlachten von Tieren. Lorenz (*538*) beschreibt seine Skrupel, die er nach dem notwendigen Töten *junger* Ratten empfand; Bilz (*263*) geht der Tötungshemmung und ihrer Durchbrechung am Beispiel des Tiertöter-Skrupulantismus nach. Sehr viele Opferbräuche, Jagdzeremonien und andere Riten haben dieses urmenschliche „Du-sollst-nicht-töten" zur Grundlage. Dem Töten-Müssen im Kampf ums Dasein steht die Tötungshemmung entgegen. *Der Ritus ist ein Kompromiß.* Die Hemmung kommt deutlich in der Erlebnisanalyse von Frauen heraus, die in einer Konfliktsituation abgetrieben haben. Sehr eigenartig und mich immer wieder überraschend ist die nicht seltene Äußerung von endogen Depressiven, „mir ist, als ob ich jemanden getötet hätte". Bilz sagt im Zusammenhang mit den *primären Schuldgefühlen* sehr treffend: „. . . und so kramen die Depressiven ihre alten ‚Tabu-Brüche' aus" (*263*). Im modernen Krieg scheint die Tötungshemmung nahezu unwirksam geworden zu sein. Die Schergen sehen das Lächeln des zu tötenden Kindes nicht mehr (vgl. S. 322) oder — um wölfisch zu sprechen — der dargebotene Hals, die Demutsgebärde, die die Hemmung auslösenden Signale können dem Töter nicht mehr in Erscheinung treten. Das Töten ist *anonym* geworden.

2. Familien- und Gemeinschaftsleben

Das Familien- und Gruppenleben der Tiere (*168, 732*) verwirklicht sich in einer solchen Mannigfaltigkeit, daß in unserem Zusammenhang grobe Schematisierungen und Vernachlässigung auch wichtiger Funktionskreise nicht zu vermeiden sind. Um irreführenden Simplifizierungen vorzubeugen, wählen wir nach kurzer Orientierung statt generalisierender Aussagen lieber einige Beispiele, die engere Vergleiche zum Menschen erlauben.

Tinbergen (*198*) hat die Formen sozialen Zusammenlebens verschiedenen Hauptthemen untergeordnet: Paarung, Brutpflege, Organisation von Familien- und Gruppenverband.

Für das *Paarungsverhalten* der meisten Tiere, vor allem auch der Säugerwildformen, ist besonders wichtig zu wissen, daß *mit Aktivierung des Geschlechtstriebes gleichzeitig auch Angriffs- und Fluchtbereitschaft aktiviert* werden. Welcher dieser drei Funktionskreise die Oberhand gewinnt, hängt stets von einer Kette ineinandergreifender Handlungsglieder ab. Das unerhört variationsreiche und differenzierte Balzverhalten ist meist die „kunstreichste" unter den Handlungsketten, die eine Art als Verhaltensinventar zur Verfügung hat. Als plausibelsten Grund dafür kann man den hohen Selektionswert ansehen, der dem Balzverhalten zukommt. Ein rein geschlechtlich erregtes, aber nicht kampfbereites Männchen würde nicht mit anderen rivalisierenden Männchen fertig, ein nicht gleichzeitig auch fluchtbereites Tier würde seinen Feinden unterliegen. Tatsächlich sind bei jedem Tier diese drei Triebe wohl gegen einander ausgewogen, und der *Sexualtrieb* ist — wie wir hier schon betonen wollen (vgl. S. 374) — *besonders leicht störbar.* Für die in der Psychoanalyse oft vertretene Ansicht, daß Aggression und Sexualität dem *gleichen* Funktionskreis angehören, finden sich *keine* ausreichenden Anhaltspunkte. Andererseits gehen dem Sexualverhalten oft Aggression oder Flucht voran. Sexualverhalten setzt Annäherung und enge Berührung voraus, etwas, was die meisten Tiere nur in besonderen sozialen Situationen und in besonderer Gestimmtheit dulden.

Ein gutes *Beispiel*, das sich in komplizierterer Weise auch auf Säugetiere übertragen läßt, gibt der wintersüber alleinlebende *Fischreiher* ab. Im Frühjahr (Außenfaktor) besetzt jedes Männchen sein vorjähriges Nest oder einen neuen Nistplatz. Wenn auf seinen Ruf (Auslöser) ein Weibchen kommt, beginnt er mit Balzbewegungen (weitere Auslöser). Nähert sich nun das Weibchen, wehrt er es ab, und es kann vom Geplänkel bis zum wütenden Kampf kommen. Fliegt das Weibchen davon, beginnt er sogleich wieder zu rufen. Falls es zurückkommt, geht das Geplänkel von neuem los, und erst allmählich schwindet die Angriffslust, und der Geschlechtstrieb gewinnt die Oberhand. Je später im Jahr die Partner zueinanderfinden, um so weniger streiten sie sich. Männchen, die schon 2 Wochen auf ein Weibchen gewartet haben, können das erste beste, das sich ihnen zugesellt, annehmen (*198*). Gut analysierte Beispiele ähnlicher Art geben MOYNIHAN und HALL (*607*). In Fällen verlangerter „Wartezeiten" kann schließlich, wie bei sehr „heißen" Katzen, das ganze Paarungsvorspiel mit Kokettierflucht, Wälzen, Umherschauen usw. einfach fortfallen. Die Begattung erfolgt unmittelbar (*126*).

Ein merkwürdiges Verhalten bei nicht rechtzeitig zur Abfuhr kommendem Geschlechtstrieb beschreibt EISENTRAUT (*336*) bei einem *Igelweibchen*, dessen Brunst am Hervortreten der Geschlechtsteile deutlich erkennbar war. Ein hinzugesetztes Männchen, das aber nicht paarungsbereit war, wehrte das Weibchen ab. Das Weibchen wurde immer erregter und bespuckte schließlich durch Hervorschnellen der Zunge zweimal sein Stachelkleid. Danach zeigte es kein Interesse mehr für den Partner. Einen Monat später wurde ein anderes, *brünstiges* Männchen zum selben Weibchen gesetzt, jedoch wieder fortgenommen, als das Weibchen erregt wurde. Darauf lief die Spuckhandlung wieder zweimal ab. Die Beziehung des Sich-selbst-Bespuckens zum Geschlechtstrieb ist in diesem Fall deutlich. Doch üben auch schon ganz junge, noch blinde und nackte Igelsäuglinge das Selbstbespucken aus.

ULLRICH (*787*) beschreibt ein recht ähnliches Verhalten bei einem männlichen *Wollaffen*, der sich unter Zeichen starker sexueller Erregung folgendermaßen bespuckt: Auch ohne erkennbare Ursache — etwa Nahrungsreize oder andere Duftstoffe, die offenbar bei den Igeln als Auslöser wirken — sammelt der Affe unter heftigen Kaubewegungen Speichel, den er an der Käfigwand mit dem Mund abstreicht. Unmittelbar danach reibt er seine Brust an der bespeichelten Wand, ergreift mit beiden Händen das Gitter über sich, beugt und streckt abwechselnd die Arme, so daß die Brust auf der Wand Kreisbögen beschreibt. Zugleich erreicht die Erregung den Höhepunkt, und der Affe masturbiert.

Für die engen Beziehungen zwischen *oralen und sexuellen Verhaltensweisen*, auf die wir im zweiten Teil dieses Beitrages noch ausführlicher zu sprechen kommen (s. S. 378 ff.), kann man noch eine Reihe anderer Beobachtungen anführen. Affen verschiedener Arten, z. B. auch Schimpansen und die schon erwähnten Totenkopfäffchen (*659*), onanieren oft mit Hilfe ihres Mundes. Zwei 4 Monate alte kleine Bärenmädchen sogen vor dem Einschlafen je an einem Ohr eines gleichaltrigen Männchens, während dieses an seinem Penis sog. Dabei summten alle drei wie beim Milchtrinken, ein Verhalten, das alle drei Bären noch mit drei Jahren nach Eintritt der Geschlechtsreife zeigten. Der Saugtrieb ist bei Bären außerordentlich stark und geht weit über das bloße Nahrungsbedürfnis hinaus. Das Lutschen ist, ähnlich wie bei Menschenkindern (*366*), besonders *vor dem Einschlafen* beliebt. — Erwachsene, sexuell erregte Bärinnen können sich mit den Tatzen an den Geschlechtsteilen kratzen oder mit der Aftergegend auf dem Boden hin- und herrutschen (*146*).

Haben die Auslöser des Spielers und die antwortenden, wiederum auslösenden Signale des Gegenspielers die Hemmungen, die der Annäherung entgegenstehen, beseitigt, so hat die Balz weitere Aufgaben zu erfüllen, nämlich die Synchronisierung der Partner. Ist z. B. das Männchen schon bereiter zur Paarung, so kann es durch hartnäckiges Werben das „Reifen" des Weibchens beschleunigen. Setzt man zwei Tauben isoliert in zwei nebeneinanderstehende Käfige so, daß sie einander sehen und sich berühren, aber nicht paaren können, legt das Weibchen, wenn das Männchen lange genug gebalzt hat, schließlich die Eier ab, was ein einsames Taubenweibchen niemals tut. Fehlen in der Gefangenschaft Männchen, können auch zwei Weibchen ein Paar bilden. Dann verhält sich eins von ihnen in allen Stücken wie ein Männchen, und auch wenn sie anfangs verschieden reif gewesen sein mögen, so legen doch beide gleichzeitig Eier. Ihre Rhythmen haben sich angeglichen (*198*).

Homosexuelle Handlungen (*573*) gibt es auch unter Säugern, speziell unter Affen. KUMMER (*113*) beobachtet in seiner Pavian-Gruppe häufig unter den geschlechtsreifen Weibchen homosexuelle Handlungen, die vom Pavian-Pascha geduldet wurden.

Ein sexuell sehr aktives Totenkopfäffchen habe ich oft dabei beobachtet, wie es mit erigiertem Penis andere Mannchen von hinten in typischer Stellung umklammerte; es machte wenige Begattungsbewegungen und gab dann auf. Nie kam es zur Ejakulation. Im Kafig befand sich ein Weibchen, das sich ihm standig verweigerte, so daß alle Aufsteigeversuche scheiterten. Naherte sich diesem Weibchen ein Rivale, drängte das Männchen ihn vom Weibchen fort, ja, es stieß ihn gelegentlich sogar mit den Handen weg, auch wenn es selbst sich nicht in sexueller Erregung befand. In anderen Fällen beobachtete ich, daß einzelne mannliche Affen einer Gruppe einen mannlichen Neuankömmling als Sexualpartner „ausprobierten" (*657, 659*).

Ob es eine echte Homosexualität, d. h. auf den gleichgeschlechtlichen Partner *fixiertes* Sexualverhalten, unter Tieren gibt, ist m. E. nicht genügend erwiesen. Bei gleichgeschlechtlichen Vogelpaaren, z. B. Graugänsen, handelt es sich offenbar eher um ein „Verkennen" des Geschlechtspartners als um echte Homosexualität. Am Institut von LORENZ werden die Ehegeschichten von Graugänsen, insbesondere auch solche gleichgeschlechtlicher Gespanne, verfolgt.

Besonders dann, wenn zur Befruchtung eine Begattung erforderlich ist, müssen Mann und Weib ihr Verhalten genau synchronisieren, oft bis auf Sekundenbruchteile. Die fein auf einander abgestimmten Auslöser des Balzritus haben im fortgeschrittenen Stadium der Balz nicht nur die sexuelle Stimmung zu synchronisieren, sondern sie geben auch die richtenden Reize ab, welche die Partner so orientieren, daß die oft komplizierte Zusammenfügung der Geschlechtsorgane möglich wird. Diese Orientierungsreaktionen (vgl. S. 299f.) sind also ein Teil des Synchronisierungsvorganges.

Vergewaltigung soll es nur bei wenigen Arten geben (*198*), doch scheint sie bei Säugetieren, z. B. bei männlichen See-Elefanten (*149*) und Lamas (*644*) häufiger, sogar an gleichgeschlechtigen Jungtieren, vorzukommen.

Manchmal haben Balzbewegungen noch eine andere Funktion. Weibchen, die sich durch ihr Aussehen nicht vom Männchen unterscheiden, müssen das aggressive, in ihnen einen Rivalen vermutende Männchen beschwichtigen. Die Methoden sind je nach Art recht verschieden. Bei manchen Vogelarten „bettelt" das Weibchen und spricht wahrscheinlich mit diesem kindlichen Verhalten den Pflegetrieb des Männchens an. Deshalb füttern auch die Männchen ihre Weibchen in der Balz.

Bei Säugetieren dauern die Paarungsvorspiele verschieden lange, bei Braunbären z. B. etwa 8 Tage. Häufige Verhaltensweisen sind das Belecken der Gesichtspartien und der Geschlechtsteile, seitliche Umarmungen des Hinterkörpers ohne Aufreiten, Kopfschwenken in einer vis-à-vis-Stellung, Flankenreiben, Kopfstoßen in die Flanken u. a. m. Auch regelrechte *Tänze* kommen vor (*146, 149, 537, 644, 659*).

In Untersuchungen über das Sozial- und Sexualverhalten der Totenkopfaffen (s. Abb. 13) haben wir zeigen können, daß sich die sexuellen Verhaltensweisen dieses Primaten durchaus nicht nur in Paarungsvorspielen und im Begattungsakt manifestieren, sondern daß sie in andere, verschiedenartige soziale Beziehungen eingebaut sind und die Funktion von sozialen Auslösern haben, die sowohl die soziale Struktur der Gruppe als auch die Aktivität ihrer Mitglieder entscheidend beeinflussen (*657, 659, 661*) [s. S. 340].

Über das *Brutpflegeverhalten* gibt es eine ausgedehnte Literatur (*360, 362, 499, 501, 606, 690, 691, 728, 729, 730*). Allein schon unter den Säugetieren ist es recht unterschiedlich (*50, 72, 126, 127, 146, 149, 158, 328, 329, 350, 352, 644*).

Eine lebenserhaltende angeborene Verhaltensweise ist das *Zerbeißen der Nabel-schnur und der Eihüllen* durch die Mutter sofort nach dem Partus (*72, 126, 146, 565*). Die Nase des Neugeborenen wird freigeleckt, die Nachgeburt mit dem abgebissenen Nabelschnurrest hervorgezogen und sogar von Nicht-Fleisch-Fressern verzehrt. Tote oder schwache Junge, die sich nicht bewegen, werden ebenfalls häufig gefressen (*126*). GAFFREY beobachtete bei einer Afghanen-Hündin, wie die ebenfalls hochtragende Mutter der erstgebärenden und unruhigen Tochter „*Hebammendienste*" leistete: Sie leckte ihrer Tochter „massierend" die Weichen und wartete neben ihr stehend die Geburt ab, riß die Fruchtblasen der ersten drei Welpen auf und leckte die Kleinen trocken. Die unerfahrene Erstgebärende „lernte" schnell, besorgte bei den etwas später folgenden Welpen alles selbst und wollte die Mutter nicht mehr dulden (*352*). Bei Hündinnen kann man nach erfolgloser Deckung gelegentlich *Scheinträchtigkeit* beobachten (Anschwellen der Gebärmutter mit Zunahme des Leibesumfanges, Milchdrüsenschwellung bis zur Lactation, Ausgraben des Wurflagers, Suche nach Jungen, Unruhe, ja, schließlich Nahrungsverweigerung). Die „hysterischen" Erscheinungen verteilen sich ent-sprechend der normalen Tragzeit auf 9 Wochen und eine mehrwöchige Säugezeit (*350*). Setzt man Welpen oder auch z. B. verwaiste Rehkitze zu, können solche Jungen gesäugt und aufgezogen werden; das vorher abnorme Verhalten der scheinträchtigen Hündin normalisiert sich dann schnell (*565*).

Bei sehr vielen Säugetieren setzt der Suchautomatismus zum Auffinden der mütterlichen Brustwarze sofort nach der Geburt ein, bei manchen aber fehlt er auch ganz (*644*); dagegen kann man die Saugbewegungen im Leerlauf wohl stets beobachten. Das Auffinden der mütterlichen Brustwarze ist teils von engeren Schlüsselreizen, z. B. von haarlosen Stellen im Fell, teils aber auch von allgemei-neren Schlüsselreizen abhängig. Lamas, Alpakas und andere Kameliden suchen in allen senkrecht und waagerecht begrenzten Winkeln. Durch Versuch und Irrtum lernen sie, dieses Schema auszufüllen, so daß nach einigen Tagen keine „Irrtümer" mehr vorkommen (*644*). Hat ein Junges den Kontakt mit Mutter und Geschwi-stern verloren, wird die Mutter häufig allein durch „Weinen" alarmiert, während sie stumme Junge nicht beachtet (*126, 149*). Zum Transport der Jungen dienen verschiedene „Griffe": Katzen- und Hundeartige wenden den vorsichtigen Nacken-biß an, Bären nehmen den ganzen Babykopf ins Maul, Eisbären und Affen tragen ihre Jungen am Bauch. Gerade die Affen sind allesamt tatsächlich Affenmütter; sie hätscheln ihre Kinder mit den Händen, schmiegen sich an, umarmen sie, tragen sie in den ersten Wochen fortgesetzt mit sich herum und füttern sie regel-mäßig. Ältere Affenkinder, aber auch Koala-Bärchen und das junge Opossum werden auf dem Rücken getragen (*36*). Fledermaussäuglinge beißen sich im Bauch-fell der Mutter so fest, daß sie mit auf den Flug genommen werden können.

Die Beteiligung des Vaters an der Aufzucht ist je nach Art recht verschieden. Füchse und Koyoten sind besonders gute Väter und bereiten etwas älteren Kindern im Übergang von der Milch zur Fleischnahrung die Bissen durch Kauen vor. Auch Affenmütter tun das. BILZ berichtet von einer Orang-Mutter, die ihren älteren Säug-ling mit Breikost ernährte, die sie von Mund zu Mund weitergab (*261*). Das kann man auch bei Menschenkindern machen und wurde vor etwa 30 Jahren noch in Holstein geübt, wo Großmütter dem Säugling Buttermehlklöße vorkauten! Kommt die Mutter ihrem dreimonatigen Säugling mit dem Mund nahe, so stülpt er schon bei Annäherung seine Lippen vor. Ist der Mund-zu-Mund-Kontakt vollzogen, schiebt das Kind seine Zunge vor und macht Leckbewegungen. Dieses Experiment wiederholten wir mit gleichem Resultat bei unseren eigenen Kindern. BILZ hat diese und viele andere Instinktbewegungen, wie z. B. den Suchautomatismus, schon 1940 und auch später beschrieben (*15, 259, 262*); er zählt diese „Kußhandlung" zu den

„Urszenen" des Menschen, in denen die Rollen des *Spielers* und *Gegenspielers* —
Ausdrücke, die Tinbergen (*198*) später auch verwendete — nach Art eines Text-
buches festgelegt sind. „Diese Rollen sind immer zugleich auch emotionale Rollen!"
(*262*).

Auch im *Familien- und Sippenleben* sind die Rollen verteilt (*359, 361, 534,
570, 755*). Nicht alle Säuger führen ein eigentliches Familienleben, bei anderen ist
es dagegen recht ausgeprägt (*126, 146, 230, 242, 571, 609, 644*).

Die *Walrosse* geben ein instruktives Beispiel. Unter den Robben führen sie das am meisten
entwickelte Gemeinschaftsleben in gemischten Gruppen aller Altersstufen, deren Oberhaupt
oft ein von allen respektierter alter Bulle ist. Die noch saugenden Jungen dürfen sich selbst dem
Alten gegenüber Dinge erlauben, die bereits bei Halbwüchsigen bestraft würden. Kann ein
Junges nicht selbst aus dem Wasser klimmen, so hilft ihm irgendein anderes der Tiere, das die
vergeblichen Bemühungen beobachtet hat, auch dann, wenn es selbst schon auf dem Trockenen
ist. Junge, die ihre Mutter verloren haben, werden vom Sippenverband aufgezogen. Zur Erziehung der Walroß-Jugend gehört es auch, daß die Kleinen zwar noch nicht selbst an den Ver-
teidigungs- und Angriffskämpfen des Familienverbandes teilnehmen dürfen, jedoch unter Auf-
sicht eines halbwüchsigen „Kindermädchens" dem Kampfe aus sicherer Entfernung folgen
können und müssen. Die Walrosse sind beherzte Tiere und greifen in Gruppen sogar Ruderboote
an. Sie stehen für einander ein. Selbst verwundete Tiere werden nicht im Stich gelassen: Junge
werden von der Mutter „unter den Arm geklemmt", ältere, gleichgültig welcher Rangordnung,
von einem stärkeren Tier unterschwommen und auf den Nacken geladen. Ist aber ein altes,
schweres Tier außerhalb der Nähe eines gleichstarken betroffen, stützen mehrere Jüngere den
Kranken von allen Seiten und sorgen dafür, daß sein Kopf über Wasser bleibt. Dieser soziale
Zusammenhalt trägt dazu bei, daß das *Walroß das ranghöchste Tier in den arktischen Gewässern*
ist, dem selbst der Eisbär weicht.

Die *Ohrenrobben* leben in großen Harems, in denen ein Riesenbulle so viele Weibchen wie
möglich um sich schart. Ähnlich ist es auch beim See-Elefanten, während andere Arten, wenn
nicht monogam, so doch in Paaren leben. Ein Harems-Pascha hat es nicht leicht: Durch seine
eifersüchtige Wach- und Kampfbereitschaft kommt er manchmal 2 Monate und länger kaum
zum Schlafen, Fressen und Trinken; am Ende der Paarungszeit hat er bis zu zwei Zentnern an
Gewicht verloren. Bei See-Elefanten kommt während der Brunstzeit eine sehr eigentümliche
Form von „Exhibitionismus" vor. Wenn sich den an Land liegenden Elefanten-Robben ein
Mensch nähert, zwingt der Bulle eines seiner Weibchen zur Kopulation. Robben, die kein
matures Weibchen erringen konnten, vergreifen sich sogar an Jährlingen und vergewaltigen
sie (*149*).

Die *Wale* (*185*), besonders die Familien der *Delphine* und *Tümmler*, sind in den letzten
Jahren wegen ihrer erstaunlichen Hirnentwicklung, die in vielem die des Menschen übertrifft,
wegen ihrer hohen Intelligenz und Lernfähigkeit, wegen ihrer überraschenden stimmlichen
Kommunikationsfähigkeit („Sprache") und wegen ihres differenzierten Sozialverhaltens in
den Vordergrund des Interesses von Anatomen, Neurophysiologen, Verhaltensforschern und
Technikern getreten. Schon im Altertum erwähnte Berichte über sinnvolle Begebenheiten
zwischen Mensch und Delphin dürfen nach den neuen Erkenntnissen nicht mehr als reine
Fabeln betrachtet werden. Die beim Tümmler festgestellte Orientierungsleistung durch Echo-
lotung mit Stimmfrequenzen bis in den Ultraschallbereich sowie die Fähigkeit des Delphins,
mit zunehmender Geschwindigkeit die Oberflächenbeschaffenheit seiner Haut so zu verändern,
daß deren Reibungswiderstand beträchtlich herabgesetzt wird, hat Neurophysiologen und
Techniker fasziniert (*3, 293, 448, 783*).

Seit den Arbeiten Schjelderup-Ebbes (*198, 722*) hat die *soziale Rangordnung*
unter den in Gruppen lebenden Tieren zunehmend an Beachtung gewonnen. Besonders ausgeprägt ist sie bei vielen Vögeln und wurde von Lorenz an Dohlen (*129,
530*) eindrucksvoll beschrieben. Aber auch bei Fischen (*198*) und bei vielen Säugetieren einschließlich der obenerwähnten Pinnipedier und Cetaceen (*126, 130, 146,
149, 158, 185, 198, 242, 721, 792*) wurde die Rangordnung eingehend studiert.
Bei diesen Untersuchungen ist es besonders wichtig, einen „Verhaltenskatalog"
aufzustellen, der Auskunft über die überhaupt möglichen sozialen Beziehungen
gibt (*113, 657, 659*).

Die Tiere kämpfen nicht nur um ihre Weibchen und ihr Revier, sie zanken sich
auch um Futter oder den Futterplatz, um einen Lieblingsplatz oder um ihren

Ruhe- oder Schlafplatz. Mitunter kann sich für jede der mit diesen „Vorlieben" zusammenhängenden Verhaltensweisen eine eigene Rangordnung ausbilden, oft gilt aber die „Hackordnung" durchgehend, so daß das Alphatier in jedem Fall an erster und das Omegatier stets an letzter Stelle rangiert. Fremden, ja, selbst dem Menschen als Freund gegenüber kann das Omegatier verteidigt werden, wenn es Notsignale aussendet (538).

Die Rangordnung ist oft, aber durchaus nicht immer von der körperlichen Stärke abhängig. „Schneidige", aber schwächere Tiere können unter Umständen den starken „Alten" aus seiner Spitzenstellung für immer vertreiben. Manchmal dankt er ab und wird zum Einzelgänger, manchmal begnügt er sich mit dem zweiten oder dritten Platz. Dohlen-Weibchen, die sich mit einem Männchen hohen Standes verloben oder verheiraten, können sofort und ohne Kämpfe zum Rang ihres Erwählten aufsteigen und werden von allen ihnen vorher überlegenen Genossen als ranghöher respektiert (529).

Wie schon öfter erwähnt, bildet sich die Rangordnung im Zusammenwirken von Instinkt und Dressur aus. Ein Artgenosse „versteht" den anderen angeborener-

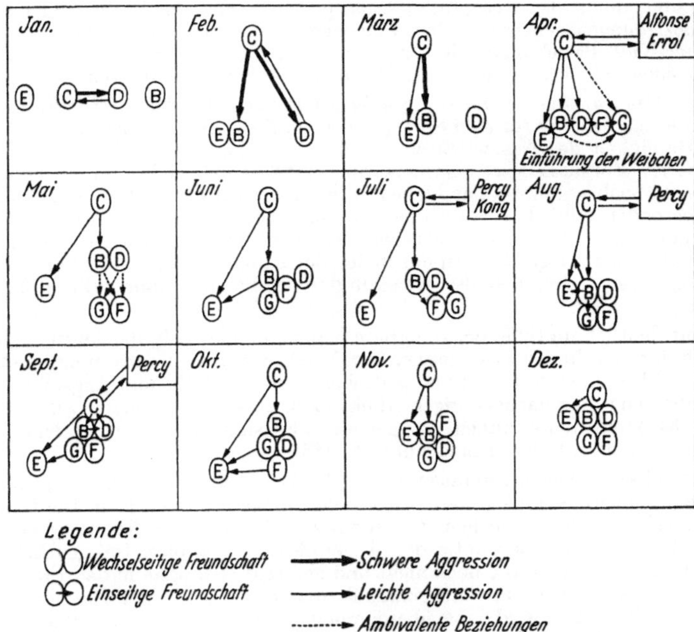

Abb. 13. *Entwicklung der sozialen Struktur und Rangordnung in einer Gruppe von Totenkopf-Affen (Saimiri sciureus).* Die Diagramme fußen einerseits auf der numerisch erfaßten Häufigkeit und Verteilung einer größeren Anzahl von typischen Verhaltenselementen, andererseits auf fortlaufenden qualitativ-descriptiven Beobachtungen. Jedes Oval stellt ein Tier mit der Initiale seines Namens dar. B, C, D, E sind männliche, F und G weibliche Affen. Man sieht, wie C seine Alpha-Stellung aufbaut, indem er ein Mannchen nach dem anderen unter Kontrolle bekommt. Nach Festigung seiner Alpha-Position verteidigt er seine Gruppe gegen Feinde (s. Apr., Juli, Aug., Sept.), bleibt aber dabei isoliert von der Gruppe. Auch das Omega-Tier E ist stärker isoliert, während die Tiere der Kern-Gruppe mannigfaltige und wechselvolle Beziehungen untereinander austauschen. Nach 3-monatigem Zusammensein spielen härtere Kämpfe keine Rolle mehr. Leichte Aggression wird vorwiegend durch Imponieren, ein sehr wirksames soziales Signal, gezeigt, nämlich durch frontale Annäherung an den Partner und Präsentieren des erigierten Penis mit abgewinkeltem Bein. Im Laufe der Zeit lernt jedes Mitglied, seine Gruppenrolle zu erfüllen. Alpha- und Omega-Tier sind weniger isoliert, und die Gruppe lebt spannungsloser als zu Beginn. Bei gelegentlichen Streitereien brechen alte Animositäten wieder auf [PLOOG et al. (*657, 659, 661*)]

maßen, aber er hat zu lernen, wer der Überlegene ist. Wer nicht rasch genug lernt, dem Stärkeren aus dem Wege zu gehen, bekommt erstens mehr Prügel und zweitens verbraucht er seine Kraft unnötig, so daß er anderen artfremden Feinden leichter zur Beute fällt. Auf Abb. 13 ist die *Entwicklung der sozialen Struktur und Rangordnung* in einer Gruppe von 6 Totenkopfaffen schematisch dargestellt (*657, 659*).

Ein, auch in methodischer Hinsicht, schönes Vorbild für die Untersuchungen des *Sozialverhaltens von Affen* hat HANS KUMMER (*113*) gegeben. Er knüpft an das klassische Buch von ZUCKERMAN (*216*) und an die Untersuchungsmethoden CARPENTERs (*26, 27, 309*) an und beschreibt seine auch quantitativ erfaßten Ergebnisse unter ethologischen Gesichtspunkten.

In der Gruppe von 15 Mantelpavianen des Zürcher Zoos (Papio hamadryas: ein adultes Mannchen, vier adulte Weibchen, zehn zum Teil geschlechtsreife Jungtiere im Alter von 1—5 Jahren) ließen sich rund 70 stets wiederkehrende Verhaltenselemente rein descriptiv unterscheiden, wie z. B. Brauenziehen, Bodenschlag oder Mundkontakt. Dieser Katalog bildete die Grundlage fur die Untersuchung der sozialen Gruppenstruktur. Die Beziehung eines jeden Individuums zu jedem anderen lieferte das Bild der Gesamtgruppe. Auf diese Weise erkennt man die verschiedenen Rollen. die jedem Tier der Gruppe zugewiesen sind und seine Stellung im Netzwerk der Beziehungen für jede Situation festlegen. Die Häufigkeit eines Verhaltenselementes wurde mit Hilfe des von MORENO (*178*) beschriebenen *Soziogrammes* quantitativ dargestellt. Darin erscheint fur jede Verhaltensweise jedes Individuum einmal als ,,Aktor" (Spieler) und einmal als ,,Receptor" (Gegenspieler), so daß die Partnerrollen und die Intensitat der Beziehungen sichtbar werden. Eingehend dargestellt wurden die Verhaltensgruppen der Mutter-Kind-Beziehungen, der Angst und der Drohung. Eine Herde von Babuinen (Papio papio), einer nahe verwandten Art, diente zu Vergleichen und Kontrollen.

Ergebnisse: Das Jungtier ist frei von den harten Regeln der Adult-Beziehungen. Erst nach und nach tritt es ins Feld der sozialen Spannungen ein. Die Zunahme solcher Spannungen läßt sich an der Haufigkeit des Nasewischens verfolgen, das im Sozialkontakt als Übersprungbewegung auftritt. Erstmals ist es als Übersprung mit 2 Jahren und dann mit zunehmendem Alter häufiger zu beobachten. — Die kleinen Jungen werden nur sachte ins Handgelenk gebissen. Diese besonders milde Form der Zurechtweisung (Drohung) erzeugt kein Angstverhalten. Die Alters- und Geschlechtsunterschiede zeigen sich im allgemeinen nicht in Verschiedenheiten der Verhaltenselemente selbst, sondern nur in der Bevorzugung bestimmter Verhaltensweisen, im Ausschluß gewisser Individuen als Partner und in der Beschränkung auf bestimmte Rollen in Zeremonien.

Das kommt deutlich im Spiel der Jungtiere heraus, in dem z. B. die Angst- und Drohelemente frei von den Regeln der Erwachsenen kombiniert werden. Mature Jungtiere lassen sich im Spiel von viel kleineren verfolgen und bedrohen. Gewisse Droh- und Angstelemente scheinen sich offenbar von dem dazugehorigen Affekt losen zu konnen, andere, wie z. B. Brauenziehen (vgl. S. 340) und Haarstrauben, dagegen nicht. Sie sind aufs engste mit dem ,,Ernstfall" verkoppelt und treten im Spiel niemals auf (s. S. 343).

Bei den erwachsenen Tieren vereinigen sich *18 Droh- und Angstelemente* zu einem reichhaltigen *Zeremoniell.* Größere Konflikte werden vor dem Alphatier ausgetragen. Die Rangordnung der übrigen, die sich bei den Weibchen oft erst zur Zeit der ersten Ovulation herausstellt, entscheidet sich also gewissermaßen unter den Augen des Oberhauptes. Gelegentlich kennt ein jüngeres Tier seinen eigenen Rang noch nicht und vergreift sich dann in den Einzelheiten des Zeremoniells. — Drohung eines Pavians veranlaßt andere nahebei befindliche zu gleichem Tun. Die allgemeine Drohrichtung wird dabei übernommen, doch richtet sich die induzierte Drohung häufig auf andere Objekte, vor allem auf rangtiefe Weibchen. Das rangtiefste Weibchen wurde einmal nach einem Konflikt dabei beobachtet, wie es eine Mauer androhte, ein anderes Mal trat das Drohelement ,,Brauenziehen" (niedrige Intensitätsstufe des Drohens, vgl. S. 301 f) sogar im Schlaf auf.

Bekommt ein Affe auf eine Drohung hin *Angst*, entfernt er sich fluchtartig vom Bedroher und sucht bei großer Angst stets ein möglichst ranghohes Tier auf, unter Umstanden sogar den Verursacher selbst, wenn dieser gerade der Ranghochste unter den Anwesenden ist. Angstäußerungen sind z. B. Keckern, Schwanzheben, Beinflexion, Kreischen, Pressen, Harnen. Die *Entladung der Angst* ist dem Alphatier gegenuber streng von der Rangordnung abhangig. Sie findet ihre Abfuhr im Durchsuchen seines Felles oder dementsprechenden Ersatzhandlungen. Erwachsene Weibchen untersuchen stets mit beiden Handen; jungere, rangtiefere, aber schon mature Weibchen beruhren nur mit dem Zeigefinger einer Hand die außersten Haarspitzen von Alpha. Wahrend sie das Fell anderer Genossen normal mit beiden Handen durchstobern, wagen sie das beim Alphatier selbst ein Jahr nach der Pubertat noch nicht. Die alteren Mannchen beruhren Alpha uberhaupt nicht, sondern setzen sich hinter seinen Rücken und betrachten sein Fell aus 10—30 cm Abstand. Dreht der Herrscher seinen Kopf, fahren sie zurück. Das Felldurchsuchen als Angstentladung unterscheidet sich in Frequenz und Bewegungsart eindeutig von der normalen sozialen Hautpflege, bei der auch stets Hautteilchen mit dem Munde aufgenommen werden. Das fehlt bei der *Felldurchsuchung im Übersprung*. Gerade bei solchen Tieren, denen nur das „Zeigefingerrühren" gestattet ist, genügen diese gehemmten Bewegungen nicht zur vollen Angstentladung. Sie wischen dann mit erhöhter Frequenz auf dem blanken Fels oder graben in Spalten, führen die Bewegungen des Felldurchsuchens an toten Objekten aus, welche ihrer Motorik keine sozialen Hemmungen auferlegen, oder sie rühren mit dem Zeigefinger auf dem Boden herum (s. Abb. 13a).

Ähnlich entwickelt sich die *Individualdistanz*. Babies und Jungtiere kennen sie noch nicht. Je jünger sie sind, desto mehr suchen sie die Nähe der Mutter auf. Die erwachsenen Weibchen

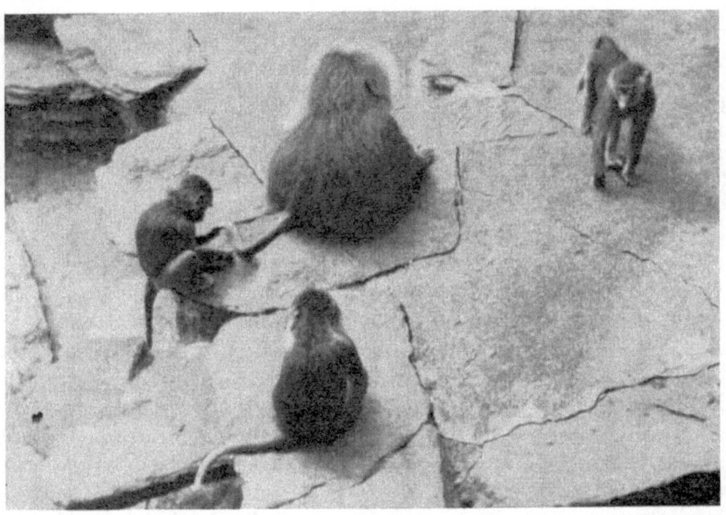

Abb. 13a. *Rangordnung*. Zeigefinger-Rühren eines maturen Pavian-Weibchens am Schwanz des Alpha-Tieres nach erfolgloser Drohung gegen ein ranghöheres matures Weibchen (rechts im Bilde). [Aufnahmen von KUMMER (*113*)]

nähern sich Alpha ohne Scheu bis zur Berührung, die jüngeren halten sich ohne Scheu noch in einem halben Meter Abstand von ihm auf. Die älteren Männchen dagegen geraten schon in 1—2 m Abstand in Angst; das Aufsuchen des Fürsten ist für sie eine Ausnahmesituation.

Auch die *soziale Hemmung* entwickelt sich spät. Zuerst beobachtet man die Hemmung, Futter und Gegenstände im Besitze eines älteren Partners zu ergreifen. Sie werden stattdessen berochen. Größere Junge nehmen kleineren niemals Futter weg. Der Mundkontakt bekommt eine rein soziale, vom Objekt gelöste Bedeutung. Die Berührungshemmung gegenüber dem Alphatier ist erst mit drei Jahren voll ausgebildet. Nun erscheint mit der Geschlechtsreife die typische Entladungs-Hautpflege am Fell des alten Männchens nach Angst und Bedrohung. Der Konflikt dieses Verhaltens mit der Berührungshemmung führt zur geschlechtsspezifischen Bewegungsreduktion beim Felldurchsuchen. Jungtiere kennen die soziale Hautpflege nicht.

Bei den 4 in der Gruppe vorhandenen Weibchen konnte festgestellt werden, daß die *Schlafbewegungen* pro Stunde mit absteigendem Rang regelmäßig zunehmen.

Das *Sexualverhalten* ist streng an die Rangordnung gebunden. Ranghohe, adulte Weibchen treten auf eigene Initiative vor allem mit Alpha in Beziehung. Rangtiefe Weibchen sind fast nur mit jungen Männchen zu beobachten, wobei die Männchen die Initiative ergreifen. Dabei ist bemerkenswert, daß die jüngeren Männchen den Weibchen gegenüber eine stärkere Aktivität entwickeln als die älteren mit ihrem primär höheren Rang, so daß also die Frequenz sexueller Verhaltensweisen umgekehrt zur primären Altersrangordnung steht.

Innerhalb der vom Alpha-Tier überragend beherrschten Gruppe sondert sich häufig das älteste mature Männchen mit einer *Gruppe von Jungtieren* ab. Dazu gehörten in dieser Mantelpavian-Gesellschaft alle Männchen außer Alpha und die noch nicht geschlechtsreifen Weibchen. Das Verhalten des Anführers gleicht bis in einzelne Elemente demjenigen des Oberhauptes; nur das *Sexualverhalten fällt fast vollkommen weg*. Die Weibchen treten nach der Geschlechtsreife zum Harem des Oberhauptes über. Der Aufenthaltsort der Jungengruppe liegt möglichst weit vom Harem entfernt und stets außerhalb des Sichtbereiches von Alpha. Dieser erhebt sich, gefolgt von seinem Harem, alle 3—30 min und wechselt seinen Standort so, daß er die Jungengruppe in den Blick bekommt. Nach etwa einer Minute löst sich dann die Jungengruppe auf; der Anführer entzieht sich Alphas Blick. Erst nach einer Weile wandern die andern wie zufällig nacheinander in die Nähe des Anführers ab. Meist sind es zuerst zwei spielende kleine Junge, die dem Anführer kraft der Anziehung des „großen vertrauten Tieres" folgen. Die Zweierteilung der gesamten Gruppe ist nicht starr und kann unter gewissen Umständen aufgegeben werden. Das Zentrum bleibt — im Beobachtungszeitraum von mehr als 3 Monaten — stets Alpha. — Nach neuesten Freilandbeobachtungen (*796*) ist die soziale Struktur der Paviangruppen komplizierter. Die Trupps zahlen durchschnittlich 40—80 Mitglieder und werden von einer Gruppe dominanter Mannchen gefuhrt.

Auch die *Mutter-Kind-Beziehungen* der Zoo-Gruppe sind höchst interessant. Bei quantitativer Auswertung dominieren die hierzu gehörigen Verhaltensweisen der Weibchen zahlenmaßig erheblich. Vorherrschend ist die lang andauernde Umarmung des Kindes im Sitzen. *Bei Angst suchen die Kleinen Schutz* in den Armen oder auf dem Rücken der Mutter. Ein verwaister Zweijahriger fand hierin Ersatz beim altesten maturen Männchen. Die Mütter üben das Umarmen und Tragen am Bauch und auf dem Rucken oft langdauernd und mit geringer Affektbeteiligung aus. Mit 2—2$^1/_2$ Jahren lost sich die Mutter-Kind-Beziehung; Umarmen und Tragen horen nach und nach auf, das Bauchtragen beträchtlich eher als das Rückentragen. Jungtiere unter sich dagegen umarmen und tragen sich kurzdauernd und mit starker Affektbeteiligung bis weit über die Geschlechtsreife hinaus bei Angst und im Spiel. Junge und Erwachsene mit intensiven Tagesbeziehungen schlafen in gegenseitiger Umarmung ein.

Die zahlreichen Parallelen zum menschlichen Sozialverhalten liegen auf der Hand (*118, 268*). Exakt vergleichende Untersuchungen müßten allerdings erst im einzelnen erweisen, welche Verhaltensweisen als *echte* Homologien aufzufassen sind. Sicher sind die Mutter-Kind-Beziehungen (*383*) homolog. Das *Schutz- und Hilfesuchen* im Arm der Mutter oder beim „großen Vertrauten" gehört in denselben Funktionskreis. Das Umarmen und Tragen der Jungen untereinander kann man bei Menschenkindern, die sich selbst nur noch unter besonderen Umständen hätscheln lassen, recht gut beobachten; mit großer Affektbeteiligung umarmen und tragen sie kleinere Geschwister oder jüngere Spielgefährten und lassen bald darauf auch wieder von ihnen ab. Die Freude, die das Auf-dem-Arm-Getragenwerden bei älteren Säuglingen auslöst, ist ebensowenig durch Erfahrung und Lernen zu erklären wie die Wonne, die etwa das erste Huckepack-Getragenwerden (Rückentragen, bei weniger zivilisierten Völkern auch in Tüchern) bei den meisten Kindern im 2. Lebensjahr bewirkt. Primär ängstliche Kinder scheinen das „Arm-Bauch-Tragen" länger zu lieben und das „Rückentragen" nicht so zu schätzen.

Für besonders wichtig halten wir die Feststellung KUMMERs, daß die Alters- und Geschlechtsunterschiede sich im sozialen Zusammenleben *nicht* in Verschiedenheiten der Verhaltenselemente selbst zeigen (s. Abb. 13). Auch beim Menschen sind die meisten Verhaltenselemente schon längst vor der Pubertät entwickelt. *Die Alters- und Geschlechtsunterschiede kommen vor allem — wie bei den Affen (659) — durch andere Häufigkeitsverteilung und andere Kombination heraus.* Zum Beispiel lassen sich die sexuellen Spielereien älterer Kinder und die sexuellen Bewegungen von Kindern aller Altersstufen sehr wohl mit dem entsprechenden Verhalten der Erwachsenen vergleichen, und es besteht kein hinreichender Grund, den Bereich der Sexualität für den Erwachsenen zu reservieren. Das volle Bild des integrierten Sexualverhaltens entwickelt sich erst von der Pubertät ab bis zum Erwachsenenalter; die *Elemente* dieses Verhaltens sind in verschiedener, variabler Kombination und Intensität aber längst vorher da. Erektionen z. B. kommen bereits beim Säugling vor, doch besagt dies für die „normale" oder „anormale" sexuelle Entwicklung ebensowenig wie spätere Spielereien, die Eltern oft in Aufregung versetzen. Der tatsächliche Entwicklungszustand kann im sexuellen Bereich ebensowenig nach Einzelsymptomen beurteilt werden wie die Entwicklung der gesamten Persönlichkeit (*790*). Diese Feststellung entbindet freilich nicht von einer gründlichen Analyse des jeweiligen Persönlichkeitsbildes, sondern fordert

vielmehr auch zu einer quantitativen Erfassung der Kombination von Verhaltenselementen auf (2, 25, 357).

Der heute noch bestehende Meinungsunterschied zwischen Psychoanalytikern
und deren Gegnern hinsichtlich der Anerkennung und Bewertung frühkindlicher
Sexualität hat unter ethologischen Gesichtspunkten keine prinzipielle Bedeutung.
Weder läßt sich die frühkindliche Sexualität leugnen, noch kommt *einzelnen*
Ereignissen ohne Berücksichtigung des jeweiligen Entwicklungsstatus eine

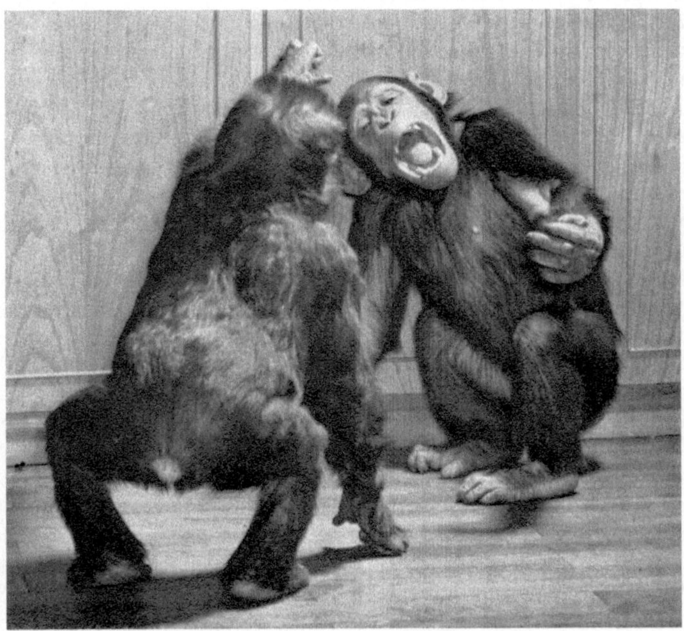

Abb. 14. *Kampfspiel* in der Phase der Scheindrohung zwischen Schimpansen- und Gorillajungem. (Aufnahme
von Prof. Dr. GRZIMEK, Zoologischer Garten, Frankfurt a. M.)

besondere Bedeutung zu. Aber auch für viele andere Bereiche menschlichen Sozial-
lebens ist der Gesichtspunkt der Häufigkeitsverteilung, der Kombination und
des Heranreifens von Verhaltensweisen viel zu wenig berücksichtigt worden. Wenn
man heute gern mehr von der Besonderheit der Menschen gegenüber den Tieren als
von deren Gemeinsamkeiten spricht, sollte man sich die große Variabilität der
Verhaltensweisen mindestens der Säugetiere vor Augen halten und sich eingestehen,
daß wir von den Tieren viel zu wenig wissen, um in prinzipiell vergleichende und
unterscheidende Betrachtungen eintreten zu können. Das gilt ganz besonders für
das auch die Menschen bestimmende emotionale Verhalten (*367, 382, 383, 506,
507, 509*).

Die freie Kombinierbarkeit von verschiedenartigen Verhaltenselementen, die
im „Ernstfall" zu fest geordneten Verhaltensabläufen zusammengefügt sind, zeigt
sich vor allem im *Spiel der Säugetiere (145)*. Darin fehlt z. B. bei den Pavianen die
Kopplung von Angst- und Drohelementen im Sinne streng eingehaltener Auf-
einanderfolge. Die Verhaltensweisen verschiedener Intensitätsstufen — sonst
wohl abgestuft — mischen sich durcheinander, und wenn man einen klaren
Intensitätsanstieg beobachten kann, dann ist das Spiel zum Ernst geworden. Auch
bei spielenden Hunden sieht man diesen Übergang oft. Nur im Spiel ist es möglich,
daß ein kleines Junges ein großes verfolgt und „bedroht". Die Hauptspielform der

Paviangruppe ist der frontale Beißkampf; Kampfspiele überhaupt werden bevorzugt von Gleichaltrigen ausgeführt (s. Abb. 14). Dabei wechseln die Rollen, wobei der jeweilige Angreifer „Imponiergehabe" und der Unterlegene „Demuthaltung" zeigen. Kreischen eines Spielpartners bricht das Spiel sofort ab. Ein nur zwischen Jungen und Erwachsenen vorkommendes Spiel der Paviane ist der Tragtanz, wobei das erwachsene Tier das junge mit den Armen in die Horizontale hochhebt, sich selbst auf die Hinterbeine stellt und sich auch noch oft um sich selbst dreht (*113*).

Über das Spiel ist viel Interessantes und Wichtiges beobachtet, geschrieben (*145, 149, 158, 569*) und diskutiert worden (*539*). Eine allgemeinverbindliche Definition kann man nicht geben. Wirkliches Spiel gibt es wohl nur bei Säugetieren und Vögeln, also den beiden höchsten Wirbeltierklassen. Neugierverhalten, Leerlaufaktivität, Jugendlichkeit, Lernen nach Versuch und Irrtum und das „Ausprobieren" reifender angeborener Verhaltensweisen sind Komponenten, die das Spiel konstituieren, das ganze Phänomen aber nicht hinreichend erklären können. Man muß sich vorläufig mit der Feststellung begnügen, daß das Spiel ein wichtiger und integrierender Bestandteil höchstorganisierten Verhaltens ist, welches zahlreiche Vergleiche zwischen Mensch und Tier erlaubt.

Gemeinsame Wurzeln menschlichen und tierischen Verhaltens finden wir auch im *Anspruch auf Territorium und Besitz*. Das Territorium oder Revier ist der Aktionsraum eines Tieres, den es im allgemeinen für lange Zeit, manchmal zeitlebens nicht verläßt. Auch innerhalb dieses Raumes bewegt sich das Tier nicht beliebig, sondern nur auf bestimmten Wegen und auf diesen nach einem von der Jahreszeit abhängigen ziemlich festliegenden Zeitplan. Im Revier gibt es Schlafplätze, die für Wildsäugetiere „die Stelle maximaler Geborgenheit" und von einer „Schonzone" umgeben sind, in der sie auf Nahrungserwerb verzichten (*393*). Diese sicherste und bequemste Ruhestelle wird besonders bevorzugt und ist zur gegebenen Zeit das Ziel des Appetenzverhaltens für *triebbedingte Ruhezustände*. Die Absperrung vom „Heim" versetzt das Tier in Erregung (*420*). Oft ist das Jagdrevier an einem anderen Ort als der „Wohnraum". Es gibt Tränken, Nahrungs-, Ausgucks-, Schwimm- und Tummelplätze, Scheuer- oder Wälz-, Harn- und Kotstellen. Manche Säuger kennzeichnen ihr Revier durch „Duftmarken" (*50, 126, 146, 149, 158, 393, 641, 644*); anderen, z. B. den Brüllaffen, dient die Stimme zur Kennzeichnung (*26, 617*).

Höhere Säuger, besonders die in Herden lebenden Arten, haben im ganzen gesehen weniger scharf abgegrenzte Reviere als Vögel und Fische. Gerade bei letzteren kann man Revierkämpfe gut beobachten und dabei feststellen, daß der Herr im eigenen Hause bedeutend mutiger ist als in nachbarlichen Gefilden (*197, 198*). Gleiches gilt cum grano salis von Säugetieren (*334*). Auch kann es zu gut nachbarlichem Frieden kommen, wo sich die Anrainer Grenzüberschreitungen erlauben dürfen, die einem Fremden verboten sind (*508*). Die Eigenschaften, die ein Revier haben muß, um als Heimat des betreffenden Tieres dienen zu können, „weiß" das Tier angeborenermaßen. Gegenden mit Anhäufungen der für eine Art günstigen Revier-Eigenschaften sind dichter bevölkert als andere. Hier sind die Reviere kleiner und die *Revierkämpfe* heftiger. Doch ist die Wohndichte begrenzt und wird bei manchen Arten, z. B. Ratten, so geregelt, daß die Geburtenziffer der betreffenden Population nicht weiter steigt, ohne daß man bisher genügende Erklärungen für diese Geburtenregulierung hätte (*316*)[1]. Die Revierverteidigung als solche ist ebenfalls angeboren und findet auch dort statt, wo das betreffende

---

[1] Hier wäre der Ort, einen sehr wichtigen und interessanten Zweig der Verhaltensforschung, die *Ökologie*, zu behandeln. Die Ecology macht in Nordamerika einen großen Teil der Verhaltensforschung aus und beschäftigt sich mit dem Verhalten bzw. den Verhaltensveränderungen unter Einfluß der, auch experimentell, veränderten *Umwelt* (*304—308, 496, 711, 757, 758, 759*).

Individuum den Kampf sozusagen gar nicht nötig hätte, da es alles hat, was es braucht.

Vom *Freiland-Leben der Affen* wissen wir trotz zahlreicher Studien noch wenig, wenn sich auch der Wissensstand gerade in den letzten Jahren beträchtlich vermehrt hat (*24a, 26, 27, 96, 166a, 176, 226, 346, 486a, 617, 774, 792, 796*). Familiengruppen oder größere Banden behaupten im allgemeinen ein bestimmtes Wohngebiet, das z. B. bei den mittelamerikanischen Klammeraffen oft durch schwer passierbare Gebirgshänge begrenzt wird. Unter günstigen Verhältnissen können mehrere Trupps dicht nebeneinander wohnen, ohne einander merklich anzufeinden oder sich zu vermischen (*792, 796*). Schimpansen wandern in kleineren oder größeren Verbänden durch ihr Gebiet. Abends baut sich jedes Mitglied der Bande ein Schlafnest in einem Baum; Mütter nehmen ihre Säuglinge mit ins Nest (*24a, 617*).

Trotz der wenigen Angaben, die wir vom Freileben der Menschenaffen (*176, 486a, 617*) haben, ergeben sich doch einige auffällige Übereinstimmungen mit dem *Sozialleben primitiver Jäger- und Sammlervölker*. Auch bei ihnen ist der wesentliche Sozialverband die Familie oder die Sippe von drei bis vier Familien, die in einem abgegrenzten „Schweifgebiet" ihren Lebensunterhalt gewinnen. Die Beziehungen zu den Nachbarsippen sind, wie bei Affen und speziell bei Pongiden, im allgemeinen durchaus freundlich, Gebietsübertretungen allerdings werden sofort mit der Waffe bekämpft. Auf den Wanderungen werden von den einzelnen Familien Windschirme für die Nacht errichtet, oder es kommt unter Bedingungen, die ein längeres Verweilen am Ort erlauben, auch zum Hüttenbau, der aus dem Zusammenrücken von einzelnen Windschirmen entsteht. Innen grenzt jede Familie ihren Teil durch Steine oder Holzstücke ab (*508*). Dieses Verhalten erinnert sehr an die eifersüchtig überwachten Platzansprüche und Raumeinteilungen von auf engstem Raum zusammengepferchten Kriegsgefangenen. Jedermann, der solche ungewöhnlichen Bedingungen des Zusammenlebens mitgemacht hat, weiß, welche nichtigen Anlässe zu schweren Auseinandersetzungen führen können, die unter denselben Menschen in normalen „Wohnplatz"-Verhältnissen niemals vorkommen würden. Neben offenen Streitereien wachsen Spannungen und paranoide Verdächtigungen, eine Entwicklung, die ebenso im angespannten sozialen Konkurrenzkampf beobachtet werden kann. Aber auch Fehden unter Nachbarn in bürgerlichen Verhältnissen ziehen sich durch die menschliche Geschichte und Literatur.

Unter den heutigen beengten Wohnverhältnissen stoßen wir immer wieder auf Affekte gegen Hausgenossen, die nur dann „verständlich" werden, wenn man berücksichtigt, daß der *individuelle und der soziale Raumanspruch zur Stammesgeschichte der Menschheit* gehören. Die Nicht-Befriedigung dieses Bedürfnisses erweckt Affekte, die in der heutigen Gesellschaftsordnung nicht mehr direkt abreagiert werden können. Die abgrenzenden Mauern in engen Wohngebieten sind im Laufe der Zeit immer höher geworden, und jene Menschen, die in dünnbesiedelten Gebieten noch mit herzlicher Gastfreundschaft empfangen werden, sind in der Stadt längst zu „Unbefugten" geworden. Das oft unverständlich schikanöse Verhalten Einheimischer gegenüber Vertriebenen, die in deren Wohnungen eingewiesen wurden, beweist nur allzu deutlich, mit welcher Kraft sich die Abwehr gegen „Eindringlinge", nicht selten wider bessere Einsicht und Vernunft durchsetzt. Kurz: *Raumanspruch und Besitzverteidigung* gehören zum Instinktverhalten der Menschheit (*508*).

Manche überspitzten Rangordnungskämpfe in unserer heutigen Gesellschaft lassen sich mit denen bei soziallebenden Tieren in Gefangenschaft vergleichen: Mitglieder einer freilebenden Wolfsfamilie sind miteinander freundlich, und die erkennbare Rangordnung wird nur wenig betont. Beißereien kommen fast nie vor, und Futter wird bereitwillig geteilt. Bei den Tieren in Gefangenschaft hingegen herrscht schärfste Rangordnung, die nur dem Spitzentier volle Entfaltung erlaubt (*721*).

Menschenkinder und Schimpansen zeigen überraschende Ähnlichkeiten in ihrem *Verhalten gegenüber Objekten*, die sie besitzen oder besitzen möchten. Triebhafte Verschränkung von Betteln und Füttern erwähnten wir beim Brutpflegeverhalten der Vertebraten (s. S. 336, S. 337). Weil alles von Schlüsselreizen, nicht aber von freiwilliger Entscheidung abhängt, kann man noch nicht von einem Verschenken sprechen; anders ist es beim Schimpansen (*144, 617*). Der bettelnde Schimpanse streckt die nach oben gekehrte Handfläche aus, Handgelenk und Finger werden in rascher Folge gebeugt und gestreckt. Dazu kommen lautliche Äußerungen, auch Fußstampfen oder Rütteln am Käfiggitter. Der angebettelte Schimpanse *muß* nun keineswegs hergeben; er benimmt sich so, als habe er die Wahl. Bald gibt er dem Bettelnden die Nahrung in den Mund oder in die Hand, bald wirft er sie einfach dem anderen hin; er kann auch gleichgültig bleiben oder gar die begehrten Objekte — durchaus nicht immer Nahrung — außer Reichweite räumen. Grzimek (*378*) erzählt von seinem kleinen Schimpansenmädchen, das er in seiner Familie aufzog, daß es mit Vorliebe Speisen, die es selbst nicht mochte, dem Dackel schenkte, ein Verhalten, das man auch bei $1^{1}/_{2}$—5 jährigen Kindern feststellen kann. Manchmal wird eine solche Gabe sogar „scheinheilig" als Opfer verbrämt. Die Fähigkeit zu echter Opferbereitschaft entwickelt sich beim Menschen sehr langsam, und es ist recht lustig, sich Mütter über ihre „unmoralischen" Kinder empören zu sehen: Jedes der Kinder liegt mit umgreifenden Armen über einem Haufen von gleichartigem Kleinspielzeug, keines will etwas abgeben. Läßt man solche kleinen Sozialpartner in Ruhe, beginnt nach einer Phase des Hortens oder auch Versteckens — beides wie bei den Affen stark triebhaft verankert — der Austausch, das Abwägen und „Handeln", etwas, was es erst bei primitiven Völkerstämmen, jedoch bei keinem Tier einschließlich der Pongiden gibt.

Wolfgang Köhler (*110, 482, 483*) hat bei seinen berühmten Studien an Schimpansen die Verwendung von Objekten als *Werkzeug* beschrieben, und Heinrich Klüver (*107*) konnte in subtilen Experimenten neben anderen hochstehenden Leistungen dasselbe auch bei anderen Affen zeigen. Die beliebten Gegenstände — Nahrung, Büchsen, Hölzer, Steine, Lappen — werden vom Schimpansen oft zwischen Bauch und Oberschenkel herumgetragen. Die Tiere drapieren sich gerne und wirken so geschmückt geradezu naiv-selbstgefällig. Man kann beim Schimpansen eine gewisse Differenzierung des Objektbesitzes in Gegenstände mit Werkzeug-, Schmuck- und Spielbedeutung feststellen (*144*).

Wir müssen uns mit diesen wenigen Beispielen begnügen. Sie alle zeigen, daß *die besitzartigen Bindungen sicher biologischen Notwendigkeiten entspringen.* Die Besitzformen des Menschen wären im einzelnen zu vergleichen und zahlreiche ethnologische Beobachtungen (*124, 143, 144, 564*) dazu heranzuziehen. Die menschlichen *Besitzgefühle*, eingeschlossen solche, die sich auf Weib und Kinder, auf Eltern und Freunde beziehen, zeigen die triebhaften Wurzeln an. Der lange Weg der Menschen vom rein physischen Besitzstreben — z. B. dem Erwerb der Ehefrau als einem gekauften Wertobjekt — bis zum Verlangen, auch über die Seele eines geliebten Menschen zu verfügen, ist nur im Rahmen einer stammesgeschichtlich vergleichenden Betrachtung zu verstehen. Der Vergleich der intellektuellen Leistungen von Mensch und Tier zeigt uns die großen Unterschiede, der Vergleich der triebhaften Verhaltensweisen die engen Gemeinsamkeiten auf (*144*). Wie merkwürdig ist es in diesem Zusammenhang, daß Völker mit betont emotionalem Erleben den Tieren in ihrer Religion einen großen Platz einräumen, während diese in anderen Kulturkreisen ein kaum beachtetes Dasein führen.

3. Domestikation

CHARLES DARWIN (*33*) widmete zwei gewichtige Bände dem Studium der Domestikation von Tieren und Pflanzen und gründete einen guten Teil seiner Abstammungslehre auf den Veränderungen, die wildlebende Stammesarten im Laufe der Haustierwerdung durchmachen. Die Domestikation bestimmter Tierarten ist das älteste biologische Experiment, das Menschen machten, und ist wie kein anderes geeignet, der Synthese zwischen Abstammungs- und Erblehre zu dienen (*131, 132*).

Als „domestiziert" bezeichnet man herkömmlicherweise eine Rasse von Tieren, wenn sie sich von der wildlebenden Stammart in einigen typischen, erblichen Merkmalen unterscheidet, die sich im Laufe der Haustierwerdung herausgebildet haben. Bei fast allen Haustieren finden sich Scheckigkeit, Verkürzung der Extremitäten und der Schädelbasis, Verminderung der Straffheit des Bindegewebes mit Ausbildung von Wammen, Hängeohren, Herabsetzung des Muskeltonus, Neigung zum Fettwerden, vor allem aber eine ganz allgemeine und erhebliche Zunahme der Variationsbreite in allen möglichen Artcharakteren (*131, 134*). Die Domestikationserscheinungen sind mit Abnahme des Hirngewichtes verbunden (*75, 701*). An einigen domestizierten Arten kann man zeigen, daß nicht etwa die veränderten Lebensbedingungen (Futter, Licht, Bewegung usw.) für die Artabwandlung verantwortlich gemacht werden können, sondern das *Fortfallen der natürlichen Auslese* (*75*).

Zum Beispiel hat das nordeuropaische Ren, wenn auch nicht in extremer Ausbildung, so doch ziemlich alle typischen Domestikationserscheinungen, obwohl es im ursprünglichen Lebensraum und praktisch in völliger Freiheit lebt, so daß sich seine Lebensbedingungen von denen der Wildform ausschließlich in einem — nicht einmal sehr gründlichen — Schutz vor Wolfen und in einer bestimmten Auswahl der Zuchthirsche unterscheiden; die Lappen kastrieren gerade die starksten Hirsche, um ihre Bösartigkeit zu vermindern (*75*).

LORENZ (*131, 134, 532*) faßt die domestikationsbedingten Veränderungen angeborenen Verhaltens in drei Gruppen zusammen: Erstens unterliegt *die endogene Reizerzeugung* (s. S. 296) mancher Instinktbewegungen erheblichen *quantitativen Veränderungen,* so daß es einerseits zur Hypertrophie, andrerseits zur Atrophie des Instinktverhaltens kommen kann.

Zum Beispiel läßt der Bewegungsantrieb bei fast allen Haustieren in Korrelation zum Schwinden des Muskeltonus und der Neigung zum Fettwerden erheblich nach. Das Tier ist ärmer an entsprechenden Instinktbewegungen; Flucht- aber auch Aggressionstendenzen schwinden, was nicht allein mit der Gewohnung an den Menschen und seine Umgebung erklärt werden kann. Auch die feiner spezialisierten Instinkte, z. B. die Tötungshemmung oder andere soziale Hemmungen atrophieren. Das Brutpflegeverhalten wird undifferenzierter und weniger intensiv, während Freß- und Begattungstrieb erheblich gesteigert sind.

Zweitens geht bei den meisten Haustieren *die spezifische Selektivität der angeborenen Auslösemechanismen* (s. S. 303) *weitgehend verloren* (*131*).

Reaktionen, die bei der Wildform nur auf Reizsituationen voll intensiv ansprechen, die durch eine ganze Reihe von Bestimmungsstücken gekennzeichnet sind, konnen beim Haustier durch viel einfachere und genereller wirkende *Ersatzreize* ausgelöst werden. Auf diese Weise lassen sich z. B. recht verschiedene Haustierrassen — man denke an Hunde — miteinander kreuzen, was bei ähnlich verschiedenen Wildformen nicht möglich wäre.

Drittens können funktionell zusammengehörige Verhaltensweisen völlig unabhängig von einander werden. Kreuzt man Haus- und Wildformen miteinander, kann man diese *Dissoziation funktionell zusammengehöriger Verhaltensweisen* experimentell studieren.

Zum Beispiel entstehen unter den Nachkommen der Kreuzung von Hausgans und Wildgans eigenartige „Mißverständnisse" im Paarungszeremoniell dadurch, daß die Kette aufeinanderfolgender Handlungsglieder zerbricht und die Bruchstücke (Verhaltenselemente) anders in den Verhaltenszusammenhang eingebaut sind als bei der Wildform. Bei der Hausgans dissoziieren die Instinkthandlungen des „Sich-Verliebens" (Paarbildung und monogamer

Zusammenhalt) von denen der Begattung. Oft fallen auch einfach Glieder in der Kette aus oder die Kette bricht vorzeitig ab (*131, 532*). Beispielsweise haben viele Haustiere (u. a. Hunde, Rinder) „verlernt", die Eihüllen unmittelbar nach dem Partus zu zerreißen, so daß das Neugeborene ohne menschliche Hilfe in den Embryonalhüllen ersticken würde (s. S. 337) (*72, 565*).

Schon Whitman (*205*) hat klar gesehen, daß diese domestikationsbedingten Ausfälle durchaus keinen Rückschritt in bezug auf die höheren Leistungen des Lernens und der Intelligenz bedeuten. Diese „Instinktfehler", so sagt er, sind das offene Tor, durch das Erfahrung und Lernen in das starre Aktionssystem eines Tieres eindringen und alle Wunder der Intelligenz bewirken können. Dissoziationen in diesem Sinne sind die ersten Zeichen einer größeren Plastizität innerhalb der angeborenen Koordinationen und führen zu Neubildungen von Handlungskombinationen, die eine Wahlfreiheit des Handelns mit sich bringen. Mit anderen Worten: *Die Freiheitsgrade des Handelns nehmen mit Abnahme instinktiver Koppelungen zu.*

Wir wollen die Beweisführung übergehen, nach der auch der *Mensch ein domestiziertes und ein sich ständig weiter selbst domestizierendes Wesen* ist. In Heberers Handbuch über „die Evolution der Organismen" (*70*) kann man sich über dieses Gebiet im Zusammenhang mit der Abstammungslehre des Menschen informieren. Auch Gehlen (*60*) baut seine Anthropologie wesentlich darauf auf. Nehmen wir also die Selbstdomestikation des Menschen als gesicherte Tatsache hin und sehen zu, wie dieser morphologisch-genetische Vorgang auch die Verhaltensweisen beeinflußt.

Der Mensch verdankt seiner Selbstdomestikation zwei Eigenschaften, die als wichtigste konstitutive Merkmale seines Wesens anzusehen sind, nämlich erstens das Erhaltenbleiben der Neugier — ein Jugendmerkmal, wie schon erwähnt (s. S. 326f.) — für nahezu das ganze Leben und zweitens sein Nicht-spezialisiert-Sein (*131, 134*). Die konstitutive Freiheit des menschlichen Handelns ist die unmittelbare Folge domestikationsbedingter Reduktion des starr instinktiven Verhaltens (*134*).

Bei Betrachtung der ontogenetischen Entwicklung des Menschen können wir den phylogenetischen Prozeß der Instinktverwandlung gleichsam skizzenhaft verfolgen. Ausreichend ausgestattet mit einem relativ starren System angeborener Verhaltensweisen kommt der Säugling zur Welt. Erfahrung und Lernen spielen eine zunehmend größere Rolle, während die Bausteine angeborenen Verhaltens mehr und mehr eingebaut und verdeckt werden, bis sie schließlich nach Erreichung der vollen Freiheitsgrade des Handelns nicht mehr isoliert herausgelöst werden können. Die ursprünglich recht spezifischen Schlüsselreize werden mehr und mehr unspezifisch, die auslösenden Mechanismen zunehmend erweitert, und schließlich ist eine *Fülle von Ersatzreizen an die Stelle der ursprünglichen Auslöser* getreten. Nur in pathologischen Zuständen wird vom ursprünglichen Konstruktionsplan manches wieder sichtbar, und die erfahrungsfreien, angeborenen Verhaltensweisen treten in verändertem Gesamtzusammenhang wieder in Erscheinung. Die experimentellen und klinischen Daten, die zu dieser Auffassung berechtigen, haben wir im Kapitel III dargestellt.

Die Freiheit des Menschen hat Gefahren mit sich gebracht, mit denen sich die Kulturvölker mehr und mehr auseinanderzusetzen haben (*435, 503, 701*). Eine fast ins Unvorstellbare gehende Anpassungsfähigkeit des Menschen an von ihm selbst hervorgerufene Umweltveränderungen geht parallel mit einem nahezu völligen Schwinden der natürlichen Selektion, dem wichtigsten biologischen Regulationsprinzip. Instinktausfälle, denen der Mensch sein Kulturdasein verdankt, stehen dicht neben solchen, die ihn ernsthaft bedrohen. Gehlens Aussage (*60*), daß der Mensch das „riskierte Wesen", das Wesen „mit einer konstitutionellen Chance zu verunglücken" ist, gilt sowohl für die gesamte Species Mensch als auch für die Individuen, deren anlagemäßige Verschiedenheit nicht zuletzt aus der Variationsbreite der Instinktausfälle resultiert.

V. Psychopathologie und Verhaltensforschung

1. Neurosen

Zwar führten uns die ausgewählten Ergebnisse der Verhaltensforschung immer wieder auf menschliches Verhalten und auf die Grenze zu menschlichem pathologischen Verhalten hin, doch wäre nun der Augenblick gekommen, in klare Beziehungssetzungen und Vergleiche zwischen Verhaltensforschung und Psychopathologie einzutreten. Nach reiflicher Überlegung habe ich mich entschlossen, dieser Versuchung nur in einzelnen Punkten nachzugeben, da mir die Zeit für generalisierende Vergleiche verfrüht scheint. Müßte man doch z. B. — um den Stier bei den Hörnern zu packen — in längere theoretisierende Erörterungen über psychoanalytische Triebtheorien eintreten, ehe man im einzelnen präzise Aussagen über neurotische Störungen und deren Beziehungen zur ethologischen Trieblehre machen kann. STIERLIN (*776*) hat einen solchen Vergleich zwischen der Freudschen und der Lorenzschen Trieblehre versucht und sich als Psychiater, was die *allgemeine* Triebtheorie anbelangt, für FREUD entschieden, ohne dabei die Entdeckungen der Ethologie, auch hinsichtlich psychosomatischer Krankheitsbilder (*777*), geringzuachten.

Der Kernpunkt des Vergleichs liegt in FREUDs Libidotheorie, die auf dem „Lustprinzip" aufbaut, und LORENZ' physiologischem Triebmodell von der Aufspeicherung und Entladung endogen erzeugter „aktionsspezifischer Energie" (s. S. 296). FREUD selbst hat sich vorgestellt, daß der Trieb die „psychische Repräsentanz einer kontinuierlich fließenden innersomatischen Reizquelle" ist, und der Hoffnung Ausdruck gegeben, daß seine Triebpsychologie — in seinen eigenen Augen ein bloßer Überbau — eines Tages auf ein organisches Fundament aufgestockt werde (*54*)[1]. Bemerkenswerte Übereinstimmung herrscht in diesem entscheidenden Punkte zwischen FREUD und JASPERS (*93*), der klar ausspricht, daß ohne ein intaktes Funktionieren der „außerbewußten Mechanismen", diesem „Unterbau des Seelischen", sich verständliche Zusammenhänge niemals verwirklichen können.

„Den Begriff des seelischen Mechanismus als einer außerbewußten Bedingung seelischer Erscheinungen und seelischer Wirkungen auf körperliche Funktionen sich klarzumachen, ist für das Begreifen des abnormen Seelenlebens von fundamentaler Wichtigkeit. Diese Mechanismen sich körperlich oder physiologisch genauer vorzustellen, ist bisher unfruchtbar; sie sind ein *rein psychologischer und theoretischer Hilfsbegriff* (vom Verf. kursiv), der uns zur Ordnung von Tatsachen dient (wie z. B. der hysterischen Tatsachen) ..." JASPERS betont mehrfach, daß seine Darstellung der sich *in den verständlichen Zusammenhängen* zeigenden Mechanismen lediglich eine Ordnung der mannigfaltigen Erscheinungen anstrebt, nicht aber „die Enge einer Theorie, die doch immer falsch ist".

Die Feststellung, daß eine Theorie „doch immer falsch ist", würde man für sich genommen als trivial ansehen. Das methodische Denken, das hinter dieser Aussage steht, nämlich *die Trennung kausaler und verständlicher Zusammenhänge*, verdient aber größte Beachtung. Wenn wir z. B. die absonderlichen Appetenzen gravider Frauen zu begreifen suchen, haben wir irgendwie eine kausale Beziehung im Sinn, daß nämlich die Schwangerschaft diese Gelüste bewirkt. Im Sinne der Ethologie (s. S. 306) kann man von zentraler Gestimmtheit, von "appetitive behavior" (s. S. 296) sprechen. Wenn wir aber sagen, daß uns beim Essen der

---

[1] LASHLEYs (*492*) scharfe Kritik der Libidotheorie aus dem Jahre 1924 ist auch heute noch unübertroffen hinsichtlich der Präzisierung des physiologischen Standpunktes.

Appetit vergangen ist, weil wir während der Mahlzeit an eklige Dinge erinnert
worden sind, dann gehen wir primär von Erlebnissen aus, die zunächst nichts
mit dem Mechanismus der zentralen Gestimmtheit zu tun haben. Wir können
den ekelerregenden Erlebnisbereich untersuchen, und es werden sich Erlebniszusammenhänge ergeben, die uns einen hinreichenden Grund liefern, uns das
Vergehen des Appetits als Folge verständlich zu machen. Wird uns durch
die Ekelerinnerung beim Essen bis zum Erbrechen übel, schiebt sich der
Kausalmechanismus in den Vordergrund: Wir haben uns *so* geekelt, *daß* wir
erbrechen mußten. Der Ekel verursachte eine zentrale Umstimmung mit dem
Effekt einer vegetativen Notfallsreaktion, dem Erbrechen. In allen drei Fällen,
dem Gelüste der Schwangeren, dem Ekel und dem Erbrechen, sind beide Fragen,
nämlich die nach dem „Mechanismus" wie die nach dem verständlichen Zusammenhang möglich, aber verschieden relevant und methodisch streng zu trennen. Die
Ethologen untersuchen kausale Mechanismen des Triebverhaltens und möchten
damit einen Beitrag zum Verstehen von Erlebnissen liefern, die Psychoanalytiker
untersuchen Erlebniszusammenhänge und möchten zu den Kausalmechanismen
menschlichen Trieblebens vorstoßen. „Kausalforscher" und „Erlebensforscher"
sollten sich aber stets bewußt bleiben, daß ihre Folgerungen vom Mechanismus
auf das Erleben oder umgekehrt vom Erleben auf den Mechanismus indirekt und
darum nicht für generalisierende Theoriebildungen geeignet sind (*654*).

LORENZ, der selbst auf die Beziehungen der Verhaltensphysiologie zur Psychoanalyse hinweist (*132*), ist hinsichtlich der Einzelheiten menschlichen Verhaltens,
die schon heute einen Vergleich erlauben, zurückhaltender als viele Tiefenpsycho-
logen, die vom „Übersprungharnen" beim Bettnässen, von „Übersprungonanie"
oder „Übersprungerbrechen" sprechen [vgl. (*654*)], so als sei damit der Vorgang erklärt. STIERLIN (*776*) warnt mit Recht vor einem unberechtigten Homo-
logisieren im Bereich neurotischer Phänomene. „Das feine psychologische Stell-
werk, das beim Menschen die ungewöhnlich komplizierten Verwandlungen und
Verschiebungen seiner Libido ermöglicht, wird uns nur wenig einsichtiger, wenn
wir seine Wurzel etwa in Übersprungbewegungen suchen." Denn bedenken wir,
jedem menschlichen Trieb wohnt ein Bedürfnis inne, und wohl nahezu jedes
menschliche Bedürfnis erwächst aus ursprünglich Triebhaftem. Dies berechtigt
uns aber nicht dazu, die menschlichen Bedürfnisse mit den Trieben und Bedürfnisspannungen mit Triebspannungen ohne weiteres gleichzusetzen. Im Gegensatz zu
allen Tieren ist das menschliche Verhalten stets durch Einsicht in die Zwecke des
Handelns mitbestimmt (*655*). Schon „im 2. Lebensjahr ist das Menschenkind so
weit, daß es nicht nur über eine Fülle von bedingten Reflexen, von Dressaten und
Gewöhnungen verfügt, sondern daß es auch schon einfache freie Entscheidungen
trifft, die durch erwägende, also das Ziel und die Wirkung der Handlung vor-
stellende Überlegungen geleitet sind", sagt VILLINGER (*790*).

Bereits zu diesem Zeitpunkt menschlicher Entwicklung sind also erworbene
und, wie wir früher gesehen haben (s. S. 319ff.), angeborene Verhaltensweisen aufs
engste miteinander verschmolzen, und gar beim Erwachsenen gibt es kaum eine
Situation, in der nicht ein Bündel von Erfahrungen, einst erlebten Bedeutungs-
gehalten oder auch automatisierten erworbenen Reaktionen enthalten ist, so
daß die Fundamentbausteine angeborenen Verhaltens normalerweise nicht heraus-
zulösen sind. Bekanntlich sind in Kinderneurosen sowohl die äußeren Bedingungen,
die zur Neurose führen, als auch die „Mechanismen", die zur Abwehr und Bewälti-
gung dienen, leichter durchschaubar als beim Erwachsenen. Wie schwer ist es aber
schon in diesem frühen Alter, Instinktverhalten von Dressurverhalten zu trennen.
Aus diesen und anderen Gründen (*654, 655*) haben wir Bedenken, die Neurosen
zum Angelpunkt des Vergleichs zwischen Ethologie und Psychopathologie zu

machen (*656*). Daß man auch auf dem Neurosengebiet intuitiv viele Einzelvergleiche durchführen und in eine biologisch gedachte Anthropologie aufnehmen kann, ohne mit dem Anspruch einer alles erklärenden Triebtheorie aufzutreten, hat Bilz gezeigt (*260, 264, 265, 266*). Ihm verdanken wir zahlreiche Einzelbeobachtungen, auf die es unseres Erachtens im Augenblick noch vor allem ankommt. Kretschmer (*112*) hat in der letzten Auflage seines bekannten Hysterie-Buches die Ergebnisse der Verhaltensforschung zwar nicht berücksichtigt, aber seine Beobachtungen an Hysterikern im ersten Weltkrieg tragen doch ebenso wie R. Bruns (*21, 22*) Neurosenlehre, E. Bleulers (*17*) und v. Monakows (*150*) Psychopathologie Wesentliches zu einer vergleichenden menschlichen Trieblehre bei.

2. Psychosen

Merkwürdigerweise gibt es bisher nur wenige ethologisch orientierte Untersuchungen, die sich mit *psychotischem Verhalten* beschäftigen, obwohl unseres Erachtens gerade hier der methodisch günstigste Ansatz liegt. Besonders in der akuten Psychose tritt das spezifisch Menschliche, nämlich die Einsichtsmöglichkeit in Zweck und Ziel alles Handelns, weitgehend in den Hintergrund. Seelenkräfte werden in einer sonst nie vorhandenen Einfachheit offenbar, die ungebrochen durch Erfahrung und Urteil, ungeleitet von Einsicht und geistigen Maximen in Erscheinung treten. In solchen Zuständen primitivierter seelischer Struktur bietet sich unseres Erachtens die beste Gelegenheit, präformiertes, angeborenes Verhalten in ähnlicher Weise zu studieren wie motorische Schablonen (*487*) während hirnorganischer Störungen (s. S. 315 ff.).

a) Stereotype Bewegungen

Beginnen wir wie im III. und IV. Kapitel wieder mit der Motorik, speziell mit den *motorischen Stereotypien der Katatonen*. Diese dem Beobachter unmotiviert und unverständlich erscheinenden Bewegungsstörungen wurden von den „Somatikern" unter den Psychiatern auf einen nicht faßbaren hirnorganischen Prozeß zurückgeführt, während die „Psychiker" (*243, 814*) denselben Vorgang für ein psychopathologisch ableitbares, verstehend zu interpretierendes seelisches Geschehen halten [vgl. (*652*)].

Bei Beobachtung der Kranken sehen wir bestimmte Bewegungen, die ganz überwiegend mit Tätigkeitsworten beschrieben werden können, wie z. B. streichen, wischen, schütteln, schlenkern, bohren, fingern, nesteln, kauen, kratzen, reiben, wälzen, greifen; zu einem geringeren Teil sind es mimische Bewegungen mit Ausdruckscharakter und solche, die Gesten oder ritualisierte Bewegungen (s. S. 330 ff.) kennzeichnen, wie z. B. nicken, winken, zeigen, drohen oder sich bekreuzigen. In vielen Stereotypien vereinigen sich mehrere dieser Bewegungsweisen zu einem einfachen Ablauf mit geringen Modifikationen oder sie wechseln miteinander ab wie bei dem Kranken auf Abb. 15, der entweder nestelte oder kaute. Eine andere Patientin neigte ihren Körper rhythmisch nach vorne und hinten oder sie wechselte diese Bewegung mit einer Kratzbewegung gleicher Frequenz ab, wobei sie im Takt Satzbruchstücke bis zu 10 min Dauer verbigerierte (*649*). Meist bleiben Frequenz und Amplitude oder auch der Rhythmus solcher Bewegungen recht einförmig.

Diese uniformierten Bewegungsweisen haben häufig den Charakter von *Grundbewegungen*, wie wir sie auch beim Kleinkind beobachten können, wenn es etwa ausdauernd reibt, wischt, schüttelt oder fingert. Die Bewegungen sind verglichen mit z. B. dem primitiven Greifen (s. S. 311 ff.) komplexer und nicht mehr so schablonenhaft. Sie sind wie kleine einfache Melodien, die sich gern wiederholen. Diese elementaren Weisen des Bewegens haben beim Kinde Funktionswert, und zwar sowohl eine explorierende Funktion wie etwa der in verschiedensten Situationen angewandte Schnabelhieb des jungen Kolkraben (s. S. 327) als auch eine „Ausprobier"- und Übungsfunktion, wie wir sie z. B. im Spiel der Säugetiere (s. S. 343f.) beobachten können. Wie eng in diesem Zusammenhang Ausdruck und Bewegung, ja, auch emotionales Verhalten miteinander verknüpft sind, haben wir beschrieben (s. S. 330ff.).

Welchen Funktionswert haben aber nun die motorischen Stereotypien der Katatonen? Wir wollen das an zwei Beispielen zeigen:

1. W. B., 1888 geboren, erstmals 1944 aufgenommen. Der Patient hat ein unstetes Leben mit haufigem Berufswechsel gefuhrt. Im ersten Weltkrieg wurde er wegen verschiedentlich aufgetretener Erregungszustande militärisch bestraft und kam wegen Hysterie in nervenarztliche Lazarettbehandlung. 1933 wurde er wegen eines religiosen Wahns, in dem er sich von einem Christusbild in einer Kirche beeinflußt fühlte und Erregungszustande bekam, in eine Heilanstalt gebracht. Wegen impulsiver Akte war er zeitweise gemeingefährlich. — In der Klinik zeigte er 1944 über lange Zeit folgende motorische Stereotypien: Liegend, in selig-euphorischer Stimmung, ansprechbar, aber nicht zu fixieren, hob er abwechselnd die Beine, die Arme oder je ein Bein und einen Arm im Wechsel. Das Heben und Senken einer Extremitat wurde mit immer den gleichen Worten: Heil (rechtes Bein hoch, linkes Bein runter) — Hitler (linkes Bein hoch, rechtes Bein runter) usw. begleitet. Zu anderen Zeiten wurden die Worte bei gleichen Bewegungen durch das Singen eines Vierklanges ersetzt, also z. B.: Do (rechtes Bein hoch, linkes Bein runter), Mi (linkes Bein, rechtes Bein), So (rechter Arm, linker Arm), Do (linkes Bein, rechtes Bein). Nach einer Pause wurde der Vierklang gelegentlich bei gleichen Bewegungen von oben nach unten gesungen. Mitunter kamen Bewegungen des Kopfes nach links und rechts im Takt dazu. Diese Verhaltensweisen wurden bis zu 15 min durchgehalten. — Ohne Übergang konnte der Pat. ohne erkennbaren Anlaß plötzlich Kontakt zu einem anderen Kranken aufnehmen, indem er z. B. seinen Nachbarn mit den Worten ansprach: „Sag mal Deutschland!" (Keine Antwort von seiten des stuporosen Mitpatienten.) „Sag Deutschland, sonst mußt du sterben!" (in humoristischem Tonfall). Nach weiteren, vergeblichen Bemühungen: „Sag nur einmal D., sonst kriegst Du nichts zu fressen!" (Schweigen). Der Pat. laßt nun ab, wendet sich einem Pfleger zu, bemerkt: „Der Satan sagt partout nicht Deutschland, der kriegt nichts zu fressen, da muß er sterben", legt sich aufs neue hin und beginnt unablenkbar mit den oben beschriebenen Stereotypien. Am anderen Tage versucht er auf die gleiche (ebenfalls stereotype Weise) mit dem gleichen Nachbarn zum Ziel zu kommen; ohne Erfolg. — Im Laufe der Elektroschockbehandlung verschwinden die motorischen Stereotypien, es kommt eine Reihe anderer psychotischer Symptome heraus (Reden mit abnormem Bedeutungsgehalt: „Ich bin das liebe, gute Hitlerchen und Gottes lieber Sohn …" o. a., Beeinflussung durch elektrische Strome usw.). Drei Monate nach der Entlassung wurde der Pat. nachuntersucht: Antriebsmangel, einige Klagen über körperliche Beschwerden, keine psychotischen Erlebnisinhalte oder Verhaltensweisen. — 1953 kommt der Pat. wiederum zur Aufnahme. Diesmal zeigte er — neben vielen anderen Verhaltensweisen im Verlaufe der Psychose — während längerer Zeit eine *Bartstreich-Stereotypie*: Abwechselnd mit dem linken und rechten Fingerrucken streicht er sich in ziemlich schnellem Rhythmus die linke bzw. rechte Wangenseite. Dabei wendet er den Kopf in unbestimmten Abständen hin und her. Diese Bewegungen sind unbeeinflußbar und ohne Bezug zur jeweiligen Situation. Der Pat. läßt sich, ohne sich daran zu kehren, auch filmen (*653*).

Diesem 1. Fall mit einer noch relativ großen Variabilität seiner Verhaltensweisen stellen wir nun einen 2. Fall gegenüber, bei dem das Verhalten starrer, „festgestellter" und in höherem Maße automatenhaft ist als bei dem ersten Patienten:

2. H. St., 1913 geboren (s. Abb. 15). Der Pat. war ein sehr guter Volksschüler. Mit 23 Jahren begann die ebenfalls schizophrene Erkrankung. St. bekam Angst, er versteckte sich aus Furcht, abgeholt zu werden, und hielt sich die Ohren zu. Nach etwa einem Jahr sprach er gelegentlich nur noch zu sich selbst und verstandigte sich im übrigen durch Gesten. Zur Arbeit war er ab 1937 nicht mehr zu bringen; er wurde sterilisiert, aber *nie behandelt*. Im ganzen wird er als gutmütig-stumpf geschildert, verübte aber gelegentlich ebenfalls impulsive Akte. — Nach der Aufnahme (August 1955) in die Klinik kommt er einfachen Aufforderungen (z. B. aufstehen, gehen, stehenbleiben) nach, kann aber fortlaufende Handlungen (z. B. An- und Ausziehen) nicht zu Ende führen. Er fällt alsbald in seine statuenhafte Haltung zurück, in der nun fast unentwegt — außer im Schlaf — folgende *motorische Stereotypien* ablaufen: Entweder macht der Kranke

bei sonst unbewegtem Gesichtsausdruck und nahezu vollständiger Regungslosigkeit des ganzen Körpers *Kaubewegungen* oder aber er *nestelt* mit den Fingern abwechselnd an seinen drei Jackenknopfen. Seltene abrupte sprachliche Äußerungen sind unverständlich und gleichen einem bellenden Schimpfen. Gemütsbewegungen sind weder dabei noch sonst irgendwann festzustellen.

In einem Film haben wir festgehalten, daß man diesen Kranken nach vielen Mühen über einen aufgezwungenen Rhythmus vorübergehend zum *Mitagieren* und zu *motorischer Anpassung* bringen kann, also beispielsweise beim Marschieren zu zweit im Gleichschritt (der nur kurze Zeit vom Pat. eingehalten wird), beim gegenseitigen In-die-Hand-Schlagen, wobei er sich an eine langsamere oder schnellere Schlagfolge anzupassen, oder beim Sägen, bei dem er in variiertem Tempo gegenzuziehen hat. *Während einer solchen vorgegebenen Handlungsfolge horen die stereotypen Bewegungen auf.* Sobald der Kranke aber wieder in seine Statuen-Haltung zurückfällt, beginnen die motorischen Stereotypien erneut mit immer der gleichen Frequenz. Gewohnlich wendet der Patient sich nicht mit Kopf oder Blick zu irgendeinem Partner. Wenn man seinem Munde jedoch den Finger oder Füllhalter nahert, wendet er Kopf, Mund und Augen diesem sich nähernden Objekt zu, macht einige Schnappbewegungen oder stülpt die Lippen rüsselartig mit gelegentlich einigen Saugbewegungen vor. Zu anderen Malen wird das Objekt nach dem Vorstülpen der Lippen fortgepustet, oder die Lippen werden fest aufeinander gepreßt. Auch ohne optische Kontrolle nur bei Berührung des Mundes oder seiner nachsten Umgebung sind die oralen motorischen Schablonen auslosbar und mit unbedeutenden Variationen in gewissen Zeitabständen wiederholbar (s. Abb. 15). (Neurologisch o. B. Im Luftencephalogramm Ventrikelsystem nicht gefüllt. Soweit zu beurteilen keine grobere Hirnrindenatrophie.) *(653)*.

Fassen wir das Kennzeichnende der beiden Fälle zusammen: Im ersten Falle kommt den Verhaltensweisen eine relativ große Variabilität zu. Doch fehlt dem Verhalten der Bezug zur jeweiligen Situation. Auch das *Ziel des Handelns ist weitgehend verlorengegangen.* Könnte man im Falle der Kontaktnahme mit dem Mitpatienten noch von einem Ziel sprechen — nämlich den Nachbarn zu etwas zu bringen —, so zeigt doch die Stereotypie dieser wie nach einem Schema wiederholten Versuche, daß es sich um eine *starre* Zielsetzung handelt. — Die Möglichkeit des Subjektes, dasselbe Ziel auf verschiedene Weise des Handelns zu erreichen, ist verlorengegangen. Immerhin scheint bei der „Bein-Arm"-Stereotypie das

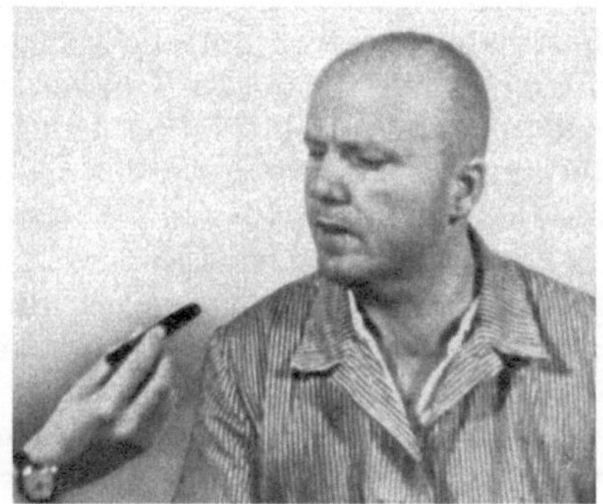

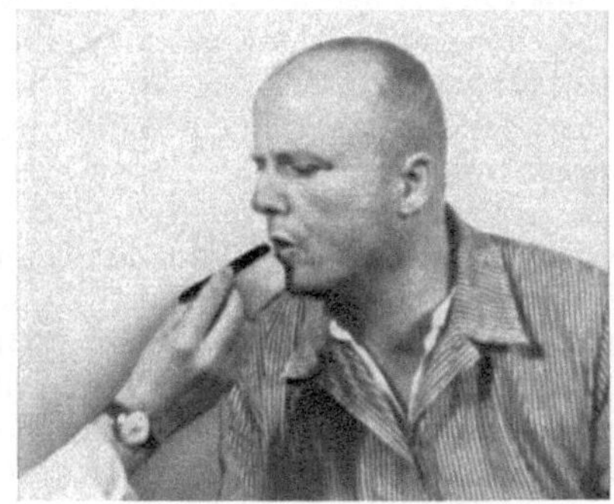

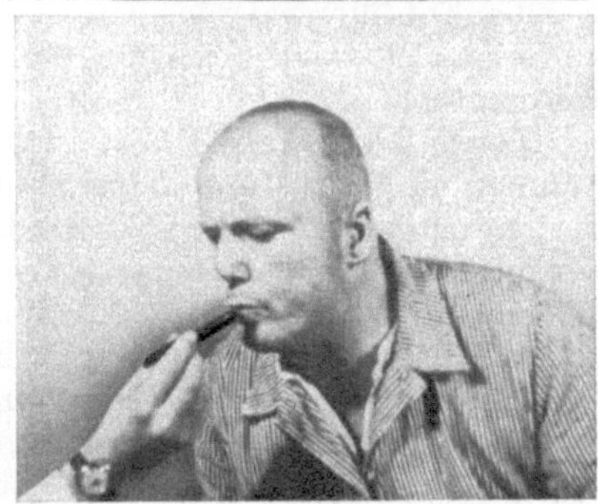

Abb. 15a—c. *Optisch orientiertes orales Greifen* bei einem Defektschizophrenen mit motorischen Stereotypien. (Filmaufnahmen des Verfassers aus der Universitats-Nervenklinik Marburg)

Handeln noch in — zwar unverständlicher — Beziehung zum Erleben des Kranken zu stehen. Bereits die Bartstreich-Stereotypie bedeutet aber eine weitgehende *Festlegung des Verhaltens.* Dies wird vor allem im zweiten Fall deutlich. Die Verhaltensweisen bekommen den Charakter des Automatenhaften, der nahezu unbedingten Zwangsläufigkeit, die man nur durch das Einbeziehen der kranken Persönlichkeit in eine vorgegebene Handlungsfolge vorübergehend durchbrechen kann. Dieses stereotype Verhalten hat den Charakter des freien Handelns verloren, wirkt völlig determiniert, läßt keine Beziehungen zum Erleben des Subjektes mehr erkennen, und die einförmig ablaufenden Grundbewegungsweisen (z. B. kauen, nesteln) erscheinen als Relikt der ehemaligen Bewegungsmannigfaltigkeit. Die Determinierung wird wohl am deutlichsten bei Auslösung der oralen Automatismen.

Es gibt noch eine weitere, von diesen zwei Mustern abweichende Situation, in der motorische Stereotypien auftreten, nämlich auf einen bestimmten Anlaß hin. Meist handelt es sich um solche Situationen, die auch im täglichen Leben der Gesunden einen „Komment" haben, wie z. B. die Essensmanieren oder das Begrüßungszeremoniell. Während aber normalerweise solche Zeremonien weitgehend abwandlungsfähig sind, werden sie durch die Stereotypie fast gänzlich festgelegt. Andere Kranke entwickeln die Stereotypie nur dann, wenn sich aus dem Einerlei des Tages ein besonderes Ereignis heraushebt, wie z. B. bei der Arztvisite oder bei einem ungewohnten Angesprochenwerden. Solch einem auslösenden „Reiz" folgt dann die stereotype Reaktion als einzig verbliebene Antwortmöglichkeit auf eine Anpassung erfordernde Situation.

Für die motorischen Stereotypien zusammengenommen kann man im Vergleich zu normalen Handlungs- und Bewegungsweisen eine *Rangordnung nach ihrem Grade von Freiheit und Zwangsläufigkeit* aufstellen. Danach käme den Handlungen und Bewegungen des Gesunden eine optimale Freiheit zu, die nur in besonderen, beispielsweise affektbesetzten Situationen eingeschränkt wäre. In den unteren Abschnitten eines solchen Ordnungssystems stehen die katatonen Verhaltensweisen mit nur noch geringen Freiheitsgraden und unter ihnen schließlich die Stereotypien mit nahezu gänzlicher Zwangsläufigkeit weniger Grundbewegungsweisen, die dissoziiert von der Gesamt-Bewegungsmöglichkeit ablaufen. Solche Bewegungen haben kein adaptives, sondern ein konstantes Verhältnis zur Umwelt und antizipieren kein Ziel mehr (652).

Vergleichen wir diese Kriterien mit den motorischen Schablonen im cerebralorganischen Abbau (s. S. 315), ergibt sich eine prinzipielle Übereinstimmung. Auch dort auf dieser gleichsam unteren, reflexartigen Ebene kommt es zu einer zunehmenden Entdifferenzierung der Schlüsselreize, zu einer schablonenhaften Reaktion auf eine sich wandelnde Umwelt und zu einem Hervortreten des „motorischen Kernbestandes".

Dieser Kern enthält die erfahrungsfreien, angeborenen Verhaltensweisen, während die durch Gewöhnung erworbenen, bedingten oder sekundär automatisierten sensomotorischen Vollzüge der Dissolution anheimfallen. Ob man nun die von uns als *Grundbewegungsweisen* charakterisierten Bewegungen auf der gleichsam höheren Ebene der motorischen Stereotypien auch als schlechthin erfahrungsfrei und angeboren betrachten kann, wollen wir nicht entscheiden, weil die zu diesem Vergleich notwendigen Untersuchungen noch fehlen. Viele dieser einfachen Bewegungsmelodien, wie z. B. kratzen, wischen, reiben, bohren mit dem Finger, kommen jedenfalls sowohl bei Klein-Kindern als auch bei den Primaten regelmäßig vor (s. S. 341). So stellen sie mindestens etwas sehr Ursprüngliches im Aufbau der Motorik dar. Gerade, daß viele dieser Bewegungen Ausdruckscharakter haben und auch mit Vorliebe in ritualisierten Situationen auftreten, spricht für deren ursprüngliche Primitiv-Koordination (s. S. 330 ff.).

Für den Abbau der Bewegungsweisen und das *Hervortreten von Primitiv-Koordinationen* führen wir weitere Gründe an. Unser zweiter Fall H. St. zeigt klar die enge funktionale Verbindung von Hand und Mund. Stereotypes Nesteln an der Kleidung wechselt mit Kauen ab. Gerade zu einer Zeit, wo das Klein-Kind seine Grundbewegungen entwickelt, steht der Mund als „Tätigkeitsorgan" noch gleichberechtigt neben der Hand und exploriert wie diese die Umwelt. Diese

Primitiv-Koordination ist auch beim Patienten vorhanden, wie die Abb. 15 zeigt. Das dargestellte orale Verhalten kann man von den oralen motorischen Schablonen im cerebralorganischen Abbau nicht unterscheiden (*233, 234*) (vgl. Abb. 6, S. 315). Orales Greifen ohne visuelle Orientierung zeigt Abb. 16 bei einem anderen Defektschizophrenen. Gewiß finden wir unter den motorischen Stereotypien nur selten eine so tiefgreifende lokale Dissolution (s. S. 318), daß nachweisbar angeborene Verhaltensweisen, wie die oralen Mechanismen, herauskommen. Von den Grundbewegungsweisen vermuten wir, daß sie ebenfalls angeboren sind. Für die Abstufung der motorischen Stereotypien von komplexen Bewegungsweisen über Grundbewegungen bis zu Schablonen-Bewegungen kann man in Übereinstimmung mit JACKSON die Regel aufstellen: *Je stärker die Dissolution der Verhaltensweisen, desto automatischer wird das Geschehen.* Oder anders ausgedrückt: *Je geringer die Freiheitsgrade des Handelns, desto einfacher ist es determiniert.*

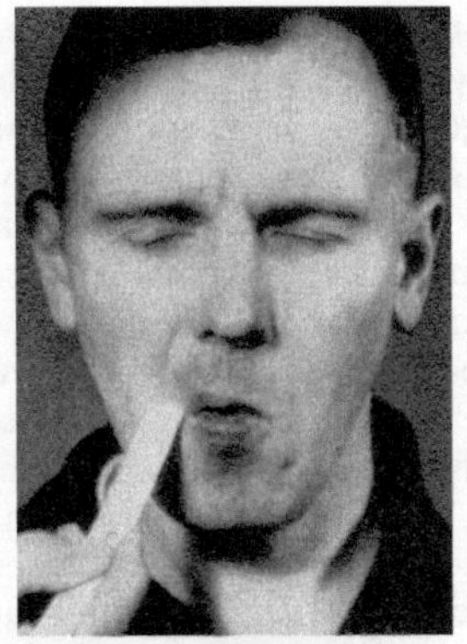

LORENZ (*132*) z. B. hält die Handbewegung, die man macht, um ein lästiges Insekt abzuschütteln, für angeboren, eine Bewegung, die wir ebenfalls als Stereotypie gesehen haben. HOLZAPFEL (*419*) führt für die Entstehung von Bewegungsstereotypien bei gehaltenen Säugern und Vögeln drei Ursachen auf: 1. Die Tendenz zur Gewohnheitsbildung, etwas, was nach allen Erfahrungen auch bei den motorischen Stereotypien der Schizophrenen eine wichtige Rolle spielt. 2. Ein Affekt. 3. Eine Stauung dieses Affektes durch Behinderung der normalen Affektentladung. Wir haben kürzlich eine solche Stereotypie bei einem Affen während der Einübung einer bedingten Reaktion regelmäßig herbeiführen können. Nur in dieser Situation wiegte das Tier seinen Körper im Sitzen hin und her. Sobald die Angst erzeugende Versuchssituation vorüber war, verschwand die Stereotypie. Die normale Entladung wäre die Flucht gewesen; diese war aber behindert. Auch bei den motorischen Stereotypien der Schizophrenen dürfen wir Erregungen (im Verhalten z. B. erkenntlich an Impulsivhandlungen, s. Fall 2) annehmen, die sich aus uns unbekannten Gründen nicht normal entladen können. Doch bietet es unseres Erachtens keine Erklärung der Stereotypie, wenn man deren symbolischen Gehalt aufdecken kann (*814*). Jede Handlung, die noch genügend bewußt ist oder doch bewußt gemacht werden kann, kann vom Subjekt als inhaltlich bestimmt erlebt werden, ohne daß aber dieses Erlebnis eine hinreichende Erklärung für Art und Verlauf der Handlung abgibt. Ein gutes Beispiel dafür bietet die epileptische Dämmerattacke, nach deren Abklingen viele Patienten über ihre gerade abgelaufenen Erlebnisse berichten können. Niemand

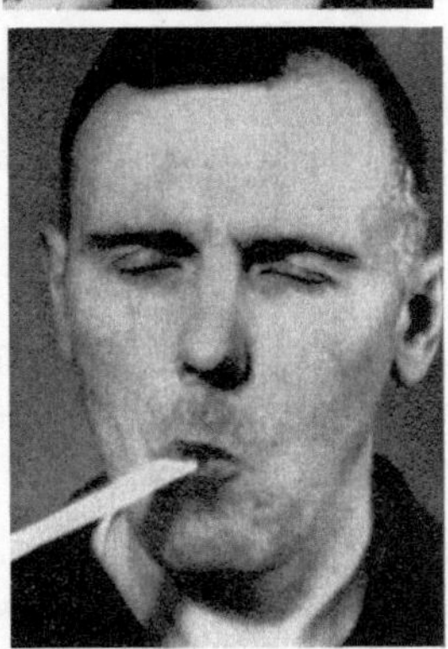

Abb. 16a u. b. *Taktiles orales Greifen* bei einem Defektschizophrenen mit mimischer Desintegration. (Filmaufnahmen des Verfassers aus der Universitäts-Nervenklinik Marburg)

wird aber auf den Gedanken kommen, diese Erlebnisse für die Ursache der Attacke zu halten. Wir stoßen auch hier wieder auf die methodische Trennung von Verstehen und Erklären.

In *epileptischen Dämmerattacken* sehen wir gelegentlich Grundbewegungsweisen, die in diesem Zusammenhang als *Automatismen* bezeichnet werden. Wohl alle automatischen Bewegungen, die in solchen Attacken vorkommen, kann man auch als motorische Stereotypien bei Schizophrenen beobachten. Selbst recht komplexe Bewegungsweisen, wie das abwechselnde Beinanziehen (s. Fall 1), sind beschrieben worden (*575*). Die Ursache für die Dämmerattacke kennen wir, für die motorischen Stereotypien kennen wir sie nicht; doch liegt es nahe, aus der klinischen Übereinstimmung der Bewegungsphänomene auch für die Stereotypien einen hirnphysiologisch begründbaren Mechanismus anzunehmen (vgl. S. 416 ff.). Natürlich ist damit nichts über die spezielle, neurophysiologische Vergleichbarkeit beider Mechanismen ausgesagt (*652*).

23*

b) Ausdrucksverhalten

Im III. und IV. Kapitel (S. 319; 330) war bereits vom Ausdruck die Rede. Wir legten z. B. dar, daß das Lächeln eine angeborene Ausdrucksbewegung ist und daß Ausdrucksbewegungen schlechthin als Verständigungsmittel fungieren, die zur Steuerung des sozialen Zusammenlebens beitragen. Der Ausdruck des „Spielers" löst Antwortverhalten des „Gegenspielers" aus. Im Ausdrucksverhalten ist die Gestimmtheit erkennbar, und gleichzeitig wird Stimmungsübertragung möglich.

Der Ausdruck in endogenen Psychosen ist seit altersher (73) Gegenstand des Interesses gewesen, und es mangelt weder an Theorien über das Wesen der Psychosen noch an diagnostischen Einteilungen, die auf dem Ausdrucksverhalten aufgebaut sind. Die Verhaltensforschung gibt uns Material genug, um auch auf diesem Gebiet neue Ansätze zu versuchen.

Heimann und Spoerri (395, 396, 769) haben sich in den letzten Jahren systematischer mit der Analyse des Ausdrucks von Schizophrenen, vergleichweise auch mit dem von Debilen, Hysterischen und neurologischen Kranken beschäftigt und bei den Schizophrenen verschiedene Ausdruckssyndrome aufgestellt. Nach ihren Filmuntersuchungen unterscheiden sie die Syndrome des „Maskenhaft-Natürlichen", des „Versunken-Bedrängten" (769), des „Magisch-Verwirrten", des „Ekstatisch-Obszönen" und das der „mimischen Desintegrierung" (396). Das Verkoppeltsein von Ausdruckssyndrom und Gestimmtheit kommt besonders gut in folgender Beschreibung des „Versunken-Bedrängten" zum Ausdruck:

„Den Pfleger abwehrend, geht der Pat. unruhig und getrieben, nachtwandlerisch tappend und gespannt zugleich auf und ab. Der rasch hin und her irrende *Blick wirkt wie das angstvolle Auge eines gestellten Tieres* (von mir kursiv); aufgewühlt und staunig kommt der Blick von irgendwoher und stößt erschreckt an den Beobachter an. Fur kurze Zeit verschwindet dann der Eindruck des äußeren und inneren Bedrängtseins; der Blick wird passiv und doch sprechend, die Spannung weicht, und der Pat. wirkt abwesend versunken. Wahrend der Körper sich langsam hin und her wiegt, zucken die Augen in rascherem Tempo; der Pat. verharrt in rhythmischem Schaukeln" (769).

Wir sehen aus dieser Beschreibung, wie das Bedrängtsein in ein Versunkensein hinübergleitet. Die Doppelworte in den einzelnen Syndromen meinen offensichtlich nicht nur Pole eines Ausdruckssyndroms, sondern auch Stimmungen, die sich von einem Pol zum anderen verschieben können. Unwillkürlich fließt den Autoren bei Beschreibung des angstvollen Blickes der Vergleich mit einem bedrängten Tier in die Feder, womit irgendwie das Bare dieses Ausdruckes, das schlechthin Typische beschrieben werden soll. Nicht der normal bedrängte Mensch symbolisiert das Bedrängtsein, sondern der Ausdruck des Tieres. Zweifellos zielen die Ausdruckssyndrome auf spezifisch menschliche Daseinskategorien ab, und es mag deswegen auch berechtigt sein, daß die Verfasser eine philosophisch-anthropologische Deutung im Sinne Buytendijks (395, 652) und Plessners vorziehen — eine Richtung der Verhaltensforschung, die wir auf Grund der biologischen Orientierung dieses Beitrages unberücksichtigt lassen —, doch drängt sich die Beziehung zu ethologischen Ergebnissen geradezu auf. Für Triebkonflikte, die sich im Ausdruck verraten, wählt z. B. Klaesi (104), von dem die Verfasser angeregt wurden (395), das treffende Wort „Ausdruckshader". An anderer Stelle bezeichnet er alle Erscheinungen als Ausdrucksphänomene, die letzte, *anlagebedingte Antriebe des Menschen* verdeutlichen. Die Stimmungsüberlagerung haben wir schon beim Lächeln besprochen (s. Abb. 8, S. 320), und sie kommt auch besonders schön in den Ausdrucksstudien an Wölfen (721) und Katzen (127) heraus (vgl. S. 330 ff.).

Ähnlich wie wir bei den motorischen Stereotypien (652, 653), beschreiben Heimann und Spoerri ein Desintegrationssyndrom im Ausdruck chronisch Schizophrener (vgl. Abb. 16). Das sind „isolierte Bewegungen relativ eng umschriebener einzelner Gesichtsteile; das Heraustreten dieser Bewegungen aus einem mimischen

Gesamtablauf; der fehlende Ausdruckswert der für sich allein genommenen Einzelbewegungen . . ." (*396*). Solche „Paramimien" vermitteln dem Beobachter, ähnlich wie die Stereotypien, den Eindruck des Automatenhaften. Die Ausdrucksbewegungen sind nicht unterdrückbar, nicht voluntativ gesteuert und wirken „sinnlos". Aber — und das ist bedeutsam — sie können plötzlich verschwinden, wenn der volle emotionale Kontakt zum Partner sich vorübergehend herstellt. Das bestätigen auch HEIMANN und SPOERRI, wenn sie schreiben, „für Augenblicke eint ein warmes Lächeln die Mimik". Mit dem Zerfallen oder „Anderssein" der Ausdrucksbewegungen zerbricht der soziale Kontakt! Die Steuerung des sozialen Zusammenlebens, der wichtigsten Funktion von Ausdrucksbewegungen, hört auf, und der Kranke fällt in sich — *partnerlos* — zurück. Damit ist knapp das Wesen der schizophrenen Erkrankung (unseres Erachtens *eine* Erkrankung mit den verschiedenartigsten Symptomverbindungen) gekennzeichnet. Das veränderte Ausdrucksverhalten ist es denn auch vornehmlich, an dem wir den Defektkranken intuitiv erkennen. Und wenn in der Psychiatrie von verschiedenen Seiten zu verschiedenen Zeiten und mit verschiedenen Ausdrücken (*17, 213, 214*) immer wieder das Zerbrechen oder Anderssein der „zwischenmenschlichen Beziehungen" als besonders charakteristisches, *einigendes* Symptom hervorgehoben wurde, so erweist sich an Bewegung und Ausdruck, daß es sich um eine ganz *elementare Störung* handelt, die *in das Fundament unserer angeborenen menschlichen Ausstattung* hineingreift. Wieso gerade Bewegung und Ausdrucksverhalten biologisch fundamental sind, zeigt uns die vergleichende Verhaltensforschung mit ihren Untersuchungen über den Aufbau des Verhaltens (*7*) (vgl. Kapitel II).

c) Gemeinschaftsleben

An einer ethologisch orientierten psychiatrischen Studie wollen wir zeigen, wie sich die „zwischenmenschlichen Beziehungen" unter Geisteskranken gestalten. Es ist merkwürdig, daß die schönen Beobachtungen, die BALTHASAR STAEHELIN (*770, 771*) an einer Gruppe schwer und zumeist chronisch Geisteskranker während anderthalb Jahren auf einer geschlossenen Abteilung gemacht hat, nicht schon früher beschrieben worden sind, da vermutlich jeder, der längere Zeit mit solchen Kranken enger zusammengelebt hat, Ähnliches kennt. Die Beziehungen zur vergleichenden Verhaltensforschung drängen sich geradezu auf.

Bei STAEHELIN dominierte in der Gruppe von etwa 50 Patientinnen eine mutistisch Katatone so, daß sie die Funktion einer Alpha-Person hatte. Dies zeigte sich auf folgende Weise:

Die Pat., Frau S. A., hält streng darauf, daß der seit Jahren von ihr besetzte Eß- und Sitzplatz in Tagesraum und Garten von keiner anderen Person eingenommen wird. Wer diesen *Platzanspruch* nicht respektiert oder sich diesem „*Territorium*" auch nur auf weniger als 20 cm zu nähern wagt, setzt sich brutalen Aggressionen aus. Die Stärke der Aggression, die eindeutig durch die Verteidigung oder Zurückeroberung des beanspruchten „Territoriums" (vgl. S. 344) motiviert ist, hängt ganz von der „Rangstellung" ab, welche die Person einnimmt, gegen die sich die Aggression richtet. Gegen schwächliche oder autoritätslose Mitpatientinnen ist die Aggression heftiger als gegen „ranghöhere" Personen. Es spielt dabei keine Rolle, ob die „Tabu-Vorschrift" der Frau S. A. absichtlich oder unabsichtlich verletzt wird. Da die *Alpha-Stellung* der Pat. nie ernsthaft angetastet wurde, kommt es nur selten zu „Kämpfen" (handfesten Schlägereien). Dem Arzt gegenüber, den Frau S. A. als eindeutig überlegenen *Rivalen* empfindet, reagiert sie, als dieser ganz und gar nicht vom angestammten Platz weichen will, mit einer *stereotypen Umkreisung* des geraubten Territoriums. Ihren *Schlafplatz* verteidigt Frau S. A. über viele Jahre fast noch heftiger. Das Bett darf in ihrer Anwesenheit selbst von einer Pflegerin nicht berührt werden.

Eine andere Pat. nimmt die *Stellung einer „kleinen Königin"* ein und meidet Alpha vollständig. Ihr in den Weg laufende Patientinnen werden verbal oder mit Ohrfeigen zurechtgewiesen, und zwar wiederum besonders dieselben drei ärmlichen Geschöpfe, die auch von den anderen Kranken am meisten eingeschüchtert und hie und da geschlagen werden. Sie nehmen durch Schwäche und Krankheit den *untersten Platz in der sozialen Rangordnung* ein und können mit Omega-Tieren verglichen werden. *Beta* hat im Gegensatz zu vielen anderen

Kranken keinen festen Sitzplatz, nimmt sich aber heraus, über die meisten Sitzplätze nach
Belieben zu verfügen. Manche Patientinnen, die sich in dieser Beziehung gegen sie behauptet
haben, werden nur selten von ihr belästigt.

Wieder andere Patientinnen stehen hinsichtlich ihrer Autorität und Eigentumsansprüche
(Sitz-, Arbeits-, Eß- und Schlafplatz) auf gleicher Rangstufe und genießen hohe Anerkennung,
die hauptsächlich darauf gegründet ist, daß die anderen *Angst* vor ihnen haben. Unter solchen
Gleichgeordneten kommt es gelegentlich zu Aggressionen, die stark an *Rangordnungskämpfe*
erinnern. Manche dieser Patientinnen wurden leukotomiert, genießen aber nach wie vor unter
ihren Mitpatientinnen eine hohe Stellung (vgl. dazu den Einfluß von experimentellen Hirnläsionen auf die Rangordnung von Rhesusaffen: S. 408).

Die Ranggleichen befreunden sich nicht miteinander. Manche von ihnen halten auf genaue
„Individualdistanzen"; Annäherung mit Überschreiten dieser „kritischen Distanz" wird ge-
ahndet. Eine dauernde freundschaftliche Empfindung scheint die Stellung zu gefährden, da sie
zur Aufhebung der Mißtrauensschranke verpflichten würde. Stark und Schwach dagegen gesellt sich gern, so daß die Häufigkeit erotisch-zartlicher Annäherung (Umarmungen, korper-
liche Kontaktsuche, Sich-Einhängen, Anschmiegen usw.) umgekehrt proportional der Rangordnung ist.

Staehelin beschreibt besonders eindrucksvoll eine katatone Kranke mit stereotypem
Hin- und Hergehen vor der Gartenpforte, dem Weg zur Freiheit und zugleich zu dem Orte, der
sie am sinnfälligsten an der Flucht hindert, einer Situation also, die mit ihren negativen und
positiven Valenzen schon bei den motorischen Stereotypien (s. S. 353) beschrieben wurde.
Rückte dieser Kranken nun eine Ranghöhere auf den Leib, geriet sie in ängstliche Erwartung,
unterbrach ihr stereotypes Wandern und wich bei Überschreitung einer 3 m-Grenze nach
der Seite der besten Fluchtmöglichkeit aus, dabei ängstlich die Gartenture im Auge behaltend,
zu der sie nach vorübergegangener „Gefahr" sofort zurückkehrte, um das Gitter-Pendeln
wieder aufzunehmen. Staehelin trieb die Kranke planmäßig in die Enge eines Hauswinkels
unweit der Gartenpforte. Bei Annäherung auf 5 m suchte sie, ihre Wanderung unterbrechend,
mit den Augen nach der erfolgreichsten Fluchtrichtung; nach Erreichen der 3 m-Grenze wich
sie aus. Schließlich in die Enge getrieben, drückte sie sich an die Mauer, drehte sich verzweifelt
um ihre eigene Achse und verbarg stark zitternd den Kopf in beide Arme. Dann aber, beim
allmahlich-langsamen Überschreiten der Distanz von 30 cm geschah das Unerwartete: Trotz
freundlich dargebotener Hand und beruhigendem Sprechen schlägt die aufgestaute Angst um,
und die Pat. stürzt sich aggressiv auf den ranghohen Artgenossen.

Schließlich noch eine mehrfach gemachte, wichtige Beobachtung: Die beschriebenen Verhaltensweisen — Einhalten der Rangordnung durch Drohung oder Aggression, Platz- oder
Revierverteidigung, Individual- oder Fluchtdistanz — sind abhängig von der Grundstimmung
der Patienten. Dies ließ sich bei solchen Patienten verfolgen, die periodisch oder episodisch aus
ihrer Psychose auftauchten. Die Versklavung an das rigide Reglement lockerte sich erheblich
auf oder verschwand ganz, so daß wahrend solcher Zeiten Verlegung auf die ruhige Abteilung
möglich wurde. Ein vorher brutales Verhalten wandelte sich in eine liebenswürdig-zuvorkom-
mende und hilfsbereite Art, ohne Anspruch auf Ansehen und Rang. Der Spielraum für differenzierte menschliche Beziehungen eröffnete sich.

Anderen Patientinnen, die hin und wieder versuchsweise auf die ruhige Abteilung verlegt
wurden, gelang die Anpassung nicht. Sie trachteten einesteils danach, ihre in der Primitiv-
Gemeinschaft durchgesetzten Ansprüche auch im neuen Milieu aufrechtzuerhalten; andrerseits
strebten sie an den gewohnten Ort zurück. Ihre „Sprache" wurde in einer Gemeinschaft, die
mehr in spezifisch-menschlichem Verhalten begründet ist, nicht verstanden, mit dem Ergebnis,
daß die in größere Freiheit gelassenen Kranken sich in ihrem Sozialverhalten verschlechterten
und zurückverlegt werden mußten.

Auch auf der Ebene des Gemeinschaftsverhaltens finden wir also, wie schon
bei den Stereotypien und im Ausdrucksverhalten, eine strikte *Reduktion der beim
Gesunden unübersehbar großen Verhaltensmöglichkeiten*. Territorium, Besitz, Rangordnung, Individualdistanzen, Aggression, Angst, Flucht — das alles sind Situationen und Zuständlichkeiten, die auch im normalen menschlichen Leben eine
Rolle spielen (s. S. 345). Auch der Gesunde hat es nicht gerne, wenn man ihm „zu
nahe auf den Pelz rückt"![1]; er tritt zurück und sucht zu seinem Gesprächspartner
eine gemäße Distanz zu gewinnen. Doch schlägt oder flieht er nicht, wenn er
sich unterlegen fühlt. In der chronischen schizophrenen Psychose wird das Gerippe
des Gemeinschaftslebens bloßgelegt. *Die Partnerschaft ist auf das Schema Gestimmtheit und Situation reduziert.* Nach diesem Schema läuft das Sozialverhalten

---

[1] Bereits sprachlich ist mit dem „Pelz" eine Parallele zum tierischen Verhalten ausgedrückt.

ab und ist in viel höherem Maße als beim Gesunden voraussagbar, da die Handelnsmöglichkeiten des kranken Individuums bis auf wenige Aktionen und Reaktionen eingeschränkt sind.

Betrachtet man sich nun diesen Torso, so zeigt er Grundzüge, die auch das Zusammenleben sozialer Tiere (*570, 571*) (Säuger, Vögel und mancher anderer Vertebraten) gestalten. Wie schon an den motorischen Schablonen gezeigt, sind die Auslöser stärker vom Abbau betroffen als die angeborenen Reaktionen. Das kommt sehr schön in dem einen der von STAEHELIN beschriebenen Fälle heraus: Freundliches Zureden und eine dargebotene Hand vermögen nicht die Angst zu durchbrechen. Dazu läßt sich gut eine ontogenetische Parallele ziehen: Kinder bilden ihre Individualdistanzen zur selben Zeit aus, wenn sich auch das Besitzgefühl zu entwickeln beginnt. Das jedem bekannte Verhalten eines Kindes, das von einem Fremden mit freundlichen Worten und ausgestreckter Hand begrüßt wird, hat mit dem der beschriebenen Patientin gemeinsame Züge: Das Kind drückt sich zur Seite, womöglich mit dem Rücken an der Wand entlang, es wendet sich ab und macht allerhand Bewegungen, die manchmal wie ,,Verrenkungen'' aussehen und an Stereotypien erinnern. Schließlich, wenn der wohlmeinende Besucher gar nicht ,,verstehen'' will und weiter zudringlich wird, kann das Kind auch beide Hände vors Gesicht halten, zu weinen beginnen oder sogar plötzlich dreinschlagen, dem höchstüberraschten Menschenfreund mitten ins Gesicht.

Das starre Festhalten an Gewohnheiten und Reglements ist für Kinder bis zum Schulalter charakteristisch. Dazu gehören auch allerhand ,,Tabu-Vorschriften'', welche Geschwister, Gespielen und eigentlich auch Eltern zu beachten haben, wenn nicht Wutausbrüche riskiert werden sollen. Die ,,Grausamkeiten'' von Kindern untereinander sind bekannt. Ein Kind in einer Gemeinschaft kann schon dann zum Prügelknaben werden, wenn es in einer, für die Begriffe der Erwachsenen, geringfügigen Weise anders als die anderen ist. Kleidung und sonstige Äußerlichkeiten geben meist den Grund zum ,,Anstoß-Nehmen''. F. GOETHE (*359*) hat amüsante Parallelen zum vergleichbaren Verhalten von Vögeln gezogen. Die Rangordnung unter Kindern und Jugendlichen ist noch weitaus klarer auf ,,Imponieren'', ,,Drohen'', Einschüchtern und Angst aufgebaut als beim Erwachsenen.

Gerade am Beispiel der Rangordnung von chronisch Geisteskranken (*816*) kann man zeigen, wie auch hier das Lernen die jeweilige Ordnung ausbildet. Neuankömmlinge haben die Rangordnung zu lernen; Patienten z. B. mit amnestischen Syndromen, die das nicht können, beziehen Prügel. Bezeichnenderweise waren die Omega-Personen STAEHELINs verblödete Patienten. Mit der Lerntheorie (bedingte, erworbene Angstreaktion, s. S. 396 ff.) kann die jeweilige Rangordnung bezüglich ihrer Abhängigkeitsverhältnisse bis zu einem gewissen Grade erklärt werden, aber die Rangordnung als solche beruht auf angeborenen Grundlagen des Verhaltens; denn es gibt auch lernfähige Tierarten, bei denen sich keine Rangordnung ausbildet.

Zusammengefaßt darf man wohl sagen, daß das Gemeinschaftsleben chronisch Schizophrener vom Instinktverhalten gesteuert und geregelt wird. Die tierischen Komponenten sozialen Lebens kommen unverhüllt und klar zum Vorschein. Daß es sich bei diesem Vorgang nicht um eine bloße Umkehr der phylogenetischen oder ontogenetischen Entwicklung handeln kann, haben wir früher in anderem Zusammenhang (vgl. S. 318 f.) betont. Meistens ist das Gemeinschaftsleben auf psychiatrischen Stationen verwickelter aufgebaut; die akuten Psychosen bilden den größeren Teil der Gruppe, die Behandlungen greifen in das Stimmungsgefüge ein (*647*), so daß die individuellen Züge der Psychose das hier bloßgelegte Skelet des Gemeinschaftslebens verdecken.

d) Komplexe individuelle Reaktionsformen

Stereotypien, Ausdrucksbewegungen und die Verhaltensweisen der Schizophrenen im Gemeinschaftsleben mögen dem Psychiater vielleicht allzusehr am Rande des prozeßpsychotischen Geschehens stehen. Er wird darin nicht das Wesen der Psychose sehen, das sich doch letztlich im Erleben der Kranken am deutlichsten auszudrücken scheint. Obwohl wir daran erinnern müssen, daß Verhaltensforschung nicht primär Erlebensforschung ist (s. S. 293), wollen wir doch versuchen, den Ablauf von endogenen Psychosen so zu beschreiben, daß sich auch das Erleben in eine biologisch orientierte Verhaltenstheorie einbeziehen läßt. Daß die Mannigfaltigkeit menschlichen Verhaltens nicht schlechtweg auf angeborenes Verhalten zu reduzieren ist, haben wir mehrfach betont. Selbstverständlich gilt das auch für psychotische Verhaltensweisen, in denen sich stets das ganze Individuum mit seiner einmaligen Lebensgeschichte ausspricht (243).

An „reichen" Krankengeschichten können wir die Vielfalt und Verschlungenheit menschlichen Erlebens studieren; das spezifisch Menschliche tritt in den Vordergrund und wird durch seine „Verstiegenheit", seine Zuspitzung oder Verzerrung gerade erst recht deutlich gleich Bildnissen des menschlichen Antlitzes in Trauer, Haß, Verzweiflung oder Verklärung, Darstellungen, die auf das typisch Menschliche abzielen.

Unsere kleinen Krankengeschichten verfolgen indessen die entgegengesetzte Absicht: Verhaltens- und Erlebensweisen, in denen das spezifisch Menschliche in den Hintergrund tritt, sind uns wichtig für Vergleiche, die auf präformiertes Verhalten abzielen. Nicht die Blüten, sondern die Wurzeln der Species Mensch sollen beachtet werden. Krankengeschichten jugendlicher Schizophrener fanden wir als Modelle am geeignetsten. In dieser Phase menschlicher Entwicklung scheinen die „Instinktmelodien" noch ungebrochen, in geordnetem Verband hervorzutreten, so daß angeborenes Verhalten sichtbar werden kann.

Ein fast 13jähriger Junge (Dieter K.) wurde u. a. zuerst dadurch auffällig, daß er in vorgebeugter Haltung den Kopf einzog, die Schultern anhob und gleichzeitig scheu und überangstlich wurde. Gelegentlich wurde diese Schreck- und Schutzhaltung von frecher Aufsässigkeit durchbrochen. Der Junge begann übermäßig zu onanieren und näherte sich dem Pflegerpersonal mit der Tendenz zu sexuellen Handlungen. Zu anderen Zeiten machte er Umarmungsgebarden und streichelnde Bewegungen. Er zeichnete stereotyp neben 3 oder 4 anderen Themen immer wieder eine Onanie-Symbolik, nämlich einen Spieß mit Blutstropfen, der von Armen umfaßt und von einem Hut oder einer Hose teilweise bedeckt wurde. Im Garten trat er über Wochen täglich stundenlang monoton rhythmisch von einem Fuß auf den anderen und schlug im gleichen Takt der Füße mit einem Stock auf den Zaun. Oder er wiegte im Knien oder Sitzen den Oberkorper rhythmisch nach vorn und hinten. Versuchte man, diese motorischen Stereotypien irgendwie eingreifend zu durchbrechen, wurde er aggressiv. Zum Zeichen seiner Kontaktnahme hakte er seinen Arm — auch wieder in stereotyper Weise — in den des Partners. Besonders eindrucksvoll war das fluktuierende oder auch ganz abrupt schwankende Verhalten zwischen kalbernd-erotisch-sexuell getönter körperlicher Kontaktnahme und plötzlichem Furchtverhalten mit schrillem Schreien und aggressiver Abwehr mit weit von sich gestrecken Handen. Im Tagesraum der Station beanspruchte er stets den gleichen Sitzplatz und verteidigte ihn hartnäckig. Er entwickelte ganz spezifische Appetenzen und verlangte begierig nach Süßigkeiten, später nach Salzig-Saurem und besonders nach sauren Gurken, die er hastig schlingend fur sich allein verzehrte. Außerdem wurden periodisch auftretend regressive, kleinkindhafte Verhaltensweisen beobachtet. Zum Beispiel spielte er „Hund" und näßte nachts und auch tagsüber ein. Zu anderen Malen wollte er nach Art eines 2—3jährigen kuschelnd in die Betten anderer kriechen (656).

In diesem Beispiel sehen wir viele der bereits bekannten Verhaltensweisen wiederkehren, nämlich eine fixierte Schreck- und Schutzhaltung (s. S. 313 f.), einige Grundbewegungen und Stereotypien, Platzverteidigung und Aggression. Handelnsbereitschaften, also Stimmungen im ethologischen Sinne, wechseln abrupt und sind nicht durch die äußere Situation bestimmt. Flucht, Aggression und Sexualverhalten stehen dicht beieinander, so wie wir es im Balz- und Paarungsverhalten vieler Tiere kennengelernt haben. Die Nahrungsappetenzen (*412*) sind einförmig festgelegt und richten sich für längere Zeit nur auf Süßes, dann wieder auf Salzig-Saures, eine Art von Bevorzugung, wie man sie zeitweilig bei kleinen Kindern antrifft. Auch andere kleinkindhafte Verhaltensweisen kehren periodisch wieder. Die einzige inhaltlich bestimmte Aussage, die der fast völlig mutistische Junge trotz intensiver ärztlicher Bemühungen über mehr als ein Jahr hindurch zu machen imstande war, spiegelte sich in seinen stereotypen Malereien wider, die hauptsächlich sexuelle Erlebnisinhalte, aber auch Erlebnisse der Angst und Aggression zum Gegenstand hatten.

In der zweiten Krankengeschichte erhalten wir etwas mehr Auskunft über die Erlebnisse und können verschiedene, miteinander abwechselnde Episoden unterscheiden.

Ein 14jähriger Junge (Wulf T.) kam im Juli 1954 zum erstenmal in die Klinik, nachdem er Anfang 1953 erstmals kürzere psychotische Episoden durchgemacht hatte. Er klagte damals über Sterbensangst und das Gefühl, von Erdstrahlen durchdrungen zu werden. Zeitweilig beklagte er sich, schlecht zu verstehen, horte die Stimmen anderer Menschen wie aus weiter Ferne, lauschte in sich hinein und hatte wahrscheinlich akustische Halluzinationen. Im Winter 1955/56 kam W. erneut in akut psychotischem Zustand zur Aufnahme. Sein Verhalten, das dem während der Beobachtung 1954 sehr ähnlich war, läßt drei Stadien erkennen:

a) Stadium der Schutzsuche: W. klammert sich an alle Autoritätspersonen, und zwar besonders an diejenige, die ihm als die einflußreichste bzw. mit der größten „Macht" ausgestattet erscheint, redet in monotonen, sich immer wiederholenden Wendungen auf sie ein, sieht ihr tief in die Augen, schlingt nach Möglichkeit den Arm um sie, legt den Kopf an die Schulter und birgt das Gesicht an der Brust. Diese ausdrucksvolle Geste kann knabenhaft, aber auch wie die eines erschöpften Kindes wirken. Eine solche Situation wird von W. aus nie abgebrochen; er könnte beliebig lange darin verharren. Das geschilderte Verhalten kann sich in zwei Richtungen abwandeln. Entweder tritt zu dem bittend-beschwörenden Schutz- und Hilfesuchen ein zärtlich gefärbtes, liebesuchendes Verhalten, wobei W. mehr als sonst den körperlichen Kontakt herbeiführt, oder er bedrängt einen unentwegt mit stereotypen Fragen, ohne die Antwort aufzunehmen noch auch sie nur abzuwarten.

b) Stadium der Erregung: W. läuft stunden- und tagelang in wechselndem, aber meist forciertem Tempo auf und ab. Er wirkt dabei wie manche höheren Säuger in Gefangenschaft. Bei seinem Hin- und Herwandern spielt er gelegentlich an seinem erigierten Penis und onaniert mitunter auch öffentlich, ohne Notiz von seiner Umgebung zu nehmen. Versucht man, ihn am Umherlaufen zu hindern, wird er gereizt, ja, entgegen dem oben geschilderten anschmiegsamen Verhalten, richtig böse. Aber auch ohne jeglichen erkennbaren Anlaß schlägt er beim Wandern plötzlich und blitzschnell auf einen gerade in seiner Bahn stehenden Pfleger ein. Als Ziel des Schlages wird das Gesicht bevorzugt. Nach Art des geführten Schlages und im Hinblick auf das aktive Aufsuchen des Aggressionszieles ist deutlich, daß es sich nicht um ein Abwehr- oder Verteidigungsverhalten, sondern um ein aktives Angriffsverhalten handelt. An manchen solchen Tagen redet W. auf seinem Marsch, meist unverständlich, monoton vor sich hin, wobei sich gewisse banale Inhalte immer wiederholen. Ob W. in solchen Zuständen halluziniert, ist nicht sicher auszumachen.

c) Stadium des „Leerlaufes": W. liegt in seinem Bett, wirkt von seiner Umgebung „abgeschaltet" und onaniert sehr häufig, mitunter halbstündig. Wenn man ihn rapportsuchend oder beruhigend anspricht, reagiert er, obwohl wach, manchmal überhaupt nicht, manchmal wie jemand, der Lästige abschütteln will. Da W. mit offenen Augen und abwesendem Blick daliegt, ist es möglich, daß er halluziniert, ohne daß aber von ihm darüber etwas zu erfahren wäre.

Die drei beschriebenen Stadien sind nun nicht starre Zuständlichkeiten, sondern stellen häufig beobachtete Extremvarianten seines Verhaltens dar. Es gab Zeiten, in denen sich die Verhaltensweisen miteinander mischten, einander rascher ablösten oder in abgemilderter und mannigfaltig abgewandelter Form auftraten. Besonders während der mit Erfolg durchgeführten Elektroschockbehandlung, der andere erfolglose Behandlungsversuche vorangingen, änderten sich die beschriebenen Verhaltensweisen rasch.

Bemerkenswert ist bei W., daß er wohl immer im üblichen Sinne orientiert ist, d. h. er weiß, wo er ist, kann, soweit er zum Rapport zu bringen ist, über sich sogar mit einer gewissen Krankheitseinsicht Auskunft geben und über seine Vorgeschichte detailliert und zeitlich geordnet berichten. Dennoch ist er während der oben beschriebenen Stadien in seiner Bewußtheit hochgradig eingeengt. Er ist vom eigenen Erleben so besessen, fasziniert oder getrieben, daß weder die „Umgebung" noch die „Welt" irgendeinen Einfluß auf ihn bzw. sein Verhalten hat. Dafür noch ein drastisches Beispiel: Als die alte und erfahrene, doch häufig freundlich moralisierende Stationsschwester W. am Onanieren hindern will, sagt er ganz unbeteiligt und beziehungslos, die Schwester solle es dann doch bei ihm machen. In gesundem Zustand hat W. ein höflich-wohlerzogenes, etwas altkluges Auftreten und entspricht in seinem Denken, Fühlen, Urteilen und Verhalten der Altersnorm. Die geschilderten Verhaltensweisen empfindet er als fremd; sie sind ihm peinlich, und er steht ihnen verständnislos gegenüber. Das Wachrufen der mit seinem Verhalten verbundenen Erlebnisse, uber die er keine rechte Auskunft geben kann, hat den Charakter einer Traumerinnerung (654).

Nehmen wir uns das „*Stadium der Schutzsuche*" nochmals vor: Das Werben des Schwachen und Hilflosen um Gunst und Hilfe des Starken, das Beschwören seiner Macht, glauben wir als angeborene Verhaltensweise — oder vielleicht besser als angeborene Verhaltensbereitschaft — erkennen zu können, die hier in der Psychose bar zum Ausdruck kommt (vgl. S. 333f.; 340 ff.). Daß es sich um etwas Präformiertes handelt, geht z. B. daraus hervor, daß die für diese Situation symbolische Geste, nämlich das „Gesicht an der Brust des Starken bergen", stets von einer affektiven Antwort des „Starken" gefolgt ist: er fühlt sich *gedrängt*, den Schutzsuchenden anzunehmen, und legt ihm zum Zeichen dafür z. B. die Hand auf den Kopf oder schließt ihn — je nach Art der Beziehung — in den Arm. Dieses Doppel, Gebärde und Reaktion, Schlüsselreiz und Antwort darauf, hat ganz den Charakter eines Verhaltens auf dem Boden eines angeborenen Auslösemechanismus. Will der Starke den Flehenden aus irgendeinem Grunde nicht annehmen, kann er dies nur unter Überwindung eines stärkeren inneren Widerstandes tun; Unlustgefühle sind die Folge.

Im „*Stadium der Erregung*" sieht man sehr schön, wie in motorischer Unruhe sexuelle Erregung und blanke Aggressionen miteinander abwechseln, ohne daß es zu einer Triebverzehrung kommt. Die Stimmung ist gereizt. Es besteht ein starker Erregungsdruck, und die Instinkthandlungen — Aggression und sexuelles Verhalten — gehen einfach los, ohne daß sich eine adäquate Auslöser-Situation anbietet. Man darf dieses Verhalten wohl als Übersprungverhalten auffassen.

Etwas anders ist die Situation im „*Leerlaufstadium*". W. liegt „abgeschaltet" da und realisiert immer wieder die sexuelle Triebhandlung. Ob er sich den Sexualpartner in seinem traumartigen Zustand vorstellt oder ihn regelrecht halluziniert, ist nicht auszumachen. Diese unerhört starke sexuelle Triebabfuhr trägt ja allein durch ihre Dauer pathologischen Charakter und ist nicht mit den üblichen masturbatorischen Akten Jugendlicher zu vergleichen. Es besteht ein derartiger Erregungsdruck, daß wir glauben, den Vorgang am besten zu erfassen, wenn wir ihn als Leerlaufaktivität ansehen (vgl. S. 304).

Die letzte Krankengeschichte zeigt das Auseinanderbrechen des Stimmungsgefüges. Ein zunächst noch angepaßtes Appetenzverhalten bahnt sich an; die Schwelle für Auslösereize erniedrigt sich; es entsteht ein erheblicher Erregungsdruck, und schließlich entlädt sich eine Instinkthandlung spontan, als sich nach vergeblichem Suchen keine adäquate Auslösersituation finden ließ:

Erika P., ein 14jähriges, von jeher auffällig scheues, korperlich retardiertes, noch sehr kindliches Mädchen offenbarte eine zarte Schwärmerei für einen jungen Gehilfen ihres Vaters. Einige Zeit darauf las sie bis tief in die Nacht hinein Bücher über Liebesprobleme; deswegen hielt sie sich für schlecht. Später besuchte sie ihren Lehrer in seiner Wohnung, drangte sich an ihn und versuchte ihn zu küssen. Dabei war sie — wie der Lehrer berichtete — sehr aufgeregt. Der Vater brachte sie daraufhin zur Großmutter. In der Bahn sprach das Mädchen einen Mitreisenden mit dem Namen des Lehrers an. Am Reiseziel war E. nachts sehr unruhig und schlief überhaupt nicht. Schließlich in die Klinik eingeliefert, glaubte sie, 10 Jahre auf der Bahn gefahren zu sein, hielt sich für 24 Jahre alt und sprach von ihrer Schwiegermutter. Den Arzt hielt sie für den Gehilfen ihres Vaters oder zu anderen Zeiten für ihren Lehrer und versuchte, nach deutlich wahrnehmbarer Steigerung des Erregungsdruckes bei der Visite ihn unbekleidet zu umschlingen. Wenige Zeit danach lag sie unansprechbar, sozusagen abgeschaltet von der Umgebung, im Bett und führte unter erregtem Gefluster onanierend fertig ausgeprägte Begattungsbewegungen aus.
Einige Tage spater drängte sich das Mädchen durch ein Fenster und sprang vom 1. Stock in den Stationsgarten. Inzwischen wieder rapportfahig, gab es als Motiv fur sein Verhalten an:

„Es wird höchste Zeit, daß ich hinunterspringe, sonst wird es immer höher. — Ich wollte in die Freiheit, ein freies Herz haben. Der enge Raum erdrückt mich so. Ich dachte, ich könnte bei jemandem Zuflucht suchen. — In den See möchte ich, da ist es mir so heimatlich." Ich fragte, ob sie sich denn ertränken wolle. „Nein, ich möchte dort sein und dort bleiben."

Dieser Episode folgte ein halluzinatorisches Stadium der Psychose, in dem das Mädchen oft die Augen schloß und sagte, es sei so schön wie im Traum. Nach ihrer Genesung gewann sie ihre kindlich scheue Wesensart vollkommen wieder zurück, erkrankte aber nach Jahren des Wohlbefindens und der Unauffälligkeit erneut, diesmal an einer stärker paranoid gefärbten Psychose (*654*).

Die kleine Patientin erlebt also einen pathologischen Einbruch in ihr bis dahin intaktes, noch ganz kindliches Persönlichkeitsgefüge. Ihr anfänglich noch angepaßt wirkendes Liebes*appetenzverhalten* richtet sich schließlich auf jedes in den Blickpunkt rückende männliche Wesen. Unter höchstem Erregungsdruck verhält sich die Kranke dann so wie ein ohne menschlich geprägte Konvention und Sitte aufgewachsenes Menschenweibchen und versucht in gänzlich unangepaßter Situation die Endhandlung, die Cohabitation, zu realisieren. Als dieser Versuch mißlingt, verliert sie jeden Rapport, und die als *Leerlaufaktivität* zu erklärenden Begattungsbewegungen setzen ein. Jedoch läßt der Erregungsdruck nur vorübergehend nach; die leerlaufende Endhandlung zehrt den Trieb nicht auf, sondern es kommt zu einer anderen Abfolge von Verhaltensweisen, nämlich zum *Zuflucht- und Ruhesuchen im Übersprung* als Folge einer nicht realisierbaren Triebhandlung. „Eine echt endogene Motivation liefert die Energie für ganz andere als ihr normalerweise zugeordnete Verhaltensweisen" (*131*). Nachdem die Patientin auch hier ihr Ziel nicht erreicht, setzt ein halluzinatorisches Stadium ein, in dem sie sich glücklich fühlt. Die Motorik ist gleichsam „abgehängt" (*60*), und die ersehnte innere Ruhe tritt ein (*572*).

Auch diese drei akuten Fälle lassen die gleichen Prinzipien der Dissolution auf der Ebene komplexen individuellen Handelns erkennen: Dem Normal-Gestimmten steht eine optimale Handlungsfreiheit zur Verfügung. Mit dem Aufkommen spezifischer Handelnsbereitschaften, wie wir sie von Tieren kennen, schränkt sich die Handlungsfreiheit ein. Je intensiver eine solche Partialstimmung hervortritt, je eindeutiger sie sich in angeborenem Verhalten entlädt, desto zwangsläufiger ist das Handlungsgeschehen. In gleichem Grade wandelt sich das Realitätsbewußtsein der Kranken. Eine spezifische Handelnsbereitschaft geht mit einer Änderung der Bedeutungsgehalte der Objekte einher; die Objekte ändern je nach Stimmung ihre Physiognomie. Für die kleine Erika (Fall 3) sind zuerst Lehrer und Gehilfe — Vater- und Jünglingsfigur — die Liebesobjekte. Später werden die Auslöser für das Sexualverhalten immer unspezifischer, es treten „Personenverwechslungen" männlicher Wesen ein, bis schließlich jede reale Partnerschaft erlischt und die Triebobjekte irreal werden. An ihnen vollziehen sich schließlich die Instinkthandlungen. — Wulf (Fall 2) kann dem gleichen Menschen, je nach Stimmung, aggressiv oder schutzsuchend begegnen. Ein noch eben erstrebter Partner wird angsterfüllt von sich gestoßen (Fall 1). Zwei Instinkthandlungen liegen miteinander in Konkurrenz. Die gleiche Umgebung ist in der Psychose freundlich oder feindlich, nah oder fern, heimatlich oder fremd, abstoßend oder anziehend, kurz, irgendwie „anders" getönt. Diesem Bedeutungswandel der Objekte unter dem Einfluß verschiedener Stimmungen sind wir bei der Verhaltensanalyse der Tiere immer wieder begegnet (s. S. 306, 309, 328, 330 ff., 334 ff.).

3. Ethologischer Deutungsversuch des endogen psychotischen Verhaltens

In der Klinik wird der Ausdruck „endogene Verstimmung" alltäglich benutzt. Die heute gerne als klassisch bezeichnete Richtung in der Psychiatrie betont das Endogene, vermutet darin bekanntlich eine Somatose, einen Krankheitsprozeß, entstehend aus bisher unbekannten körperlichen Ursachen. Die Kranken werden entsprechend dieser Hypothese mit körperlichen Methoden — und wohl unbestritten mit guten Teilerfolgen — behandelt. Bei den „Psychikern" unter den Psychiatern verschiebt sich der Akzent dieses klinischen Ausdrucks auf das Wort „Verstimmung", womit der phänomenologisch faßbare psychische Zustand des Kranken gemeint ist. Die seelischen Störungen werden als Folge erlebnisbedingter Fehlentwicklung oder Fehlanpassung begriffen. Auch hier gibt es bei konsequenter seelischer Behandlung ausgewählter Fälle gewisse Teilerfolge, vor allem aber unbestreitbar eine intimere Kenntnis der Psychopathologie der Psychosen.

Sieht man einmal von den fast stets nachzuweisenden Prodromen der klinisch manifesten Verstimmung ab [Schlafstörungen und andere vegetative Beeinträchtigungen des Befindens (*322, 649, 658*)], so ist eine sich anbahnende Veränderung der Lebensgrundstimmung als allgemeinstes und kaum je fehlendes Symptom herauszustellen (*647*). Noch ehe im engeren Sinne psychotische Symptome auftreten, bemerken Angehörige, Lehrer, Arbeitskameraden und andere „Sozialpartner" eine Änderung des „Sozialverhaltens" und der Lebensgewohnheiten des Kranken. Sein Verhalten ändert sich, ohne daß er dafür hinreichende Motive angeben kann (*655*).

Man setzt also beim Gebrauch des Wortes „Verstimmtheit" voraus, daß der Normale sich im Zustand der Gestimmtheit befindet, und zwar infolge des Zusammenwirkens einer Vielfalt von inneren und äußeren Faktoren. Die Untersuchung solcher Faktoren auf der Ebene des Verhaltens war Gegenstand der vorangegangenen Kapitel, die Einblicke in den Aufbau des Verhaltens vermitteln und zeigen sollten, daß prinzipiell auch höheres Verhalten der Kausalanalyse zugänglich ist. Zwar wandelt sich der einfache Modellfall „Schlüsselreiz — Ansprechen des angeborenen Auslösemechanismus (AAM) — Freisetzung der Instinkthandlung" mit zunehmender Organisationshöhe der Lebewesen in zunehmend komplizierterer Form ab, doch kann kein Zweifel darüber bestehen, daß auch die menschliche Gestimmtheit im strikten Vergleich zum Tiere auf dem physiologischen Gesamtzustand des Organismus basiert. In diesem Sinne kann man von einer Verhaltensphysiologie sprechen und den Ausdruck Stimmung im Sinne der Ethologie, nämlich als Kennzeichen eines zentralnervösen Zustandes benutzen.

Die Stimmungshierarchie (s. S. 306) ist in niederorganisierten Organismen so aufgebaut, daß die einzelnen Funktionskreise, wie z. B. Beutefang, Paarungsverhalten usw., in sich hierarchisch gegliedert sind. Ist ein Funktionskreis wirksam, werden damit andere Funktionskreise mit den dazugehörigen Handelnsbereitschaften (Stimmungen) ausgeschlossen. Je höher organisiert, desto größer die Zahl der determinierenden inneren und äußeren Faktoren, desto mehr Überschneidungen der Funktionskreise, desto höher integriert das Gesamtverhalten, desto ausbalancierter die Stimmungen. Das heißt zugleich: Mit zunehmender Organisationshöhe steigt die Handlungsfreiheit und damit die Anpassungsfähigkeit an eine sich wandelnde Umwelt. Wie sehr selbst noch beim hochentwickelten Säugetier spezifische Handelnsbereitschaften das jeweilige Handeln bestimmen, haben wir gesehen. *Beim Menschen* hingegen besteht normalerweise eine *Integrationsstufe höchster Art*, auf der *spezifische Handelnsbereitschaften*, im Sinne der Realisierung angeborenen Verhaltens, *nicht in Erscheinung treten*[1]. Das heißt, mit Ablauf einer Handlung werden andere Handelnsbereitschaften nicht ausgeschlossen. Die Stimmungen sind gewissermaßen frei „konvertierbar". Es besteht eine vergleichsweise unbegrenzte Handlungsfreiheit. Daß diese Stimmungsintegration aber doch störbar ist, wenn willkürlich in die „Triebregulierung" (s. S.375 ff.) eingegriffen wird,

---

[1] Ausnahmen machen die sog. physiologischen Bedürfnisse wie z. B. Schlaf und Nahrungsaufnahme. Doch ist deren Befriedigung nur im Kleinkindalter imperativ und kann später abgewandelt oder hinausgeschoben werden.

sehen wir im Schlafentzug (*159*), im chronischen Hunger- oder Durstzustand, im hypoglykämischen Schock und in der experimentellen Psychose (*123, 504, 654*), wie vor allem LEUNER gezeigt hat.

Beim gesunden Menschen sind die zahlreichen, am Aufbau der Stimmungshierarchie beteiligten Faktoren so komplex und vielgestaltig, daß damit eine Fähigkeit zur Umweltanpassung und -bewältigung erreicht worden ist, wie sie sonst in der Natur nicht vorkommt.

Anders in der endogenen Psychose: Hier, so mögen die Beispiele des vorigen Kapitels gezeigt haben, treten spezifische Handelnsbereitschaften hervor, die Stimmungshierarchie gerät aus den Fugen, und die sonst nicht aus dem Gesamtverhalten herauslösbaren Bausteine angeborenen Verhaltens treten bar und unangepaßt in Erscheinung. Wie bei den Instinkthandlungen der Tiere scheinen unter dem Einfluß spezifischer Handelnsbereitschaften andere mögliche Verhaltensweisen ausgeschlossen zu werden. Gerade diese Ausschließlichkeit des Verhaltens ist aber für die psychotische „Verrückung" charakteristisch. Nicht die Umwelt ist realitätsbestimmend, sondern die spezifische Stimmung. Aus dieser Verschiebung der Subjekt-Objekt-Beziehung kann man versuchen, das magische Bezugssystem der Psychose-Kranken abzuleiten. Eine endogen depressive Bauersfrau z. B. ließ ein Schwein schlachten, obwohl man ihr den bis oben gefüllten Rauchschrank zeigte. Der Ausruf: „Ja, aber wir müssen *doch alle* verhungern!", zeigt die bekannte subjektive Gewißheit der Wahnkranken, entgegen aller Überzeugungskraft der objektiven Tatsachen. Die „Mangelstimmung", eine normalerweise in das gesamte Handlungsgefüge eingebettete Handelnsbereitschaft, löst sich heraus, wird dominierend und ist realitätsbestimmend, nicht aber das wahrgenommene Objekt. Und die gleiche Frau verschenkt in ihrer anschließenden manischen Phase wahllos ihre gerade verfügbare Habe.

Wie bei den motorischen Schablonen im cerebralorganischen Abbau können angeborene Grundweisen des Verhaltens die Oberhand gewinnen, während die übrigen Verhaltensweisen graduell der Dissolution anheimfallen. Die Dissolution ist erkennbar an der Einbuße von Freiheitsgraden des Handelns, an der Abnahme voluntativer Funktionen, an der einfacheren Determinierung des Handlungsgeschehens und an dem Vorherrschen von vergleichsweise starren „Mechanismen", wie z. B. der Leerlaufaktivität und dem Übersprungverhalten (s. S. 304). Diesen Prozeß haben wir entsprechend dem Aufbau tierischen Verhaltens in vier Stufen zu zeigen versucht, nämlich an der Bewegung (motorische Stereotypien; s. S. 351), am Ausdrucksverhalten (mimische Desintegration; s. S. 356), am Gemeinschaftsleben (S. 357) und im komplexen Individualverhalten (S. 360).

Sollten nicht die großen, im Grunde unwandelbaren Themen der Depressiven, oben am Beispiel der Mangelstimmung angedeutet, der Ausdruck eines angeborenen Bestandteiles menschlicher Veranlagung sein? In ihnen scheint sich die Species Mensch noch klarer und „verständlicher" auszudrücken als in der vergleichsweise tiefer greifenden Dissolution im schizophrenen Prozeß. BILZ (*265*) hat das, wenn auch in anderem Zusammenhang, am Beispiel einer Umzugsdepression gezeigt. Wir nehmen diese Form der Auslösung einer Depression — auch BILZ spricht ausdrücklich von Auslösung — zum Anlaß, um die Ergebnisse der Ethologie auch für das Problem *Anlage-Umwelt* (*795*) heranzuziehen.

Schlüsselreize klinken bei Tieren angeborenes Verhalten aus. Solche Schlüsselreize gibt es sicherlich auch beim Menschen noch. Für die ersten Monate unseres Lebens kann man das schon recht gut nachweisen, im Erwachsenenalter wird die Beweisführung schwieriger, und es ist nicht möglich, etwa einen Katalog von Schlüsselreizen aufzustellen, wie man das bei einem Fisch z. B. tun kann. Dennoch gibt die alte psychiatrische Erfahrung zu denken, daß bestimmte Situationen, wie

z. B. ein Umzug, der Verkauf eines Hauses, der „Erwerb" eines Weibes (s. S. 346) u. a. m., eine endogene Psychose auslösen können. Andererseits können besondere Situationen, die das Sozialverhalten ansprechen, eine Psychose, meist vorübergehend, zum Verschwinden bringen. In einem Fall wird ein pathologisches Verhalten in Gang gesetzt, im anderen Fall kommt eine Re-Integration des Verhaltens zustande. Bilz betont mit Recht, daß ein gesunder Mensch von einem Umzug nicht derartig beeinträchtigt wird, daß er seine Geborgenheit verliert und depressiv wird. Bei Menschen mit der Anlage zu psychotischem Reagieren können aber offenbar „Schlüsselreize" spezifische Handelnsbereitschaften oder ganze Funktionskreise ausklinken, die dann eine dominierende, unkontrollierte und das *ganze* Handeln bestimmende Wirkung entfalten.

Welche Antwort kann uns die Verhaltensforschung auf die Frage geben, wie es zum Zerbrechen der Stimmungshierarchie, zum Hervortreten angeborener Verhaltensweisen, d. h. in unserem Deutungsversuch, wie es zur Psychose kommt? Im IV. Kapitel wurde gezeigt, daß die *Domestikation* imstande ist, entscheidend in das Gefüge angeborener Verhaltensweisen einzugreifen. Sie kann die endogene Reizproduktion verändern, sie kann funktionell zusammengehörige angeborene Verhaltensweisen aufsplittern und die Selektivität der angeborenen Auslösemechanismen schwächen, so daß an ihre Stelle einfachere und genereller wirkende Ersatzreize treten können. Der Gewinn der Domestikation liegt in der Zunahme der Freiheitsgrade des Handelns, die durch Abnahme instinktiver Koppelungen erreicht wird; dieser Vorteil wird durch Instinktausfälle erkauft. An der Tatsache, daß der Mensch selbst ein domestiziertes und ein sich weiter selbst domestizierendes Wesen ist, kann man nicht zweifeln. Für ihn treffen alle Auswirkungen der Domestikation — positive und negative — in erhöhtem Maße zu. Nicht die veränderten Lebensbedingungen bewirken die Domestikationsmerkmale der Artabwandlung, sondern ganz vorwiegend das Fortfallen der natürlichen Auslese. *Die Domestikation wirkt sich also genetisch aus und greift in das Gefüge angeborener Verhaltensweisen ein.*

So schwer nun angeborenes Verhalten beim gesunden Erwachsenen als solches isolierbar ist, so darf man es doch als das tragende Fundament im Aufbau des Verhaltens ansehen. Phylogenetische und ontogenetische Verhaltensentwicklung lassen jedenfalls keinen anderen Schluß zu. Eingriffe an diesem Fundament können die hochintegrierte Stimmungshierarchie empfindlicher treffen als Störungen auf anderen Funktionsebenen. Jacksons Lehre ist unseres Erachtens auch hier anwendbar und läßt sich durch moderne neurophysiologische Vorstellungen (*138, 418*) präzisieren und erweitern. Die höchsten „Zentren" — den Ausdruck gebraucht Jackson ebenso wie die Verhaltensphysiologen in rein funktionellem Sinne (s. S. 318) — sind am wenigsten fest organisiert und fallen am ehesten der Dissolution anheim, während die fester organisierten, mehr automatisch funktionierenden resistenter sind. Eine Veränderung im Fundament, z. B. die Veränderung der endogenen Reizproduktion, die Aufsplitterung funktionell zusammengehöriger Verhaltensweisen oder die Veränderung ihrer Auslösemechanismen, können die Stimmungshierarchie umstürzen. Die Bausteine angeborenen Verhaltens kommen dann zum Vorschein und springen als primitive Verhaltens-Regulationen ein (*649, 654—656*).

Auf diese Weise kann man zu begreifen versuchen, warum ureigen menschliche Grundhaltungen uns bar und unangepaßt, gleichsam in „Verrückung" entgegentreten. Die oft und vor allem von C. G. Jung (*97*) hervorgehobenen archaischen Erlebensweisen der Psychose-Kranken (*488*) würden sich mit Hilfe dieses Konzeptes biologisch begründen lassen, und es ergeben sich enge Beziehungen zu den von

Klaus Conrad (*30*) und Henry Ey (*45*) entwickelten, psychopathologisch fundierten Auffassungen (s. a. Ey und Conrad in Band I/2, S. 720 bzw. Bd. II, S. 369).

Die durch Domestikation von Generation zu Generation ermöglichten Veränderungen der Anlagen könnten die Tatsache begreiflich machen, daß ein bestimmter Prozentsatz der Menschen an endogenen Psychosen erkrankt, ohne daß in der Familien-Vorgeschichte eine erbliche Disposition zur Krankheit nachweisbar ist. Die Verhaltensforschung gibt uns Beispiele für die kompensatorische Funktion, die innere und äußere Faktoren für das effektive Verhalten haben (s. S. 301). Ein starker Signalreiz kann eine schwach ausgeprägte Handelnsbereitschaft so anfachen, daß der gleiche Handlungseffekt eintritt, wie er bei schwachem Signalreiz in schwellennaher Handelnsbereitschaft zustande kommt. Für die endogenen Psychosen würde dies bedeuten, daß verschieden starke Signalreize von Fall zu Fall notwendig sein können, um das Hervortreten angeborener Verhaltensweisen auszulösen; es kommt darauf an, wie weit die Reaktion durch „innere Faktoren" *vorbereitet* ist. Solche Faktoren wären z. B. Pubertät, Klimax und Senium, Schwangerschaft und Stillzeit, also Episoden im menschlichen Leben, in denen die Psychosebereitschaft erhöht ist.

Für das Problem Anlage—Anpassung sind folgende Ermittlungen der Weltgesundheitsorganisation von Bedeutung und weiterer Nachprüfung wert: Manisch-depressive und schizophrene Erkrankungen sollen sich bei Vergleich von weißen Amerikanern und Negern am seltensten bei bäuerlichen Negern in Afrika finden. Mit zunehmender Erkrankungshäufigkeit folgen bäuerliche Neger in den USA — Weiße in den USA — in den Städten lebende Neger in den USA. Bei den letzteren nimmt die Erkrankungshäufigkeit mit zunehmender Anpassung an die zivilisatorischen Verhältnisse im Laufe der Generationen ab und gleicht sich der Quote der weißen Bevölkerung wieder an (*654*). Wie sehr scheinen diese Ergebnisse für die Bestrebungen der amerikanischen Psychiatrie zu sprechen, die Psychosen als Reaktion auf eine „pathogene" Umgebung aufzufassen. In der Tat kann man sich wohl keine gründlichere Veränderung der Umgebung vorstellen als die Versetzung vom afrikanischen Land in eine amerikanische Stadt. Der Neger verlor sein „Heim", sein „Territorium", seine „Objekte" und sah sich einer Welt von Objekten und Sozialpartnern gegenübergestellt, die ihm fremd, wenn nicht sogar feindlich erscheinen mußte. Aber nur bei einem Teil der Neger wird die psychotische Defensive ausgelöst, der andere paßt sich an.

Stellen wir diesem „Experiment" der Versetzung einer Rasse andere zur Seite, die in vergleichbarer Weise eine völlige Veränderung der Umwelt herbeiführen (*517, 518*): Von 135 Schiffbrüchigen in Rettungsbooten überlebten vier. Im Bericht heißt es, daß viele Personen halluziniert und andere Selbstmord verübt haben, wobei sie versuchten, das ganze Boot mit den anderen Insassen mitzuversenken. Wieder andere mordeten. Einer halluzinierte einen über Bord kletternden Helfer. Andere hatten destruktive Halluzinationen. Nach Beendigung dieser Situation hatten die Überlebenden Angst zu sprechen, bis sie ihres normalen Realitätsbewußtseins wieder sicher waren.

Lassen sich Menschen freiwillig oder sogar gegen Belohnung isolieren, z. B. im Bett mit stark eingeschränkter Bewegungsfähigkeit und in homogenisiertem Gesichtsfeld (Milchglasbrillen), wird nach einigen Stunden folgerichtiges Denken unmöglich. Danach tritt ein intensiver Wunsch nach Reizen und Aktion auf. Schließlich wird die Grenze zwischen Wachen und Schlafen unscharf; die Bewußtseinsinhalte ähneln denen im Traum. Nach etwa 2 Tagen entwickeln sich dann Wahnbildungen und Halluzinationen, die dem Mescalin-Rausch nahestehen (*69, 392*).

Diese zur Zeit in Amerika recht aktuellen Isolierungsexperimente (*186a, 382a*) kann man in Beziehung zu religiösen Erfahrungen und Exerzitien setzen. Jesus ging 40 Tage in die Wüste, bevor er zu lehren begann, Buddha versenkte sich in der Einsamkeit des Gebirges. Die weitgehende Abschaltung von der Außenwelt bringt Funktionen in Führung, die unter gewohnlichen Bedingungen nicht frei zum Zuge kommen können. C. G. JUNG hat seine Psychologie auf dieser Erkenntnis aufgebaut, und KLAGES' Konzeption fußt auf ahnlichem Boden.

Weniger radikal als die religiosen Versenkungen wirken sich manche heutigen Isolierungen aus. Die Mannschaft des amerikanischen U-Bootes, das die Eiskappe des Nordpoles unterquerte, war 60 Tage unter Wasser und lange Zeit von jeder Radioverbindung abgeschnitten. Die Matrosen lasen zu Anfang Wildwest-Romane, am Ende Shakespeare und philosophische Werke, obwohl noch reichlich ungelesene, leichte Lektüre zur Auswahl stand (*327*).

Aus den Isolierungs-Versuchen wird geschlossen, daß das Hirn auch bei sehr geringer Afferenz und Efferenz nicht einfach seine Aktivität einstellt, sondern im Gegenteil Energie kumuliert, die zur Entladung drängt (*518*). Diese Vorstellung kann man neurophysiologisch, informationstheoretisch, libido-theoretisch oder — wie wir schon zu Beginn zeigten — ethologisch formulieren. Jede Formulierung kann neue Aspekte liefern, sie kann aber auch zum Dogma werden, wenn sie nicht empirisch nachprüfbar ist. Der junge GOLGI bekannte sich vor bald 100 Jahren zu einer Psychiatrie, die auf den Funktionen des Nervensystems aufbaut. Nur dadurch laufe die Psychiatrie keine Gefahr, eine Pseudowissenschaft zu bleiben. Die Geisteskrankheiten seien auch nach anatomischen und zoologischen Prinzipien zu systematisieren (*640*).

Wir wollen im folgenden zweiten Teil einen Eindruck davon geben, was über die Hirnorganisation triebhaften Verhaltens bekannt ist.

B. Gehirnorganisation und triebhaftes Verhalten

I. Hirnstruktur, Hirnphysiologie und emotionales Verhalten

1. Zwischenhirn und Mittelhirn

a) Experimentelle Grundlagen triebhaften Verhaltens

Wir beschränken uns auf solche experimentellen Ergebnisse, die triebhaftes Verhalten oder solchem Verhalten nahestehende vegetativ-motorische Äußerungen und Ausdrucksfunktionen zum Gegenstand haben. Dabei sollen in diesem Abschnitt fast ausschließlich die Untersuchungen von W. R. HESS (*76, 77*) und seinen Mitarbeitern Berücksichtigung finden, weil diese Ergebnisse wegen der einheitlich angewandten Reiz-, Ausschaltungs- und Lokalisationstechnik bei ein und demselben Versuchstier (Katzen) unter sich vergleichbar sind. Andere Experimente kommen erst in den folgenden Kapiteln zur Sprache.

Da das bewundernswürdige Lebenswerk von HESS leicht zuganglich ist und sowohl in monographischer Form (1954; dort auch Auseinandersetzung mit Ergebnissen anderer Autoren) als auch in knapper Gestalt eines Atlas (1956) mit vollstandiger Bibliographie vorliegt, können wir auf die Darstellung der Versuchstechnik, auf die Dokumentation der Lokalisationen und im allgemeinen auch auf Literaturhinweise verzichten. Auf Abb. 17, S. 369, ist in vereinfachter Form die Lokalisation der Reizpunkte schematisch eingezeichnet, von denen aus die meisten der im folgenden besprochenen Verhaltensweisen induziert werden konnen. Zur Orientierung dient außerdem Abb. 19, S. 371, in der speziell die Affektreaktionen symbolisiert sind, und Abb. 26, S. 382, als topographisch-schematische Übersicht.

Eine für den Verhaltensphysiologen wertvolle, zusammenschauende Darstellung hat E. v. HOLST (*86*) 1958 gegeben, worin er die Ergebnisse von HESS zugleich für seine eigenen Hirnstamm-Reizversuche an Huhnern (*416, 417*) nutzbar macht[1]. Eine lebendige Diskussion der HESSschen Ergebnisse ist weiterhin anlaßlich eines Symposiums uber das Zwischenhirn (*79*)

---

[1] Über diese Versuche liegt inzwischen ein ausführlicherer Bericht vor (*417*), in dem neue Anschauungen uber das „Wirkungsgefuge der Triebe" entwickelt werden; naheres s. bei R. JUNG, ds. Bd. Teil A.

zustande gekommen, an dem Physiologen, Neurologen, Psychiater und andere medizinische Fachvertreter teilnahmen (s. auch das Symposium: Brain Mechanisms and Consciousness 1954) (*35*).

Seit 1925 hat W. R. Hess in bisher unerreichter Vollständigkeit viele Orte des Zwischenhirns und benachbarter Zonen elektrisch gereizt bzw. ausgeschaltet, das so erzielte Verhalten im Film festgehalten und die Reizorte bzw. Defekte durch histologische Schnittserien lokalisiert. Abgesehen von den uns hier besonders in-

teressierenden Studien über das Instinktverhalten soll wenigstens erwähnt werden, daß Hess durch seine Reizversuche schon 1931 das heute von anglo-amerikanischer Seite (*92, 137, 181, 528*) gründlich bearbeitete Projektionssystem aus Thalamus und Formatio reticularis entdeckt hat. Die späteren Untersuchungen über die elektrophysiologischen Wirkungen dieses Systems auf die Hirnrinde bedeuten eine Bestätigung und Ergänzung der Hessschen Konzeption einer vegetativ-diencephalen Beeinflussung des Cortex (*407*).

Eine Fülle diencephal auslösbarer Bewegungsakte bezieht sich auf *Ernährung und Säuberung*, z. B. sind rhythmisch-automatische *Leckbewegungen* hauptsächlich von Punkten im mittleren Thalamus zu erzielen. Die Reizpunkte ziehen sich bis in pericommissurale und septale Regionen hinauf und korrespondieren dann mehr mit einem *Kau-Leck-Automatismus*, teils mit Herausschleudern der Zunge, und schließlich tritt eine Kau-Leck-Bewegung auf, die so aussieht, als wolle das Tier etwas Störendes aus dem Maul befördern.

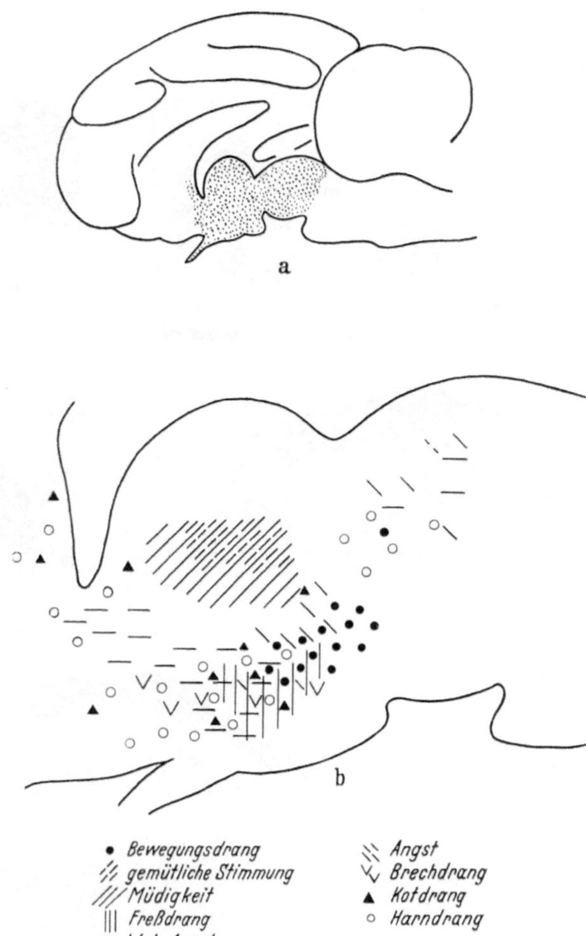

Abb. 17a u. b. *Verhaltensweisen, die durch elektrische Reizung des Zwischenhirns ausgelöst werden.* a Katzenhirn schematisch; die von W. R. Hess gereizte Gegend des Stammhirns ist schraffiert. b Die gleiche Hirngegend stärker vergrößert. Durch die eingetragenen Symbole sind die Orte und die von dort aus hervorgerufenen verschiedenen Stimmungen gekennzeichnet. [Nach W. R. Hess, durch v. Holst (*416*) etwas vereinfacht]

Wie wir im nächsten Kapitel sehen werden, gibt es auch bei Reizung im Hippocampus und im mediobasalen Cortex einen Leck-Automatismus mit feiner nuancierten Bewegungen. In engem funktionalen und lokalisatorischen Zusammenhang mit dem Lecken steht die *Fellreinigung*, eine Verhaltensweise, die stark von der Umweltsituation abhängig ist und daher leicht überdeckt wird. Dieses Verhalten scheint wie das *Schnurren* zum *triebbedingten Ruheverhalten* (s. S. 344) zu gehoren und hat lokalisatorische Beziehungen zur somnogenen Zone im unteren Anteil des mittleren Thalamus. Ist es einmal im Gange, kann es — ähnlich dem durch Reizung induzierten Fressen und Schlafen — den Reizschluß erheblich überdauern (*409*).

Der durch Reizung im basalen Hypothalamus ausgelöste *Freßtrieb* zeigt sich besonders schön an einer satten Katze. Das gierige Fressen und Trinken setzt nach

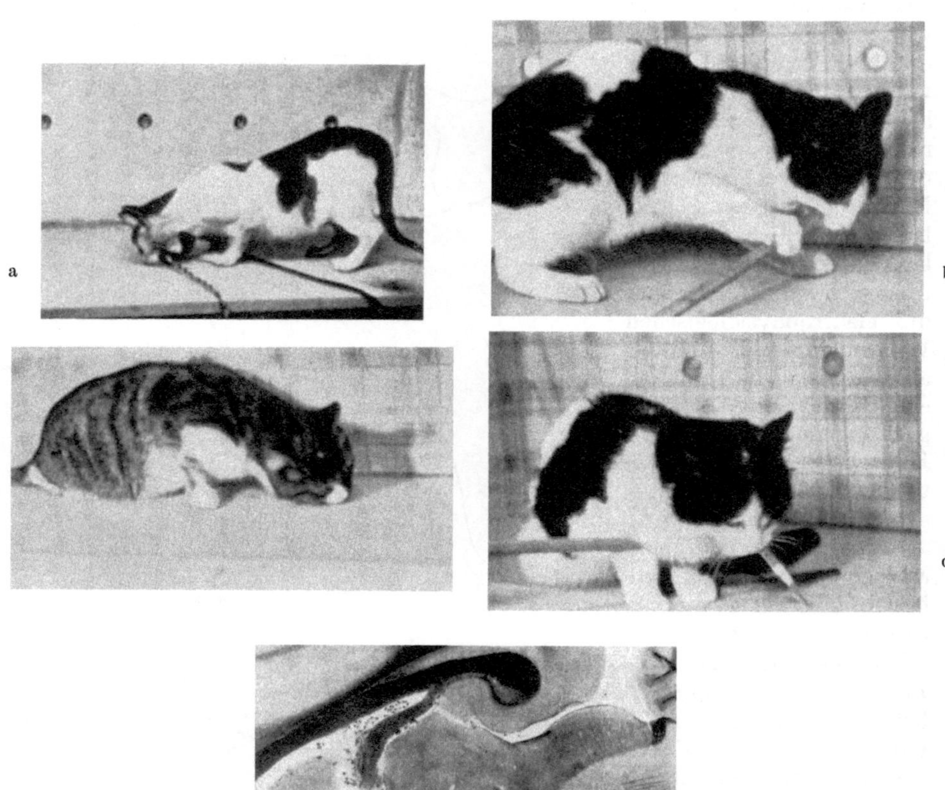

Abb 18a—e. *Freßtrieb*. Das vorher ruhige Tier außert wahrend und im Anschluß an die Reizung ein triebhaftes Anbeißen und Benagen ungenießbarer Gegenstande (a, b, d) Ein hingeworfenes Fleischstuck wird mit Gier verschlungen (c). Vorher verschmahte Milch leckt die Katze eifrig auf *Lokalisation* e Caudaler Hypothalamus, unterhalb der Zone der affektiven Abwehrreaktion (s. Abb 19 u 20), z. T sich mit dieser uberschneidend. Die mit a, b, d gekennzeichneten Orte beziehen sich auf gleichartige, nicht abgebildete Reizeffekte. [Nach W. R HESS (77)]

längerer Latenzzeit ein und kann erheblich länger als der Reiz anhalten. Der induzierte Trieb kann so stark sein, daß es gar nicht erst zur Kontrolle durch den Geruchs- oder Tastsinn kommt. Sogar für die Ernährung untaugliche Gegenstände werden ins Maul genommen und bekaut, wenn sich nichts anderes bietet (Abb. 18). Von caudal anschließenden Reizpunkten läßt sich ein unruhiges Umhersuchen auslösen. Nach Ausschaltungsversuchen anderer Autoren (*90, 431, 563*) ist für die Appetitregulation der ventromediale und laterale Hypothalamuskern verantwortlich (s. Abb. 26, S. 382).

Die variabelsten Instinktbewegungen, die vom Zwischenhirn aus zu aktivieren sind, entsprechen den Stimmungen von *Wut und Angst, Gemütlichkeit und Müdigkeit.*

In affektive *Wut-Angst-Stimmung (408, 423)* gerät die Katze bei Reizung von zusammenhängenden Strukturen grauer Substanz in einem Gebiet, welches sich von der intermediären Zone der Area praeoptica und des vorderen Hypothalamus über den hinteren Hypothalamus bis ins zentrale Höhlengrau des Mittelhirns erstreckt (Abb. 19). Innerhalb dieses Gebietes können zwei zentrale Zonen größter Reizempfindlichkeit abgegrenzt werden, von denen aus mit schwellennaher Reizung eine *affektive Abwehrreaktion,* charakterisiert durch Fauchen, Anlegen der Ohren, starke Pupillendilatation, Haarsträuben und Andeutung von Katzenbuckel, zu erhalten ist (Abb. 20, S. 372). Die eine dieser Zonen liegt perifornical im vorderen Hypothalamus, die andere im mittleren Abschnitt des zentralen Höhlengraus des Mittelhirns (Abb. 19). In dem diese Zonen umgebenden Reizgebiet erhält man bei schwellennaher Reizung eine einfache *Flucht-Reaktion* oder ein *Flucht-Abwehr-Verhalten.* Die Art der Reaktion richtet sich danach, ob der Fluchtweg versperrt ist oder nicht. Behinderung der Flucht kann zu Fauchen führen. Bei Reizung in der hypothalamischen Zone ist die Latenzzeit für das Fauchen größer, das *orientierende Umherschauen* vor der Flucht und das *gezielte Angreifen* ausgeprägter. Bei starker Reizung im Bereich der zentralen Zonen

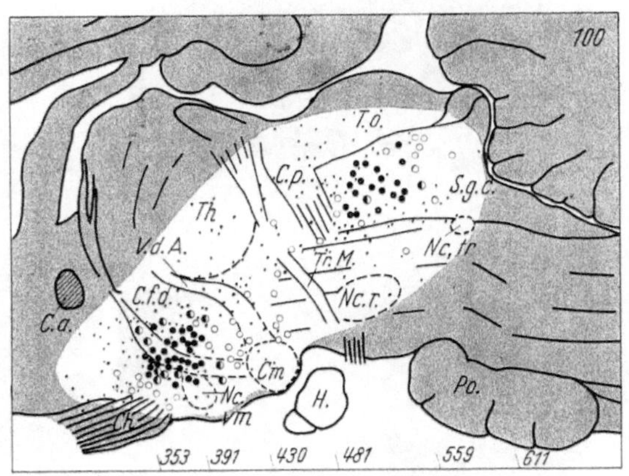

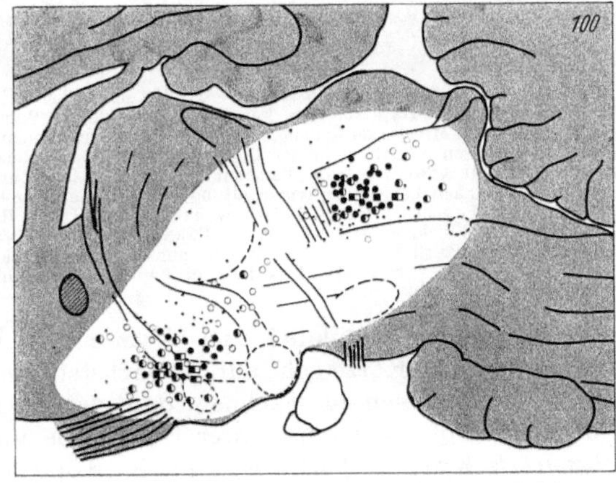

Abb. 19. *Affektreaktionen im Zwischen- und Mittelhirn* (schematische Darstellung der Reizstellen auf paramedianem Sagittalschnitt, HESSsche Leitserie: S. 100). Reizstellen sind von maximal 1 mm mehr medial oder mehr lateral auf Sagittalschnitt 100 projiziert. Bezeichnung der Strukturen s. unten. ● affektive Abwehrreaktion, ◗ Fluchtreaktion; ○ Flucht mit Abwehr; ■ Angriffsreaktion; ▣ Schreckreaktion oder alternierendes Auftreten von Angriffs- und Schreckreaktion; ● negative Reizstellen. Oben: Schwache Reizung 0,75—1,5 Volt, 8,5 sec Zwei zentrale Zonen· Affektive Abwehrreaktion. Eine periphere Zone: Fluchtreaktion. Unten: Starke Reizung 1,5 bis 3 Volt, 8,5 sec oder 1,5 Volt, 17/sec. Ausdehnung des Reizgebietes und Weiterentwicklung der Reaktionen. *C. a.:* Commissura anterior; *C. f d.:* Columna fornicis descendens; *C. m.:* Corpus mamillare; *C. p.:* Commissura posterior; *Ch.:* Chiasma; *H.:* Hypophyse; *Nc om ·* Nucleus oculomotorius, *Nc. r.:* Nucleus ruber, *Nc. tr.:* Nucleus trochlearis; *Nc. vm.:* Nucleus ventromedianus hypothalami (Tuberkern); *Po.:* Pons; *S. g. c.:* Substantia grisea centralis mesencephali (zentrales Höhlengrau des Mittelhirns); *T. o:* Tectum opticum; *Th.:* Thalamus; *Tr. M.:* Tractus Meynert; *V. d'A.:* Tractus Vicq d'Azyr. [Nach HUNSPERGER (*423*)]

geht die affektive Abwehr nicht selten in *Angriff* über, der wiederum plötzlich in *Flucht* umschlagen kann. HUNSPERGER (*423*) hat eindeutig bewiesen,
daß die Zone im zentralen Höhlengrau des Mittelhirns nicht einfach den deszen-
dierenden neuronalen Weg des affektiv wirksamen Substrats im Hypothalamus
darstellt, sondern daß diesem Areal eine selbständige Wirkung innerhalb des im
Hirnstamm gelegenen Ursprungsgebietes für Affektreaktionen zukommt. Allerdings zeigen die Versuche, daß bei Reizung dieses Gebietes die Reaktionen der
Katzen weniger objektbezogen, aber schneller einsetzen. *Es scheint, daß die Integration der situationsbezogenen Leistung von caudal nach rostral zunimmt.* Dafür
werden wir im nächsten Kapitel noch Bestätigungen finden.

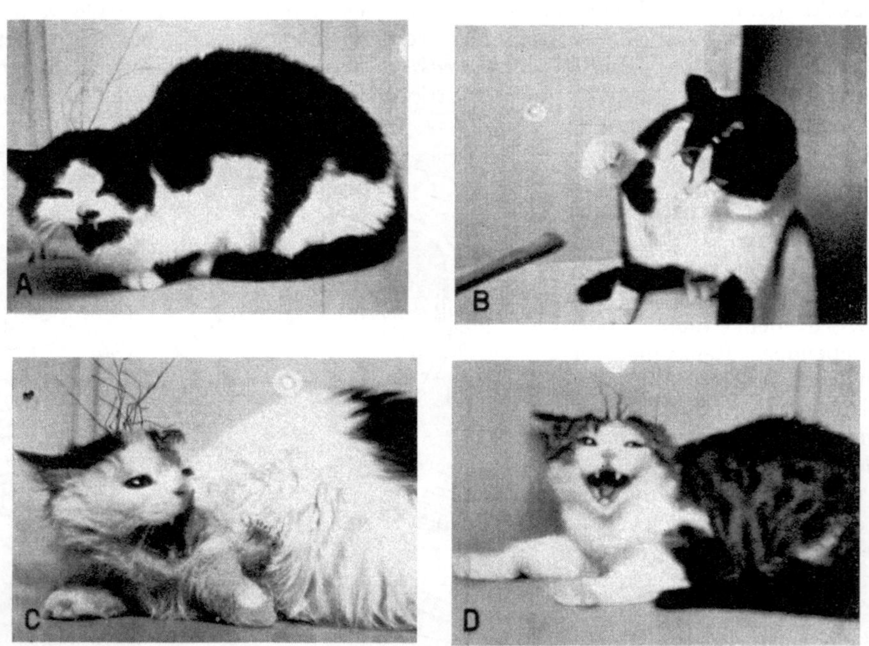

Abb. 20 A—D. *Abwehr- und Angriffsreaktionen.* A Mit schwacher Reizung erhaltene affektive Abwehrreaktion aus
der zentralen Zone des *Hypothalamus.* Fauchen, Buckelbildung, Piloerektion. Die Reaktion ist auf den Filmopera-
teur ausgerichtet. B Mit starker Reizung ausgeloste Angriffsreaktion aus der gleichen Zone Ausholen mit der Vorder-
pfote zum gezielten Angriff auf einen Stab. C Mit schwacher Reizung aus der zentralen Zone des *Mittelhirns*
erhaltene affektive Abwehrreaktion. Fauchen, Pupillendilatation, Zurucklegen der Ohren, Piloerektion. D Affektive
Abwehrreaktion nach beidseitiger Ausschaltung der zentralen Zone im Hypothalamus und Reizung in derjenigen
des Mittelhirns Fauchen, Anlegen der Ohren, Piloerektion. [Nach HUNSPERGER (*423*)]. Weitere Untersuchungen
zur Abwehr- und Fluchtreaktion wurden von FERNANDEZ DE MOLINA und HUNSPERGER (*344*) durchgefuhrt. Danach wird Abwehrverhalten auf drei Ebenen zunehmender funktionaler Bedeutung integriert, namlich durch
Amygdala, Hypothalamus und zentrales Hohlengrau des Mittelhirns

    Gleichsam spiegelbildlich zur abweisenden Aggression steht die *zutrauliche
Annäherung.* Die Katze geht auf die nächststehende Person zu, schnurrt und gibt
durch ihr Benehmen zu erkennen, daß man sie streicheln und kraulen soll. Sie
reibt den Kopf am Objekt ihrer Sympathie und zeigt ein Verhalten, das als
Schmeicheln bezeichnet wird und durch „Köpfchen-Geben", Flanken-Reiben und
steile Schwanzstellung charakterisiert ist. Schon unter natürlichen Bedingungen
ist es schwer, die sexuelle Werbephase der weiblichen Katze von nicht sexuell
orientiertem Schmeicheln zu unterscheiden (*126, 127, 509*). *Schmeicheln und Sexualverhalten* sind jedenfalls eng miteinander verwandt. Im gesamten Material von
HESS finden sich nur 10 Beobachtungen über reizbedingte Symptome des Sexualverhaltens und der Schmeichelstimmung, Symptome männlichen Sexual-

verhaltens wurden überhaupt nicht beobachtet. Die zur Auslösung verwendeten
Reizspannungen sind niedrig und die Latenzzeiten lang. Oft wird die Wirkung
erst nach Reizschluß sichtbar und besonders dann, wenn vorher nach stärkerer
Reizdosierung u. a. affektive Abwehr und offensives Verhalten beobachtet worden
waren (vgl. dazu S. 390). Reproduzierbarkeit der Symptome ist nur ausnahmsweise möglich und die Dauer dieser Instinkthandlungen kürzer als andere schon
beschriebene. Die Schmeichelstimmung scheint noch leichter unterdrückbar zu
sein als die der Fellreinigung.

Sieht man sich die Lokalisationen für das Schmeicheln an, so finden sich
einige nahe der Massa intermedia des Thalamus und in unmittelbarer Nachbarschaft zum Tractus mamillo-thalamicus oder zum Tractus habenulo-peduncularis.
Andere Reizstellen finden sich im Septum und ebenso viele im Stria-terminalis-
Bett (566); zur Orientierung vgl. Abb. 19, S. 371, und Abb. 26, S. 382. Wir werden
später sehen, daß es sich hier um das Ansprechen von Faserzügen handelt, die mit
dem limbischen System (s. S. 383) zusammenhängen.

Beachtenswert ist, daß eine größere Zahl dieser Reizpunkte in der unmittelbaren Nähe des unteren Teiles der Massa intermedia liegt, also in Beziehung zur
somnogenen Zone[1], innerhalb derer mit einiger Latenz, mit niedrigen Spannungen
und nach mehrfachen umstimmenden Reizungen mit Zwischenpausen der *natürliche Schlaf* induziert werden kann: Die Katze beginnt zu blinzeln, schließt mit
Unterbrechungen die Augen, die Nickhaut kommt allmählich nach vorne, und die
Pupillen werden eng. Schließlich schläft das Tier ein. HESS hat viel Mühe darauf
verwandt, um gegenüber anderen Autoren zweifelsfrei zu beweisen, daß nur in
diesem Gebiet des unteren Thalamus *echter* Schlaf auszulösen ist und nicht im
Hypothalamus, wie im Zusammenhang mit Ausschaltungsversuchen und unter
anderen pathologischen Bedingungen mehrfach behauptet worden ist (403). Die
auch für die Verhaltensforschung wichtige Physiologie und Pathologie des Schlafes
wurde andernorts (159, 212) zusammenfassend dargestellt[2]. Wir wollen uns hier
mit einigen Feststellungen begnügen, die für das *triebbedingte Ruheverhalten*
(s. S. 344) von Bedeutung sind. Daß es sich um natürlichen Schlaf bzw. um ein
zwar reizbedingtes, aber *physiologisches Einschlafen* handelt, beweisen zunächst
die Verhaltensweisen bis zum Eintritt des Schlafes: Gelegentliches Schnurren,
Gähnen und andere vegetativ-motorische Anzeichen von Müdigkeit, wie z. B.
Vorrücken der Nickhaut, Aufsuchen einer bequemen Stellung u. a. Weitere
Beweise wurden durch corticale, thalamische und andere subcorticale hirnelektrische Ableitungen der natürlichen Schlafpotentiale erbracht (410, 481). Der
induzierte Schlaf überdauert einerseits den Reizschluß ganz erheblich, andererseits ist er reversibel, d. h. Sinnesreize führen zum Erwachen. Hält man der
schlafenden Katze ein Stück rohes Fleisch vor die Nase, so schickt sie sich rasch
dazu an, das Stück zu fressen, selbst wenn sie sich danach aufrichten muß, um
dann alsbald wieder einzuschlafen (Abb. 21, S. 374). Charakteristisch ist ferner,

---

[1] Zur somnogenen Zone gehören die Kerne der Lamella medialis, der Nucl. parafascicularis
und das Centre médian. Dies sind Stammhirnanteile, d. h. sie bleiben auch nach Rindenabtragung erhalten und funktionsfähig (386, 387).

[2] Inzwischen hat JOUVET bei Katzen ein zweites Schlafsteuerungssystem entdeckt, das
in der Formatio reticularis pontis gelegen ist. Die rhombencephale Schlafphase führt zu einer
völligen Erschlaffung des Muskeltonus und ist von einem schnellen corticalen EEG-Rhythmus
begleitet. JOUVET nennt diesen Schlaf „Archisleep" und nimmt Abhängigkeit von neurohumoralen Mechanismen an.— Durch systematische extracellulare Einzelzellableitungen im
akuten (CREUTZFELDT u. JUNG) und chronischen Tierversuch (EVARTS) beginnt jetzt auch
Licht in die Frage zu kommen, welche neuronalen Veränderungen dem geheimnisvollen
Phänomen des Schlafes tatsächlich zugrunde liegen. — Biochemische Untersuchungen am
schlafenden Menschen (S. S. KETY) zeigen einen leichten Anstieg der cerebralen Durchblutung
und einen arteriellen Anstieg des Kohlendioxyddruckes (212).

daß ein Kitzeln der Ohrmuschel wie bei der wachen und auch normal schlafenden
Katze mit dem bekannten Abwehrreflex, dem kurzen, raschen Vibrieren der Ohrmuschel, beantwortet wird. Zum experimentellen Einschlafen gehört außerdem
eine Umgebung, die das Tier nicht stört; z. B. verhindert eine nasse Unterlage das
Wiedereinschlafen, und vorher aufgeregte Tiere schlafen erst nach Beruhigung ein.
Bei Überschreitung einer bestimmten Reizintensität schlägt die einschläfernde
Wirkung ins Gegenteil um. Die schlafende Katze wird geweckt und unter Umständen sogar erregt, vermutlich als Folge der Aktivierung des unspezifisch aktivierenden Systems der Formatio reticularis des Mittelhirns.

Die enge Beziehung zwischen Funktion und Lokalisation, die sich aus den
Untersuchungen über die Fellreinigung, das Schmeicheln, Schnurren und Einschlafverhalten ergibt, verdient großes triebphysiologisches Interesse, sehen wir

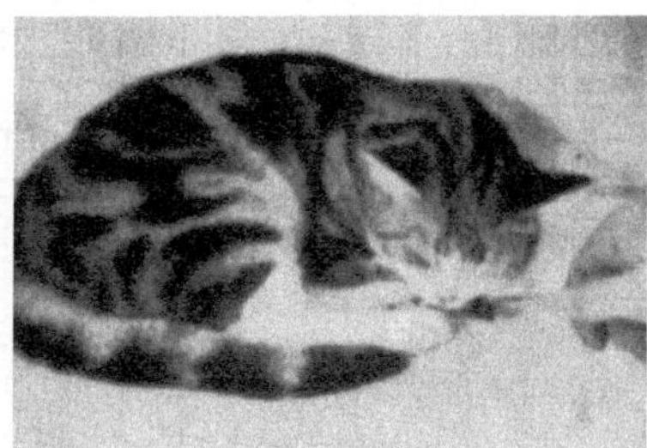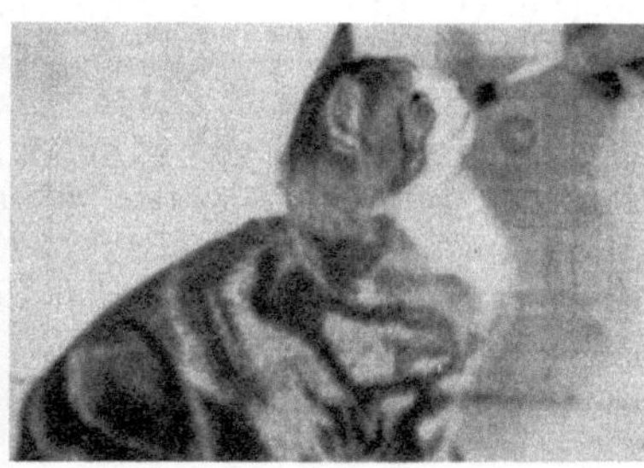

Abb. 21. *Induzierter Schlaf.* Links· Die Katze hat sich als Folge vorangegangener Reizung (lateral der Massa
intermedia) in typische Schlafstellung begeben. Rechts: Jetzt wird ihr Fleisch vor die Nase gehalten. Der Geruch
des Futters wirkt als ausgesprochener Weckreiz, die Katze erhebt sich und läßt sich futtern. Hernach legt sie sich
wieder nieder und schlaft weiter. [Nach W. R. HESS (*76*)]

doch daraus, daß sich „Triebe" nicht stets nur in Verhaltensweisen zeigen, die
sich auf äußere Objekte richten (z. B. Aggression, Nahrungssuche, Annäherung,
Paarungsverhalten) oder diese meiden (z. B. Verteidigung, Abwehr, Flucht),
sondern daß diese „Triebe" ihr notwendiges Gegenstück im gleichermaßen triebbedingten Ruhesuchen haben (s. S. 363). Die Ablösung des Interesses von der
Umwelt wird erstrebt, und dieser Zustand bringt, wenn er erreicht ist, Befriedi-
gung. Man kann in diesem Sinne durchaus von extratensivem und introversivem
Instinktverhalten sprechen. Dabei ist bedeutsam, daß das Sexualverhalten oder
auch die nicht sexuell gefärbte Annäherung am leichtesten störbar ist und auf der
„Stimmungs-Skala" extratensiv-introversiv gerade in der Mitte zu stehen scheint.
Sicher ist es eine Simplifizierung, wenn Sexualverhalten so häufig schlechtweg mit
Aggression gleichgesetzt wird. Agressions- und Sexualverhalten oder Flucht- und
Sexualverhalten oder auch alle drei können zu *einer* Stimmung (s. S. 334f.) integriert sein, müssen es aber nicht. In diesem Zusammenhang haben wir mehrfach
die Ansicht vertreten, daß das Schlafen am äußersten Pol introversiver Gestimmtheit steht und als Verhaltensweise — so paradox dies klingen mag — zu bewerten
ist, nämlich als extremes *Sich-nicht-Verhalten,* das in der besonders für Säugetiere
jeweils typischen Schlafhaltung geradezu Ausdruckscharakter gewinnt (*649, 655*).

Wir legen auf den Schlaf als Instinkt (*197, 649*) so großen Wert, weil der Mensch
diese Verhaltensweise am augenfälligsten mit den übrigen Säugetieren gemeinsam
hat. So darf man denn auch die Schlafexperimente an Katzen im Prinzip auf den
Menschen übertragen, wie Ergebnisse anläßlich stereotaktischer Hirnoperationen
zeigen (*388, 441*).

Die These der Ethologie, daß Handelnsbereitschaft und Gestimmtheit,
Instinkthandlung und Stimmung einander entsprechen, kann durch HESS' Versuche glänzend gestützt werden. Ohne auf funktionale und lokalisatorische

Einzelheiten eingehen zu können, sei auf die *enge Verflechtung der Motorik mit diencephal ausgelösten vegetativen Symptomen und triebhaften Reaktionen* hingewiesen. Jüngst noch haben HASSLER und HESS dies an Dreh- und Wendebewegungen gezeigt (*389*). Wie eng schließlich *Ausdrucksbewegungen mit triebhaften Reaktionen* verknüpft sind, geht aus den wiedergegebenen Abbildungen dieses Kapitels genügend hervor. Dabei können bei Säugetieren auch solche Verrichtungen wie Kot- und Harnentleerung — beides diencephal induzierbar — Ausdrucksfunktionen haben, wie die Verhaltensforschung z. B. für die „Duftmarken" (s. S. 332, 344) gezeigt hat. Wie sehr diese Verrichtungen bei Kleinkindern noch Ausdrucksfunktion und für größere Kinder noch Ausdruckscharakter haben, ist den Entwicklungspsychologen gut bekannt.

b) Psychiatrische Bemerkungen

W. R. HESS hat schon 1924 auf die Beziehungen zwischen psychischen und vegetativen Funktionen hingewiesen und deren Bedeutung für die endogenen Psychosen betont (*402*).

Betrachtet man die endogenen Psychosen einmal unabhängig von der speziellen Diagnose gemeinsam unter dem Gesichtspunkt pathologischer Stimmungen, so kann man einerseits nach Art der Ethologie die Ausdrucksqualitäten und das affektive Verhalten auch hinsichtlich der Umweltverschränkung beobachten und andererseits die Stimmung bzw. den pathologischen Stimmungswechsel physiologisch zu erfassen versuchen.

Beginnen wir wieder mit dem Schlaf (*159, 212*). Im Zusammenhang mit den HESSschen Versuchen hat R. JUNG (*79, 439, 440*) auf die Beziehung zwischen Schlaf und Affekt und deren Bedeutung für die manisch-depressiven Erkrankungen hingewiesen. Das Sich-in-den-Schlaf-Bringen ist ein Instinktverhalten (*655*). Das Nicht-Schlafen-Können — hartnäckig wie es in der Depression und mindestens auch in den Prodromalstadien der Schizophrenie nun einmal ist — ist eine Störung dieses Verhaltens, eine Verstimmung. Oft genug sehen wir einen komplexen Bedingungszusammenhang zwischen depressiv-psychotischer oder erregt-psychotischer Verstimmung und Schlafstörung. Im Elektroschock-Experiment kann es gelingen, psychotische Verstimmung und Schlafstörung gemeinsam zu beseitigen. Setzt man in der Psychose einen Testreiz mit einem Sympathicomimeticum (Sympatol), bekommt man eine andere Reaktion des diencephal gesteuerten Blutdrucks als in equilibrierter Stimmung mit tiefem Nachtschlaf (Abb. 22). Das Beispiel zeigt den Bedingungszusammenhang von psychischem Befinden, Schlaffunktion und physiologischer Stimmung des Organismus. Derartige klinische Beobachtungen sind mit den HESSschen Ergebnissen in guten Einklang zu bringen (*649, 658*).

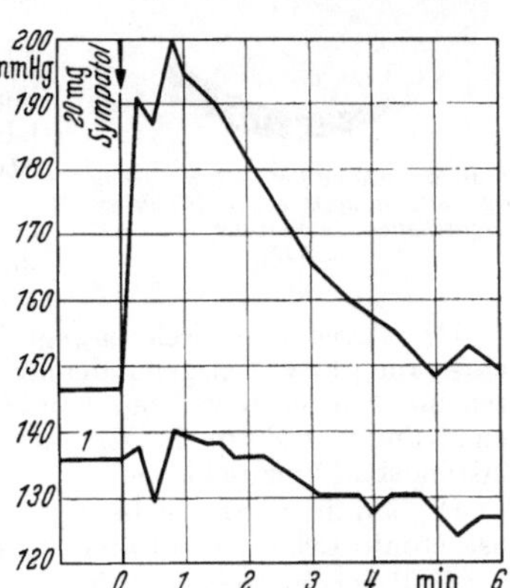

Abb. 22. *Agitiert depressive Verstimmung.* Blutdruckverhalten auf jeweils 20 mg Sympatol intravenös. Kurve *1* vor der Umstimmung während wochenlang anhaltender schwerer Schlafstörung; Kurve *2* nach der Umstimmung (*1* Elektroschock) und darauffolgendem tiefen Nachtschlaf (*649*)

Analysiert man mit psychopathologischen Mitteln den Wandel der Stimmungen in akuten Psychosen, so lassen sich aus der Mannigfaltigkeit psychotischen Erlebens und Handelns bestimmte, immer wiederkehrende Extremvarianten menschlicher Handelns-(und Erlebens-)bereitschaften herausarbeiten (*647*).

Wir greifen auf den Begriff der Stimmungshierarchie zurück (s. S. 364). Der kleine dunkle Kreis (Abb. 23) in der Mitte soll die hochintegrierte Stimmungshierarchie des nicht psychotischen Menschen darstellen. Ihm ist in diesem equilibrierten Zustand von allen Lebewesen die größte Handlungsfreiheit gegeben. Spezifische Handelnsbereitschaften treten nicht in Erscheinung und können, soweit sie sich bemerkbar machen (z. B. Nahrungs-, Schlaf-, Liebesbegehren, soziale Kontaktsuche, Aggression, Aversion, Scheu, Flucht usw.), unterdrückt, verändert oder angepaßt ausgelebt werden. Die sich aus diesem Kreis herausdrehende Spirale deutet das zunehmende Aus-den-Fugen-Geraten der Stimmungshierarchie an. Mehr und mehr treten spezifische Handelnsbereitschaften hervor, womit eine Primitivierung des Handlungsgefüges und eine Vereinheitlichung sonst differenzierter Erlebnisse verbunden ist (s. S. 351). Auf diese Weise kann es zu spezifischen, „exzentrischen", Stimmungen (= Handelnsbereitschaften) kommen, die das Wesen der Psychose ausmachen. Je tiefere „Schichten" der Persönlichkeit bei diesem Desintegrierungsprozeß (s. S. 363) ergriffen werden, desto stärker drängen sich triebhafte und angeborene Verhaltensweisen her-

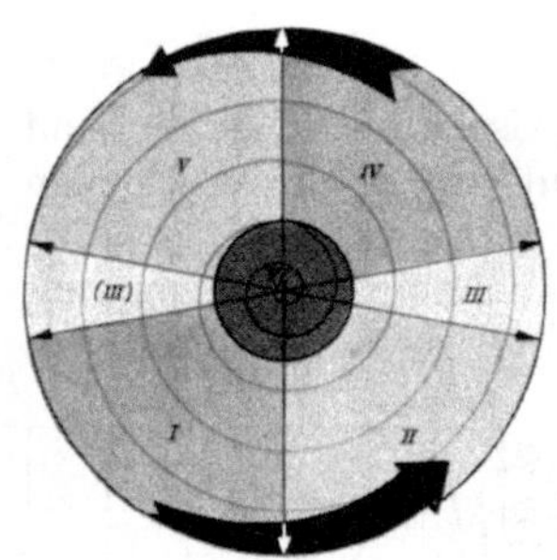

Abb. 23. *Schema für die Regulierung von Stimmungen bzw. Handelnsbereitschaften.* Erklärung im Text, *(647)*

vor (angedeutet durch die Pfeile im Kreisdurchmesser). Die an- und abschwellenden Pfeile auf der Kreisperipherie sollen Zustände der psychomotorischen und psychischen Spannung symbolisieren. Die Sektoren I—V kennzeichnen spezifische Stimmungen bzw. Handelnsbereitschaften, die durch reine Verhaltensbeobachtung erfaßt werden können. Mit anderen Worten: Es wird aus dem Verhalten, der Psychomotorik und dem Ausdruck auf die Stimmung geschlossen, ohne daß Erlebensqualitäten in die Klassifizierung eingehen.

I. Psychomotorische Ruhe und Spannungslosigkeit, „eingefrorener" Ausdruck, Umweltverschränkung aufgehoben (kontaktlos). Dem Ausdruck nach unlustbetonte Erlebnisqualitäten. Klinisches Musterbeispiel: Depressiver Stupor.

II. Psychomotorisch bewegt bis erregt, ausdrucksreich, eingleisige Umweltverschränkung mit geringen Freiheitsgraden, unlustbetont, ängstlich. Klinisches Musterbeispiel: Depressiver Erregungszustand.

III. Psychomotorisch bewegt bis erregt, ausdrucksreich, wechselnd starke Umweltverschränkung bzw. Reizgebundenheit, Lachen und Weinen in raschem Wechsel, im Wettstreit stehende Antriebstendenzen, Konkurrenz von Aggressions- und Aversions- bzw. Fluchtverhalten. Klinisches Beispiel: Depressiver Erregungszustand, der im Begriff ist, in ein manisches Zustandsbild umzuschlagen.

IV. Psychomotorisch bewegt und erregt, ausdrucksreich, starke Umweltsverschränkung, lustbetonte Erlebnisqualitäten. Klinisches Beispiel: Manisches Zustandsbild.

V. Psychomotorisch einförmig bewegt, Verlust der Umweltverschränkung (kontaktlos). Klinische Beispiele: Motalitätspsychosen, halluzinatorische Zustandsbilder, motorische (und sprachliche) Stereotypien *(647)*.

Freilich ist eine solche Klassifizierung grob und unvollständig, aber sie reicht aus, um Stimmungen durch Verhaltensbeobachtung voneinander abzugrenzen. Dabei ist wichtig, sich gleichzeitig auch Rechenschaft darüber abzulegen, welche Handelnsbereitschaften damit *ausgeschlossen* sind, wenn eine bestimmte spezifische Stimmung besteht. Während der Gesunde in hochintegrierter Stimmung vergleichsweise volle Handlungsfreiheit besitzt, bleibt dem Psychotiker in spezifischer Gestimmtheit stets nur ein Sektor von Handlungs- und Erlebnismöglichkeiten übrig. Praktisch machen wir in der Psychiatrie von dieser Erkenntnis täglichen Gebrauch, wenn wir z. B. einzuschätzen haben, ob von einem Kranken aggressive Handlungen zu erwarten sind, ob er sich selbst gefährlich ist, wie er eine — ihn normalerweise wahrscheinlich erschütternde — Nachricht aufnehmen wird usw. Im Vergleich dazu können wir bei Kenntnis der Stimmung eines Tieres ebenfalls Aussagen über seine Handelnsbereitschaften machen. Je intimer die Kenntnis der Ausdrucksbewegungen, desto präziser die Aussage über die Wahrscheinlichkeit, mit der eine Handlung eintreten kann. LORENZ gibt dafür geradezu verblüffende Beispiele. Aber auch der ungeschulte Beobachter wird von einem fremden, ihn leckenden und wedelnd umspringenden Hund nicht erwarten, daß er ihn beißt. Laien als Besucher psychiatrischer Unruhigen-Abteilungen haben Angst vor fast jedem Patienten, während geschultes Pflegepersonal auf Grund genauerer Stimmungsbeurteilung gelassen bleibt.

Nach den Hessschen Untersuchungen ist zu erwarten, daß einer aus dem Verhalten ersichtlichen spezifischen Stimmung auch ein physiologisch von anderen Stimmungen unterscheidbarer Zustand entspricht. In dieser Beziehung wissen wir, was psychotische Stimmungen anbetrifft, noch nicht viel. Wir geben zwei Beispiele, die zeigen sollen, daß der hier verwandte verhaltensphysiologische Begriff der Stimmung — nämlich ein psychophysiologisch definierbarer Zustand — auch für psychotische Verstimmungen zutrifft (Abb. 24 u. Abb. 25).

Wieder verwenden wir sympathicomimetische, standardisierte Testreize (Sympatol) in verschiedenen spezifischen Stimmungen während des Verlaufes einer Psychose. Die jeweiligen Umstimmungen werden durch den Elektroschock erzwungen.

In Abb. 24 sieht man auf dem oberen Abschnitt den psychopathologischen Verlauf einer Psychose eingetragen. Die waagerechte Linie symbolisiert die gedachte Normal-Stimmung. Auf der Senkrechten sind die um die Waagerechte schwankenden spezifischen Stimmungen eingetragen, die entsprechend unseren oben angegebenen Klassifizierungen unterschieden wurden (Katatonie im Stupor: I; im Erregungszustand: II; im „Wettstreit" bzw. in der Labilität: III; in der Euphorie: IV. Die obere Reihe von Pfeilen zeigt die Elektroschocks (3 Dreierblocks innerhalb von 3 Wochen), die untere Pfeilreihe die Zahl und zeitliche Verteilung

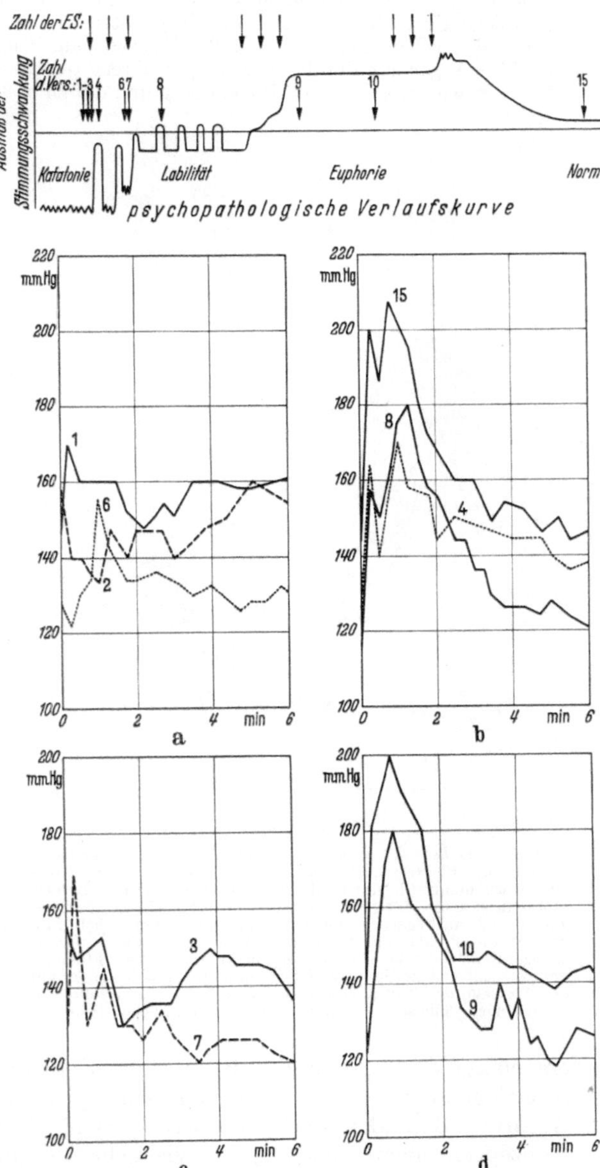

Abb. 24 a—d. *Psychophysiologische Umstimmungen im Verlaufe einer Elektroschockbehandlung.* Die Kurven a—d zeigen 10 verschiedene Blutdruckreaktionen auf jeweils 20 mg Sympatol intravenös. Die Nummern der Kurven entsprechen den Versuchen, die im Verlaufe der katatonen Psychose vorgenommen wurden, und sind oben auf der Verlaufskurve, die sich über 30 Tage erstreckt, in ihrer zeitlichen Reihenfolge eingetragen. Die Kriterien für das Ausmaß der Stimmungsschwankungen sind im Text angegeben. Die Kurven *1* und *2* wurden vor Beginn der ES-Behandlung gewonnen. Die Kurven *3* und *7* stammen von Messungen unmittelbar nach dem ES, die übrigen Kurven von Messungen vor dem jeweiligen ES. Die hier nicht eingezeichneten Kurven *11—14* fallen in den Reaktionsbereich zwischen den Kurven *9* und *10* (*648*)

der Testreize an. In den 4 Koordinatensystemen sind die Ergebnisse der Testreize eingetragen, wobei die Nummern der Kurven den Nummern der Testreizpfeile entsprechen. Ohne auf Einzelheiten einzugehen, sieht man klar die *sehr unterschiedlichen Blutdruckreaktionen auf den Standardreiz.* Die Untersuchungen von SLOANE u. a. im Anschluß an FUNKENSTEIN beweisen, daß solche Unterschiede auch statistisch bestehen (*751—754*). Im Stupor (Kurve 1—2 vor Beginn der ES-Behandlung) sind die Kurven ganz flach oder der sympathicomimetische Reiz führt sogar zur Blutdrucksenkung, während die Kurven im Zuge der Umstimmung eine größere Fläche zwischen Blutdruckanstieg und -abfall bestreichen (*648, 658*).

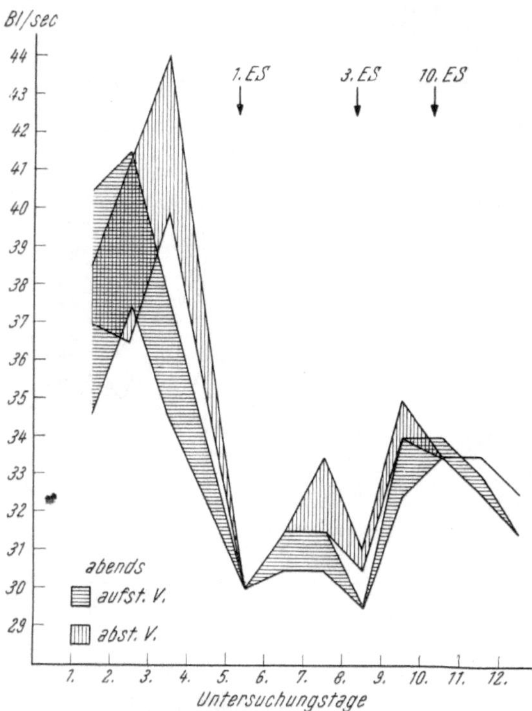

Abb. 25. *Wechsel der visuellen Flimmer-Verschmelzungsfrequenz* während der Elektroschockbehandlung als Ausdruck der zentralen Umstimmung. Die Ränder des waagerecht schraffierten Bandes repräsentieren die extremen Meßwerte von 9 Einzelmessungen bei zunehmend ansteigender Lichtblitzzahl (sog. Verschmelzungsgrenze), die Ränder des senkrecht schraffierten Bandes die entsprechenden Werte bei absteigender Lichtblitzzahl (sog. Flimmergrenze). Auf der Ordinate sind die Blitzreize pro Sekunde, auf der Abszisse die Untersuchungstage, über 7 Wochen verteilt, eingetragen. Klinische Diagnose: Involutionsdepression (*650*)

Zu dem gleichen Ergebnis, daß der psychischen Umstimmung eine physiologische entspricht, kommt man auch, wenn man die visuelle Flimmerverschmelzungsfrequenz im Laufe der ES-Behandlung verfolgt, wie auf Abb. 25 gezeigt wird. Die Verschmelzungsfrequenzen schwanken von Tag zu Tag stark und stabilisieren sich erst mit zunehmender Integration der Stimmung (*650*). Daß die Flimmerverschmelzungsfrequenz tatsächlich ein empfindlicher Indicator für die zentrale Erregungslage ist, zeigen neurophysiologische Untersuchungen mit Mikroelektroden im optischem Cortex (*224, 313, 376*). Wir konnten auch den Nachweis führen, daß nicht der Elektroschock, sondern die Psychose die spezifische Stimmung bedingt (*647, 648, 650, 658*). Diese psycho-physiologischen Ergebnisse besagen aber vorläufig nur,*daß* einer spezifischen Handelnsbereitschaft auch physiologisch gesehen eine spezifische Stimmung entspricht. Neurophysiologisch läßt sich vorläufig über die Beschaffenheit des physiologischen bzw. pathophysiologischen Zustandes nichts aussagen. Wir werden später zeigen, daß man mit Hilfe der intrakraniellen Selbstreizung diesem Problem näher kommt (s. S. 409).

W. R. HESS hat sich in den letzten Jahren mit den Beziehungen zwischen psychischen Vorgängen und der Organisation des Gehirnes auseinandergesetzt und auf der Basis seiner Experimente eine Psychophysiologie in Angriff genommen (*78*). In einem neuen psychophysischen Konzept kommt zum Ausdruck, daß „das psychische Geschehen in einer bloß energetisch orientierten Konzeption nicht aufgeht", daß vielmehr die „im Kräftegefüge zum Ausdruck kommende *Ordnung* den gemeinschaftlichen Nenner von neuronalem und psychischem Geschehen darstellt" (*404, 406*). „Ordnung ist weder Kraft, noch Energie, noch Stoff. Sie bedarf aber dieser, um sich zu manifestieren" (*406*). NORBERT WIENER (*206*) kommt zu einem grundsätzlich vergleichbaren Schluß: "Information is information, not matter or energy."

2. Das limbische System

a) Experimentelle Hirnläsionen und emotionales Verhalten

Die berühmten, aus dem Jahre 1870 stammenden, ersten elektrischen Hirnreizversuche von HITZIG (*81*), der seine Hunde aus Mangel an Arbeitsraum im Schlafzimmer operieren mußte, und seines großen Gegners GOLTZ' (1876) bahnbrechende Experimente mit großhirnlosen Hunden (*364, 365*) werden heute wenig beachtet. Sie stehen am Anfang eines Weges, der neuerdings zu internationalen Symposien führte, deren Gegenstand das Thema Hirnorganisation und Verhalten war (*35, 67, 92, 172, 181, 211*). Die deutsche Wissenschaft hat während der letzten 25 Jahre kaum noch Anteil an der Fortsetzung dieses Weges gehabt. Vornehmlich in den Laboratorien der angelsächsischen Länder ist ein experimentell fundiertes Werk entstanden, dessen Darstellung ein Handbuch für sich allein fordern würde (*61, 62*). Um überhaupt nur einiges zu erwähnen, denken wir an das Werk FULTONs und seiner Mitarbeiter (*56*) über die Verbindungen des Frontalhirnes und seine Beziehungen zum affektiven Verhalten, an die Studien von MAGOUN (*137, 138*) über das unspezifisch aktivierende System, von PENFIELD über den Temporallappen, das centrencephale System und die Bewußtseinsfunktion (*73, 630, 631, 633, 635—637*) oder die fundamentalen Arbeiten von KLÜVER über die vom Occipitallappen-System vermittelte „externe Homeostase" unserer Sehwelt (*161, 456, 458—462*). KLÜVERs erstmals 1933 erschienenes Buch „Behavior Mechanisms in Monkeys", wohl die gediegendste und umfassendste experimental-psychologische Arbeit mit Affen, ist in Deutschland kaum bekannt geworden (*107*).

Wir schenken nun jenen Ergebnissen besondere Aufmerksamkeit, die das emotionale Verhalten, seine Hirnorganisation und Hirnfunktion betreffen (*10, 115*). PAPEZ schrieb 1937 (*626*) eine sehr bekannt gewordene Arbeit, in der er eine vergleichend hirnanatomisch fundierte Theorie der emotionalen „Mechanismen" aufstellte, die sich in der Folgezeit als fruchtbar erwies und in zahlreichen Punkten ihre experimentelle Bestätigung fand. Das von ihm herausgestellte Funktionssystem, welches er sowohl für unsere Gefühlserlebnisse als auch für unseren Gefühlsausdruck verantwortlich machte, betraf den Hypothalamus, den Nucl. thalam. ant., den Gyrus cinguli, den Hippocampus und deren Verbindungen untereinander, also phylogenetisch alte Hirnteile der medio-basalen Hirnmittellinie. Der Kernpunkt seiner Theorie steht KLEISTs schon 1934 entwickelter Vorstellung (*105, 106*) nahe, daß das sog. Schmeck- und Riechhirn im Unterschied zu den anderen exteroceptiven Systemen nicht allein als exteroceptives, sondern auch als enteroceptives System anzusehen ist, das Zustände der Leibeshöhlen zur Wahrnehmung bringt.

Einige Monate vor PAPEZ' Publikation demonstrierte KLÜVER zusammen mit dem Chirurgen BUCY (*465*) vor der amerikanischen Physiologischen Gesellschaft im Film Ergebnisse, die die *zentrale Rolle von rhinencephalen Strukturen für das emotionale Verhalten* nahelegten. Den Affen wurden beiderseits Hippocampus, Uncus und Amygdalum, aber auch ein großer Teil des temporalen Neocortex (BRODMANNs Areae 20, 21 und 22) fortgenommen, und die Folge waren schwere Verhaltensstörungen, schwerer, als sie bis dahin durch vergleichbare Hirnoperationen an anderen Hirnteilen erzielt worden waren. Die Affen bekamen (*466*) eine „optische Agnosie"; sie nahmen alles ohne Unterschied in den Mund, um erst nach dieser Examinierung der Objekte Eßbares von nicht Eßbarem zu unterscheiden, so, als ob sie erst dann in der Lage seien, die Bedeutung des Gegenstandes zu erkennen. Gleich darauf begannen sie aber wieder und immer wieder dieselben ausrangierten, nicht eßbaren Gegenstände verschiedenster Art, ob es nun lebendige Schlangen, Faeces oder auf Papier gezeichnete Figuren waren, so intensiv wie eßbare Gegenstände zu untersuchen. Sie behandelten in dieser Form auch solche Objekte, deren Anblick präoperativ zu schweren emotionalen Reaktionen (Schreie, Flucht u. a.) geführt hatte. Dies Verhalten war nun aber nicht nur visuellen, sondern auch akustischen und taktilen Eindrücken gegenüber festzustellen. Alle wahrgenommenen Objekte wurden zuerst mit den Lippen berührt, in den Mund genommen, beleckt, sanft „bebissen" und an die Nasenlöcher gehalten. Selbst, wenn man den Tractus olfactorius beiderseits entfernte, änderten sich diese gänzlich das Verhalten beherrschenden *oralen Tendenzen* — bis auf das Beriechen — nicht. Die Tiere zeigten eine hochgradige visuelle Reizgebundenheit: Geradezu zwanghaft wendeten sie sich jedem Objekt unmittelbar nach seinem Auftauchen zu und nahmen oralen Kontakt (*466*).

Die Affen (9 männliche, 5 weibliche Rhesus-Affen, 1 männlicher Cebus- und 1 weiblicher Java-Affe) wurden Monate vor und nach der doppelseitigen Temporallappen-Operation beobachtet (*467*). Die umwälzende Veränderung des emotionalen Verhaltens der vorher kaum zähmbaren und sehr aggressiven Tiere war höchst eindrucksvoll: Die „wilden" Affektreaktionen schwanden dahin. Ob es nun Katzen, Hunde, Schlangen oder fremde Personen waren oder ein anderer Genosse, der sie gerade gebissen hatte, die Affen zeigten ihnen gegenüber keine emotionale Reaktion. Die Tiere, besonders die männlichen, wurden einige Wochen nach der Operation hypersexuell und betätigten sich onanierend, heterosexuell und homosexuell, die weiblichen Tiere sogar trotz der vor der Hirnoperation vorgenommenen Ovarektomie. Auch nahmen die Affen — abweichend von ihrer sonstigen Gewohnheit, nur Früchte zu fressen — allerlei denaturierte Fleischsorten in ungewohnten Quantitäten zu sich; sie ruminierten und kauten wieder.

Die *histologische Untersuchung* der Affenhirne mit den bilateralen Temporalhirn-Resektionen brachte ein Ergebnis, das die Theorie von Papez experimentell stützte. Es waren nämlich degeneriert: Der Fornix, und zwar so, daß die Faserdegeneration in der Septum-Gegend oder in den Corpora mamillaria endete, die vordere Commissur, die Stria terminalis, der Fasciculus uncinatus, der temporale Pulvinar-Anteil, Fasern, die durch das hintere Cingulum und durch den hinteren Anteil des Corpus callosum liefen, sowie temporo-olfactorische, cortico-tectale und cortico-nigrale Faserverbindungen. Auf die Degenerationen im Hor- und Sehsystem wollen wir hier nicht eingehen.

Klar ist jedenfalls, daß der von Papez geforderte „Neuronenkreis für Emotionen" (Hippocampus → Fornix → Corpora mamillaria → vorderer Thalamuskern → Gyrus cinguli → Cingulum → Hippocampus) in den Klüverschen Affenexperimenten unterbrochen wurde. Man kann die Verhaltensstörungen der Tiere nicht auf einfache oder kombinierte sensorische Defekte zurückführen. Andererseits beweisen die bis zu 7 Jahren nach der Operation durchgeführten Reaktions- und Leistungsprüfungen (*453—455*) klar, daß *keine Demenz* im Sinne einer Allgemeinstörung vorlag; denn die Affen waren in der Lage, neue Probleme zu lösen, und konnten neue bedingte Reaktionen auf Sinnesreize ausbilden. Selbst die höchste Form tierischer Intelligenz, nämlich der einsichtige Geräte- und Werkzeuggebrauch (*107*) war nicht gestört, so daß sich die Frage erhebt, wieso dann ein Affe, der sich so verhält, als ob er eßbare nicht von anderen Objekten, Harmloses nicht von Gefährlichem unterscheiden kann, doch in der Lage ist, auf der Stufe des Werkzeuggebrauches einsichtig zu handeln.

Um nur ein Beispiel für die Art dieser Intelligenzleistungen zu nennen: Der schlauste von Klüvers Affen — ein mannlicher Cebus, der nicht operiert wurde und kein „Klüver-Bucy-Syndrom" zeigte, bei dessen Hirnsektion sich aber eine beiderseitige, ausgedehnte Destruktion der Temporallappen einschließlich rhinencephaler Strukturen fand (infektioses Granulom) — wußte sich ohne fremde Hilfe dadurch Futter zu verschaffen, daß er nacheinander 3 Geräte einsetzte, um sein Ziel zu erreichen. Der Cebus war an der Leine, hatte aber Bewegungsraum genug, um auf eine Mauer zu klettern, wo ein großer Metallring in einer Schachtel lag. Mit dem Ring [1] konnte er sich einen außer Reichweite gelegenen Stock angeln; den Stock [2] benutzte er, um einen größeren Stock [3], der an der Wand hing, herunterzuschlagen, und dieser wiederum diente ihm dazu, das von der Decke herabhängende Futter zu erreichen (*108*). Das ist in dieser Beziehung eine hoher strukturierte Aufgabe, als sie Wolfgang Kohlers Schimpansen (*110, 482, 483*) zu losen vermochten. — (Vergleiche hinsichtlich anatomischer Befunde *301, 462*.)

Fassen wir das *Klüver-Bucy-Syndrom* kurz zusammen: Affen, denen man beide Temporallappen einschließlich Uncus, Amygdala und größere Hippocampus-Teile entfernt hat, verhalten sich so, als ob sie (1.) eine *optische Agnosie* hätten. Sie zeigen (2.) intensive *orale Tendenzen*, (3.) eine *extreme Reizgebundenheit*, (4.) einen ausgeprägten *Mangel an Angst und emotionalen Reaktionen* überhaupt,(5.) eine *Hypersexualität* und (6.) eine Veränderung der Futtergelüste (*463*).

Daß tatsächlich das Betroffensein rhinencephaler Strukturen für das Zustandekommen des Syndroms entscheidend ist, beweisen andere Ablationsexperimente am Temporallappen: Beiderseitige Entfernung nur der 1. Windung oder der 2. und 3. Windung oder beiderseitige Durchtrennung allein temporofrontaler oder temporo-occipitaler (*672*) Verbindungen können das Syndrom nicht hervorrufen (*467*).

Die Folge dieser bahnbrechenden Experimente war eine große Zahl von anatomischen, neurophysiologischen und Verhaltensuntersuchungen mit dem Ziel, die Bedeutung des Rhinencephalon, gerade auch in Verbindung mit dem seit W. R. HESS und P. BARD (*9, 240, 241*) besser bekannten Hypothalamus und Thalamus, hinsichtlich des Verhaltens näher kennenzulernen.

In den letzten Jahren hat man sich darum bemüht, das Klüver-Bucy-Syndrom aufzuschlüsseln, indem man die an seinem Zustandekommen beteiligten Hirnstrukturen einzeln zu lädieren versucht hat (*175, 373*). Vor allem galt es, die neocorticalen von den rhinencephalen Anteilen zu trennen. Zerstört man allein die neocorticalen (lateralen und inferioren) Anteile des Temporallappens, kommt es zu visuellen Störungen ohne emotionale Beteiligung (*338, 591, 592,684*, abweichend davon *222*), werden nur rhinencephale Anteile lädiert, sieht man ausschließlich emotionale Störungen, während perceptive fehlen (*166, 794, 797*). Im Anschluß an die Versuche von BARD und MOUNTCASTLE (*241*) gelang es anderen Untersuchern, isolierte Läsionen am Amygdaloid-Komplex durchzuführen (*299, 345, 348, 484, 591, 734, 794, 797, 798*).Untersucht wurden Luchse, Katzen, Hunde und Affen. Die meisten Tiere wurden zahm und zeigten nur noch geringe Reaktionen auf Angst und Wut erzeugende Reize, andere aber wurden wild-aggressiv, ohne daß Unterschiede im Ausmaß der Läsion gefunden werden konnten. Auch das Sexualverhalten war unterschiedlich. Viele, aber nicht alle Katzen entwickelten wie KLÜVERs Affen starke orale Tendenzen und eine markante Hypersexualität, die durch Kastration beseitigt und durch Hormon-Substitution wiederhergestellt werden konnte (*735*).Wurde zusätzlich der Nucl. ventromedialis hypothalami (s. Abb. 26, S. 382) lädiert, wandelte sich das zahme in ein bösartiges und zorniges Tier (*734*). Im einzelnen decken diese und andere nicht genannte Untersuchungen (*108, 373*) manche bisher nicht gelosten Widersprüche auf. Es bleibt die Frage, ob es sich bei diesen isolierten Schädigungen mit ihren Folgen tatsächlich um „Teile" des Klüver-Bucy-Syndroms handelt (*193*), und es erscheint mindestens verfrüht, es in seine neocorticalen und rhinencephalen Komponenten aufzuspalten (*794*). Die Ergebnisse sind bei den verschiedenen Species, ja, selbst bei näher verwandten Affenarten, nicht gleich und werden durch Alter und Geschlecht, durch das Ausmaß der betroffenen Hirnstrukturen und nicht zuletzt auch durch die bei der Verhaltensanalyse benutzten Methoden beeinflußt (*457, 464*).

Angesichts der komplizierten Verhältnisse ist es nicht verwunderlich, daß die bisher vorliegenden *Beobachtungen am Menschen* (*217, 736*) uneinheitlich sind. Daß es auch beim Menschen ein dem Klüver-Bucy-Syndrom mindestens sehr ähnliches Verhalten gibt, ist kaum noch zu bezweifeln. Es ist bei Temporallappen-Tumoren und -Epilepsien mehrfach beschrieben worden (*227, 494, 514, 693, 720*). PILLERI veröffentlichte entsprechende Ergebnisse bei hirnatrophischen Prozessen mit neuropathologischen Befunden (*643*). TERZIAN und DALLE ORE (*784*) sahen bei bilateraler Temporallappen-Resektion ein Klüver-Bucy-Syndrom, während SCOVILLE, MILNER (*587, 737*), PENFIELD (*157, 632, 635, 638*) und WALKER (*793*) das Syndrom nicht sahen, hingegen schwere Merkfähigkeitsstörungen fanden, deren Ausmaß von der Größe der Hippocampus-Läsion abhing (*737*). Bisher liegen über diese Fälle keine ausreichenden anatomischen Kontrollen vor, so daß man über das tatsächlich geschädigte Gebiet einschließlich der durch retrograde Degeneration lädierten Strukturen nichts aussagen kann. Zudem ist es fraglich, ob die angewandten psychologischen Untersuchungen der Fragestellung angemessen waren (*67, 186, 211, 457*).

Trotz vieler ungeklärter Fragen führen doch alle vorliegenden Untersuchungen zu dem *Ergebnis*, daß Hippocampus und Area piriformis, Fornix, Corpora mamillaria, Nucl. ant. thalami, Gyrus cinguli und Cingulum, Amygdaloid-Komplex, Stria terminalis, vordere Commissur und Pulvinar sowie Faserverbindungen verschiedener Regionen mit Beziehungen zu diesen Strukturen eine *fundamentale Rolle für das emotionale Verhalten* spielen (s. Abb. 26—28). Diese Hirnstrukturen sind inzwischen von sehr zahlreichen Autoren neurophysiologisch auf ihre motorischen,

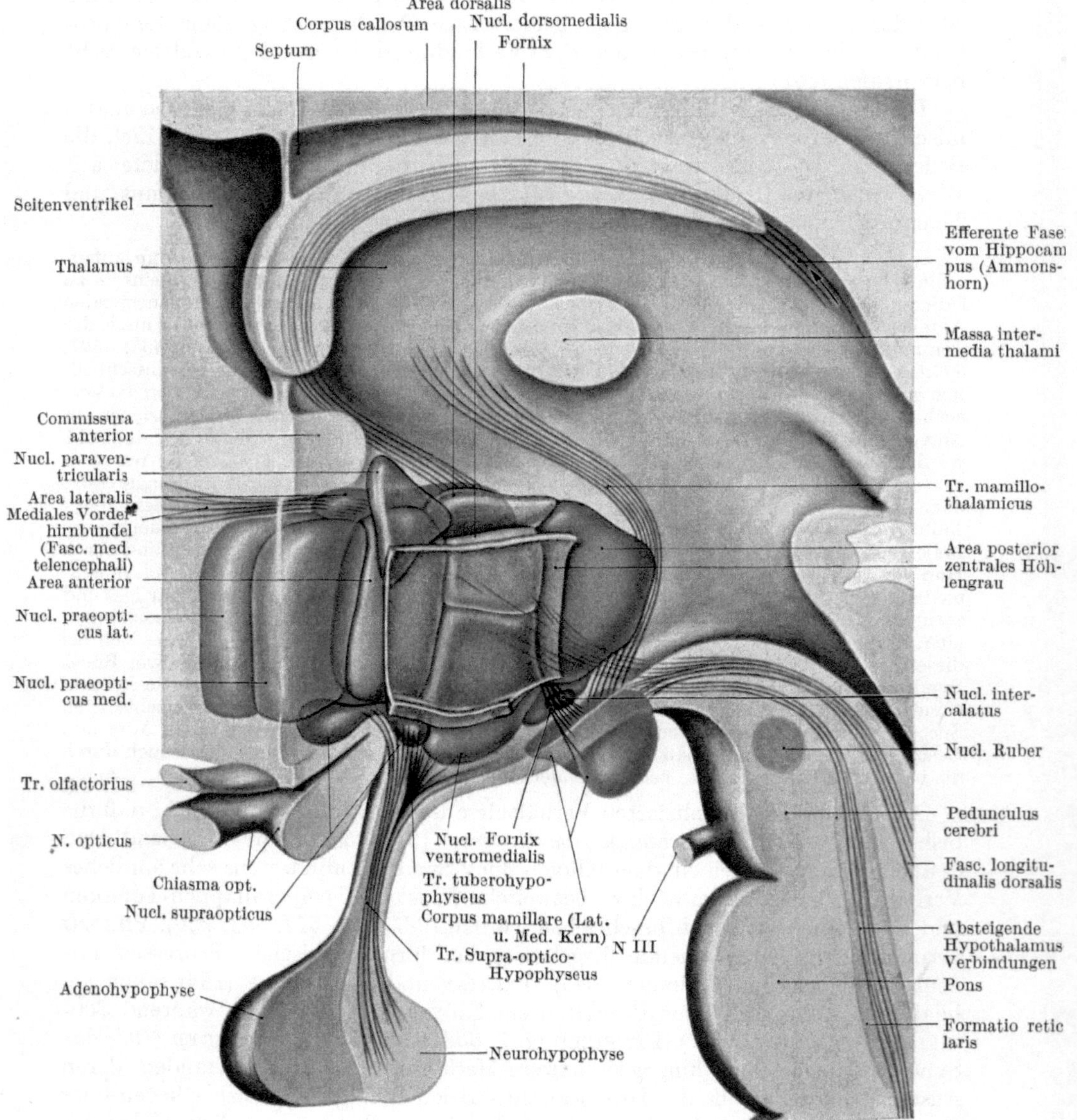

Abb. 26. *Hypothalamus mit Hauptverbindungen.* Dreidimensionales Schema (*90*)

sensorischen und vegetativen Reaktionen untersucht worden (*1, 63, 65, 102, 175, 219, 220, 239, 311, 318, 339, 340, 372, 385, 468, 484, 546, 554, 595*).

Manche Vorstellungen älterer vergleichender Neuroanatomen über das Rhinencephalon scheinen sich zu bestätigen, so z. B. wenn HERRICK (*400*) davon spricht, daß das Rhinencephalon als "the internal apparatus of general bodily attitude, disposition and affective tone" fungiert, oder wenn KLEIST (*105*, S. 1166f.) vom „Innenhirn" spricht, das „aufs engste mit den Innenempfindungen und den Gefühlen bei der Nahrungssuche, den Körperausscheidungen und den Geschlechtsvorgängen" verknüpft ist. GRÜNTHALs (*375*) Vorstellung vom Hippocampus als dem aktivierenden Katalysator gehört ebenfalls hierher.

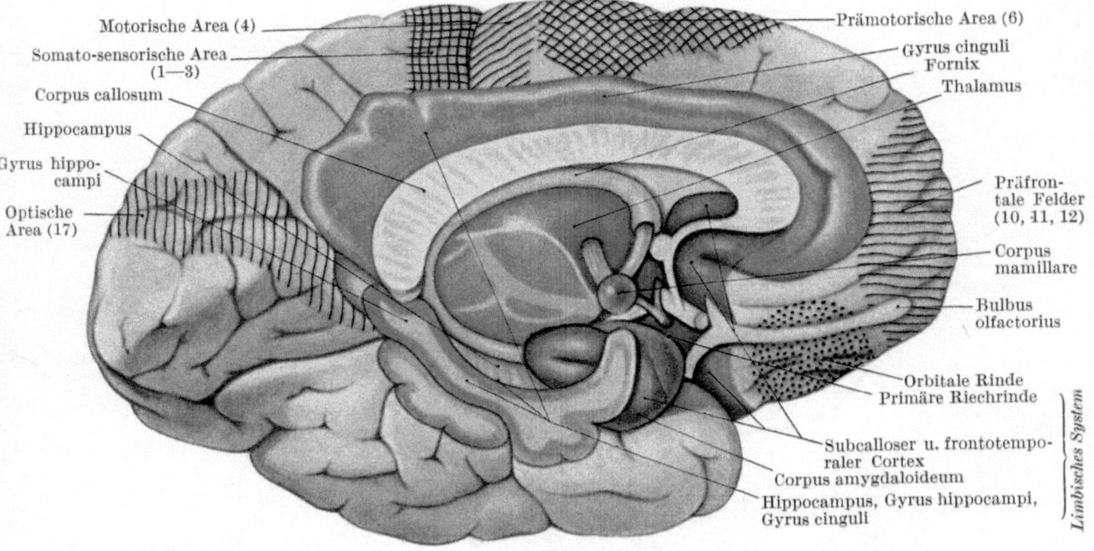

Abb. 27. *Das limbische System.* [Nach Ciba Clinical Symposia 8, S. 127 (1956); etwas verändert]

Heute weiß man, daß das sog. Riechhirn beim Menschen und auch bei anderen Mikrosmatikern so gut wie keine Riechfunktion hat, eine Erkenntnis, die MAXIMILIAN ROSE (*786*) schon 1926/27 auf Grund seiner ausgedehnten Studien des „Allocortex bei Tier und Mensch" gewann.

Seine homologisierenden Studien von niederen Vertebraten bis zum Menschen deckten u. a. auf, daß z. B. die Area entorhinalis beim Menschen bedeutend ausgedehnter als beim Schimpansen und sogar dreimal so groß wie beim makrosmatischen Hund ist. Eine Anzahl von Einzelfeldern dieser Area sind spezifisch nur dem Menschen eigen.

Wir können uns nicht eingehend mit der in den letzten 15 Jahren sehr gründlich bearbeiteten Anatomie des sog. Rhinencephalon befassen. Jedoch kommt diesen Hirnstrukturen, die den am weitesten vorgeschobenen Teil des schon erwähnten gesamten „Mittellinien-Systems" ausmachen, für das emotionale Verhalten eine so entscheidende Bedeutung zu, daß wir die beteiligten Strukturen wenigstens im einzelnen benennen und in Abb. 27 und 28, S. 384, anschaulich machen wollen.

b) Anatomische Bemerkungen über das limbische System

BROCA[1] bezeichnete in seiner 1878 erschienenen Arbeit «Le grand lobe limbique» (*295*) diesen Hirnteil, der sich wie ein Saum (Limbus) um den Hirnstamm legt, als „Generalnenner" des Säugerhirns. Daran anknüpfend schlug PAUL D.

---

[1] BROCA (1879) nimmt bereits eine sehr differenzierte, vergleichend phylogenetisch orientierte Einteilung der „Centres olfactifs" vor und belegt seine Ergebnisse mit eindrucksvollen Zeichnungen der Riechhirne von Delphin, Schaf, Pferd, Fuchs, Tapir, Halbaffen, Schimpansen, Menschen u. a. (*296*).

MacLean vor, den irreführenden Namen Rhinencephalon durch "visceral brain" (*541*) oder "limbic system" (*542*) zu ersetzen. Sein Ausdruck *Limbisches System* hat sich seither durchgesetzt (*349, 543*). Folgende Strukturen gehören dazu (s. Abb. 27, S. 383):

1. Rindenanteile. Für die phylogenetisch alten und älteren Rindenanteile des limbischen Systems gibt es vorläufig weder eine einheitliche Nomenklatur noch

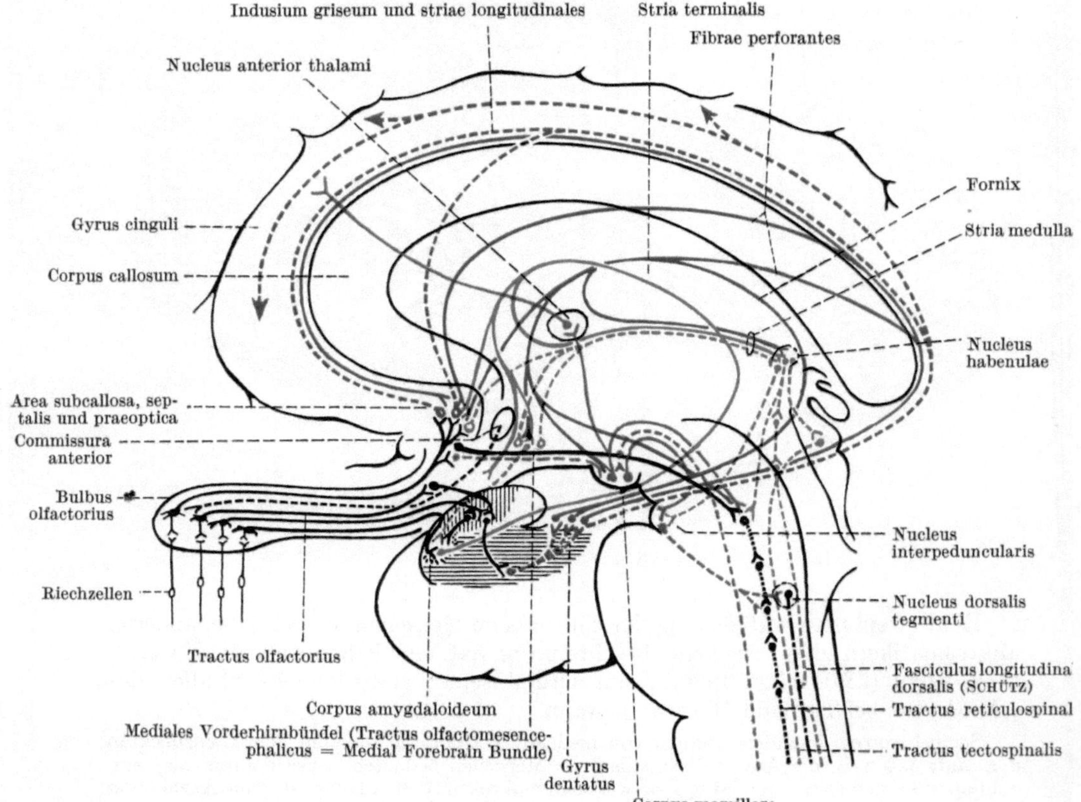

Abb. 28. *Die hauptsächlichen Bahnen des limbischen Systems.* Periphere Riechleitung und die aus den sog. sekundaren Riechzentren entspringenden Bahnen schwarz. Primare Riechrinde senkrecht, sog. sekundare Riechrinde waagerecht schraffiert. — Bahnen der Hippocampusformation blau: efferente Bahnen ausgezogene, afferente gestrichelte Linien. — Bahnen der Corpora mamillaria grun: efferente ausgezogene, afferente gestrichelte Linien. — Bahnen des Corpus amygdaloideum rot: efferente ausgezogene, afferente gestrichelte Linien. — Efferente Bahnen der Habenula rot, efferente Bahnen des Nucleus interpeduncularis grun gestrichelt. — Weitere, hier nicht dargestellte, aber funktional wichtige afferente Bahnen entspringen in der Formatio reticularis des paramedianen Mittelhirns und folgen weitgehend dem medialen (basalen) Vorderhirnbundel. Dieses empfangt, neben den hier dargestellten, zahlreiche Fasern vom Septum, der praoptischen Region und dem Hypothalamus. Das Fornix-System ist vereinfacht wiedergegeben und weist weit mehr Verbindungen auf. Direkte Verbindungen vom Hippocampus zu den Habenula uber den Fornix existieren offenbar nicht. (Nach M. CLARA: Das Nervensystem des Menschen, 3. Aufl. 1959)

eine übereinstimmende cytoarchitektonische Einteilung. Zu diesen allocorticalen (archi- und pallaeocorticalen) und juxtallocorticalen (meso-corticalen) Strukturen gehören:

a) Bulbus und Tuberculum olfactorium; Regio praepiriformis und Regio periamygdalaris (lila in Abb. 27);

b) Subcalloser und fronto-temporaler Cortex (grün in Abb. 27);

c) Hippocampus oder Ammonshorn mit Gyrus dentatus, Subiculum und Fimbria hippocampi;

d) das Praesubiculum als „Nabel" des ganzen Systems und die anschließende Area entorhinalis mit der nachfolgenden Area retrosplenialis; Regio periamygdalaris, Praesubiculum und Area entorhinalis zusammengenommen werden als Gyrus hippocampi oder besser als Gyrus parahippocampalis bezeichnet. Dieser bildet zusammen mit dem Ammonshorn die Hippocampus- oder Ammonsformation.

e) Der Gyrus cinguli (limbischer Cortex), teils schon mit Area 24 zum Neocortex (Isocortex) gehörig (c—e orange in Abb. 27).

2. *Subcorticale Anteile* in enger anatomischer und funktionaler Verbindung zum Allo- und Juxtallocortex: Der Nucleus amygdalae mit seinen verschiedenen Einzelkernen (Corpus amygdaloideum); das Septum mit seinen Kernen und dem Brocaschen Diagonalband; der Epithalamus (Trigonum habenuale mit seinen Kernen, dem paraventriculären Zellkomplex und der praetektalen Kerngruppe); der Nucleus anterior thalami, der ja fast ausschließlich zum Gyrus cinguli projiziert und seine Hauptafferenzen vom Hippocampus und den Corpora mamillaria bekommt (*386, 387, 708* u. a.); auch das intralaminäre unspezifische System des Thalamus hat Verbindungen zu allo- und juxtallocorticalen Strukturen (*663*), ebenso sämtliche Hypothalamus-Anteile und das Infundibulum; schließlich sind auch Teile der Basalganglien, insbesondere der „olfactorische" Anteil des Caudatum, in die Funktionen des limbischen Systems einbezogen.

Wohl das wichtigste Projektionssystem innerhalb des limbischen Systems ist der Fornix (in Abb. 27 gelb, in Abb. 28 blau) mit seinen efferenten Fasern von der Hippocampusformation zu den Corpora mamillaria, zum Epithalamus, zum zentralen Höhlengrau und zum Nucleus reticularis tegmenti sowie seinen afferenten Fasern, z. B. ZUCKERKANDELs Bündel (Tractus olfacto-hippocampicus), das einen Hauptteil im EDINGERschen medialen (basalen) Vorderhirnbündel (siehe Abb. 26 u. 28) einnimmt.

Dazu noch folgende *Erklärungen:*

Der Terminus Tuberculum olfactorium wird bei Primaten synonym mit Substantia perforata anterior gebraucht.

Der Lobus piriformis ist eine allocorticale Rindenformation, in der drei Abschnitte unterschieden werden können, und zwar von vorne nach hinten die Regio praepiriformis, die größere Regio periamygdalaris (Uncusgebiet der menschlichen Anatomie) und die Area entorhinalis (der anschließende Rest des Gyrus hippocampi). Regio praepiriformis und Regio periamygdalaris bilden die primäre Riechrinde, während die Area entorhinalis keine direkten Verbindungen mit dem Bulbus olfactorius hat und offenbar enger mit dem Hippocampus zusammenhängt.

Die Area entorhinalis und das mit ihr verbundene Praesubiculum bilden den größeren Teil des Gyrus hippocampi (Uncus ausgenommen) und liegen zwischen Hippocampus und temporalem Isocortex.

Die Area retrosplenialis und der Gyrus cinguli sind mit dem Gyrus hippocampi kontinuierlich verbunden und bilden zusammen den supracallosen Teil des Juxtallocortex. Nach vorn geht dieses Gebiet durch Vermittlung der subcallosen Area in den medialen fronto-temporalen Cortex über.

Das Corpus amygdaloideum liegt medio-caudal von der Area praepiriformis und kann in eine cortico-mediale und eine baso-laterale Hälfte eingeteilt werden. Die erstere empfängt direkte Fasern aus dem Bulbus olfactorius, während die basolaterale Gruppe keinen direkten Zusammenhang mit dem Riechsystem und wahrscheinlich mehr mit dem temporalen Neocortex zu tun hat (*803*).

Der fronto-temporale Cortex ist ein bandförmiges Gebiet zwischen der Area praepiriformis und der Regio periamygdalaris einerseits und dem orbito-frontalen und temporo-polaren Isocortex andererseits.

Das Brocasche Diagonalband (oft als septale Struktur angesehen) ist ein sub-
corticales Kerngebiet, das sich vom Septum basal und lateralwärts bis zum
Corpus amygdaloideum ausdehnt. Dieser diagonale Nucleus hat reziproke Verbindungen sowohl mit dem Corpus amygdaloideum als auch mit der Hippocampusformation und stellt einen Schaltkern zwischen diesen beiden Strukturen dar.

Die Area septalis hat gegenseitige Verbindungen mit der Ammonsformation
und dem Corpus amygdaloideum. Andererseits steht das Septum durch zahlreiche
Fasern mit dem Hypothalamus und paramedianen Mittelhirnregionen in Verbindung.

Die subcallose Area ist ein juxtallocorticales Übergangsgebiet zwischen Septum
und medio-frontalem Isocortex (*1, 5, 166, 188, 202, 300, 310, 452, 637, 680*).

Dieses weitverzweigte *limbische System (59)* hat zahlreiche projektive *Faserverbindungen zum Mittelhirn (302)*. Nauta (*615*) konnte kürzlich mit einer von ihm
und Gygax entwickelten, eleganten Fein-
faser-Silberimprägnationstechnik alte Untersuchungen von Gudden, Koelliker,
Bechterew u. a. bestätigen und neue Verbindungen finden, die zeigen, daß es einen
Neuronenkreis zwischen dem limbischen
System und einer paramedianen Zone des
Mittelhirns gibt. Dieses Gebiet wurde von
Nauta *limbische Mittelhirn-Area* genannt
(s. Abb. 29).

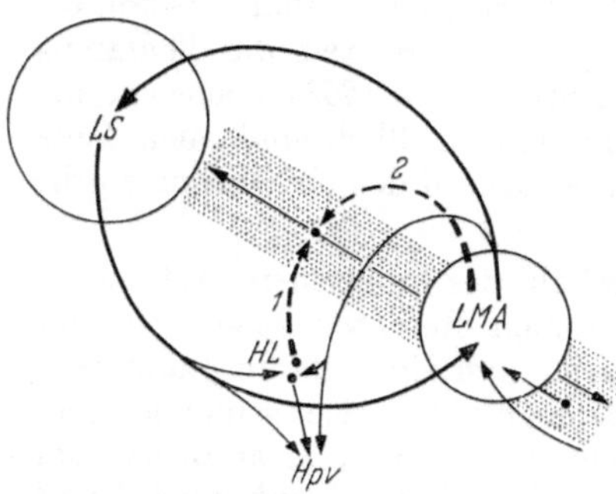

Abb. 29. *Diagramm uber den Neuronenkreis zwischen limbischem System und der limbischen Mittelhirn-Area* (Nauta). Gleichzeitig ein Diagramm
des sog. Mittellinien-Systems. Die gebrochenen
Pfeillinien bezeichnen Kollateralen zu lateralen
und zentralen Regionen der Mittelhirnhaube
(punktiert). Pfeil *1* laterale limbische Faserverbindungen, Pfeil *2* „Radiatio grisea tegmenti“
(Weisschedel) aus dem zentralen Hohlengrau.
Weiteres s. Text, S. 386.) *LMA* Limbische Mittelhirn-Area; *LS* Limbische Vorderhirnstrukturen
(Hippocampus, Septum-Region, Amygdala); *HL*
Lateraler Hypothalamus; *Hpv* Mediale und peri-
ventriculare Hypothalamus-Regionen.
[Nach Nauta (*615*)]

Direkte Projektionen vom Hippocampus gelangen bis zum rostralen Teil dieser
Zone, nämlich in das zentrale Höhlengrau.
Indirekte, transsynaptische Fasersysteme
aus Hippocampus und Corpus amygdaloideum erreichen das Mittelhirn in drei
Fasersystemen, nämlich durch das mediale
Vorderhirnbündel (Fasciculus medialis
telencephali, s. Abb. 26, S. 382), den
Tractus retroflexus (Meynert) und das
Guddensche Haubenbündel (Tractus ma-
millo-tegmentalis). Diesen Verbindungen
zur limbischen Mittelhirn-Area entsprechen reziproke Verbindungen, die im Hippocampus und im Corpus amygdaloideum enden. Ausgedehnte Kollateralen zum
Hypothalamus und zum auf- und absteigenden reticulären System des Mittelhirns
(*616*) verschmelzen das ganze *Mittellinien-System* (s. Abb. 28, S. 384, und Abb. 29,
S. 386) zu einem geschlossenen Funktionssystem. Durch diese Untersuchungen
bekommen die neurophysiologischen Ergebnisse über die Affektreaktionen im
Zwischen- und Mittelhirn (s. S. 368ff. und Abb. 19, S. 371) auch eine gesicherte
anatomische Grundlage.

c) Neurophysiologische Experimente und Verhalten

Neurophysiologische Reizversuche und neuronographische Untersuchungen
(*65, 102, 108, 555, 683*) zeigen, daß man einen Unterschied zwischen den Funktionen des medio-basalen Cortex und den übrigen limbischen Strukturen machen
kann (*1, 65, 128, 219*).

Reizversuche am medio-basalen Cortex (64, 542, 546, 553, 554, 675) führen zu großen
koordinierten Körperbewegungen, oralen motorischen Phänomenen, Oculomoto-
rius-Effekten mit Pupillenveränderungen, Blutdruckveränderungen, Verände-

rungen der Atmung und der Darmmotilität. Im großen und ganzen erhält man diese Phänomene bei Reizung des medio-basalen, temporo-frontalen Cortex(Abb.27, grün) und weniger regelmäßig auch von den am weitesten rostral gelegenen Teilen der Hippocampusformation und des Gyrus cinguli. Es scheint so, als ob diese vorderen limbischen Strukturen eine Art von altem „motorischen Cortex", vergleichbar dem präzentralen Neo-Cortex (*682*), darstellen. Während bei dessen Reizung Einzelbewegungen entstehen, kommt es bei Reizung jener zu komplexen Bewegungen.

Alle Antworten, die man bei Reizung dieses alten Cortex erhält, sind unspezifisch und nicht topographisch zuzuordnen. Ein Reiz mag das eine Mal hemmend, ein anderes Mal fördernd auf autonom innervierte Organe oder auf gerade ablaufende Extremitätenbewegungen wirken. Dabei können benachbarte Reizpunkte am selben Tier durchaus verschiedene Wirkungen auslösen, aber es gelingt keine konstante Zuordnung von Reiz und Reaktionsort bzw. Reaktionsqualität. Auch wenn man umgekehrt im peripheren Nervensystem reizt — sei es sensibel, sensorisch oder -vegetativ —, die abgeleiteten Potentialveränderungen sind unspezifisch. Die Einheitlichkeit in der Reaktion auf verschiedenartige periphere Reize scheint in diesem Gebiet sogar für die Einzel-Nervenzelle zu gelten (*675, 676*).

Reizungen des übrigen limbischen Cortex (Abb. 27, orange), i. e. Ammonsformation, Regio retrosplenialis und Gyrus cinguli, führen zu *keinen* somato-viscero-motorischen Reaktionen. (Eine Ausnahme machen, wie schon erwähnt, die rostralen Anteile der Ammonsformation und des Gyrus cinguli.) Bei isocorticaler Ableitung am narkotisierten Tier erhält man diffuse Reizantworten in Form von schnellen, niedrig gespannten Aktivierungen, obgleich auch andere Effekte, wie z. B. eine Drosselung der Spontanaktivität, vorkommen können. Die corticalen Aktivierungsformen ähneln denen, die man bei Reizung der Formatio reticularis im medialen Mesencephalon und des hinteren Hypothalamus erhält. Die Potentialveränderungen breiten sich leicht auf das ganze limbische System, besonders auch auf Amygdaloidkomplex und Septum aus und beziehen am ehesten die frontale Convexität ein (*102, 675*).

Registriert man im Ammonshorn periphere Sinnesreize, und zwar besonders solche, die Qualität und Intensität vermitteln (Geruchs-, Geschmacks- und Schmerzreize), findet man charakteristische, hochamplitude, sinusoidale Wellen, die sich von der gleichzeitig im Isocortex auftretenden Abflachung, der Weck- oder "arousal" Reaktion unterscheiden, wie Jung und Kornmüller (*442*) zuerst feststellten. Der elektrischen Aktivität in der Ammonsformation wurde in den letzten Jahren besondere Aufmerksamkeit geschenkt (*370, 371, 543, 554*), wobei neurophysiologisch wichtige Fragen der Reizausbreitung, der Projektion, der Erregbarkeit und Krampfausbreitung (*312, 438*) im Vordergrund standen.

Auch *Reizwirkungen auf Diencephalon und Mesencephalon* sind eingehend studiert worden (*1, 65, 128, 220, 431, 434, 544, 675*). Grob zusammengefaßt können Reizantworten vor allem im Nucleus anterior und im intralaminären Thalamuskern, im antero-medialen und posterioren Hypothalamus registriert werden. Subthalamus (Corpus Luysi), Nucleus ruber und Substantia nigra sind einbezogen. Man kann die Reizwirkungen bis hinunter ins zentrale Höhlengrau und in die reticuläre Substanz des Mittelhirns verfolgen.

Dieser Überblick, bei dem wir die speziellen funktionalen Zuordnungen von bestimmten limbischen Strukturen zu bestimmten Zwischen- und Mittelhirnkernen ganz unberücksichtigt ließen, soll vor allem die reziproke Verknüpfung der limbischen Strukturen untereinander und — im Gegensatz zum Neocortex — mit den genannten Stammhirn-Anteilen unterstreichen (Abb. 28 und Abb. 29).

Pribram (*675*) kommt angesichts dieser Ergebnisse sowie auf Grund faseranatomischer und synapsen-physiologischer Details zu folgendem heuristischen Schluß: Das limbische System mit seinen polysynaptischen, mehrfach parallel geschalteten Verbindungen zum Zwischen- und Mittelhirn dient der Modulation des zentralen Erregungszustandes, jedoch nicht, um momentane Impulsmuster zu formen, sondern um Erregungszuständlichkeiten dauerhaft aufrechtzuerhalten und zu modulieren. Großhirn, Zwischen- und Mittelhirn zeigen in ihrer Funktion einen Gradienten derart, daß von der Mittellinie (vom Ependym) zu den Außengrenzen hin die komplexe *Momentan*funktion zunimmt, während die *dauerhafte* unspezifische Funktion abnimmt. Das limbische System als der am weitesten vorgeschobene Teil dieses ganzen Mittelliniensystems (Abb. 29, S. 386) stellt das neuronale Korrelat für folgende Verhaltensweisen dar: Nahrungssuche und -aufnahme, Kämpfen, Fliehen, Paaren und solche Verhaltensweisen, die mit der Aufzucht der Jungen zusammenhängen (*676, 677, 678, 772, 773*). Das sind angeborene Verhaltensweisen, wie sie im ersten Teil dieses Beitrages dargestellt wurden.

Eine gute Stütze dieser Hypothese ist die Arbeit von MacLean und Delgado (*553*), in der nachgewiesen wird, daß durch elektrische oder chemische Reizung des alten temporo-frontalen Cortex Freß-Automatismen, Angriffs-, Flucht- und Verteidigungshaltungen induziert werden können. Aus den detaillierten Hirn-Reizkarten geht das Vorwiegen oraler Aktivität, verbunden mit autonomen Symptomen, eindrucksvoll hervor.

MacLean (*549—552*) unterscheidet zwei anatomisch-neurophysiologische Funktionskreise, denen er jeweils Funktionskreise des Verhaltens (vgl. S. 295) zuordnet.

Der *Amygdaloid-Zirkel* umfaßt den frontotemporalen Cortex, der in unmittelbarer funktionaler Beziehung zu den Amygdala steht und in sie „hineinfeuert". Dieser Funktionskreis empfängt zwei sich hier vereinigende Afferenzen, nämlich einerseits vom lateralen Tractus olfactorius und andererseits vom Hirnstamm, wahrscheinlich über Teile des medialen Vorderhirnbündels. Am sich frei bewegenden und wachen Tier können durch Reizung Verhaltensweisen der Nahrungssuche und -aufnahme (Suchen, Schnüffeln, Lecken, Kauen, Fressen, Würgen) und Verteidigungs- und Angriffsverhalten mit den dazugehörigen Lautgebungen ausgelöst werden. Dieser Teil des limbischen Systems ist für die *Selbsterhaltung des Individuum* im Kampf ums Dasein verantwortlich. Wie wir am Klüver-Bucy-Syndrom gesehen haben, werden die eben aufgezählten Verhaltensweisen durch Zerstörung der entsprechenden Hirnpartien erheblich verändert oder sie verschwinden ganz und gar (s. S. 380f.).

Der *Septumzirkel* schließt Hippocampus, Gyrus hippocampi (bis auf seinen vorderen Anteil), den Gyrus cinguli und das Septum ein. Im letzteren vereinigen sich Meldungen, die über den Tractus olfactorius medialis und vom Hirnstamm her einströmen. Nach der ganzen Topographie dieser Septumregion ist es durchaus möglich, daß sich hier somato-genitale, Seh- und Geruchsreize vereinigen. Die durch elektrische oder chemische Reizung hervorgerufenen Symptome betreffen das Sexualverhalten im engeren und weiteren Sinne, worauf wir noch näher eingehen werden. Dieser Funktionskreis gewährleistet die *Erhaltung der Art*.

Das Konzept hat für Verhaltensforschung und Psychiatrie große Bedeutung. Legt es doch nahe, daß orales Verhalten (Amygdaloid-Zirkel) und Sexualverhalten (Septum-Zirkel) anatomisch-neurophysiologisch getrennten Funktionskreisen zugeordnet sind. Beide aber sind durch ihre Hirnorganisation eng zusammengeschlossen, und zwar so, daß sie sowohl agonistisch als auch antagonistisch miteinander ins Spiel kommen können. Damit wird anatomisch-neurophysiologisch verständlich, warum orales Verhalten, Angriffs-, Flucht- und Sexualverhalten so häufig gemeinsam aktiviert werden (s. S. 334f., 374). Die weitere Entwicklung des Instinktverhaltens hängt dann von zahlreichen inneren und äußeren Faktoren ab (s. S. 297), die bestimmen, welches Verhalten sich schließlich durchsetzt. Dieses Zusammenspiel wird im Laufe der Phylogenese fraglos immer komplizierter. Jedoch sollte man sich vor Augen halten, daß sich das limbische System im Gegensatz zu jüngeren telencephalen Strukturen der Säuger sehr konservativ verhält. Es bleibt also mit anderen Worten bis zum Menschen hinauf vergleichsweise primitiv.

Die anatomischen Strukturen, die in die beiden Funktionskreise verwickelt sind, üben gleichzeitig auch *neuro-endokrine Kontrollfunktionen* aus (*64, 544*). Reizung der Amygdala führt zu einem beträchtlichen Anstieg der 17-Hydroxy-corticosteroide, vergleichbar der Wirkung, die sich durch Reizung des Infundibulums erzielen läßt. Über das Hippocampus-Fornix-System kann man dagegen die Hypophysen-Nebennieren-Funktion nachhaltig hemmen. Das System scheint den Rhythmus der ACTH-Ausscheidung mitzubestimmen (*560*). Reizung des Septums führt bei Kaninchen zu Ovulationen (*64*). Zerstört man bei Ratten den Gyrus cinguli, sind sie nicht mehr fähig, ihre Jungen aufzuziehen (*772, 773*).

Kehren wir zu den unter „Septum-Zirkel" erwähnten Verhaltensweisen zurück. MacLean (*547, 548*) hat in experimentell reizvoller Weise Untersuchungen der Hippocampus-Funktion mit Verhaltensstudien gekoppelt.

Durch stereotaktisch eingeführte feine Kanülen, die zugleich als Ableite-Elektroden dienten, ließ er radiummarkierte Phosphatverbindungen diffundieren (Diffusions-Radius innerhalb von 40 min 1 mm). Das waren vor allem Metacholin, Acetylcholin in Kombination mit Physostigmin und Doryl (ein Cholin-chlorid-carbamat), welches sich unter den cholinergischen Stoffen als besonders reizwirksam erwies. Außer der chemischen Reizung wurde auch elektrisch gereizt und die Elektrodenlage histologisch bestimmt. Auf Abb. 30, S. 389, sieht man die Ausbreitung der Nachentladungen schematisch eingezeichnet. Die Verhaltensänderungen der Katzen waren bei Doryl-Reiz mit den hirnelektrischen Potentialveränderungen gut korreliert.

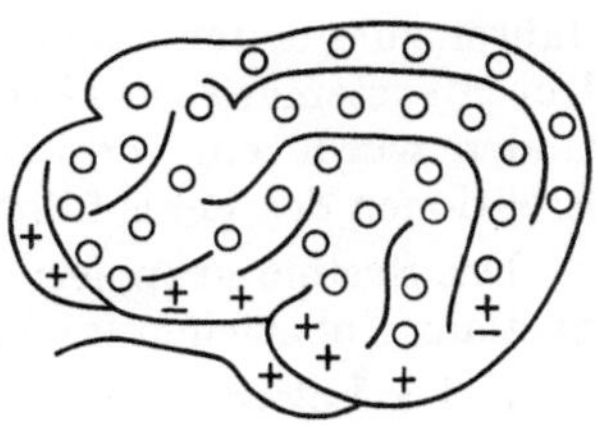

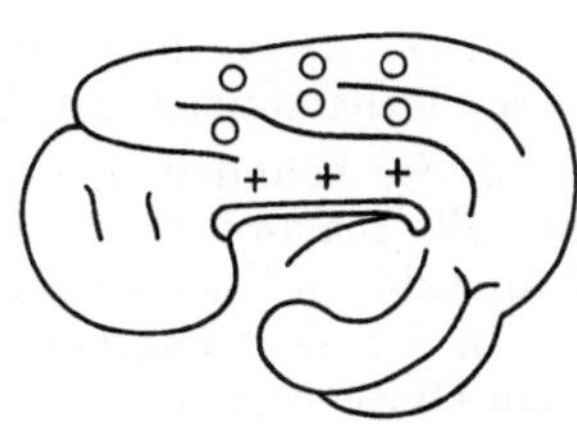

Abb. 30. *Hirnelektrische Ausbreitung von Krampfentladungen im Hippocampus* auf den Cortex von Katzen nach chemischer und elektrischer Hippocampus-Reizung. Oben laterale, unten mediale Hirnoberfläche. + stark positive Punkte; ± noch deutliche hirnelektrische Veränderungen; ○ negative Punkte. [Nach MacLean (*547*)]

In den ersten 15 min nach dem cholinergischen Reiz zeigen die Katzen nur geringe Verhaltensänderungen. In Korrelation zur heftig zunehmenden bioelektrischen Aktivität geraten sie in ein stuporöses Verhalten, zeigen keine Spontanbewegungen, verharren gleichsam kataton in abnormer Haltung, weichen unangenehmen Reizen (Licht, Rauch) höchstens mit einer leichten Kopfbewegung aus, reagieren aber auf heftige, schmerzhafte Reize dramatisch mit einem großen Sprung. Hält der schmerzhafte Reiz an, faucht die Katze, gerät in rasende Wut oder beißt in das erste beste Objekt, ohne die Quelle des Schmerzes ausfindig machen zu können. Währenddessen sind die Pupillen erweitert, Speichel fließt, und die Pulsfrequenz steigt. Sobald der Reiz aufhört, fällt das Tier wieder in den katatonieartigen Zustand, und die vegetativen Veränderungen gehen zur Ausgangslage zurück. Der Muskeltonus ändert sich nicht.

In der zweiten und dritten Stunde, während die bioelektrische Aktivität abklingt, kommen selbst vor Versuchsbeginn noch sehr aggressive Katzen in eine träge Stimmung des Wohlbehagens, in der sie schnurren, das Fell reinigen, dem Experimentator die Hand lecken und ihn zart beißen. Während dieser "pleasure reactions" zeigen besonders die Kater eine abnorm leichte genitale Erregbarkeit:

schon geringe Reize rufen eine Erektion hervor. Ganz ähnliche "pleasure reactions" mit gesteigerter sexueller Erregbarkeit findet man vergleichsweise bei Ratten.

Sieht man diese Verhaltensstudien mit dem bioelektrischen Ausbreitungsgebiet der Erregungen (s. Abb. 30, S. 389) und den histologischen Kontrollen im Zusammenhang, so liegt der Schluß nahe, daß Teile der Ammons-Formation, des Gyrus cinguli und der Septum-Region als das *neuronale Substrat für die beschriebenen Stimmungen* (im Sinne der Definition S. 306ff.; 364) zu betrachten sind. Dieser Befund stimmt gut mit dem von W. R. Hess und A. E. Meyer (*409, 566*) überein (s. S. 369f.; 372f.).

Die *cerebrale Repräsentation des Sexualverhaltens* (*557*) ist in den vergangenen Jahren zum erstenmal von MacLean und seinen Mitarbeitern untersucht worden. Durch systematische Hirnreizungen an Affen mit chronisch implantierten Elektroden wurde ein verzweigtes System entdeckt, dessen elektrische Reizung zu Erektionen des Penis führt (Abb. 31, S. 391 u. Abb. 31a, S. 392—393).

Das System gruppiert sich um drei Hauptabschnitte, die Teile des limbischen Systems einbeziehen (s. Abb. 31a):

1. Die Lokalisationen für Erektionen fallen zusammen mit der bereits bekannten Distribution der Hippocampusprojektion (*789*) zu Septum-, Thalamus- und Hypothalamus-Anteilen.

2. Sie liegen in solchen Strukturen, die die Corpora mamillaria, den Tractus mamillothalamicus, den Nucl. anterior thalami und den Gyrus cinguli umfassen.

3. Sie befinden sich im Gyrus rectus und im medialen Teil des Nucl. mediodorsalis thalami wie auch in solchen Regionen, die als deren Verbindungen und Projektionen bekannt sind.

In den Hirndiagrammen (Abb. 31a) folgt man den Symbolen für Erektionen vom Gyrus rectus (A 16) in den medialen Septumanteil (A 13.5) und dann in die mediale präoptische Region (A 12.5). Ungefähr auf halbem Wege durch die vordere Commissur beginnen die positiven Punkte (siehe Legende) zu divergieren (A 11). Medial folgt man ihnen in den antero-medialen Teil des Hypothalamus; dort ist die Lokalisation inmitten des Nucl. paraventricularis besonders erwähnenswert (A 10.5; A 10). Lateralwärts ziehen die positiven Punkte über den Nucl. supraopticus hinweg und in den ventrolateralen Hypothalamus hinein. Auf der Ebene A 9.5 häufen sich die Loci oberhalb des Tractus opticus und lateral vom Fornix; aus den folgenden Diagrammen (A 9; A 8.5) ist zu ersehen, daß sie dem medialen Vorderhirnbündel (vgl. Abb. 26 u. 28) folgen. Weiter caudalwärts finden sich positive Punkte in den Corpora mamillaria und den medialen Anteilen des Nucl. subthalamicus und der Hirnschenkel (A 7.5; A 7). Für die Corpora mamillaria wurden positive Reizantworten in nicht weniger als 11 Tieren gefunden (*557, 660*). Während man am hinteren Pol der Corpora mamillaria noch positive Reaktionen erhält, sind unmittelbar caudal davon gelegene Punkte der Mittellinie negativ. Die positiven Orte verschieben sich dann lateral und folgen tangential dem Verlauf der austretenden Oculomotoriusfasern durch den mittleren Teil der Substantia nigra ziehend (A 6). Das weiter caudalwärts davon ziehende System ist noch nicht dokumentiert.

Die Befunde an den Corpora mamillaria lenken auf die positiven Loci entlang dem Tractus mamillo-thalamicus (A 9; A 8.5) und im vorderen Thalamus (A 10; A 7.5; A 7). Wie man auf A 10 sieht, können positive Reizantworten im Tuberculum thalami und im rostralen Thalamuspol ausgelöst werden. Andere Punkte finden sich an einer Stelle, wo die anteroventralen und anterodorsalen Kerne gerade caudalwärts auslaufen (A 7). Besonders zu beachten sind die Lokalisationen im medialen Anteil des Nucl. dorsomedialis thalami, die bei sieben Tieren gefunden wurden (A 7.5 bis A 6); Teile intralaminärer Kerne scheinen einbezogen zu sein.

Wie auf Ebene A 8.5 und A 7 zu sehen, entstanden starke Erektionen bei Reizung nahe dem Dach des dritten Ventrikels; diese Area greift auf den Nucl. reuniens und die Gegend des dorsalen und posterioren Hypothalamus über. Auf A 10 sieht man positive Symbole auf der ganzen vertikalen Länge des Ventrikelwalles in der Ebene des Nucl. paraventricularis eingetragen. Eben caudal davon erhält man hochgradig aversive Reizeffekte (ängstliches Gekreische usw.) sobald der Nucl. ventromedialis hypothalami einbezogen ist. Wiederum weiter caudalwärts und rostral zu den Corpora mamillaria stößt man im Wall des 3. Ventrikels nochmals auf positive Punkte, die man bis in die Tubergegend[1] verfolgen kann. Nach den Befunden ist wahrscheinlich, daß Teile der periventriculären Strukturen (mit deren Fortsetzung im Schützschen Bündel) in das Gesamtsystem einbezogen sind.

Schließlich sieht man auf A 12.5 und A 7.5, daß gelegentlich schwach positive Reizantworten im (oder gerade oberhalb vom) vorderen supracallosen Gyrus cinguli auszulösen waren. In späteren, hier noch nicht dokumentierten Versuchen fanden sich stark positive Punkte eben rostral vom Corpus-callosum-Knie und in der Gegend des Gyrus subcallosus.

Der phylogenetisch jüngere Anteil des ganzen Systems, vor allem der Nucl. dorsomedialis thalami mit seinen Projektionen zum orbitofrontalen und präfrontalen Cortex, spielt wahrscheinlich für die spezielle Entwicklung des Sexualverhaltens der Primaten eine entscheidende Rolle. Auch

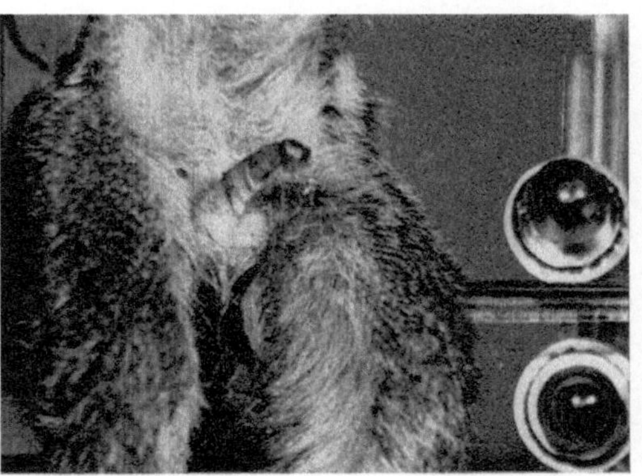

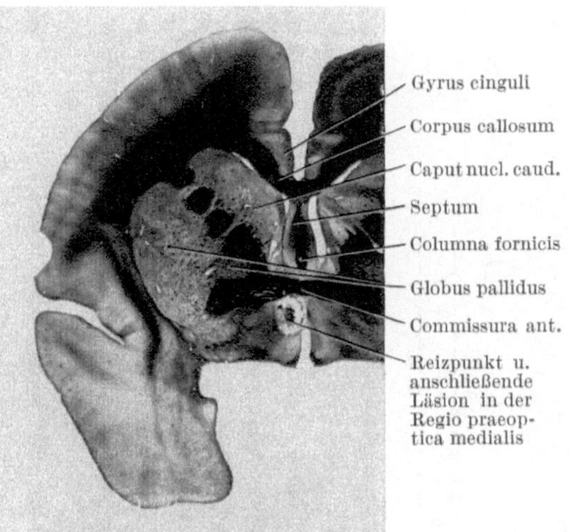

Abb. 31. *Zur cerebralen Repräsentation der Genitalfunktion* (*556—559*). Hirnreizversuche am Totenkopfäffchen (Saimiri sciureus). Oben: Das wache Tier sitzt für die Dauer des Versuches ruhig im Untersuchungsstuhl (vgl. Abb. 40) und hat während der Hirnreizung eine Erektion des Penis bekommen, die nach Beendigung des Reizes wieder verschwindet. Mit Hilfe der chronisch implantierten, kombinierten Reiz- und Ableite-Elektroden kann die Reaktion über Wochen nachgeprüft und auf ihre spezifischen Reizcharakteristica untersucht werden. (Filmaufnahme aus dem Department of Neurophysiology, National Institutes of Health, Bethesda, Maryland, USA.) Unten: Frontalschnitt (Gefrierschnitt-Markfaserfärbung) mit Darstellung einer der gefundenen Regionen, von denen Erektionen ausgelöst werden können. Nach Beendigung der Versuche wurde in diesem Falle eine kleine Elektrocoagulation vorgenommen. [Nach MacLean, Ploog und Robinson]

die anteriore Kerngruppe des Thalamus, die wiederum ein Teil des Hippocampus-Corpus mamillare-Cingulum-Systems ist, entwickelt sich bei den Primaten

---

[1] Siehe hierzu Spatz, H.: Das Hypophysen-Hypothalamus-System in seiner Bedeutung für die Fortpflanzung sowie frühere Arbeiten dieses Autors zum gleichen Thema (*761*).

bis zum Menschen hinauf progressiv, während sich das Septum regressiv
verändert.

Das die Erektionen begleitende Verhalten ist je nach Elektrodenlage verschieden. Strukturen, deren Reizung Angriffs-, Angst- oder Fluchtverhalten auslöst,

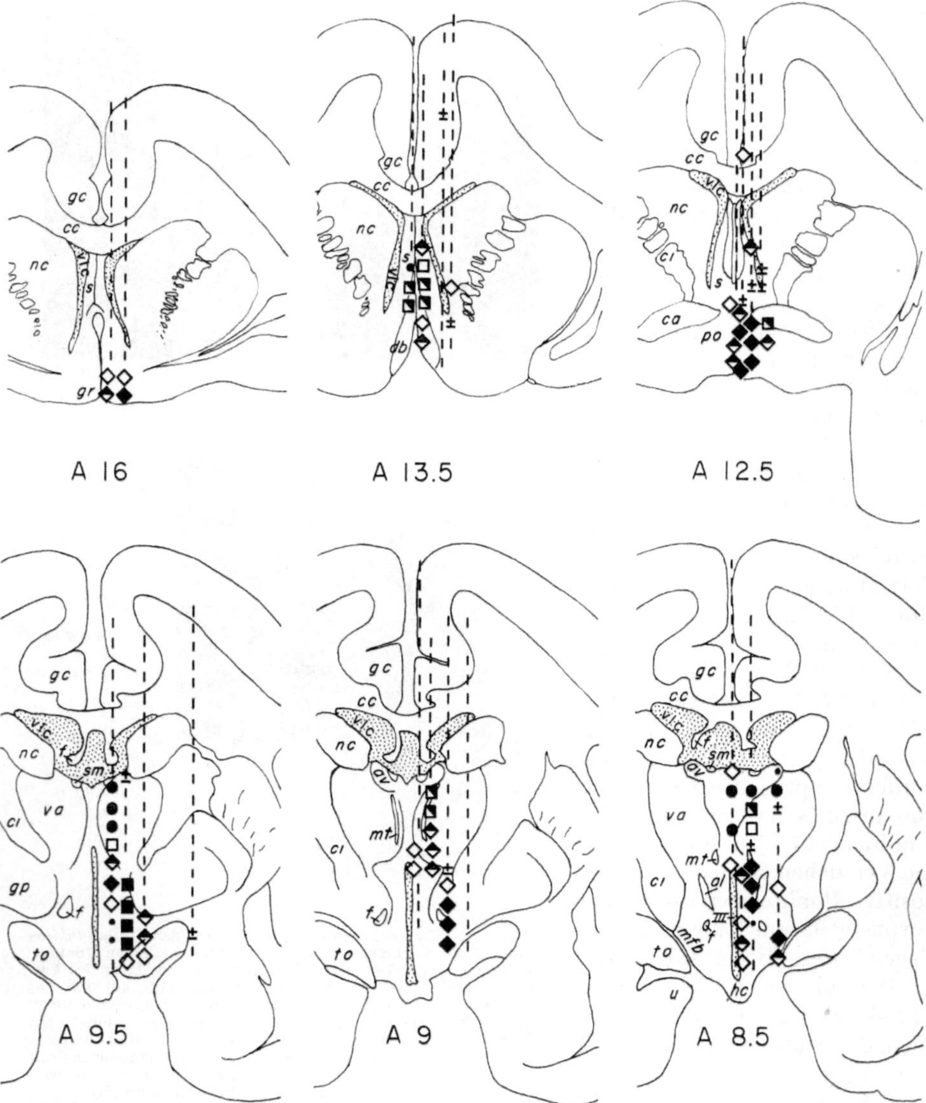

Abb. 31a. *Hirnkarten der cerebralen Reprasentation der mannlichen Genitalfunktion von Saimiri sciureus* [MACLEAN
und PLOOG (557)]. In 12 Diagrammen sind die Orte eingetragen, von denen an 29 erwachsenen Totenkopfaffen
Erektionen durch elektrische Reizung ausgelost werden konnten. Die schematischen Frontalschnitte entsprechen
Ebenen der stereotaktischen Koordinaten A 16 bis A 6. Diese Werte zeigen in Millimetern an, wie weit der jeweils
reprasentative Schnitt oral von der Null-Linie (Zentrum der Ohrbolzen des stereotaktischen Gerates) entfernt liegt.
Buchstabe A (Anterior) und die zugehorige Zahl sitzen stets einer Linie auf, die 4 mm oberhalb der Null-Linie
gelegen ist, womit neben der *a-p*-Ebene auch die Horizontalebene gekennzeichnet ist. Außerdem reprasentiert die
Entfernung von aufeinanderfolgenden senkrechten Strichen jeweils 1 mm. Auf diese Weise konnen die stereotaktischen Koordinaten fur die einzelnen Symbole geschatzt werden. — *Senkrechte Striche* entsprechen Orten, die
bei der Hirnreizung negativ bezuglich der Erektionsauslosung waren. ◇ und □ entsprechen Orten, von denen
Erektionen ausgelost wurden (positive Punkte). ◇ Positive Punkte ohne Nachentladungen im Hippocampus.
□ Positive Punkte mit begleitender oder folgender Hippocampus-Nachentladung. ◇ und □ schwach ausgepragte

können denen, die zur Erektion führen, ganz eng benachbart sein. Die entsprechenden Verhaltensweisen können sich durch Reizung überlagern. Die angewandte Technik erlaubte jedoch in den meisten Fällen, Elektrodenlage und Reizparameter

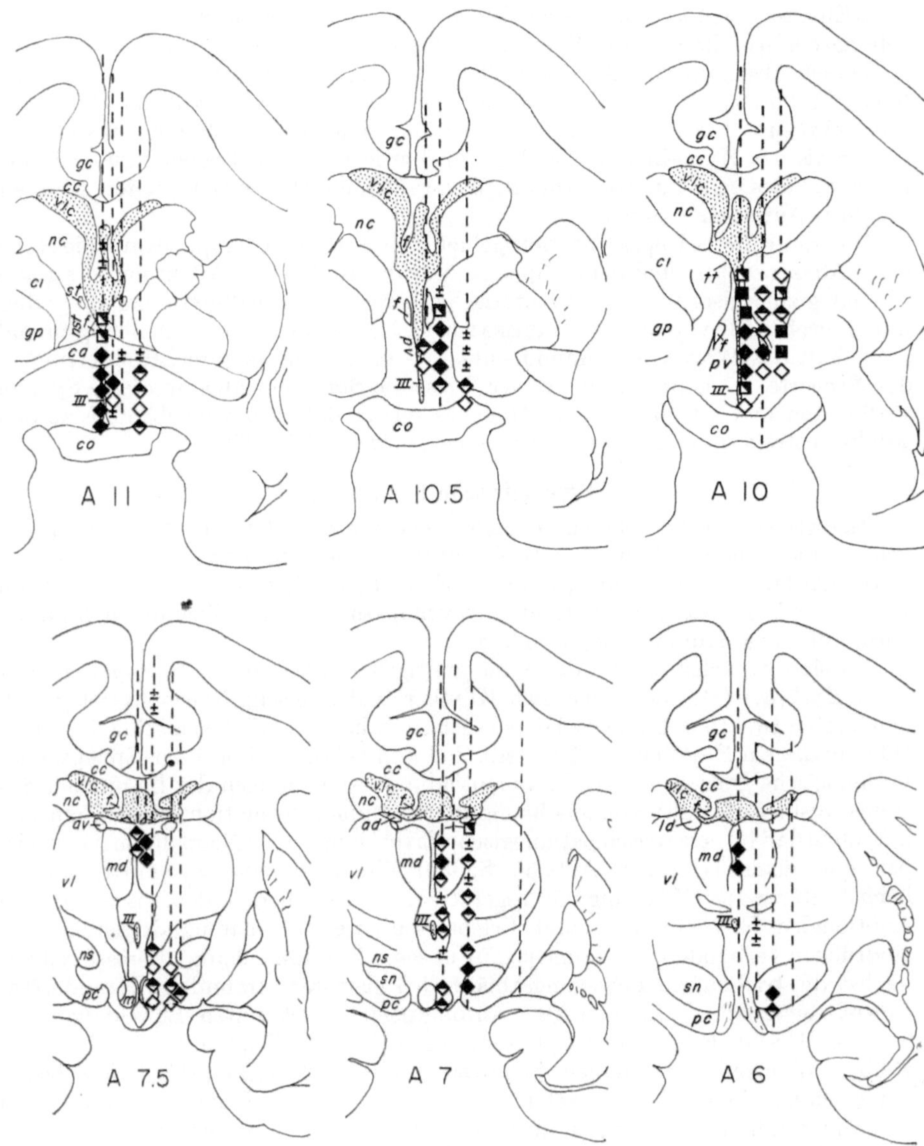

Erektion. ◇ und ◻ mittelstark ausgepragte Erektion. ◆ und ■ starke bis maximale Erektion. ± Schwellung der Glans mit Vortreten des Penis aus dem Praeputium. ● Erektionen nach Reizbeendigung in Verbindung mit Nachentladungen, die bioelektrische Aktivitatsveranderungen im Hippocampus nach sich ziehen. • Erektionen als Rebound-Phänomen nach Reizende ohne begleitende Hippocampus-Nachentladungen. — *Abkurzungen: ad* Nucl. anterodorsalis thalami, *al* Ansa lenticularis, *av* Nucl. anteroventralis, thalami, *ca* Commissura anterior, *cc* Corpus callosum, *ci* Capsula interna, *co* Chiasma opticum, *db* Diagonalband von BROCA, *f* Fornix, *gc* Gyrus cinguli, *gp* Globus pallidus, *gr* Gyrus rectus, *hc* Hypophysis cerebri, *ld* Nucl. lateralis dors. thalami, *m* Corpus mamillare, *md* Nucl. medialis dors. thalami, *mfb* Fasciculus medialis telencephali (medial forebrain bundle), *mt* fasciculus mamillothalamicus, *nc* Nucl. caudatus, *ns* Nucl. subthalamicus, *nst* Nucl. stria terminalis, *p* Putamen, *pc* Pedunculus cerebri, *po* Area praeoptica, *pv* Nucl. paraventricularis hypothalami, *s* Septum pellucidum, *sm* Stria medullaris, *sn* Substantia nigra, *st* Stria terminalis, *to* Tractus opticus, *tt* Tuberculum thalami, *u* Uncus gyri hippocampi, *va* Nucl. ventralis anterior thalami, *vl* Nucl. ventralis lateralis thalami, *vlc* Ventriculus lateralis cerebri, *III* Ventriculus tertius so zu verändern, daß derartige Überlagerungen ausgeschaltet werden konnten. Aus den bisher vorliegenden Ergebnissen darf man bereits schließen, daß es außer dem Erektionen auslösenden System auch ein Erektionen hemmendes System gibt, das in Narkose früher ausfällt als das Erregungssystem. Nach Kastration bleiben die Reiz-Effekte offenbar im wesentlichen unverändert erhalten. Störende Umgebungseinflüsse können die Erektionen empfindlich hemmen (556—559).

Diesen Abschnitt beschließend wollen wir die Arbeitshypothese wagen, daß das *limbische System als zentrale Repräsentation von Triebhandlungen und Handelnsbereitschaften (Stimmungen)* anzusehen ist und nach Art eines *Modulators* differenzierter als der Hypothalamus wirkt, dem hinsichtlich der Triebhandlungen eine mehr exekutorische Funktion zufällt. Wir werden im Abschnitt II weitere Stützen für diese Auffassung finden.

Innerhalb dieses Repräsentationsgebietes mag dem Gyrus hippocampi die Rolle eines Affektozeptors und dem Hippocampus die Rolle eines Affektomotors (791) — analog zur sensorischen und motorischen Area des Neopallium — zufallen; dies nur als grobe Hilfsvorstellung. MacLean (541) hat in diesem Zusammenhang einmal scherzhaft das Wort vom „Animunculus" — im Gegensatz zum „Homunculus", des Neocortex — geprägt. In welcher Weise die Stammganglien in dieses System verflochten sind, ist noch unklar. Manches spricht dafür, daß sie ebenfalls zu den Funktionsträgern instinktiven Verhaltens gehören (101, 707).

d) Psychiatrische Bemerkungen

Zu diesen experimentellen und vergleichend anatomisch fundierten Ergebnissen gehört eine Fülle von klinischen Beobachtungen. Doch müssen wir uns in der Erwartung, daß der Leser im weiteren Verlauf dieses Beitrages selbst die für ihn sinnvollen Verbindungen zu klinisch-psychopathologischen Zuständen knüpfen wird, auf einige Hinweise beschränken:

Da sind zunächst einmal die mannigfaltigen *Erscheinungen der psychomotorischen Epilepsie (8)*, mit denen sich Kliniker und klinische Neurophysiologen in den letzten 10—15 Jahren besonders beschäftigt haben (vgl. die einschlägigen Beiträge in diesem Handbuch). Man weiß, daß sich bei dieser Form der Epilepsie der pathologische Prozeß — die Krampfentladung — im Bereich des limbischen Systems ausbreitet und besonders häufig in der Ammonsformation seinen Ursprung hat, ohne daß hirnelektrisch pathologische Erscheinungen im Neopallium nachweisbar sein müssen (vgl. dazu Abb. 30, S. 389). Wir finden eine psychopathologisch höchst interessante Mischung von vegetativen, motorischen, oralen, visceralen und emotionalen Erscheinungen und Erlebnissen, die mit mannigfaltigen Sinneseindrücken verbunden sein können. Für unseren Zusammenhang interessieren zunächst die triebhaften Bewegungsabläufe bei gleichsam traumhaft verändertem Bewußtseinszustand. Zu den als „Automatismen" bekannten Bewegungen gehören z. B. Schnalzen, Kauen, Spucken, Pusten, Nesteln, Rupfen, Zupfen, Kratzen, Reiben, Wischen, Händereiben, Scharren, Trippeln, Tänzeln (575). Ohne bisher ein pathophysiologisches Korrelat aufgespürt zu haben, findet man diese und andere Grundbewegungsweisen auch bei den motorischen Stereotypien der Katatonen, ein Zusammenhang, der uns für das pathogenetische Begreifen der Katatonie wichtig erscheint (652) (s. S. 351 ff.; 363 ff.).

Wir erinnern weiter an die psychopathologisch aufschlußreichen abnormen Gefühlserlebnisse in der Aura und während der psychomotorischen Anfälle. Hier kann nahezu alles in bunter Durchmischung vorkommen, was es an Gefühlserlebnissen gibt: Glücks- und Angstgefühle, Depersonalisationserlebnisse, Veränderungen der Leibgefühle und Gefühlsempfindungen, eigenartige Kontrastgefühle, Intensivierung und Veränderung von sinnlichen Gefühlen oder Sinneserlebnissen sowie Störungen der Gefühlsbezogenheit (*11*), aber auch das plötzliche Aufsteigen von gegenstandslosen Gefühlen und Stimmungen. Sexuelle Reizzustände sind im Rahmen des Uncinatus-Syndroms beschrieben worden: Eine Patientin von BENTE und KLUGE (*252*) führte im Anfall bei leicht angezogenen Beinen rhythmische, auf- und abschaukelnde Bewegungen mit dem Becken aus, eine andere masturbierte. In diesen Fällen war die Verschränkung olfactorischer Störungen mit Reizzuständen in der oralen und anal-genitalen Sphäre bei gleichzeitiger Veränderung der Bewußtseinslage besonders eindrucksvoll. LIDDELL und NORTHFIELD (*514*) beschrieben 2 Patienten mit temporaler Epilepsie, deren Verhalten außerhalb der Attacken sehr stark einem Klüver-Bucy-Syndrom glich, das nach der einseitigen temporalen Lobektomie verschwand. Während der Attacken hatten die Patienten typische Aura-Erlebnisse und Automatismen. Andererseits trat bei 5 chronisch Schizophrenen, wie SAWA und Mitarb. beschreiben (*720*), nach bilateraler Amygdalektomie ein ähnliches Syndrom auf, bei dem das abnorme orale Verhalten während monatelanger Beobachtung im Vordergrund stand. Vor der Operation handelten die Kranken impulsiv-destruktiv.

Im ganzen gesehen sind aus diesen psychopathologischen Phänomenen für die endogenen Psychosen bisher erstaunlich geringe Konsequenzen gezogen worden, obwohl nahezu alle in Dämmerattacken und Dämmerzuständen oder auch in der Aura und im psychomotorischen Anfall beschriebenen Erlebnisse in schizophrenen Psychosen, gerade auch bezüglich des Verflochtenseins von abnormen Sinneserlebnissen und Gefühlszuständen, vorkommen können. Es scheint, als scheue man sich, für die Symptomatologie der Psychosen hirnphysiologische und verhaltensphysiologische Ergebnisse heranzuziehen (*654*). Die Tatsache, daß menschliches affektives Verhalten durch ein — im Vergleich zum Neocortex — relativ primitives Hirnsystem bestimmt wird, sollte für die Lehre von den endogenen Psychosen zu denken geben. Der Unterschied zwischen dem, was wir „*fühlen*", und dem, was wir „*wissen*", ist jedem aus der Selbstbeobachtung bekannt. Hinsichtlich der Psychosen scheint uns dieser Unterschied ein zentrales Problem zu sein (vgl. S. 365). "A crazy man would be crazy not to believe in the reality of his crazy feelings" (*549*). MacLEAN (*544, 545*) hat in ähnlichem Zusammenhang von einer „Schizophysiologie" des limbischen und neocorticalen Systems gesprochen.

II. Hirnfunktionen und erworbene Verhaltensweisen

1. Über die Theorien und Methoden des sog. Behaviorismus

Bisher war von einer für das Verhalten der meisten Lebewesen (insbesondere der Säuger) entscheidend wichtigen Fähigkeit, dem Lernen, noch kaum die Rede (*195, 196*). Die Theorie, daß alles Verhalten auf Erfahrung, d. h. Erlerntem, beruhe, daß also ein Menschen- oder Tierbaby als Tabula rasa zu denken sei, hat neben vielen Mißverständnissen und manchem Schaden (s. S. 293) zahlreiche Früchte gebracht. Das Verhalten wird auf ein Reiz-Reaktions-Modell entsprechend einem „Reflex" reduziert, und das Nervensystem ist in diesem Lehrgebäude ein Instrument, das durch Sammeln von Erfahrungen zum Funktionieren gebracht wird, eine Art Matrix, welche durch Erfahrungen geformt wird. Die radikalste Formulierung einer solchen Milieutheorie hat wohl J. B. WATSON gegeben, der glaubte, aus Kleinkindern ohne Rücksicht auf deren Veranlagung durch ausgewählte Umwelteinflüsse je nach Wunsch Künstler, Ärzte, Rechtsanwälte, Landstreicher oder Diebe machen zu können (*84*). Wegen solcher und anderer extremistischer Thesen, z. B. auch der Verbannung des „Bewußtseins", der Aufmerksamkeit, der Introspektion, des Willens, der Gefühle und Empfindungen, ja, sogar der Wahrnehmung aus der Psychologie, ist der Behaviorismus in Deutschland mehr berüchtigt als berühmt, und seine in den letzten 30 Jahren erzielten wissenschaftlichen Ergebnisse sind kaum bekannt geworden.

Der Einfluß bedeutender Forscher, wie z. B. des genial-kritischen Karl S. Lashley (*14, 114—117, 492*), hat sich auf die deutsche Verhaltensforschung, sei es nun in Zoologie, Psychologie oder Neuropsychiatrie, kaum ausgewirkt, in Amerika hingegen das Denken und Experimentieren nachhaltig bestimmt. In der jüngeren anglo-amerikanischen Psychologie hat die Bezeichnung "Behaviorismus" ihre scharfe Prägung weitgehend verloren und wird kaum noch benutzt. Die naturwissenschaftlich eingestellte Psychologie hat den Namen comparative physiological psychology (*139, 203, 204*). Verschiedene Schulen sind entstanden, deren Hauptgegenstand der Forschung das *Lernen* ist (*44, 47, 68, 69, 80, 84, 88, 89, 116. 152, 183, 184, 190, 199, 323, 381*). So unterschiedlich die daraus entstandenen Verhaltenstheorien[1] im einzelnen sind, so tragen sie doch alle den gemeinsamen Zug des streng empirischen Vorgehens in ihrer Beweisführung. Als wissenschaftlich sinnvoll gelten nur solche Aussagen, die unter genau festgelegten Bedingungen von unabhängigen Beobachtern empirisch bestätigt oder widerlegt werden können. Lassen sich zur Überprüfung einer Hypothese keine „Operationen" angeben, die zur Verifizierung führen können, ist die Hypothese als „sinnlos" zu bezeichnen. Die Einflüsse des großen amerikanischen Psychologen und Philosophen W. James (Pragmatismus), des logischen Positivismus (R. Carnap u. a.) und des sog. Operationismus (P. W. Bridgman) sind wirksam geblieben.

Drei Quellen sind es, aus denen der sog. Behaviorismus schöpft: Die Assoziationspsychologie von Wundt und Thorndike, Pawlows Lehre von den Bedingten Reflexen (*155, 160*) und Freuds Lust-Unlust-Prinzip im Zusammenhang mit seiner Libido-Theorie[2]. Die folgende Darstellung verzichtet auf eine Wiedergabe der für die theoretische Psychologie wichtigen formalen Lerntheorien (*80*) und ist mehr auf klinisch-psychiatrische Gesichtspunkte abgestellt (*154, 215*).

Der *Klassische Bedingte Reflex* von Pawlow wird zum Studium der Lernvorgänge auch jetzt noch viel benutzt. Daneben hat sich das *Lernen am Erfolg* durchgesetzt. Das Verdienst von Pawlow (*155*) bleibt es, unter der Unmenge von erworbenen komplexen Verhaltensweisen das einfachste Phänomen ausgesondert zu haben. Zwar hat sich klar herausgestellt, daß man den Bedingten Reflex nicht als „Element" betrachten darf, aus dem das Verhalten „aufgebaut" zu denken wäre, jedoch schien der Bedingte Reflex zunächst mindestens eine Bestätigung der assoziationspsychologischen Theorien zu sein.

Fassen wir kurz den ursprünglichen Vorgang ins Auge: Pawlow arbeitete mit Hunden und maß zunächst die Magensaft-, später fast ausschließlich die Speicheldrüsensekretion. Futter, der *natürliche Auslöser* für die Speichelsekretion, bildete den sog. *Unbedingten Reiz* (Unconditioned Stimulus), hier durchwegs mit US abgekürzt; ein Geräusch, ein Ton, ein Lichtreiz u. a. bildete den sog. *Bedingenden Reiz* (Conditioning Stimulus), durchwegs CS abgekürzt[3]. Wenn nun erstens der US dem CS in kurzem Zeitabstand folgt und wenn dieses Ereignis zweitens Gegenstand wiederholter Erfahrung geworden ist — bei uns Dressur, englisch "training" genannt —, dann bildet sich der Bedingte Reflex aus, d. h. in Pawlows Schul-

---

[1] Manche dieser Theorien hatten ursprünglich gar nichts mit dem Behaviorismus zu tun. wie z. B. die Theorie von Tolman (*199*), welche der Zweckpsychologie entstammt und als Antithese zur behavioristischen Theorie von Hull (*89*) aufzufassen ist.

[2] Dies gilt nicht generell für die vergleichende physiologische Psychologie; s. Fußnote S. 349, Lashley (*490*).

[3] Wir bevorzugen die anglo-amerikanisch-romanischen Abkürzungen, da sie in der Literatur fest eingebürgert sind. Bei Wahl der deutschen Abkurzungen. die man wegen Mangel an neueren einschlägigen experimentellen Arbeiten kaum mehr findet, würden zudem Verwechslungen zwischen *R*eiz und *R*eaktion zu häufig vorkommen.

beispiel, die Speichelsekretion schießt bereits auf das Glockenzeichen (CS) ein, ohne daß der Hund Futter (US) bekommen oder wahrgenommen hat. Mithin hat der CS die Funktion des US übernommen oder anders ausgedrückt: der CS ist an die Stelle des US getreten. Es hat sich gezeigt, daß nahezu jeder natürliche „Reflex" mit Bedingten Reizen verknüpft werden kann, wenn auch die Bedingte Reaktion (CR) der Unbedingten Reaktion (UR) nicht vollständig zu gleichen braucht. Zum Beispiel verengt sich nach der Dressur die Pupille (CR) nicht erst auf Lichteinfall (US), sondern schon auf ein Geräusch (CS), das ursprünglich keine Pupillenverengung hervorzurufen imstande war. Ein Bedingter Reflex erlischt, wenn stets nur noch der CS, nicht aber hin und wieder auch der US geboten wird.

Man nennt diesen Vorgang *Löschung* (extinction) im Gegensatz zur *Verstärkung* oder *Bekräftigung* (reinforcement) des CS durch gelegentliche Wiederholung des US.

Eine Bestätigung der Assoziationstheorie hat sich durch das Studium der Klassischen Bedingten Reflexe insofern nicht ergeben, als es für die Ausbildung eines Bedingten Reflexes nötig ist, daß der US dem CS während der Dressur in kleinem Zeitabstand folgt (Optimum 0,5 sec), was aber für Assoziationen keine notwendige Bedingung ist.

Als *Selbstdressur durch Eigentätigkeit* (instrumental oder operant conditioning) bezeichnet man mit SKINNER (*183*) eine Dressurweise, bei der das Tier durch eigene Tätigkeit behält, was Erfolg bringt, und Erfolgloses unterläßt. Die so erzielten Bedingten Reaktionen werden von den sog. Klassischen Bedingten Reflexen streng unterschieden und spielen in den Lern-Theorien des Verhaltens eine wichtige Rolle (*111*).

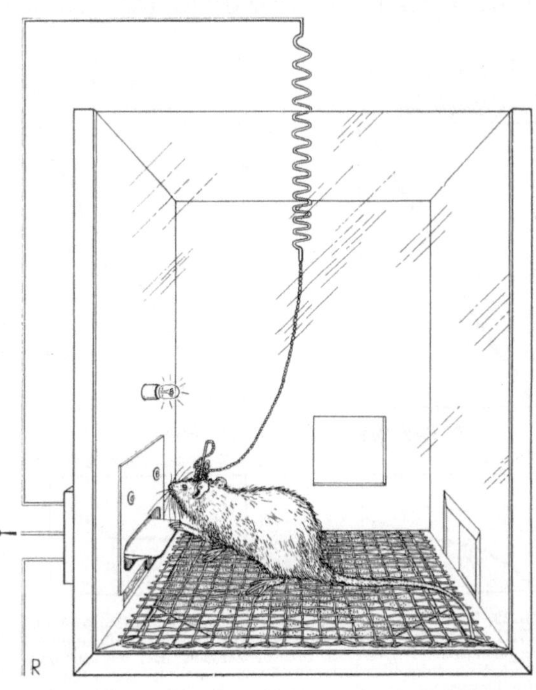

Abb. 32. *Schema eines Skinner-Käfig. — Versuchsanordnung zur intracraniellen Selbstreizung* (vgl. Abb. 40). Jeder Druck auf den Hebel liefert dem Versuchstier Futter und wird gleichzeitig automatisch registriert. Über das Drahtgitter am Boden des Käfigs kann ein schmerzhafter elektrischer Schlag ausgelöst werden. Wird der Skinner-Käfig zu Selbstreizungsversuchen benutzt, bekommt das Tier *statt* Futter einen elektrischen Hirnreiz, der durch den Hebeldruck über die in das Hirn implantierte Elektrode ausgelöst wird. [Nach OLDS (*623*)]

Das *Lernen am Erfolg* benutzte im Grunde schon THORNDIKE (*80, 84*): Wenn seine Katzen an einem Rädchen zu drehen gelernt hatten, wurde der Weg zur Nahrung frei. Um Strafschläge austeilen zu können, war der Käfigboden ganz oder teilweise mit einem elektrifizierbaren Drahtrost belegt. Im *Skinner-Käfig* befindet sich außerdem eine Drucktaste, deren Betätigung zu Futter- oder Wassererwerb führt (s. Abb. 32, S. 397). Das eingesetzte Versuchstier (Ratte, Katze, Affe, Vogel) hat meist schon nach kurzer Zeit den Zusammenhang erfaßt. Da jeder Hebeldruck graphisch registriert wird, schreibt das Tier seine Protokolle selbst (*337*).

Die Häufigkeit des Hebeldrückens hängt u. a. vom Hunger bzw. Durst und von der Art der Belohnung ab, ob nämlich z. B. jeder 2., 5. oder 10. Hebeldruck nach

Art einer Akkordarbeit oder aber jede 2., 5. oder 10. Sekunde („Stundenlohn") Futter bringt. Skinner (*47, 183, 184*) hat gezeigt, daß eine Belohnung nach Leistung die Tätigkeit weitaus mehr anreizt als die nach Zeit. Sogar bei starker „Erhöhung der Norm", wenn nur noch auf — sagen wir — jeden 150. Hebeldruck Futter kommt, läßt sich eine Ratte nicht entmutigen. Unter anderem gestattet die Methode, die Stärke des Nahrungstriebes an einer mit dem Nahrungserwerb bedingt verknüpften Tätigkeit zu messen.

Nachdem bei einem bestimmten Belohnungsschema die Zahl der Hebeldrucke je Zeiteinheit konstant geworden ist, folgt eine zweite Dressur: Auf einen akustischen Reiz (rasch wiederholtes Geräusch) folgt in festgelegtem Zeitabstand ein elektrischer, schmerzhafter Schlag (*425*). Nach einigen Wiederholungen von Reiz (CS) und darauf folgendem Schlag (US) unterbricht das Tier beim Ertönen des CS seine nahrungsbringende Tätigkeit und zeigt alle Anzeichen der Angst oder, korrekter ausgedrückt, emotionaler Gestörtheit. Bei der Ratte sind dies Kriechen, Defäzieren und Urinieren (*380, 733*). Wenn der US vorüber ist, nimmt das Tier seine Hebeldruck-Tätigkeit wieder auf. Auf diese Weise gelingt es also, das *Angstverhalten graphisch sichtbar* zu machen, es zu quantifizieren und *Anfang und Ende der Bedingten Emotionalen Reaktion* (Conditioned Emotional Reaction; CER) festzulegen (s. Abb. 33).

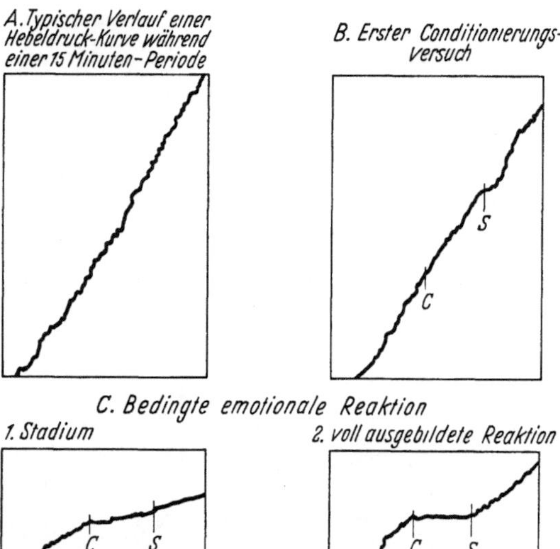

Abb. 33. *Typische Ausbildung einer Bedingten Emotialen Reaktion (CER). A* Normale Registrierkurve für die Hebeldrücke einer 15 min-Periode. *B* Der erste Dressur-Versuch: Bei *c* ertont das Gerausch (bedingender Reiz) für 5 min, bei *s* wird der schmerzhafte elektrische Schlag ausgelost (unbedingter Reiz). *C* Im 1. Stadium bildet sich die CER aus: Nach dem Gerausch (*c*) drückt das Versuchstier noch mit stark verminderter Geschwindigkeit den Hebel und erreicht nach dem Schmerzreiz seine anfängliche Aktivität nicht wieder. Im voll ausgeprägten Stadium der Bedingten Reaktion hört das Hebeldrücken nach dem Einsetzen des Geräusches auf und setzt nach dem Schmerzreiz ungefahr mit der anfanglichen Frequenz wieder ein. [Nach Hunt und Brady (*424*)]

An diesem Beispiel können wir kurz die *Theorie von Bedarf und Bedürfnis* erläutern, die für den *Begriff der primären Triebe* (primary drives) von Bedeutung ist. Seit Cannon verstehen wir unter Homeostase die Konstanthaltung des „inneren Milieus" (Claude Bernard). Dazu haben die Organismen im Laufe der Evolution Organsysteme entwickelt, die diese Homeostase gewährleisten, wenn die *primären Bedürfnisse* befriedigt werden. Diese Bedürfnisse bestehen z. B. in Hunger (im Sinne von Appetenzen), Durst, Verlangen nach Schlaf, Sauerstoff-Aufnahme und Wärme, Vermeidung von Schmerz. Darüber, ob auch das geschlechtliche Verlangen zu den primären Bedürfnissen zu rechnen ist, gehen die Meinungen auseinander. Die Verhaltensweisen, die zur Deckung dieser primären Bedürfnisse dienen, nennt man *primäre Triebe*. Die Störung der Homeostase führt zu Verhaltensänderungen, die die Wiederherstellung des gestörten Gleichgewichtes zum Ziel haben. Beim *Menschen* besteht zwischen Bedarf und Bedürfnis kein festes Kopplungsverhältnis mehr. Es gibt — auch bei höheren Tieren — Bedarfslagen, denen kein spezifisches Bedürfnis zugeordnet ist und umgekehrt vor allem auch viele Bedürfnisse, die primär keinen organischen Bedarf decken. Diese theoretische Basis hat für verschiedene Hypothesen über die Sucht Bedeutung bekommen (*82, 209, 250, 276, 278, 279, 579, 582, 748, 749*).

Die *sekundären Bedürfnisse*, auch „sekundäre Motivationen" (*20, 88*) oder „lernbare Antriebe" (*190*) genannt, sind an die Deckung eines organischen Bedarfes assoziativ gekoppelt. An diesem Punkt tritt in der Theoriebildung eine Verschmelzung der Lehre Sigmund Freuds von den „großen organischen Bedürfnissen" (im Zusammenhang mit Lustprinzip und Libidotheorie) und der Assoziationstheorie ein. Sekundäre Bedürfnisse sind erlernt. Unter Lernen werden mit Wahrscheinlichkeit auftretende Veränderungen des Verhaltens in definierten Reizsituationen verstanden. Für das Lernen ist der Erfolg, den die Verhaltensänderung herbeiführt, entscheidend. *Mit Eintritt des Erfolges verringert sich die Bedürfnisspannung.* Dies bedeutet die Befriedigung des sekundären Bedürfnisses.

Fassen wir das Gesagte am Beispiel des Skinner-Verfahrens zusammen: Ihr primäres Bedürfnis Hunger lernen die Tiere durch das Hebeldrücken zu decken. Das Hebeldrücken ist assoziativ an dieses Bedürfnis gekoppelt und wird zum sekundären Bedürfnis. Je nach Reizsituation (Belohnungsschema) kann das Bedürfnis größer oder kleiner gehalten werden. Die Anzahl der Hebeldrucke pro Zeiteinheit ist ein indirektes Maß für die Bedürfnisspannung.

In diese quantifizierende Versuchssituation ist nun eine zweite Situation, nämlich eine „Angst"-erzeugende Konfliktsituation, eingebaut. Das Skinner-Verfahren soll uns nunmehr noch Modell stehen zur Skizzierung der *Konflikttheorie*, die von der anglo-amerikanischen Verhaltensforschung entwickelt worden ist. Wohl alle derartigen Theorien gehen auf die scherzhafte Geschichte von Buridans Esel zurück, der, gleich weit von zwei gleich beschaffenen Heuhaufen entfernt, zwischen ihnen verhungerte. Angeregt durch Freuds triebdynamische Vorstellungen haben Kurt Lewin (*125, 505*) unter gestaltpsychologischen und N. E. Miller (*576—578, 583, 586*) unter behavioristischen Gesichtspunkten das buridanische Modell weiter ausgebaut.

Lewins grundlegende Untersuchungen zur Handlungs- und Affektpsychologie fanden durch Conrad (*29, 30*) und andere (*451, 647, 651*) Eingang in die deutsche Psychopathologie. Um N. E. Millers Theorie [s. in (*190*)] darzulegen, wäre ein großer Aufwand an recht abstrakten Begriffen der Hullschen Lerntheorie nötig (Reaktionspotential, Zielgradient, Appetenz- und Aversionsgradient, Generalisierung usw.), ohne daß damit für unseren Zusammenhang viel gewonnen wäre.

Im Prinzip lassen sich alle Konfliksituationen aus dem *gleichzeitigen Ablaufen von mindestens zwei Verhaltenstendenzen* erklären. Man unterscheidet daher zwischen Tendenzen, die sich auf Erreichung eines Zieles richten (Appetenz), und solchen, die zur Vermeidung gefürchteter Situationen führen (Aversion). Buridans Esel befand sich im Konflikt zwischen zwei Hinstrebungen (Appetenz-Appetenz-Konflikt); wer zwischen zwei Übeln wählen muß, sieht sich in einem Aversions-Aversions-Konflikt (zwei Wegstrebungen), und wer für die Erfüllung eines Wunsches einen großen oder allzu großen Preis zahlen muß, steht in einem Appetenz-Aversions-Konflikt, der wahrscheinlich am häufigsten ist.

Kehren wir zum Skinner-Verfahren zurück, das uns in den nächsten Kapiteln mehrfach wieder begegnen wird: Durch die graphische Aufzeichnung des Hebeldrückens kann man, so sagten wir, die durch den Hunger entstehende Bedürfnisspannung des primären Triebes „messen". Die Tätigkeit des Hebeldrückens ist durch den primären Trieb bedingt. Die dann ausgebildete Bedingte Emotionale Reaktion (CER), die zugleich auch einen Aversions-Appetenz-Konflikt darstellt, verhindert für eine Weile die bedingte Tätigkeit des Hebeldrückens. An dem Grad des daraus entstehenden Leistungsabfalles läßt sich die CER messen.

Nach den drei oben erwähnten Konflikttypen sind nun die Experimente N. E. Millers und anderer (*148, 190, 576, 577, 584, 585, 610*) aufgebaut:

Ein Beispiel: Ein Angestellter, der Angst vor seinem Chef hat und gehemmt ist, seine Aggressionen gegen ihn auszudrücken, nimmt den Laufjungen als Sündenbock und gibt ihm eine Ohrfeige. In dieser Beobachtung steckt die psychoanalytisch relevante Behauptung, daß die Aggression sich überträgt (Generalisierung). Dagegen kann man einwenden, daß sich ebenso wie die Aggression auch die dem Chef gegenüber gezeigte Hemmung generalisieren müßte. Wenn das so wäre, würde der Laufjunge seine Ohrfeige nicht beziehen. DieVersuchsplanung zielt daher darauf ab zu prüfen, ob die Hemmung der Aggression schneller abnimmt als die Aggression oder, anders ausgedrückt, ob die Aversion (Vermeidung der Aggression) sich rascher vermindert als die Appetenz (eine Ohrfeige zu geben).

Versuch: Hungrige, in drei Gruppen eingeteilte Ratten laufen durch einen weißen, weiten Gang zum Futter. Nach einigen Tagen erhalten sie auf halbem Wege einen elektrischen Schlag, so daß sich rasch ein Aversions-Appetenz-Konflikt ausbildet und nur noch ein Teil der Ratten zum Futterplatz vorstößt. Der kritische Test — ohne elektrischen Schlag — findet für die erste Gruppe in einem weiten weißen, für die zweite Gruppe in einem schmaleren grauen und für die dritte Gruppe in einem engen dunkelgrauen Gang statt. 23% der ersten, 37% der zweiten und 70% der dritten Gruppe erreichen den Futterplatz (*584, 585*).

Aus diesen und ähnlich aufgebauten Versuchen wird geschlossen, daß sich die Aversion weniger auf eine neue Situation überträgt als die Appetenz (*148*). Die unter psychoanalytischen Gesichtspunkten entwickelten Arbeiten verfolgen weiterhin die Frage, ob die primären und sekundären Bedürfnisse sich hinsichtlich ihrer Bedürfnisspannungen unterscheiden und wie sich diese Unterschiede in den drei Konflikttypen bemerkbar machen. Eine wesentliche Hypothese besagt schließlich, daß stets nur die *Reduktion* von Bedürfnisspannungen zur Befriedigung führe (*323, 576*). Gerade dies ist allerdings fraglich, wie wir noch sehen werden (s. S. 416ff.).

Ein anderer Versuchstyp ist nach dem Modell von Pawlow (*155*) ausgebildet worden: Hunde lernen, daß sie beim Anblicken eines Kreises Futter bekommen, bei Darbietung einer Ellipse hingegen nicht und bilden infolgedessen nur auf den Kreis einen Bedingten „Nahrungsreflex" aus. Gleicht man nach und nach die Ellipsenform dem Kreis an, so treten an einem kritischen Punkt hinreichender Ähnlichkeit „neurotische" Verhaltensstörungen auf (Versuch von Schenger-Krestownikowa; s. Pawlow, Bd. III/2, S. 314). Die so oder auf andere Weise neurotisierten, vorher zutraulichen Tiere bellen, beißen, verweigern die Nahrung, zeigen Kreislaufstörungen, mitunter auch Lähmungserscheinungen oder sexuelle Erregung. Dem Studium dieser experimentellen Neurosen bei Tieren (*515, 516*) sind sehr viele Arbeiten gewidmet, die auch dem Problem psychosomatischer Erkrankungen nachgehen (*53, 235, 289, 493, 516, 576, 715, 745—747*).

J. H. Masserman hat in dieser Richtung auf experimenteller Basis eine Art „bionomer" psychoanalytischer Psychiatrie entwickelt, die originelle, aber umstrittene Einsichten vermittelt (*140, 562*) und von ihm auch nach der praktisch psychiatrischen und psychotherapeutischen Seite hin ausgebaut wurde (*141, 142*). Weiteres dazu findet man bei Elkes, ds. Bd., Teil A.

Nach dieser Einführung wenden wir uns jetzt speziellen Ergebnissen zu, die uns für die Psychiatrie wertvoll erscheinen. — Über die Theorien, Methoden und Ergebnisse des sog. Behaviorismus wird man ausführlich durch Stevens (*190*) unterrichtet. Eine sehr gedrängte, aber gut ausgewählte und klare Übersicht gibt Hofstätter (*84*).

2. Elektrokrampf und bedingtes emotionales Verhalten

Von den zahlreichen experimentellen Untersuchungen, die sich mit der Wirkung des Elektrokrampfes (EK) auf das Verhalten von Tieren befassen, stellen wir eine Versuchsserie als Modell dar. Die meisten der im folgenden mitgeteilten Ergebnisse stammen von J. V. Brady (*19*) u. Mitarb.

Versuchsanordnung:

Die Tiere — meist Ratten —, mit denen zuerst das Hebeldruckverfahren im Skinner-Käfig eingeübt wurde, haben vor Versuchsbeginn eine bestimmte Zeit (zwischen 22 und 48 Std.) gehungert oder gedurstet. Dann beginnt die *Dressur*, wie schon geschildert, und wird in jedem Falle so lange fortgesetzt, bis nahezu 100% der Versuchstiere die „Bedingte Emotionale Reaktion" (CER) zeigen (s. S. 398). Bei 8 Versuchen pro Tag von jeweils 15 min Dauer ist das 90—100%-Kriterium in wenigen Tagen erreicht (Abb. 33, S. 398).

48 Std. nach der letzten CER beginnt die *Elektrokrampfbehandlung.* Innerhalb von 7 Tagen werden 21 Elektrokrämpfe gesetzt, und zwar 3mal täglich 1 Krampf. Während dieser Zeit bewegen sich die Tiere frei und erhalten genügend Nahrung. 4 Tage nach dem letzten EK und somit 13 Tage nach der letzten CER wird der sog. *Erinnerungsversuch* (retention test) angestellt, d. h. man prüft, wieviel Prozent der Tiere die CER auf den Sinnesreiz zeigen oder, anschaulicher ausgedrückt, wieviel Tiere *behalten* haben, daß auf den Sinnesreiz Schmerz folgt. Die Angst der Tiere wird, das sei nochmals hervorgehoben, durch das Hebeldruckverfahren quantifiziert (*337*). Außerdem wird das qualitativ sichtbare, Angst ausdrückende Verhalten (*380*) (Kriechen, Defäzieren usw.) protokolliert.

Die Versuchsergebnisse:

Die mit EK behandelten Tiere zeigten im *Erinnerungsversuch* ausnahmslos *keine* Bedingte Emotionale Reaktion (CER), d. h. sie reagierten nicht auf das Geräusch (CS), sondern bedienten im Skinner-Käfig mit unverminderter Häufigkeit den Hebel, um Wasser zu erhalten. Die auf das den elektrischen Schlag ankündigende Geräusch dressierten, aber *nicht* mit EK behandelten Kontrolltiere hingegen hatten ausnahmslos Angst, d. h. die Hebeldrucktätigkeit setzte aus und man beobachtete Immobilität, Kriechen, Defäzieren (*424*) (s. Abb. 34, S. 401). Die behandelten Tiere „behielten" also die zuerst eingeübte Methode, mit der sie ihren Durst stillen können, „vergaßen" hingegen die nach dem Hebeldruckverfahren erlernte, Schmerz ankündigende Bedeutung des Bedingten Reizes. Somit war zu prüfen, ob die Reihenfolge der gesammelten Erfahrungen einen Einfluß auf das Ergebnis hat. Wenn die Dressur auf den elektrischen Schlag der Dressur auf das Hebeldrücken voranging, änderten sich die Ergebnisse nicht: Die gleiche EK-Serie löschte die Angst aus, ohne das Hebeldruckverhalten zu beeinträchtigen (*356*). Somit sind frühere Untersuchungen widerlegt, nach denen der EK spezifisch auf das zuletzt erlernte Verhalten wirken soll (*326*).

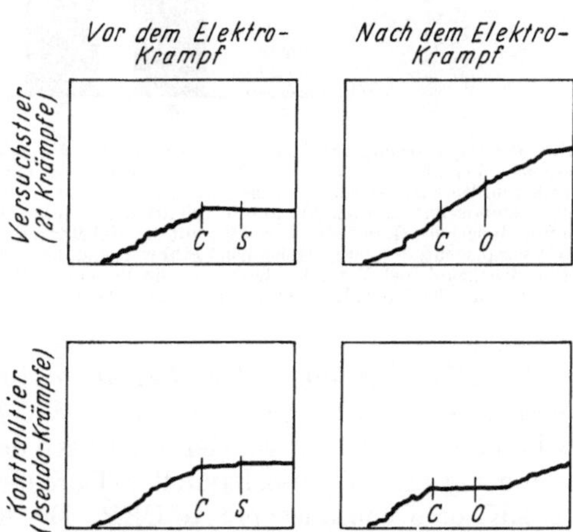

Abb. 34. *Typische Wirkung einer Elektrokrampfbehandlung auf die Bedingte Emotionale Reaktion (CER.)* Kurven von 2 Ratten, die nach dem Schmerzreiz (*s*) eine Weile warten, bis sie die Hebeldrucktätigkeit wieder aufnehmen. Das Geräusch (*c*) ertönt für 3 min. Die linken Felder zeigen Versuchs- und Kontrolltier vor der Behandlung. Im rechten Feld oben ist das Ergebnis des Erinnerungsversuches nach 21 Elektrokrämpfen dargestellt. Das Tier reagiert nicht auf das Geräusch und fahrt unbeeinflußt mit dem Hebeldrucken fort. Bei (*o*) hört das Gerausch auf; ein Schmerzreiz wird im Erinnerungsversuch nicht gegeben. Im unteren rechten Feld die ausgebildete CER des zum Schein behandelten Kontrolltieres. [Nach HUNT und BRADY (*424*)]

Führt man nun 30, 60 oder 90 Tage nach dem letzten EK weitere — für jede Zeitspanne in gesonderten Tiergruppen — Erinnerungsversuche durch, sieht man bei allen behandelten Tieren das Angstverhalten zurückkehren, d. h. die Ratten erwarten zwischen dem 30. und 90. Tage nach dem letzten EK beim Ertönen des Geräusches wieder ängstlich das schmerzhafte Ereignis, den Unbedingten Reiz, ohne daß in der Zwischenzeit eine erneute Dressur stattgefunden hat (*271*).

Im *Löschungsversuch* (extinction) — das ist die Darbietung des CS ohne nachfolgenden US — unterscheiden sich die behandelten Tiere jedoch noch von den
unbehandelten Kontrolltieren: Bei letzteren bleibt nämlich das Angstverhalten
während der Löschungsversuche, die nach 90 Tagen 8 Tage lang vorgenommen
wurden, hartnäckiger bestehen. Bereits beim 5. Löschungsversuch verloren 58%
der EK-behandelten Ratten die CER, während sich nur 17% der Kontrolltiere
angstfrei verhielten.Erst nach weiteren 2—3 Löschungsversuchen waren auch die
Kontrolltiere frei von Angst (*271*).

Diese statistisch signifikanten Versuchsergebnisse wurden durch eine Reihe von Neben-
versuchen gesichert. Zum Beispiel wurde entkraftet, daß die EK-Serie zu einer Überempfindlichkeit gegenuber akustischen Reizen fuhre (*271*) oder daß der EK Taubheit verursache (*284*).

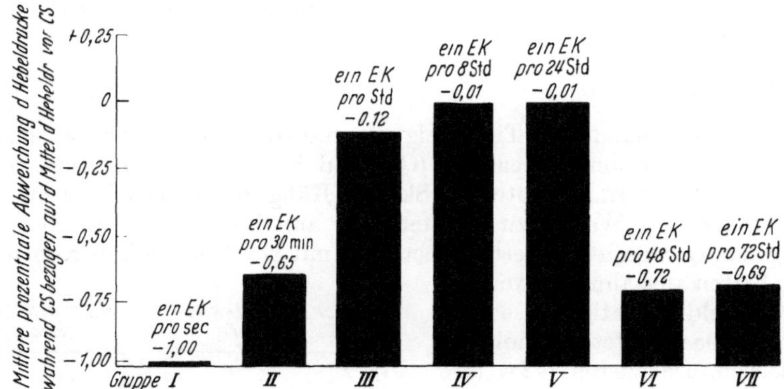

Abb 35. *Die Wirkung des Elektrokrampfes auf die Bedingte Emotionale Reaktion (CER) in Abhangigkeit von der
zeitlichen Verteilung der Krampfe.* Die 8—24stundliche Anwendung des Elektrokrampfes beeinflußt die CER am
starksten. Die Tiere zeigen bei dieser Anwendungsweise keine „Angst" mehr. *Abszisse* 7 Gruppen von je 12 Ratten,
jede Gruppe hat 21 Elektrokrampfe erhalten. *Ordinate* Die Hebeldruckzahl wahrend des bedingenden Reizes
(3 min dauerndes Gerausch = *cs*) wird mit der Hebeldruckzahl der 3 min-Periode verglichen, die dem bedingenden
Reiz vorausgeht. —1,00 = Hebeldruckzahl wahrend des bedingenden Reizes gleich Null. 0 = keine Differenz der
Hebeldruckzahl bei Vergleich beider 3 min-Perioden. Positivere Werte geben dementsprechend die relative
Zunahme der Hebeldrucke wahrend des bedingenden Reizes an. [Nach Brady, Hunt und Geller (*286*)]

Die Frage ist nun, welche *Bedeutung der Zeitspanne* zukommt, die *von der Ausbildung der CER bis zum Beginn der EK-Behandlung* verstreicht. Setzt die EK-
Behandlung erst 30 Tage oder mehr nach der Dressur ein, haben sowohl die behandelten wie auch die unbehandelten Tiere im Erinnerungsversuch, 4 Tage nach dem
21. EK, eine voll ausgeprägte CER. Die EK-Serie hat also unter sonst gleichen
Versuchsbedingungen die CER weder ausgelöscht noch auch nur verändert. Bei
der Löschung der CER zeigen sich jedoch Unterschiede, und zwar wieder derart,
daß das Angstverhalten bei den behandelten Ratten schneller verschwindet als bei
den unbehandelten. Dieser Unterschied gleicht sich aber mit zunehmendem Zeitraum zwischen vollendeter Dressur und Einsetzen der EK-Behandlung aus:
Beträgt der Zeitraum 30 Tage, gelingt die Löschung bei den behandelten Tieren
2—3mal schneller, sind es 60 Tage, geht die Löschung nur noch 1—2mal schneller,
und bei 90 Tagen kommt kein signifikanter Unterschied mehr heraus (*272*). Verwendet man statt des akustischen Bedingten Reizes intermittierendes Licht, erhält
man die gleichen Ergebnisse (*284*).

Die Schwächung oder Tilgung der CER durch die EK-Behandlung hängt von
weiteren Faktoren ab, denen auch unter praktisch klinischen Gesichtspunkten
Bedeutung zukommt. Die *Zeitspanne zwischen den Einzelkrämpfen* ist für die
Wirkung entscheidend (*286*) (s. Abb. 35, S. 402). Werden die Elektroschocks im
Abstand von einer Sekunde gegeben, ist kaum eine Wirkung festzustellen, wäh-

rend sich eine solche schon beim Abstand von einer halben Stunde von Krampf zu Krampf zeigt. Beim einstündigen Intervall ist die Wirkung schon nahezu optimal und erreicht zwischen dem 8—24 Std.-Intervall ihren Höhepunkt. Eine längere Zeitspanne von 48 oder 72 Std. wirkt sich auf die Schwächung der CER bereits wieder recht ungünstig aus (286).

Natürlich spielt auch die *Gesamtzahl der Krämpfe* eine Rolle (292, 355). Bei weniger als 15 Krämpfen wird der Tilgungseffekt zunehmend und signifikant geringer.[1] Übrigens wirkt sich auch die Stärke des Strafschlages auf die Stabilität der CER aus und ist eine wichtigere Variable als die Anzahl der Dressurversuche (173, 185, 449).

Die Wirkung der EK-Behandlung auf die CER ist erheblich geschwächt, wenn der Krampf durch eine kurz vor dem Schock gegebene Äthernarkose verhindert wird (427). Dies führte zu der Frage, ob der elektrisch erzeugte Krampf oder der Krampfanfall überhaupt das Entscheidende ist.

Unter genau definierten Bedingungen wurden bei Ratten *audiogene Krampf-anfälle* erzeugt. Die Versuche ergeben eindeutig, daß sowohl der Krampfanfall als solcher, unanbhängig von seiner Genese, als auch die Anzahl der Krämpfe sowie die Zeit von Anfall zu Anfall entscheidend sind (291). Akustisch erzeugte Krampf-anfälle unterscheiden sich nicht prinzipiell von den elektrischen: Ratten, bei denen audiogen kein Krampf hervorgerufen werden konnte, behielten die CER komplett, während bei audiogen krampfenden Tieren die CER genauso wie durch den EK getilgt werden konnte (285).

Ein überraschendes und besonders interessantes Ergebnis lieferte folgende Versuchsserie:

1. Ratten werden in der beschriebenen Weise dressiert und unter den Standard-Bedingungen mit der EK-Serie behandelt. Sie zeigen im Erinnerungsversuch, wie schon beschrieben, keine CER. Nunmehr folgt unmittelbar anschließend an 13 aufeinander folgenden Tagen je ein Löschungsversuch.

2. Dasselbe geschieht bei einer Kontrollgruppe von Ratten, die keine EK-Serie erhalten und infolgedessen im Erinnerungsversuch eine komplette CER zeigen, die dann während der 13 Löschungsversuche verschwindet.

3. Eine weitere Kontrollgruppe wird nach der Dressur mit der EK-Serie behandelt, ohne daß hernach Löschungsversuche angeschlossen werden.

Prüft man die 1. Gruppe nach 30 Tagen auf ihr Angstverhalten, so kehrt dies (im Gegensatz zu den oben beschriebenen Versuchen *ohne* Löschungsversuche) überraschenderweise gar nicht oder gerade nur angedeutet zurück, d. h. die an den Erinnerungsversuch angeschlossene Löschung ist wirksam geworden, obwohl die Tiere nach beendeter EK-Behandlung keine CER gezeigt hatten. Anders ausgedrückt: Die Tiere haben beim Erinnerungsversuch „vergessen", daß das Geräusch Schmerz ankündigt und reagieren entsprechend auch bei der Löschungsprozedur nicht darauf. Dennoch ist die Löschung „unbewußt" wirksam, denn bei der 3. Gruppe, bei der unter sonst gleichen Bedingungen keine Löschungsversuche vorgenommen wurden, kommt die CER nach 30 Tagen wieder zum Durchbruch. Die 2. Gruppe beweist, daß allein die Löschungsversuche und nicht irgendwelche anderen Umstände für die Tilgung der CER verantwortlich zu machen sind (280, 285, 426).

---

[1] Diese tierexperimentellen Ergebnisse hinsichtlich der Zeitspanne zwischen den Einzelkrämpfen und der Gesamtzahl der Krämpfe stimmen gut mit klinischen Erfahrungen überein (647, 658).

Dieses Ergebnis wirft die Frage auf, ob man zwei voneinander unabhängig störbare Funktionen annehmen muß, nämlich das sensorische Unterscheidungsvermögen von Reizen (akustischer bzw. visueller CS) und das motorische Verhalten, welches die Angst ausdrückt. Eine ähnliche Unterscheidung trifft Rioch, der die Unabhängigkeit antizipierender Hirnfunktionen von solchen des expressiven Verhaltens annimmt (703). Man könnte vermuten, daß die Tiere zwar durchaus auch nach der EK-Behandlung „wissen", was der CS „bedeutet", daß sie sich darüber aber nicht „aufregen". Dann würde das Vermögen, sich „aufzuregen", innerhalb von 30 Tagen wiederkehren und damit auch der motorische Ausdruck für die Emotion. Im Falle der Löschung im Sinne einer Gedächtnistilgung würde gewissermaßen der „Beweggrund", sich aufzuregen, fortfallen und somit auch der motorische Ausdruck für diese Emotion nicht wiederkehren. — Dem gleichen

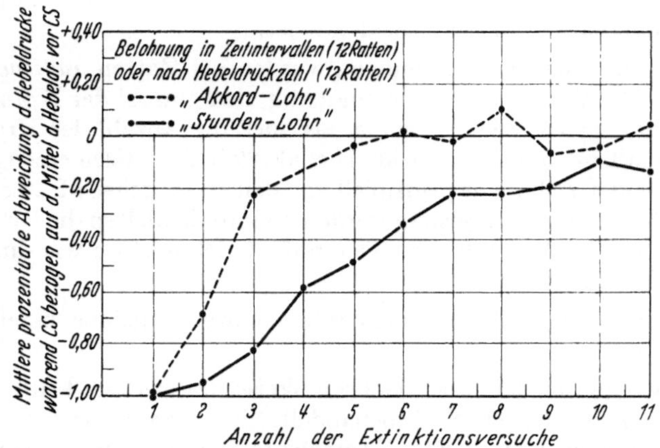

Abb. 36. *Der Löschungseffekt in Abhängigkeit vom Belohnungsschema.* Die bedingte „Angst" kann schneller getilgt werden, wenn die Tiere nach Leistung (nach einer bestimmten Anzahl von Hebeldrücken) anstatt in fortgesetzten Zeitintervallen (untere Kurve) belohnt werden. Zur Erklärung der Skala auf der Ordinate vgl. Abb. 35. *CS* = bedingender Reiz (Conditioning Stimulus). [Nach Brady (274)]

Problem werden wir später bei der Erörterung der anatomischen Substrate bedingten emotionalen Verhaltens nochmals begegnen.

Erwerb und Löschung des bedingten ängstlichen Verhaltens hängen von weiteren Bedingungen ab. Es kommt nämlich auch darauf an, welches Belohnungsschema angewendet wird. Jede Belohnung bedeutet ja bekanntlich eine Bekräftigung der Bedingten Reaktion. Wählt man ein regelmäßig periodisches Belohnungsschema, z. B. so, daß auf jeden 10. Hebeldruck Wasser kommt, bildet sich die Angst-Reaktion der Tiere langsamer aus, als wenn man z. B. jede Minute oder gar in wechselnden Zeitabständen belohnt. Ebenso wird die „Angst" schneller wieder gelöscht, wenn man nicht in Zeitabständen, sondern regelmäßig nach bestimmter Hebeldruckzahl belohnt, so als ob also die Tiere den Schmerz des elektrischen Schlages bei Belohnung nach Art eines Wettbewerbs gleichsam in Kauf nehmen (274, 280). Es kommt somit nicht auf die seit der letzten Belohnung verstrichene Zeit an, sondern auf die positive Leistung, die das Tier vollbringen muß, um zu seiner Belohnung zu gelangen (s. Abb. 36, S. 404). Wenn solche an Ratten gewonnenen Ergebnisse auch noch nicht zur Übertragung auf klinisch psychopathologische oder psychotherapeutische Phänomene ausreichen, so sollten die in den Experimenten steckenden Fragestellungen doch bei klinischen Untersuchungen berücksichtigt und unter angemessenen Bedingungen nachgeprüft werden.

3. Experimentelle Hirnläsionen und bedingtes emotionales Verhalten

Die folgenden Versuche beschäftigen sich mit der Wirkung von experimentellen Hirnverletzungen auf das bedingte emotionale Verhalten. Ort und Ausmaß der Läsionen wurden histologisch kontrolliert.

Ausgedehnte corticale Läsionen rufen bei *Ratten* (*14*) keinen oder kaum einen Effekt auf Erwerb, Behalten oder Löschung der Bedingten Emotionalen Reaktion (CER) hervor. Zerstörung tiefer liegender subcorticaler Anteile (*288, 786*) innerhalb des limbischen Systems (s. S. 383) führt jedoch zu erheblichen Veränderungen. Besonders Läsionen der Septum-Region, des Fornix und des Hippocampus bewirken eine signifikante Verminderung der CER, d. h. die Tiere haben nach der Operation eine viel schwächere CER als die nicht lädierten Kontrolltiere (*287*). Wird der Habenula-Komplex des Thalamus von der Läsion betroffen, kann man eine signifikant schnellere Löschung der CER erzielen, ohne daß deren Erwerb oder Behalten gestört zu sein scheint (*288*).

Katzen mit beiderseitiger Zerstörung der Mandelkerne brauchen, um eine CER zu bekommen, signifikant mehr Dressurversuche als solche, bei denen das Cingulum oder der Hippocampus zerstört wurden.

Bei diesen Versuchen wurden 28 Katzen darauf trainiert, in einer sog. Double Grill Box durch eine offene Tür zu gehen, wenn ein akustischer Reiz ertönte. Versäumte das Tier, dies zu tun, bekam es einen schmerzhaften elektrischen Schlag. Die Bedingte Reaktion besteht hier also darin, daß das Tier durch eine Handlung etwas vermeidet, was ihm unangenehm ist. Diese *Ausweich-Reaktionen* (conditioned avoidance reaction) spielen beim Studium der Bedingten Reaktionen eine große Rolle und werden häufig als Modell für solche Situationen im menschlichen Leben benutzt, in denen man etwas meidet, sich etwas versagt oder auch einem Bedürfnis entsagt, um keine Unbill (Unlust) zu erleiden.

Führt man die Amygdala-Zerstörung erst nach der Dressur durch, behalten die Katzen ihre Ausweich-Reaktion bei, genauso wie die nicht operierten Kontrolltiere. Dagegen verlieren Katzen, bei denen die orbito-frontale Region zerstört wird, die Ausweich-Reaktion vollständig, und es gelingt auch innerhalb von 150 erneuten Dressurversuchen (reconditioning) nicht, ihnen die Reaktion wieder beizubringen. BRADY u. Mitarb. folgern aus ihren Versuchen, daß nur der Erwerb und nicht das Behalten der Ausweich-Reaktion durch die Amygdala-Läsion beeinträchtigt wird (*290*).

Ob man diese Folgerung in der Form aufrechterhalten kann, müssen weitere Versuche zeigen. Mindestens kann man ausschließen, daß amygdalektomierte Tiere sensorisch gestört sind (*591, 592, 797*).

Diese und die folgenden Versuche passen zu KLÜVERs früheren Ergebnissen (vgl. S. 379 ff.). Mit Hilfe verschiedener psychotechnischer Methoden (*107, 455, 458*) hatte er an Affen nach Ausbildung Bedingter Reaktionen auf verschiedenen Sinnesgebieten bereits festgestellt, daß die Reaktionen nach bitemporaler Resektion verschwanden, sich aber mit größerem Aufwand von Wiederholungsversuchen neu ausbilden ließen und dann noch nach Jahren recht stabil waren (*108*).

PRIBRAM und WEISKRANTZ (*688*) führten bei 14 Rhesus-Affen Resektionen am medio-basalen und vergleichsweise am lateralen Frontal-Cortex durch und prüften die Wirkungen dieser Läsionen auf Bedingtes Ausweich-Verhalten (s. Abb. 37 und 38, S. 406—407).

Die 2 Jahre alten Affen müssen von einem in einen anderen Raum über eine Rampe springen, wenn der Raum, in dem sie sich gerade befinden, verdunkelt wird. Tun sie das nicht, bekommen sie einen elektrischen Schlag. Wenn alle Affen gelernt haben, den Schlag zu vermeiden, werden sie operiert. Eine Woche später folgen die 1. Löschungsversuche, wobei die Zahl der Versuche, die zur Löschung des Ausweich-Verhaltens nötig ist, als Maß für den Operationseffekt galt. Dann folgt die Neudressur, d. h. die operierten Tiere müssen wieder lernen, den plötzlich verdunkelten Raum innerhalb einer bestimmten Zeit durch Sprung über die Rampe zu verlassen. Haben alle Affen das von neuem gelernt, folgt die 2. Loschungsserie.

a) Tiere, bei denen der medio-frontale Cortex einschließlich des vorderen Cingulum zerstört ist, verlieren die Ausweich-Reaktion während der 1. Loschungsserie abnorm schnell innerhalb von 20 min, benotigen aber mindestens dreimal so viele Ruckdressurversuche wie die nur zum Schein operierten, d. h. nicht hirnverletzten Kontrolltiere. Haben sie schließlich erneut gelernt, den dunklen Raum zu vermeiden, gelingt die 2. Loschung wiederum rapide, d. h. signifikant schneller als bei den Kontrolltieren, bei denen die volle Loschung nicht vor dem dritten Versuchstage eintrat (s. Abb. 37).

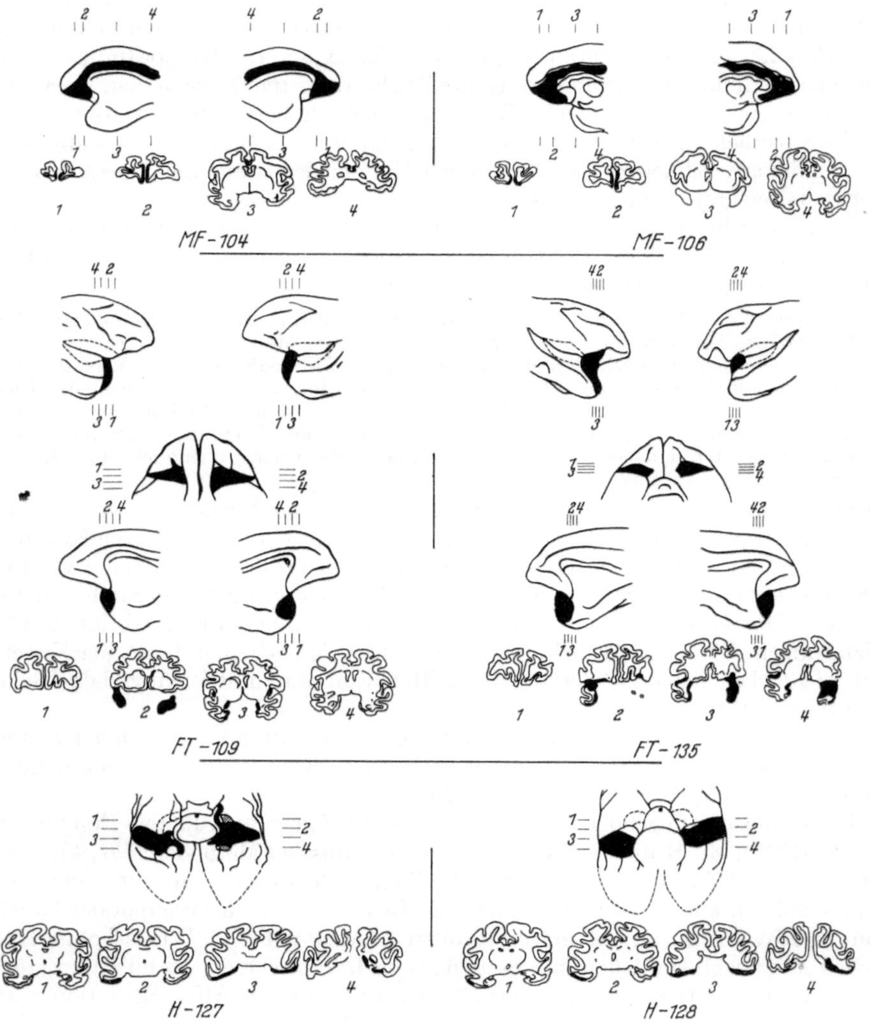

Abb. 37. *Hirnrinden-Abtragungen und Bedingte Emotionale Reaktion. I.* Rekonstruktionen (schwarze Flachen und fette Linien) der abgetragenen *mesocorticalen* Hirnregionen in sagittaler, horizontaler und transversaler Schnittebene. Die mehrstelligen Ziffern sind Kenn-Nummern der fur die Versuche verwendeten Rhesus-Affen. Die ubrigen Zahlen bezeichnen die korrespondierenden Hirnsektionen in den dargestellten zwei oder drei Schnittebenen. *MF* Medio-frontale Rindenabtragung; *FT* Fronto-temporale Abtragung; *H* Hippocampus-Resektion. Psychologische Versuchsergebnisse im Text [Nach Pribram und Weiskrantz (688)]

b) Bei Lasion der fronto-temporalen Region gelingt die 1. Loschung wiederum rapide, aber beim erneuten Lernen benotigen die Tiere mindestens 13 mal soviel Dressurversuche wie die Kontrolltiere. Die 2. Loschung nach diesem Wiederlernen gelingt ebenfalls schnell (s. Abb. 37).

c) Bei Läsion der Ammonsformation gelingt die 1. Löschung rasch. Zur Rückdressur brauchen die Tiere dreimal so lange und verlieren das wiedererlernte Verhalten bei der 2. Löschung abnorm schnell (s. Abb. 37.

d) Wird die antero-frontale Region (Stirnhirnpol und -konvexität) lädiert, gelingt die 1. Löschung sehr schnell, das Wiederlernen dauert 13 mal länger als bei den Kontrolltieren. Die 2. Löschung dauert normal lange (s. Abb. 38).

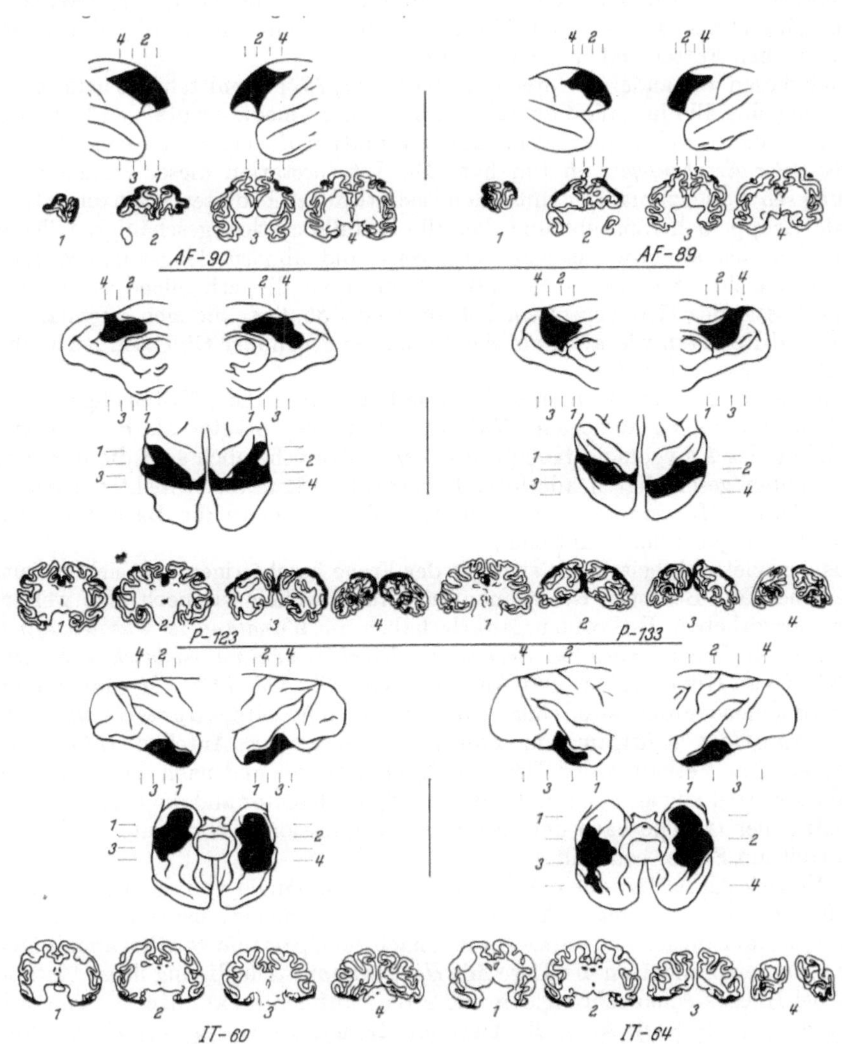

Abb. 38. *Hirnrinden-Abtragungen und Bedingte Emotionale Reaktion. II.* Rekonstruktionen der abgetragenen *isocorticalen* Regionen. Im übrigen s. Legende zu Abb. 37. *AF* Antero-frontale Abtragung; *P* Parieto-occipitale Abtragung; *IT* Infero-temporale Abtragung. [Nach PRIBRAM und WEISKRANTZ (*688*)]

e) Tiere, bei denen parieto-occipitale oder (f) temporo-inferiore Regionen zerstört werden, verhalten sich bei allen Prozeduren so wie die normalen, scheinoperierten Kontrolltiere (s. Abb. 38).

Bei der ersten Löschung verhalten sich also die Gruppen *e* und *f* normal. Alle anderen vergessen abnorm rasch (Gruppe *a—c* siehe Abb. 37, Gruppe *d—f* siehe Abb. 38).

Bei der Rückdressur verhalten sich die Gruppen *e* und *f* wieder normal; bei den Gruppen *a* und *c* gelingt das Wiederlernen dreimal langsamer. Besonders bemerkenswert sind die Gruppen *b* und *d*, bei denen die Rückdressur 13 mal so lange, ja, bei *b* sogar meist noch länger dauerte; die so geschädigten Tiere lernen also sehr schwer.

Bei der 2. Löschung verhalten sich alle Tiere, bei denen der Isocortex lädiert ist (Gruppen *d, e, f*), wie die normalen. Diejenigen Tiere, bei denen eine allo-juxtallo-corticale Hirnschädigung (s. S. 406) vorliegt (Gruppen *a, b, c*), vergessen rapide, kümmern sich schon nach 15—20 min nicht mehr um das Signal, sondern spielen, suchen Futter und springen herum.

Nach diesen und anderen Untersuchungen (*681, 797*) vermitteln die neuronalen Strukturen des allo-juxtallo-Cortex an der temporo-medio-frontalen Fläche des Hirns also eine recht komplexe gemeinsame Funktion, die etwas mit dem *Erinnern affektbesetzter Erfahrungen* zu tun hat. Die Interpretation dieser Funktion ist vorläufig schwierig, zumal sich unter den isocortical geschädigten Affen die antero-frontale Gruppe *d* heraushebt und den allo-juxtallo-cortical geschädigten Tieren hinsichtlich des abnorm raschen Vergessens und abnorm langsamen Wieder-erlernens gleicht. Für dieses Verhalten kann man die erhebliche motorische Hyperaktivität der Tiere verantwortlich machen (*686, 688*), die sich offenbar auf Lernen und Behalten wie auch auf das Verhalten gegenüber Objekten bei Wahl-handlungen auswirkt (*685*).

Sicher ist, daß die fronto-temporal geschädigten Affen die gröbsten allgemeinen Verhaltensänderungen aufzeigen (*679*), und zwar ausgeprägter als bei isolierter Schädigung des Amygdaloid-Komplexes (*797*). Wahrscheinlich sind die in diesen Experimenten geschädigten allo-juxtallo-corticalen Strukturen nicht die neuro-nalen Substrate für emotionales Verhalten allein, sondern die Basis für recht verschiedene psychische Funktionen.

Aus den vielen Arbeiten, die sich mit der Frage beschäftigen, wie sich gezielte Hirnläsionen auf Bedingte Reaktionen auswirken, wollen wir noch eine weitere Gruppe hervorheben. Rosvold u. Mitarb. haben die *Wandlung der sozialen Rang-ordnung* (s. S. 339ff.) *nach umschriebenen Hirnläsionen im limbischen System* (s. S. 378ff.) an Hunden (*348*) und Rhesus-Affen (*297, 590, 713, 714*) untersucht.

Die Läsionen wurden jeweils bilateral im vorderen Anteil des *Gyrus cinguli* (*590*), in den *Amygdala* (*713*) und in größeren *Hippocampus*-Anteilen (*714*) vor-genommen. Das Verhalten der Tiere wurde Monate vor und nach der Operation sowohl im Einzelkäfig als auch im Gruppenkäfig beobachtet und die Rangordnung innerhalb einer Gruppe nach der Anzahl der Aggressionen und Unterwerfungen beim Streit um Futter beurteilt.

Im Einzelkäfig hatten alle operierten Tiere, unabhängig von der Lokalisation der Hirnschädigung, weniger Angst vor dem Untersucher, beurteilt nach der Anzahl von Nahrungsbissen, die sie vor und nach der Operation von ihm annahmen. In der Gruppe veränderten die Tiere mit *Hippocampus*-Schädigung ihren Platz in der — bei Rhesus-Affen sehr rigiden und streng aufrechterhaltenen — Rangord-nung nicht (vgl. S. 339). Auch die Tiere mit Läsion des *Gyrus cinguli* behielten ihren Rangordnungsplatz, ein Ergebnis, das mit Experimenten von Pribram und Fulton (*641*) übereinstimmt.

Anders dagegen bei Schädigung der *Amygdala:* Drei von vier Affen, die vor der Operation Alpha-Tiere waren, sanken bis zum Omega-Tier oder bis zum vor-letzten Platz ab (vgl. S. 339). Der vierte Makak kam in einer Vierergruppe von dem 3. auf den 4. Platz. Diese 4 Tiere nahmen auch im Einzelkäfig weniger Nah-rung vom Untersucher an als vor der Operation, obwohl sie im übrigen weniger Angst zeigten.

Diesem Verhalten nach Verletzungen im limbischen System ist das nach prä-frontaler Lobotomie gegenüberzustellen (*593, 594, 673, 674*). Die so geschädigten

Tiere rückten, ohne etwa aggressiver geworden zu sein, in der sozialen Rangordnung auf (*297*).

Die Verfasser erklären die Ausbildung der sozialen Rangordnung in einer Gruppe damit, daß sich im Laufe einer gewissen Zeit eine von Tier zu Tier verschieden starke Angst (avoidance behavior) (s. S. 397f.) ausbildet. Das rangtiefere Tier hat schließlich gelernt, das ranghöhere zu meiden. Während die präfrontal lobotomierten Tiere nicht in der Lage sind, ihren Rangordnungsplatz kennenzulernen oder — anders ausgedrückt — keine Ausweich-Reaktion ausbilden, haben die amygdalektomierten Tiere ihren Rang nach der Operation vergessen und lernen nun, von kräftigeren Tieren attackiert, die Unterwerfung, d. h. die Ausweich-Reaktion.

Zur Stütze dieser Hypothese wurden weitere drei Affen amygdalektomiert und nach der Operation zunächst mit jüngeren, schwächeren Tieren zusammengetan. Als diese drei nach einer Weile wieder zu ihren alten Genossen zurückkehrten, verloren sie nun nicht wie die anderen Amygdalektomierten an Rang, ja, einer gewann sogar für dauernd, ein anderer vorübergehend eine höhere Rangstufe, der dritte sank nicht ab, und alle waren gegen die nachgeordneten Tiere aggressiv. Diese drei Affen hatten also nach der Operation im Zusammenleben mit den schwächeren Tieren neu gelernt, daß sie zu den „Oberen" gehörten, und verhielten sich später dementsprechend ihren alten Gruppengenossen gegenüber.

4. Intrakranielle Selbstreizung

Die von OLDS und MILNER 1954 (*625*) erstmals publizierte Methode der intrakraniellen Selbstreizung darf man wohl mit Recht als eine wichtige Entdeckung bezeichnen, ermöglicht sie uns doch neue Einblicke in die Zusammenhänge zwischen Hirnfunktion und emotionalem Verhalten.

Zwei bereits bekannte und besprochene Methoden wurden zu einer neuen Methode vereint: Die Technik von W. R. HESS mit chronisch implantierten, die Bewegungsfreiheit des Tieres nicht behindernden Elektroden und die Technik der Hebeldruck-Dressur von B. F. SKINNER (s. S. 397). Anstatt daß die Tiere nun aber durch Hebeldrücken Futter oder Wasser erhalten, lösen sie durch diese Tätigkeit einen elektrischen Reiz in ihrem eigenen Hirn aus (s. Abb. 32, S. 397).

Der elektrische Hirnreiz übt, bestimmte Lokalisationen vorausgesetzt, eine solche Wirkung auf die Tiere aus, daß sie sehr bald vorziehen, immer wieder den Hebel zu drücken, anstatt die im Käfig bereit stehende Nahrung zu fressen. Auf diese Weise entstehen Hebeldruckkurven, wie wir sie schon kennenlernten (s. S. 398ff.). Nachdem die Ratten sich Tage hindurch (in anderen Experimenten auch über Wochen und Monate) selbst gereizt haben, kann das Hebeldruckverhalten wieder gelöscht werden: Wenn die Ratten den Hirnreiz-Effekt vermissen, geben sie das Hebeldrücken auf, gerade so, wie sie es beim Ausbleiben der Nahrungsbelohnung im üblichen Skinner-Verfahren unterlassen, den Hebel weiterhin zu betätigen.

Die bisher vorliegenden Untersuchungen von OLDS (*621, 622, 625*) und anderen Autoren (*277, 280—282, 523, 580, 750, 775*) erlauben bereits, Hirnkarten aufzustellen, die zeigen, von welchen Hirnstrukturen aus das Hebeldrücken durch elektrische Selbstreizung gefördert oder gehemmt werden kann. — Die Versuchstiere sind zumeist Ratten; aber auch Katzen und Affen sind bereits untersucht worden.

Die ersten Versuchsergebnisse von OLDS (*621*) an 76 Ratten sind auf der Hirnkarte in Abb. 39 (S. 410) schematisch eingezeichnet. Hohe Selbstreizungs-Frequenzen (Hebeldrucke/Stunde) werden bei folgendem Elektrodensitz erreicht: In der ganzen Septumgegend von oben bis hinunter zur Area praeoptica, in den Amygdala und in vorderen bis mittleren Hypothalamus-Anteilen. Mittelhohe Frequenzen finden sich bei der Reizung des Hippocampus, des Gyrus cinguli, des Thalamus anterior und retrosplenialer, entorhinaler und periamygdaloider Areale, mit anderen Worten in weiten Teilen des limbischen Systems und benachbarter Funktionsgebiete (s. S. 383ff.). Sitzt die Elektrode in einem der genannten Orte, lernt die Ratte nach wenigen — zunächst zufälligen — Hebeldrucken und innerhalb einiger Minuten, dies Verhalten fortgesetzt zu wiederholen. Während sie ohne elektrischen Reiz oder bei indifferentem Elektrodensitz das Pedal 15—20mal in der Stunde zufällig herunterdrückt, gibt sie sich bei „positiver" Elektrodenlage bis zu 7000 Selbstreizungen (*153, 623*).

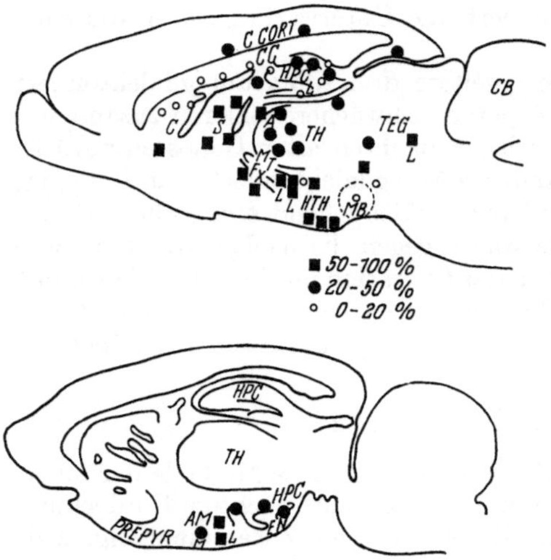

Selbstreizung innerhalb kleiner Mittelhirnbezirke und mit diesen in funktionellem Zusammenhang stehenden Teilen des Hypothalamus und Thalamus führt dagegen zu einem ausgesprochen gehemmten Verhalten (s. Abb. 42, punktierter Bereich): Die Tiere vermeiden, den Hebel zu drücken; der Hirnreiz schreckt sie geradezu ab, und die Hebeldruckzahl pro Stunde sinkt bis auf 0—5. Solch ein negativ akzentuiertes Verhalten in diesen Bereichen entdeckten zuerst DELGADO, ROBERTS und MILLER bei Katzen, die, obgleich ausgehungert, nach solcher „Bestrafungsreizung" ihr Futter nicht mehr anrührten (*320*). Die Area, von der aus ein „negatives" Verhalten (avoidance behavior) erzeugt wird, ist im Vergleich zu der mit positiver, die Handlung fördernder Wirkung (approach behavior) recht klein. Sie entspricht übrigens derjenigen von W. R. HESS und HUNSPERGER, in der Wut und Flucht bei Katzen ausgelöst werden konnten (s. Abb. 19; s. S. 371). Im Hippocampus-Gebiet liegen negative und positive Reizpunkte vermischt nahe beieinander (*621*).

Abb. 39. *Hirnkarte zu den Selbstreizungsversuchen an Ratten*. Rekonstruktion der Reizpunkte nach Gefrierschnitten durch das Rattenhirn. Repräsentativer schematischer Sagittalschnitt. Schwarze Quadrate stellen Punkte mit maximaler, schwarze Kreise solche mit mittelstarker Selbstreizungswirkung dar. Offene Kreise zeigen neutrale oder negative Lokalisationen an. Aus Gründen der Übersichtlichkeit sind nicht alle neutralen oder negativen Punkte eingetragen. Positive Punkte, denen ein *L* hinzugefugt ist, befinden sich etwa 2 mm lateral, solche mit einem *M* etwa 2 mm medial von der dargestellten Sagittalebene. *A* Thalamus anterior; *AM* Amygdala; *C* Ncl. caudatus; *CB* Cerebellum; *CC* Corpus callosum; *C* Cort, Gyrus cinguli; *FX* Fornix; *HPC* Hippocampus; *HTH* Hypothalamus; *MB* Corpora mamillaria; *MT* Tractus mamillothalamicus; *PREPYR* Regio praepiriformis; *S* Septum-Area; *TEG* Tegmentum; *TH* Thalamus. Zur Methodik der Selbstreizung s. Abb. 32 u. 40. [Nach OLDS (*621*)]

Die höchsten Hebeldruckzahlen (7000/h) werden bei Selbstreizungen in der Gegend eines kleinen Kerngebietes (Ncl. interpeduncularis tegmenti; s. Abb. 28, S. 384) im basalen Mittelhirn erreicht. Aber auch im hinteren Hypothalamus gerade vor den Corpora mamillaria lassen sich Reizungen um 5000/h erzielen, im vorderen Hypothalamus solche von 400—1100/h. Weiter zum Endhirn hin gibt es in der Area praeoptica nochmals eine hohe Quote um 3000/h; dann nehmen die Reizungen zum vorderen Telencephalon hin ab (200/h). Je weiter also die Elektroden im Mittel- und Zwischenhirn nach vorn gerückt werden, desto geringer wird die Selbstreizungshäufigkeit. So ist es auch im Telencephalon; nur sind dort die Quoten im ganzen niedriger als im hypothalamischen Bereich (*153*).

Steigert man die Stromstärke des Reizes stufenweise um 10 Mikro-Ampere von 0—150 µA, ergeben sich je nach Sitz der Elektroden Veränderungen der

Selbstreizungsfrequenz. Die so gereizten Neurone gehorchen dem Alles-oder-nichts-Gesetz und haben offenbar annähernd gleiche Schwellen: Je größer die Stromstärke, desto ausgedehnter das elektrische Reizfeld an der Elektrodenspitze und desto mehr schwellig gereizte Zellen. Die Hebeldruckkurven steigen bei dieser Versuchsanordnung stetig im vorderen Telencephalon und im hinteren Hypothalamus an, während sie im mittleren Hypothalamus trotz stufenweise steigender Reizstärke wellenförmig verlaufen. Im mittleren Endhirn, in der Gegend des Brocaschen Diagonalbandes, kommt es rasch zu einer mäßigen Reizungssteigerung um etwa 500/h, die dann mit steigender Stromstärke nicht mehr zunimmt. Die

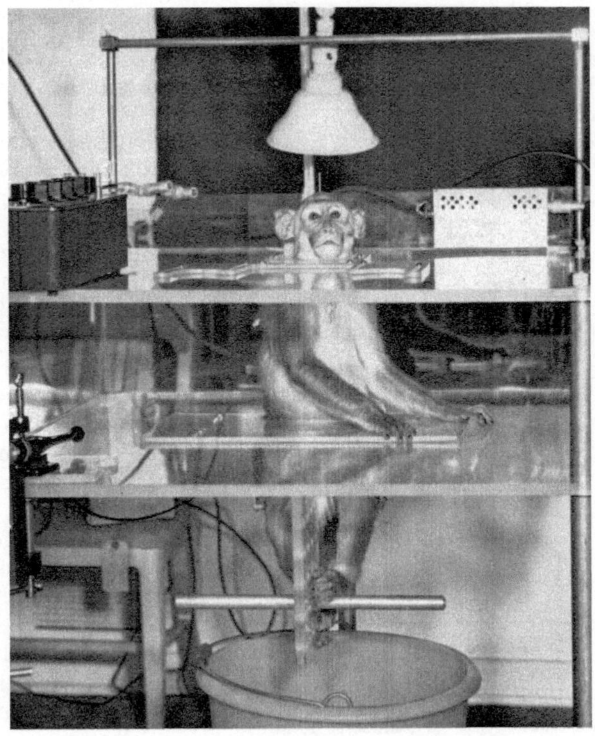

Abb. 40. *Rhesus-Affe im Stuhl.* Unter der Kopfhaut befindet sich der auf der Calotte befestigte Elektrodenhalter mit zahlreichen Führungskanälen, durch welche die Reizelektroden bei Versuchsbeginn in die gewünschten Hirnregionen stereotaktisch eingeführt werden können. Vor den Händen des Affen wird eine Morsetaste befestigt, mit der das Tier elektrische Reize im eigenen Hirn auslösen kann. [Aufnahme Dr. J. C. LILLY. — Technik s. LILLY (*521, 522*)]

Erklärung für diese Differenzen der Reizungshäufigkeit in verschiedenen Hirnbereichen darf man darin suchen, daß in den Arealen mit stetig steigender Hebeldruckfrequenz zunehmend mehr Zellelemente mit positivem Belohnungs-Effekt einbezogen werden, während die wellenförmig verlaufenden Kurven im Zusammenhang mit anderen Versuchsergebnissen nahelegen, daß hier im mittleren Hypothalamus außer den positiven (fördernden) auch negative (hemmende) Areale miterregt werden. Die nach mäßigem Anstieg gleichbleibenden Hebeldruckkurven im mittleren Vorderhirn hingegen dürften ein Ausdruck dafür sein, daß die positiv fördernde Area in diesem Hirnabschnitt recht klein ist, so daß das sich mit zunehmender Stromstärke vergrößernde elektrische Feld keine weiteren „positiven" Neurone erfaßt. Selbst wenn die Tiere dieses Zellareal täglich während

8 Monaten mit einem 15 fachen Schwellenreiz (150 μA) stimulieren, ändert sich an den Hebeldruckkurven nichts, ein Zeichen dafür, daß die „positiven" Neurone durch den Strom nicht geschädigt werden.

Bei den bisher an *Rhesus-Affen* durchgeführten *Selbstreizungsversuchen* (Abb. 40, S. 411) liegen die Verhältnisse offenbar komplizierter, und die verschiedenen Hirnregionen zugeordneten Reizungsfrequenzen verteilen sich anders.

Den Affen wird ein Elektrodenhalter, in dem 20 und mehr Elektroden Platz haben, so implantiert, daß die Tiere sich außerhalb des Versuches frei bewegen können, ohne daß sich der Elektrodensitz über Monate hindurch verandert. Während des Versuches kommen die Affen in einen Spezialstuhl, der den Tieren Bewegungsfreiheit für Kopf und Extremitäten laßt. Vorrichtungen zur Entnahme von Blut und Urin sind angebracht (Abb. 40).

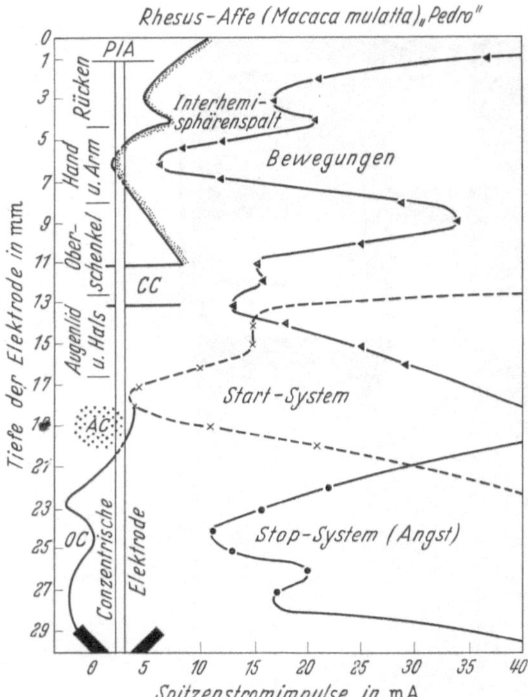

Abb. 41. *Start- und Stop-System ermittelt durch Selbstreizungsversuche am Rhesus-Affen.* Diagramm fur die Reizergebnisse entlang eines Elektroden-Traktes. Die konzentrische Elektrode wurde in der Hirn-Mittellinie von der Hirnoberflache bis auf den Hypophysenstiel (schwarze Balken unten links) hinunter gesenkt. Die Reizschwellen (Abscisse) fur die eingetragenen Phanomene wurden millimeterweise absteigend (Ordinate) bestimmt. Das *Start-System* ist dadurch gekennzeichnet, daß sich der Affe nach einmal erlebtem Fremdreiz durch Hebeldrucken selbst weiter stimuliert. Im *Stop-System* unterbricht das Tier ihm gegebene Reize durch Hebeldrucken selbst. [Technische Einzelheiten s. LILLY et al. (526, 527)]. CC Corpus callosum, AC Commissura anterior; OC Chiasma opticum. [Nach LILLY (523)]

Bei Elektrodensitz in der orbito-frontalen Region, im medialen Vorderhirn-Bündel, in den Amygdala, in der Area entorhinalis und in der Formatio reticularis werden hohe Frequenzen erzielt (900—1000 in 45 min). Bei Hypothalamus-Reizen (genauere Lokalisation der Hypothalamus-Anteile fehlt vorläufig) sind die Quoten niedrig (um 50 in 45 min), aber konstant. Bei Reizung des Ammonshorns vermeidet der Affe das Hebeldrücken sofort nach den ersten Reizen ängstlich. Es scheint bei diesen Affenversuchen nicht gleichgültig zu sein, in welcher Reihenfolge verschiedene Hirnstrukturen gereizt werden. Zum Beispiel fällt die Selbstreizung deutlich ab, wenn *vor* einer Reizungs-Periode des medialen Vorderhirnbündels der Hypothalamus oder die Amygdala gereizt werden, während eine vorherige Reizung der Area entorhinalis keinen Einfluß auf die nachfolgende Reizung des Vorderhirnbündels hat. Andererseits hat eine vorangehende Reizung des Vorderhirnbündels oder der Orbito-frontal-Region eine Senkung der nachfolgenden Reizungshäufigkeit in den Amygdala zur Folge, während eine vorherige Reizung der entorhinalen Area nichts ausmacht (275).

LILLY (*519, 520, 524, 525*) verwendet für die Selbstreizungsexperimente an Rhesus-Affen eine ausgeklügelte Technik (*521, 522, 526, 527*), mit der Reizfolgen und Reizdauer stark variiert werden können, ohne daß eine Hirnschädigung einzutreten scheint. LILLYs Affen können sich nicht nur selbst reizen, sie können auch einen ihnen gegebenen Reiz selbst unterbrechen, eine Methode, die N. E. MILLER (*581*) schon an Ratten verwendete. Auf diese Weise ist es möglich, „Start"- und „Stop"-Regionen (*523*) im Hirn zu unterscheiden (Abb. 41, S. 412). Liegt die Elektrode in der Start-Region, lernt der Affe sehr schnell, sich selbst zu reizen, liegt sie in der Stop-Region, unterbricht das Tier einen gegebenen Hirnreiz, oft unter Anzeichen heftiger Angst, die sich zur Panik steigern kann. Läßt man den Affen länger unter solchen Reizbedingungen, in denen er von Zeit zu Zeit immer wieder einen Panik erzeugenden Reiz erhält, kommt es zu schweren Nachwirkungen: Das Tier ist verstört, verweigert die Nahrung und bricht Sondennahrung wieder aus, Haut und Schleimhäute werden weißlich-grau, und die Herzfrequenz steigt. Läßt man das Tier nicht zu lange in diesem Zustand und schaltet einen Hirnreiz im „Startsystem" ein, wandelt sich die Verfassung in wenigen Minuten: Das Verhalten normalisiert sich, der Appetit kehrt wieder, die Selbstreizungs-Tätigkeit wird aufgenommen, das Tier handelt wieder „cooperativ".

LILLY (*523*) betont mit Recht, daß es heute nicht mehr angängig ist, von „Schein-Affekten" zu sprechen. Es kann kein Zweifel über die „Echtheit" solcher induzierten Affekte mehr bestehen, wovon sich jeder überzeugen wird, der die untersuchten Tiere persönlich kennt und derartige Experimente selbst vorgenommen hat.

Die anatomischen Daten sind noch nicht ausgearbeitet. Die bisher angegebenen Lokalisationen gründen sich auf Messungen mit dem Zielgerät (Horsley-Clark-Apparat) und geben wahrscheinlich recht gute Annäherungswerte. Die Zone, in der Panik erzeugt wurde, liegt in den Wänden des 3. Ventrikels oberhalb des Hypophysenstiels. Eine sehr wirkungsvolle „Startzone" findet sich im Kopf des Caudatum. Bei Anwendung sehr kurz dauernder Reize stimulierte sich ein Affe 200000mal innerhalb von 20 Std. bis zur Erschöpfung. 18000 Reize innerhalb 24 Std. mehrere Wochen hindurch kommen vor.

Es wäre nun zu beweisen, daß die durch Selbstreizung erregten Neuronengruppen auch tatsächlich mit jenen identisch sind, die normalerweise in die Triebregulation einbezogen sind. Dazu liegen folgende Untersuchungen vor:

In einem Labyrinth rennen Ratten z. B. genauso schnell zum Futter wie zum Selbstreizungshebel. In einem einfachen Laufkäfig rennen sie um elektrischer Belohnung willen sogar schneller als nach 24stündigem Nahrungsentzug um Futter (*622*). In einem Hinderniskäfig können sich die Ratten an einem Ende des Käfigs dreimal selbst reizen, dann aber keinen Strom mehr mit dem Hebeldrücken auslösen. Am anderen Ende des Käfigs können sich die Tiere wiederum dreimal reizen, erhalten aber auf dem Wege dorthin eine im Laufe des Versuchs zunehmende Zahl von schmerzhaften elektrischen Schlägen. Die so hin- und herlaufenden Ratten überwinden um der Hirnreize willen mehr Schmerz als 24 Std. lang hungernde Ratten des Futters wegen. Bei dieser Art von Triebmessung ist der Drang zur Selbstreizung in manchen Fällen mindestens doppelt so stark wie der Drang nach Futter (*153*). Andere Versuche im T-Labyrinth oder im Vier-Ecken-Futter-Kasten brachten ähnliche Ergebnisse (*623*). Offenbar sind also die durch die Selbstreizungsversuche ermittelten Hirnstrukturen mit denen identisch, die unter natürlichen Bedingungen das neuronale Substrat für die „primären" Belohnungseffekte abgeben.

Eine weitere interessante Frage ist nun, ob eine *Sättigung* des Dranges zur Selbstreizung, vergleichbar der Nahrungssättigung, herbeizuführen ist.

Wird hoch überschwellig gereizt, bleibt die Hebeldrucktätigkeit bei täglich einer Stunde Selbstreizung über Monate nahezu gleich. Wenn *jeder* Hebeldruck einen Reiz auslöst, betätigen Ratten mit Hypothalamus-Elektroden die Taste so lange, wie es ihre Kräfte erlauben, nämlich ununterbrochen je 2000mal in der Stunde 24 Std. lang. Dagegen begnügen sich Tiere mit Septum-Elektroden mit einer gewissen, konstant bleibenden Anzahl von Hirnreizen, gleich ob man ihnen 1 oder

24 Std. Zeit zur Selbstreizung läßt. Sie zeigen eine „natürliche" Sättigung, die bei den Hypothalamus-Tieren offensichtlich nicht besteht.

Bei unterschwelliger Reizung mit Elektroden längs der Hirn-Mittellinie (s. S. 386, Abb. 29) im ventro-medialen Hypothalamus und in der Septum-Gegend reizen sich die Tiere, je hungriger sie sind, desto öfter (277, 283). Beginnt man aber stufenweise ansteigend mit unterschwelligen Reizen, kann man so etwas wie eine „Hungerschwelle" abtasten und ein Gebiet abgrenzen, innerhalb dessen satte Tiere gerade eben einen „Hungereffekt" (das ist das Ansteigen der Selbstreizungs-frequenz) zeigen und kann so ein „Hunger-Befriedigungs-Zentrum" (hunger reward center) nachweisen. Das gesamte Gebiet der positiven Reizeffekte läßt sich auf diese Weise in Untergruppen aufgliedern, die verschiedenen primären Trieben [z. B. auch dem Sexualtrieb (211, 580)] zugeordnet sein sollen. Innerhalb des gesamten Systems haben verschiedene Reizstärken verschiedene Wirkungen, wie ja schon aus den Hessschen Versuchen hervorging (s. S. 374). Am besten scheint das Hungerareal untersucht und abgegrenzt zu sein. Es liegt nach Oldss Unter-suchungen (153) unmittelbar rostral vom Corpus mamillare 1,25 mm lateral der Mittellinie.

Überraschende Veränderungen der Bereitschaft, sich selbst zu reizen, erhält man bei *Kastration* und nachfolgender *Behandlung mit männlichem Sexualhormon.*

Nachdem Ratten die Selbstreizung kennengelernt haben, werden sie kastriert; während der nächsten 14 Tage registriert man bei fallendem Hormonspiegel die Hebeldruckkurven. Dann injiziert man den Tieren in steigenden Dosen (1—5 mg) Sexualhormon und beobachtet während der folgenden Tage, in denen der Hormonspiegel steigt und wieder fällt, das weitere Verhalten der Ratten.

Zwei Ergebnisse sind besonders instruktiv:

Bei Lokalisation der Elektroden im dorso-medialen Caudatum fand sich nach dem Alles-oder-nichts-Gesetz eine feste Korrelation zwischen Höhe des Androgen-spiegels und Höhe der Selbstreizungsraten: Bei hohem Androgenspiegel reizte sich das Tier schon bei der niedrigsten der gestuft angewandten Stromstärken (15 μA), während umgekehrt bei niedrigem Hormonspiegel, selbst bei der höchsten Stromstärke (55 μA), keine Selbstreizung errreicht werden konnte.

Es besteht ferner eine feste reziproke Beziehung von Androgenspiegel und Hungerzustand in ihrer Wirkung auf die Selbstreizungsfrequenz: Wenn Hunger die Selbstreizung förderte, wurde sie durch Testosteron vermindert, aber wenn die Elektrode anderswo im Hypothalamus oder Endhirn lag und Androgen fördernd wirkte, senkte Hunger die Reizfrequenz. Daraus wird der Schluß gezogen, daß es eine anatomisch definierbare Differenzierung zwischen solchen neuronalen Syste-men geben muß, die auf den Hungerzustand, und solchen, die auf den Hormon-spiegel ansprechen (153).

Reizt man *Rhesus-Affen* in der Gegend des Tuber cinereum und Infundibulum, so steigt der Blut-Steroid-Spiegel plötzlich stark an (560, 561). Kurz vor dem Anstieg der Steroide scheinen unlustbetonte Emotionen aufzutreten; die Affen lassen vom Hebeldrücken ab, urinieren und defäzieren (275).

Auch frühere Untersuchungen von Delgado und Anand (319) können durch Selbstreizungs-Experimente gestützt werden. Bei Elektroden etwa 1,5 mm lateral der Mittellinie im vorderen Anteil des hinteren Hypothalamus reizen sich Ratten gewöhnlich außerordentlich häufig; das ist derselbe Bereich, in dem durch Hirnreizung vermehrter Futterkonsum ermittelt wurde (319). Setzt man die Elektroden mehr zur Mittellinie, sinken die Selbstreizungen beträchtlich; das ist dieselbe Lokalisation, bei der auch — allerdings nicht so konstant — ein vermin-derter Futterkonsum festgestellt wurde. Es gibt aber auch im Telencephalon Bereiche, in denen ähnliche Beziehungen zwischen Nahrungsverbrauch und

Selbstreizungshäufigkeit zu beobachten sind, so daß man nicht im engeren Sinne von einem Appetit-*Zentrum* sprechen sollte.

Diese experimentellen Ergebnisse beginnt man dafür zu nutzen, die *Wirkung moderner Neuroplegica* (*87, 582*) und z. B. auch den *Lysergsäure-Serotonin-Antagonismus* zu studieren (*153*); (vgl. ELKES, ds. Bd. Teil A).

Wieder werden Ratten mit verschiedenem Elektrodensitz in gestuften Reizstärken auf ihre Selbstreizungsrate getestet. Der gerade wirksame Reiz gilt als Schwellenreiz und die so innerhalb eines 8 min-Intervalls gewonnene Rate als Vergleichszahl für den nachfolgenden pharmakologischen Test. Die Selbstreizungsrate unter Drogenwirkung wird in Relation zur Vergleichszahl gesetzt.

Die *Ergebnisse* zeigen, daß Chlorpromazin die Selbstreizung am stärksten drosselt, wenn die Elektroden im vorderen Anteil des *hinteren* Hypothalamus liegen. Das Tier reizt sich dann überhaupt nicht mehr. Bei Elektrodensitz im *mittleren* Hypothalamus ist die Chlorpromazin-Wirkung geringer und vermindert die Hebeldrucktätigkeit, je nach Reizstärke, nur um $21-25\%$. Im *vorderen* Hypothalamus hat die Droge kaum noch Einfluß, so daß die Selbstreizungsfrequenz nahezu gleich bleibt. In der Area praeoptica ist ein nur gering drosselnder Effekt feststellbar, während sich bei Elektrodenlokalisation in Teilen der Septumgegend wieder eine recht kräftige Drosselung zeigt (*153*).

Da Chlorpromazin die Selbstreizung bei Elektrodensitz im vorderen Hypothalamus kaum beeinträchtigt, scheint es also nicht auf dieses Verhalten selbst zu wirken. Bei Berücksichtigung der starken Drosselungswirkung im hinteren Hypothalamus darf man aber folgern, daß dieses Mittel selektiv wirkt, und zwar entweder auf diesen Zwischenhirnteil oder auf solche Projektionsfelder des hinteren Hypothalamus, die das Verhalten vermitteln helfen. Diese für Chlorpromazin empfindlichen Hirnteile konnen zudem nicht für jegliche mit Lustgewinn verknüpften Verhaltungsweisen verantwortlich sein, denn sonst würde die Selbstreizung im vorderen Hypothalamus nicht trotz der Droge funktionieren.

Bei Untersuchungen der *Beziehungen zwischen Serotonin und Lysergsäure-Diäthylamid* (LSD 25) finden sich wiederum zwei von einander zu trennende Wirkungen (s. Abb. 42, S. 416):

a) Eine intraperitoneale LSD-Injektion hemmt die Selbstreizung beträchtlich (während Brom-LSD, das die Blut-Hirn-Schranke wahrscheinlich schwerer passiert, unwirksam bleibt). Wenn man nun aber vor der LSD-Gabe Serotonin einspritzt, wird die Selbstreizung nicht beeinflußt.

b) Bei anderer Elektrodenplazierung wirkt LSD wiederum hemmend, aber Serotonin hat keinen antagonistischen Effekt, und Brom-LSD wirkt genauso wie LSD.

Diese Ergebnisse bringen einen weiteren Beweis für die chemische Differenzierung der untersuchten Hinstrukturen.

Früher hatten wir schon dargelegt, daß die Hebeldruckfrequenz vom Schema der Belohnung abhängt (s. S. 404). Ein genau vergleichbares Verhalten kann man auch bei der Selbstreizung erzielen (s. Abb. 43, S. 416).

Eine *Katze* mit einer Elektrode im *Nucl. caudatus* produziert in 15 min etwa 200 Selbstreizungen, wenn der Hebeldruck in wechselnden Zeitabständen, durchschnittlich alle 16 sec, einen Hirnreiz auslöst. Kommt jedoch auf je 7 Hebeldrucke ein Reiz, steigt die Rate auf nahezu 1000 an (*280*). In Abb. 43 sind die Ergebnisse für 3 Katzen mit Elektroden im Caudatum-Kopf wiedergegeben. Die Katzen reizen sich also häufiger bei Belohnung nach Leistung als nach Zeit. Auch Hunger und Durst wirken fördernd auf die Reizungshäufigkeit (vgl. auch ELKES, ds. Bd., Teil A).

Dressiert man durstigen *Ratten* im Skinner-Käfig eine Bedingte Angst-Reaktion an und belohnt sie mit Wasser, so wird das durstlöschende Hebeldrücken, wie wir wissen (s. S. 398), beim Ertönen des Bedingten Reizes unterdrückt. Liefert nun der

Hebeldruck statt Wasser einen elektrischen Hirnreiz im Septum, kümmert sich die Ratte kaum um den Bedingten Reiz und setzt die Selbstreizung fort, obwohl dem Bedingten regelmäßig ein Unbedingter Reiz (schmerzhafter elektrischer Schlag) folgt. Stellt man die Belohnung wieder auf Wasser um, kehrt die Angst-Reaktion sofort voll ausgeprägt zurück. Ja, die Ratten bekommen sogar keine Angst-Reaktion, wenn sie von vornherein mit Selbstreizung belohnt werden. Geht man dann zur Wasserbelohnung über, prägt sich sehr rasch die bedingte Angst aus (*280*).

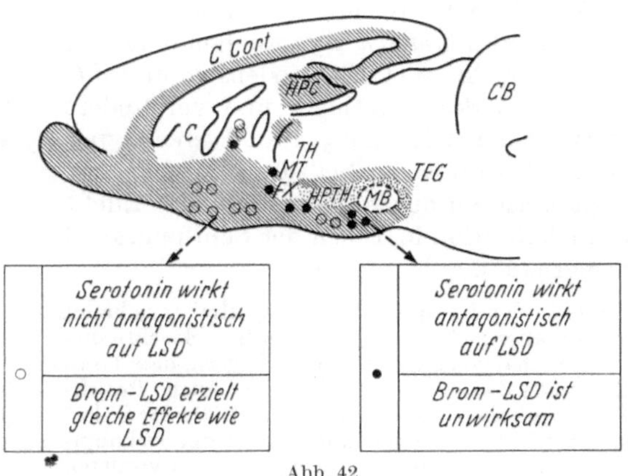

Abb. 42

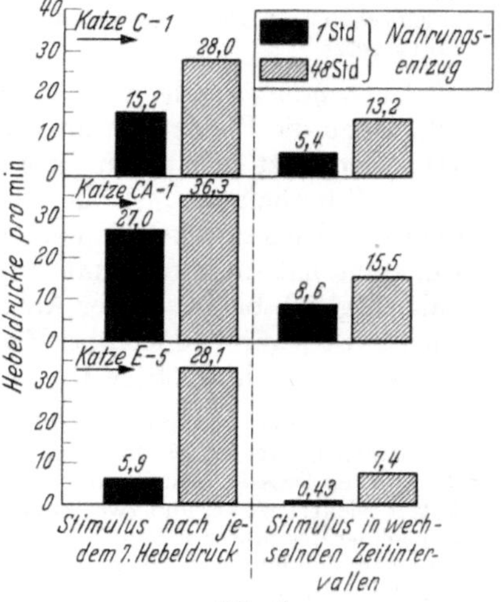

Abb. 43

Abb. 42. *Die Wirkung von Lysergsaure-Diathylamid (LSD) und Serotonin auf die Selbstreizung.* Die schraffierten Flachen entsprechen Hirnarealen, in denen die Ratte sich selbst reizt, die punktierte Flache solchen Arealen, in denen sie die Selbstreizung vermeidet (s. Abb. 39). LSD setzt die Haufigkeit der Selbstreizung significant herunter. Die offenen Kreise entsprechen Arealen, in denen der LSD-Effekt nicht durch Serotonin aufgehoben werden kann. In diesen Bereichen hat Brom-LSD die gleiche herabsetztende Wirkung wie LSD. Die soliden Kreise entsprechen solchen Arealen, in denen Serotonin die LSD-Wirkung aufhebt, auch Brom-LSD ist dann unwirksam. [Nach Olds (*153*)]

Abb. 43. *Abhangigkeit der Selbstreizungs-Haufigkeit vom Reiz-Belohnungsschema und vom Hungerzustand.* 1. Die *Katzen* C-1, CA-1 und E-5 mit Elektroden im Caudatum-Kopf reizen sich haufiger selbst, wenn sie nach jedem 7. Hebeldruck einen elektrischen Hirnreiz auslosen konnen, als wenn dieser Reiz in unregelmaßigen Zeitabstanden (durchschnittlich alle 16 sec) auslosbar ist. 2. Die Lust der Katzen, sich elektrisch selbst zu reizen, ist nach 48stundigem Nahrungsentzug betrachtlich großer als nach einstundigem. [Nach Brady et al. (*283*)]

Abschließende Bemerkungen über die Selbstreizungsversuche

Die sich selbst reizenden Ratten, Katzen und Affen verhalten sich im Skinner-Verfahren (s. S. 397 und Abb. 32) so wie hungrige oder durstige Tiere, die mit Nahrung belohnt werden, vorausgesetzt, daß die Elektroden in bestimmten Hirnstrukturen liegen. Diese Hirnareale gruppieren sich um die Hirnmittellinie (s. Abb. 29, S. 386) vom Mittelhirn durch den Hypothalamus und mediane Thalamus-Anteile bis zum limbischen System (s. S. 382, Abb. 26—28). Innerhalb dieses „Mittellinien-Systems" kann man kleinere Areale abgrenzen, in denen die Selbstreizung genauso wirkt, als ob man die Tiere bestraft. Die Areale mit Belohnungs- und Bestrafungseffekt stehen in enger funktionaler Beziehung, die weiterer neurophysiologischer Untersuchung bedarf. Dieses gesamte „*Lust- und Unlust-System*" — die amerikanischen Autoren nennen es entsprechend ihrer Lehre von den primären Trieben „primäres Belohnungssystem" (primary reward system) — ist unterteilt in Areale, die spezifische Triebe wie Hunger oder Sexualverhalten vermitteln.

Olds (*624*) sah bei etwa einem Drittel der sich reizenden Ratten Erektionen; N. E. Miller (*580*) fand unter 146 Elektroden 18mal solche, deren Reizung zur

Ejaculation führt, ein Effekt, der stark „belohnend" wirkte. Lilly sah bei einem sich selbst reizenden Affen Erektionen.

Ob tatsächlich anatomische Unterabteilungen in dem von verschiedenen Autoren beschriebenen Sinne vorgenommen werden können oder ob es sich um Funktionseinteilungen auf rein neurophysiologisch-neurochemischer Basis handelt, scheint uns noch nicht genügend gesichert (*704, 705*). Wichtig ist jedenfalls, daß erstens Selbstreizung der Amygdala und der Tuber cinereum-Infundibulum-Gegend zu blutchemischen Veränderungen des Steroid-Spiegels führt, daß zweitens verschiedene Pharmaka (z. B. Chlorpromazin, Lysergsäure, Serotonin) in verschiedenen Arealen verschiedene Wirkungen auf das Selbstreizungsverhalten haben und daß drittens der Testosteronspiegel unter gewissen Bedingungen die Selbstreizungstätigkeit beeinflußt.

Der *Vorzug der Selbstreizungsmethode* gegenüber anderen Reizexperimenten mit Verhaltenseffekten und gegenüber dem Skinner-Verfahren allein ist darin zu sehen, daß *quantifizierbares triebhaftes Verhalten unter lokalisatorischer und neurophysiologischer Kontrolle auf das Verhalten selbst zurückwirkt.* Unter diesem Gesichtspunkt sind die weiteren Ergebnisse von Bedeutung: Bei Reizung telencephaler Hirnregionen, z. B. des Septums, sieht man „*Sättigung*" eintreten, d. h. das Tier macht von der Möglichkeit, sich zu reizen, begrenzten Gebrauch, während es sich bei Elektrodensitz im Hypothalamus unbegrenzt bis zur physischen Erschöpfung reizt. Stellt man die Tiere unter Bedingungen nach Art einer „Akkord-Arbeit" (z. B. Hirnreiz nach jedem 7. Hebeldruck), treiben sie ihre Leistung sehr hoch, offensichtlich zur Steigerung des Lustgewinnes; im „Stundenlohn" (Hirnreiz in Zeitabständen) sinkt die Leistung beträchtlich (Abb. 43).

Dressiert man den Tieren eine Bedingte Angst-Reaktion an, so macht der Hirnreiz den Bedingten und sogar auch schmerzhaften Unbedingten Reiz nahezu unwirksam. Die Bedingte Emotionale Reaktion kehrt aber wieder, sobald statt des Hirnreizes ein natürlicher Triebanreiz (Futter- oder Wasserbelohnung) gegeben wird.

Gerade diese Ergebnisse legen den Vergleich zum Suchtverhalten (*209*) nahe: Eine unangenehme, Angst erzeugende Situation, der sich das Tier nicht entziehen kann, wird durch den selbst beigebrachten Hirnreiz gleichsam für ungültig erklärt, überwunden oder nicht in Rechnung gestellt, oder — wie andere Versuche zeigen — die normale Triebbefriedigung, der Nahrungserwerb, wird zugunsten der Selbstreizung unterlassen. Und schließlich fällt bei Selbstreizung im Hypothalamus die sonst für viele Triebhandlungen typische Triebsättigung weg; erst die physische Erschöpfung setzt der sich eintönig wiederholenden Tätigkeit ein Ende. Werner (*802*) gewöhnte 4 Cebus-Affen an Morphium und stellte fest, daß die Selbstreizfrequenz in der Entziehungsphase erheblich höher lag als vor der Gewöhnung (*98*). Rado (*689*) und Jung (*98*) haben Parallelen zwischen Selbstreizung von Tieren und dem Suchtverhalten des Menschen gezogen. Sicherlich kann man mit den Selbstreizungsversuchen allein nicht das komplexe Phänomen der menschlichen Süchte erklären. Soweit aber in unsere Vorstellungen vom Zustandekommen einer Sucht physiologische und pharmakologische Vorgänge einbezogen sind und soweit psychopathologischerseits Triebvorgänge und Bedingte Reaktionen zur Erklärung einer Sucht beitragen, sind diese Experimente bedeutsam.

Wenn bei den Tieren besonders hohe Selbstreizungsfrequenzen beobachtet werden, scheinen sie sich selbst in einen lokalen epileptischen Anfall hineinzubringen und dann das Hebeldrücken in einer Art Automatismus fortzuführen. Wenn sich diese bisher vereinzelten Beobachtungen als richtig erweisen, findet die von Jung (*98*) gezogene Parallele zu bestimmten Fällen mit photogener Epilepsie auch in den Tierversuchen eine Bestätigung. Es handelt sich um meist jugendliche Patienten mit vorwiegend kleinen Anfällen, die zufällig entdeckt haben, daß

Flackerlicht ihre Attacken auslöst. Die Anfälle werden, im Gegensatz zur ganz überragenden Mehrzahl sonstiger epileptischer Anfallszustände, lustbetont erlebt und können mit sexueller Erregung einhergehen. Die Patienten rufen ihre Anfälle willkürlich hervor, indem sie in Sonnenlicht oder andere helle Lichtquellen blicken und durch schnelles Hin- und Herbewegen der gespreizten Finger vor den Augen Flimmerlicht erzeugen.

Mit Bezug auf den ersten Teil dieser Abhandlung wollen wir uns nochmals auf die *Verschränkung von Instinkthandlung und Lernen* konzentrieren. Das alte, oft kritisierte und in Philosophie und Psychologie häufig in neuem Gewande wiederkehrende hedonische Prinzip hat wohl niemals vorher eine so klar nachprüfbare, naturwissenschaftlich unterbaute Grundlage erhalten wie durch die Selbstreizungsversuche. Die Ergebnisse zeigen aber auch gleichzeitig eindeutig, daß das Lustprinzip in einer bestimmten, heute in der Psychoanalyse häufig angenommenen Fassung zumindest einseitig ist. Lust oder Befriedigung entsteht nicht stets sekundär durch Vermeidung von Unlust oder Entspannung eines Bedürfnisses, sondern Lust und Unlust kommen von Anbeginn als gleichwertige Partner ins Spiel und treten als Antagonisten auf. Daß dieser Antagonismus physiologischen Regelkreisgesetzen folgt, wie sie in der Psychiatrie vor allem Selbach (*738*) vertreten hat, ist anzunehmen; spezielle neurophysiologische Formulierungen fehlen vorläufig.

Für die von der Ethologie entwickelten Funktionstheorien ist von großer Bedeutung, daß nun auch vom neurophysiologischen Blickwinkel von Appetenz-Verhalten, von zentralnervöser Stimmung und von stimmenden Faktoren (s. S. 300 ff) gesprochen werden kann. Vermutlich wird sich der Begriff der Zentrenhierarchie (s. S. 306) in Zukunft auch neurophysiologisch-neuroanatomisch formulieren lassen. Die Präzisierung des Triebbegriffes durch Precht (s. S. 309) erfährt durch die Selbstreizungs-Experimente eine schöne Bestätigung; denn es konnte gezeigt werden, daß der Hungerzustand und der Hormonspiegel entscheidend auf das triebhafte Verhalten der Selbstreizung einwirken. Ein interessantes Phänomen, daß nämlich Selbstreizungen mit Elektroden im Hypothalamus zu keiner „Sättigung", Reizung im Septum [oder anderen Strukturen im limbischen System (s. S. 383)] dagegen zur „freiwilligen" Beschränkung der Selbstreizung führen, kann vielleicht zum Problem der Ermüdbarkeit und Unermüdbarkeit von Triebhandlungen in Beziehung gesetzt werden. Offenbar sind die unermüdbaren, „automatischen" Triebhandlungen mit niedereren, die ermüdbaren dagegen mit komplizierter regulierten, höheren Zentren verknüpft. Bei den Hypothalamus-Tieren wird gleichsam eine Art Kurzschluß hergestellt, so daß komplexe Regulative ausgeschaltet werden. Auch darin mag man Parallelen zum Suchtverhalten sehen.

Entsprechend der Anlage des Selbstreizungsversuches sehen wir nur *ein* Verhalten des Tieres, nämlich das Hebeldrücken. Dieses Verhalten ist erlernt. Angeborene Verhaltensweisen, also Instinktverhalten im engeren Sinne, treten selbst bei der mit solchen Verhaltensweisen gut ausgestatteten Katze nicht in Erscheinung, wenn man von Sexual-Reizantworten (Erektionen) absehen will. Der Lusteffekt des Hirnreizes ist größer als die natürliche Triebbefriedigung, wie Versuche, in denen Futtererwerb und Selbstreizung wahlweise angeboten werden, zeigen. Hier zeigt sich besonders deutlich die von den Ethologen oft betonte Wirkung der „endogenen" Motivation auf den raschen Neuerwerb erlernten Verhaltens. Fällt die „endogene" (freilich im Versuch durch Hirnreiz induzierte) Motivation fort, verlieren die Tiere das Interesse an der erlernten nicht artgemäßen, aber zum Lustgewinn führenden Handlung.

Der Haupteinwand (den man immer wieder hört, wenn es sich um die Anwendung von tierexperimentellen Ergebnissen auf den Menschen handelt), daß wir ja keineswegs wissen, was das Tier *erlebt* — ob Lust, ob Unlust, Schmerz oder Angst —

ist nicht recht überzeugend. Freilich erlebt das Tier nicht menschliche Lust oder Unlust; wie schon eingangs gesagt, werden wir nie wissen, was ein Tier erlebt. Die Menschen benutzen hauptsächlich die Sprache zur Erlebnismitteilung, und doch weiß jedermann, daß dadurch nur ein schwacher Abglanz des Erlebens vermittelt wird.

Die 18 Patienten von SEM-JACOBSEN (*741, 742*), in deren Hirn aus neuro-chirurgisch-diagnostischen Gründen die Selbstreizung durchgeführt wurde, beschreiben ganz eindeutig „positive" und „negative", lustbetonte und unlust-betonte Erlebnisse. Die positiven Erlebnisse waren Gefühle der Befriedigung, Behaglichkeit und Entspannung, ja, der Freude mit Lächeln (wie man auch im Film sehen kann). Die negativen Erlebnisse werden als Angst, Ruhelosigkeit, Niedergeschlagenheit, als Furcht und Schrecken beschrieben. Manche Patienten wünschten, sich selbst wiederholt reizen zu dürfen, und gaben verschiedene Motive dafür an, z. B. aus Neugier, wegen des „ulkigen" Gefühls, wegen der erlebten Ent-spannung oder wegen des Vergnügens, das sie dabei empfanden.

Die höchsten Selbstreizungsfrequenzen kamen bei veränderter Bewußtseins-lage zustande. Bei Elektrodensitz in Regionen, die bei Reizung starkes Vergnügen erzeugten, reizten sich Patienten in einen Krampfanfall hinein und lagen danach entspannt und glücklich lächelnd im Bett, im Gegensatz zu Patienten nach der üblichen Elektrokrampfbehandlung, wie der Autor schreibt.

In der zitierten Arbeit wird nur über 18 Patienten berichtet. Jedoch wurden bei 120 Pa-tienten — meist Parkinson-Kranke — mehr als 6000 Elektroden eingeführt. Andere Autoren (*256, 257, 391*) berichten über ähnliche Operationen. — Von den 18 Patienten SEM-JACOB-SENs hatten 15 eine Schizophrenie, 2 eine Epilepsie und 1 eine schwere Psychopathie; 14 waren Männer, 4 Frauen, im Alter zwischen 21 und 54 Jahren. Über die ärztliche Indikation des Ein-griffes wird nichts Detailliertes ausgesagt. Die Technik wird hier und auch von BICKFORD (*257*) genauer beschrieben.

SEM-JACOBSEN stellt fest, daß das „positive" und „negative" System eng benachbart liegen, daß man, mit anderen Worten, in einer Distanz von 0,5 bis 1,0 cm gegenteilige Erlebnisse auslösen kann. Beide Systeme scheinen zwar eng benachbart zu sein, sich aber streng zu unterscheiden, gleich einem Hemmungs- und Erregungssystem. Das antagonistische System wurde im ventro-medialen Frontalhirn, in Teilen des Parietal- und Temporallappens, im Hypothalamus und in anderen Mittellinienstrukturen gefunden. Im Frontallappen konnten, ohne daß Krampfanfälle erzeugt wurden, so stark entspannende Effekte von Behaglichkeit er-zielt werden, daß psychotische Episoden aufhörten. Der therapeutische Erfolg wird dem einer Elektrokrampfbehandlung gleichgestellt.

Die stärksten positiven und negativen Reizeffekte fanden sich um den 3. Ven-trikel herum. Zum Mittelhirn hin kam es zu euphorischem Lachen und zu Freu-densäußerungen, aber auch zu Depressionen, Angst und Schrecken. Die Daten über die negativen Areale sind klein, da diese Reizungen nicht wiederholt wurden.

Diese Untersuchungen, wie man sie ärztlich auch beurteilen mag, beweisen im Zusammenhang mit vielen anderen besprochenen Ergebnissen eindeutig, daß *im Prinzip keine naturwissenschaftlichen Unterschiede von emotionalem Verhalten und Hirnfunktion zwischen Tier und Mensch* bestehen. Auch in dieser Hinsicht sind Tiere und Menschen in derselben Weise vergleichbar wie ihre Organe in der vergleichen-den Morphologie und Physiologie. Vergleichbarkeit heißt auf diesem Gebiete eben-sowenig wie in anderen vergleichenden Wissenschaften Gleichsetzung. Die Ver-gleichbarkeit gibt der Psychiatrie und der experimentellen Psychopathologie Me-thoden in die Hand, die zu der Hoffnung berechtigen, psychiatrische Probleme — ähnlich wie in der übrigen Medizin — naturwissenschaftlich zu lösen (*48*). Ein gutes Beispiel für eine solche Arbeitsweise gibt die neurophysiologische Unter-suchung der Bedingten Emotionalen Reaktion.

5. Über die Neurophysiologie der Bedingten Emotionalen Reaktion

Über die Bedingten Reflexe und Reaktionen gibt es inzwischen zahlreiche elektroencephalographische (*58, 162*) und auch im engeren Sinne neurophysiologisch-experimentelle Studien (*52, 303, 324, 353, 369, 598, 662, 815*). Wir wollen nur wenige Daten herausgreifen, um das Prinzipielle in bezug auf emotionales Verhalten und seine neurophysiologischen Beziehungen zum limbischen System darzustellen, und können im übrigen auf Jung (ds. Bd., Teil A) verweisen.

Nach Andressur eines Bedingten akustischen Reizes (CS) und chronisch implantierten Ableite-Elektroden im Katzenhirn folgen dem Klangreiz ziemlich klar abgegrenzte Potentiale innerhalb des limbischen Systems, wie z. B. dem Hippocampus, und, weniger gesichert, im Amygdaloid-Komplex, im Nucl. caudatus und in der Septum-Gegend. Dabei wird der in Serien gegebene CS mehr und mehr unwirksam, d. h. *nach* dem 1. Reiz nimmt die Reizantwort zunehmend ab, und zwar bei Reizabständen von 1 sec schneller als bei einem Abstand der Reizgeräusche von 3 sec. Setzt man aber nach einer solchen CS-Serie einen schmerzhaften Unbedingten Reiz, so bleiben die elektrischen Reizantworten auf die akustische Reizserie schon nach ein paar Versuchen, speziell im Hippocampus, gleich stark ausgeprägt. Hier finden wir also ein, wenn auch sehr komplexes, neurophysiologisches Korrelat zu dem Phänomen der Löschung einer Bedingten Reaktion und ihrer Wiederbelebung. Die mit Wiederholung des CS abnehmende bedingte elektrische Antwort entspricht der Löschung des bedingten Verhaltens, und die nach Bekräftigung durch den Unbedingten Reiz sich erneut ausbildende bedingte Reaktion entspricht der nunmehr gleichbleibend kräftigen bedingten elektrischen Antwort (*57, 744*). Diesen Ergebnissen kommt für die Lerntheorie des Verhaltens eine große Bedeutung zu, wie sich auch bei anderen Untersuchungen zeigt, in denen bedingte elektrische Potentiale in der Formatio reticularis mesencephali bereits dann aktiviert werden, wenn man die Katzen lediglich in die Umgebung bringt, in welcher die Dressur vorgenommen wurde, ohne daß ein Bedingter oder Unbedingter Reiz gegeben wird (*815*). Von den bedingten hirnelektrischen Potentialen ist die Abnahme von Reizantworten zu unterscheiden, die durch einfache Wiederholung von Sinnesreizen (ohne nachfolgenden Unbedingten Reiz) entsteht (*57, 399, 437, 743*). Hier handelt es sich um das neurophysiologische Korrelat der Gewöhnung (habituation), der einfachsten Form des Lernens (*195*) (vgl. S. 395). Nach den bisher vorliegenden EEG-Untersuchungen am Menschen darf man die Vermutung aussprechen, daß hier prinzipiell die gleichen neurophysiologischen Korrelate bedingten Verhaltens angenommen werden können (*353*).

Mikrcelektroden-Ableitungen an einzelnen Ganglienzellen während der Bedingten Reaktion von Affen verfeinern die Erkenntnisse über die sehr komplizierten neurophysiologischen Grundlagen des bedingten Verhaltens (*699*). Die oben kurz erwähnten Untersuchungen über die hirnelektrischen Korrelate der Gewöhnung zeigten, daß die bloße Wiederholung eines Reizes nicht notwendig zur Bedingten Reaktion führen muß. Dafür ist außer der herausgehobenen Signifikanz des Reizes auch die gespannte Erwartung dieses Reizes erforderlich (*369*).

Nach den neurophysiologischen Versuchen zum bedingten Verhalten kann man den Dressurvorgang nicht einfach als eine „Stiftung neuer Verbindungen" zwischen verschiedenen corticalen Feldern betrachten (*597*). Komplizierte Hemmungs- und Enthemmungsprozesse scheinen dafür verantwortlich zu sein, daß eine begrenzte Reizantwort zustande kommen kann, ohne daß man diesen Vorgang aber in Ausdrücken der lokalen Erregung oder Hemmung beschreiben könnte. Nicht nur die Erregung und Erregbarkeit vieler corticaler Areale, sondern auch spezifischer und unspezifischer Hirnstammteile ändern sich. Im Zusammenhang mit anderen Mikroelektrodenstudien ist sogar anzunehmen, daß bereits periphere (sensorische) Neurone am Gesamtvorgang beteiligt sind (*100, 224, 313, 376, 377, 699*).

Schluß

Warum eigentlich, so mag man zum Schluß noch einmal fragen, soll die Verhaltensforschung eine der geeigneten Grundlagen für die Psychiatrie sein? Niemand zweifelt daran, daß Neuroanatomie, Neurophysiologie und Biochemie zu den biologischen Grundpfeilern der Psychiatrie gehören. Auf diesen Gebieten sind mit Erfolg und in methodischer Übereinstimmung mit der übrigen Medizin vergleichende Forschungen getrieben und die an Tieren gewonnenen Ergebnisse für den Menschen ausgewertet worden.

Anders steht es mit dem Verhalten. Das Niveau der Verhaltensweisen, in denen sich Psychisches ausdrückt, scheint von den organischen Grundvorgängen so weit entfernt zu sein, daß es mit deren Analyse allein nicht getroffen werden kann. Wir müssen daher nach niveauadäquaten Fragestellungen und Grundlagen suchen. Zwar gibt es seit langem eine vergleichende Psychologie. Aber erst der Leitsatz, daß man Verhaltensweisen ebenso vergleichen kann wie Organe in der Morphologie, ja, daß Verhaltensweisen sich oft konstanter durch die Stammesgeschichte ziehen als manche Organe, stellt den rechten Bezug zu den biologischen Wissenschaften her. Ein wesentliches Merkmal dieser Verhaltensweisen ist ihre Formstarrheit, wie z. B. am Kratz-„Reflex" ersichtlich, einer sehr einfachen Verhaltensweise, die sich von den Amphibien bis zu den Säugern erhalten hat. Solche formstarren Verhaltenseinheiten — von den Reflexen wohl zu unterscheiden — machen den Kernbestand des „Verhaltensinventars" der Arten und Gattungen aus. Sie gehören zu ihnen wie deren art- und gattungsspezifische Organe. Um es in einem Beispiel nochmals zu sagen: Zu den jeweils arttypischen Geschlechtsorganen gehört die Bewegung, die sie zusammenführt, zu den Flügeln die Flugbewegung, zur Hand das Greifen usw. Die formstarren Verhaltensweisen sind angeboren wie Organe, und unter ihnen scheinen die Instinkte eine besondere Gruppe zu bilden, die wir näher charakterisiert haben.

A. Theorie, Methoden und Ergebnisse der Ethologie (i. e. vergleichende Erforschung angeborenen Verhaltens) wurden zunächst systematisch in Kapitel I und II und später speziell in bezug auf menschliches Verhalten in Kapitel III und IV dargestellt. Im V. Kapitel behandelten wir psychopathologische Probleme unter ethologischen Gesichtspunkten.

Die Ethologie bietet eine noch im Werden begriffene Lehre vom Aufbau des Verhaltens an, die sich erstens vom Reiz-Reaktionsmodell im Sinne der Reflexologie und zweitens von reinen Lern- und Milieutheorien freimacht. Die Beteiligung von Reflexen am Aufbau des Verhaltens, von Lernprozessen und Umgebungseinflüssen wird nicht etwa bestritten, doch bekommen alte Begriffspaare wie Reiz-Reaktion, Begabung-Lernen, Anlage-Umwelt neue Inhalte. Das erste Begriffspaar ist z. B. in die Lehre von den Auslösermechanismen eingegangen und kann dort — ähnlich wie der Reflex — einen Spezialfall darstellen. Das 2. Paar erscheint unter dem Aspekt des angeborenen Lernvermögens, des Wachstums und Reifens von Verhaltensweisen. Der Lernprozeß als solcher interessiert den Ethologen weniger als vielmehr die Frage, wie angeborenes und erlerntes Verhalten miteinander verschränkt sind. Das 3. Paar tritt überhaupt nicht mehr in dieser Alternative auf, sondern unter dem Thema des Eingepaßtseins in eine artspezifische Umwelt. Diese drei und andere in diesem Beitrag behandelte Themen sind Bestandteile des Generalthemas, nämlich einer Triebtheorie auf vergleichend verhaltensphysiologischer Grundlage. Diese Theorie ist durchaus noch nicht geschlossen und wird sich im

Gange der weiteren Forschung noch ändern. Sie hat aber den großen Vorteil, daß sie induktiv korrigierbar ist, ja, daß mit ihrer Hilfe z. B. die psychoanalytische Triebtheorie aus einem dogmatischen Stadium befreit zu werden verspricht und eine biologische Grundlage gewinnen kann, die Sigmund Freud selbst erhofft hat.

Das für den Psychiater fruchtbare Element in dieser Theorie sehen wir vor allem in der Vereinigung von ,,statischen'' und ,,dynamischen'' Funktionen, von formstarren Mechanismen einerseits und Regeln der Verhaltensentwicklung andererseits. Die Modeworte ,,statische'' oder ,,dynamische'' Psychiatrie verlieren bei dieser Betrachtungsweise ihren Sinn.

Die Ethologie nennt sich auch Verhaltensphysiologie. Sie kann dies mit Recht tun, nämlich einmal im Hinblick auf Experimente, die eine physiologische Analyse des Verhaltens im strengen Sinne darstellen, zum anderen aber in bezug auf das von ihr aufgestellte Forschungsprogramm.

B. Dieses Programm hat die Ethologie mit ihrer älteren Schwester, der ,,vergleichenden physiologischen Psychologie'' (Comparative Physiological Psychology) gemeinsam. Hier vereinigen sich manche Gegensätze in dem Bemühen um eine naturwissenschaftliche Grundlage des Verhaltens.

Das I. Kapitel handelte von den Hirnstrukturen und -funktionen, die triebhaftem Verhalten zugrunde liegen. Sowohl Triebhandlungen als auch Handelnsbereitschaften (Stimmungen) haben auf verschiedenen Integrationsstufen im Mittelhirn, Zwischenhirn und limbischen System ihr anatomisch-physiologisches Substrat. Die Ergebnisse stammen vornehmlich von Experimenten an Katzen und Affen. Entsprechend den Unterschieden im Verhaltensinventar der verschiedenen Tiergattungen und -arten können Einzelresultate nicht verallgemeinert, sondern nur vergleichend übertragen werden. Nach den vorliegenden klinischen Erfahrungen, Operationen und Hirnreizungen am Menschen dürfen für ihn homologe Gesetzmäßigkeiten angenommen werden.

Im II. Kapitel wurde am Beispiel der Bedingten Reaktion verfolgt, wie triebhaftes und emotionales Verhalten in Lernprozesse verflochten ist und welche Hirnstrukturen für Erwerb und Verlust von Bedingten Reaktionen von Bedeutung sind. Elektrische Selbstreizungen des Gehirns, durchgeführt an Säugetieren einschließlich Affen und Menschen, zeigen klar, daß es triebabhängige handlungsfördernde und handlungshemmende Hirnstrukturen gibt. Das alte, regulative Prinzip von Lust und Unlust findet eine hirnphysiologische Begründung und kann spezieller formuliert werden.

Um den ersten und zweiten Teil dieses Beitrages noch enger zu verschmelzen, hätte ein weiteres Kapitel geschrieben werden müssen, für das uns die Voraussetzungen fehlten. Nahezu hundert Jahre sind vergleichend hirnanatomische Studien getrieben worden, die für die Verhaltensforschung weithin ungenutzt blieben. Diese Ergebnisse mit der vergleichenden Verhaltensforschung zu konfrontieren, beide zu ergänzen und nachzuprüfen, wäre notwendig, um zu einer evolutionistisch fundierten Verhaltenstheorie zu kommen, die weder einseitig von der Hirnstruktur noch allein vom Verhalten her aufgebaut ist.

Rufen wir in Erinnerung, daß bei niederen Tieren ohne Großhirnmantel der Einbau von Erfahrungen in die artspezifischen und arterhaltenden Verhaltensweisen bereits in erstaunlichem Ausmaße möglich ist. Formstarre Verhaltensweisen und die Fähigkeit, das Verhalten den Erfahrungen anzupassen, entwickeln sich *gleichzeitig*. Dasselbe gilt für Tiere, bei denen sich ein Großhirn ausbildet. Erfahrungsorientierte Verhaltensweisen können nicht schlechthin der Entwicklung eines Neopalliums und formstarre (instinktive) Verhaltensweisen nicht einfach dem Paläo- und Archipallium zugeschrieben werden. *Jeder* Teil des Endhirns hat alte *und* neue Unterformationen. Jeder Schritt in der Verhaltensentwicklung schließt das *ganze* Verhalten ein. Evolution des Verhaltens kann nicht als additiver Zuwachs von Fähigkeiten verstanden werden.

Unter allen Lebewesen ist beim Menschen die Fähigkeit, Unterscheidungen zu treffen und das Verhalten diesen „Urteilen" anzupassen, am kompliziertesten aufgebaut. Auf dieser Stufe der hochentwickelten Diskriminationsfähigkeit sind gleichzeitig aber auch die spezifischen Handelnsbereitschaften (Stimmungen) am höchsten integriert. Formstarre Verhaltensweisen treten nur im Beginn der ontogenetischen Entwicklung und unter pathologischen (neuropsychiatrischen) Bedingungen als isolierbare Bestandteile hervor. Unter diesen Umständen ist dann gleichzeitig auch die diskriminative Fähigkeit vermindert bzw. verändert.

Faßt man die Psychopathologie als eine Lehre von den Störungen des Verhaltens in dem hier gemeinten Sinne auf, läßt sich ein biologisches Konzept der Psychiatrie erarbeiten, das die Dichotomie somatischer und psychischer Vorgänge im Ansatz vermeidet und mit naturwissenschaftlichen Methoden vorangetrieben werden kann.

Der Beitrag ist Herrn Professor KONRAD LORENZ zum 60. Geburtstag gewidmet.

Für wertvolle Kritik am Manuskript, das im März 1960 erstmals abgeschlossen wurde, danke ich den Herren HEINRICH KLÜVER, OTTO KOEHLER, PAUL MACLEAN, WALLE NAUTA und den Herausgebern.

Literatur

Übersichtsarbeiten

1. ADEY, W. R.: The Rhinencephalon: A review of recent studies of its interrelations with brain stem structures. J. anat. Soc. India 4, 27—36 (1955). — 2. ALLPORT, G. W.: Persönlichkeit, eine psychologische Interpretation. Stuttgart: Klett 1949. — 3. ALPERS, A.: Delphine, Wunderkinder des Meeres (Dolphins, The Myth and the Mammal), Bern und Stuttgart: Scherz Verlag 1962. — 4. ANDERSON, E. et al.: Disturbances in blood sugar regulation in animals subjected to transsection of the brain stem. Acta neuroveg. (Wien) 5, 132—164 (1952). — 5. ARIENS KAPPERS, C. U., G. C. HUBER and E. C. CROSBY: The comparative anatomy of the nervous system of vertebrates, including man. 3 Vol. New York: Hafner Publishing Comp. 1960. — 5a. ASCHOFF, J.: Spontane lokomotorische Aktivität. Hdb.Zool. Bd. VIII, 11 (4) 1—74 (1962). — 6. AUTUORI, M., M.-P. BENASSY et al. (Eds.): L'instinct dans le comportement des animaux et de l'homme. Paris: Masson & Cie. 1956.

7. BAERENDS, G. P.: Aufbau des tierischen Verhaltens. Handb. Zool. Bd. 8, 10 (3) 1—32 Berlin: Walter de Gruyter 1956. — 8. BALDWIN, M., and P. BAILEY (Eds.): Temporal lobe epilepsy. Springfield/Ill.: Ch. C. Thomas Publisher 1958. — 9. BARD, P.: Central nervous mechanisms for emotional behavior patterns in animals. Res. Publ. Ass. nerv. ment. Dis. 19, 190—218 (1939). — 10. BARD, P.: Central nervous mechanisms for the expression of anger in animals. In: Feelings and Emotions (Ed. M. L. REYMERT). New York-Toronto-London: McGraw-Hill Book Comp. Inc. 1950.— 11. BASH, K. W.: Lehrbuch der allgemeinen Psychopathologie. Stuttgart: Thieme 1955. — 12. BEACH, F. A.: Hormones and Behavior. New York: P. B. Hoeber 1948. — 13. BEACH, F. A.: Evolutionary aspects of Psychoendocrinology. In: Behavior and Evolution (Eds. A. ROE and G. G. SIMPSON). Yale University Press 1958. — 14. BEACH et al. (Eds.): The neuropsychology of Lashley. Selected papers of K. S. Lashley. New York-Toronto-London: McGraw-Hill 1960. — 15. BILZ, R.: Pars pro toto. Ein Beitrag zur Pathologie menschlicher Affekte und Organfunktionen. Leipzig: Thieme 1940. — 16. BILZ, R.: Lebensgesetze der Liebe. 4. Beih. Zbl. Psychotherapie. Leipzig: Hirzel 1943. — 17. BLEULER, E.: Naturgeschichte der Seele. Berlin: Springer 1921. — 18. BLEULER, M.: Endokrinologische Psychiatrie. In: Psychiatrie der Gegenwart Bd. I/1, Berlin-Göttingen-Heidelberg: Springer 1963. — 19. BRADY, J. V.: The paleocortex and behavioral motivation. In: HARLOW and C. WOOLSEY (Eds.): s. Nr. 67. — 20. BROWN, J. S.: The motivation of behavior. New York-Toronto-London: McGraw-Hill 1961. — 21. BRUN, R.: Gehirn. Handb. Innere Medizin, Bd. V/1, 4. Aufl., S. 704—903, Berlin-Göttingen-Heidelberg: Springer 1953. — 22. BRUN, R.: Allgemeine Neurosenlehre, 3. Aufl. Basel u. Stuttgart: Benno Schwabe 1954. — 23. BUDDENBROCK, W. v.: Vergleichende Physiologie. 5 Bde. Basel: Birkhäuser 1950—61. — 24. BÜNNING, E.: Die physiologische Uhr. Berlin-Göttingen-Heidelberg: Springer 1958. — 24a. BUETTNER-JANUSCH et al. (Eds.): The relatives of man: modern studies of the relation of the evolution of nonhuman primates to human evolution. Ann. N. Y. Acad. Sci. 102, Art. 2, p. 181—514 (1962).

25. CARMICHAEL, L.: Manual of child psychology. 2nd ed. New York: J. Wiley 1954. — 26. CARPENTER, C. R.: A field study of the behavior and social relations of howling monkeys. Comp. Psychol. Monogr. Bd. 10, Nr. 2. Baltimore: 1934. — 27. CARPENTER, C. R.: A field

study in Siam of the behavior and social relations of the gibbon. Comp. Psychol. Monogr. Bd. 16, Nr. 5. Baltimore: 1940. — 28. COBB, S.: Emotions and clinical medicine. New York: Norton 1950. — 29. CONRAD, K.: Die Gestaltanalyse in der Psychiatrie. Studium Generale 5, 503—514 (1952). — 30. CONRAD, K.: Die beginnende Schizophrenie. Stuttgart: Thieme 1958. — 31. CRAIG, W.: Appetites and aversions as constituents of instincts. Biol. Bull. (Woods Hole) 34, 91—107 (1918).

32. DARWIN, CH.: The origin of species. 6. Aufl. London: J. M. Dent & Sons Ltd. 1947. — 33. DARWIN, CH.: The variation of animals and plants under domestication. 2. Aufl., 2. Bde. New York: D. Appleton & Co. 1892. — 34. DARWIN, CH.: Der Ausdruck der Gemütsbewegungen bei Menschen und Tieren. (Übersetz. TH. BENGFELDT) Halle: 1896. — 35. DELAFRESNAYE, J. F. (Ed.): Brain mechanisms and consciousness (Symposium). Oxford: Blackwell scientific publications 1954. — 36. DEVOE, A.: Animal children. National Audubon Society, Nelson Doubleday, Inc. 1958.

37. EBBECKE, U.: Angeborene Verhaltensweisen des Menschen. Dtsch. med. Wschr. 1950, 54—57; 88—91. — 38. EBBECKE, U.: Physiologie des Bewußtseins in entwicklungsgeschichtlicher Betrachtung. Stuttgart: Thieme 1959. — 39. EIBL-EIBESFELDT, I.: Fortschritte der vergleichenden Verhaltensforschung. Naturwiss. Rsch. 1956, 86—90; 136—142. — 40. EIBL-EIBESFELDT, I.: Ausdrucksformen der Säugetiere. Handbuch der Zoologie VIII, 10 (6), 1—26. Berlin: Walter de Gruyter 1957. — 41. EIBL-EIBESFELDT, I.: Technik der vergleichenden Verhaltensforschung. Handb. Zool. VIII, 10 (2), 11—34, 1962. — 42. EICKSTEDT, E. Frh. v.: Vom Wesen der Anthropologie. Homo 1, 1—13 (1949). — 43. ELKES, J.: Behavioral pharmacology in relation to psychiatry. In: Psychiatrie der Gegenwart, Bd. I/1, Berlin-Göttingen-Heidelberg: Springer 1963. — 44. ESTES, W. K., S. KOCH et al.: Modern learning theory. New York: Appleton-Century-Crofts 1954. — 45. EY, H.: Grundlagen einer organodynamischen Auffassung der Psychiatrie. Fortschr. Neurol. Psychiat. 20, 195 (1952).

46. FABRE, J. H.: Aus der Wunderwelt der Instinkte. Meisenheim/Glan: Westkulturverlag 1950. — 47. FERSTER, C. B., and B. F. SKINNER: Schedules of reinforcement. New York: Appleton-Century-Crofts, Inc. 1957.—48. FESSARD, A., R. GERARD and J. KONORSKI (Eds.): Brain mechanisms and learning. Oxford: Blackwell 1961.—49. FIELDS, W. S., et al. (Eds.): Hypothalamic-Hypophysial Interrelationships. Springfield, Ill.: Thomas 1955.—50. FISCHEL, W.: Haushunde. Handbuch der Zoologie. VIII, 10 (16), 1—16. Berlin: Walter de Gruyter 1957. — 51. FISCHEL, W.: Methoden der tierpsychologischen Forschung nebst Anleitung zu einem tierpsychologischen Praktikum. Bonn: H. Bouvier & Co. 1953. — 52. FISCHGOLD, H., et H. GASTAUT (Herausgeber): Conditionnement et réactivité en électroencéphalographie. Paris: Masson et Cie. 1957. (Electroenceph. clin. Neurophysiol. Suppl. Nr. 6, 475 Seiten.) — 53. FREMONT-SMITH, F.: The central nervous system and behavior. (Translation from the Russian medical literature). Princeton, N. J.: The Josiah Macy, Jr. Foundation, The National Science Foundation 1959. — 54. FREUD, S.: Ges. Werke, Bd. V, S. 67; Bd. XI, S. 403. London: Imago Publ. 1940/1942. — 55. FRISCH, K. v.: Aus dem Leben der Bienen, 5. Aufl., Berlin-Göttingen-Heidelberg: Springer 1953. — 56. FULTON, J. F.: Frontal lobotomy and affective behavior. New York: Norton & Co. 1951.

57. GALAMBOS, R.: Electrical correlates of conditioned learning. In: The Central Nervous System and Behavior. First (1958) Conference, The Josiah Macy, Jr. Foundation, Madison, N. J.: Madison Printing Co. 1959. — 58. GASTAUT, H. (Herausgeber): L'électro-encéphalographie du conditionnement. (Symposium.) 1. Internationaler Kongreß für Neurologie. Acta med. belg. Brüssel: 1957. — 59. GASTAUT, H., et H. J. LAMMERS: Anatomie du Rhinencéphale. In: Les grandes activités du rhinencéphale (Ed. TH. ALAJOUANINE), Paris: Masson et Cie 1960. — 60. GEHLEN, A.: Der Mensch. 3. Aufl. Bonn 1950. — 61. GELLHORN, E.: Autonomic imbalance and the hypothalamus; implications for physiology, medicine, psychology, and neuropsychiatry. Minneapolis: University of Minnesota Press 1957. — 62. GELLHORN, E.: Physiological foundations of neurology and psychiatry. Minneapolis: University of Minnesota Press 1953. — 63. GLEES, P.: Morphologie und Physiologie des Nervensystems. Stuttgart: Thieme 1957. — 64. GLOOR, P.: Telencephalic influences upon the hypothalamus; s. Nr. 49, S. 74—113. — 65. GREEN, J. D.: The rhinencephalon: Aspects of its relation to behavior and the reticular activating system. In: Symposium on the reticular formation, Detroit 1957. Boston, Mass.: Little, Brown & Co. 1958.

66. HALL, C. S.: The genetics of behavior. In: Handbook of experimental psychology; s. Nr. 190. — 67. HARLOW, H., and C. WOOLSEY (Eds.): Biological and biochemical bases of behavior. Madison, Wisconsin: University of Wisconsin Press 1958. — 68. HEBB, D. O.: The organization of behavior. New York: J. Wiley 1949. — 69. HEBB, D. O.: A textbook of psychology. Philadelphia: W. B. Saunders Co. 1958. — 70. HEBERER, G.: Die Evolution der Organismen. 2. Aufl. Stuttgart: Fischer 1954.—71. HEBERER, G., u. F. SCHWANITZ (Herausgeb.): Hundert Jahre Evolutionsforschung. Stuttgart: Fischer 1960.—72. HEDIGER, H.: Brutpflege bei Säugetieren. Ciba-Z. 59, 1965—1973 (1953).—73. HEIBERG, J. L.: Geisteskrankheiten im klassi-

schen Altertum. Berlin und Leipzig: de Gruyter 1927. — 74. HEMPELMANN, F.: Tierpsychologie vom Standpunkte des Biologen. Leipzig: Akademische Verlagsgesellschaft m. b. H. 1926. — 75. HERRE, W.: Einflüsse der Umwelt auf das Säugetiergehirn. Dtsch. med. Wschr. 1958 II, 1568—1574. — 76. HESS, W. R.: Das Zwischenhirn. Basel: Schwabe & Co. 1954. — 77. HESS, W. R.: Hypothalamus und Thalamus. Experimental-Dokumente. Stuttgart: Thieme 1956. — 78. HESS, W. R.: Psychologie in biologischer Sicht. Stuttgart: Thieme (1962). — 79. HESS, W. R., u. K. AKERT: Symposium über das Zwischenhirn. Helv. physiol. pharmacol. Acta, Suppl. VI (1950). — 80. HILGARD, E. R.: Theories of learning. New York: Appleton-Century-Crofts, Inc. 1948. — 81. HITZIG, E.: Physiologische und klinische Untersuchungen über das Gehirn. Gesammelte Abhandlungen. Berlin: A. HIRSCHWALD 1904. — 82. HOCH, P., and J. ZUBIN (Eds.): Experimental Psychopathology. New York: Grune & Stratton 1957. — 83. HOFER, H., A. H. SCHULTZ u. D. STARCK (Hrsg.): Primatologia, Bd. I. Basel-New York: Karger 1956. — 84. HOFSTÄTTER, P. R.: Psychologie. Frankfurt: Das Fischer-Lexikon, Bd. 6, Fischer-Bücherei KG 1957. — 85. HOLST, E. v.: Zentralnervensystem. Fortschr. Zool. 10, 381—390 (1956). — 86. HOLST, E. v.: Die Funktionsstruktur des Zwischenhirns (ZH). Fortschr. Zool. 11, 245—275 (1958). — 87. HOTOVY, R.: Die „Neuroplegica" und ihre psychopharmakologische Prüfung. Mercks Jber. Pharm. 1956/57, 1—23. — 88. HULL, C. L.: Principles of behavior. New York: Appleton-Century-Crofts 1943. — 89. HULL, C. L.: A behavior system. New Haven: Yale University Press 1952.

90. INGRAM, W. R.: The hypothalamus. Ciba Clinic. Symp. 8, 117—153 (1956).

91. JACKSON, J. H.: Selected writings of John Hughlings Jackson. Vol. 1—3, New York: Basic Books, Inc. 1958. — 92. JASPER, H., L. PROCTOR et al. (Eds.): Reticular formation of the brain. Boston, Mass.: Little, Brown & Comp. 1958. — 93. JASPERS, K.: Allgemeine Psychopathologie. 4. Aufl., S. 303ff. Berlin-Heidelberg: Springer 1946. — 94. JEFFRESS, L. A. (Ed.): Cerebral mechanisms in behavior. New York: John Wiley & Son, Inc. 1951. — 95. JENNINGS, H. S.: The behavior of the lower organisms. New York: Columbia University Press 1906. — 96. J. Primatology 1, (1959). Japan Monkey Center. Kurisu, Inuyama City, Japan. — 97. JUNG, C. G.: Wandlungen und Symbole der Libido. Leipzig-Wien: F. Deuticke 1912. — 98. JUNG, R.: Selbstreizung des Gehirns im Tierversuch. Dtsch. med. Wschr. 1958, 1716—1721. — 99. JUNG, R.: Nervensystem und Umwelt. In: Allgemeine Neurophysiologie. Handb. Innere Med. Bd. V/1, 145—159 (Lit. S. 180). Berlin-Göttingen-Heidelberg: Springer 1953.— 100. JUNG, R., O. CREUTZFELDT u. O.-J. GRÜSSER: Die Mikrophysiologie kortikaler Neurone und ihre Bedeutung für die Sinnes- und Hirnfunktion. Dtsch. med. Wschr. 1957, 1050—1059. — 101. JUNG, R., and R. HASSLER: The extrapyramidal motor system. Handbook Physiol. Neurophysiol. II, 863—927. Washington, D. C. 1959.

102. KAADA, B.: Somato-motor, autonomic and electrocorticographic responses to electrical stimulation of "rhinencephalic" and other structures in primates, cat and dog. Acta physiol. scand. 24, Suppl. 83, 1—285 (1951). — 103. KALLMANN, F. J.: Heredity in health and mental disorder. New York: Norton 1953.— 104. KLAESI, J.: Über Neurosenlehre und Psychotherapie. Handb. Innere Med. Bd. V/3, 1260. Berlin: Springer 1953.— 105. KLEIST, K.: Gehirnpathologie. Leipzig: Barth 1934.— 106. KLEIST, K.: Bericht über die Gehirnpathologie in ihrer Bedeutung für Neurologie und Psychiatrie. Z. Neurol. 158, 159—193 (1937).—107. KLÜVER, H.: Behavior mechanisms in monkeys. 2. Aufl. Chicago-Illinois: The University Press of Chicago 1957.— 108. KLÜVER, H.: Brain mechanisms and behavior with special reference to the rhinencephalon. Journal-Lancet 72, 567—577 (1952).— 109. KOEHLER, O.: Die Analyse der Taxisanteile instinktartigen Verhaltens. 4. Symposion of the society for experimental biology: Physiological mechanisms in animal behaviour. S. 269—302. Cambridge: University Press 1950. — 110. KÖHLER, W.: Intelligenzprüfungen an Menschenaffen. Unveränd. Nachdruck der 2. Aufl. Berlin-Göttingen-Heidelberg: Springer 1963. — 111. KONORSKI, J.: Conditioned reflexes and neuron organization. Cambridge University Press 1948. — 112. KRETSCHMER, E.: Hysterie, Reflex und Instinkt. 6. Aufl. Stuttgart: Thieme 1958. — 113. KUMMER, H.: Soziales Verhalten einer Mantelpavian-Gruppe. Bern und Stuttgart: Huber 1957.

114. LASHLEY, K. S.: Experimental analysis of instinctive behavior. Psychol. Rev. 45, 445—471 (1938). — 115. LASHLEY, K. S.: Persistent problems in the evolution of mind. Quart. Rev. Biol. 24, 28—42 (1949). — 116. LASHLEY, K. S.: In search of the engram, s. Nr. 192, S. 454—482. — 117. LASHLEY, K. S.: Cerebral organization and behavior. In: s. Nr. 14 u. 186, S. 1—18. — 118. LEHMANN, F. E. (Hrsgeb.): Gestaltungen sozialen Lebens bei Tier und Mensch. Bern: Francke 1958. — 119. LEHRMAN, D. S.: Comparative Physiology (Behavior). Ann. Rev. Physiol. 18, 527—542). — 120. LEHRMAN, D. S.: Ethology and Psychology. In Recent Advances in Biological Psychiatry. Vol. 4, p. 86—94, 1962. — 121. LEHRMAN, D. S.: Interaction of hormonal and experiential influences on development of behavior. In: Roots of Behavior (Ed. E. L. BLISS), Hoeber Medical Division of Harper & Brothers, 1962. — 122. LEHRMAN, D. S.: Hormonal regulation of parental behavior in birds and infrahuman mammals. In: Sex and internal secretion. (Ed. W. C. YOUNG), William and Wilkins Comp., 3. ed., Baltimore 1961. — 123. LEUNER, H.: Die experimentelle Psychose. Ihre Psychopharma-

kologie, Phänomenologie und Dynamik in Beziehung zur Person. Berlin-Göttingen-Heidelberg: Springer 1962. — 124. LEVY-BRUHL, L.: Die Seele der Primitiven. Düsseldorf: Diederichs 1956. — Die geistige Welt der Primitiven. Darmstadt: Wissenschaftl. Buchgesellschaft 1958. — 125. LEWIN, K.: A dynamic theory of personality. New York-London: McGraw-Hill 1935. — 126. LEYHAUSEN, P.: Das Verhalten der Katzen. Handb. Zool. Bd. VIII, 10 (21), 1—34 (1956). — 127. LEYHAUSEN, P.: Verhaltensstudien an Katzen. Berlin und Hamburg: Parey 1956. — 128. LINDSLEY, D. B.: Physiological Psychology. Ann. Rev. Psychol. 7, 323—348 (1956). — 129. LORENZ, K.: Er redete mit dem Vieh, den Fischen und den Vögeln. Tiergeschichten. Wien: Borotha-Schoeler 1949. — 130. LORENZ, K.: So kam der Mensch auf den Hund. Wien: Borotha-Schoeler 1950. — 131. LORENZ, K.: Die angeborenen Formen möglicher Erfahrung. Z. Tierpsychol. 5, 235—409 (1943). — 132. LORENZ, K.: Über angeborene Instinktformeln beim Menschen. Dtsch. med. Wschr. 1953 II, 1566, 1600. — 133. LORENZ, K.: Gestaltwahrnehmung als Quelle wissenschaftlicher Erkenntnis. Z. exp. angew. Psychol. 6, 118—165 (1959). — 134. LORENZ, K.: Psychologie und Stammesgeschichte: In: G. HEBERER: s. Nr. 70. — 135. LORENZ, K.: Methoden der Verhaltensforschung. Handb. Zool. Bd. VIII, 10. Teil, 1—22 (1957). — 136. LORENZ, K.: Phylogenetische Anpassung und adaptive Modifikation des Verhaltens. Z. Tierpsychol. 18, 139—187 (1961).

137. MAGOUN, H. W.: An ascending reticular activating system in the brain stem. A. M. A. Arch. Neurol. Psychiat. 67, 145 (1952). — 138. MAGOUN, H. W.: The waking brain. Springfield, Ill.: Thomas 1958. — 139. MAIER, N. R. F., and T. C. SCHNEIRLA: Principles of animal psychology. London-New York 1935.— 140. MASSERMAN, J. H.: Principles of dynamic psychiatry. Philadelphia: Saunders Comp. 1946.— 141. MASSERMAN, J. H.: The practice of dynamic psychiatry. Philadelphia-London: Saunders Comp. 1955.— 142. MASSERMAN, J. H., and J. L. MORENO: Progress in psychotherapy. Vol. II: Anxiety and Therapy. New York-London: Grune & Stratton 1957.— 143. MEAD, MARGARET: Mann und Weib. Das Verhältnis der Geschlechter in einer sich wandelnden Welt. Rowohlts deutsche Enzyklopädie 1958. — 144. MEYER-HOLZAPFEL, MONIKA: Die Bedeutung des Besitzes bei Tier und Mensch. Biel: Institut f. Psycho-Hygiene 1952.— 145. MEYER-HOLZAPFEL, MONIKA: Das Spiel bei Säugetieren. Handb. Zool. Bd. VIII, 10 (5) 1—36 (1956). — 146. MEYER-HOLZAPFEL, MONIKA: Das Verhalten der Bären (Ursidae). Handb. Zool. Bd. VIII, 10 (17), 1—28 (1957). — 147. MILL, J. ST.: A system of logic, 3. Aufl. London: Parker 1851. Bd. 2: Of ethology, or the science of formation of character. S. 432—448. — 148. MILLER, N. E.: Theory and experiment relating psychoanalytic displacement to stimulus-response generalization. J. abnorm. soc. Psychol. 43, 155—178 (1948). — 149. MOHR, ERNA: Das Verhalten der Pinnipedier. Handb. Zool. Bd. VIII 10 (1), 1—16 (1956). — 150. MONAKOW, C. V., u. R. MOURGUE: Biologische Einführung in das Studium der Neurologie und Psychopathologie. Stuttgart und Leipzig: Hippocrates Verlag 1930. — 151. MONTAGU, M. F. A.: The direction of human development. Biological and social bases. New York: Harper & Brothers 1955. — 152. MOWRER, O. H.: Learning theory and behavior. New York-London: John Wiley & Sons 1960.

153. OLDS, J.: Self-stimulation of the brain. Science 127, 315—324 (1958).

154. PASCAL, G. R., and W. O. JENKINS: Systematic observation of gross human behavior. New York-London: Grune & Stratton: 1961. — 155. PAWLOW, I. P.: Sämtliche Werke. Bd. III/2. Berlin: Akademie Verlag 1953. — 156. PEIPER, A.: Die Eigenart der kindlichen Hirntätigkeit. 2. Aufl. Leipzig: Thieme 1956. — 157. PENFIELD, W.: The role of the temporal cortex in recall of the past experience and interpretation of the present. In: WOLSTENHOLME et al. (Eds.): s. Nr. 211, S. 149—174. — 158. PILTERS, HILDE: Das Verhalten der Tylopoden. Handb. Zool., Bd. VIII, 10 (27), 1—24 (1956). — 159. PLOOG, D.: Physiologie und Pathologie des Schlafes. Fortschr. Neurol. Psychiat. 21, 16—56 (1953). — 160. PODKOPAEW, N. A.: Die Methodik der Erforschung der bedingten Reflexe. München: Bergmann 1926. — 161. POLYAK, ST. (Ed. H. KLÜVER): The vertebrate visual system. The University of Chicago Press 1957. — 162. POPOV, C.: Contribution à l'étude du mécanisme d'élaboration des connexions corticales dans le conditionnement électroencéphalographique sonlumière chez l'homme. Paris 1955. — 163. PORTMANN, A.: Zoologie und das neue Bild vom Menschen. Biologische Fragmente zu einer Lehre vom Menschen. Rowohlts deutsche Enzyklopädie Nr. 20. — 164. PRECHTL, H. F. R.: Neurophysiologische Mechanismen des formstarren Verhaltens. Behaviour 9, 243—319 (1956). — 165. PRECHTL, H. F. R.: Die Entwicklung und Eigenart frühkindlicher Bewegungsweisen. Klin. Wschr. 1956, 281—284. — 166. PRIBRAM, K. H., and L. KRUGER: Functions of the "olfactory brain". Ann. N. Y. Acad. Sci. 58, 109—138 (1954). — 166a. Primatologia. Handbuch der Primatenkunde. (Eds. H. HOFER, A. H. SCHULTZ, D. STARCK.) Band I ff. Basel-New York: S. Karger 1956.

167. REMANE, A.: Die Grundlagen des natürlichen Systems, der vergleichenden Anatomie und der Phylogenetik. Leipzig: Akademische Verlagsgesellschaft Geest & Portig K.-G. 1952. — 168. REMANE, A.: Das soziale Leben der Tiere. Hamburg: Rowohlts deutsche Enzyklopädie Bd. 97, 1960.— 169. RENSCH, B.: Das Problem der Residuen bei Lernvorgängen. Arbeitsgemein-

schaft für Forschung des Landes Nordrhein-Westfalen.H.29,7—41 (1955).—170.Rensch,B.: Die biologischen Beweismittel der Abstammungslehre, S. 57—85. In: G. Heberer: s. Nr. 70. — 171. Rensch, B.: Die stammesgeschichtliche Sonderstellung des Menschen. Arbeitsgemeinschaft für Forschung des Landes Nordrhein-Westfalen. H. 64, 7—47 (1956). — 172. Reymert, M. L. (Ed.): Feelings and emotions. (The Mooseheart Symposium). New York-Toronto-London: McGraw-Hill Comp., Inc. 1950. — 173. Roe, A., and G. G. Simpson (Eds.): Behavior and Evolution. Yale University Press 1958. — 174. Roeder, K. D.: Insect Physiology. New York: J. Wiley 1953. — 175. Rosvold, H. E.: Physiological Psychology. Ann. Rev. Psychol. 10, 415—454 (1959). — 176. Ruch, T. C.: Bibliographia primatologica. A classified bibliography of primates other than man. Part I. Springfield: Thomas 1941. — 177. Russell, E. S.: The behaviour of animals. London: Arnold & Co. 1938, 2nd ed.

178. Schaffner, B. (Ed.): Group processes. New York: The Josiah Macy Jr. Foundation, Columbia University 1954. — 179. Schelsky, H.: Soziologie der Sexualität. Hamburg: Rowohlts deutsche Enzyklopädie, Nr. 2 (1955). — 180. Schiller, P. H.: Innate motor action as a basis of learning. In: Instinctive behavior. New York: International Universities Press, Inc. 1959. — 181. Sheer, D. E. (Ed.): Electrical stimulation of the brain. Houston, Texas: University of Texas Press 1958. — 182. Singh, J. A. L., and R. M. Zingg: Wolf-children and feral men. IV. Contribution of the University of Denver. New York-London: Harper & Brothers 1942. Ref. Z. Tierpsychol. 7, 148—160 (1950). — 183. Skinner, B. F.: The behavior of organisms. New York: Appleton-Century-Crofts 1938. — 184. Skinner, B. F.: Science and human behavior. New York: MacMillan 1953. — 185. Slijper, E. J.: Das Verhalten der Wale (Cetacea). Hdb. Zool. (Ed. Kükenthal) 8, 10 (14), 1—32. Berlin: W. de Gruyter 1958. — 186. Solomon, H. C., St. Cobb and W. Penfield: The brain and human behavior. Ass. Res. nerv. Dis. Proc. Vol. 36 (1958). — 186a. Solomon, Ph. et al.: Sensory Deprivation. Cambridge, Mass.: Harvard University Press 1961. — 187. Spencer, H.: First Principles. London: Williams and Norgate 1862. — 188. Sperling, E., u. O. Creutzfeldt: Der Temporallappen. Fortschr. Neurol. Psychiat. 27, 296—344 (1959). — 189. Spitz, R. A.: Die Entstehung der ersten Objektbeziehungen. Stuttgart: Klett 1957. — 190. Stevens, S. S. (Ed.): Handbook of experimental psychology. New York: John Wiley & Sons, Inc. 1951. — 191. Stirnimann, F.: Psychologie des neugeborenen Kindes. Zürich: Rascher 1940. — 192. Symposia of the society for experimental biology, Nr. IV: Physiological mechanisms in animal behaviour. Cambridge: University Press 1950.

193. Teuber, H.-L.: Physiological psychology. Ann. Rev. Psychol. 6, 267—296 (1955). — 194.Teuber,H.-L.: Perception. Handb. of Physiology. Neurophysiol. III,Washington,D.C.1960. — 195. Thorpe, W. H.: Learning and instinct in animals. London: Methuen and Co. Ltd. 1956. — 196. Thorpe, W. H., and O. L. Zangwill (Eds.): Current problems in animal behavior. Cambridge: University Press 1961. — 197. Tinbergen, N.: Instinktlehre. Vergleichende Erforschung angeborenen Verhaltens. Berlin und Hamburg: Parey 1952. — 198. Tinbergen, N.: Tiere untereinander. Berlin und Hamburg: Parey 1955. — 199. Tolman, E. C.: Purposive behavior in animals and men. New York: Appleton-Century-Crofts 1932.

200. Uexküll, J. v.: Bedeutungslehre. Hamburg: Rowohlts deutsche Enzyklopädie. Nr. 13 (1956). — 201. Uexküll, J. v., u. G. Kriszat: Streifzüge durch die Umwelten von Tieren und Menschen. Hamburg: Rowohlts deutsche Enzyklopädie, Nr. 13 (1956). — 202. Ule, G.: Über das Ammonshorn. Fortschr. Neurol. Psychiat. 22, 510—530 (1954).

203. Warden, C. J., T. N. Jenkins and L. H. Warner: Comparative Psychology, 3 Vol. New York: Ronald Press Co. 1935, 1936, 1940. — 204. Waters, R. H. et al. (Eds.): Principles of comparative psychology. New York-Toronto-London: McGraw-Hill 1960. — 205. Whitman, C. O.: Animal behavior. Biol. Lect. Mar. Biol. Lab. Wood's Hole, S. 285—338.Boston: Ginn & Comp. 1899. — 206. Wiener, N.: Cybernetics, or control and communication in the animal and the machine. New York: John Wiley & Sons, Inc. 1948. — 207. Wieser, St.: Die motorischen Schablonen des Oralsinnes. Fortschr. Neurol. Psychiat. 23, 94—124 (1955). — 208. Wieser, St.: Pathologie des Greifens. Fortschr. Neurol. Psychiat. 25, 317—341 (1957). — 209. Wikler, A.: The relation of psychiatry to pharmacology. Baltimore, Md.: Williams & Wilkins Comp. 1957. — 210. Windle, W. F.: Genesis of somatic motor function in mammalian embryos: A synthesizing article. Physiol. Zool. 17, 247—260 (1944). — 211. Wolstenholme, G. E. W. et al. (Eds): Neurological basis of behaviour. (Ciba Found. Symposium) London: J. and A. Churchill 1958. — 212. Wolstenholme, G. E. W., and M. O'Connor (Eds.): The nature of sleep. (Ciba Found. Symposium). London: J. and A. Churchill 1961. — 213. Wyrsch, J.: Zur Geschichte und Deutung der endogenen Psychosen. Stuttgart: Thieme 1956. — 214. Wyrsch, J.: Die Person des Schizophrenen. Bern: P. Haupt 1949.

215. Young, P. T.: Motivation and emotion. A survey of the determinants of human and animal activity. New York-London: Wiley & Sons 1961.

216. Zuckerman, S.: The social life of monkeys and apes. London: Kegan Paul 1932.

Einzelarbeiten

217. ADAMS, R. D. et al.: Some observations on disturbances in learning and memory in man and their relationship to lesions in the rhinencephalon and diencephalon. In: Physiologie de l'hippocampe. Paris: CNRS 1962. — 218. ADEY, W. R.: The neuroanatomical basis of mental disorder. Aust. Ann. Med. **5**, 153—162 (1956). — 219. ADEY, W. R., N. C. R. MERRILLEES and S. SUNDERLAND: The entorhinal area; behavioural, evoked potential, and histological studies of its interrelationship with brain-stem regions. Brain **79**, 414—439 (1956). — 220. ADEY, W. R., S. SUNDERLAND and C. W. DUNLOP: The entorhinal area: electrophysiological studies of its interrelations with rhinencephalic structures and the brain-stem. Electroenceph. clin. Neurophysiol. **9**, 308—324 (1957). — 221. AHRENS, R.: Beitrag zur Entwicklung des Physiognomie- und Mimikerkennens. Z. exp. angew. Psychol. **2**, 412—454; 599—633 (1954). — 222. AKERT, K. et al.: Klüver-Bucy syndrome in monkeys with neocortical ablations of temporal lobe. Brain **84**, 480—498 (1961). — 223. AKERT, K. et al.: Learned behavior of rhesus monkeys following neonatal bilateral prefrontal lobotomy. Science **132**, 1944—1945 (1960).— 224. AKIMOTO, H., u. O. CREUTZFELDT: Reaktionen von Neuronen des optischen Cortex nach elektrischer Reizung unspezifischer Thalamuskerne. Arch. Psychiat. Nervenkr. **196**, 494—519 (1958). — 225. ALFORD, L. B.: Localization of consciousness and emotion. Amer. J. Psychiat. **12**, 789—799 (1933). — 226. ALTMANN, S. A.: Field observations on a Howling Monkey society. J. Mammalogy **40**, 317—330 (1959). — 227. ANASTASOPOULOS, G.: Hypersexualität, Wesensänderung, Schlafstörungen und akute Demenz bei einem Tumor des rechten Schläfenlappens. Psychiat. et Neurol. (Basel) **136**, 85—108 (1958). — 228. ANDERSON, E. et al.: The influence of the central nervous system on metabolic and endocrine activity as based on transection of the brain-stem in dogs. Acta neuroveg. (Wien) **12**, 53—94 (1955). — 229. ANDERSON, E., et al.: The effects of midbrain and spinal cord transection on endocrine and metabolic functions with postulation of a mid-brain hypothalamic-pituitary activating system. Recent Progr. Hormone Res. **13**, 21—66 (1957). — 230. ANTONITIS, J., and A. J. SHER: Social regression in the white rat. J. Psychol. **33**, 99—111 (1952). — 231. ANTONITIS, J., and G. B. KISH: Reactions of C57 black male mice to active and inactive social stimuli. J. genet. Psychol. **86**, 115—130 (1955). — 232. ANTONIUS, O.: Über die Schlangenfurcht der Affen. Z. Tierpsychol. **2**, 293—296 (1938). — 233. ARIETI, S.: The "placing-into-mouth" and coprophagic habits. J. nerv. ment. Dis. **99**, 959—964 (1944). — 234. ARIETI, S.: Primitive habits and perceptual alterations in the terminal stage of schizophrenia. A. M. A. Arch. Neurol. Psychiat. **53**, 378—384 (1945). — 234a. ASCHOFF, J.: Aktivitätsmuster der Tagesperiodik. Naturwissenschaften **44**, 361—367 (1957). — 234b. ASCHOFF, J., u. R. WEVER: Beginn und Ende der täglichen Aktivität freilebender Vögel. J. Ornithol. **103**, 1—27 (1962). — 234c. ASCHOFF, J., u. R. WEVER: Spontanperiodik des Menschen bei Ausschluß aller Zeitgeber. Naturwissenschaften **49**, 337—342 (1962).

235. BABKIN, B. P.: The conditioning of emotions. In: Feelings and emotions, s. Nr. 172.— 236. BAERENDS, G. P.: The contribution of ethology to the study of the causation of behaviour. Acta physiol. pharmacol. neerl. **7**, 466—499 (1958). — 237. BAERENDS, G. P.: Comparative methods and the concept of homology in the study of behaviour. Arch. neerl. Zool. **13**, Supp. 1, 401—417 (1958). — 238. BAERENDS, G. P., R. BOUWER and H. TJ. WATERBOLK: Ethological studies on Lebister reticulatus (Peters). Behaviour 8, 249—334 (1955). — 239. BAGSHAW, M. H., and K. H. PRIBRAM: Cortical organization in gustation (macaca mulatta). J. Neurophysiol. **16**, 499—508 (1953). — 240. BARD, P.: A diencephalic mechanism for the expression of rage with special reference to the sympathetic nervous system. Amer. J. Physiol. **84**, 490 to 515 (1928). — 241. BARD, P., and V. B. MOUNTCASTLE: Some forebrain mechanisms involved in expression of rage with special reference to suppression of angry behavior. Ass. Res. nerv. Dis. Proc. **27**, 362—404 (1947). — 242. BARON, A., C. N. STEWART and J. M. WARREN: Patterns of social interaction in cats (Felis domestica). Behaviour 11, 56—66 (1957). — 243. BASH, K. W.: Descensus ad inferos. Psyche 9, 505—525 (1957). — 244. BASTOCK, M., and A. MANNING: The courtship of Drosophila melanogaster. Behaviour 8, 85—111 (1955). — 245. BEACH, F. A.: Instinctive behavior: Reproductive activities. In: Stevens Handbook of experimental psychology, s. Nr. 190. — 246. BEACH, F. A.: The descent of instinct. Psychol. Rev. **62**, 401—410 (1955). — 247. BEACH, F. A.: Normal sexual behavior in male rats isolated at fourteen days of age. J. comp. physiol. Psychol. **51**, 37—38 (1958). — 248. BEACH, F. A., and LISBETH JORDAN: Sexual exhaustion and recovery in the male rat. Quart. J. exp. Psychol. 8, 121—133 (1956). — 249. BEACH, F. A., A. ZITRIN and J. JAYNES: Neural mediation of mating in male cats: I. Effects of unilateral and bilateral removal of the neocortex. J. comp. physiol. Psychol. **49**, 321—327 (1956). — 250. BEACH, H. D.: Morphine addiction in rats. Canad. J. Psychol. **11**, 104—112 (1957). — 251. BECKER, A. M.: Möglichkeiten und Grenzen des Vergleichens von menschlichem und tierischem Verhalten. Psyche 11, 170—198 (1958). — 252. BENTE, D., u. E. KLUGE: Sexuelle Reizzustände im Rahmen des Uncinatus-Syndroms. Arch. Psychiat. Nervenkr. **190**, 357—376 (1953). — 253. BENTE, D., u. ST. WIESER: Motorische Schablonen bei stufenweiser cerebraler Restitution.

Psychiat. et Neurol. (Basel) 1, 13—18 (1953). — 254. BERKUN, M. M., M. L. KESSEN, and N. E. MILLER: Hunger reducing effects of food by stomach fistula versus food by mouth measured by a consummatory response. J. comp. physiol. Psychol. 45, 550—554 (1952). — 255. BETTELHEIM, B.: Feral children and autistic children. Amer. J. Sociol. 64, 455—467 (1959). — 256. BICKFORD, R. G.: Electrical rhythms recorded from the depth of the frontal lobes during operations on psychotic patients. Proc. Mayo Clin. 28, 135—143 (1953). — 257. BICKFORD, R. G.: A multielectrode lead for intracerebral recordings. Electroenceph. clin. Neurophysiol. 11, 165—169 (1959). — 258. BIERENS DE HAAN, J. A.: Über den Begriff des Instinktes in der Tierpsychologie. Folia biotheoret. 2, 1—16 (1937). — 259. BILZ, R.: Zur Biologie und Psychologie der Mutterrolle. Zbl. Psychother. 14, 277—298 (1942). — 260. BILZ, R.: Die Stimmung als leib-seelisches Phänomen. Dargestellt am Beispiel der Magenneurose. Dtsch. med. Wschr. 1942, 640. — 261. BILZ, R.: Zur Grundlegung einer Paläopsychologie. I. Paläophysiologie. Schweiz. Z. Psychol. 3, 202—212 (1944). — 262. BILZ, R.: Zur Grundlegung einer Paläopsychologie. II. Paläopsychologie. Schweiz. Z. Psychol. 3, 272—280 (1944). — 263. BILZ, R.: Tiertöter-Skrupulantismus. Jb. Psychol. Psychother. 3, 226—244 (1955). — 264. BILZ, R.: Die Intention zur motorischen Verkürzung und zur Elevation der Extremitäten im Angsterleben. Nervenarzt 27, 104—108 (1956). — 265. BILZ, R.: Pole der Geborgenheit. Eine anthropologische Untersuchung über raumbezogene Erlebnis- und Verhaltensbereitschaften. Studium Generale 10, 552—563 (1957). — 266. BILZ, R.: Die Tat und das Motiv-Objekt. Jb. Psychol. Psychother. 1958, 208—224. — 267. BILZ, R.: Faszination und Scheu. Eine Untersuchung über elementare Zuordnungen im Erleben und Verhalten des Menschen. Homo 9, 91—100 (1958). — 268. BILZ, R.: Biologische Radikale. Eine Untersuchung über homologisch-emotional begründete Erlebens- und Verhaltensweisen des Menschen. Die Heilkunst, H. 5 (1961). — 269. BIRCH, H. G.: The pertinence of animal investigation for a science of human behavior. Am. J. Orthopsychiat. 31, 267—275 (1961). — 270. BIRKMAYER, W., E. FRÜHMANN u. H. STROTZKA: Motorische Schablonen im Erwachen nach dem Elektroschock. Arch. Psychiat. Nervenkr. 193, 513—525 (1955). — 271. BRADY, J. V.: The effect of electro-convulsive shock on a conditioned emotional response: The permanence of the effect. J. comp. physiol. Psychol. 44, 507—511 (1951). — 272. BRADY, J. V.: The effect of electro-convulsive shock on a conditioned emotional response: The significance of the interval between the emotional conditioning and the electro-convulsive shock. J. comp. physiol. Psychol. 45, 9—13 (1952). — 273. BRADY, J. V.: Experimental analysis of emotional behavior. Proc. 14. International Congress of Psychology, Montreal, June 1954. — 274. BRADY, J. V.: Exstinction of a conditioned "fear" response as a function of reinforcement schedules for competing behavior. J. Psychol. 40, 25—34 (1955). — 275. BRADY, J. V.: Motivational-emotional factors and intracranial self-stimulation. Amer. J. Psychol. 10, 396 (1955). — 276. BRADY, J. V.: Assessment of drug effects on emotional behavior. Science 123, 1033 to 1034 (1956). — 277. BRADY, J. V.: Emotional behavior and the nervous system. Trans. N. Y. Acad. Sci. 18, 601—612 (1956). — 278. BRADY, J. V.: Comparative Psychopharmocology: Animal experimental studies on the effects of drugs on behavior. In: J. COLE and R. GERARD (Eds.): Psychopharmacology: Problems in evaluation. Publication 583, National Academy of Sciences-National Research Council, Washington, D. C. 1959. — 279. BRADY, J. V.: A comparative approach to the evaluation of drug effects upon affective behavior. Ann. N. Y. Acad. Sci. 64, 632—643 (1956). — 280. BRADY, J. V.: A comparative approach to the experimental analysis of emotional behavior. In: HOCH and ZUBIN (Eds.): Experimental Psychopathology, s. Nr. 82. — 281. BRADY, J. V.: Temporal and emotional effects related to intracranial electrical self-stimulation. In: E. R. RAMEY and D. S. O'DOHERTY (Eds.): Electrical Studies on the Unanesthesized Brain. New York: P. E. Hoeber 1960. — 282. BRADY, J. V.: Temporal and emotional factors related to electrical self-stimulation of the lin bic-system. In: H. JASPER, L. PROCTOR et al. (Eds.): Reticular formation of the brain, s. Nr. 92. — 283. BRADY, J. V., et al.: The effect of food and water deprivation upon intracranial self-stimulation. J. comp. physiol. Psychol. 50, 134—137 (1957). — 284. BRADY, J. V., and H. F. HUNT: The effect of electro-convulsive shock on a conditioned emotional response: A control for impaired hearing. J. comp. physiol. Psychol. 45, 180—182 (1952). — 285. BRADY, J. V., and H. F. HUNT: An experimental approach to the analysis of emotional behavior. J. Psychol. 40, 313—324 (1955). — 286. BRADY, J. V., H. F. HUNT, and I. GELLER: The effect of electro-convulsive shock on a conditioned emotional response as a function of the temporal distribution of the treatments. J. comp. physiol. Psychol. 47, 454—457 (1954). — 287. BRADY, J. V., and W. J. H. NAUTA: Subcortical mechanisms in emotional behavior: affective changes following septal forebrain lesions in the albino rat. J. comp. physiol. Psychol. 46, 339—346 (1953). — 288. BRADY, J. V., and W. J. H. NAUTA: Subcortical mechanisms in emotional behavior: The duration of affective changes following septal and habenular lesions in the albino rat. J. comp. physiol. Psychol. 48, 412—420 (1955).— 289. BRADY, J. V. et al.: Avoidance behavior and the development of gastroduodenal ulcers. J. exp. anal. Behav. 1, 69—72 (1958). — 290. BRADY, J. V. et al.: Subcortical mechanisms in emotional behavior: The effect of rhinencephalic injury upon the acquisition and retention of a conditioned avoidance response in cats. J. comp. physiol. Psychol. **47**, 179—186 (1954). — 291. BRADY, J. V. at al.: The effect of audiogenic convulsions on a conditioned emotional response. J. comp. physiol. Psychol. **46**, 363—367 (1953). — 292. BRADY, J. V. et al.: The effect of electroconvulsive shock (ECS) on a conditioned emotional response: the effect of additional ECS convulsions. J. comp. physiol. Psychol. **46**, 368—372 (1953). — 293. BREATH-NACH, A. S.: The cetacean central nervous system. Biol. Rev. **35**, 187—230 (1960).— 294. BRIL-MAYER, H., u. F. MARGUTH: Störungen im Zwischenhirn-Hypophysensystem. Dtsch. Z. Nervenheilk. **176**, 441—448 (1957). — 295. BROCA, P.: Le grand-lobe limbique et la scissure limbique dans la série des mammifères. Rev. d'anthropol. Jg. 7, Bd. 1, 385—498 (1878). — 296. BROCA, P.: Recherches sur les centres olfactifs. Rev. d'anthropol. Jg. 8, Bd. 2. 385—455 (1879). — 297. BRODY, E. B., and H. E. ROSVOLD: Influence of prefrontal lobotomy on social interaction in a monkey group. Psychosom. Med. **14**, 406—415 (1952). — 298. BRUTKOWSKI, S.: Comparison of classical and instrumental alimentary conditioned reflexes following bilateral prefrontal lobectomies in dogs. Acta Biol. exp. (Warszawa) **19**, 291—299 (1959).— 299. BRUT-KOWSKI, S. et al.: Aphagia and adipsia in a dog with bilateral complete lesion of the amygdaloid complex. Acta Biol. exp. (Warszawa) **22**, 43—50 (1962). — 300. BUCY, C., and H. KLÜVER: Anatomic changes secondary to temporal lobectomy. A. M. A. Arch. Neurol. Psychiat. **44**, 1142—1146 (1940). — 301. BUCY, C., and H. KLÜVER: An anatomical investigation of the temporal lobe in the monkey (macaca mulatta). J. comp. Neurol. **103**, 151—252 (1955). — 302. BÜRGI, S., u. VERENA M. BUCHER: Über einige rhinencephale Verbindungen des Zwischen- und Mittelhirns. Dtsch. Z. Nervenheilk. **174**, 89—106 (1955). — 303. BUREŠ et al.: Experimental study of the role of hippocampus in conditioning and memory functions. In: Physiologie de l'hippocampe. Paris: CNRS 1961.

304. CALHOUN, J. B.: The social aspects of population dynamics. J. Mammal. **33**, 139 to 159 (1952). — 305. CALHOUN, J. B.: A comparative study of the social behavior of two inbred strains of house mice. Ecol. Monogr. **26**, 81—103 (1956). — 306. CALHOUN, J. B.: Behavior of house mice with reference to fixed points of orientation. Ecology **37**, 287—301 (1956). — 307. CALHOUN, J. B.: Social welfare as a variable in population dynamics. Cold Spr. Harb. Symp. quant. Biol. Vol. **22**, 339—356 (1957). — 308. CALHOUN, J. B., and J. U. CASBY: Calculation of home range and density of small mammals. Publ. Health Monogr. **55**, 1—24 (1958). — 309. CARPENTER, C. R.: Sexual behavior of free ranging Rhesus monkeys. J. comp. Psychol. **33**, 113—162 (1942). — 310. CHOW, KAO LIANG, and K. H. PRIBRAM: Cortical projection of the thalamic ventrolateral nuclear group in monkeys. J. comp. Neurol. **104**, 57—75 (1956). — 311. CORRELL, R. E., and W. R. INGRAM: Variations in after-discharge from the hippocampus. Proc. Soc. exp. Biol. (N. Y.) **93**, 240—245 (1956). — 312. CREUTZ-FELDT, O.: Die Krampfausbreitung im Temporallappen der Katze. Die Krampfentladungen des Ammonshorns und ihre Beziehungen zum übrigen Rhinencephalon und Isocortex. Schweiz. Arch. Neurol. Psychiat. **77**, 163—194 (1956). — 313. CREUTZFELDT, O., u. H. AKIMOTO: Konvergenz und gegenseitige Beeinflussung von Impulsen aus der Retina und den unspezifischen Thalamuskernen an einzelnen Neuronen des optischen Cortex. Arch. Psychiat. Nervenkr. **196**, 520—538 (1958).

314. DANDY, W. E.: Seat of consciousness. In: D. LEWIS: Pract. surg. Bd. 12, 57. Hagertown, Md.: W. F. Prior Comp., Inc. 1931. — 315. DAVIS, D. E.: Aggressive behavior in castrated starlings. Science **126**, 253 (1957). — 316. DAVIS, D. E., and J. J. CHRISTIAN: Changes in Norway rat populations induced by introduction of rats. J. Wildl. Manag. **20**, 378—383 (1956). — 317. DAVIS, D. R.: Recovery from depression. Brit. J. med. Psychol. **25**, 104—113 (1952). — 318. DAVIS, H.: Space and time in the central nervous system. Electroenceph. Neurophysiol. **8**, 185—191 (1956). — 319. DELGADO, J. M. R., and B. K. ANAND: Increase of food intake induced by electrical stimulation of the lateral hypothalamus. Amer. J. Physiol. **172**, 162—168 (1953). — 320. DELGADO, J. M. R., W. W. ROBERTS and N. E. MILLER: Learning motivated by electrical stimulation of the brain. Amer. J. Physiol. **179**, 587—593 (1954). — 321. DENNIS, W.: The significance of feral man. Amer. J. Psychol. **54**, 425—432 (1941). — 322. DITFURTH, H. v.: Die affektiv-vegetative Kommunikation. (Versuch einer psychosomatischen Theorie der vitalen Stimmung.) Nervenarzt **2**, 70—80 (1957). — 323. DOLLARD, J., and N. E. MILLER: Personality and Psychotherapy. An analysis in terms of learning, thinking and culture. Psychol. Rev. **1**, 47—49 (1951). — 324. DOTY, R. W. et al.: Conditioned reflexes established to electrical stimulation of cat cerebral cortex. J. Neurophysiol. **19**, 401—415 (1956). — 325. DUENSING, F.: Schreckreflex und Schreckreaktion als hirnorganische Zeichen. Arch. Psychiat. Nervenkr. **188**, 162—192 (1952). — 326. DUNCAN, C. P.: Habit reversal induced by electroshock in the rat. J. comp. physiol. Psychol. **41**, 11—16 (1948).

327. EBERSOLE, J. H. (Lt. Cdr.): Long submergence on nuclear submarines. Vortrag auf der 115. Jahresversammlung der American Psychiatric Association, Philadelphia 1959. — 328. EIBL-EIBESFELDT, I.: Zur Ethologie des Hamsters (Cricetus cricetus L.) Z. Tierpsychol.

10, 204—254 (1953). — 329. Eibl-Eibesfeldt, I.: Angeborenes und Erworbenes im Nestbauverhalten der Wanderratte. Naturwissenschaften **42**, 633—634 (1955). — 330. Eibl-Eibesfeldt, I.: Über die ontogenetische Entwicklung der Technik des Nüsseöffnens vom Eichhörnchen (Sciurus vulgaris L.). Z. Säugetierk. **21**, 132—134 (1956). — 331. Eibl-Eibesfeldt, I.: Angeborenes und Erworbenes in der Technik des Beutetötens (Versuche am Iltis, Putorius putorius L.) Z. Säugetierk. **21**, 135—137 (1956). — 332. Eibl-Eibesfeldt, I.: Einige Bemerkungen über den Ursprung von Ausdrucksbewegungen bei Säugetieren. Z. Säugetierk. **21**, 29—43 (1956). — 333. Eibl-Eibesfeldt, I.: Darwin und die Ethologie. In: s. Nr. 71. — 334. Eibl-Eibesfeldt, I.: The fighting behavior of animals. Sci. Amer. **205**, No. 12, 112—121 (1961). — 335. Eibl-Eibesfeldt, I.: The interactions of unlearned behavior patterns and learning in mammals. In: s. Nr. 48. — 336. Eisentraut, M.: Vergleichende Beobachtungen über das Sichbespucken bei Igeln. Z. Tierpsychol. **10**, 50—55 (1953). — 337. Estes, W. K., and B. F. Skinner: Some quantitative properties of anxiety. J. exp. Psychol. **29**, 390—400 (1941). — 338. Ettlinger, G.: Visual discrimination following successive unilateral temporal excisions in monkeys. J. Physiol. **140**, 38—39 (1957).— 339. Euler, C. v. et al.: The role of hippocampal dendrites in evoked responses and after-discharges. Acta physiol. scand. **42**, 87—111 (1958). — 340. Evarts, E. V.: Neurophysiological correlates of pharmacologically induced behavioral disturbances. In: The Brain and human behavior, Ass. Res. nerv. Dis. Proc. **36**, Kap. 14 (1958).

341. Fabricius, E.: Zur Ethologie junger Anatiden. Acta Zool. Fenn. **51**, 1—178 (1950). — 342. Fabricius, E.: Some experiments on imprinting phenomena in ducks. Proc. Xth Intern. Ornithol. Congress, Uppsala Juni 1950, Uppsala-Stockholm: Almquist & Wiksells Boktrickery AB 1951. — 343. Fabricius, E., and H. Boyce: Experiments of the following-reaction of ducklings. Wildf. Trust Ann. Rep. **6**, 84—89 (1954). — 344. Fernandez de Molina, A., and R. W. Hunsperger: Organization of the subcortical system governing defence and flight reactions in the cat. J. Physiol. **160**, 200—213 (1962).— 345. Fonberg, E. et al.: Defensive conditioned reflexes and neurotic motor reactions following amygdalectomy in dogs. Acta Biol. exp. (Warszawa) **22**, 51—57 (1962). — 346. Frisch, J. E.: Research on primate behavior in Japan. Amer. Anthropol. **61**, 584—596 (1959). — 347. Frisch, K. v., u. M. Lindauer: Himmel und Erde in Konkurrenz bei der Orientierung der Bienen. Naturwissenschaften **41**, 245—253 (1954). — 348. Fuller, J. R. et al.: The effect on affective and cognitive behavior in the dog of lesions of the pyriformamygdala-hippocampal complex. J. comp. physiol. Psychol. **50**, 89—96 (1957). — 349. Fulton, J. F.: The limbic system: a study of the visceral brain in primates and man. Yale J. Biol. Med. **26**, 107—118 (1953).

350. Gaffrey, G.: Scheinträchtigkeit bei einer Afghanen-Hündin. Zool. Garten (NF) **19**, 261—262 (1952). — 351. Gaffrey, G.: Ortsgebundene Scheinjagd bei einer afghanischen Windhündin. Z. Tierpsychol. **11**, 144—146 (1954). — 352. Gaffrey, G.: Zur Fortpflanzungsbiologie bei Hunden. Zool. Garten (NF) **23**, 251—252 (1957). — 353. Gastaut, H. et al.: Etude topographique des réactions électroencéphalographiques conditionées chez l'homme. Electroenceph. clin. Neurophysiol. **9**, 1—34 (1957). — 354. Gauthier-Pilters, Hilde: Quelques observations sur l'écologie et l'éthologie du dromadaire dans le Sahara nordoccidental. Mammalia **22**, 140—151 (1958). — 355. Geller, I., and J. V. Brady: The effect of electroconvulsive shock on a conditioned emotional response as a function of a number of ECS treatments. Res. Rep. **93**, 1—6 (1956). Washington, D. C.: Walter Reed Army Institute of Research. — 356. Geller, I. et al.: The effect of electroconvulsive shock on a conditioned emotional response: a control for acquisition recency. J. comp. physiol. Psychol. **48**, 130—131 (1955). — 357. Gesell, A.: Emotion from the standpoint of a developmental morphology. In: Feelings and emotions (Ed. M. L. Reymert) s. Nr. 172. — 358. Ghent, L.: Perception of overlapping and embedded figures by children of different ages. Amer. J. Psychol. **69**, 575—587 (1956). — 359. Goethe, F.: Über das „Anstoß-Nehmen" bei Vögeln. Z. Tierpsychol. **3**, 371—374 (1940). — 360. Goethe, F.: Experimentelle Brutbeendigung und andere brutethologische Betrachtungen bei Silbermöven. J. Ornithol. **94**, 160—174 (1953). — 361. Goethe, F.: Über soziale Hierarchie im Aufzuchtschwarm der Silbermöwen. Z. Tierpsychol. **10**, 44—50 (1953). — 362. Goethe, F.: Vergleichende Beobachtungen zum Verhalten der Silbermöwen (Larus argentus) und der Heringsmöwe (Larus fiscus). Acta XI. Congr. Int. Ornithol. 1954, 577—582. — 363. Goldstein, K. et al.: Moro reflex and startle pattern. A. M. A. Arch. Neurol. Psychiat. **40**, 322—327 (1938). — 364. Goltz, F.: Über die Verrichtungen des Großhirns. Pflügers Arch. ges. Physiol. **13**, 1—44 (1876). — 365. Goltz, F.: Der Hund ohne Großhirn. Pflügers Arch. ges. Physiol. **51**, 570—614 (1892). — 366. Gött, H.: Über das Einschlafverhalten des Kindes. Homo **5**, 60—63 (1954). — 367. Gottschaldt, K.: Handlung und Ausdruck in der Psychologie der Persönlichkeit. Riv. psicol. **4**, 161—175 (1956). — 368. Grabowski, U.: Prägung eines Jungschafes auf den Menschen. Z. Tierpsychol. **4**, 326—329 (1940/41). — 369. Grastyán, E., and G. Karmos: The influence of hippocampal lesions on simple and delayed instrumental conditioned reflexes. In: Physiologie de l'hippocampe. Paris: CNRS 1961.—370. Green, J. D., and W. R. Adey: Electrophysiological studies of

432   DETLEV PLOOG: Verhaltensforschung und Psychiatrie

hippocampal connections and excitability. Electroenceph. clin. Neurophysiol. 8, 245—262. (1956). — 371. GREEN, J. D., and A. A. ARDUINI: Hippocampel electrical activity in arousal. J. Neurophysiol. 17, 533—557 (1954). — 372. GREEN, J. D. et al.: Experimentally induced epilepsy in the cat with injury of cornu ammonis. A. M. A. Arch. Neurol. Psychiat. 78, 259 to 263 (1957). — 373. GREEN, J. D. et al.: Rhinencephalic lesions and behavior in cats. J. comp. Neurol. 108, 505—545 (1957). — 374. GREEN, J. D., et R. NAQUET: Etude de la propagation locale et à distance des démarches épileptiques. Intern. Congr. Sci. neurol. 1957, Brüssel. — 375. GRÜNTHAL, E.: Über das klinische Bild nach umschriebenem, beiderseitigem Ausfall der Ammonshornrinde. Mschr. Psychiat. Neurol. 113, 1 (1947). — 376. GRÜSSER, O.-J., u. O. CREUTZFELDT: Eine neurophysiologische Grundlage des Brücke-Bartley-Effektes: Maxima der Impulsfrequenz retinaler und corticaler Neurone bei Flimmerlicht mittlerer Frequenzen. Pflügers Arch. ges. Physiol. 263, 668—681 (1957). — 377. GRÜSSER, O.-J., u. A. GRUTZNER: Neurophysiologische Grundlagen der periodischen Nachbildphasen nach kurzen Lichtblitzen. Albrecht v. Graefes Arch. Ophthal. 160, 65—93 (1958). — 378. GRZIMEK, B.: Beobachtungen an einem kleinen Schimpansenmädchen. Z. Tierpsychol. 4, 295—306 (1940/41). — 379. GRZIMEK, B.: Totung von Menschen durch befreundete Hunde. Z. Tierpsychol. 11, 147—149 (1954).

380. HALL, C. S.: Emotional behavior in the rat. I. Defecation and urination as measures of individual differences in emotionality. J. comp. Psychol. 18, 385—403 (1934). — 381. HARLOW, H. F.: The development of learning in the Rhesus Monkey. Amer. Scientist 47, 459 bis 479 (1959). — 382. HARLOW, H. F.: Primary affectional patterns in primates. Amer. J. Orthopsychiat. 30, 676—684 (1960). — 382a. HARLOW, H. F., and MARGARET HARLOW: Social deprivation in monkeys. Sci. Amer. 207, Nr. 5, 136—146 (1962). — 383. HARLOW, H. F., and R. R. ZIMMERMANN: Affectional responses in the infant monkey. Science 130, 421—432 (1959).— 384. HARRIS, G. W., R. P. MICHAEL and PATRICIA P. SCOTT: Neurological site of action of stilboestrol in eliciting sexual behavior. In: Neurological Basis of Behaviour, s. Nr. 211. — 385. HARRISON, J. M., and M. LYON: The role of the septal nuclei and components of the fornix in the behavior of the rat. J. comp. Neurol. 108, 121—128 (1957). — 386. HASSLER, R.: Über die Rinden- und Stammhirnanteile des menschlichen Thalamus. Psychiat. Neurol. med. Psychol. 1, 181—187 (1949). — 387. HASSLER, R.: Die Anatomie des Thalamus. Arch. Psychiat. Nervenkr. 184, 249 (1950). — 388. HASSLER, R.: Weckeffekte und delirante Zustande durch elektrische Reizungen bzw. Ausschaltungen im menschlichen Zwischenhirn. Ier Congrès international de neurochirurgie, Acta Med. Belg. Bruxelles 1957, 179—181. — 389. HASSLER, R., u. W. R. HESS: Experimentelle und anatomische Befunde über die Drehbewegungen und ihre nervösen Apparate. Arch. Psychiat. Nervenkr. 192, 488—526 (1954). — 390. HASSLER, R., u. T. RIECHERT: Wirkungen der Reizungen und Koagulationen in den Stammganglien bei stereotaktischen Hirnoperationen. Nervenarzt 32, 97—109 (1961). — 391. HEATH, R. G., R. R. MONROE and W. A. MICKLE: Stimulation of the amygdaloid nucleus in a schizophrenic patient. Amer. J. Psychiat. 111, 862—863 (1955). — 392. HEBB, D. O., et H. MAHUT: Motivation et recherche du changement perceptif chez le rat et chez l'homme. J. Psychol. norm. path. 52, 209—221 (1955). — 393. HEDIGER, H.: Säugetierterritorien und ihre Markierung. Bijdragen tot dierkde 28, 172—184 (1949). — 394. HEIMANN, H.: Ausdrucksphänomenologie der Modellpsychosen (Psilocybin). Psychiat. et Neurol. (Basel) 141, 69—100 (1961). — 395. HEIMANN, H., u. TH. SPOERRI: Zur Ausdrucksphänomenologie. Psychiat. et Neurol. (Basel) 134, 203—214 (1957). — 396. HEIMANN, H., u. TH. SPOERRI: Das Ausdruckssyndrom der mimischen Desintegrierung bei chronischen Schizophrenen. Schweiz. med. Wschr. 1957, 1126. — 397. HEINROTH, O.: Beiträge zur Biologie, insbesondere Psychologie und Ethologie der Anatiden. Verh. V. internat. Ornithol. Kongreß 1910. — 398. HENRY, CH., and W. B. SCOVILLE: Suppression-burst activity from isolated cerebral cortex in man. Electroenceph. clin. Neurophysiol. 4, 1—22 (1952). — 399. HERNÁNDEZ-PEÓN, R., H. SCHERRER and M. JOUVET: Modification of electric activity in cochlear nucleus during "attention" in unanesthetized cats. Science 123, 331—332 (1956). — 400. HERRICK, C. J.: The functions of the olfactory parts of the cerebral cortex. Proc. nat. Acad. Sci. (Wash.) 19, 7 (1933). — 401. HESS, E. H.: Imprinting: An effect of early experience, imprinting determines later social behavior in animals. Science 130, 133—141 (1959). — 402. HESS, W. R.: Über die Wechselbeziehungen zwischen psychischen und vegetativen Funktionen. Schweiz. Arch. Neurol. Psychiat. 15, 260—277 (1924); 16, 36—55; 285—306 (1925). — 403. HESS, W. R.: Das Schlafsyndrom als Folge diencephaler Reizung. Helv. physiol. pharmacol. Acta 2, 305—344 (1944). — 404. HESS, W. R.: Prinzipien organischer Ordnung am Beispiel des vegetativen Nervensystems. Klin. Wschr. 1951, 105—111. — 405. HESS, W. R.: Vom Lichtreiz zur bildhaften Wahrnehmung. Helv. physiol. pharmacol. Acta 10, 395—402 (1952). — 406. HESS, W. R.: Beziehungen zwischen psychischen Vorgängen und Organisation des Gehirns. I. und II. Teil. Studium Generale 9, 467—479 (1956); 10, 327—339 (1957). — 407. HESS, W. R.: Die Formatio reticularis des Hirnstammes im verhaltenspsychologischen Aspekt. Arch. Psychiat. Nervenkr. 196, 329—336 (1957). — 408. HESS, W. R., u. M. BRÜGGER:

Das subcorticale Zentrum der affectiven Abwehrreaktion. Helv. physiol. pharmakol. Acta 1, 33—52 (1943). — 409. HESS, W. R., u. A. E. MEYER: Triebhafte Fellreinigung der Katze als Symptom diencephaler Reizung. Helv. physiol. pharmacol. Acta 14, 397—410 (1956). — 410. HESS, R. JUN., K. AKERT et W. KOELLA: Les potentiels bioélectriques du cortex et du thalamus et leur altération par stimulation du centre hypnique chez le chat. Rev. neurol. 83, 537—544 (1950). — 411. HINDE, R. A.: Ethological models and the concept of "drive". Brit. J. philos. Sci. 6, 321—331 (1956). — 412. HIRSCHMANN, J.: Instinktmechanismen im menschlichen Nahrungsverhalten. Studium Generale 7, 285 (1954). — 413. HOLST, E. v.: Versuche zur Theorie der relativen Koordination. Pflügers Arch. ges. Physiol. 237, 93—121, 356—378 (1936). — 414. HOLST, E. v.: Über relative Koordination bei Säugern und Menschen. Pflügers Arch. ges. Physiol. 240, 44—59 (1938). — 415. HOLST, E. v.: Zentralnervensystem und Peripherie in ihrem gegenseitigen Verhältnis. Klin. Wschr. 29, 97—105 (1951). — 416. HOLST, E. v.: Die Auslösung von Stimmungen bei Wirbeltieren durch „punktförmige" elektrische Erregung des Stammhirns. Naturwissenschaften 44, 549—551 (1957). — 417. HOLST, E. v., u. URSULA V. SAINT PAUL: Vom Wirkungsgefüge der Triebe. Naturwissenschaften 47, 409—422 (1960). — 418. HOLST, E. v., u. H. MITTELSTAEDT: Das Reafferenzprinzip. Naturwissenschaften 37, 464—476 (1950). — 419. HOLZAPFEL, MONIKA: Die Entstehung einiger Bewegungsstereotypien bei gehaltenen Säugern und Vögeln. Rev. Suisse Zool. 46, 18 (1939). — 420. HOLZAPFEL, MONIKA: Triebbedingte Ruhezustände als Ziel von Appetenzverhalten. Naturwissenschaften 28, 273 (1940). — 421. HOOGLAND, R., D. MORRIS and N. TINBERGEN: The spines of sticklebacks (Gasterosteus and Pygosteus) as means of defence against predators (Perca and Esox). Behaviour 10, 205—236 (1957). — 422. HÖRMANN, S. v.: Über den Erbgang von Verhaltensmerkmalen bei Grillenbastarden. Naturwissenschaften 42, 470—471 (1955). — 423. HUNSPERGER, R. W.: Affektreaktionen auf elektrische Reizung im Hirnstamm der Katze. Helv. physiol. pharmacol. Acta 14, 70—92 (1956). — 424. HUNT, H. F., and J. V. BRADY: Some effects of electro-convulsive shock on a conditioned emotional response ("Anxiety"). J. comp. physiol. Psychol. 44, 88—98 (1951). — 425. HUNT, H. F., and J. V. BRADY: Some effects of punishment and intercurrent "Anxiety" on a simple operant. J. comp. physiol. Psychol. 48, 305—310 (1955). — 426. HUNT, H. F., P. JERNBERG and J. V. BRADY: The effect of electroconvulsive shock (ECS) on a conditioned emotional response: The effect of post-ECS extinction on the reappearance of the response. J. comp. physiol. Psychol. 45, 589—599 (1952). — 427. HUNT, H. F., P. JERNBERG and W. G. LAWLOR: The effect of electro-convulsive shock on a conditioned emotional response: The effect of electro-convulsive shock under ether anesthesia. J. comp. physiol. Psychol. 46, 64—68 (1953). — 428. HUNT, W. A., and C. LANDIS: The overt behavior pattern in startle. J. exp. Psychol. 19, 309—315 (1936).

429. IERSEL, J. J A. VAN and A. C. ANGELA BOL: Preening of two tern species. A study of displacement activities. Behaviour 12, 13—88 (1957). — 430. INGRAM, W. R.: Brain stem mechanisms in behavior. Electroenceph. clin. Neurophysiol. 4, 397—406 (1952). — 431. INGRAM, W. R. et al.: Physiological relationships between hypothalamus and cerebral cortex. Electroenceph. clin. Neurophysiol. 3, 37—58 (1951).

432. JACKSON, J. H.: Croonian lectures on the evolution and dissolution of the nervous system. Lancet 1884, 555—558; 649—652; 739—744. — 433. JACKSON, J. H.: The Bowman Lecture: Ophthalmology and diseases of the nervous sytem. Lancet 1885, 935—938. — 434. JASPER, H. H. et al.: Corticofugal projections to the brain stem. A. M. A. Arch. Neurol. Psychiat. 67, 155—166 (1952). — 435. JENNINGS, H. S.: Public health progress and race progress—Are they incompatible? Science 66, 45—50 (1927). — 436. JOUVET, M.: Telencephalic and rhombencephalic sleep in the cat. In Nr. 212, S. 188—206. — 437. JOUVET, M., et R. HERNÁNDEZ-PEÓN: Méchanismes neurophysiologiques concernant l'habituation, l'attention et le conditionnement. Electroenceph. clin. Neurophysiol. Supp. 6, 39—49 (1957). — 438. JUNG, R.: Hirnelektrische Untersuchungen über den Elektrokrampf: Die Erregungsabläufe in corticalen und subcorticalen Hirnregionen bei Katze und Hund. Arch. Psychiat. Nervenkr· 183, 206—244 (1949). — 439. JUNG, R.: Zur Klinik und Pathogenese der Depression. Zbl. ges. Neurol. Psychiat. 119, 163 (1951). — 440. JUNG, R.: Diskussionsbemerkung. In: Symposion über das Zwischenhirn, S. 42—43, s. Nr. 79. — 441. JUNG, R.: Tierexperimentelle Grundlagen und EEG-Untersuchungen bei Bewußtseinsveränderungen des Menschen ohne neurologische Erkrankungen. Ier Congrès Int. Neurol. Bruxelles 1957, II, 148—180. — 442. JUNG, R., u. A. E. KORNMÜLLER: Eine Methodik der Ableitung lokalisierter Potentialschwankungen aus subcorticalen Hirngebieten. Arch. Psychiat. Nervenkr. 109, 1—30 (1939).

443. KAGAN, J., and F. A. BEACH: Effects of early experience on mating behavior in male rats. J. comp. physiol. Psychol. 46, 204—208 (1953). — 444. KAILA, E.: Die Reaktionen des Säuglings auf das menschliche Gesicht. Ann. Univ. Aboensis, Ser. B., 17, 114 (1932). — 445. KARSTEN, ANITRA: Psychische Sättigung. Psychol. Forsch. 10, 142—254 (1928). — 446. KEITER, F.: Das Instinktproblem in der Anthropologie. Z. Morph. Anthropol. 45, 147 bis 194 (1953). — 447. KEITER, F.: Kunstwerke als reaktionsauslösende Attrappen und Überattrappen. Homo 5, 81—87 (1954). — 448. KELLOGG, W. N.: Echo ranging in the porpoise. Science

128, No. 3330, p. 982—988 (1958). — 449. KISH, G. B.: Avoidance learning to the onset and cessation of conditioned stimulus energy. J. exp. Psychol. 50, 31—38 (1955). — 450. KISKER, K. P.: Sprachliche Stereotypien bei Temporallappenepilepsie. Nervenarzt 28, 366—368 (1957). — 451. KISKER, K. P.: Dynamische Topologie und Psychopathologie der Schizophrenien. Nervenarzt 28, 199—206 (1957). — 452. KLINGLER, J.: Die makroskopische Anatomie der Ammonshornformation. Denkschr. Schweiz. Naturforsch. Ges. 78, 1—78 (1948). — 453. KLÜVER, H.: A tachistoscopic device for work with sub-human primates. J. Psychol. (Princetown) 1, 1—4 (1935). — 454. KLUVER, H.: Use of vacuum tube amplification in establishing differential motor reactions. J. Psychol. (Princetown) 1, 45—47 (1935). — 455. KLÜVER, H.: An auto-multi-stimulation reaction board for use with sub-human primates. J. Psychol. (Princetown) 1, 123—127 (1935). — 456. KLÜVER, H.: An analysis of the effects of the occipital lobes in monkeys. J. Psychol. (Princetown) 2, 49—61 (1936). — 457. KLÜVER, H.: The study of personality and the method of equivalent and non-equivalent stimuli. Charact. Personal. 5, 91—112 (1936). — 458. KLÜVER, H.: Certain effects of lesions of the occipital lobes in Macaques. J. Psychol. (Princetown) 4, 383—401 (1937). — 459. KLUVER, H.: Visual functions after removal of the occipital lobes. J. Psychol. (Princetown) 11, 23—45 (1941). — 460. KLÜVER, H.: Functional significance of the geniculo-striate system. Biol. Symposia VII, 253—299 (1942). — 461. KLÜVER, H.: Mechanisms of hallucinations. In: Studies in Personality, S. 175—207. New York and London: McGraw-Hill Book Comp., Inc. 1942. — 462. KLÜVER, H.: Functional differences between the occipital and temporal lobes. In: Cerebral Mechanisms in Behavior, s. Nr. 94. — 463. KLÜVER, H.: The temporal lobe-syndrome. s. Nr. 8, S. 504—506. — 464. KLÜVER, H.: "The temporal lobe syndrome" produced by bilateral ablations. s. Nr. 211, S. 175—186. — 465. KLÜVER, H., and P. C. BUCY: "Psychic blindness" and other symptoms following bilateral temporal lobectomy in rhesus monkeys. Amer. J. Physiol. 119, 352 (1937). — 466. KLÜVER, H., and P. C. BUCY: An analysis of certain effects of bilateral temporal lobectomy in the rhesus monkey with special reference to "psychic blindness". J. Psychol. (Princetown) 5, 33—54 (1938). — 467. KLÜVER, H., and P. C. BUCY: Preliminary analysis of functions of the temporal lobes in monkeys. A. M. A. Arch. Neurol. Psychiat. 42, 979—1000 (1939). — 468. KNOTT, J. R., W. R. INGRAM and W. D. CHILES: Effects of subcortical lesions of cortical electroencephalogram in cats. A. M. A. Arch. Neurol. Psychiat. 73, 203—215 (1955). — 469. KNOWLTON, KATHRYN, et al.: Metabolic changes following transection of the spinal cord in dogs. Acta neuroveg. (Wien) 15, 374—403 (1957). — 470. KOEHLER, O.: Kritik an SINGH und ZINGG. Z. Tierpsychol. 7, 148—160 (1950). — 471. KOEHLER, O.: „Wolfskinder", Affen im Haus, und vergleichende Verhaltensforschung. Folia phoniat. (Basel) 4, 29—53 (1952). — 472. KOEHLER, O.: Vom unbenannten Denken. Verh. dtsch. zool. Ges. 1952, 99—108. — 473. KOEHLER, O.: Vom Erbgut der Sprache. Homo 5, 97—104 (1954). — 474. KOEHLER, O.: Das Làcheln des Sauglings. Umsch. Wiss. Techn. 11, 321—324 (1954). — 475. KOEHLER, O.: Das Làcheln als angeborene Ausdrucksbewegung. Z. menschl. Vererb. u. Konstit.-Lehre 32, 390—398 (1954). — 476. KOEHLER, O.: Vorformen menschlicher Ausdrucksmittel im Tierreich. Universitas 7, 759—770 (1954). — 477. KOEHLER, O.: Antwort auf die Kritik von D. S. LEHRMAN an K. LORENZ' Theorie des instinktiven Verhaltens. Z. Tierpsychol. 11, 330—334 (1954). — 478. KOEHLER, O.: Referat zur Arbeit von A. KORTLANDT, s. Nr. 486, Z. Tierpsychol. 12, 332—335 (1955). — 479. KOEHLER, O.: Tierische Vorstufen menschlicher Sprache. Erste Arbeitstagung über zentrale Regulation der Funktionen des Organismus, Leipzig 1.—3. Dez. 1955. — 480. KOEHLER, O.: Kritik an PORTMANN. Z. Tierpsychol. 13, 176—182 (1957). — 481. KOELLA, W., R. HESS JR. u. K. AKERT: Zur Technik der Registrierung hirnelektrischer Erscheinungen im Rahmen des subcorticalen Reizversuches bei der Katze. Helv. physiol. pharmacol. Acta 9, 316—325 (1951). — 482. KÖHLER, W.: Intelligenzprüfungen an Anthropoiden. I. Abhandl. Kgl. Preuß. Akad. Wiss. 1917. Physik. math. Klasse. — 483. KÖHLER, W.: Zur Psychologie der Schimpansen. Psychol. Forsch. 1, 2 (1922). — 484. KOIKEGAMI, H., et al.: Contributions to the comparative anatomy of the amygdaloid nuclei of mammals with some experiments of their destruction or stimulation. Folia psychiat. neurol. jap. 8, 336 (1955). — 485. KORTLANDT, A.: Eine Übersicht der angeborenen Verhaltensweisen des mitteleuropaischen Kormorans, ihre Funktion, ontogenetische Entwicklung und phylogenetische Herkunft. Arch. néerl. Zool. 4, 401—442 (1940). — 486. KORTLANDT, A.: Aspects and prospects of the concept of instinct. Vicissitudes of the hierarchy theory. Arch. néerl. Zool. 11, 156—284 (1955); Ref. Z. Tierpsychol. 12, 332—335 (1955). — 486a. KORTLANDT, A.: Chimpanzees in the wild. Sci. Amer. 206, Nr. 5, 128—138 (1962). — 487. KRETSCHMER, E.: Der Begriff der motorischen Schablonen und ihre Rolle in normalen und pathologischen Lebensvorgàngen. Arch. Psychiat. Nervenkr. 190, 1—3 (1953). — 488. KRETSCHMER, W., u. R. HARDER-MENZEL: Über archaische Erlebnisweisen bei Schizophrenen. Z. Psychother. med. Psychol. 2, 55—64 (1954).

489. LANSDELL, H. C.: Effect of brain damage on intelligence in rats. J. comp. physiol. Psychol. 46, 461—464 (1953). — 490. LARSSON, K.: Neurol basis of sexual behavior. Vortrag vor der Western Psychol. Ass., San Diego, California, 1959. — 491. LARSSON, K.: Conditioning

and sexual behavior in the male albino rat. Acta psychol. Gothoburgens. 1, 3—269 (1956). — 492. LASHLEY, K. S.: Contributions of Freudism to psychology. III. Physiological analysis of the libido. Psychol. Rev. 31, 192—202 (1924). — 493. LEBIDINSKIAIA, S. I., and J. S. ROSENTHAL: Reactions of a dog after removal of the cerebral hemispheres. Brain 58, 412—419 (1935). — 494. LECHNER, H.: Über das Auftreten von postoperativen Störungen des Gedächtnisses nach einseitiger Temporallappenresektion unter Einschluß von Teilen des Hippocampus wegen psychomotorischer Epilepsie. Wien. Z. Nervenheilk. 15, 183 bis 194 (1958). — 495. LEHMANN, E. v.: Zwei Leerlaufbeobachtungen im Freien. Z. Tierpsychol. 9, 120—121 (1952). — 496. LEHMANN, E. v.: Heimfindeversuche mit kleinen Nagern. Z. Tierpsychol. 13, 485—491 (1956). — 497. LEHRMAN, D. S.: A critique of K. LORENZ's theory of instinctive behavior. Quart. Rev. Biol. 28, 337—363 (1953). — 498. LEHRMAN, D. S.: Parental behavior in birds and the problem of "instinct". Proceedings of the 14th Int. Congress of Psychology, Montreal, June 1954. — 499. LEHRMAN, D. S.: The physiological basis of parental feeding behavior in the ring dove (Streptopelia risoria). Behaviour 7, 241—286 (1955). — 500. LEHRMAN, D. S.: Nurture, nature and ethology. Ref. über W. H. THORPE: Learning and instinct in animals. Contemp. Psychol. 2, 103—104 (1957). — 501. LEHRMAN, D. S.: On the organization of maternal behavior and the problem of instinct. Aus: L'instinct dans le comportement des animaux et de l'homme, S. 475—520; s. Nr. 6. — 502. LEHRMAN, D. S., and PH. BRODY: Oviduct response to estrogen in the ring dove (Streptopelia risoria). Proc. Soc. exp. Biol. (N. Y.) 95, 373—375 (1957). — 503. LENZ, F.: Die soziologische Bedeutung der Selektion. In: s. Nr. 71. — 504. LEUNER, H.: Psychotherapie in Modellpsychosen. In: Kritische Psychotherapie (Herausg. E. SPEER) München: Lehmann 1959. — 505. LEWIN, K.: Vorsatz, Wille und Bedürfnis. Untersuchungen zur Handlungs- und Affektpsychologie II (fortlaufend in der gleichen Zeitschr. bis 1936). Psychol. Forsch. 7, 330—385 (1926). — 506. LEYHAUSEN, P.: Einführung in die Eindruckskunde. Schola (Mschr. Erziehung u. Unterricht) 6, 895—900 (1951). — 507. LEYHAUSEN, P.: Das Verhältnis von Trieb und Wille in seiner Bedeutung für die Pädagogik. Schola (Mschr. Erziehung u. Unterricht) 7, 521—542 (1952). — 508. LEYHAUSEN, P.: Vergleichendes über die Territorialität bei Tieren und den Raumanspruch des Menschen. Homo 5, 68—76 (1954). — 509. LEYHAUSEN, P.: Über die Wahl des Sexualpartners bei Tieren. Beitr. Sexualforsch. 6, 47—56 (1955). — 510. LEYHAUSEN, P.: Die Entdeckung der relativen Koordination: Ein Beitrag zur Annäherung von Physiologie und Psychologie. Studium Generale 7, 45—60 (1957). — 511. LHOTSKÝ, J.: Der „Auslösermechanismus" in der Psychotherapie. Prakt. Arzt 7, 200—202 (1953). — 512. LHOTSKÝ, J.: Gespräche mit dem Unbewußten. Die Fortpflanzungstriebe und die Auslösermechanismen im Lichte der vergleichend-analytischen Psychologie. Nervenarzt 24, 217 (1953). — 513. LHOTSKÝ, J.: Der Begriff „Prägung" in der vergleichend-analytischen Psychologie. Beitr. Sexualforsch. 6, 57—67 (1955). — 514. LIDDELL, D. W., and D. W. C. NORTHFIELD: The effect of temporal lobectomy upon two cases of an unusual form of mental deficiency. J. Neurol. Neurosurg. Psychiat. 17, 267—275 (1954). — 515. LIDDELL, H. S.: The experimental neurosis and the problem of mental disorder. Amer. J. Psychiat. 94, 1035 to 1041 (1938). — 516. LIDDELL, H. S.: Animal origins of anxiety. In: Feelings and emotions, s. Nr. 172. — 517. LILLY, J. C.: Some thoughts on brain-mind, and on restraint and isolation of mentally healthy subjects. (Comments on "Biological roots of psychiatry" by C. E. BENDA.) Scientific staff meeting, National Institute of Mental Health, Bethesda, Md., 10. November 1955. — 518. LILLY, J. C.: Mental effects of reduction of ordinary levels of physical stimuli on intact, healthy persons. Psychiat. Res. Rep. Amer. psychiat. Ass. 5, 1—28 (1956). — 519. LILLY, J. C.: Distribution of "motor" functions in the cerebral cortex in the conscious intact monkey. Science 124, 937 (1956). — 520. LILLY, J. C.: A state resembling "fear-terror-panic" evoked by stimulation of a zone in the hypothalamus of the unanesthetized monkey. Excerpta med. IV. intern. Congr. Electroenceph. clin. Neurophysiol., Brüssel 1957. — 521. LILLY. J. C.: Development of a double-table-chair method of restraining monkeys for physiological and psychological research. J. appl. Physiol. 12, 134—136 (1958). — 522. LILLY, J. C.: Electrode and cannulae implantation in the brain by a simple percutaneous method. Science 127, 1181—1182 (1958). — 523. LILLY, J. C.: Learning motivated by subcortical stimulation: The start and stop patterns of behavior. In: Reticular Formation of the Brain, S. 705—727 (s. Nr. 92). — 524. LILLY, J. C.: Some considerations regarding basic mechanisms of positive and negative types of motivations. Amer. J. Psychiat. 115, 498—504 (1958). — 525. LILLY, J. C.: Correlations between cortical neurophysiological activity and short-term behavior in the monkeys. In: Biological and Biochemical Bases of Behavior, Univ. of Wisconsin Symposion, Madison, Wis. Aug. 1955. — 526. LILLY, J.C., J. R. HUGHES et al.: Production and avoidance of injury to brain tissue by electrical current at threshold values. Electroenceph. clin. Neurophysiol. 7, 458—459 (1955). — 527. LILLY, J. C., et al.: Brief, noninjurious electric waveform for stimulation of the brain. Science 121, 468—469 (1955). — 528. LINDSLEY, D. B.: The reticular activating system and perceptual integration. In: Electrical Stimulations of the Brain, s. Nr. 181. — 529. LORENZ, K.: Beobachtungen an Dohlen. J.

Ornithol. **75**, 511—519 (1927). — 530. LORENZ, K.: Der Kumpan in der Umwelt des Vogels. J. Ornithol. **83**, 137—213; 289—413 (1935). — 531. LORENZ, K.: Über die Bildung des Instinktbegriffes. Naturwissensch. **25**, 289—300; 307—318; 324—331 (1937). — 532. LORENZ, K.: Durch Domestikation verursachte Störungen arteigenen Verhaltens. Z. angew. Psychol. Charakterk. **59**, 2—81 (1940). — 533. LORENZ, K.: The comparative method in studying innate behavior patterns. Symp Soc. exp. Biol. New York: Academic Press 1950. — 534. LORENZ, K.: Ganzheit und Teil in der tierischen und menschlichen Gesellschaft. Studium Generale **3**, 455—499 (1950). — 535. LORENZ, K.: Ausdrucksbewegungen höherer Tiere. Naturwissensch. **38**, 113—116 (1951). — 536. LORENZ, K.: Über die Entstehung auslösender „Zeremonien". Vogelwarte **16**, 9—13 (1951). — 537. LORENZ, K.: Über tanzähnliche Bewegungsweisen bei Tieren. Studium Generale **5**, 1—9 (1952).— 538. LORENZ, K.: Moral-analoges Verhalten geselliger Tiere. Forsch. u. Wirtsch. **4**, 1—23 (1954). — 539. LORENZ, K.: Plays and vacuum activities. In: L'instinct dans le comportement des animaux et de l'homme, S. 633—645, s. Nr. 6. — 540. LORENZ, K.: The objectivistic theory of instinct. In: L'instinct dans le comportement des animaux et de l'homme, S. 51—76, s. Nr. 6.

541. MACLEAN, P. D.: Psychosomatic disease and the "visceral brain". Psychosom. Med. **11**, 338—353 (1949). — 542. MACLEAN, P. D.: Some psychiatric implications of physiological studies on fronto-temporal portion of limbic system (visceral brain). Electroenceph. clin. Neurophysiol. **4**, 407—418 (1952). — 543. MACLEAN, P. D.: The limbic system and its hippocampal formation: studies in animals and their possible application to man. J. Neurosurg. **11**, 29—44 (1954). — 544. MACLEAN, P. D.: The limbic system ("visceral brain") in relation to central gray and reticulum of the brain stem. Psychosom. Med. **17**, 355—366 (1955). — 545. MACLEAN, P. D.: The limbic system ("visceral brain") and emotional behavior. A. M. A. Arch. Neurol. Psychiat. **73**, 130—134 (1955). — 546. MACLEAN, P. D.: Hippocampal function: Tentative correlations of conditioning, EEG, drug, and radioautographic studies. Yale J. Biol. Med. **28**, 380—395 (1955/56). — 547. MACLEAN, P. D.: Chemical and electrical stimulation of hippocampus in unrestrained animals. I. Methods and electroencephalographic findings. A. M. A. Arch. Neurol. Psychiat. **78**, 113—127 (1957). — 548. MACLEAN, P. D.: Chemical and electrical stimulation of hippocampus in unrestrained animals. II. Behavioral findings. A. M. A. Arch. Neurol. Psychiat. **78**, 128—142 (1957). — 549. MACLEAN, P. D.: Contrasting functions of limbic and neocortical systems of the brain and their relevance to psycho-physiological aspects of medicine. Amer. J. Med. **25**, 611—626 (1958). — 550. MACLEAN, P. D.: The limbic system with respect to self-preservation and the preservation of the species. J. nerv. ment. Dis. **127**, 1—11 (1958). — 551. MACLEAN, P. D.: The limbic system with respect to two basic life principles. In: The central nervous system and behavior. Trans. 2nd Conference, Febr. 1959. The Josiah Macy, Jr. Foundation and the National Science Foundation. — 552. MACLEAN, P. D.: Psychosomatics. Handbook of Physiology, Neurophysiology, Vol. III, p. 1723—1744. Washington, D. C. 1960. — 553. MACLEAN, P. D., and J. M. R. DELGADO: Electrical and chemical stimulation of frontotemporal portion of limbic system in the waking animal. Electroenceph. clin. Neurophysiol. **5**, 91—100 (1953). — 554. MACLEAN, P. D., H. HORWITZ and F. ROBINSON: Olfactory-like responses in pyriform area to non-olfactory stimulation. Yale Biol. Med. **25**, 159—172 (1952). — 555. MACLEAN, P. D., and K. H. PRIBRAM: Neuronographic analysis of medial and basal cerebral cortex. I. Cat. J. Neurophysiol. **16**, 312—323 (1953). — 556. MACLEAN, P. D., and D. W. PLOOG: Cerebral loci involved in penile erection. Fed. Proc. **19**, part I, 288 (1960). — 557. MACLEAN, P. D., and D. W. PLOOG: Cerebral representation of penile erection. J. Neurophysiol. **25**, 29—55 (1962). — 558. MACLEAN, P. D., D. W. PLOOG and B. W. ROBINSON: Circulatory effects of limbic stimulation, with special reference to the male genital organ. Physiol. Rev. **40**, Suppl. No. 4, 105 —112 (1960). — 559. MACLEAN, P. D., B. W. ROBINSON and D. W. PLOOG: Experiments on localization of genital function in the brain. Trans. Amer. neurol. Ass. **1959**, 105. — 560. MASON, J. W.: The central nervous system regulation of ACTH secretion. In: Reticular formation of the brain; s. Nr. 92. — 561. MASON, J. W., and J. V. BRADY: Plasma 17-Hydroxycorticosteroid changes related to reserpine effects on emotional behavior. Science **124**, 983—984 (1956). — 562. MASSERMAN, J. H.: A biodynamic psychoanalytic approach to the problems of feeling and emotion. In: Feelings and emotions (Ed. M. L. REYMERT), s. Nr. 172. — 563. MCCRUM, W. R., and W. R. INGRAM: The effect of morphine on cats with hypothalamic lesions. J. Neuropath. exp. Neurol. **10**, 190—203 (1951). — 564. MEAD, MARGARET: Anthropological considerations concerning guilt. In: Feelings and Emotions (Ed. M. L. REYMERT), s. Nr. 172. — 565. MENZEL, R., and R. MENZEL: Einiges aus der Pflegewelt der Mutterhündin. Typisches und atypisches Verhalten von Hündinnen unter Einwirkung des Brutpflegetriebes. Behaviour **5**, 289—304 (1953). — 566. MEYER, A. E., u. W. R. HESS: Diencephal ausgelöstes Sexualverhalten und Schmeicheln bei der Katze. Helv. physiol. pharmacol. Acta **15**, 401—407 (1957). — 567. MEYERHARDT, O.: Phylogenetische Grundlagen einiger Verhaltensweisen. Schweiz. Z. Psychol. **15**, 184—195 (1956). — 568. MEYER-HOLZAPFEL, MONIKA: Unsicherheit und Gefahr im Leben hoherer Tiere. Schweiz Z. Psychol.

14, 171—194 (1955). — 569. MEYER-HOLZAPFEL, MONIKA: Über die Bereitschaft zu Spiel und Instinkthandlungen. Z. Tierpsychol. 13, 442—462 (1956). — 570. MEYER-HOLZAPFEL, MONIKA: Gruppenbildung bei Wirbeltieren. In: s. Nr. 118, S. 66—85. — 571. MEYER-HOLZAPFEL, MONIKA: Soziale Beziehungen bei Säugetieren. s. Nr. 118, S. 86—109. — 572. MEYER-HOLZAPFEL, M.: Geborgenheit in tierpsychologischer Sicht. In: Seelische Gesundheit, S. 3199 bis 3330. Bern u. Stuttgart: Huber 1959. — 573. MEYER-HOLZAPFEL, M.: Homosexualität bei Tieren. Praxis 1961, 1266—1272. — 574. MEYER-HOLZAPFEL, M.: Psychoreaktive Verhaltensstörungen bei Tieren. Die Heilkunst, H. 5 (1961). — 575. MEYER-MICKELEIT, R.: Die Dämmerattacken als charakteristischer Anfallstyp der temporalen Epilepsie (psychomotorische Anfälle, Äquivalente, Automatismen). Nervenarzt 24, 331—346 (1953). — 576. MILLER, N. E.: Studies of fear as an acquirable drive: I. Fear as motivation and fear reduction as reinforcement in the learning of new responses. J. exp. Psychol. 38, 89—101 (1948). — 577. MILLER, N. E.: Comments on theoretical models illustrated by the development of a theory of conflict behavior. J. Personality 20, 82—100 (1951). — 578. MILLER, N. E.: Shortcomings of food consumption as a measure of hunger; results from other behavioral techniques. Ann. N. Y. Acad. Sci. 63, 141—143 (1955). — 579. MILLER, N. E.: Effects of drugs on motivation; the value of using a variety of measures. Ann. N. Y. Acad. Sci. 65, 318—333 (1956). — 580. MILLER, N. E.: Learning and performance motivated by direct stimulation of the brain. In: Electrical stimulation of the brain (Ed. D. E. SHEER), s. Nr. 181. — 581. MILLER, N. E., and J. R. ANGELL: Objective techniques for studying motivational effects of drugs on animals. Int. Symposium on psychotropic drugs, Mailand, Mai 1957. — 582. MILLER, N. E., and H. BARRY: Motivational effects of drugs: Methods which illustrate some general problems in psychopharmacology. Psychopharmacologia 1, 169—199 (1960). — 583. MILLER, N. E., and M. L. KESSEN: Reward effects of food via stomach fistula compared with those of food via mouth. J. comp. physiol. Psychol. 45, 555—564 (1952). — 584. MILLER, N. E., and D. KRAELING: Displacement: Greater generalization of approach than avoidance in a generalized approach-avoidance conflict. J. exp. Psychol. 43, 217—221 (1952). — 585. MILLER, N. E., and E. J. MURRAY: Displacement and conflict: Learnable drive as a basis for the steeper gradient of avoidance than of approach. J. exp. Psychol. 43, 227—231 (1952). — 586. MILLER, N. E., et al.: Thirst-reducing effects of water by stomach fistula versus water by mouth measured by both a consummatory and an instrumental response. J. comp. physiol. Psychol. 50, 1—5 (1957). — 587. MILNER, BRENDA: Psychological defects produced by temporal lobe excision. In: The brain and human behavior. S. 244—257; s. Nr. 186. — 588. MINER, R. W.: The regulation of hunger and appetite. Ann. N. Y. Acad. Sci. 63, 1—144 (1955). — 589. MIRSKY, A. F.: The influence of sex hormones on social behavior in monkeys. J. comp. physiol. Psychol. 48, 327—335 (1955). — 590. MIRSKY, A. F., H. E. ROSVOLD and K. H. PRIBRAM: Effects of cingulectomy on social behavior in monkeys. J. Neurophysiol. 20, 588—601 (1957). — 591. MISHKIN, M.: Visual discrimination performance following partial ablations of the temporal lobes: II. Ventral surface versus hippocampus. J. comp. physiol. Psychol. 47, 187—193 (1954). — 592. MISHKIN, M., and K. H. PRIBRAM: Visual discrimination performance following partial ablations of the temporal lobe: I. Ventral versus lateral. J. comp. physiol. Psychol. 47, 14—20 (1954). — 593. MISHKIN, M., and K. H. PRIBRAM: Analysis of the effects of frontal lesions in monkey. II. Variations of delayed response. J. comp. physiol. Psychol. 49, 36—40 (1956). — 594. MISHKIN, M., H. E. ROSVOLD and K. H. PRIBRAM: Effects of nembutal in baboons with frontal lesions. J. Neurophysiol. 16, 155—159 (1953). — 595. MONROE, R. R., et al.: Correlation of rhinencephalic electrograms with behavior. Electroenceph. clin. Neurophysiol. 9, 623—642 (1957). — 596. MONTAGU, A.: Natural selection and the origin and evolution of weeping in man. Science 130, 1572—1573 (1959). — 597. MORRELL, F., and H. H. JASPER: Electrographic studies of the formation of temporary connections in the brain. Electroenceph. clin. Neurophysiol. 8, 201—215 (1956). — 598. MORRELL, F., and M. ROSSI: Central inhibition in cortical conditioned reflexes. A. M. A. Arch. Neurol. Psychiat. 70, 611—616 (1953). — 599. MORRIS, D.: The markings of the cut throat finch. Birds illustr. 1, 182—183 (1955). — 600. MORRIS, D.: The fighting postures of finches. Birds illustr. 1, 232—234 (1955). — 601. MORRIS, D.: The causation of pseudofemale and pseudomale behavior: a further comment. Behaviour 8, 46—56 (1955). — 602. MORRIS, D.: The feather postures of birds and the problem of the origin of social signals. Behaviour 9, 75—113 (1956). — 603. MORRIS, D.: "Typical intensity", and its relation to the problem of ritualisation. Behaviour 11, 1—12 (1957). — 604. MOYNIHAN M.: Notes on the behaviour of some North American gulls. I. Aerial hostile behaviour. Behaviour 10, 126—178 (1956). — 605. MOYNIHAN, M.: Behaviour of a pratincole. The Auk 73, 268 to 271 (1956). — 606. MOYNIHAN, M.: California Gulls and Herring Gulls breeding in the same colony. The Auk 73, 453—454 (1956). — 607. MOYNIHAN, M., and M. F. HALL: Hostile, sexual and other social behaviour patterns of the spice finch (Lonchura punctulata) in captivity. Behaviour 7, 33—76 (1954). — 608. MÜLLER-USING, D.: Über einige bisher unbeachtete Übersprunghandlungen bei höheren Säugern. Z. Tierpsychol. 9, 479—481 (1952). — 609. MÜLLER-USING, D.: Zum Verhalten des Murmeltieres (Marmota marmota L.). Z. Tierpsychol.

13, 135—142 (1956). — 610. Murray, E. J., and N. E. Miller: Displacement: Steeper gradient of generalization of avoidance than of approach with age of habit controlled. J. exp. Psychol. 43, 222—226 (1952). — 611. Meyers, A. K., and N. E. Miller: Failure to find a learned drive based on hunger; evidence for learning motivated by "exploration". J. comp. physiol. Psychol. 47, 428—436 (1954). — 612. Myers, R. E., and R. W. Sperry: Interhemispheric communication through the corpus callosum. Arch. Neurol. Psychiat. (Chic.) 80, 298—303 (1958).

613. Nachtsheim, H.: Vergleichende und experimentelle Erbpathologie in ihren Beziehungen zur Humangenetik. Acta genet. (Basel) 6, 223—239 (1956). — 614. Nachtsheim, H.: Umwelteinflüsse und Erbgut. Dtsch. Univ.-Ztg. Gottingen 1957, 15. — 615. Nauta, W. J. H.: Hippocampal projections and related neural pathways in the mid-brain in the cat. Brain 81, 319—340 (1958). — 616. Nauta, W. J. H., and H. G. J. M. Kuypers: Some ascending pathways in the brain-stem reticular formation. In: Reticular formation of the brain; s. Nr. 92. — 617. Nissen, H. W.: A field study of the chimpanzee. Observations of chimpanzee behavior and environment in Western French Guinea. Comp. Psychol. Monogr. 8, Nr. 1, 1—122 (1931). — 618. Nitschke, A.: Über Eigenart und Ausdrucksgehalt fruhkindlicher Motorik. Dtsch. med. Wschr. 1953, 1787—1792. — 619. Nolte, A.: Beobachtungen über das Instinktverhalten von Kapuzineraffen (Cebus apella L.) in der Gefangenschaft. Behaviour 12, 183—207 (1958). — 620. Nolte, A., u. G. Ducker: Jugendentwicklung eines Kapuzineraffen (Cebus apella L.) mit besonderer Berucksichtigung des wechselseitigen Verhaltens von Mutter und Kind. Behaviour 14, 335—373 (1959).

621. Olds, J.: A preleminary mapping of electrical reinforcing effects in the rat brain. J. comp. physiol. Psychol. 49, 281—285 (1956). — 622. Olds, J.: Runway and maze behavior controlled by basomedial forebrain stimulation in the rat. J. comp. physiol. Psychol. 49, 507—512 (1956). — 623. Olds, J.: Pleasure centers in the brain. Sci. Amer. 195, No. 4, 105—116 (1956). — 624. Olds, J.: Selective effects of drives and drugs on "reward" system of the brain. In: Neurological basis of behaviour, S. 124—148; s. Nr. 211. — 625. Olds, J., and P. Milner: Positive reinforcement produced by electrical stimulation of septal area and other regions of rat brain. J. comp. physiol. Psychol. 47, 419—427 (1954).

626. Papez, J. W.: A proposed mechanism of emotion. Arch. Neurol. Psychiat. (Chicago) 38, 725—743 (1937). — 627. Peiper, A.: Die Schreitbewegungen des Neugeborenen. Mschr. Kinderheilk. 45, 444 (1929). — 628. Peiper, A.: Instinkt und angeborenes Schema beim Säugling. Z. Tierpsychol. 8, 449 (1951). — 629. Peiper, A.: Schreit- und Steigbewegungen des Neugeborenen. Arch. Kinderheilk. 147, 135 (1953). — 630. Penfield, W.: The cerebral cortex in man I. The cerebral cortex in consciousness. Arch. Neurol. Psychiat. (Chicago) 40, 417—442 (1938). — 631. Penfield, W.: Epileptic automatism and the centrencephalic integrating system. In: Patterns of organization in the central nervous system. Ass. Res. nerv. Dis. Proc. 30, 513—528 (1952). — 632. Penfield, W.: Memory mechanisms. Arch. Neurol. Psychiat. (Chicago) 67, 178—191 (1952). — 633. Penfield. W.: The permanent records of the stream of consciousness. Proc. 14th Int. Congr. Psychol. Montreal, June 1954, p. 47—69. — 634. Penfield, W.: Mechanisms of voluntary movement. Brain 77, 1—17 (1954). — 635. Penfield, W.: Some observations on the functional organization of the human brain. Proc. Amer. philos. Soc. 98, 293—297 (1954). — 636. Penfield, W.: The role of the temporal cortex in certain psychical phenomena. J. ment. Sci. 101, 451—465 (1955). — 637. Penfield, W., and M. E. Faulk, jr.: The insula: Further observations on its functions. Brain 78, 445—470 (1955). — 638. Penfield, W., and B. Milner: Memory deficit produced by bilateral lesions in the hippocampal zone. A. M. A. Arch. Neurol. Psychiat. 79, 475—497 (1958). — 639. Perdeck, A. C.: The isolating value of specific song patterns in two sibling species of grasshoppers (Chorthippus brunneus Tunb. and Ch. biguttulus L.). Behaviour 12, 1—75 (1958). — 640. Pilleri, G.: Camillo Golgi. In: Große Nervenarzte (Herausg. K. Kolle), Bd. 2, Stuttgart: Thieme 1959.— 641. Pilleri, G.: Zum Verhalten der Paka. Z. Säugetiere 25, 107—111 (1960). — 642. Pilleri, G.: Kopfpendeln („Leerlaufendes Brustsuchen") bei cinem Fall von Pickscher Krankheit. Arch. Psychiat. Nervenkr. 200, 603—611 (1960). — 643. Pilleri, G.: Orale Einstellung nach Art des Klüver-Bucy-Syndroms bei hirnatrophischen Prozessen. Schweiz. Arch. Neurol. 87, 286—298 (1961)—644. Pilters, Hilde: Untersuchungen über angeborene Verhaltensweisen bei Tylopoden, unter besonderer Berücksichtigung der neuweltlichen Formen. Z. Tierpsychol. 11, 213—303 (1954). — 645. Pilters, Hilde: Observations éthologiques sur les tylopodes. Mammalia 19, 399—415 (1955). — 646. Pilters, Hilde: Quelques observations sur le comportement des dromadaires Camelus dromaderius L. relevés dans le Sahara nord-occidental. Bull. Soc. vét. Zootechn. Algér. 3, 9—13 (1955). — 647. Ploog, D.: „Psychische Gegenregulation", dargestellt am Verlaufe von Elektroschockbehandlungen. Arch. Psychiat. Nervenkr. 183, 617—663 (1950). — 648. Ploog, D.: Der Sympatol-Test im Verlauf endogener Psychosen. Nervenarzt 24, 102—107 (1953). — 649. Ploog, D.: Über den Schlaf und seine Beziehungen zu endogenen Psychosen. Munch. med.

Wschr. **1953**, 897—900. — 650. PLOOG, D.: Über den Einfluß der Elektroschockbehandlung auf die Flimmerverschmelzungsfrequenz (FVF). Acta neuroveg. (Wien) **12**, 405—420 (1955). — 651. PLOOG, D.: Über den Abbau des Gedächtnisses und seine Beziehungen zum Unbewußten. Gestaltanalyse eines amnestischen Symptomenkomplexes. Schweiz. Arch. Neurol. Psychiat. **76**, 259—297 (1955). — 652. PLOOG, D.: Motorische Stereotypien als Verhaltensweisen. Nervenarzt **28**, 18—22 (1957). — 653. PLOOG, D.: Über den Abbau menschlichen Verhaltens am Beispiel motorischer Stereotypien. Dtsch. med. J. **8**, 261—262 (1957). — 654. PLOOG, D.: Endogene Psychosen und Instinktverhalten. Fortschr. Neurol. Psychiat **26**, 83—98 (1958). — 655. PLOOG, D.: Angeborenes Verhalten in endogenen Psychosen. In: Psychiatrie und Gesellschaft (Herausg. H. EHRHARDT et al.). S. 133—145. Bern und Stuttgart: Huber 1958. — 656. PLOOG, D.: Über das Hervortreten angeborener Verhaltensweisen in akuten schizophrenen Psychosen. Psychiat. et Neurol. (Basel) **136**, 157—164 (1958). — 657. PLOOG, D.: Vergleichend quantitative Verhaltensstudien an zwei Totenkopfaffen-Kolonien. Z. Morph. Anthr. **53**, 92—108 (1963). — 658. PLOOG, D., u. H. SELBACH: Über den Funktionswandel des vegetativen Systems im Sympatolversuch während der Elektroschockbehandlung. Dtsch. Z. Nervenheilk. **167**, 270—302 (1952). — 659. PLOOG, D. et al.: Studies on social and sexual behavior of the squirrel monkey (Saimiri sciureus). Folia primatologica **1**, 28—63 (1963). — 660. PLOOG, D., and P. D. MacLEAN: On functions of the mamillary bodies in the squirrel monkey. Exp. Neurol. **7**, 76—85 (1963) — 661. PLOOG, D., and P. D. MacLEAN: Display of penile erection in squirrel monkey (Saimiri sciureus). Animal Behaviour **11**, 32—39 (1963). — 662. POPOV, N. A.: Etudes électroencéphalographiques du problème des réflexes conditionés. I—IV Année psychologique 1947—1950. — 663. POWELL, T. P. S.; The organization and connexions of the hippocampal and intralaminar systems. Recent Progr. Psychiat. **3**, 54—74 (1958). — 664. PRECHT, H., u. G. FREYTAG: Über Ermüdung und Hemmung angeborener Verhaltensweisen bei Springspinnen (Salticidae). Zugleich ein Beitrag zum Triebproblem. Behaviour **13**, 143—211 (1958). — 665. PRECHTL, H. F. R.: Das Verhalten von Kleinkindern gegenüber Schlangen. Wien. Z. Psychol. Philos. **2**, 68—70 (1949). — 666. PRECHTL, H. F. R.: Die Kletterbewegungen beim Säugling. Mschr. Kinderheilk. **12**, 519—521 (1953). — 667. PRECHTL, H. F. R.: Zur Physiologie der angeborenen auslösenden Mechanismen. I. Quantitative Untersuchungen über die Sperrbewegung junger Singvögel. Behaviour **5**, 32—50 (1953). — 668. PRECHTL, H. F. R.: Die Physiologie der angeborenen auslösenden Mechanismen. Proc. XIV. Int. Congr. Zool. Copenhagen 1953; Copenhagen, 1956, S. 263 bis 265. — 669. PRECHTL, H. F. R., u. A. R. KNOL: Der Einfluß der Beckenendlage auf die Fußsohlenreflexe beim neugeborenen Kind. Arch. Psychiat. Nervenkr. **196**, 542—553 (1958). — 670. PRECHTL, H. F. R., u. W. M. SCHLEIDT: Auslösende und steuernde Mechanismen des Saugaktes. I. Mitt. Z. vergl. Physiol. **32**, 257—262 (1950). — 671. PRECHTL, H. F. R., u. W. M. SCHLEIDT: Auslösende und steuernde Mechanismen des Saugaktes. II. Mitteilung. Z. vergl. Physiol. **33**, 53—62 (1951). — 672. PRIBRAM, H. B., and J. BARRY: Further behavioral analysis of parieto-temporo-preoccipital cortex. J. Neurophysiol. **19**, 99—106 (1956). — 673. PRIBRAM, K. H.: Some physical and pharmacological factors affecting delayed response performance of baboons following frontal lobotomy. J. Neurophysiol. **13**, 373—382 (1950). — 674. PRIBRAM, K. H.: Lesions of "frontal eye fields" and delayed response of baboons. J. Neurophysiol. **18**, 105—112 (1955). — 675. PRIBRAM, K. H.: Concerning the neurophysiological correlates of limbic system stimulation. In: Electrical stimulation of the brain, s. Nr. 181. — 676. PRIBRAM, K. H.: Comparative neurology and the evolution of behavior. In: Behavior and Evolution, p. 140—164; s. Nr. 173. — 677. PRIBRAM, K. H.: Neocortical function in behavior. In: Biological and biochemical bases of behavior, S. 151—172; s. Nr. 67. — 678. PRIBRAM, K. H.: The intrinsic systems of the forebrain. Handbook of Physiology, Neurophysiol. II, 1323—1344. Washington, D. C. 1960. — 679. PRIBRAM, K. H., and M. BAGSHAW: Further analysis of the temporal lobe syndrom utilizing frontotemporal ablations. J. comp. Neurol. **99**, 347—375 (1953). — 680. PRIBRAM, K. H., et al.: Limit and organization of the cortical projection from the medial thalamic nucleus in monkey. J. comp. Neurol. **98**, 433—448 (1953). — 681. PRIBRAM, K. H., and J. F. FULTON: An experimental critique of the defects of anterior cingulate ablations in monkey. Brain **77**, 34—44 (1954). — 682. PRIBRAM, K. H., et al.: The effects of precentral lesions on the behavior of monkeys. Yale J. Biol. Med. **28**, 428—443 (1955/56). — 683. PRIBRAM, K. H., and P. D. MacLEAN: Neuronographic analysis of medial and basal cerebral cortex. II. Monkey. J. Neurophysiol. **16**, 324—340 (1953). — 684. PRIBRAM, K. H., and M. MISHKIN: Simultaneous and successive visual discrimination by monkeys with inferotemporal lesions. J. comp. physiol. Psychol. **48**, 198—202 (1955). — 685. PRIBRAM, K. H., and M. MISHKIN: Analysis of the effects of frontal lesions in monkeys. III. Object alternation. J. comp. physiol. Psychol. **49**, 41—45 (1956). — 686. PRIBRAM, K. H., et al.: Effects on delayed-response performance of lesions of dorsolateral and ventromedial frontal cortex of baboons. J. comp. physiol. Psychol. **45**, 565—575 (1952). — 687. PRIBRAM, K. H., et al.: Electrical responses to acustic clicks in monkey: Extent of neocortex activated. J. Neurophysiol. **17**, 336—344 (1954). — 688. PRIBRAM, K. H., and L. WEISKRANTZ: A comparison of the effects of medial and lateral cerebral resections on conditioned avoidance behavior of monkeys. J. comp. physiol. Psychol. 50, 74—80 (1957).

689. Rado, S.: Narcotic bondage. A general theory of the dependence on narcotic drugs. Amer. J. Psychiat. 114, 165—170 (1957). — 690. Ramsay, A. O.: Variations in the development of broodiness in fowl. Behaviour 5, 51—57 (1953). — 691. Ramsay, A. O.: Seasonal patterns in the epigamic displays of some surface-feeding ducks. Wilson Bull. 68, 275—281 (1956). — 692. Ramsay, A. O., and E. H. Hess: A laboratory approach to the study of imprinting. Wilson Bull. 66, 196—206 (1954). — 693. Reeth, P. C. van, et al.: L'hypersexualité dans l'épilepsie et les tumeurs du lobe temporal. Acta neurol. belg. 1958, 194—218. — 694. Reeth, P. C. van: Un cas d'épilepsie temporale autoprovoquée et le problème de l'autostimulation cérébrale hédonique. Acta neurol. belg. 4, 490—495 (1959). — 695. Rensch, B.: Probleme der gerichteten Entwicklung und der Bauplanentstehung. Verh. anat. Ges. auf der 49. Versammlung in Heidelberg 1951, S. 3—16. Jena: G. Fischer 1951. — 696. Rensch, B.: Tatsachen und Probleme der Evolution. In: Vom Unbelebten zum Lebendigen. Stuttgart: Enke 1956. — 697. Rheingold, Harriet L., and E. H. Hess: The chicks "preference" for some visual properties of water. J. comp. physiol. Psychol. 50, 417—421 (1957). — 698. Rheingold, H. L. et al.: Social conditioning of vocalizations in the infant. J. comp. physiol. Psychol. 52, 68—73 (1959). — 699. Ricci, G., et al.: Microelectrode studies of conditioning: technique and preliminary results. IV. Congrès Int. Electroencéph. Bruxelles 1957. — 700. Richter, C. P.: Total selfregulatory functions in animals and human beings. Harvey Lect. Ser. 38, 63—103 (1942/43).— 701. Richter, C. P.: Rats, man, and the welfare state. Amer. Psychologist 14, 18—28 (1959).— 702. Richter, C. P.: Biological clocks in medicine and psychiatry: Shockphase hypothesis. Proc. nat. Acad. Sci. (Wash.) 46, No. 11, 1506—1530 (1960). — 703. Rioch, D. Mck.: Certain aspects of "conscious" phenomena and their neural correlates. Amer. J. Psychiat. 3, 810—817 (1955). — 704. Roberts, W.W.: Rapid escape learning without avoidance learning motivated by hypothalamic stimulation in cats. J. comp. physiol. Psychol. 51, 391—399 (1958).—705. Roberts, W. W.: Both rewarding and punishing effects from stimulation of posterior hypothalamus of cat with same electrode at same intensity. J. comp. physiol. Psychol. 51, 400—407 (1958). — 706. Roberts, W. W.: Fear-like behaviour elicited from dorsomedial thalamus of cat. J. comp. physiol. Psychol. 55, 191—197 (1962). — 707. Rogers, F. T.: Studies of the brain stem. VI. An experimental study of the corpus striatum of the pigeon as related to various instinctive types of behavior. J. comp. Neurol. 35, 15—59 (1922). — 708. Rose, J. E., and C. N. Woolsey: Structure and relations of limbic cortex and anterior thalamic nuclei in rabbit and cat. J. comp. Neurol. 89, 279 (1948). — 709. Rose, M.: Der Allocortex bei Tier und Mensch. J. Psychol. Neurol. (Lpz.) 34, H. 1/2 (1926).—710. Rose, M.: Die sog. Riechrinde beim Menschen und beim Affen. J. Psychol. Neurol. (Lpz.) 34, H. 6 (1927).— 711. Ross, S., et al.: The hoarding of non-relevant material by the white rat. J. comp. physiol. Psychol. 43, 217—225 (1950). — 712. Ross, S., et al.: Benzedrine and social behavior in mice. Behaviour 3, 167—173 (1951).— 713. Rosvold, H. E., et al : Influence of amygdalectomy on social behavior in monkeys. J. comp. physiol. Psychol. 47, 173—178 (1954). — 714. Rosvold, H. E.: Persönl. Mitt. — 715. Russel, R. W.: Experimentelle Neurose. Fortschr. Neurol. Psychiat. 21, 78—93 (1953). — 716. Russel, W. M. S., et al.: A basis for the quantitative study of the structure of behaviour. Behaviour 6, 153—205 (1954). — 717. Russell, E. S.: The stereotypy of instinctive behaviour. With an appendix on valence as "meaning for action". Proc. Linn. Soc. London, Session 155, Part 2, 186—208 (1942/43). — 718. Russell, E. S.: Biological adaptedness and specialization of instinctive behaviour. Proc. Linn. Soc. London, Session 153, 250—268 (1940/41).

719. Sauer, F.: Die Entwicklung der Lautäußerungen vom Ei ab schalldicht gehaltener Dorngrasmücken (Sylvia c. communis Latham) im Vergleich mit später isolierten und mit wildlebenden Artgenossen. Z. Tierpsychol. 11, 10—93 (1954). — 720. Sawa, M., et al.: Preliminary report on the amygdalectomy on the psychotic patients, with interpretation of oral-emotional manifestation in schizophrenics. Folia psychiat. neurol. jap. 7, 309—329 (1954). — 721. Schenkel, R.: Ausdrucksstudien an Wölfen. Behaviour 1, 81—130 (1947). — 722. Schjelderup-Ebbe, T.: Beitrage zur Sozialpsychologie des Haushuhnes. Z. Psychol. 88, 225—252 (1922). — 723. Schleidt, Margret: Untersuchungen über die Auslösung des Kollerns beim Truthahn. Z. Tierpsychol. 11, 417—435 (1954). — 724. Schleidt, W. M.: Reaktionen auf Töne hoher Frequenz bei Nagern. Naturwissenschaften 39, 69—70 (1952). — 725. Schleidt, W. M.: Über die Auslösung der Flucht vor Raubvögeln bei Truthühnern. Naturwissenschaften 48, 141 (1961). — 726. Schleidt, W. M.: Reaktionen von Truthühnern auf fliegende Raubvögel und Versuche zur Analyse ihrer AAM's. Z. Tierpsychol. 18, 534—560 (1961). — 727. Schleidt, W. M., u. M. Schleidt: Kurven gleicher Lautstarke beim Truthahn (Meleagris gallopavo). Naturwissenschaften 45, 119 (1958).—728. Schmidt, R. S.: The evolution of nest-building behavior in Apicotermes (Isoptera). Evolution 9, 157—181 (1955). — 729. Schmidt, R. S.: Termite (Apicotermes) nests-important ethological material. Behaviour 8, 344—356 (1955). — 730. Schmidt, R. S.: The nest of Apicotermes Trägårdhi (Isoptera)

new evidence on the evolution of nest-building. Behaviour 12, 76—94 (1958). — 731. SCHNEIDER, D.: Beiträge zu einer Analyse des Beute- und Fluchtverhaltens einheimischer Anuren. Biol. Zbl. 73, 225—282 (1954). — 732. SCHNEIRLA, T. C., and J. ROSENBLATT: Behavioral organization and genesis of the social bond in insects and mammals. Amer. J. Orthopsychiat. 31, 223—253 (1961). — 733. SCHOENFELD, W. N.: An experimental approach to anxiety, escape, and avoidance behavior. In: P. H. HOCH and J. ZUBIN (Eds.): Anxiety. New York: Grune & Stratton 1950. — 734. SCHREINER, L., and A. KLING: Behavioral changes following rhinencephalic injury in the cat. J. Neurophysiol. 16, 643—659 (1953). — 735. SCHREINER, L., and A. KLING: Effects of castration on hypersexual behavior induced by rhinencephalic injury in cat. A. M. A. Arch. Neurol. Psychiat. 72, 180—186 (1954). — 736. SCOVILLE, W. B.: The limbic lobe in man. J. Neurosurg. 11, 64—66 (1954). — 737. SCOVILLE, W. B., and B. MILNER: Loss of recent memory after bilateral hippocampal lesions. J. Neurol. Neurosurg. Psychiat. 20, 11—21 (1957). — 738. SELBACH, C., u. H. SELBACH: Das Rekelsyndrom als Wirkungsfolge eines biologischen Regelsystems. Mschr. Psychiat. Neurol. 125, 671—682 (1953). — 739. SELBACH, C., u. H. SELBACH: Krisenanalyse. Studium Generale 9, 394—404 (1956). — 740. SEITZ, A.: Untersuchungen über angeborene Verhaltensweisen bei Caniden. III. Teil. Beobachtungen an Marderhunden (Nyctereutes procyonoides Gray). Z. Tierpsychol. 12, 463—489 (1955). — 741. SEM-JACOBSEN, C. W.: Effects of electrical stimulation on the human brain. Electroencephal. clin. Neurophysiol. 11, 379 (1959). — 742. SEM-JACOBSEN, C. W., and A. TORKILDSEN: Depth recording and electrical stimulation in the human brain. In: E. R. RAMAY and D. S. O'DOHERTY (Eds.): Electrical studies on the unanesthetized brain. New York: P. E. Hoeber 1960. — 743. SHARPLESS, S., and H. H. JASPER: Habituation of the arousal reaction. Brain 79, 655—680 (1956). — 744. SHEATZ, G. C., et al.: An EEG study of conditioning. Amer. J. Physiol. 183, 660 (1955). — 745. SIDMAN, M.: Avoidance conditioning with brief shock and no exteroceptive warning signal. Science 118, 157—158 (1953). — 746. SIDMAN, M.: Some properties of the warning stimulus in avoidance behavior. J. comp. physiol. Psychol. 48, 444—450 (1955). — 747. SIDMAN, M.: On the persistance of avoidance behavior. J. abnorm. soc. Psychol. 50, 217—220 (1955). — 748. SIDMAN, M.: Technique for assessing the effects of drugs on timing behavior. Science 122, 925—955 (1955). — 749. SIDMAN, M.: Drug-behavior interaction. Ann N. Y. Acad. Sci. 65, 282—302 (1956). — 750. SIDMAN, M., et al.: Reward schedules and behavior maintained by intracranial self-stimulation. Science 122, 830—831 (1955). — 751. SLOANE, R. B. N., and D. J. LEWIS: Prognostic value of adrenaline and mecholyl responses in electroconvulsive therapy. J. psychosom. Res. 1, 273—286 (1956). — 752. SLOANE, R. B. N., et al.: Diagnostic value of blood pressure responses in psychiatric patients. A. M. A. Arch. Neurol. Psychiat. 77, 540—542 (1957). — 753. SLOANE, R. B. N., et al.: Reliability of epinephrine-methacholine (Mecholyl) testing. A. M. A. Arch. Neurol. Psychiat. 78, 294—300 (1957). — 754. SLOANE, R. B. N., et al.: Prognostic value of adrenaline and mecholyl responses in electroconvulsive Therapie-II. J. psychosom. Res. 2, 271—273 (1958). — 755. SMITH, W.: Social "learning" in domestic chicks. Behaviour 11, 40—55 (1957). — 756. SMITH, W., et al.: Hoarding behavior of adrenalectomized hamsters. J. comp. physiol. Psychol. 47, 154—155 (1954). — 757. SMITH, W., and S. ROSS: Hoarding behavior in the golden hamster (mesocricetus auratus auratus). J. genet. Psychol. 77, 211—215 (1950). — 758. SMITH, W., and S. ROSS: The role of activity in hoarding. — Some observations on the foetal behavior of the hamsters. Anat. Rec. 117, Abstract No. 87 and 165 (1953). — 759. SMITH, W., and S. ROSS: The hoarding behavior of the mouse: 1. The role of previous feeding experience. 2. The role of deprivation, satiation, and stress. 3. The storing of "non-relevant" material. J. genet. Psychol. 82, 279—316 (1953). — 760. SPALDING, D.: Instinct, with original observations on young animals. Brit. J. Anim. Behav. 2, 1—11 (1954); Neudruck aus dem Jahre 1873. — 761. SPATZ, H.: Das Hypophysen-Hypothalamus-System in seiner Bedeutung für die Fortpflanzung. Verhandlungen der Anatom. Gesellschaft, 51. Vers. 1953. — 762. SPERRY, R. W.: Preservation of high-order function in isolated somatic cortex in callosum-sectioned cat. J. Neurophysiol. 22, 78—87 (1959). — 763. SPINDLER, P.: Die Bedeutung des menschlichen Verhaltens für die physische Anthropologie. Homo 5, 63—64 (1954). — 764. SPINDLER, P.: Ausdruck und Verhalten erwachsener Zwillinge. Acta Genet. med. (Roma) 4, 32—61 (1955). — 765. SPINDLER, P.: Einige Filmerfahrungen bei Verhaltensstudien am Menschen. Res. Film 2, 180—184 (1956). — 766. SPINDLER, P.: Zur Vererbung von Verhaltensweisen. Ber. 5. Tagung, Dtsch. Ges. Anthropol. 5.—7. April 1956, Freiburg 1956. — 767. SPINDLER, P.: Studien zur Vererbung von Verhaltensweisen. 1. Verhalten auf einen starken akustischen Reiz. Anthropol. Anz. 22, 137—155 (1958); 2. Verhalten gegenüber Schlangen. Anthrop. Anz. 23, 187—218 (1959); 3. Verhalten gegenüber jungen Katzen. Anthrop. Anz. 25, 60—80 (1961). — 768. SPITZ, R. A., and K. M. WOLF: The smiling response; a contribution to the ontogenesis of social relations. Genet. Psychol. Monogr. 34, 57—125 (1946). — 769. SPOERRI, TH., u. H. HEIMANN: Ausdruckssyndrome Schizophrener. Nervenarzt 28, 364—366 (1957). — 770. STAEHELIN, B.: Gesetzmäßigkeiten im Gemeinschaftsleben schwer Geisteskranker. Schweiz. Arch. Neurol. Psychiat. **72**, 277—298 (1953). — 771. STAEHELIN, B.: Soziale Gesetzmaßigkeiten im Gemeinschaftsleben Geisteskranker, verglichen mit tierpsychologischen Ergebnissen. Homo **5**, 113—116 (1954). — 772. STAMM, J. S.: The function of the median cerebral cortex in maternal behavior of rats. J. comp. physiol. Psychol. **48**, 347—356 (1955). — 773. STAMM, J. S.: Effects of cortical lesions upon the onset of hoarding in rats. J. genet. Psychol. **87**, 77—88 (1955). — 774. STARCK, D., u. H. FRICK: Beobachtungen an äthiopischen Primaten. Zool. Jb. Syst. **86**, 41—70 (1958). — 775. STEIN, L.: Secundary reinforcement established with subcortical stimulation. Science **127**, 466—467 (1958).—776. STIERLIN, H.: Zwei Trieblehren: LORENZ und FREUD. Nervenarzt **25**, 407—410 (1954). — 777. STIERLIN, H.: Probleme der Ätiologie psychosomatischer Erkrankungen im Lichte moderner Erkenntnisse der vergleichenden Physiologie des Verhaltens. Psyche **8**, 605—623 (1955). — 778. STIRNI-MANN, F.: Das Kriech- und Schreitphänomen des Neugeborenen. Schweiz. med. Wschr. **1938**, 1374—1379. — 779. STRAUS, E.: Formen und Formeln. In: Psychiatrie und Gesellschaft. (Herausg. H. EHRHARDT et al.) Bern-Stuttgart: Huber 1958. — 780. STRAUSS, H.: Das Zusammenschrecken. Experimentell-kinematographische Studie zur Physiologie und Pathophysiologie der Reaktivbewegungen. J. Psychol. Neurol. (Lpz.) **39**, 111—231 (1929).

781. TALLAND, G.: Confabulation in the Wernicke-Korsakoff-Syndrome. J. nerv. ment. Dis. **132**, 361—381 (1961). — 782. TASAKI, I., and J. J. CHANG: Electric response of gliacells in cat brain. Science **128**, 1209—1210 (1958). — 783. TAVOLGA, MARGARET C., and F. S. ESSAPIAN: The behavior of the bottle-nosed dolphin (Tursiops truncatus): Mating, pregnancy, parturition and mother-infant behavior. Zoologica **42**, part I, 11—31 (1957). — 784. TERZIAN, H., and G. DALLE ORE: Syndrome of KLÜVER and BUCY reproduced in man by bilateral removal of the temporal lobes. Neurology (Minneap.) **5**, 373—380 (1955). — 785. TISCHLER, H.: Schreien, Lallen und Sprechen in der Entwicklung des Säuglings. Z. Psychol. **160**, 210—263 (1957). — 786. TRACY, W. H., and J. N. HARRISON: Aversive behavior following lesions of the septal region of the forebrain in the rat. Amer. J. Psychol. **69**, 443—447 (1956).

787. ULLRICH, W.: Zur Frage des Sichselbstbespuckens bei Säugetieren. Z. Tierpsychol. **11**, 1 (1954). — 788. ULLRICH, W.: Das Verhalten des Schimpansen, Pan tr. troglodytes (BLUMENBACH, 1799), beim Sprung. Säugetierkundl. Mitt. **2**, 124—126 (1954).

789. VALENSTEIN, E. S., and W. J. H. NAUTA: A comparison of the distribution of the fornix system in the rat, guinea pig, cat and monkey. J. comp. Neurol. **113**, 337—363 (1959). — 790. VILLINGER, W.: Vom anthropologischen Hintergrund der seelisch-geistigen Situation unserer Jugend. Jb. Jugendpsychiat. Bern und Stuttgart: Huber 1956. — 791. VOTAW, CH. L.: Certain functional and anatomical relations of the cornu ammonis of the macaque monkey. J. comp. Neurol. **112**, 353—382 (1959); **114**, 283—293 (1960).

792. WAGNER, H. O.: Freilandbeobachtungen an Klammeraffen. Z. Tierpsychol. **13**, 302—313 (1956). — 793. WALKER, A. E.: Recent memory impairment in unilateral temporal lesions. A. M. A. Arch. Neurol. Psychiat. **78**, 543—552 (1957). — 794. WALKER, A. E., et al.: Behavior and the temporal rhinencephalon in the monkey. Bull. Johns Hopk. Hosp. **93**, 65—93 (1953). — 795. WALTHER-BÜEL, H.: Die soziale Problematik gestörten Seelenlebens. In: Gestaltungen sozialen Lebens bei Tier und Mensch. Bern: Francke-Verlag 1958. — 796. WASHBURN, S. L., and I. DE VORE: The social life of Baboons. Sci. Amer. June 1961, p. 62—71. — 797. WEISKRANTZ, L.: Behavioral changes associated with ablation of the amygdaloid complex in monkeys. J. comp. physiol. Psychol. **49**, 381—391 (1956). — 798. WEISKRANTZ, L., and W. A. WILSON JR.: The effects of reserpine on emotional behavior of normal and brain-operated monkeys. Ann. N. Y. Acad. Sci. **61**, 36—55 (1955). — 799. WEISKRANTZ, L., and W. WILSON JR.: Effect of reserpine on learning and performance. Science **123**, 1110—1118 (1956). — 800. WEISS, P.: Autonomous versus reflexogenous activity of the central nervous system. Proc. Amer. philos. Soc. **84**, 53—64 (1941).— 801. WEISS, P.: Experimental analysis of coordination by the disarrangement of central-peripheral relations. Symp. Soc. exp. Biol. **4**, 92—111 (1950). — 802. WERNER, G.: Die neurophysiologischen Grundlagen der Wirkung von Tranquillisatoren. Klin. Wschr. **1958**, 404—408. — 803. WHITLOCK, D. G., and W. J. H. NAUTA: Subcortical projections from the temporal neocortex in Macaca mulatta. J. comp. Neurol. **106**, 183—212 (1956). — 804. WIESER, ST.: Zur Pathophysiologie der Greifphänomene. Arch. Psychiatr. Nervenkr. **194**, 315—328 (1956). — 805. WIESER, ST.: Schlüsselreize raumorientierender Zuwendungsreaktionen. Arch. Psychiat. Nervenkr. **195**, 373—382 (1957). — 806. WIESER, ST.: Der Abbau der oralen Leistungen. Ein Beitrag zum Problem der Evolution und Dissolution nervöser Leistungen. Ann. Univ. Saraviensis Med. **5**, Fasc. 3 (1957). — 807. WIESER, ST., u. K. DOMANOWSKY: Das Schreckverhalten des Sauglings. Arch. Psychiat. Nervenkr. **198**, 257—266 (1959). — 808. WIESER, ST., u. K. DOMANOWSKY: Zur Ontogenese und Pathologie des Schreckverhaltens. Arch. Psychiat. Nervenkr. **198**, 267—273 (1959). — 809. WIESER, ST.: Das Schreckverhalten des Menschen. Beiheft schweiz. Z. Psychol. u. Anwendg. Nr. 42, 1961. — 810. WIESER, ST., u. K. DOMANOWSKY: Greifreflex und Stellmechanismus beim Säugling. Dtsch. Z. Nervenheilk. **175**, 520—527 (1957). — 811. WIESER, ST. et al.: Moroscher Reflex und Schreckreaktion beim Säugling. Arch. Kinderheilk. **155**, 17—23 (1957).—

812. Wieser, St., u. T. Itil: Die Aufbaustufen der primitiven Motorik. Arch. Psychiat. Nervenkr. **191**, 450—462 (1954). — 813. Winkelsträter, K. H.: Das Betteln der Zoo-Tiere. Bern u. Stuttgart: Huber 1960. — 814. Winkler, W. Th.: Dynamische Phänomenologie der Schizophrenien als Weg zur gezielten Psychotherapie. Z. Psychother. med. Psychol. **7**, 192 bis 204 (1957).

815. Yoshii, N., et al.: Electrographic activity of the mesencephalic reticular formation during conditioning in the cat. Electroenceph. clin. Neurophysiol. **9**, 595—608 (1957). —

816. Zbinden, H.: Zur Verhaltensweise stark abgebauter epileptischer Persönlichkeiten in vergleichend-psychologischer Betrachtung. Mschr. Psychiat. Neurol. **125**, 769—776 (1953). — 817. Zingg, R. M.: Feral man and extreme cases of isolation. Amer. J. Psychol. **53**, 487—517 (1940); **54**, 432—435 (1941). — 818. Zippelius, Hanna-M., u. W. M. Schleidt: Ultraschall-Laute bei jungen Mäusen. Naturwissenschaften **43**, 502 (1956).— 819. Zitrin, A., et al.: Neural mediation of mating in male cats. III. Contributions of occipital, parietal and temporal cortex. J. comp. Neurol. **105**, 111—122 (1956).— 820. Zutt, J.: Sexualität, Sinnlichkeit und Prägung. Beitr. Sexualforsch. **6**, 1—9 (1955).

Die Lehre von den bedingten Reflexen
und ihre Entwicklung in der russischen Psychiatrie

Von

W. A. Giljarowsky †, Moskau

Inhalt

I. Die bedingten Reflexe und die Physiologie des Zentralnervensystems

1. Einleitung: Historisches, Setschenow* und Pawlow

Die Lehre von den bedingten Reflexen ist von dem großen russischen Physiologen Pawlow geschaffen worden und ist das Resultat einer 36jährigen gründlichen und zielstrebigen Arbeit.

Nach seiner Lehre sind die bedingten Reflexe eine *zentrale physiologische Funktion in der normalen Tätigkeit der Rinde beider Großhirnhemisphären*. Es sind *Lernvorgänge*, die durch *zeitweilige neuronale Erregungsverbindungen* von ungezählten, durch Receptoren aufgenommenen Reizwirkungen der Umwelt mit bestimmten Tätigkeiten des Organismus hervorgerufen werden. Die physiologische Hauptbedeutung dieser Verbindungen wird von Pawlow folgendermaßen präzisiert: Bei höheren Tieren, z. B. dem Hunde, der gewöhnlich als Forschungsobjekt dient, werden die hauptsächlichen kompliziertesten Beziehungen des Organismus zur Umwelt, die zur Erhaltung des Individuums und der Art notwendig sind, vor allem durch die Tätigkeit der den Hirnhemisphären nächstgelegenen *subcorticalen*

---

* Die Rechtschreibung der Namen wurde der in Deutschland üblichen Transkription des Russischen angepaßt, also: Setschenow (statt Ssetschenoff oder Sečenov) und Wedensky (statt Wwedenskij).

Teile sichergestellt. Diese Tätigkeiten: Nahrungssuche = Tätigkeit, die der Ernährung dient, und Sichfernhalten von Schädlichkeiten = Abwehrhandlungen, werden gewöhnlich als *Instinkte* bezeichnet. PAWLOW bezeichnete sie mit einem physiologischen Terminus: *komplizierteste unbedingte Reflexe.*

Zur Bildung eines bedingten Reflexes ist es notwendig, daß ein indifferenter Reizerreger zeitlich ein- oder mehrmals mit einem unbedingten Reflex zusammenfällt oder ihm vorausgeht. Nach demselben Prinzip des zeitlichen Zusammenfallens synthetisieren sich alle möglichen Reize zu Gruppen — gleichzeitige wie auch aufeinanderfolgende Vorgänge in der Natur. In Anbetracht der ständigen Bewegungen und Schwankungen der Naturerscheinungen, müssen natürlich auch die bedingten Reflexe Veränderungen erfahren. Wenn der bedingte Reizerreger ständig dem unbedingten zeitlich wesentlich vorausgeht, so bleibt sein entfernter Teil wirkungslos, da er quasi vorzeitig einsetzt und das Prinzip der Ökonomie stört. Wenn ein bedingter Reizerreger, der ständig mit einem anderen indifferenten Reizerreger verbunden ist, nicht von einem unbedingten Reizerreger begleitet wird, so bleibt er in dieser Kombination ohne Wirkung. Wenn nahe Reize, die einem gegebenen Reizerreger, der sich gebildet hat, verwandt sind, z. B. einander nahe Töne, nicht von einem unbedingten Reizerreger begleitet werden, also ohne Verstärkung bleiben, so verlieren sie allmählich ihre Wirkung.

Diesen Tatsachen entsprechend vollzieht sich die Differenzierung der Reizerreger der Umwelt, die Analyse der Umwelt mit allen ihren Elementen und Zeitmomenten. Auf diese Weise vollbringen die Großhirnhemisphären ständig in verschiedenstem Ausmaß sowohl die Analyse als auch die Synthese der auf sie einwirkenden Reize. PAWLOW sah es nicht nur als möglich, sondern als notwendig an, diesen Prozeß als *elementares konkretes Denken* zu bezeichnen. Das Denken bedingt eine vollkommene Anpassung, ein feineres Gleichgewicht des Organismus mit der Umwelt. Diese Tätigkeit der Großhirnhemisphären zusammen mit den nächstgelegenen subcorticalen Teilen, welche die normalen komplizierten Beziehungen des ganzen Organismus zur Außenwelt sicherstellen, rechnet man nach PAWLOW zur „*höchsten Nerventätigkeit*". Die Funktionen des Hirnstamms und Rückenmarks, die vorwiegend das Zusammenspiel und die Integration der Teile des Organismus untereinander lenken, werden dieser als „niedere Nerventätigkeit" gegenübergestellt. Die bedingten Reflexe werden durch die Tätigkeit der Rinde der Hemisphären verwirklicht, deren Unversehrtheit, die allerdings nicht vollkommen zu sein braucht, eine Voraussetzung dafür ist. Die Lehre von den bedingten Reflexen ist Physiologie, und das versteht sich von selbst, da ihr Schöpfer ein Physiologe war, ein ehemaliger Schüler LUDWIGs und HEIDENHAINs, der aber später seine eigene Physiologie mit einer Reihe verschiedener Schulen aufbaute, in denen unter seiner Führung seine Mitarbeiter und Schüler tätig waren.

Die wissenschaftliche Tätigkeit PAWLOWs war vielseitig. Es interessierten ihn allgemeine Fragen der Philosophie, das Problem „Naturkunde und Gehirn", das Problem der Evolution; doch an alle Fragen, die ihn beschäftigten, trat er als Physiologe heran.

Um sich eine bestimmte Vorstellung von den bedingten Reflexen zu machen, muß man die Situation kennen, in der die Lehre entstanden ist; man muß wissen, wer darüber oder über ähnliche Fragen gearbeitet hat. Die Lehre von den bedingten Reflexen von PAWLOW ist neu und in höchstem Maße originell, aber in ihrer Entwicklung ging sie von dem aus, was andere Physiologen erarbeitet hatten. Besonders bezieht sich das auf SETSCHENOW, den anerkannten „Vater der russischen Physiologie".

Zwischen den bedingten Reflexen Pawlows und den „Reflexen des Gehirns", wie Setschenow 1863 seine Monographie benannte, besteht fraglos ein Zusammenhang im Sinne einer Nachfolge. Es muß hier vermerkt werden, daß auch Setschenow in der Erfassung der Rolle der Reflexe beim Entstehen psychischer Erscheinungen einen Vorgänger gehabt hat, und zwar W. Griesinger, nach dessen Gedankengängen das psychische Leben seinen Anfang in den Sinnesorganen nimmt und seine endgültige Äußerung in der Bewegung findet. Aber Ssetschenoff gab als erster eine entwickelte Lehre von den Reflexen des Gehirns heraus.

Die Verdienste Setschenows sind auch in anderer Hinsicht beachtlich. Er stellt die Tatsache des hemmenden Einflusses der Nervenzentren auf die Reflexe fest (als Setschenows Hemmung bekannt). Als entgegengesetzte Tatsache entdeckte er die erregende Wirkung der höchsten Nervenzentren auf die niedrigsten und ebenso die Trägheit der Nervenprozesse, derzufolge das Nervensystem langsam in Bewegung kommt und ebenfalls langsam in den Zustand der Beruhigung zurückkehrt. Die Entdeckung der Tatsache des zentralen hemmenden Einflusses wurde für Setschenow der Schlüssel sowohl zum Verständnis vieler komplizierter Erscheinungen in der Tätigkeit des Nervensystems als auch der psychischen Tätigkeit, welche nach seiner Meinung durch Einflüsse, die auf die hoheren Sinnesorgane einwirken, als auch durch Reizung der sensiblen Nervenendigungen in den inneren Organen unterhalten und stimuliert wird. Wie Setschenow gezeigt hat, verfügt der Organismus über Nervenimpulse, die die Reflexe nicht nur verstärken, sondern auch hemmen können. Als die wichtigste Errungenschaft im individuellen Leben des Menschen sah Setschenow die Fähigkeit der Bildung besonderer reflektorischer Akte an, die hinhaltend und hemmend auf die äußere Manifestierung des reflektorischen Aktes hinwirken. Diese Fähigkeit liegt dem komplizierten Prozeß zugrunde, der die Bezeichnung: Gedanke, Absicht, Wunsch trägt. Wie er in seinen „Reflexen des Gehirns" sagt, „ist der Gedanke das Ergebnis von zwei Dritteln eines psychischen Prozesses, eines psychischen Reflexes ... Im Gedanken hat der Anfang eines Reflexes und seine Fortsetzung Platz, nur das Ende nicht — die Bewegung." Nach Setschenow kann es besondere Reflexe geben, „solche mit verstärktem Endstadium, wie man es am Beispiel des Affektes sehen kann ..." Die von Setschenow vermerkten Gesetzmäßigkeiten konnen in der Entwicklung der psychischen Tätigkeit von Anfang an verfolgt werden.

Auf den untersten Stufen der psychischen Entwicklung, wie sie den Tieren und auch den Neugeborenen eigen sind, beschränkt sich das psychische Leben darauf, was Pawlow als komplizierteste unbedingte Reflexe und vegetative Prozesse bezeichnet. Das Neugeborene befindet sich ständig in einem schläfrigen Zustand mit Unempfindlichkeit gegenüber äußeren Eindrücken und mit schwach ausgeprägten reflektorischen Bewegungen. Seine Psyche befindet sich im Zustand eines „fetalen Schlafes" (Heckel). Die Verbindung des Schreiens mit dem Gefühl des Hungers oder der Verunreinigung stellt einerseits einen reflektorischen Akt reinster Art dar — andererseits ist dies eine gewisse Etappe in der Evolution des psychischen Lebens. Die bestimmende Rolle der äußeren Reize ersieht man aus den Fällen, wo infolge irgendeines pathologischen Prozesses die Aufnahmefähigkeit eines Sinnesorganes sich nicht entwickelt oder ganz im Anfang zerstört wird. Als Regel wird man in solchen Fällen eine bestimmte Stufe des intellektuellen Zurückbleibens konstatieren, die um so tiefer sein wird, je stärker die Kontakte zur Außenwelt zerstört wurden. So führt eine angeborene oder eine in einer frühen Periode, wo das Sprechvermögen noch nicht voll entwickelt war, erworbene Taubheit zur Stummheit. Wenn ein solches Kind keine Spezialschule für Taube besucht, so wird es schwachsinnig. Der Schwachsinn wird besonders in den Fällen sehr ausgeprägt, wo nicht nur das Gehör, sondern auch die Sehkraft und vielleicht noch andere Sinnesorgane geschädigt sind. Wie man annehmen muß, stellen die Außenwelteindrücke nicht nur das Material für die psychische Arbeit, sondern sind an sich ein mächtiger Stimulus für das Funktionieren der Psyche.

Wie die Fälle zeigen, die Setschenow in seinen „Reflexen des Gehirns" beschreibt, führt bei Kranken, die beinahe vollkommen der Möglichkeit eines Kontaktes mit der Außenwelt beraubt sind und denen sozusagen nur ein kleines Fenster für diese Kontakte geblieben ist (z. B. in Gestalt eines Restes des Gehörs auf einer Seite oder der nicht gestörten Sensibilität der Hand, so daß man auf ihr mit einem Finger Buchstaben malen kann), die Schließung dieses kleinen Fensters, d. h. die volle Unterbrechung der Reize, dazu, daß diese Kranken in einen Schlafzustand verfallen, der dem fetalen Schlaf sehr ähnlich ist.

Die Analyse der Handlungen und der ihnen zugrunde liegenden psychischen Vorgänge eines erwachsenen Menschen bietet bedeutende Schwierigkeiten, aber zweifelsohne ist das vielseitige und komplizierte psychische Leben, das sich in voller Entfaltung befindet, nach denselben Prinzipien aufgebaut wie das Leben eines kleinen Kindes, es stellt nur eine weitere Evolution desselben dar. Das Studium des kindlichen Verhaltens jedoch gibt klare Hinweise auf das Reflektorische daran, auf die Bedingtheit durch die Reize, die von der Außenwelt ausgehen oder sich innerhalb des Organismus bilden. Das Ausstrecken des Händchens nach einem glänzenden Gegenstand, das Ergreifen des sich Bietenden mit dem Trieb, alles in den Mund zu stecken, das Hinstreben zur Mutter und das Abweisen alles Unbekannten — das alles sind Reflexhandlungen reinster Art. Im weiteren Verlauf, mit Komplizierung des psychischen Lebens und der Entwicklung hemmender Einflüsse, wird die Verbindung eines einzelnen psychischen Vorganges und des daraus resultierenden motorischen Aktes mit dem ursprünglichen Reiz weniger klar, um so mehr, als Anfang und Ende, d. h. der äußere Reiz und der motorische Akt, voneinander durch einen mehr oder weniger großen Zeitraum getrennt sein können; aber das Wesentliche des Vorgangs wird dadurch nicht geändert. Im Hinblick auf diese und analoge Vorgänge, kam Setschenow zu der Schlußfolgerung, daß das psychische Leben im ganzen eine *Reihe von Reflexen auf die Reize der Außenwelt* darstellt und insofern, als entsprechende physiologische Prozesse im Gehirn verlaufen müssen, zog er den Schluß, daß die Reflexe des Gehirns dem psychischen Leben zugrunde liegen.

In bezug auf die Monographie von Setschenow „Reflexe des Gehirns", sprach Pawlow vom genialen Schwung seiner Gedanken. Von ihm ausgehend, schuf Pawlow eine Lehre von den bedingten Reflexen, in deren Licht sowohl die psychischen Prozesse als auch ihre Abweichungen vom normalen Verlauf, die Psychosen, verständlich werden.

Von größter Wichtigkeit ist es, daß der Forscher es hier nicht mit spekulativen, wenn auch vielleicht scharfsinnigen, aber willkürlichen Konstruktionen zu tun hat, wie das bei vielen psychologischen Konzeptionen der Fall ist, sondern mit fundierten Schlußfolgerungen aus genau durchgeführten Erforschungen physiologischer Prozesse, die im Nervensystem ablaufen. Pawlow und seine Mitarbeiter erforschten die Bedingungen der Entstehung einer Erregung, ihrer Weiterleitung im Nervensystem, ihrer Irradiation und der Hemmung der Endreaktion, d. h. des letztes Gliedes des Reflexbogens.

Das psychische Leben wird von ihm und seiner Schule nicht vom subjektiven Erleben her erforscht, das keiner genauen Nachprüfung zugänglich ist, sondern durch streng objektive Methoden, denen eine genaue Beobachtung und Registrierung der motorischen und sekretorischen Vorgänge zugrunde liegt, die eine Antwort auf verschiedene in ihrem Charakter und ihrer Intensität wechselnden Reize darstellen. Diese als Antwort erfolgenden Bewegungen sind, wie Pawlow gezeigt hat, Reflexe; aber zum Unterschied von den gewöhnlichen unbedingten Reflexen, sind sie von ihm als *bedingte Reflexe* bezeichnet worden. Von den unbedingten Reflexen, die mit einer mechanischen Regelmäßigkeit und Beständigkeit nach einem entsprechenden, genügend starken Reiz entstehen, unterscheiden sie sich dadurch, daß sie anfänglich auf der Grundlage eines unbedingten Reflexes entstehen, falls der zufällige Reiz sich einige Male zusammen mit dem Reizerreger des unbedingten Reflexes wiederholt und dabei eine für denselben charakteristische Reflexbewegung hervorruft. Sie führen aber nicht zu diesen Reaktionen, wenn der zufällige Reiz nicht von dem unbedingten Reizerreger begleitet wird.

Wenn man, wie es in den Versuchen von Pawlow geschehen ist, einen Hund, dem man Hopfenöl — einen unbedingten Reizerreger für die Absonderung von Speichel — eingeflößt hat, gleichzeitig einem anderen Reiz aussetzt, z. B. einem Ton von einer gewissen Höhe, dann kann dieser Ton nach einigen Wiederholungen ebenfalls die Speichelabsonderung hervorrufen.

Zur Entwicklung eines bedingten Reflexes bedarf es einer gewissen Anzahl von Wiederholungen, die in Abhängigkeit vom Charakter des Reizes, der Eigenart des Tieres und anderen zufälligen Momenten variieren. Die bedingten Reflexe können nicht nur auf der Basis von unbedingten Reflexen, sondern auch auf derjenigen anderer bedingter Reflexe anerzogen werden. Auf diese Weise entstehen *Superreflexe, bedingte Reflexe II., III. usw. Ordnung.*

Zur besseren Erklärung des Wesens der höchsten Nerventätigkeit muß man die Resultate der Forschungen von Wedensky und Uchtomsky über die Bedingungen der Weiterleitung (Übertragung) von Erregungen in Betracht ziehen. Sie wurden hauptsächlich am peripheren Nerven studiert, erwiesen sich aber als gleichartig im zentralen Nervensystem.

Eine Unzahl nach Charakter und Intensität verschiedener Reize wirken in jedem gegebenen Moment auf die Sinnesorgane ein. Viele von diesen wirkten auch schon früher, manchmal zu wiederholten Malen, auf das Nervensystem, wobei sie so oder anders am Spiel der neuerlich entstehenden und wieder erlöschenden bedingten Reflexe beteiligt waren.

Eine jede von diesen scheinbar auf das Nervensystem nicht einwirkenden Erregungen ruft in ihm den einen oder anderen physiologischen Prozeß hervor und strebt ihre Manifestierung in irgendeinem abschließenden motorischen Akt an, aber auf dem Wege dazu entstehen viele Hindernisse. Die Anzahl der äußeren Reize ist unermeßlich groß im Vergleich zur Anzahl der Wege, auf denen die Erregung weitergegeben werden kann, und der Anzahl der möglichen motorischen Akte.

Diese Beziehung stellen die Physiologen bildlich in der Form eines riesigen Trichters dar, durch dessen enge Öffnung die in ihm in großer Menge gestauten Erregungen sich durchzuzwängen suchen. Hier, um bei der Sprache der Physiologen zu bleiben, findet ein intensiver *Kampf der verschiedenen Erregungen um ein und dasselbe Bewegungsfeld* statt. Auch spielt es eine Rolle, daß die Wege, auf denen die Erregung sich fortzupflanzen strebt, nicht frei zu sein brauchen. Die Physiologen weisen darauf hin, daß die Weiterleitung der Erregung und ihre Richtung im Nervensystem nicht allein durch anatomische Beziehungen bestimmt werden, sondern auch durch die Anwesenheit von Erregungsherden auf dem Wege und durch den Zustand, in dem sich die peripheren Apparate befinden.

Im zentralen Nervensystem befindet sich stets eine große Anzahl von Erregungsherden, sie irradiieren nach verschiedenen Richtungen und wechseln ihren Ort, eine Zone herabgeminderter Erregung hinterlassend. Die einander berührenden Erregungsherde führen zu verschiedenen Prozessen der Wechselwirkung. Gewöhnlich beobachtet man, daß verschiedenartige Erregungen einen hemmenden Einfluß aufeinander ausüben. Nach dem von Uchtomsky aufgestellten *Gesetz der Dominanz* sind beim Vorhandensein von Herden intensiver Erregung geringfügige Erregungen nicht in der Lage, einen entsprechenden Effekt hervorzurufen, und fließen mit dem Herd der intensiven Erregung zusammen, wobei sie den von ihm ausgehenden Effekt verstärken. So schließt eine durch schweres Unglück ausgelöste Schwermut die Möglichkeit freudiger Erlebnisse aus, und alle Versuche der Beschwichtigung verstärken sie nur.

Ein bestimmtes Niveau der Entwicklung des Nervensystems ist für das Zustandekommen bedingter Reflexe notwendig. Zum Beispiel fehlen sie bei schweren Fällen von angeborenem Schwachsinn. Im Alter und nach Exstirpation der Schilddrüse wird das Anerziehen von bedingten Reflexen schwierig. Bei ausgeprägten, destruktiven Gehirnprozessen wird die Bildung der bedingten Reflexe stark herabgesetzt, oder sie unterbleibt, da dabei die Analysatoren zerstört werden; wenn aber die Zerstörung nicht stark ist, so wird auch der Prozeß der Bildung bedingter Reflexe nicht sonderlich gestört, da ein Analysator bis zu einem gewissen Grade durch einen anderen ersetzt werden kann. Diese äußerst wichtige und genau festgestellte Tatsache harmoniert vollkommen mit einigen Daten der Pathologie, welche schon längst bekannt waren, aber keine genügende Erklärung fanden. So haben auch früher gewisse klinische Ergebnisse die Annahme nahegelegt, daß die Funktionen zerstörter Gehirnbezirke durch andere übernommen werden können. Es erregte auch Aufmerksamkeit, daß in einigen Fällen, ungeachtet der verhältnismäßig großen Zerstörung des Gehirns, das psychische Funktionieren sich als wenig verändert erwies.

Aus der großen Anzahl von Reizen, von denen die Sinnesorgane getroffen werden, führen die wenigsten im Enderfolg zur Auslösung irgendeines motorischen Aktes. Aber wie wir sahen, bedeutet das nicht, daß die durch sie hervorgerufenen Erregungsprozesse sofort spurlos verschwinden. Im Grunde sind es dieselben Prozesse, die sich nur dadurch unterscheiden, daß ihr letztes Glied — die Bewegungsreaktion — durch andere konkurrierende Prozesse unterdrückt, gehemmt wird. Wie SETSCHENOW dachte, wird das psychische Leben auf Reflexe zurückgeführt, aber es sind nicht unbedingte Reflexe, sondern solche, die an eine große Anzahl allerverschiedenster Bedingungen geknüpft sind.

Wie man aus allem Dargelegten ersieht, hat die Analyse der von den russischen Physiologen gewonnenen Ergebnisse eine große Bedeutung bei der Erfassung des Wesens psychischer Erscheinungen und weist auf die Einstellung zu ihnen als unteilbaren, einheitlichen Prozessen hin. Auch die einfachste Bewegungsreaktion ist das Ergebnis sehr komplizierter Prozesse, die sich nicht nur auf irgendein einzelnes begrenztes System der Nervenelemente beschränken. Jeder neue Reiz wird in einen komplizierten Kampf verschiedener Erregungen und Hemmungen eingekeilt, und das Endresultat hängt von sehr vielen Bedingungen ab, unter denen das Vorhandensein des einen oder anderen Prozesses der Erregung im ganzen Nervensystem eine große Rolle spielt, ebenso wie der Zustand der Erregbarkeit desselben in Abhängigkeit von vegetativen Prozessen und vom Allgemeinzustand des Gesamtorganismus. Auf diese Weise muß jeder psychische Prozeß, sogar der scheinbar einfachste, als eine Ganzheitsreaktion nicht nur des Nervensystems, sondern des Gesamtorganismus angesehen werden.

Das bezieht sich auch auf die *Emotionen*. Sie werden, wie auch alle Reaktionen des Organismus, von allen drei Instanzen geliefert — vom subcorticalen Bereich und von den beiden Signalsystemen. In die emotionalen Reaktionen werden verschiedene mimische und pantomimische Komponenten einbezogen, in Abhängigkeit von der Irradiation des Erregungsprozesses auf die subcorticalen Zentren. Eine charakteristische Besonderheit der emotionalen Reaktionen besteht darin, daß dabei irgendein bedingter Reflex übermäßig stark angespannt wird, durch welchen dann die ganze Tätigkeit der Rinde und des Subcortex dirigiert wird, während die bedingte Tätigkeit anderer Bezirke unterdrückt wird, was sogar eine geraume Zeit andauern kann.

Die physiologische Bedeutung der bedingten Reflexe besteht in ihrer Rolle als *Signale*. Die Signale haben die Aufgabe, indem sie eine Tätigkeit mal stimulieren und mal hemmen, den Organismus für entsprechende Veränderungen vorzubereiten. Auf diese Weise entsteht zwischen einem komplexen Organismus und seiner Umwelt das feinste und genaueste Gleichgewicht.

2. Unbedingte Voraussetzungen zur Bildung bedingter Reflexe. Hemmungserscheinungen und Phasen

Zum besseren Verständnis des Zustandekommens der *Signaltätigkeit der Großhirnhemisphären* muß man feststellen, was zur Bildung der bedingten Reflexe erforderlich ist. Erstens, wie schon oben erwähnt, ist es das zeitliche Zusammenfallen des vordem indifferenten Reizerregers mit der Tätigkeit des unbedingten Agens, welches einen bestimmten, unbedingten Reflex hervorruft, wobei das indifferente Agens der Tätigkeit des unbedingten Reizerregers zeitlich ein wenig vorausgehen muß. Dabei ist es notwendig, daß der indifferente Reizerreger eine gewisse minimale Stärke besitzt, unter der er nicht mehr in der Eigenschaft eines bedingten Reizerregers funktionieren kann. Der bedingte Reizerreger braucht auch nicht im Moment zu bestehen, es genügen die Reste seiner Einwirkung im Nervensystem, nach seiner Unterbrechung. Das bildet die Grundlage zur Unterscheidung zwischen bestehenden bedingten Reflexen und nachfolgenden bedingten Reflexen = Reflexspuren.

Jede Einwirkung, auf welche ein bedingter Reflex erfolgt, veranlaßt zunächst eine verallgemeinernde Reaktion, z. B. bei der Anwendung eines Tones haben anfänglich auch andere Töne dieselbe bedingte Wirkung, aber nach Ausarbeitung des bedingten Reflexes wird die nur angenäherte verallgemeinernde Verbindung durch eine genaue und spezielle ersetzt. Diese Differenzierung kann durch Anwendung von Reizerregern, die dem bedingten Reizerreger nahestehen, aber von keinem unbedingten Reizerreger begleitet werden, erreicht werden. So erreicht man die Abgrenzung eines Reizerregers von einem ihm nahen anderen. Pawlow maß dieser differenzierenden Hemmung in der allgemeinen Arbeit der Analyse große Bedeutung bei.

Es besteht die Notwendigkeit, zwischen der äußeren (unbedingten, passiven) und der inneren (aktiven) *Hemmung* zu unterscheiden.

Pawlow nahm an, daß alle Arten der Hemmung ihrer physikalisch-chemischen Grundlage nach einen und denselben, aber unter verschiedenen Bedingungen entstehenden Prozeß darstellen. Die äußere, unbedingte Hemmung ist ohne Ausnahme allen Teilen des Nervensystems eigen, während die innere, bedingte Hemmung eine Funktion der Rinde der Großhirnhemisphären darstellt. Die äußere, unbedingte Hemmung entsteht sofort, ohne jede Vorbereitung, während die innere sich allmählich, bei Wiederholung der Bedingungen ihres Eintretens, entwickelt. Vom Standpunkt der Evolution stellt die unbedingte Hemmung die ältere Form dar. Zur unbedingten Hemmung gehören: Hemmung bei den Erscheinungen der negativen Induktion, bei konkurrierender Wirksamkeit verschiedener Reizerreger und die überschießende Hemmung (wörtlich: jenseits der Grenzen liegende Hemmung).

Als *Induktion* bezeichnete Pawlow die Einwirkung eines Prozesses auf einen anderen. Diese Einwirkung ist gegenseitig und reziprok: die Anwendung des Reizes führt zur Hemmung und umgekehrt die Hemmung zur Erregung — die sog. negativen und positiven Induktionen.

Die überschüssige Hemmung entsteht bei der Wirkung eines außerordentlich starken Reizerregers oder bei gleichzeitiger Wirkung im einzelnen nicht sonderlich starker Reizerreger. Diese letztere Art der Hemmung, die sich bei pathologischen Bedingungen entwickelt, nannte Pawlow *schützende Hemmung*.

Wenn man von der Hemmung spricht, muß auf Pawlows Konzeption des Schlafes hingewiesen werden. *Der Schlaf ist eine Hemmung, die sich über die Hemisphären ergießt und entlang dem Gehirn bis zu einer gewissen Tiefe vordringt.*

Eine derartige Hemmung kann eine verschiedene Tiefe haben und verschiedene Phasen der Veränderung der Rindentätigkeit durchlaufen. Zwischenzustände zwischen Schlaf und Wachen. Die Übergangsphasen zwischen Erregung und Hemmung stellen verschiedene Stufen der Intensität des Hemmungsprozesses dar. Diese Zwischenzustände treten besonders deutlich bei der Entwicklung des Schlafes hervor. Pawlow nannte sie „hypnotische Phasen". Bei der Vertiefung der Hemmung werden die regelmäßigen Wechselbeziehungen zwischen Erregung und Reaktion geändert. Wenn alle Reizerreger, unabhängig von der Intensität, ganz gleichmäßig einwirken, so haben wir es mit einer ausgleichenden Phase zu tun. Wenn aber ein starker Reizerreger untätig oder schwach wirksam ist, während ein schwacher Reizerreger einen Effekt hervorruft, der sogar die Norm übersteigt, so haben wir eine paradoxe Phase. Als eine ultraparadoxe Phase bezeichnete Pawlow einen Zustand, bei dem der bedingte positive Reizerreger seine Wirksamkeit verliert, während umgekehrt der negative Reizerreger eine deutliche positive Wirkung ausübt.

Mit Zuständen, die verschiedenen physiologischen Phasen entsprechen, hat man es oft in der Pathologie zu tun, besonders wo es sich um *Halluzinationen* und Fieberdelirien handelt. Seit Bayarget ist es eine feststehende klinische Tatsache, daß Halluzinationen besonders oft in den Übergangszuständen vom Wachen zum Schlafen beobachtet werden; gerade diese Periode ist durch das Bestehen der soeben beschriebenen Phasenzustände charakterisiert, jeder von ihnen hat seine Eigentümlichkeiten, denen man diese oder jene Halluzination gegenüberstellen kann.

Die Entwicklung des *Wahns* wurde von PAWLOW als eine Erscheinung der ultraparadoxen Phase erklärt.

Wir ersehen dies aus seinem Brief an PIERRE JANET aus Anlaß von dessen Hervorhebung des „Gefühls der Bemächtigung" — welches aber seinem Wesen nach der Verfolgungswahn ist. Nach der Definition von PAWLOW sind es zwei physiologische Prozesse, die dem Wahn zugrunde liegen: pathologische Trägheit (wörtlich: pathologisches Inertsein) und die ultraparadoxe Phase. Entsprechend der ultraparadoxen Phase erscheinen die vorher gehemmten Vorstellungen im Bewußtsein. So entwickelt sich aus eifersüchtigen Befürchtungen, die im normalen Zustand abgelehnt und unterdrückt werden, in pathologischen Zuständen der Eifersuchtswahn.

Wie man aus den Untersuchungen der Aktionsströme, die von mir und LIWANOW durchgeführt wurden, ersieht, können die Herde der inerten Erregung bei der Entstehung der Halluzinationen eine Rolle spielen. POPOW hält das Vorhandensein eines Hemmungsprozesses für das Zustandekommen von Halluzinationen für notwendig. Das ersieht man daraus, daß sie oft nachts oder abends auftreten oder sich verstärken, wenn der Hemmungsprozeß eine relative Vorherrschaft erlangt hat. Die Rolle der Hemmung ersieht man daraus, daß Coffein durch die Verstärkung des Erregungsprozesses eine zeitweilige Abschwächung oder das Verschwinden der Halluzinationen bewirkt.

Wie wir oben sagten, sind dem Nervensystem die Funktionen der *Analyse und der Synthese* eigen. Nach PAWLOW bestehen die großen Hemisphären aus einer Ansammlung von Analysatoren. Außer den Analysatoren, die die Erscheinungen der Außenwelt aufnehmen, verlangt PAWLOW die Annahme des Vorhandenseins besonderer Analysatoren, deren Aufgabe im Empfangen und Differenzieren der großen Menge von Empfindungen bestehen soll, die aus der inneren Sphäre, aus den Prozessen, die innerhalb des Organismus ablaufen, stammen. Eine große Anzahl solcher Analysatoren der inneren Sphäre wurden nach dem Tode von PAWLOW detaillierter erforscht. Es stellte sich heraus (BYKOW u. a.), daß die somatischen Organe sehr reich mit Baro-, Osmo-, Mechano- und Proprioreceptoren versehen sind, die man unter dem Allgemeinbegriff Interoreceptoren zusammenfaßt.

Die Tätigkeit der Großhirnrinde, wie auch anderer Teile des Gehirns, wird durch die Prozesse der Erregung und der Hemmung bestimmt. Diese Prozesse können von ihrem Ausgangspunkt aus in die Masse der Hemisphären irradiieren oder auch sich konzentrieren. PAWLOW nahm an, daß gerade die Prozesse der Erregungskonzentration der Bildung von Verbindungen zugrunde liegen, d. h. den bedingten Reflexen.

Das Auftreten bald positiver, bald negativer bedingter Reflexe in der Großhirnrinde, die die Tätigkeit und das Verhalten des Organismus bestimmen, wird durch die Einwirkung verschiedener Faktoren der Um- und Innenwelt bedingt. Jeder Reflex hat in der Hirnrinde seinen Ansatzpunkt, seine Zelle oder Zellgruppe. Gewisse Rindeneinheiten sind mit gewissen Tätigkeiten, andere mit anderen verbunden.

Auf diese Weise muß die Gehirnrinde einem riesigen Mosaik gleichen. Dieses funktionelle Mosaik befindet sich im Zustand ununterbrochener Bewegung, es stellt ein *dynamisches System* dar, das ständig zur Vereinheitlichung, zur Integration und Stereotypie strebt. Unter letzterer verstand PAWLOW eine bestimmte physiologische Beständigkeit der in der Hirnrinde entstehenden Prozesse bei Wiederholung durch ein und denselben Reizerreger.

3. Das Gehirn und das Denken. Die Typen des Nervensystems

Dem Denken liegt die analytisch-synthetische Tätigkeit der Großhirnrinde zugrunde. Die wechselseitigen Beziehungen zwischen dem Organismus und der Umwelt werden beim Menschen durch die Tätigkeit der Rinde der Hemisphären so vielseitig und vollkommen wahrgenommen, daß ihm dadurch eine führende Rolle in der Natur zugefallen ist. Das gestattet dem Menschen in seinen Wechselbeziehungen zur Umwelt, dieselbe aktiv umzugestalten und sie zu zwingen, seinen Interessen zu dienen. Nach Engels liegt die Ursache für die ungewöhnliche Entwicklung des Gehirns beim Menschen in der Arbeit und der artikulierten Sprache. Die qualitativen Besonderheiten der Entwicklung des menschlichen Gehirns führten zur Bildung des menschlichen Denkens; es kommt dank dem Erscheinen eines *zweiten Signalsystems* zustande, anders ausgedrückt, das Denken wird auf der Grundlage der *Sprache* durch die Gehirnrinde realisiert.

Das genaue Erfassen des *Begriffs des zweiten Signalsystems* und seine Abgrenzung vom ersten ist sehr wichtig.

Das zweite Signalsystem, nach der Definition von Pawlow eine außerordentliche Zugabe zu den Mechanismen des Nervensystems, stellt eine spezifische *Besonderheit der höchsten Nerventätigkeit des Menschen* dar.

Den Tieren wird die Wirklichkeit durch unmittelbare Gehör-, Gesichts- und andere Reize signalisiert; beim Menschen hat sich — durch das Wort — eine neue Signalisation herausgebildet. Durch das Wort wird etwas verallgemeinert, dadurch werden allgemeine Begriffe möglich. Die Begriffe der Zeit, des Raumes, der Ursache — auf die Analyse der Wirklichkeit angewendet — erweitern in hohem Maße die Möglichkeiten der Orientierung des Menschen in seiner Umwelt.

Die Wechselbeziehungen zwischen Mensch und Umwelt werden, wie schon oben erwähnt, durch drei Instanzen realisiert: durch den Subcortex mit seinen unbedingten Reflexen und durch die Rinde mit ihrem ersten und zweiten Signalsystem. Das zweite Signalsystem ist dabei der höchste Regulator des menschlichen Verhaltens. Durch dasselbe wird auch die subcorticale unbedingte Tätigkeit in erheblichem Maße reguliert. Nach Pawlow besteht das erste Signalsystem aus: „Eindrücken, Empfindungen und Vorstellungen von der umgebenden Außenwelt, d. h. sowohl der Natur als auch unserer sozialen Umwelt, mit Ausnahme des Wortes, des Sichtbaren und des Hörbaren." Das führt zur Schlußfolgerung, daß die Prozesse im Nervensystem, und sogar solche im subcorticalen Bereich, nicht als rein biologisch angesehen werden dürfen.

Die Lehre von den Signalsystemen führte zur These der *Einheit von Sprache und Denken*. Den Begriff des letzteren hält Pawlow in den Fällen für anwendbar, wo in der Rinde neue bedingte Verbindungen entstehen, eine Wechselwirkung des Alten mit dem Neuen als schöpferischer Vorgang stattfindet und das sich so Bildende Einschluß in der Rinde findet.

Wie schon erwähnt, hatte für Pawlow die Idee der Entwicklung, der *Evolution*, die von Darwin ausging und von Setschenow und Botkin entwickelt wurde, große Bedeutung. Diese Ideen sind auch für das Verständnis der Erscheinungen der Vererbung in der klinischen Forschung von Bedeutung. In dieser Hinsicht haben große Veränderungen in den Anschauungen der sowjetischen Forscher stattgefunden.

Lange Zeit sprachen sie im Gefolge von Weismann, Mendel, Morgan von einer besonderen Substanz, die unverändert von einer Generation der anderen übergeben wird und die Entstehung von Krankheiten und ihren Ausgang bestimmt — sozusagen ein Fatum darstellt. Dabei wurde den äußeren Umständen nur so viel Bedeutung beigemessen, als sie in der Lage waren, „eine Erkrankung zu provozieren".

Es ist für die zeitgenössischen sowjetischen Psychiater sehr charakteristisch, daß sie die Rolle der Vererbung nicht überschätzen, sondern den Einflüssen der Umwelt eine große Bedeutung einräumen. Die Gesetzmäßigkeiten der Vererbung werden im Licht neuer Daten überprüft. Solche Daten sind die von Mitschurin festgestellten Tatsachen. Er weist auf die Möglichkeit der *Vererbung erworbener Merkmale* hin. Diese Tatsachen wurden von ihm an Pflanzen erarbeitet, haben aber auch Bedeutung für den Menschen.

Auch das Wesen der *Konstitution* muß man im Lichte neuer Daten anders sehen. Zur Zeit der Überbewertung der Bedeutung der Erblichkeit wurde auch das Wesen der Konstitution falsch gesehen. Sie wurde als die Gesamtheit der erblichen Eigentümlichkeiten des Organismus definiert, die die Art seiner Reaktion auf äußere Schädlichkeiten bestimmten. In Gedanken verband man diese Eigentümlichkeiten mit bestimmten somatischen Anlagen, mit anderen

Worten, mit somatischen Konstitutionen. Letztere, ebenso wie die Erblichkeit, wurden als ein Fatum angesehen, das das Schicksal des Menschen und seine Neigung zu Erkrankungen vorausbestimmte. Solch eine Einstellung zur Definition des Begriffes Konstitution war das Resultat einer fälschlichen Loslösung des Organismus aus seiner Umwelt, ein Ignorieren des Prinzips der Entwicklung. Im Lichte der Lehre von MITSCHURIN stellt die Konstitution nichts Stabiles dar, sondern verändert sich im Laufe des Lebens unter dem Einfluß äußerer Faktoren. Dementsprechend müßte man die Konstitution als Reaktionseigentümlichkeiten des Organismus definieren, die sich auf der Grundlage der angeborenen und der besonders in frühen Perioden des Lebens erworbenen Eigenschaften entwickelt haben und die durch das Nervensystem bestimmt werden. Eine große Bedeutung kommt der Einwirkung *intrauteriner Schädigungen* zu.

Die sowjetischen Psychiater stellen den Einfluß der Eigentümlichkeiten der somatischen Anlage in Rechnung, aber sie geben ihnen nicht die Bedeutung, die KRETSCHMER ihnen zuerkennt. PAWLOW verurteilte seinen Versuch, eine Klassifikation der Konstitutionstypen zu schaffen, die einzelnen psychischen Erkrankungen entsprechen. Als falsche Interpretation von KRETSCHMERs Lehre sah er es an, daß man somatische Typen, ebenso wie die Erblichkeit, als ein die Erkrankung an einer bestimmten Psychose bedingendes Fatum betrachtete.

Um das Wesen der Konstitution zu verstehen, ist es sehr wichtig, die Lehre von den Typen des Nervensystems und der *Temperamente*, wie PAWLOW sie sah, zu berücksichtigen.

Er wandte seine Aufmerksamkeit vom Beginn der Erforschung der höchsten Nerventätigkeit an der Tatsache zu, daß Ergebnisse, die man unter gleichen Bedingungen bei verschiedenen Tieren erhält, durchaus verschieden sind. Auf dieser Grundlage entstand seine Lehre von den Typen des Nervensystems. Drei Merkmale liegen ihrer Klassifikation zugrunde: Kraft, Ausgeglichenheit und Lebhaftigkeit der Nervenprozesse. Auf diese Weise lassen sich *vier Grundtypen* bestimmen:

1. kräftig, unausgeglichen, hemmungslos,
2. kräftig, ausgeglichen, lebhaft,
3. kräftig, ausgeglichen, ruhig, zögernd,
4. schwach.

Ihnen entsprechen die vier Temperamente nach Hippokrates: das cholerische, sanguinische, phlegmatische und melancholische Temperament.

Nach PAWLOW ist der Begriff des Typus dynamisch. Unter dem Einfluß ungünstiger Faktoren kann ein starker Typus geschwächt und umgekehrt kann bei entsprechenden Bedingungen ein schwacher Typ des Nervensystems gefestigt werden. Ein starker Typus kann ausgeglichen und unausgeglichen, lebhaft und inert sein. Es gibt sowohl zahlreiche Variationen des starken wie auch verschiedene des schwachen Typus, die voneinander abweichen.

Die vier angeführten Typen erscheinen als die ausgeprägtesten und grundlegenden. Diese *Grundtypen* lassen sich nicht nur bei Tieren, sondern auch beim Menschen aussondern. Doch werden beim Menschen als Resultat der Entwicklung der Hemisphärenrinde und im Zusammenhang mit der Entwicklung des Denkens und der Sprache die Typen der Nerventätigkeit durch neue Züge und Eigentümlichkeiten bereichert, so daß man sie nicht immer streng unterscheiden kann. Der Mensch ist der Besitzer eines zweiten Signalsystems. Im Zusammenhang damit kann man bei ihm auch Persönlichkeitstypen feststellen, die hauptsächlich durch die Verschiedenartigkeit der Beziehungen zwischen dem ersten und zweiten Signalsystem unterschieden sind. So dominiert beim künstlerischen Typ das erste, beim Denker das zweite Signalsystem. Bei einem mittleren Typ befinden sich beide Systeme im Gleichgewicht.

II. Psychiatrie und bedingte Reflexe

Die *Annäherung der Psychiatrie an die Psychologie* gab den Klinikern die Möglichkeit zur volleren Charakterisierung der Typen in ihrer Anwendung auf den Menschen, wobei sie den Reichtum und die Vielseitigkeit seiner Psyche sowie die Entwicklung der Sprache, die sich im Einklang mit dem Denken befindet, in Betracht zogen. Die Persönlichkeit ist etwas Größeres als was durch die physiologischen Methoden der Forschung erfaßt werden kann. In diesem Zusammenhang unterstreicht Mjassischtscheff, daß die von den Psychiatern häufig gebrauchten Begriffe „Persönlichkeit", „Erlebnisse" psychologische Kategorien darstellen. Dementsprechend muß die Festlegung der Typen beim Menschen nicht bloß auf Grund von Experimenten sondern nach dem Studium der Persönlichkeit als Ganzem und der Geschichte ihrer Entwicklung erfolgen. Der erwähnte Reichtum und die Vielseitigkeit der psychischen Äußerungen des Menschen lassen annehmen, daß die Anzahl der Persönlichkeitstypen sich nicht auf die drei besprochenen begrenzen lassen kann.

1. Die Rolle des Nervensystems bei der Herausbildung der Krankheitserscheinungen und ihrer Rückbildung im Gesundungsprozeß

Pawlow brachte den Prozessen der Pathogenese große Aufmerksamkeit entgegen. Seiner Ansicht nach stellt die Krankheit immer einen Kampf des Organismus mit schädigenden Faktoren dar. Dementsprechend kann man in einem Krankheitsbild immer zwei Gruppen entgegengesetzter Erscheinungen feststellen. Die einen werden durch die unmittelbare Einwirkung schädigender Momente hervorgerufen, die anderen erweisen sich als Ausdruck des Kampfes des Organismus mit der Krankheit und stellen physiologische Schutzmaßnahmen dar. Dasselbe findet natürlich auch bei psychischen Erkrankungen statt, wenn das Nervensystem die ihm eigenen Funktionen des Schutzes des Organismus und der Wiederherstellung normaler Verhältnisse ausübt. Das Zentralnervensystem reguliert alle Prozesse im Organismus und hat natürlich eine große Bedeutung bei der Entwicklung der Krankheitserscheinungen, abgesehen davon, daß die Schwächung des Nervensystems die Kampffähigkeit gegen die äußeren Schädlichkeiten herabsetzt. Als Resultat somatischer Störungen, besonders unter dem Einfluß langdauernder psychischer Traumen bildet sich in der Rinde der Hemisphären das, was Pawlow als isolierte *pathologische Punkte* oder Zonen bezeichnete.

Sie werden dadurch charakterisiert, daß der reizerregende Prozeß in ihnen zu einem unnormal inerten und beständigen wird. Das Wesen dieser isolierten Punkte wurde in Tierexperimenten studiert, sie spielen aber auch in der menschlichen Pathologie eine Rolle: sie sind dynamisch und verändern sich in Abhängigkeit vom Allgemeinzustand der Rindenprozesse. Bei schwacher Ausprägung der Erscheinungen brauchen solche begrenzten Punkte nicht auf die Rinde im ganzen einzuwirken, was die Möglichkeit der kritischen Einstellung zu den Störungen, die mit ihnen verbunden sind, erklärt; so auch insbesondere die kritische Einstellung zu den Erscheinungen der fixen Idee. Doch die Veränderungen im isolierten Punkt können in das nächste pathologische Stadium übergehen, wo seine Reizung zur Störung der Tätigkeit der ganzen Rinde führt und dadurch die Bedingungen für die Entwicklung solcher Erscheinungen wie den Wahn geschaffen werden.

Bei der Aufstellung des *Behandlungsplanes* tragen die sowjetischen Psychiater diesen beiden Momenten Rechnung — dem Kampf mit der schädigenden Ursache und der Verstärkung der physiologischen Abwehrmaßnahmen, über die der Organismus verfügt. Die Behauptung Pawlows, daß das Nervensystem eine große Rolle in den Prozessen der Wiederherstellung normaler Beziehungen spielt, war kein einfaches Erraten oder eine zufällige Entdeckung, sondern basierte, wie alles bei ihm, auf den Resultaten der wissenschaftlichen Forschung, der genauen Beobachtung und dem Experiment.

Die Experimente von Asratjan sind ein Beispiel dafür, worauf Pawlow seine Schlußfolgerungen gründete. Asratjan führte eine teilweise Beinamputation bei Hunden durch und beobachtete die Wiederherstellung der Funktion in den verbleibenden Extremitäten, speziell in den Fällen, wo die Rinde unbeschädigt blieb. In den Fällen von Asratjan und einer Reihe analoger anderer besteht kein Zweifel daran, daß das Zentralnervensystem, und insbesondere die Rinde, bei der Wiederherstellung gestörter Funktionen eine Rolle spielt.

PAWLOW blieb vom Anfang bis zum Ende Physiologe; aber die theoretischen Schlußfolgerungen, zu denen er kam, eröffneten neue Möglichkeiten für die praktische Behandlung, die von seinen Mitarbeitern und Nachfolgern wahrgenommen wurden. Folgendes verdient in dieser Hinsicht Beachtung: die erste Hälfte seiner 36 jährigen wissenschaftlichen Arbeit war aufs rein Physiologische gerichtet, erst später wandte er sich der Neurologie und Psychiatrie zu. Sein bekanntes Werk: „Probeexkursion eines Physiologen in das Gebiet der Psychiatrie" gehört in das Jahr 1930. Es ist kein Zufall, daß er selbst, beim Kennenlernen seiner Kranken, die Resultate der bei ihnen angewandten speziellen Untersuchungen außer acht ließ und zur Entscheidung der Frage nach dem Charakter der bei ihnen beobachteten Störungen von den Ergebnissen ausging, die er im Tierexperiment gewonnen hatte.

Der Hinweis PAWLOWs, daß bei der Wiederherstellung normaler Beziehungen im Krankheitsfalle der Hemisphärenrinde eine bestimmende Rolle zufällt, erwies sich als sehr wertvoll; bei der Behandlung nervös-psychischer Erkrankungen sind die russischen Psychiater bestrebt, gerade auf die Rinde einzuwirken. Die *Schlaftherapie* erweist sich als die Methode, die zur Wiederherstellung normaler Beziehungen führt und genau dem entspricht, was PAWLOW von einer Behandlung fordert. Es ist eine der Methoden der Schutztherapie. Es werden dabei unangenehme Empfindungen unterdrückt und der Stoffwechsel normalisiert sich. Nach einem zehntägigen ununterbrochenen Schlaf erweist sich der Kranke als beruhigt und von halluzinatorischen und Wahnvorstellungen befreit. In den Fällen, in denen der unterbrochene Schlaf angewendet wird, dauert die Behandlung länger. Der Schlafzustand wird durch Einnehmen von Amytal herbeigeführt.

Seine bekannte Toxicität, wie auch die anderer Schlafmittel, führte zu dem Gedanken, die Schlaferzeugung durch einen schwachen elektrischen Strom zu erreichen. Wir haben eine Methode vorgeschlagen und sie zusammen mit LIWENTSEW, SEGAL und KYRILLOWA ausgearbeitet, den sog. *Elektroschlaf.*

Als rythmischen Erreger haben wir dabei schwach dosierte Gleichstromstöße angewandt. Bei der Einwirkung von Stromstößen mit einer Frequenz von 1—10 Stößen pro Sekunde, wobei die Elektroden an Auge-Hinterkopf oder Auge-Warzenfortsatz angelegt werden, und bei einer minimalen Dosierung des Stromes, die keine besonderen Empfindungen oder sichtbaren Reaktionen hervorruft, gelingt es in vielen Fällen, unter entsprechenden Bedingungen (Stille, ruhige Lagerung des Kranken), einen Schlafzustand von gutem therapeutischen Effekt zu erreichen. Diese Methode, die auf den Ergebnissen unserer Physiologen PAWLOW und WEDENSKY begründet ist, hat den Vorzug, daß dabei keine pharmazeutischen Mittel angewandt werden, während der durch Barbiturate erzeugte Schlaf doch ein toxischer ist.

Der Elektroschlaf kann zur Behandlung leichter Formen der Schizophrenie angewandt werden, er ist aber besonders bei Neurosen und reaktiven Zuständen angezeigt. Bei der Schizophrenie wird ein durch Barbiturate erzeugter Dauerschlaf angewendet.

Wie schon gesagt, hat der Elektroschlaf im Vergleich zu dem durch Amytal erzeugten den Vorzug des Ausschlusses der Möglichkeit toxischer Erscheinungen. Eine andere und sehr wichtige Eigentümlichkeit des Elektroschlafs ist die Schnelligkeit, mit der die Heilung oder Besserung eintritt. Bei dem durch Amytal erzeugten Schlaf erfolgt sie sehr langsam und allmählich. Wenn man die mit Elektroschlaf behandelten Menschen befragt, so muß man feststellen, daß der günstige Effekt sofort auftritt, was von ihnen selbst bemerkt wird: „sofort wird es gut, wie es vor der Erkrankung war", unverzüglich stellen sich wieder froher Mut und Leichtigkeit der Gedanken ein, „es wird so frisch im Kopf, als ob man das Gehirn durchgereinigt hätte", erklären die Kranken. Die Kranken geben an, daß sie nach dem Elektroschlaf eine Munterkeit und Frische empfinden wie nach einem guten, langdauernden Schlaf. Zugleich verschwinden verschiedene unangenehme Empfindungen — die Schwere im Kopf, das Gefühl der Gedankenleere; das Befinden wird ruhig, es verschwindet die Spannung, die Kranken sprechen von einem angenehmen Rauschgefühl. Im Verlauf der Behandlung mit Elektroschlaf werden die schweren, für die Schizophrenie charakteristischen Symptome abgelegt, es verschwindet der Autismus, die Abgrenzung gegen Andere. Die Kranken sagen: „es zieht uns zu unseren Verwandten."

Wie man aus dem Obigen ersieht, wird das Bewußtsein beim Elektroschlaf nicht so tief gehemmt, und deshalb können die Kranken über ihre Erlebnisse Bericht erstatten. Das schafft günstige Bedingungen für das Studium der Psychologie dieser Art Kranker.

Die Behandlung mit Elektroschlaf hat in der Sowjetunion eine große Verbreitung gefunden und ist dabei, ins Ausland vorzudringen. Fraglos ist sie eine Errungenschaft der sowjetischen Psychiatrie.

Für die sowjetische Psychiatrie ist überhaupt das Bestreben charakteristisch, sich alles Groben, was zum psychischen Trauma oder zu gefährlichen Komplikationen führen könnte, zu enthalten. Es ist darum nur natürlich, daß sich in der Sowjetunion die *Elektroschocktherapie* nicht einbürgern konnte. Die klinische Abteilung der Akademie der medizinischen Wissenschaften der UdSSR nahm im Jahre 1953 eine Resolution des Inhalts an, daß diese Methode nur dann angewandt werden darf, wenn alle anderen sich als erfolglos erwiesen haben.

Bei der Ausarbeitung der Methoden ihrer Therapie berücksichtigen unsere Psychiater die Hinweise Pawlows, daß bei der Wiederherstellung normaler Beziehungen der Hirnrinde wie überhaupt dem Zentralnervensystem die Hauptrolle zufällt, und darum sind sie bestrebt, bei der Behandlung auf das Zentralnervensystem einzuwirken.

Außer der Behandlung durch Schlaf bietet sich die Anwendung des *Stick(stoff)-oxyduls* an. Vor der Anwendung desselben bei Kranken wurde es an Gesunden ausprobiert, die sich freiwillig dazu erboten.

Beim Einatmen eines Gemisches von Stickoxydul mit Sauerstoff im Rahmen eines Experiments, stellt sich bei Gesunden das Gefühl der Leichtigkeit im Kopf ein, die Stimmung wird gehoben, die Zunge gelöst; man will ohne Unterlaß sprechen, singen, sich bewegen. Das Bewußtsein, daß dieses das Resultat der Einatmung des Gemisches ist, bleibt bestehen; die kritische Einstellung zu den eigenen Erlebnissen bleibt erhalten, ebenso die Möglichkeit, sich von der Ausführung, der das Bewußtsein ergreifenden Wünsche und Absichten zurückzuhalten. Gegen das Ende der zweiten Minute steigern sich die Euphorie und die motorische Erregung noch mehr. Alle unangenehmen Erlebnisse treten in den Hintergrund. Die unter der Einwirkung des Stickoxyduls Stehenden erzählen laut von den sie erfüllenden freudigen Gemütsbewegungen, führen weitausholende Bewegungen aus und fangen laut zu lachen an. Nach Ablauf der zweiten Einatmungsminute beginnt die zweite Phase der Wirkung des Gemisches: „das Gefühl der Schwere in allen Körperteilen, im Kopf ist es neblig, die Zunge versagt den Dienst, die euphorische Stimmung läßt nach, der Redefluß versickert. Man will schlummern, schlafen." Schließlich werden die äußeren Reize immer gedämpfter, es tritt ein angenehmer Dämmerzustand ein, der in einen kurzdauernden Schlaf — nicht länger als 20 min — übergeht. Beim Erwachen ist die Erinnerung an das Erlebte beinahe vollständig erhalten, und es werden keine Nebenerscheinungen wie Schwäche, Kopfschmerz oder Schwindel festgestellt. Stickoxydul wurde bei Schizophrenen, zirkulär und reaktiv Depressiven und Kranken mit neurotischen Reaktionen erfolgreich zu Behandlungszwecken angewandt.

Verschiedene therapeutische Methoden haben außer dem Behandlungseffekt noch eine experimentelle Bedeutung, indem sie die Natur der krankhaften Störung dem Verständnis näherbringen können. Aus diesem Grunde wird die Behandlung durch *Insulin-Koma* von den sowjetischen Psychiatern hochgeschätzt, ebenso die Behandlung mit Schlaf. In den letzten Jahren widmen sie den Substanzen aus der Reihe der *Phenothiazine* große Aufmerksamkeit, besonders dem Aminazin (dem Largactil und Chlorpromazin ausländischer Autoren) und dem Reserpin.

Es ist eine Menge von Beobachtungen gesammelt worden, die davon zeugen, daß Aminazin sich als sehr wirkungsvoll bei Erregungszuständen, wie man sie bei der manisch-depressiven Psychose und der zirkulären Schizophrenie beobachtet, erwiesen hat. Wir sprachen oben davon, daß von der Formatio reticularis Impulse zur Rinde der Hemisphären ausgehen, die ihren Tonus erhöhen. Aminazin gehört zu den Mitteln, die die Ganglien blockieren und führt zur Blockade der aufsteigenden Stimulationen. Das führt zur Abnahme oder Verminderung der Erregung des Kranken und zu seiner Beruhigung. Die Physiologen Moschkowsky, Anochin und die Psychiater Galenko, Tarassow u. a. haben viele Beobachtungen gesammelt, die eine Vorstellung von der Wirkung des Aminazin auf den tierischen und menschlichen Organismus geben. Bei den Tierexperimenten tritt in erster Linie seine sedative Wirkung hervor, wobei bei Erhöhung der Dosis eine Abnahme der motorischen Aktivität mit der weiteren Entwicklung eines schlafähnlichen Zustandes beobachtet wird. Die Fähigkeit des Aminazin, die Körpertemperatur zu senken, was besonders klar beim Tierversuch hervortritt, verdient Beachtung.

Bei der Behandlung psychisch Kranker mit Aminazin erweist es sich, daß es nicht nur auf die Erregungszustände einwirkt, sondern daß man auch von seiner *potenzierenden Wirkung* auf andere Substanzen sprechen kann. Seine kombinierte Anwendung mit Brom läßt einen besseren Effekt bei Anwendung geringerer Dosen des letzteren erzielen. Die Behandlung hypochondrischer Zustände mit Aminazin führt zu guten Erfolgen. Aminazin bringt großen Nutzen bei depressiven Zuständen, ebenso bei rastloser Aufgeregtheit; es kann auch bei verschiedenen Krampfzuständen, besonders bei Chorea und Bronchialasthma nützen.

Der Mechanismus der Wirkung von Aminazin ist nicht geklärt. Es gibt Gründe, eine Wirkung auf den subcorticalen Bereich anzunehmen. Physiologische Untersuchungen an Tieren sprechen dafür, daß die Reizung des reticulären Systems die Tätigkeit der Gehirnrinde aktiviert, sie quasi in einen wachen Zustand versetzt. Wie Anochin erklärt, geben afferente Bahnen von der Peripherie den Gehirnstamm durchlaufend eine bedeutende Anzahl kollateraler Abzweigungen in die Formatio reticularis ab. Hier werden diese aufsteigenden Impulse für eine bestimmte, nicht immer gleich lange Zeit in den synaptischen Umschaltstellen festgehalten. Im Resultat wird das reticuläre System zu einem eigenartigen Akkumulator der Energie afferenter Impulse; es aktiviert und reguliert die Rindentätigkeit. Die Beseitigung dieser Aktivierung führt zum Verlust des Rindentonus und zu einem schläfrigen Zustand der Tiere. Das alles ist auch für die menschliche Pathologie von Bedeutung.

Alles bezüglich des reticulären Systems Gesagte befindet sich in Übereinstimmung mit der Behauptung von Pawlow, daß der Subcortex die Rinde der Großhirnhemisphären auflädt, und stellt eine weitere Entwicklung dieser Ansicht dar. Dabei muß man beachten, daß die Aufladung aus dem subcorticalen Bereich sich nicht nur auf die motorischen, sondern auch auf die neuro-endokrinen und humoralen Prozesse bezieht.

2. Die Grundzüge der Umgestaltung der klinischen Psychiatrie auf der Grundlage der physiologischen Lehre von Pawlow

Wir sahen, daß die Lehre von den bedingten Reflexen kein enges Spezialkapitel der Physiologie darstellt, sondern die Grundlage zum Verständnis der höchsten Nerventätigkeit bildet. Sie hat der gesamten sowjetischen Medizin und nicht nur der Psychiatrie viel Neues gegeben.

In einer Art Nachfolge zu den Errungenschaften der sowjetischen Gelehrten stehend, berührt sie auch die Grundfragen der Pathologie und macht uns die Notwendigkeit der Überprüfung einer Reihe allgemein angenommener Behauptungen bewußt. Eine Eigenart des Denkens von Pawlow als Physiologen bestand darin, daß er die Pathologie und die Physiologie als eine Einheit betrachtete und im einzelnen die Psychiatrie als eine Helferin in der Erforschung der Tätigkeit der Hirnrinde ansah. Das gab ihm die Möglichkeit des volleren Verstehens und besseren Erklärens des Wesens der Krankheitsprozesse im Nervensystem. Er hat viele pathophysiologische Tatsachen festgestellt, an denen kein Psychiater bei der Bearbeitung von Fragen der allgemeinen Pathologie und der psychiatrischen klinischen Forschung vorbeigehen kann. Die Untersuchungen von Pawlow und seinen zahlreichen Mitarbeitern haben vor allem sehr viel für das Verständnis des Wesens der Psychosen und der Krankheit im allgemeinen ergeben. Es ist wichtig, die allgemeinen Ideen, die Pawlow in seiner wissenschaftlichen Tätigkeit leiteten, in Betracht zu ziehen. Hierzu muß man vor allem die Ideen des „*Nervismus*" — des Einflusses des Nervensystems auf die somatischen Veränderungen und auf alle Prozesse des Organismus — rechnen. Diese Ideen waren unseren großen Klinikern Botkin, Ostroumow, Manassein eigen. Unter ihrem wie auch Ssetschenoffs Einfluß bildete sich die Weltanschauung von Pawlow heraus.

Wenn man sich das Ziel setzt, eine Quintessenz dessen aufzustellen, was Pawlows Lehre von den bedingten Reflexen der Psychiatrie gegeben hat, so muß man besonders die Lehre von den Neurosen, von der Psychotherapie und das Problem der Schizophrenie ins Auge fassen.

3. Neurosen
a) Allgemeines

Zum Verständnis der pathophysiologischen Mechanismen der Klinik der Neurosen ist es erforderlich, die Ergebnisse des Studiums der von Pawlow experimentell erzeugten Neurosen in Betracht zu ziehen. Er war immer gegen die direkte Übertragung der im Tierexperiment gewonnenen Ergebnisse auf den Menschen, aber sowohl er wie auch seine Mitarbeiter haben durch ihre Untersuchungen bewiesen, daß die allgemeinsten Grundlagen der höchsten Nerventätigkeit gleiche Gültigkeit für den Menschen wie für die höheren Tiere haben; natürlich bezieht sich das auch auf die pathologischen Störungen. Die experimentell an Tieren ausgelösten Neurosen sind unkomplizierter als die klinisch beobachteten beim Menschen. Auf diese Weise eröffnet sich der Übergang vom Einfachen zum Komplizierten, mit anderen Worten: die Ergebnisse des Studiums der tierischen Neurosen dienen als eine Vorstufe zum Erforschen derselben beim Menschen.

Unter *Neurosen* verstand Pawlow *langanhaltende Abweichungen von der normalen höchsten Nerventätigkeit.* Diese Abweichungen werden durch Überspannung des reizerregenden oder hemmenden Prozesses, der Überpannung ihrer Beweglichkeit, dem Zusammenstoß zwischen Reiz und Hemmung verursacht. Beim Vorliegen dieser Bedingungen wird die normale höchste Nerventätigkeit gestört — es kommt zum Zusammenbruch. Bei Tieren z. B. führen übermäßig starke Reizerreger, schwierige Unterscheidungen zwischen komplizierten Reizerregern, schwierige Änderungen der dynamischen Stereotypie und andere experimentelle Verfahren zum Zusammenbruch. Das Studium der Typen des Nervensystems der Tiere zeigte, daß bei verschiedenen Typen unter gleichen Bedingungen die Störungen der höchsten Nerventätigkeit ganz verschieden sein können. Das eine oder andere Bild der Störung in Verbindung mit einem bestimmten Typus des Nervensystems, und gerade in Abhängigkeit von seinen Besonderheiten, stellt eine bestimmte Form der Neurose dar. Beim Menschen als Besitzer eines zweiten Signalsystems sind alle Erscheinungen komplizierter. Er beherrscht das Wort als Mittel der Verallgemeinerung (Abstraktion), die Sprache, die ein Instrument des Denkens ist. Das ist es, was den Menschen am meisten als soziales Wesen charakterisiert. Darum erweisen sich bei ihm auch die von der sozialen Umwelt ausgehenden Reize als besonders wirksam.

Diese Tatsachen steuern viel zum Verständnis des Mechanismus der Neurosenentwicklung beim Menschen bei. Unter gewohnten Bedingungen werden ungünstige Einwirkungen ausgeglichen und rufen keine krankhaften Reaktionen hervor, d. h. sie führen nicht zum Zusammenbruch. Der Mensch besitzt eine große Widerstandskraft, sein Nervensystem ist plastisch. Aber die Intensität der Reizung, die zur Überspannung des erregenden oder hemmenden Prozesses oder ihrem Zusammenstoß führt, kann so groß sein, daß der Mensch einen Zusammenbruch erlebt und an einer Neurose erkrankt. Die Schwächung der Widerstandskraft des Nervensystems durch irgendeine somatische Erkrankung leistet dem Vorschub.

Nicht selten entstehen neurotische Reaktionen in der *Rekonvaleszenz,* nach schweren somatischen Erkrankungen, gerade weil in dieser Periode die reaktive Lage des Organismus sich verändert und der Kranke weniger stabil gegenüber äußeren Einflüssen wird. Was früher spurlos an ihm vorbeiging, erhält nun große Wirksamkeit. Man muß aber nicht außer acht lassen, daß durch somatische

Faktoren nur der Boden für die Entstehung einer Neurose bereitet wird, nicht aber die Neurose selbst verursacht wird. Für ihre Entwicklung ist das Vorhandensein *psychotraumatischer Momente* notwendig. Im ganzen entstehen Neurosen dann, wenn der Mensch Schwierigkeiten begegnet, die er aus igendwelchen Gründen nicht bewältigen kann. Solche Schwierigkeiten können sich als Resultat des Verlustes der Angehörigen oder der früheren Stellung und auf Grund schwer erträglicher Lebens- und Arbeitsbedingungen entwickeln. Das Grundsätzliche in der Entwicklung einer Neurose wird im Lichte der Lehre von PAWLOW über die dynamischen Krankheitspunkte verständlich, von der oben die Rede war. Nach dieser Lehre können sich in der Rinde der Hemisphären unter dem Einfluß verschiedener krankheitserregender Ursachen scharf umgrenzte, isolierte Punkte oder Zonen bilden. Gerade bei einer Neurose findet die Bildung solcher kranker Punkte statt. Sie sind dynamisch, da sie in Wechselwirkung mit dem allgemeinen funktionellen Zustand der Rinde stehen. Die Korrelation verschiedener Seiten in den physiologischen Veränderungen ist bei verschiedenen Neurosen nicht gleich, und die Analyse dieser physiologischen Störungen kann zum besseren Verstehen und Unterscheiden der klinischen Erscheinungen verhelfen.

Zur Klärung der Eigenart der Neurosen beim Menschen ist folgender Ausspruch PAWLOWs von Wichtigkeit: „Die Annahme zweier Signalsysteme der Wirklichkeit beim Menschen, sollte man meinen, führt zum Verständnis des Mechanismus zweier menschlicher Neurosen: der Hysterie und der Psychasthenie."

Zum Verständnis der Neurosenstruktur muß man die Besonderheiten der Typen des Nervensystems, die PAWLOW auf Grund seiner Beobachtungen abgegrenzt hat, in Rechnung stellen. Die Vertreter des schwachen und des kräftigen hemmungslosen Typus erkranken leichter als andere an Neurosen. Am ungünstigsten sind die Bedingungen für den schwachen Typus. In einer ganz besonders schwierigen Situation, unter dem Einfluß eines sehr großen psychischen Traumas, können sich auch bei den Vertretern der ausgeglichenen Typen Neurosen entwickeln.

Wie man aus dem oben Dargelegten ersieht, entstehen die Neurosen unter dem Einfluß ungünstiger psychischer Einwirkungen der Umwelt. Wie MJASSISCHTSCHEFF sagt: „Es hat seine Bedeutung, wenn keine Übereinstimmung zwischen den Schwierigkeiten der äußeren Aufgaben und den inneren Möglichkeiten des Zentralnervensystems besteht."

Im Zentralnervensystem findet ständig die Bildung neuer und das Verlöschen früherer vorübergehender Verbindungen statt. Vorübergehende Verbindungen können sich fixieren, was für die Pathologie von großer Bedeutung ist. Vereinzelte neurotische Reaktionen können sich nach dem Prinzip des bedingten Reflexes fixieren: man kann das besonders deutlich bei Kindern verfolgen, besonders bei der Analyse nächtlicher Angstzustände, die sich nach einem Erschrecken des Kindes nachts im Schlaf einstellen. Hier findet die Bildung eines bedingten Reflexes in bezug auf Zeit oder Umgebung und andere mit dem erlittenen Schrecken zusammenhängende Situationsmomente statt. Ein Kind, welches beinahe an einem Pflaumenkern erstickt wäre, fürchtet sich auch vor Birnen, Äpfeln und anderen Gegenständen, weil zwischen dem erlebten Schrecken und dem Aussehen der Pflaume eine Assoziation entstanden ist, die sich auf alle ähnlichen Gegenstände erstreckt.

Die Neurose ist eine Allgemeinerkrankung des Organismus.

Bei manchen Kranken mit neurotischen Störungen sind die nervösen Empfindungen und vegetativen Störungen an die Tätigkeit irgendeines Organs geknüpft, des öfteren des Herzens oder Magens, und diese dominieren dann im Bilde der Krankheit. Das sind die sog. *Organneurosen.* Diese Syndrome beobachtet man besonders oft bei der Neurasthenie.

Alles Gesagte bezieht sich auf die Neurosen im allgemeinen, doch ihre klinischen Manifestationen in Einzelfällen sind verschieden. Die grundlegenden, für die Neurosen charakteristischen Störungen können in verschiedenen klinischen Formen ihren Ausdruck finden in Abhängigkeit von den Besonderheiten der Persönlichkeit, ihrem somatischen und emotionalen Zustand und der Situation, die zum Zusammenbruch führt. Die Krankheitsbilder der Neurasthenie, Hysterie,

Psychasthenie und der Zwangsneurosen sind am gründlichsten erforscht worden. Den krankhaften Störungen bei jedem von diesen Zuständen entsprechen eigene pathophysiologische Mechanismen.

b) Die Neurasthenie

Die Neurasthenie wurde Ende der sechziger Jahre des vorigen Jahrhunderts vom amerikanischen Arzt Byrd beschrieben. Ungeachtet der Mannigfaltigkeit der Krankheitserscheinungen ist es vergleichsweise ein einfach gebautes Bild der Neurose, zu dessen Verständnis der Vergleich mit den experimentellen Neurosen bei Tieren viel beiträgt. Bei letzteren führt die funktionelle Überbürdung zum Zusammenbruch; dasselbe Bild beobachten wir beim Menschen bei Überspannung der Erregungs- und Hemmungsprozesse. Beim Menschen als einem sozialen Wesen spielen der Charakter der Arbeit und die Bedingungen, unter denen sie stattfindet, die Aufregungen, mit denen sie verbunden ist, eine größere Rolle als die Belastung durch die Arbeit an sich. Bei der Neurasthenie handelt es sich um eine allgemeine Schwächung der höchsten Nerventätigkeit verbunden mit einer Unzulänglichkeit der Hemmungsprozesse, um die Hauptmomente anzuführen. Die Berücksichtigung dieser physiologischen Tatsachen verhilft zur Erklärung des klinischen Bildes, dessen Wesen in der erhöhten Erregbarkeit und Erschöpfbarkeit besteht.

Auch dem Typus des Nervensystems kommt eine Bedeutung zu. Meistens ist es der schwache oder hemmungslose Typus, ohne Überwiegen des ersten oder zweiten Signalsystems. Beim schwachen Typus wird die Grenze des Erträglichen eher überschritten. Im zweiten Falle ist es die ungeregelte Arbeit, das Fehlen eines richtigen Wechsels zwischen Arbeit und Erholung und der ungeregelte Schlaf, die zu dem gleichen Resultat führen. Als ständige Erscheinungen beobachtet man klinisch die Verschlechterung des Befindens und unangenehme Gefühle im ganzen Körper. Letztere sind auch oft im Kopf lokalisiert als Gefühle der Schwere und Spannung; oft wird über den schlechten, nicht erfrischenden Schlaf geklagt. Die Kranken klagen nicht selten über das Nachlassen ihrer Arbeitsfähigkeit und ihres Gedächtnisses, aber gewöhnlich erbringt die objektive Untersuchung bei Erholung und Ruhe keine Bestätigung dieser Beschwerden. Vieles ist durch vegetative Störungen zu erklären.

Beim Vorliegen einer starken physischen und nervösen Spannung kann man oft die Entwicklung einer Erschöpfung beobachten, die sich nicht in irgendwelchen speziellen nervösen Symptomen dokumentiert, sondern in vegetativen Störungen, die dazwischen auf den ersten Blick den Eindruck einer somatischen Erkrankung machen; die Kranken klagen über Dyspnoe, Herzklopfen, Schmerzen in der Herzgegend, Appetitlosigkeit, Übelkeit und andere Erscheinungen seitens des gastro-intestinalen Traktes. Diese Störungen stehen in Verbindung mit den Störungen der Regulation der vegetativen Prozesse seitens der höchsten Bezirke des Zentralnervensystems. In manchen Fällen werden bei Neurasthenikern die nervösen Empfindungen und vegetativen Störungen an die Tätigkeit irgendeines Organs geknüpft, des öftern des Herzens oder Magens, und erweisen sich als im Krankheitsbild dominierend.

Pawlow unterscheidet *zwei Formen der Neurasthenie:* im einen Fall wird die Herabsetzung der inneren Hemmung und die Vorherrschaft des Erregungsprozesses beobachtet, im anderen die Schwächung des Erregungsprozesses. Die erste Form wird häufiger angetroffen: bei ihr wird dank der gesteigerten Erschöpfbarkeit des Erregungsprozesses, dank seiner pathologischen Labilität, der Zustand erreicht, den man klinisch als reizbare Schwäche bezeichnet. Durch diesen Zustand ist die Leichtigkeit des Entstehens affektiver Reaktionen, die Explosivität, zu erklären.

c) Die Hysterie

Die Natur der hysterischen Störungen und der Hysterie im ganzen im Lichte der Ergebnisse der Erforschung der höchsten Nerventätigkeit.

Das allen Ärzten bekannte klinische Bild der psychischen Störungen bei Hysterie schließt eine große Anzahl verschiedenartiger und gleichsam mit einander nicht verbundener Veränderungen ein. Durch Berücksichtigung der ihm zugrunde liegenden Prozesse der höchsten Nerventätigkeit erhält dieses Bild bei näherer Betrachtung doch einen ganzheitlichen und einheitlichen Charakter.

Die Abweichungen im klinischen Bild stehen im Zusammenhang mit den Besonderheiten der nervösen Organisation der betreffenden Hysteriker, dem Typus des Nervensystems und allen Erlebnissen der Vergangenheit. Die größte Bedeutung für die Entwicklung der Hysterie haben psychische Traumen. Sie führen zur Erkrankung, sie haben auch Einfluß auf ihre Gestaltung. Nicht nur Personen mit schwachem Nervensystem ("schwacher Typus" nach PAWLOW) können unter dem Einfluß ihrer Erlebnisse an Hysterie erkranken, sondern — beim Vorhandensein somatischer Schwächungen — auch Personen des ausgeglichenen Typus. Bei Hysterikern stellt man das Überwiegen des ersten Signalsystems fest. Wie PAWLOW zeigte, bildet die Schwäche des Nervensystems eine Grundlage für die Entwicklung der Hysterie. Ein schwaches Nervensystem unterliegt unter ungünstigen Umwelteinflüssen leicht der Hemmung, was sich besonders auf die Rinde der Hemisphären als den reaktivsten Teil bezieht. Diese Hemmung liegt vielen hysterischen Störungen zugrunde, wobei je nach der Intensität der Hemmung und der Bereiche, auf die sie sich erstreckt, verschiedene Bilder entstehen. Die Schwäche der Rinde bildet den Grund für die Aktivität der Tätigkeit des subcorticalen Bereichs, was die erhöhte Emotionalität und Erregbarkeit, die affektiven Ausbrüche und Anfälle erklärt. Ungünstige äußere Einwirkungen führen zur Bildung isolierter "kranker" Punkte in der Rinde oder zu ihrer verstärkten emotionalen Anspannung, wenn sie schon vorhanden waren. Bei Schwäche der Rinde rufen sie eine starke, ausgebreitete negative Induktion übriger Teile der Rinde hervor, was die Wirksamkeit anderer Momente außer denen, die zum Wesen des psychischen Traumas gehören, ausschließt und den Einfluß in der Vergangenheit erworbener Erfahrungen zunichte macht.

Das Bestehen solcher isolierter "kranker" Punkte erklärt eine gewisse Stabilität und Wiederkehr derselben nervösen Symptome sowie deren Entwicklung nach einem bestimmten Typus, entsprechend den Mechanismen des bedingten Reflexes.

Dank derselben Schwäche und leichteren Hemmbarkeit der Hemisphärenrinde erscheinen auch die gewöhnlichen Reizungen überdurchschnittlich und werden von ausgedehnter überschüssiger Hemmung begleitet. Kraft dessen muß man einen Hysteriker auch unter gewöhnlichen Umständen als einen quasi Hypnotisierten ansehen. Im Zusammenhang damit steht auch die Suggestibilität und Autosuggestibilität der Kranken.

Nach PAWLOW ist die Suggestion eine konzentrierte Reizung einzelner Punkte der Hemisphären, die durch Worte, Empfindungen oder Vorstellungen ausgelöst wird. Diese Reizung ist wirksam, weil sie bei schwacher Rinde und deren geringem Tonus von einer starken negativen Induktion begleitet wird, die, wie wir schon sagten, von anderen Einflüssen befreit. Das ist derselbe Mechanismus, durch den die Suggestion in der Hypnose herbeigeführt wird. Für die Wirksamkeit der Suggestion ist es erforderlich, daß sie vom Kranken akzeptiert wird, wozu außer dem Bestehen einer besonders veränderten Bewußtseinslage beim Kranken, ein Eingehen auf seine Stimmung und die Richtung seiner Gedanken vorliegen muß. Als den Trägern eines schwachen Nervensystems ist es solchen Kranken eigen, ihrer Krankheit große Bedeutung beizumessen, doch können ihre Gedankengänge verschieden sein. Dazwischen scheint die Krankheit sie in ihren eigenen Augen zu erhöhen, wobei sie von der eigenen Einbildungskraft hingerissen, sich öfters in ihren Behauptungen von der Wirklichkeit entfernen. In einer Reihe von Fällen übertreiben sie ihre Klagen, scheuen nicht davor zurück, ihre Temperatur künstlich zu erhöhen oder die Aufmerksamkeit auf irgendein Symptom einer bei ihnen nicht existierenden Krankheit zu lenken.

Um das Wesen dieser Krankheitsbilder der Hysterie zu verstehen, die an Simulation gemahnen, aber keine sind, muß man das physiologische Bild in Betracht ziehen. Unter dem Einfluß einer starken Reizung gerät die schwache Hirnrinde in einen Zustand überschüssiger Hemmung, analog einer solchen bei der Hypnose. In diesem Zustand können stark emotional betonte Vorstellungen entsprechende krankhafte nervöse Erscheinungen hervorrufen. Es ist eine Art Autosuggestion der Kranken. Daher sprechen die Kliniker von der erhöhten Suggestibilität und Autosuggestibilität der Hysteriker. Unter dem Eindruck schwerer Krankheitsbilder bei anderen werden Vorstellungen erweckt, die suggestiv wirken. In solchen Fällen sind die Krankheitserscheinungen psychogen; doch ihre Analyse erweist nicht die Berechtigung, von einer Simulation zu sprechen. Es ist bekannt, daß die an Hysterie Leidenden — meistens Vertreter des schwachen Typus — nicht immer genügend innere Kräfte zur Überwindung ihrer Symptome aufbringen können. Damit erklärt sich sie sog. „Flucht in die Krankheit", genauer gesagt, das Steckenbleiben in ihr.

Die Berücksichtigung der Veränderungen der höchsten Nerventätigkeit ergibt eine klare Vorstellung von der Hysterie. Im Lichte derselben physiologischen Ergebnisse können auch die Mechanismen der Entwicklung einzelner Störungen, die eine besonders große Rolle in der Klinik dieser Krankheit spielen, geklärt werden.

Der *hysterische Anfall* hat die Hemmung zur Grundlage, doch die Hemmung der Rinde führt durch Induktion zur Reizung der subcorticalen Gegend; im Resultat schlagen die Kranken um sich, schreien, nehmen verschiedene, teils sexuelle, teils abwehrende Posen an. Das Bild des hysterischen Anfalls steht nicht nur unter dem Einfluß des soeben Erlebten, sondern auch der Erlebnisse der Vergangenheit, sofern sie eine Spur in der emotionalen Sphäre hinterlassen haben.

So war es in der Vergangenheit bei der „Kommando-Hysterie", bei der die Kranken im Zustande einer Bewußtseinsverdunklung die Bilder einer Schlacht nacherlebten. In der Vergangenheit, als der Glaube an Behexung und Zauberei verbreitet war, fanden hysterische Störungen ihren Ausdruck in der „klikuschestwo" (in hysterischen Schreianfällen). Dabei schrie der Kranke oder die Kranke im Anfall die Namen der Leute, die sie behext, „verdorben" haben sollten. Gewöhnlich konnte man solche Anfälle an öffentlichen Orten, z. B. Kirchen. beobachten, wobei zufällig anwesende andere Hysterische sich dem Anfall anschlossen.

Hysterische Dämmerzustände, wie auch andere hysterische Störungen, entwickeln sich im Zusammenhang mit psychischen Aufregungen. Als wesentlich muß man dabei die Konzentrierung des Bewußtseins auf bestimmte Vorstellungskreise ansehen, wobei alles übrige gehemmt ist. Es ist charakteristisch, daß die Umstände, unter denen das Trauma erlitten wurde, ihre Spiegelung in den Gemütsbewegungen und dem Benehmen der Patienten finden.

Sehr anschaulich ist in dieser Beziehung folgender Fall; denn alle Krankheitserscheinungen sind hier in ihrer Entwicklung eng mit den Momenten des psychischen Traumas verbunden. Das psychische Trauma wurde ständig größer und dementsprechend nahmen auch die krankhaften Störungen zu.

Es handelte sich um eine Frau von 30 Jahren, von schwacher Gesundheit und schüchternem Charakter. Sie hatte mit 20 Jahren geheiratet. Das Familienleben erwies sich als sehr unglücklich. Der Mann betrog sie ständig und kümmerte sich nicht um die Familie. In den letzten 7 Jahren konnte man bei der Kranken neben allgemeiner Nervosität mit Krämpfen in der Kehle auch des öfteren hysterische Anfälle beobachten. Vor vier Monaten verließ der Mann sie endgültig, indem er ihr in das Entbindungsheim, in dem sie lag, eine offizielle Scheidungsurkunde schickte. Unmittelbar darauf geriet sie in einen Zustand veränderten Bewußtseins vom Dämmertypus. Wie es ihr schien, war der Mann zu ihr zurückgekehrt. In ihren Halluzinationen sah sie auch ihre Tochter, der vor kurzem eine Operation gemacht worden war. — Es ist von Bedeutung, daß bei ihr im Verlauf von 16 Jahren 18 Schwangerschaften eingetreten waren, von denen drei zu Geburten führten. Die somatische Schwächung hatte fraglos eine Bedeutung, doch sie führte nicht zur Nervenerkrankung, sondern bereitete nur den Boden für die Wirksamkeit des Hauptmoments, des psychischen Traumas, vor. — Man muß auch in Betracht ziehen, daß der Mann sie zu einer Zeit verließ, in der sie besonders auf die Teilnahme eines ihr nahestehenden Menschen angewiesen war, in der Periode der Schwangerschaft, wo das Nervensystem besonders empfindlich reagiert. Hier tritt besonders deutlich die Rolle des isolierten „kranken" Punktes hervor, der sich als Ergebnis der Erlebnisse, die mit ihrem Mann verknüpft waren, herausbildete.

Wie aus allem Dargelegten zu ersehen ist, hat Pawlow eine streng wissenschaftliche Konzeption der Hysterie gegeben. Es ist in diesem Zusammenhang nicht überflüssig, sich daran zu erinnern, daß zu Anfang des 20. Jahrhunderts 50 Theorien der Hysterie von Janet gezählt wurden, die heute alle vergessen sind.

d) Die Psychasthenie

Als erster beschrieb JANET die Psychasthenie. Lange Zeit waren ihre Grenzen undeutlich und zu weit gesteckt. Das hing hauptsächlich mit der Mannigfaltigkeit des klinischen Bildes zusammen, mit der Tatsache, daß die eigentlichen neurotischen Symptome der Psychasthenie sich auf dem Hintergrunde einer eigenartigen psychischen Anlage entwickeln, die sich in manchen Fällen durch Besonderheiten auszeichnet, die die Bezeichnung Psychopathie als berechtigt erscheinen lassen. Als besonders für die Psychasthenie charakteristisch sah JANET das Vorhandensein eines eigenartigen Denkens, das er als „geistiges Wiederkäuen" bezeichnete, sowie den Verlust des Gefühls für die Realität an, weswegen die umgebende Wirklichkeit in Form von blassen blut- und körperlosen Gestalten erlebt wird.

Die Häufigkeit der Zwangszustände bei der Psychasthenie erklärte er durch primäre Schwäche des Denkprozesses.

Beobachtungen der Forscher verschiedener Länder bekräftigten die Gültigkeit seiner Ansichten, ergänzten seine Beschreibungen durch viele wesentliche Züge und gaben auf diese Weise eine vollere Vorstellung von der Psychasthenie als Ganzem.

Die Grundzüge der psychischen Anlage der Psychastheniker wurden klar. Menschen dieser Art sind immer unentschlossen, haben kein Selbstvertrauen, schwanken ständig und sind voller Zweifel in bezug auf sich und ihre eigenen Kräfte. Jede neue Situation schreckt sie; Schwierigkeiten, die, um die Lage zu meistern, überwunden werden müssen, erscheinen ihnen unüberwindlich; es erscheint ihnen alles kompliziert, über alles müssen sie grübeln. In anderen Fällen bilden Rastlosigkeit und Ängstlichkeit die grundlegenden Eigenschaften der Persönlichkeit, allem voran stehen hier das Bewußtsein der eigenen Schwäche, der Zweifel an den eigenen Kräften. Die Kranken befinden sich ständig in Aufregung und sind geneigt, das Schlimmste zu erwarten.

Auf der Grundlage der der Psychasthenie eigenen psychischen Anlage und in Verbindung mit der Verschlechterung des Allgemeinzustandes durch Übermüdung oder Schwächung infolge somatischer Erkrankungen, können sich die Erscheinungen der *Zwangsvorstellung* entwickeln, die im Zusammenhang mit den Besonderheiten der psychischen Anlage stehen. Die ausgesprochene Angst vor Verantwortung findet ihre Entsprechung in der endlosen Durchsicht von Dokumenten, dem Geldzählen, dem Zählen der Gegenstände im Zimmer; die krankhafte Ängstlichkeit äußert sich in ständigem Händewaschen oder überflüssigen Vorsichtsmaßnahmen. Diese Erscheinungen können so ausgeprägt sein, daß sie für den Kranken eine reguläre Arbeit schwierig oder sogar unmöglich machen können.

Aus diesem Grunde hat man lange Zeit die Psychasthenie und die Zwangsneurosen für Synonyme gehalten, was aber nicht zutrifft. Gerade die physiologischen Untersuchungen PAWLOWS und seiner Mitarbeiter zeigten die Richtigkeit und Notwendigkeit ihrer Abgrenzung und verhalfen zum Verständnis der Psychasthenie und des Wesens der ihr zugrundeliegenden Störungen.

Die Analyse dieser Besonderheiten beweist die Wichtigkeit der Lehre PAWLOWS von den Signalsystemen. Bei der Psychasthenie sind die subcorticale Gegend und das erste Signalsystem besonders geschwächt, es überwiegt die Tätigkeit des zweiten Signalsystems. Gerade deswegen sind alle Erlebnisse der Psychastheniker blaß, bar jeder Farbigkeit und Lebendigkeit. Diese ungenügende Lebensnähe der unmittelbaren Eindrücke bildet die Grundlage zum Verlust des Gefühls der Realität. Das Denken erweist sich bis zu einem gewissen Grade als losgelöst von den Ansprüchen des realen Lebens und nimmt den Charakter zwecklosen Tüftelns und des Steckenbleibens in Kleinigkeiten an; so wird die von JANET gegebene Charakteristik des „geistigen Wiederkäuens" bei den Psychasthenikern gerechtfertigt.

e) Die Zwangsneurosen

Es gibt sehr verschiedenartige Zwangsvorstellungen. Dazwischen kommen sie in Verbindung mit anderen psychischen Störungen vor, doch können sie auch das ganze klinische Bild beherrschen, so daß man von einer Zwangsneurose sprechen kann. Vereinzelte Zwangssymptome kann man auch bei psychisch gesunden Menschen, besonders im Zustand der Übermüdung, beobachten, aber ihr ausgeprägtes Bild entwickelt sich auf dem Boden krankhafter Vorgänge. Einen solchen Boden können die Psychasthenie, die Hysterie und depressive Zustände verschiedener Genese abgeben.

Es erweckt großes Interesse, daß Zwangszustände auch bei der Schizophrenie angetroffen werden. Diese Frage hat die Aufmerksamkeit sowohl sowjetischer als auch ausländischer Forscher erweckt. Es stellte sich heraus, daß sie bei der Schizophrenie sowohl als Prodromalzustand als auch im späteren Verlauf auftreten können. Bei ihrer klinischen Abgrenzung (Klassifizierung) muß man dazwischen mit der Schwierigkeit der Abgrenzung der Schizophrenie gegen die Neurosen rechnen. Mayer-Gross hält es für möglich, daß viele von Janets Psychasthenikern in Wirklichkeit Schizophrene waren. Zwangserscheinungen bei Zwangsneurosen entwickeln sich in typischen Fällen bei Menschen, die keine Besonderheiten des Charakters oder eine ausgeprägte Nervosität aufweisen.

Als Ausgangspunkt für die Entwicklung von Zwangsvorstellungen dient ein starkes affektives Erlebnis, das den üblichen Fluß der Vorstellungen durchbricht und in ihr Zentrum diejenigen stellt, die mit dem psychischen Trauma verbunden sind. Hierdurch ist die Konkretheit der Störungen sowie ihre Begrenzung auf vergleichsweise einige wenige Symptome der Zwangsvorstellungen erklärt, die aber von einer charakteristischen Beständigkeit sind. Die Erklärungen eines behandelnden Arztes bei einem psychisch Kranken lösen ein Trauma aus, wenn der Arzt zur Erklärung der Krankheit besondere, dem Laien unverständliche Bezeichnungen gebraucht. Einem Kranken wurde gesagt, daß sein nervus ischiadicus nicht in Ordnung sei. Der Kranke setzte sich in den Kopf, daß „ischiadicus" die Bezeichnung einer schweren Krankheit sei, und die Gedanken daran erhielten einen Zwangscharakter. Es kommt auch vor, daß ein Arzt den Ernst einer Krankheit übertreibt, um den Kranken dazu zu veranlassen, ihr mehr Beachtung zu schenken. So geschah es bei einem Kranken, der auch von Prof. Kannabich beobachtet wurde. Der Kranke hatte keine ausgesprochenen Beschwerden, wandte sich aber an einen Arzt, um seinen „Gesundheitszustand überprüfen zu lassen". Unerwartet für den Kranken teilte der Arzt ihm mit, daß bei ihm große Veränderungen am Herzen vorlagen, und sagte sogar, daß er kein Herz, sondern „irgendsoein Läppchen" statt eines Herzens hätte. Der Kranke erschrak, wurde bettlägerig und horchte an seinem „Läppchen" herum in der Erwartung, daß es ganz zu arbeiten aufhören würde. Nach einiger Zeit erholte er sich vollständig.

Als Grundlage der fixen Ideen sah Pawlow eine gestaute oder inerte Erregung an und sprach speziell von kranken Punkten. Ihr Charakter ist abhängig von den Besonderheiten der psychotraumatisch wirksamen Momente, welche auch die Richtung der Zwangsvorstellungen und ihre Symptomatik bestimmen. Diese physiologischen Daten ermöglichen das Sichdurchfinden in der klinischen Vielgestaltigkeit des Krankheitsbildes und die deutliche Abgrenzung der eigentlichen Zwangsneurosen von der Psychasthenie. Bei letzterer ist die psychische Anlage der Boden, auf dem die Zwangsvorstellung entsteht. Bei der Zwangsneurose bildet ein starkes affektbetontes Erlebnis die Grundlage, die zur Bildung eines kranken Punktes führt. Ihrem Wesen nach sind es psychische Reaktionen, die ursprünglich natürlich waren, wie z. B. ein Angstzustand bei einer gefährlichen Situation. Hier aber findet die übliche Rückentwicklung nicht statt, sondern der Zustand wird auf Grund eines schwachen Nervensystems fixiert, und es kommt zur Entwicklung einer gestauten Erregung; im weiteren Verlauf wird dieser Zustand entsprechend dem Mechanismus des bedingten Reflexes auch durch andere Reize hervorgerufen. Der *Herd einer gestauten Erregung*, der zur Zwangsvorstellung führt, kann so stabil sein, daß er nicht durch Erregungen aus anderen Bezirken gehemmt werden kann, und so wird die Zwangsvorstellung beständig. Dabei kann ein an Zwangsneurose erkrankter Mensch eine kritische Einstellung zu seinen Erlebnissen bewahren; denn der isolierte Herd einer gestauten Erregung ist nicht in der Lage, die Tätigkeit der gesamten Rinde zu stören.

f) Neurosen und Psychopathien

Wie wir schon sagten, ist die von PAWLOW geschaffene Lehre von den bedingten Reflexen keine enge Spezialdoktrin, die nur einen beschränkten Kreis klinischer Erscheinungen umfaßt. Sie stellt einen Teil der Lehre von der Physiologie des Nervensystems dar, jenes Systems, das alle Prozesse im Organismus reguliert: das betrifft insbesondere ihre Dynamik, ihre Entwicklung. Wir sahen, daß die Neurosen in einer Reihe von Fällen eine Art Persönlichkeitsentwicklung darstellten. Das bezieht sich auch auf die Psychopathien, die man als eine Art *pathologischer Entwicklung der Persönlichkeit* betrachten muß. Man kann sie in eine Reihe mit den neurotischen Persönlichkeitsentwicklungen stellen, da in beiden Fällen mit derselben Gesetzmäßigkeit zu rechnen ist. In dieser Beziehung kann man keine scharfe Grenze zwischen neurotischen und psychopathischen Erkrankungen ziehen.

Auch BECHTEREW, der sowohl auf dem Gebiet der Neurologie wie auf dem der Psychiatrie gleichermaßen kompetent war, sah keinen prinzipiellen Unterschied zwischen ihnen. So sah auch PAWLOW die Lage der Dinge an. Seine bekannten Mittwochstreffen lockten in gleichem Maße die Neuropathologen wie die Psychiater herbei. An diesen „Mittwochen" wurden verschiedene Fälle von psychischen und Nervenkrankheiten unter dem Gesichtspunkt physiologischer Konzeptionen diskutiert, die sich für die Klärung der Natur beider Krankheitsarten als gleich wichtig erwiesen. CHARCOT und BABINSKI waren große Neuropathologen und haben viel zum Studium der Hysterie beigetragen; aber für CHARCOT sie war sie eine rein neurologische Störung. Erst BABINSKI sprach vom «pithiatisme», Störungen, die durch eine Art Suggestion hervorgerufen werden.

Die Klinik der Hysterie, außer den Störungen, die unter dem neurologischen Aspekt betrachtet werden können — wie z. B. der Mutismus sowie einige Paralysen und Anaesthesien — wird durch das Vorhandensein einer bestimmten psychischen Anlage charakterisiert. Trotzdem kann der Boden, auf dem sich die Hysterie entwickelt, vollwertig sein, und die Krankheit entwickelt sich nur auf Grund extrem schwerer Erlebnisse.

Für die Psychopathie ist aber ein pathologischer Boden die Voraussetzung. Sie kommt durch angeborene oder in den frühen Perioden des Lebens erworbene Veränderungen des Nervensystems zustande. Diese Veränderungen setzen die Widerstandsfähigkeit gegen äußere Schädlichkeiten und ungünstige Einflüsse der Umwelt herab. Sie können als Resultat von Infektionen und Intoxikationen sowie traumatischen Schädigungen entstehen, auch wenn sie keine deutlichen Veränderungen des Gehirnsubstrats hinterlassen. Die Persönlichkeit entwickelt sich in solchen Fällen unter ungünstigen Bedingungen und weist psychopathische Züge auf, deren Charakter und Besonderheiten den Stempel der Umwelt und ihrer ungünstigen Einflüsse tragen. Die Klinik der Psychopathien weist eine große Mannigfaltigkeit auf. Um zu begreifen, warum eine bestimmte Form sich ausgebildet hat, muß man das ganze Leben des Betreffenden kennen, mit allen Momenten, die bei der Ausformung gerade dieser gegebenen Psychopathie eine Rolle gespielt haben. Dabei lassen sich Ansatzpunkte für eine effektive Therapie finden.

KORSAKOW sprach seiner Zeit davon, daß der Verlauf und der Ausgang einer Psychose von den Bedingungen abhängt, unter die der Kranke gestellt wird. Das trifft in noch höherem Maße auf die Psychopathien zu. In Übereinstimmung mit den Gedanken von KORSAKOW sprachen wir die Ansicht aus, daß die Menschen gewöhnlich nicht als Psychopathen geboren werden, sondern dazu erst unter dem Einfluß verschiedener ungünstiger Momente werden. Unter Umständen tritt das ein, wenn irgendein spezieller Charakterzug der betreffenden Person übermäßig ausgeprägt ist.

4. Die Schizophrenie

Seit Beginn des Jahrhunderts bewegt der Gedanke an das Wesen der Schizophrenie und ihre adäquateste Definition die Psychiater. Nacheinander entwickelten sich die Begriffe der Dysnoesie von Korsakow, der Schizophrenie von Bleuler, der dissoziativen Zustände nach Baruk, des diskordanten Irreseins nach Chasselin, der Desorganisation nach Mayer-Gross. Psychiater verschiedener Länder gelangten unabhängig voneinander zu diesen Definitionen. Sie beinhalten dasselbe: den Gedanken des Gespaltenseins, der Zersplitterung als Grundzug der Erkrankung. Jeder von den oben genannten Autoren geht auf seine Weise an die Lösung der Frage heran. Auch die sowjetischen Psychiater haben ihren eigenen Standpunkt.

Unsere Psychiatrie erfährt einen Umbau auf der Grundlage der physiologischen Lehre von Pawlow. Es ist nur natürlich, daß sie auch die Lehre von der Schizophrenie auf der gleichen Grundlage aufbaut. Als Nachfolger Pawlows stellen unsere Psychiater die Behauptung von der Einheit aller Prozesse im Organismus, von der Einheit psychischer Erlebnisse auf. Diese Einheit wird durch die Tätigkeit des Zentralnervensystems gewährleistet. Die Schwächung dieser Tätigkeit führt zur Störung der Einheit. Alle Prozesse, die früher eine Ganzheit darstellten, werden nun getrennt, und die psychische Tätigkeit wird chaotisch. Die Störung der Einheit betrifft vor allem das Bewußtsein der eigenen Persönlichkeit. Von Wichtigkeit ist auch das Bewußtsein, daß ein bestimmtes Erlebnis gerade einer bestimmten Person zugehört, d. h. ein persönliches ist. Das „Ich" der Schizophrenen ist dieser Eigenschaft und vor allem der Einheit beraubt. Es erscheint verändert, quasi ausgetauscht. Die Tatsache, daß diese Kranken manchmal in der dritten Person von sich selbst sprechen, steht damit im Zusammenhang. Dadurch wird vor allem das Vorhandensein tiefgreifender *Veränderungen im Ichbewußtsein* bestätigt. In der Weiterentwicklung können diese Störungen zum vollständigen Zerfall der Persönlichkeit führen. Die Erlebnisse des Kranken verlieren den Zugehörigkeitscharakter, vereinzelte Vorstellungen oder Gruppen von Vorstellungen erscheinen als etwas Fernes, Fremdes, von außen Eingegebenes. Ein gesunder Mensch, der etwas erörtert, wägt das pro und contra ab und findet schließlich zu einem eindeutigen Entschluß, demzufolge er dann auch handelt.

Nicht so bei der Schizophrenie; der Kranke befindet sich in der Gewalt gegensätzlicher Strebungen, Gedanken und Stimmungen. Man kann beobachten, wie der Kranke unentschlossen dasteht, sich mal nach der einen, mal nach der anderen Seite bewegt und nicht weiß, was er tun soll. Das ist das Bild des gegensätzlichen Strebens = Ambitendenz — gegensätzliche Tendenzen verhindern eine einheitliche Wirkung. Bei der *Ambivalenz* können gegensätzliche Tendenzen, Gefühle und Gedanken gleichzeitig nebeneinander bestehen. Typisch für die Schizophrenie sind der *Negativismus* und sein Gegenteil, die passive Unterordnung, wobei der Kranke ohne jeden Widerstand allen Forderungen nachkommt. Zu den Störungen der Einheit, den Erscheinungen der Dissoziation, muß man auch das Nichtübereinstimmen der intellektuellen und der emotionalen Erlebnisse rechnen, ebenso deren Abweichungen von der allgemein üblichen Verhaltensweise. Der Kranke kann mit teilnahmsloser Stimme und Gleichgültigkeit von einem tragischen Ereignis berichten, das einen ihm nahestehenden Menschen betroffen hat.

Als auf ein Beispiel besonders abweichenden Verhaltens weisen wir auf eine unserer Kranken hin, die auf der Beerdigung ihres Mannes tanzte und schrie, daß es der herrlichste Tag ihres Lebens sei; dabei hatte sie ihn vor ihrer Erkrankung heiß geliebt. Oft kann man die äußerste Gefühlskälte bei Schizophrenen gegenüber ihren Angehörigen, sogar der Mutter, beobachten. Ein Schizophrener versuchte, die Hand seiner Mutter zu verrenken, während er sie zum Abschied küßte. Ein anderer hätte beinahe seine kranke Tante erwürgt, wobei er ihr sagte: „Du hast genug gelebt, nun reicht es!" Charakteristisch für die Schizophrenen sind:

Egozentrismus, Egoismus, die Unfähigkeit, die Interessen anderer zu teilen, die Abschließung von den anderen. Die Mutter eines Kranken drückte das so aus: „Er lebt nicht mit den Leuten, er lebt ‚zwischen den Leuten'."

Ein sehr charakteristisches, wenn auch kein ständiges Symptom der Schizophrenie sind die Halluzinationen, vor allem solche des Geruchs, Gehörs und Allgemeingefühls. Sehr wesentlich ist es, daß sie hauptsächlich in den Zuständen zwischen Schlaf und Wachen beobachtet werden. Oft sprechen die Kranken von nächtlichen Erscheinungen. Die Analyse der Struktur und des Inhalts der Halluzinationen weist auf die Eigenart der Psyche der Kranken und ihr Losgelöstsein von der Umgebung hin. In dieser Hinsicht sieht man große Unterschiede zwischen schizophrenen Halluzinationen und solchen auf toxischer oder infektiöser Basis. So sind die Halluzinationen beim Delirium tremens charakteristisch grell und konkret, etwas Einheitliches, Ganzes; sie entsprechen dem, was man in der Wirklichkeit sieht, sie bestehen aus Gesichts-, Gehörs- und anderen Komponenten. Die visuellen Halluzinationen bei der Schizophrenie sind nicht immer durch Realität, Ganzheit und Greifbarkeit charakterisiert. Zum Beispiel werden von Menschen nur Teile, etwa einzelne Köpfe, gesehen — nicht ganze Figuren.

Von großem Interesse sind die *Halluzinationen von mit Dauerschlaf behandelten Schizophrenen.* In der Periode des Erwachens werden bei ihnen oft visuelle Halluzinationen besonderer Art festgestellt: oft sind es unbestimmte Figuren, Fäden, dazwischen menschliche Gestalten in geometrischer Form mit Kegeln statt Gesichtern und Pyramiden statt Extremitäten. Diese Beobachtungen wurden an Kranken, die zu Heilzwecken dem Dauerschlaf unterworfen wurden, gemacht; für eine Reihe von Fällen war es eine Art Experiment zur Klärung der Besonderheiten der schizophrenen Psyche. Unter dem Gesichtspunkt der Störung der Einheit ist es kein Zufall, daß den ganzheitlichen Visionen der toxisch und infektiös bedingten Halluzinationen im Falle der Schizophrenie ein Konglomerat verschiedener Elemente gegenübersteht, die Teile einer Figur sein könnten, den Kranken aber als Fragmente erscheinen. Bemerkenswert ist, daß die Zeichnungen der Schizophrenen dieselben Merkmale aufweisen.

Sehr viele Besonderheiten weist auch *das Denken der Schizophrenen* auf. Es ist ebenfalls unbestimmt, nicht konkret, von der Wirklichkeit abgelöst. Normalerweise befindet sich das Denken in einer Einheit mit der Sprache. Aus diesem Grunde ist es wichtig, sich mit der Sprache der Schizophrenen bekannt zu machen; dabei stellt man auch hier das Vorhandensein der Dissoziation fest. Die *Sprache* der Schizophrenen ist oft grammatikalisch richtig, dabei kann sie aber ohne Sinn sein. Man kann auch darin Hemmungserscheinungen feststellen. Sie wird oft durch Pausen unterbrochen, die an Stottern erinnern, die aber nicht durch Spasmen, sondern durch Hemmung entstehen. Die Gedanken dieser Kranken gehen merkwürdige Wege; den gewöhnlichsten Worten geben sie irgend einen besonderen Sinn. Man empfängt den Eindruck, daß den Kranken der übliche Wortschatz nicht genügt, um das, was sie fühlen und erleben, auszudrücken, und daß sie völlig neue Worte bilden. Die Rede der Schizophrenen ist oft zusammenhanglos und völlig unverständlich; diese Eigenschaften spiegeln ihr zusammenhangloses Denken wider.

Entsprechend der allgemeinen These, daß die Schizophrenie durch das Vorhandensein von Dissoziationsprozessen gekennzeichnet wird, sind auch die charakteristischen Züge der *Wahnbildung* zu verstehen. Wie bei den Halluzinationen muß man auch hierbei nicht so sehr auf Inhalt und Richtung der Wahnbildung, als auf die Formen, in denen sie sich äußert, achten. Die Wahnideen sind bei den meisten Kranken psychologisch verständlich und aus ihren Erlebnissen ableitbar. Bei der Schizophrenie erscheinen die Wahnvorstellungen ohne Bezug zu sein und sind gänzlich unverständlich. Es gibt eine Konzeption, die besonders von GRUHLE ausgearbeitet worden ist, nach der der schizophrene Wahn ein primäres Symptom ist, das für den Kranken unerwartet auftritt, der durch den Gedanken erschreckt und in Staunen versetzt wird, daß andere eine besondere Beziehung zu seinem

„Ich" besitzen. Diese Konzeption eines primären Wahns muß man als falsch ansehen. Gerade in diesem Fall ist es von Nutzen, die Errungenschaften unserer Physiologen heranzuziehen. Das psychische Leben ist mit der Bildung bedingter Reflexe verbunden; den Ausgangspunkt bilden Empfindungen; sie werden durch die höchsten Sinnesorgane wahrgenommen. Aber eine ebensolche Rolle können auch die Empfindungen spielen, die durch die Interoreceptoren vermittelt werden. Sie brauchen das Bewußtsein nicht zu erreichen, können aber trotzdem einen Einfluß auf das Befinden und den allgemeinen Fluß der psychischen Prozesse ausüben. Auf diese Weise findet das ganz Unverständliche des Denkens, gleichsam jenseits des Verstandes Liegende und unbekannt woher Entstandene, seine Erklärung.

Indem wir die Frage beiseite lassen, auf welchen Wegen sich ein Wahn bildet, können wir doch von einem besonderen schizophrenen Wahn sprechen, der sich von dem unterscheidet, was man bei anderen Erkrankungen beobachtet, und dessen Grundzüge sich in voller Übereinstimmung mit dem befinden, was wir von der Psychologie derartiger Kranker wissen, nämlich mit ihrer Isoliertheit, ihrer Loslösung aus ihrer Umgebung.

Das von uns entworfene Bild der klinischen Erscheinungen bei der Schizophrenie zeigt ihren Ganzheitscharakter. Ihre genaue Beschreibung und allgemeine Charakteristik genügen aber noch nicht. Es ist wichtig, ihre pathophysiologische Natur aufzuzeigen. Dadurch kommt man dem Verständnis des Wesens der Erkrankung als Ganzem näher und gewinnt Ausgangspunkte für eine rationelle Therapie. In dieser Beziehung ist die Lehre Pawlows eine große Hilfe, da er dem Problem der Schizophrenie große Aufmerksamkeit zuwandte.

Zwanzig Jahre sind seit seinem Tode vergangen, doch seine Schüler und Nachfolger arbeiten an der Vervollkommnung des von ihm Erreichten und Vorgezeichneten. Das Grundlegende in den Ansichten Pawlows über die Schizophrenie ist, daß er als Voraussetzung für ihre Entwicklung den Boden eines schwachen „zerbrechlichen" Nervensystems ansieht. Das schwache Nervensystem wird leicht durch innere oder äußere Reizerreger gehemmt, insbesondere trifft das auf die Rinde der Hemisphären zu. Bei der Hemmung der höchsten Gebiete des zentralen Nervensystems wird die Einheit ihrer Tätigkeit gestört: die Koordination der Arbeit ihrer Teile, die Zusammenarbeit der Hemisphärenrinde und der subcorticalen Gebiete, des ersten und zweiten Signalsystems, des animalischen und des vegetativen Nervensystems.

Das Wesen der Prozesse im Nervensystem besteht in der Erregung und Hemmung, doch können sie sich auf verschiedene Gebiete erstrecken und ihr Verhältnis zueinander kann verschieden sein. Hemmungen von verschiedener Intensität können verschiedene Gebiete betreffen, und das findet seine besondere Spiegelung in den klinischen Erscheinungen. Die Hemmung der Rinde, von der das subcorticale Gebiet freibleibt, kann zu einer chaotischen, für die *Hebephrenie* charakteristischen Erregung führen. Die Hemmung des motorischen Gebiets liegt dem *katatonen Stupor* zugrunde. Es gibt eine ansehnliche Zahl chemischer Substanzen, mit deren Hilfe man einen Modellfall der Katatonie bei Tieren erzeugen kann. Beim Menschen muß eine analoge Genese des katatonen Stupors angenommen werden, besonders da die Katatonie von außerordentlich schweren Störungen des Stoffwechsels begleitet wird.

Die Möglichkeit der Genesung von einem schweren, jahrelang andauernden Stupor spricht am meisten dafür, daß als hauptsächliche Grundlage eine Hemmung in Betracht kommt. Die den katatonen Symptomen ähnlichen Erscheinungen der wächsernen Biegsamkeit unterscheiden sich von den ersteren durch den Mechanismus ihrer Entwicklung. Man muß sie als ein Resultat der Freimachung komplexer unbedingter Reflexe ansehen, die den Körper im Gleichgewicht halten.

Pawlow legte viel Wert auf die Berücksichtigung dessen, was er als Stauung und Trägheit (Inertsein) der physiologischen Prozesse bezeichnete.

Im motorischen Bereich liegt sie der Stereotypie zugrunde und spielt in der Genese der Zwangsneurosen und Wahnideen eine Rolle.

Für das Verständnis der Psychopathologie und des Verhaltens Schizophrener ist die Beachtung der *Phasen* von großer Bedeutung. Das sind Hemmungen verschiedenen Grades, Zustände zwischen Schlaf und Wachen, hypnotische Phasen — wie PAWLOW sie nannte. Zum Verständnis der Klinik derselben haben sowohl die ausgleichende wie die paradoxe Phase Bedeutung, besonders wichtig ist aber die *ultraparadoxe Phase*. Ihre Erscheinungen können als Grundlage einer Reihe bei Schizophrenie zu beobachtender Störungen, vor allem des Negativismus und der Wahnideen, gelten. Die ultraparadoxe Phase wurde ursprünglich experimentell an Tieren studiert, hat aber auch für den Menschen Gültigkeit.

Folgende Erscheinungen sind für diese Phase charakteristisch: durch Wärmereiz werden die Gefäße gewöhnlich erweitert, im Zustand der ultraparadoxen Phase verengt. Ein im Zustand der ultraparadoxen Phase befindlicher Hund wendet sich von seinem Futternapf ab, wenn man ihn füttern will, und demselben zu, wenn man den Napf fortnehmen will. Man kann kaum bezweifeln, daß ähnliche physiologische Erscheinungen dem schizophrenen Negativismus zugrunde liegen.

Hier ein typischer Fall des Negativismus: Der Kranke zieht seine Hand zurück, wenn der Arzt ihm die Hand schütteln will, und hält seine Hand hin, wenn der Arzt die seinige zurückgezogen hat. Beim Kranken entsteht das normale Streben, die Hand auszustrecken, und es werden schon Impulse in entsprechende Teile der Rinde gesandt, doch befindet sich dieselbe in einem Zustand verminderter Arbeitsfähigkeit; dadurch erweisen sich die stimuli üblicher Stärke als zu stark, und statt einer motorischen Erregung tritt eine Hemmung ein. Wenn der Arzt die Hand zurückzieht, so gerät ein vordem gehemmtes Gebiet auf der Basis der Mechanismen der gegenseitigen Induktion in Erregung, und ein zuvor erregtes Gebiet wird gehemmt. Dabei tritt die positive Phase der negativistischen Reaktion ein, und die Hand des Kranken streckt sich dem Arzt entgegen.

Dieses Mißverhältnis des sich ergebenden Effekts im Vergleich zum Charakter der Reizung beobachtet man nicht nur bei motorischen Aktionen. Das, wovon der Kranke sich zurückzieht, was er abweist, kann sich in seinen Gedanken als Wahnidee entwickeln. Bei Schizophrenen werden im Zustand der ultraparadoxen Phase die sonst den Menschen üblichen Gedanken und Antriebe unterdrückt und das Gegensätzliche erregt. Eine unserer Kranken, eine sehr aktive Person, die ihre Selbständigkeit und Unabhängigkeit als ein großes eigenes Verdienst ansah, sagte, als sie schizophren wurde, daß sie sich in eine Puppe verwandelt hätte. „Alles, was ich sage und tue, bin nicht ich, sondern die Puppe."

Die angeführten Tatsachen weisen darauf hin, daß die Analyse physiologischer Daten zum Verständnis der Schizophrenie beitragen kann. Natürlich soll man die Situation nicht vereinfachen und annehmen, daß die ultraparadoxe Phase an sich unmittelbar zur Wahnbildung führt. PAWLOW sagte, daß im Zusammenhang damit auch das eine Rolle spielt, was er als pathologische Trägheit (Inertsein) bezeichnete. Doch befinden sich diese beiden Momente im Zusammenwirken mit einer Reihe anderer in einer Einheit mit dem allgemeinen Zustand des Nervensystems. Der Grad der Aktivität der Hemisphärenrinde befindet sich in Abhängigkeit von ihrer Aufladung durch Prozesse im subcorticalen Bereich. Bei Schizophrenie ist diese Aufladung ungenügend. In Zusammenhang damit muß man die *Abulie* stellen, eine geringe Emotionalität, die oft bis zur emotionalen Stumpfheit gehen kann, und die in vielen Fällen der Schizophrenie vorhanden ist.

Die Tätigkeit der subcorticalen Gegend wird durch die Großhirnrinde reguliert. Bei der Schizophrenie erweist sich diese Regulation als ungenügend, was sich im Mißverhältnis zwischen dem Charakter der emotionalen Erlebnisse und dem der intellektuellen und willensmäßigen zeigt. Der Typus der Persönlichkeit und ihr Temperament müssen in Rechnung gestellt werden, um die sich entwickelnden Störungen zu begreifen. Beachtlich ist, daß die Schizophrenen sich gewöhnlich in einem veränderten Bewußtseinszustand befinden. Deswegen können sie oft nicht zwischen der Wirklichkeit und ihren eigenen Traumgesichten unterscheiden. Dazwischen unterscheiden sie auch nicht zwischen den Eindrücken der Wirklichkeit und den bei ihnen selbst sich bildenden Vorstellungen.

Ein Kranker, der in der Lage war, sich über seine Erlebnisse Rechenschaft zu geben und der auch über gewisse Kenntnisse in der Psychologie verfügte, bemerkte, daß sich bei ihm „in den Prozeß der Wahrnehmung der Wirklichkeit Nebenassoziationen einkeilten". Dieselben treten in eine unlösbare Verbindung mit dem durch Wahrnehmungen Vermittelten, sind davon nicht abzugrenzen, gleichen sich dem an. So kommt es vor, daß die Kranken beim

Betrachten von Bildern oft mehr sehen, als dargestellt ist. Dazwischen „sehen" sie auch etwas, was sie überhaupt nicht sehen können, z. B. Mikroben im eigenen Gehirn.

Große Bedeutung für das Verständnis der *Wahrnehmungsstörungen* kommt der Beachtung der Spaltungsprozesse zu. Jede Wahrnehmung ist eine komplexe Wahrnehmung, sie bezieht sich auf verschiedene Seiten des in Frage stehenden Objektes. Am Gesamtkomplex beteiligen sich auch Empfindungen, die den somatischen Organen entsprechen. Ihr Vorhandensein ist nach Ssetschenoff der Grund dafür, daß ein gegebenes Erlebnis als tatsächlich uns zugehörig empfunden wird. Die Abspaltung der somatischen Empfindungen führt, wie schon oben gesagt, dazu, daß das Erlebnis als etwas Fremdes, von außen Eingegebenes erscheint. Es gibt Fälle, wo ein Schizophrener plötzlich seine eigene Hand nicht mehr als ihm zugehörig empfindet. Das Merkmal der Farbigkeit kann entfallen, und alles Wahrgenommene erscheint dann blaß und leblos.

Bei den Schizophrenen erscheint die Schwäche des Nervensystems als zentrales Moment in der Entwicklung der Erkrankung. Es gibt Anhaltspunkte dafür, daß das Nervensystem schon von Geburt an mangelhaft ist. Wir haben in unseren Arbeiten auf die Mangelhaftigkeit der Entwicklung des Herz-Gefäß-Systems, Tropfenherz, hingewiesen. In einer späteren Arbeit sprechen Hauptmann und Mayermann von der Unterentwicklung der Capillaren des Nagelbettes.

Smirnow beobachtete ungenügend entwickelte Zellen, Ablagerungen von Lipofuscin und Glykogen in den Nervenzellen. Er sah diese Veränderungen als einen Hinweis auf die Hemmung der Zelle an. Snesarew sieht auch Gliaveränderungen als typisch an, wobei er unterstreicht, daß dieselben einen regressiven und keinen progressiven Charakter tragen. Als eine ständige Erscheinung bemerkt man in den oberflächlichen Schichten der Rinde einen inselformigen Ausfall von Nervenzellen. Nach den Angaben von Surabaschwilli werden besonders die neuen, die eigentlich menschlichen Felder in den Stirn-, Schläfen- und unteren Scheitellappen betroffen.

Viel kann man von der *Elektroencephalographie* erwarten, besonders im Hinblick auf ihre neuen, verfeinerten Methoden, die die Möglichkeit eröffnen, die allerersten Veränderungen der Aktionsströme einzufangen. Diese Untersuchungen könnten auch zur Klärung der Pathogenese helfen. Oben erwähnten wir, daß bei der Schizophrenie mit großer Beständigkeit Zellen des embryonalen Typus angetroffen werden. Durch die Anwendung der Methode der Aktionsströme wird man eventuell mehr Licht in dieses Problem bringen. Es kann sein, daß der Labilität des Nervensystems der Schizophrenen eine Unterentwicklung der Nervenelemente zugrunde liegt. In den Anfangsstadien der Krankheit liegt meistens eine erhöhte Reaktionsfähigkeit auf äußere Reize vor. Aus diesem Grunde können die anfänglichen Äußerungen der Schizophrenie durch exogene Symptomatik verschleiert werden. Solches findet leicht bei dem sog. alkoholischen Beginn der Schizophrenien statt. In unserer Monographie „Alte und neue Probleme der Psychiatrie" haben wir einige Fälle unter der Bezeichnung „psychoreaktiver Beginn der Schizophrenie" beschrieben. Die Fälle beginnen als Bild einer gleichsam reinen Psychogenie, doch später verwischt sich dies, und das Bild der Schizophrenie tritt hervor.

Zu der Frage der Pathogenese hat die pathologische Histologie noch nicht das letzte Wort gesprochen. Man muß aber konstatieren, daß die mit dem Studium der Schizophrenie beschäftigten Pathohistologen keine einheitliche Meinung vertreten.

Von Jean Lhermitte stammt die Arbeit „Physiologische Anatomie schizophrener Zustände". Er spricht somit nicht von der Schizophrenie, sondern, ebenso wie Baruk, von schizophrenen Zuständen und erkennt als besondere Krankheit — außer der eigentlichen Schizophrenie — symptomatische Schizophrenien an. Er schildert einen Fall, bei dem viele kompetente Spezialisten eine Schizophrenie diagnostiziert hatten; nach dem nach einigen Jahren erfolgten Tode der Kranken stellte es sich heraus, daß es sich um eine organische Erkrankung mit einer Unzahl perivasculärer Infiltrate gehandelt hatte. Unserer Ansicht nach sprechen die Fälle falscher Diagnose nicht gegen die Existenz der Schizophrenie als einer selbständigen Krankheit. Das Wesentliche ist die Klinik, und ihre Ergebnisse geben uns das Recht, die Krankheit gegen eine Reihe anderer abzugrenzen.

Eine weitere Berechtigung ergibt sich aus den Daten des *Stoffwechsels*, die sich in Übereinstimmung mit den Veränderungen des Zentralnervensystems befinden. Bei Schizophrenie werden tiefgreifende somatische Störungen konstatiert. Die

Herabsetzung der Leberfunktion führt zu einer ungenügenden Entgiftung der giftigen Produkte des Stoffwechsels.

PROTOPOPOW schrieb den Störungen des Eiweißstoffwechsels eine große Bedeutung zu. In seiner Klinik wurden auch die Untersuchungen der 17-Ketosteroide durchgeführt. In den langwierigsten Fällen der Schizophrenie mit katatonen Erscheinungen erweist sich ihre Ausscheidung im Urin herabgesetzt. Die sowjetischen Forscher schätzen die Untersuchungen von GJESSING und BUSCAINO hoch ein. Die Reaktion nach BUSCAINO-KIMBAROWSKY fand breite Anwendung. Im ganzen sprechen die Ergebnisse der Stoffwechseluntersuchungen von der Herabsetzung desselben in mancher Hinsicht, was in Übereinstimmung mit der Schwäche des Nervensystems steht, die zur ungenügenden Regulierung der Prozesse im Organismus führt.

Da bei der Schizophrenie eine Schwächung der oxydierenden Prozesse stattfindet, sprach SNESAREW von ihr als von einer Hypoxy-Encephalopathie. Es spielen also in der Entwicklung der Krankheitserscheinungen die Störungen des Stoffwechsels eine Rolle.

III. Die derzeitige Lage der sowjetischen Psychotherapie

1. Einleitung

Die Psychotherapie — ein Teil der allgemeinen Psychiatrie — wird in Übereinstimmung mit ihren Grundthesen aufgebaut.

Die Psychotherapie wird von den sowjetischen Psychiatern als ein System von Einwirkungen verstanden, das günstige Beeinflussung des nervösen und allgemeinen Zustandes des Patienten zum Ziel hat. Ihr Vorgehen erfolgt nach dem Prinzip der Einheit des Somatischen und des Psychischen und der Einheit von Organismus und Umwelt. Das System suggerierender Maßnahmen muß in jedem Fall der Eigenart des Kranken entsprechen. Die Psychotherapeuten der verschiedensten Länder haben insofern viel Gemeinsames, als sie zur Grundlage ihrer therapeutischen Maßnahmen die *Suggestion* erwählt haben und sie entweder im hypnotischen Schlaf oder im wachen Zustand anwenden.

Viel für den Erfolg der hypnotischen Behandlung hat in unserer Medizin der Schüler von KORSAKOW — TOKARSKY — geleistet. Schon im Jahre 1887 publizierte er eine Arbeit über die Hypnose in der Medizin. Der Schöpfer der Moskauer Schule für Neuropathologie, Prof. KOSCHEWNIKOW, beschrieb um dieselbe Zeit einen Fall von Siccosisheilung durch Hypnose. Zu der Zeit wußte man noch nicht, daß die Suggestion einen Einfluß auf den gesamten Organismus haben kann, und der Fall wurde als Wunder besprochen. In der Entwicklung von Hypnose und Suggestion spielten die Untersuchungen von BECHTEREW, der Gruppenhypnose anwendete, eine große Rolle. In einer Gruppe von Kranken sind natürlich nicht alle gleich suggestibel und nicht alle gleich bereit, sich der Hypnose zu unterwerfen; es schlafen auch nicht alle gleichzeitig ein. Bei einigen tritt der hypnotische Schlaf schneller ein, was die anderen Kranken bemerken und wodurch sie suggestiv beeinflußt werden.

In den zwanziger Jahren haben wir, von denselben Ideen wie BECHTEREW geleitet, in unserer Klinik ein besonderes System *rationeller Therapie für die in Kollektiven zusammengefaßten Neurotiker* entwickelt. Die Kranken wurden so ausgesucht, daß sie alle bis zu einem gewissen Grade die gleichen Beschwerden hatten und für sie dieselben Wortsuggestionen wie auch andere Maßnahmen Gültigkeit hatten. Natürlich fanden dabei auch individuelle Unterhaltungen statt, aber ständig wurde betont, daß alle Kranken dasselbe Ziel hätten — die Genesung, die erreichbar sei und schnell eintreten könne, wenn die Kranken die Ratschläge des Arztes streng befolgten, sich an das festgesetzte Regime hielten und einander in seiner Durchführung unterstützten. Zu dem System der Behandlung gehörten Elemente des Arbeitsregimes.

Die Erfolge dieser Methode sind fraglos dadurch zu erklären, daß sie mit der für die sowjetischen Bedingungen charakteristische, auf das Kollektiv gerichtete Einstellung arbeitet, dessen Mitglieder miteinander durch Solidarität und Hilfsbereitschaft verbunden sind. Die Beseitigung irgendeines Symptoms durch die Suggestion in der Hypnose, ohne die Wiederherstellung des psychischen Gleichgewichts, kann natürlich keine dauerhafte Genesung ergeben. Die durch die Suggestion erreichten günstigen Verschiebungen werden, wenn sie ohne Festigung durch die psychische Einstellung bleiben, leicht durch Suggestionen anderer Art zunichte gemacht.

In der Arbeit mit den im Kollektiv zusammengefaßten Neurotikern wird, wie aus dem obigen erhellt, eine eigenartige rationelle Psychotherapie mit Methoden der Erklärung und Persuasion nach Dubois durchgeführt. Gerade unter den sowjetischen Bedingungen ergibt eine solche Psychotherapie, die an den Willen und das Bewußtsein appelliert, besonders gute Resultate.

Dieselben Prinzipien entwickelten unsere Psychiater auch in der Arbeit mit anderen Kranken, insbesondere mit somatisch Kranken, bei denen eine richtig eingestellte Psychotherapie sich als ganz besonders wirksam erweist.

2. Die physiologische Natur der Hypnose und ihre Anwendung für die Behandlung

Der hypnotische Zustand ist ein besonderer Zustand der *Hemmung der Hemisphärenrinde*, ein Übergangszustand zwischen Schlaf und Wachen, teilweise Schlaf, teilweise Hemmung; das gilt sowohl für die Lokalisation als auch für die Tiefe derselben.

Der wesentliche Unterschied zwischen dem gewöhnlichen und dem hypnotischen Schlaf liegt in den Bedingungen seines Eintritts, aber auch darin, daß der erste ein allgemeiner, der zweite ein teilweiser Schlaf ist. Während des hypnotischen Schlafes finden die gleichen funktionellen Veränderungen statt, doch der Schlaf tritt nicht von selbst ein, sondern unter dem Einfluß der Suggestion oder, unter bestimmten Umständen, der Autosuggestion.

Um den Mechanismus des Eintritts eines hypnotischen Zustands zu verstehen, muß man sich der Hinweise Pawlows auf die Bedingungen, unter denen er entsteht, erinnern. Das sind die Wirkungen gleichförmiger schwacher und mittlerer ununterbrochener oder rhythmischer Reize, wie z. B. Passes, Blickfixierung oder das Klopfen des Metronoms. Außerdem kann der hypnotische Zustand durch unerwartete starke Reize hervorgerufen werden. Von Bedeutung ist auch die Hervorrufung der Hypnose durch monoton wiederholte Worte, die einen Schlafzustand beschreiben. Das bestätigt Pawlows Auffassung, daß der hypnotische Zustand ein typischer bedingter Reflex ist. Sehr wichtig ist ein allgemeiner Hinweis Pawlows: „Hypnotisierend wirkt alles, was einige Male mit dem Schlafzustand zusammen erlebt worden ist." Aber der wichtigste Erreger des hypnotischen Schlafes ist das suggerierende Wort des Hypnotiseurs. Darum ist es verständlich, daß man meistens zur Herbeiführung eines hypnotischen Zustandes sich der Suggestion durch das Wort bedient.

Das Wort des Hypnotiseurs schafft eine konzentrierte Reizung eines bestimmten Punktes der Rinde. Die Konzentration der Reizung in einem begrenzten Punkt der Rinde ruft eine tiefe Hemmung in der ganzen übrigen Rinde hervor und schließt damit die Möglichkeit der Einwirkung von anderen Erregungen aus. Damit ist die Kraft der Suggestion erklärt und auch der Umstand, daß ihre Wirkung auch nach dem Aufhören des hypnotischen Zustandes weiterbesteht. Sie bleibt von deren Erregungen unabhängig, da sie im Moment der ursprünglichen Einwirkung auf die Rinde mit ihnen nicht gekoppelt war. Damit ist auch zu erklären, daß der Kontakt zum Hypnotiseur erhalten bleibt. Zwischen dem Hypnotisierten und dem Hypnotiseur stellt sich die Beziehung des Rapports ein, welche bis zur Entlassung aus dem Zustand bestehen bleibt. Der Hypnotisierte verliert mehr oder weniger die Fähigkeit der vollen Aufnahme der Umwelteindrücke, er besitzt sie nur in Beziehung zu dem, was der Hypnotiseur ihm vermittelt.

Das Wort des Hypnotiseurs ist auf Grund aller vorhergehenden Lebenserfahrungen mit allen äußeren und inneren Reizen verknüpft. Das Wort signalisiert sie, kann sie ersetzen und Reaktionen hervorrufen, welche früher durch entsprechende Erregungen zustande kamen. Die konkreten Worte des Arztes: „Ihre Arme und Beine werden schwer, die Augen fallen Ihnen zu", sind bedingte Erreger, fest verknüpft mit dem schläfrigen Zustand, und rufen ihn deshalb auch hervor.

Die Wirkung der Suggestion ist besonders stark, wenn sie kurz, isoliert und einheitlich ist. Da der Inhalt eines Wortes sehr viel umfassen kann, kann man durch die Suggestion ganz verschiedenartige Reaktionen beim Menschen hervorrufen.

Die Definition des hypnotischen Zustandes von der physiologischen Seite her präzisierend, sagt Pawlow, daß es sich um einen Hemmungsprozeß handelt, der seinen Anfang in den Hemisphären nimmt, und der verschiedene Stufen der Extension und Intensität des eintretenden schläfrigen Zustandes darstellt. Extension muß man im Sinne der Ausdehnung auf größere oder geringere Flächen der Hemisphären verstehen. Die Hemmung kann eine teilweise sein insofern, als auf dem Hintergrunde der Hemmung gewisse Bezirke verbleiben, die ihre Erregbarkeit behalten, wodurch der Rapport-Zustand sichergestellt wird. Was die Intensität betrifft, so muß man hier die verschiedenen Tiefengrade der Schlafhemmung im Sinne haben. Der Zustand des Wachseins geht nicht unmittelbar in den des Schlafes über (gemeint ist hier der gewöhnliche Schlaf), sondern durchläuft eine Reihe von Zwischenphasen. Dasselbe spielt sich auch beim Eintritt des hypnotischen Zustandes ab.

Die Ergebnisse der Physiologie der höchsten Nervenfähigkeit und die Konzeption des Nervismus gestatten ein näheres Kennenlernen der Mechanismen der Suggestionseinwirkung und der sich der Hypnose eröffnenden therapeutischen Möglichkeiten. Das Zentralnervensystem ist der Regulator aller Prozesse im Organismus. Auf dem Wege der Suggestion, der psychischen Einwirkung, kann man daher, durch die Beeinflussung der regulierenden Funktionen des Gehirns, den Verlauf sowohl der psychischen als auch der somatischen Prozesse verändern. Indem man solche emotionalen Zustände, wie z. B. Hunger oder Durst, suggeriert, kann man den Kohlenhydrat- wie auch den Wasserstoffwechsel beeinflussen. Es ist nur natürlich, daß man durch die Suggestion besonders den psychischen Zustand sehr stark beeinflussen kann.

Die Natur des hypnotischen Zustandes, besonders die charakteristische erhöhte Suggestibilität, macht es verständlich, daß man sich mit Vorteil der Hypnose zur Behandlung verschiedener krankhafter Zustände bedient. Vor allem ist der hypnotische Zustand an sich schon bedeutungsvoll. Indem er eine Art Schlaf mit Herabsetzung des Tempos und der Intensität der Tätigkeit bestimmter Teile des zentralen Nervensystems darstellt, bewirkt er eine allgemeine bedeutende Beruhigung mit dem subjektiven Empfinden der Besserung und Erholung. Die Stufe dieser Beruhigung ist um so größer, je tiefer die Intensität und Dauer des Schlafes waren. Dieser Tatsache tragen unsere Psychotherapeuten BIRMAN, PLATONOW u. a. Rechnung, indem sie den *verlängerten hypnotischen Schlaf* anwenden.

BIRMAN erreichte durch Suggestion die Verlängerung des natürlichen Schlafes bis auf 14—18 Std. täglich. Eine solche Behandlung in einer speziellen Abteilung dauerte 10—30 Tage in geräuschloser Umgebung. Der therapeutische Effekt ist natürlich größer, wenn außer der Herbeiführung des hypnotischen Zustandes auch noch irgendwelche Suggestionen angewandt werden.

Das *Anwendungsgebiet der therapeutischen Hypnose* ist recht groß und beschränkt sich nicht nur auf die Erkrankungen, in deren Genese ausschließlich psychische Momente eine Rolle spielen. Insofern als das zentrale Nervensystem alle Prozesse im Organismus reguliert, kann durch Suggestion, insbesondere im Zustand der Hypnose, auch bei solchen Erkrankungen wie der Hypertonie, den Ulcus-Krankheiten und der Coronarinsuffizienz eine Besserung des Zustandes erzielt werden. Die Hypnose kann zur Beseitigung schwerer Schmerzen beitragen, besonders wenn im Zustandekommen derselben psychische Momente eine Rolle spielen. Die Hypnose hat die Aufmerksamkeit der Chirurgen und Geburtshelfer erweckt. Die vorbereitende psychotherapeutische Behandlung der Kranken beseitigt die Angst vor der Operation und bietet die Möglichkeit, sie mit weniger Narkotica durchzuführen. Die Versuche der Durchführung kleinerer chirurgischer Eingriffe im Zustand der Hypnose erwiesen sich als erfolgreich. Man muß dabei im Auge behalten, daß jeder Schmerz, auch wenn er unmittelbar mit einer somatischen Erkrankung zusammenhängt, ein psychisches Erlebnis darstellt. Durch die Suggestion kann man auf die psychogene Komponente des Schmerzsyndroms einwirken.

Von besonderer Wichtigkeit ist die Möglichkeit der *Schmerzbeseitigung während des Geburtsaktes*. Die Schmerzlosigkeit ist für Mutter und Kind gleich wichtig. Die leichtere und schmerzlose Durchführung der Geburt bildet eine gewisse Garantie für einen komplikationslosen Verlauf.

Platonow, Welwowsky, Schagam, Plotitscher haben eine spezielle psychoprophylaktische Methode für die schmerzlose Durchführung der Geburt ausgearbeitet. Spezielle Maßnahmen zur Vorbereitung der Schwangeren für eine richtige Verhaltensweise während der Geburt liegen dieser Methode zugrunde; fraglos sind in ihr auch Momente der Suggestion enthalten. Diese Arbeiten wurden auch im Auslande, speziell in Frankreich, bekannt, doch die Einstellung zur Frage der schmerzlosen Geburt ist dort eine andere. Read kam zu dem Schluß, daß die Angst das hauptsächliche schmerzauslösende Moment sei, zu ihrer Verhinderung resp. Coupierung empfiehlt er die Suggestion im hypnotischen Zustand.

Die sowjetischen Psychiater, die auf dem Standpunkt der Einheit, gegenseitigen Verbundenheit und Bedingtheit aller Prozesse im Organismus stehen, sind bei der Anwendung der Suggestion bestrebt, ihre Wirkung durch Suggestion des Gefühls der Munterkeit, der Zuversicht in die eigene Person und die eigenen Kräfte sowie durch entsprechende Nervina und Vitamine zu verstärken. Die für den Kranken bemerkbare Besserung seines Allgemeinzustandes verstärkt die Wirkung der Suggestion und hebt den Glauben des Kranken an den Arzt. Das bezieht sich auch auf die physikalischen Methoden der Behandlung, insbesondere sind in der Wirkung der Medikamente Elemente der Suggestion verborgen. Dieselben Gedanken sind in der Arbeit des Londoner Psychiaters Denis Hill „Psychotherapie und physikalische Behandlungsmethoden in der Psychiatrie" ausgesprochen. Darin sagt er, daß die Psychotherapie der Methode der physikalischen Behandlung vorangehen, sie begleiten und beenden soll.

Wie aus dem Gesagten erhellt, muß der Psychotherapeut einem jeden Kranken gegenüber eine besondere Einstellung haben und die Eigenart des Kranken und seiner Erkrankung berücksichtigen. In hohem Maße bezieht sich das auf die Schizophrenen, deren psychische Behandlung bekanntlich große Schwierigkeiten bereitet. In Anbetracht der geringen Suggestibilität dieser Art Kranker müssen die psychischen Einwirkungen bei ihnen in irgendeiner besonderen Form erfolgen. Die Möglichkeiten hierzu eröffnen sich in der Organisation eines besonderen Regimes, insbesondere der *Arbeitstherapie*. Die Psychiatrie hat von jeher die Arbeitstherapie angewandt. Aber die Erfassung des Wesens dieser Methode, die Einstellung zu ihr im Sinne der Auswahl der am besten geeigneten Formen der Arbeit ist während der verschiedenen Etappen der Entwicklung der Psychiatrie ungleich gewesen.

Die sowjetischen Psychiater zogen aus der These, daß die Arbeit den Menschen geschaffen hat, ihre Schlußfolgerungen. Sie organisierten für ihre Kranken Arten der Arbeit, deren Nutzen durch Schaffung lebenswichtiger, notwendiger Gegenstände den Kranken selbst einleuchtete. Die Arbeit hat den Menschen erschaffen, sie kann auch die Ganzheit und Aktivität der Persönlichkeit wiedererschaffen, wenn sie durch Krankheit gestört sind. Der Effekt einer solchen Arbeitstherapie gibt dem Kranken den Glauben an seine eigenen Kräfte wieder. Der Glaube an sich selbst, seine Kräfte und Möglichkeiten ist nicht nur für die Neurotiker, sondern auch für die Schizophrenen wichtig. Die Psychotherapie ist nicht nur eine mündliche Therapie, nicht nur eine Therapie durch das Wort. Sie besitzt eine große Suggestionskraft, doch suggerierend wirkt auch manches andere: die ganze Umgebung, das Regime, das Verhältnis anderer zum Kranken, das Beispiel anderer Kranker. Es ist natürlich, daß unter den Bedingungen der Arbeitstherapie die Suggestion im Wachen eine größere Kraft besitzt; besonders klar sieht man das an den Schizophrenen.

Indem sie die Psychotherapie auf die Grundlage der physiologischen Lehre von Pawlow stellten, haben es die sowjetischen Psychiater für überflüssig gehalten, irgendwelche anderen Systeme, insbesondere die Psychoanalyse nach Freud, anzuwenden.

IV. Abschließende Bemerkungen

In dem Zeitraum, der seit dem Tode PAWLOWs vergangen ist, hat sich eine Menge physiologischer Tatsachen angesammelt, die sich auf die von ihm bearbeiteten Probleme beziehen. Er zeigte die Bedeutung der Großhirnrinde bei der Entwicklung der klinischen Störungen und der Wiederherstellung normaler Beziehungen. Er maß auch dem subcorticalen Gebiet große Bedeutung bei, dessen Prozesse, seiner Ansicht nach, die Rinde gleichsam aufladen.

Im Mittelpunkt der Aufmerksamkeit der ausländischen, namentlich der amerikanischen Gelehrten, steht zur Zeit die Frage des Formatio reticularis. MAGOUN hat das aufsteigende System im Stammhirn beschrieben, welches eine tonisierende Wirkung auf die Rinde ausübt. Es gibt auch Beweise für absteigende Einflüsse, die von den caudalen Teilen der reticulären Formation ausgehen. Die Analyse dieser und analoger Tatsachen gab dem Autor der neuen Monographie über die Morphologie und Physiologie des Nervensystems, PAUL GLEES, einen Grund, die Rinde „von ihrem Throne zu stoßen". Man muß beachten, daß die Abgrenzung des Begriffes der reticulären Formation nicht so sehr auf histologischen als auf physiologischen Untersuchungen bei Anwendung des Tierexperiments begründet ist. In der Monographie wird der Name PAWLOWs nicht erwähnt, dabei ist die Geschichte der Entdeckung der reticulären Substanz der beste Beweis der Berechtigung der von PAWLOW stets verteidigten Behauptung, daß die Struktur allein, ohne Funktion, tot ist.

In jedem Fall befinden sich die neu entdeckten Tatsachen in Übereinstimmung mit PAWLOWs Gedanken über die Aufladung der Rinde durch Prozesse in der subcorticalen Gegend. Das ist derselbe Gedanke, welcher der Idee REICHARDTs innewohnt, die in der Monographie zitiert wird, daß das subcorticale Gebiet eine Art Dynamo für die Rinde ist.

Man kann es bedauern, daß die Erforschung derselben Fragen bei uns und im Ausland in erheblicher Entfremdung voneinander vor sich geht. Von einer solchen Entfremdung kann man wohl sprechen, wenn man in Betracht zieht, wie die Lehre von den bedingten Reflexen von einigen ausländischen Autoren beleuchtet wird.

Der französische Forscher SALMON erkennt im allgemeinen die Lehre von den bedingten Reflexen an, doch bringt er Veränderungen herein, die das Wesen der Störung betreffen. Nach seiner Ansicht kann vieles als das Ergebnis des Freiwerdens chemischer Substanzen begriffen werden. Man muß aber im Auge behalten, daß PAWLOW selbst sich in dem Sinne geäußert hat, daß die endgültige Antwort über das Wesen der untersuchten Nervenprozesse von der Physik und Chemie gegeben werden könnten.

Der deutsche Forscher WEINSCHENK gibt einen Überblick über PAWLOWs Lehre von der Physiologie der Großhirnhemisphären und ihrer Beziehung zur Neurologie und Psychiatrie. Der Hauptzweck seines recht umfangreichen Überblicks ist der Wunsch, die deutschen Leser mit den Errungenschaften unseres Physiologen bekannt zu machen. Bei einer Reihe von Fragen ist er aber anderer Ansicht. Es ist ihm unverständlich, in welchem Sinne man die Schizophrenie für eine chronische Hypnose halten kann. Doch befinden sich PAWLOWs Hinweise auf das Vorhandensein einer Bewußtseinsveränderung bei den Schizophrenen, die man als hypnotisch bezeichnet, in guter Übereinstimmung mit den Ergebnissen der klinischen Beobachtung, da Kranke in diesem Zustande oft die Eindrücke der konkreten Wirklichkeit nicht von ihren Vorstellungen und dem Inhalt ihrer Traumgesichte unterscheiden können.

Es gibt viele ungelöste Fragen in der Psychiatrie. Die immer mehr zu Tage tretende wissenschaftliche Zusammenarbeit von Forschern verschiedener Länder, die verschiedene Schulen und Wissensgebiete vertreten, erfüllt uns mit der Zuversicht, daß alle diese ungeklärten Fragen eines Tages eine adäquate Lösung finden werden.

Bibliographie

1. Allgemeine Fragen der Psychopathologie und Psychiatrie

ANOCHIN, P. K.: Die innere Hemmung als Problem der Physiologie. 1958. — ASRATJAN, E. A.: Einige allgemeine Züge der Störung und Wiederherstellung der Nerventätigkeit. Akademie d. Wiss. d. UdSSR 1949.

BUDILOWA, E. A.: Die Lehre I. M. SETSCHENOWs über die Empfindungen und das Denken. Akademie d. Wiss. d. UdSSR 1954. — BYKOW, K. M.: Die Hirnrinde und die inneren Organe. MedGis 1947.

GILJAROWSKY, W. A.: Alte und neue Probleme der Psychiatrie. Moskau 1946. — GILJAROWSKY, W. A.: Die Lehre von den Halluzinationen. Moskau 1948.

JUDIN, T. I.: Abrisse der vaterländischen Psychiatrie. Moskau 1951.

KANNABICH, J. W.: Die Geschichte der Psychiatrie. Moskau 1929. — KANDINSKY, W. CH.: Über die Pseudohalluzinationen. MedGiz 1952. — KORSAKOW, S. S.: Ausgewählte Werke. MedGis 1954.

MAJOROW, F. P.: Die Geschichte der Lehre von den bedingten Reflexen. Moskau 1948. — MITSCHURIN, I. W.: Zur Frage der Erblichkeit erworbener Merkmale. Ausgewählte Werke. Moskau 1948.

PAWLOW, I. P.: Zwanzigjährige Erfahrungen in der Erforschung der höchsten Nerventätigkeit. Moskau 1938. — PAWLOW, I. P.: Ausgewählte Werke zur Frage der Physiologie der höchsten Nerventätigkeit. Moskau 1950. — POPOW, E. A.: Material zur Klinik und Pathogenese der Halluzinationen. Charkow 1941.

SETSCHENOW, I. M.: Physiologische Untersuchungea über die Hemmungsmechanismen für die Reflextätigkeit des Rückenmarks im Gehirn des Frosches. Berlin, Hirschwald, 1863 — SETSCHENOW, I. M.: Ausgewählte physiologische und psychologische Werke. Moskau 1947.

TRAUGOTT, N. N., L. J. BALONOW u. A. E. LITSCHKO: Abrisse der Physiologie der höchsten Nerventätigkeit des Menschen. 1958.

2. Klinische Probleme der Psychischen Erkrankungen

GILJAROWSKY, W. A.: Zur Frage des hypochondrischen Syndroms. Physiol. J. UdSSR **1956**, 4. — GILJAROWSKY, W. A.: Sprache und Denken der Schizophrenen. Neuropath. psychiat. J. **1957**, 11.

JANET, P.: Névroses et idées fixes I., Paris 1898.

PROTOPOPOW, W. N.: Pathophysiologische Grundlagen einer rationellen Therapie der Schizophrenie. Kiew 1946. — PROTOPOPOW, W. N.: Der Stoffwechsel bei der manisch-depressiven Psychose. 1953.

SIMSON, T. P.: Die Schizophrenie des frühen Kindesalters. Moskau 1949.

TSCHISTOWITSCH, A. S.: Lehrbuch der Psychiatrie. Moskau 1953.

3. Die Therapie der psychischen Erkrankungen. Die Psychotherapie

BECHTEREW, W. M.: Hypnose, Suggestion und Psychotherapie und ihre therapeutische Bedeutung. Bote des Wissens. 1911. — WELWOWSKY, I. Z.: Das System der Psychoprophylaxe der Geburtsschmerzen. Charkow 1957. — BIRMAN, B. N.: Die Anwendung der Schlaftherapie in der Klinik der Psychosen. Vestnik AMN SSSR **1946**, 1—5.

GILJAROWSKY, W. A.: Über Experimente und Therapie seelischer Erkrankungen (insbes. über die Behandlung mit Stickoxydul). Archiv biol. Wissenschaften 1948. — GILJAROWSKY, W. A.: Über die Psychotherapie auf den Kollektiven der Neurotiker als einer besonderen Behandlungsmethode. Moskauer med. J. **1926**, 7. — GILJAROWSKY, W. A., N. M. LIWENTSEW, J. E. SEGAL u. Z. A. KIRILLOWA: Der Elektroschlaf. Moskau 1953. Das Buch wurde in Berlin übersetzt und unter dem Titel „Electroschlaf" herausgegeben.

KOSCHEWNIKOW, A. J.: Ein geheilter Fall von Siccosis. Werke der Moskauer Universität. Moskau 1895.

4. Die Pathomorphologie der psychischen Erkrankungen

GILJAROWSKY, W. A.: Die Rolle der pathologisch-anatomischen Untersuchungen bei der Ausarbeitung der Probleme der Schizophrenie. J. Neuropath. Psychiat. **1955**, 11.

SMIRNOW, L. I.: Die pathologische Anatomie und Pathogenese der traumatischen Erkrankungen. Moskau 1949. — SMIRNOW, L. I.: Über das morphologische Studium der psychischen Erkrankungen und der Schizophrenie im besondern. J. Neuropath. Psychiat. **1955**, 11. — SNESAREW, P. E.: Theoretische Grundlagen der pathologischen Anatomie der psychischen Erkrankungen. Moskau. MedGis 1950. — SURABASCHWILLI, A. D.: Die Synapsen und die reversiblen Veränderungen der Nervenzellen. Moskau 1951.

Ausländische Autoren

BARUK, H.: Précis de psychiatrie. Paris 1950. — BELLAK, L.: Dementia praecox. New York 1948. — BELLAK, L.: Manic-depressive psychosis. New York 1952. — BLEULER, MANFRED: Endokrinologische Psychiatrie. Stuttgart 1954.

GLEES, PAUL: Morphologie u. Physiologie des Nervensystems. Stuttgart 1957.

HILL, DENIS: Psychotherapy and physical methods of treatment in psychiatry. J. ment. Sci. **100**, 360—374 (1954).

KRETSCHMER, E.: Körperbau und Charakter, Berlin, Göttingen, Heidelberg, Springer, 23. und 24. Aufl., 1961.

LHERMITTE, J.: Anatomie physiologique des états schizophréniques. Encéphale **41**, Nr. 2 (1952) — LHERMITTE, J.: Une vue nouvelle de l'anatomie physiologique cérébrale. Encéphale **40**, Nr. 6 (1951).

MAGOUN, H. W.: Caudal and cephalic influences of the brain stem reticular formation. Physiol. Rev. **30**, 459—474 (1950). — MAGOUN, H. W.: The waking brain. Springfield, Ill.: Charles C. Thomas 1958. — MAYER-GROSS, W., E. SLATER u. M. ROTH: Clinical Psychiatry. London 1954. — MELOTTE, ATHMÉE: L'Accouchement sans douleur. Presse méd. 1957.

READ, G.: Childbirth without fear. 3. ed. Harper, Heineman 1955. — REICHARDT, M.: Hirnstamm und Psychiatrie. Mschr. Psychiat. Neurol. **68**, 470 (1928).

SALMON, ALBERT: Sur le mécanisme des reflexes conditionnels. Encéphale **38** (1949). — SCHILDER, PAUL: Mind. New York 1952. — SELYE, H.: Stress. Montreal 1950.

WEINSCHENK, C.: Über PAWLOWs Lehre von der Physiol. der Großhirnhemisphären in ihrer Beziehung zur Neurologie und Psychiatrie. Nervenarzt **28**, 488—499 (1957).

Namenverzeichnis

Kursive Seitenzahlen beziehen sich auf die Literaturverzeichnisse. Die in Klammern gesetzten
kursiven Ziffern beziehen sich auf die Literaturzitate

Sachverzeichnis

Die *kursiv* gedruckten Stichwörter und Seitenzahlen beziehen sich auf den Beitrag in englischer Sprache.

The words and page numbers printed in *italics* refer to the contribution in English language.

Markennamen chemischer Präparate werden nur dort aufgeführt, wo im Text keine internationale Kurzbezeichnung angegeben ist.